a **LANGE** medical book

REVIEW OF

General Psychiatry

SECOND EDITION

a **LANGE** medical book

REVIEW OF

General Psychiatry

SECOND EDITION

Edited by

Howard H. Goldman, MD, MPH, PhD
Director of Mental Health Policy Studies
Associate Professor of Psychiatry
Department of Psychiatry
University of Maryland, Baltimore

Consultant
National Institute of Mental Health
Rockville, Maryland

Research Associate
Health Services Research and Development Center
School of Hygiene and Public Health
Johns Hopkins University, Baltimore

Prentice-Hall International Inc.

Copyright © 1988 by Appleton & Lange
A Publishing Division of Prentice Hall
Copyright © 1984 by Lange Medical Publications

Spanish Edition: Editorial El Manual Moderno. S.A. de C.V.,
Av. Sonora 206, Col. Hipodromo, 06100-Mexico, D.F.

    89 90 91 / 10 9 8 7 6 5 4 3 2

Prentice-Hall International (UK) Limited, *London*
Prentice-Hall of Australia, Pty. Limited, *Sydney*
Prentice-Hall Canada, Inc., *Toronto*
Prentice-Hall Hispanoamericana, S.A., *Mexico*
Prentice-Hall of India Private Limited, *New Delhi*
Prentice-Hall of Japan, Inc., *Tokyo*
Simon & Schuster Asia Pte. Ltd., *Singapore*
Editora Prentice-Hall do Brasil Ltda., *Rio de Janeiro*
Prentice Hall, *Englewood Cliffs, New Jersey*

ISBN (PHI): 0-8385-8419-5
ISBN (A&L): 0-8385-8420-9
ISSN: 0894-2404

PRINTED IN THE UNITED STATES OF AMERICA

Table of Contents

III. MENTAL DISORDERS

Preface

PURPOSE

Review of General Psychiatry, 2nd edition, is designed for medical students—for course adoption, to supplement course syllabus materials, to complement readings in the literature, and to use as a companion text with more comprehensive works. It has its origins in the extensive program of psychiatric education, including required courses throughout the four-year curriculum, offered by the department of psychiatry at the University of California, San Francisco. Designed with that comprehensive program in mind and written by psychiatric educators, this text should serve the needs of medical students in most settings. Furthermore, a text that meets the broadest requirements of medical student education in psychiatry should serve as a review text for psychiatric residents and other trainees and as a reference for physicians and other health and mental health practitioners.

OUTSTANDING FEATURES

- Material on basic biologic and psychosocial science as well as clinical material on diagnosis and treatment.
- Full range of disorders with complete diagnostic criteria as described in the *Diagnostic and Statistical Manual of Mental Disorders,* 3rd edition, as revised in 1987 *(DSM-III-R).*
- Clinical vignettes illustrating the features of most mental disorders and comprehensive clinical assessment.
- Glossary of psychiatric signs and symptoms.
- Seven chapters on clinical assessment in psychiatry.
- Consistent readable format, permitting efficient use in multiple clinical settings.
- Selected references for further investigation.
- Information serving the needs not only of the physician in general medical practice but also of the medical student and resident in psychiatry.

NEW TO THIS EDITION

- Revised *DSM-III-R* diagnostic criteria and terminology.
- New mental status examination format.
- New chapter on anxiety disorders.
- Updated neuroscience and psychopharmacology.
- New material on child abuse and neglect.
- Updated material on AIDS, substance abuse, and sexual disorders.

Psychiatry is a discipline of observation and probing inquiry, a basic science of behavior, and a clinical science of mental disorder and emotional responses to physiologic change, somatic illness, and life events. Critics in neuroscience characterize psychiatry as brainless; critics within psychologic medicine fear that psychiatry will become mindless. Students everywhere are concerned that the curriculum not be witless. Our aim is to present psychiatry with the proper mix of brain, mind, and wit.

ACKNOWLEDGMENTS

Review of General Psychiatry represents more than the work of its title-page editor and its named contributors. I would like to acknowledge the assistance of other contributors to our text.

The first acknowledgment goes to Judy Lusic, MD, a former student, who introduced me to Jack Lange, MD. I would like to thank our publishers, Jack Lange and Alexander Kugushev, for their support and for the assistance of the editorial and production staff of Appleton & Lange. I would like to acknowledge also the contributions of our associate authors and the various educators who organized the groundwork for this test: Ira Glick, Robert Hoffman, I.R. Feinberg, Roberta Huberman, Maleta Boatman, Herb Peterson, Robert Harris, David Rosen, Robert S. Wallerstein, Leonard S. Zegans, and the late Morton Weinstein (all MDs).

A third edition of this book is scheduled for publication in 1991. We continue to solicit comments and recommendations for future editions. Correspondence should be addressed to us at Appleton & Lange, 2755 Campus Drive, Suite 205, San Mateo, CA 94403.

Howard H. Goldman, MD
Baltimore, MD
April, 1988

Editor's Note

I am grateful for this opportunity to thank all of my students and teachers past and present for the many ways in which I have been helped by each of them. I am especially grateful to Arnold Kerzner, MD, for first stimulating my interest in psychiatry as a helping profession.

So many colleagues whose names do not appear as authors have helped me and others with the preparation of *Review of General Psychiatry, 2nd Edition*—by reviewing early drafts and contributing ideas and expert criticism—that we mention none of them rather than overlook any of them in a long list of names.

No part of this book is the product of government activity, and none of the opinions expressed necessarily reflect official views of the National Institute of Mental Health.

-HHG

To my family
four generations
but especially my wife Debra
and my children Ilana and Ari

Authors

Bruce Africa, MD, PhD
Assistant Clinical Professor of Psychiatry, Department of Psychiatry, University of California, San Francisco.

James H. Billings, PhD, MPH
Vice President, Center for Health and Preventive Medicine and Director of Psychological Services, Preventive Medicine Research Institute, San Francisco.

Renee L. Binder, MD
Associate Professor of Psychiatry, Department of Psychiatry, University of California, San Francisco.

Charles M. Binger, MD
Clinical Professor of Psychiatry and Training Director, Child and Adolescent Psychiatry, Department of Psychiatry, University of California, San Francisco.

Emmett J. Bonner, PhD
Assistant Clinical Professor of Psychiatry, Department of Psychiatry, University of California, San Francisco.

Geoffrey K. Booth, MD
Assistant Clinical Professor of Psychiatry, Department of Psychiatry, University of California, San Francisco; Associate Director of Residency Training, Veterans Administration Medical Center, San Francisco.

Carroll M. Brodsky, PhD, MD
Professor of Psychiatry, Department of Psychiatry, University of California, San Francisco.

Edward L. Burke, PhD
Clinical Professor of Psychiatry, Department of Psychiatry, University of California, San Francisco.

Frances Cohen, PhD
Associate Professor of Medical Psychology, Department of Psychiatry, University of California, San Francisco.

Kathryn N. DeWitt, PhD
Assistant Research Psychologist, Department of Psychiatry, University of California, San Francisco.

Bernard L. Diamond, MD
Clinical Professor of Psychiatry, Department of Psychiatry, University of California, San Francisco; Professor of Law Emeritus, University of California, Berkeley, California.

Stuart J. Eisendrath, MD
Assistant Professor of Psychiatry, Department of Psychiatry, University of California, San Francisco; Clinical Chief, Psychiatric Consultation/Liaison Service, Joseph M. Long Hospital and Herbert C. Moffitt Hospital, San Francisco.

Leon J. Epstein, MD, PhD
Professor of Psychiatry Emeritus, Department of Psychiatry, University of California, San Francisco.

Dennis Farrell, MD
Clinical Professor of Psychiatry, Department of Psychiatry, University of California, San Francisco; Faculty, San Francisco Psychoanalytic Institute, San Francisco.

Howard H. Fenn, MD
Assistant Clinical Professor of Psychiatry, Department of Psychiatry, University of California, San Francisco; Assistant Ward Chief, Psychiatric Intensive Care Unit, Palo Alto Veterans Administration Medical Center, Palo Alto, California.

Howard L. Fields, MD, PhD
Professor of Neurology and Physiology, Departments of Neurology and Physiology, University of California, San Francisco.

Louis M. Flohr, MD
Director, Child Psychiatry Outpatient Department, McAuley Neuropsychiatric Institute, St. Mary's Hospital and Medical Center, San Francisco.

Steven A. Foreman, MD
Assistant Clinical Professor, Department of Psychiatry, University of California, San Francisco.

Nelson B. Freimer, MD
Research Fellow, Department of Psychiatry, Columbia University College of Physicians and Surgeons, New York City.

Evalyn S. Gendel, MD
Clinical Professor of Psychiatry, Department of Psychiatry, and Director of Sex Therapy Clinic, University of California, San Francisco.

Richard Goldberg, MD
Associate Professor of Psychiatry and Human

Behavior, Department of Psychiatry and Human Behavior, Brown University, Providence, Rhode Island; Chief of Psychiatry, Rhode Island Hospital and Women and Infants Hospital, Providence, Rhode Island.

Howard H. Goldman, MD, MPH, PhD
Associate Professor of Psychiatry, Department of Psychiatry, University of Maryland, Baltimore; Consultant, National Institute of Mental Health, Rockville, Maryland; Research Associate, Center for Health Services Research and Development School of Hygiene and Public Health, Johns Hopkins University, Baltimore.

Jack A. Grebb, MD
Research Associate, Nathan S. Kline Institute for Psychiatric Research, Orangeburg, New York; Assistant Professor, Department of Psychiatry, New York University Medical Center, New York City.

John H. Greist, MD
Professor of Psychiatry, Department of Psychiatry, University of Wisconsin Medical School, Madison, Wisconsin.

Leo E. Hollister, MD
Professor of Psychiatry, University of Texas Medical School, Houston; Medical Director, Harris County Psychiatric Center, Houston.

Mardi J. Horowitz, MD
Professor of Psychiatry, Department of Psychiatry, and Director of the Center for the Study of Neuroses, Langley Porter Psychiatric Institute, University of California, San Francisco..

James W. Jefferson, MD
Professor of Psychiatry, Department of Psychiatry, University of Wisconsin Medical School, Madison, Wisconsin.

Frank A. Johnson, MD
Professor of Psychiatry, Human Development and Aging Program, Center for Social and Behavioral Sciences, University of California, San Francisco.

Nancy B. Kaltreider, MD
Clinical Professor of Psychiatry, Department of Psychiatry, University of California, San Francisco.

Nick Kanas, MD
Associate Professor of Psychiatry, Department of Psychiatry, University of California, San Francisco; Assistant Chief, Psychiatry Service, Veterans Administration Medical Center, San Francisco.

Ralph J. Kiernan, PhD
Clinical Professor of Medical Psychology, Department of Psychiatry, University of California, San Francisco.

Mim J. Landry
Clinical Information Coordinator, Training and Education Projects, Haight Ashbury Free Medical Clinics, San Francisco.

J.W. Langston, MD
Senior Scientist, Institute for Medical Research, and Director, Parkinson's Research & Clinical Programs, Institute for Medical Research, Santa Clara Valley Medical Center, San Jose, California.

Hanna Levenson, PhD
Associate Clinical Professor of Psychiatry, Department of Psychiatry, University of California, San Francisco; Director of the Brief Psychotherapy Program, Veterans Administration Medical Center, Palo Alto, California.

Roland Levy, MD
Associate Clinical Professor of Psychiatry, Department of Psychiatry, University of California, San Francisco.

Dennis P. Malinak, MD
Assistant Clinical Professor of Psychiatry, Department of Psychiatry, University of California, San Francisco.

Charles R. Marmar, MD
Assistant Professor of Psychiatry, Department of Psychiatry, and Director, Anxiety Disorders Clinic, Langley Porter Psychiatric Institute, University of California, San Francisco.

Edward L. Merrin, MD
Assistant Professor of Psychiatry, Department of Psychiatry, University of California, San Francisco; Chief, Psychiatric Inpatient Unit, Veterans Administration Medical Center, San Francisco.

Aubrey W. Metcalf, MD
Clinical Professor of Psychiatry, Department of Psychiatry, University of California, San Francisco; Clinical Professor of Health and Medical Sciences, University of California, Berkeley, California.

Joseph P. Morrissey, PhD
Associate Professor of Social and Administrative Medicine, School of Medicine, and Deputy Director Health Services Research Center, University of North Carolina, Chapel Hill, North Carolina.

Jonathan Mueller, MD
Assistant Professor of Psychiatry, Department of Psychiatry, University of California, San Francisco.

Kim Norman, MD
Assistant Clinical Professor of Psychiatry, Department of Psychiatry, University of California, San Francisco.

Herbert Ochitill, MD
Assistant Professor of Psychiatry, Department of Psychiatry, University of California, San Francisco; Chief, Psychiatric Consultation Service, Department of Psychiatry, San Francisco General Hospital, San Francisco.

Irving Philips, MD
Professor of Psychiatry, Department of Psychiatry, and Director of Child and Adolescent Psychiatry, University of California, San Francisco.

Kenneth S. Pope, PhD
Diplomate in Clinical Psychology, Los Angeles.

Stephen D. Purcell, MD
Assistant Clinical Professor of Psychiatry, Department of Psychiatry, University of California, San Francisco.

David E. Reiser, MD
Associate Clinical Professor of Psychiatry and Family Medicine, Department of Psychiatry, University of Colorado Health Sciences Center, Denver.

Victor I. Reus, MD
Associate Professor of Psychiatry, Department of Psychiatry, and Medical Director, Langley Porter Hospital, University of California, San Francisco.

Gary M. Rodin, MD
Associate Professor of Psychiatry, Department of Psychiatry, University of Toronto.

Stuart R. Schwartz, MD
Professor of Clinical Psychiatry, Department of Psychiatry, and Director of Education, University of Medicine and Dentistry of New Jersey, Piscataway, New Jersey.

Rodney J. Shapiro, MD
Clinical Professor of Psychiatry, Department of Psychiatry, University of California, San Francisco; Director, Family Therapy Program, Veterans Administration Medical Center, San Francisco.

David E. Smith, MD
Founder and Medical Director, Haight Ashbury Free Medical Clinics, San Francisco; Research Director, Merritt Peralta Institute, San Francisco; Associate Clinical Professor of Occupational Health and Clinical Toxicology, University of California, San Francisco; Visiting Associate Professor of Behavioral Pharmacology, Department of Pharmacology, University of Nevada Medical School, Reno, Nevada.

Anthony J. Trevor, PhD
Professor of Pharmacology and Toxicology, Department of Pharmacology, University of California, San Francisco.

Craig Van Dyke, MD
Professor of Psychiatry, Department of Psychiatry, University of California, San Francisco; Chief, Psychiatry Consultation/Liaison Unit, Veterans Administration Medical Center, San Francisco.

Bruce S. Victor, MD
Assistant Clinical Professor of Psychiatry, Department of Psychiatry, University of California, San Francisco.

Robert S. Wallerstein, MD
Professor of Psychiatry, Department of Psychiatry, University of California, San Francisco; Supervising and Training Analyst, San Francisco Psychoanalytic Institute, San Francisco; President, International Psychoanalytical Association.

Stephen J. Walsh, MD
Associate Clinical Professor, Department of Psychiatry, University of California, San Francisco; Consultant and Lecturer, Medicine–Psychiatry Unit, St. Mary's Hospital and Medical Center, San Francisco.

Walter L. Way, MD
Professor of Anesthesia and Pharmacology, Department of Pharmacology, University of California, San Francisco.

Daniel S. Weiss, PhD
Assistant Professor of Medical Psychology, Department of Psychiatry, and Langley Porter Psychiatric Institute, University of California, San Francisco.

Leonard S. Zegans, MD
Professor of Psychiatry, Department of Psychiatry, and Director of Education and Professional Standards, University of California, San Francisco.

NOTICE

Section I. Theory & Concepts

Review of General Psychiatry: Introduction

1

Howard H. Goldman, MD, PhD

Review of General Psychiatry undertakes to examine and discuss the 2 major domains of the medical specialty field of psychiatry: mental disorder and individual behavior in health and sickness. Both areas are characterized by a degree of scientific uncertainty that may be puzzling to students drawn to medicine by the prospect of effecting cures by extirpating tumors or disrupting bacterial cell membrane formation. The patients being treated by psychiatrists are apt to have "idiopathic" disorders, "functional" disorders, whose causes are unknown and often cannot be corrected with instruments and drugs. The patients have behavior problems, aberrations; they are "deviant" and often seen to *be* and not just *have* the diseases that will be described in the clinical chapters of this book. When, as occasionally happens, the etiologic roots of these "idiopathic" diseases are found, psychiatry loses most or at least some of its professional dominion over them, as happened when general paresis of the insane was identified as a neurologic disorder of infectious (syphilitic) origin and pellagra as a metabolic disorder attributable to niacin deficiency. Complaints with no discoverable organic cause thus always arouse a suspicion of "mental disease" and consideration of psychiatric referral. Pain or weakness with no clear pathophysiologic basis is psychogenic, hysterical, a "conversion" phenomenon. The term "residual deviance" has been applied to problems left over when "real" diseases have been ruled out.

This is not to suggest that all mental diseases are "orphans" for whom parental etiologies may yet be found, though of course that can happen in many cases and surely will in some. The affective disorders (depression, mania) are obvious examples of severe incapacitating mental diseases that are beginning to give way to conventional diagnostic and therapeutic medical management. The mental disorders are not simply "residual"; they have specific diagnostic criteria and often have biologic markers.

Just as the subject matter of psychiatry is different in kind from the subject matter of ophthalmology, rheumatology, and other medical and surgical specialties, the literature in which its concepts and theories are conveyed from teacher to student and to successive generations of readers is different in kind from the literature of medicine generally. In order to say different kinds of things, we need different kinds of communication. The writer's first task here will be to decide how best to convey the grays and off-whites of the subject matter in the plain black medium of print. Especially when writing for medical students, who are taught to anticipate documentation and distrust speculation and "anecdotalism," one is forever aware that some of the ground being covered is sandy soil. The psychiatrist with some years in practice occupies these areas comfortably enough—there is no choice, since that is where the patient is—but many times in the following pages the reader will be called on for that "willing suspension of disbelief . . . that constitutes poetic faith." A willful unbeliever will not be persuaded that a 5-year-old boy would really want to slay his father so he might lie with his mother. But the good-faith unbeliever will acknowledge the pragmatic utility of that concept when it is used successfully to help a young man tormented by career misfortunes brought on by arguments with his boss, a gray-haired man the age of his father, and by a marriage in trouble because of an affair with the boss's secretary. An unbeliever might reject the notion that medication could relieve the terrible agony of depression—after all a "natural" element of the human condition—or that a placebo could really relieve the pain of cancer, much less accomplish physiologic anesthesia by suggestion. Yet the unbeliever might be convinced by the dramatic results of clinical trials of antidepressant drugs and by the demonstration that a narcotic antagonist can block placebo-induced analgesia. These comments do not exempt the claims of psychiatry from close scrutiny or its theorists from the rigors of systematic criticism. Their purpose is rather to encourage the reader on the way with appropriate notice about what *not* to expect in the pages that follow. Much of clinical psychiatry, like much of medicine, is not a "hard science," and *it does not need to be in order to be clinically effective.*

Uncertainty may make psychiatry difficult to "understand" in the straightforward sense of that word and certainly makes it impossible to reduce psychiatry to a catechism of verified truths. But it is still possible to think clearly in psychiatry, and one may tease out the known from the unknown and certainty from conjecture. And psychiatry is undeniably a clinically effective discipline, a healing profession, a growing body of useful knowledge based on careful observation and practical research, and a capacious receptacle of *theories!* It is the *theories* that are the special language of psychiatry and the source of its growth. Fundamentally a science of individual behavior, thought, and emotion, psychiatry is often scornfully contrasted with the sciences of basic laws, empirical truths, and reductionistic categories and typologies. In psychiatry, the domain of the mental disorders *does* share a common heritage with the reductionistic "hard sciences" of fundamental laws and empirical data; but the domain of individual behavior has been a "soft science" of human motivation, personal meaning, and individual difference. Ultimately, psychiatry is a *human* science, a clinical science—seen at its best in the personal interaction between doctor and patient. Simply stated, one need not know the "truth"—the reducible facts—to be helpful, but one does need to have at hand a rich resource of theories and hypotheses and must be prepared to test them on every patient—to use them when they work and move along when they do not. Most importantly, the psychiatrist must be a good listener, waiting for the patient to suggest—in speech, affect, and behavior—what hypotheses may be tested with brighter hope of success. *The psychiatrist must know how to lead where the patient goes.*

THE BIOPSYCHOSOCIAL MODEL

The biopsychosocial model is a defense against uncertainty, an approach to thinking about mental disorder and individual behavior. The psychiatrist may view both domains from biomedical and psychosocial perspectives and consider specific problems and potential solutions from each viewpoint. The biopsychosocial model is a perspective, not a theory—a way of organizing disparate data that permits clinicians and scientists to consider various points of view and integrate them into a coherent approach to the patient. For example, the busy medical student with peptic ulcer is not viewed as the passive victim of familial defects in gastrointestinal function *or* the angry combatant in a competitive profession, living a stressful life-style. *Both* views are correct, potentially helpful, and not mutually exclusive. The model, championed by George Engel (1977) and discussed again in other chapters, is introduced below in a clinical case and in a summary of some current neuroscience research to demonstrate its breadth and utility.

What do the old couple in the illustrative case (below) and the animal model of anxiety in the snail *Aplysia* have in common? How does the biopsychosocial model help us to appreciate these shared features? There is substantial agreement that clinical biomedical problems (eg, heart attacks) are in part influenced by psychosocial factors (eg, the sudden death of a loved one) and that biomedical problems (eg, a stroke) may cause secondary behavioral and psychosocial problems (eg, loss of a job or dissolution of a marriage). It is more difficult to appreciate the specific effect of social and psychologic factors on anatomic structures and physiologic functions. The clinical case of the old couple will show how the biopsychosocial model facilitates understanding of the interactions of biomedical and psychosocial factors. The animal model of anxiety in *Aplysia* illustrates the use of the biopsychosocial model in basic research. In particular, it examines the mechanism by which *learned* responses (eg, anxiety) may cause specific neurochemical and neuroanatomic changes.

Illustrative Case

A couple in their mid 80s had been married for 65 years and continued to live together in an apartment in spite of their increasing infirmities. The husband had severe emphysema and cardiac arrhythmia and was becoming forgetful; his wife had mild hypertension and was becoming impaired by senile dementia. On the eve of his 85th birthday, the old man became acutely short of breath and anxious. Fearful that he was going to die, he called his married daughter and was taken to the hospital in acute respiratory distress. He was later found to have inoperable lung cancer for which only palliative treatment could be offered.

While the patient was hospitalized, his wife went to live with their daughter and son-in-law. At night she wandered the rooms of the house, looking for her husband. She was argumentative and confused, not seeming to know where she was or what she should do. Her children and grandchildren had been aware of her increasing mental problems, but she was much more disturbed than they had realized or perhaps had wanted to realize. Her apparently dramatic change could be explained in 2 ways. She was undergoing a period of acute situational stress, and her deteriorated functioning had not been obvious as long as she was part of a functioning couple. Her husband had been helping her at home, nursing her, and covering up her deficits so that the family would not see. He was no longer available to do these things and never would be again. Plans were made to discharge him to a nursing home where he could continue to live with his wife in a double room. Although he was depressed, he adjusted to the nursing home, accepting the fact that this was where he would live out his days. He lived to see his granddaughter married, and then he died. The wife never adjusted, and her mental condition continued to deteriorate. She still expected her husband to come home each evening from the hospital, having concluded that she never saw him because he left early each day before she awakened and returned while she was asleep.

The interaction of biomedical and psychosocial factors in disease and illness is illustrated by this case. The husband's illness had precipitated a change in the delicate balance of the couple's independence. The wife needed nursing care, and his illness kept him from providing it. Many people die or become ill upon achieving certain milestones—an anniversary, a holiday, or, as in this case, a birthday. This man's 85th birthday had special significance. His driver's license, the key to his independence and his ability to care for his wife at home, expired on his birthday. He had been preparing for the test with great difficulty and was afraid he would not pass. Going to a nursing home gave him the comfort of knowing that when he died, his wife would be taken care of without being a burden to the family. His cancer had been growing for a long time, but clinically obvious illness began on his birthday.

A keen awareness of the interplay between biomedical and psychosocial factors is the essence of clinical medicine. Knowledge of the nuances of this interaction can help to answer 2 of the most important questions in medicine: Why did the patient become ill *now* (and not yesterday or a week or month ago)? And how can we treat this *individual* with an established diagnosis (that may be incurable)?

The mechanisms by which stress precipitates and exacerbates illness, lowers host resistance, and perhaps causes some diseases are currently being investigated. It would be useful also to learn how coping and adaptation work to prevent illness or reduce its severity. Learning how symbolic events, thoughts, and feelings influence behavior and initiate pathologic processes in humans is a challenge for future research. Some early work in this area has been reported by Eric Kandel (1983) and his associates studying an animal model of anxiety in the marine snail *Aplysia,* whose nervous system is simple, well understood, and accessible to investigation.

Research Example: Animal Model of Anxiety

Using the sea snail *Aplysia* as a research subject, Kandel (1983) describes an animal model of anticipatory anxiety and chronic anxiety reflected in 2 forms of learned fear produced by classic conditioning and sensitization. Each form of fear is associated with distinguishable cellular and molecular changes.

Aplysia demonstrates a defensive "fear response" when presented with a noxious stimulus, such as an electric shock to its head. The response includes an increase in movement away from the stimulus ("escape locomotion"), an increase in other defensive behaviors (eg, withdrawal of the head and siphon into the shell, releasing ink), and a decrease in feeding behavior. This fearful response may be learned by the snail in 2 ways: *Aplysia* may be conditioned, like Pavlov's dog (see Chapter 3), to respond fearfully to a neutral stimulus, such as shrimp extract, without the electric shock. If the snail is repeatedly given an electric shock each time shrimp extract is presented to it, the snail eventually responds with fear to the shrimp extract alone. This classic conditioning is similar to human anticipatory anxiety (and phobic anxiety). *Aplysia* can also be sensitized by random, unpredictable electric shocks, resulting in generally heightened responsiveness, so that almost any stimulus produces fearful behavior, as seen in chronic anxiety in humans.

In a series of elegant experiments, Kandel and his colleagues explored the cellular and molecular mechanisms associated with these 2 forms of learned fear. The sensitization model of chronic anxiety has been studied more extensively and appears to be due to presynaptic facilitation. The repeated head shocks

lead to an "enhancement of the connections made by the sensory neurons on their target cells: the interneurons and the motor neurons . . ." (Kandel, 1983:1285), resulting in increased escape behavior. This enhancement is due to increases in a serotoninlike neurotransmitter in the presynaptic sensory neurons that produce an increase in cAMP. In turn, cAMP leads to an increase in neurotransmitter release from terminals in the synapse connecting the sensory neurons and motor neurons. The resulting neurotransmission activates "escape locomotion" and other defensive behaviors in response to a wide array of stimuli. The investigators found that the molecular mechanism involved enhanced protein phosphorylation and increased influx of calcium and resulted in morphologic changes in the presynaptic neurons, detectable by electron microscopy. They speculate that the functional and structural changes associated with sensitization may be caused by alterations in gene expression: " . . . the possibility of gene regulation by experience suggests a class of molecular regulatory defects that might be caused by learning" (Kandel, 1983:1287).

The conditioning model for anticipatory anxiety is not as well described but seems to be similar in many ways to sensitization. Also producing presynaptic facilitation, conditioned fear appears to "augment" the process by "activity-dependent enhancement." This means that the learned association between the conditioned stimulus (the shrimp extract) and the fear response is produced by the increased release of neurotransmitter when the snail senses the presence of shrimp extract. The increased neurotransmission in response to the conditioned stimulus then sets in motion the same enhanced fear response mechanism seen in the sensitization model of chronic anxiety.

This research suggests that "normal learning, the learning of anxiety and unlearning it through psychotherapeutic intervention, might involve long-term functional and structural changes in the brain . . ." (Kandel, 1983:1291). Investigations such as these demonstrate the interaction of biomedical and psychosocial phenomena, brain and behavior, in everyday life and clinical medicine.

THE PLAN OF THE TEXTBOOK

Review of General Psychiatry is divided into 4 sections: basic behavioral science, clinical assessment, the mental disorders, and treatments and special interventions.

The first section presents the basic science of psychiatry, material usually included in first-year psychiatry courses. The first 5 chapters provide a theoretical overview of psychiatry from a historical perspective (Chapter 2), in terms of 4 models of the mind (Chapter 3), and from the perspectives of mind-body relationships (Chapter 4) and stress and adaptation (Chapter 5). Chapters 6–9 present details on human development and the life cycle from birth to death. The brain, behavior, and neurochemistry are presented in Chapters 10 and 11. Psychopathology is introduced in Chapter 12. Chapter 13 discusses epidemiology and describes the mental health services system. Social and cultural aspects of psychiatry are presented in Chapters 14 and 15.

The second section concerns clinical assessment. It can serve as a basic text for introductory courses in interviewing and clinical psychiatry, including a clerkship in psychiatry. Chapter 16 is a character sketch of a patient admitted to a hospital for psychiatric evaluation and treatment. His "case" is presented formally in Chapter 22 after the intervening chapters describe the components of a complete psychiatric evaluation: psychiatric interviews (Chapter 17), mental status examination (Chapter 18), physical and laboratory examination (Chapter 19), intelligence and neuropsychologic tests (Chapter 20), and personality assessment (Chapter 21).

The third and fourth sections may be used as a text for introductory courses in clinical psychiatry and for the core clerkship in psychiatry. Many of the chapters are also designed for use in a consultation-liaison psychiatry course and for courses in the psychiatric aspects of medical practice.

The third section presents the mental disorders, for the most part as they are classified in the third edition of *Diagnostic and Statistical Manual of Mental Disorders Revised (DSM-III-R)*. Chapter 23 introduces psychiatric classification and *DSM-III-R*. Chapters 24–40 discuss the clinical manifestations, diagnostic criteria, differential diagnosis, epidemiology, etiology and pathogenesis, and treatment of each of the mental disorders. An illustrative case is provided for most of the disorders presented in each chapter. Chapter 40 discusses the personality disorders from the dual perspectives of psychiatry and general medicine. For the disorders of childhood and adolescence (Chapter 41), clinical vignettes that constitute the bulk of the chapter are presented to familiarize the reader with the wide range of childhood psychopathology.

The fourth section discusses psychiatric treatment methods and presents some material on special topics in psychiatry. Following an introduction to psychiatric treatment and a few comments on some miscellaneous treatment techniques (Chapter 42), the psychotherapies are discussed (Chapters 43–50), including psychoanalysis and its derivative techniques, behavior and cognitive therapy, group, family, and marital therapy, and psychotherapy with chronic medical patients. Techniques in behavioral medicine are presented in Chapter 51 and the psychoactive drugs in Chapters 52–54. Consultation-liaison psychiatry is the subject of Chapters 55 and 56. The final 4 chapters discuss child psychiatry (Chapter 57), forensic psychiatry (Chapter 58), emergencies—especially suicide and homicide (Chapter 59)—and occupational psychiatry (Chapter 60). A glossary of important symptoms and signs, as well as concepts, related to mental disorders is also provided.

Many chapters are of broad interest and applicability in general medicine. Almost a third of the chapters are suitable for use in a course on the psychiatric aspects of medical practice, including Chapters 4–10 on the mind and body, stress, the brain, and the human life cycle; and Chapters 24–26 on the organic mental disorders, alcoholism, and substance abuse. Parts of Chapters 30–41 include material on depression, anxiety, and stress in adults and children, on psychosexual dysfunction and its treatment, on eating disorders, physical complaints, pain, and malingering, and on the role of personality in medical management; and Chapters 48–60 deal with special psychiatric interventions in family and marital problems, in childhood problems, and in patients with chronic medical disorders.

Although the text was designed for use in general medical and psychiatric education, we hope that trainees and practitioners in other health, mental health, and social welfare disciplines will find *Review of General Psychiatry* helpful and stimulating.

REFERENCES

Dubos R: *Man Adapting*. Yale Univ Press, 1980.

Eisenberg L: Interfaces between medicine and society. *Compr Psychiatry* 1979;**20**:1.

Eisenberg L: Psychiatry and society. *N Engl J Med* 1977; **296**:903.

Engel G: The need for a new medical model: A challenge for biomedicine. *Science* 1977;**196**:129.

Foucault M: *The Birth of the Clinic*. Random House, 1974.

Goldman H: Integrating health and mental health services. *Am J Psychiatry* 1982;**139**:616.

Kandel E: From metapsychology to molecular biology: Explorations into the nature of anxiety. *Am J Psychiatry* 1983; **140**:1277.

Conceptual Issues in the History of Psychiatry

2

Leonard S. Zegans, MD, & Bruce S. Victor, MD

The story of how psychiatry became accepted as a part of medicine, inaugurated the scientific study of mental disorders, and championed the humanistic treatment of the mentally ill is a narrative of courage and resourcefulness, stagnation and doubt. Because the mind has been conceptualized both as an entity separate from the body and as entirely dependent upon somatic processes, it has been claimed as the domain of theologians, philosophers, scientists, and physicians.

Psychiatry's traditional emphasis on emotional considerations as well as on biologic factors in human behavior has set it somewhat apart from other medical specialties. As medicine grew more scientific in diagnosis and treatment and its practitioners and monitors began to insist on statistically significant observations and reproducible results, psychiatry struggled to match this progress while maintaining its humanistic concerns. Even today, because of the complexities of human thought, emotion, and behavior, conventional scientific experimentation and research are available only to a limited extent to those seeking answers to questions about the workings of the mind and the causes and cures of mental disease.

Psychiatry as a branch of medicine has sought to function within the objectives of science as Ayala (1968) has described them: It has attempted to organize knowledge in a systematic way, endeavoring to discover patterns of relationships among phenomena as well as to explain the occurrence of events. In contrast to the theologian, the scientist has not sought the authority of the Scriptures, as Galileo noted, but explanations arrived at by experimentation and demonstration. As a medical discipline, psychiatry has not been lacking in imaginative theories put forward in an attempt to explain a vast number of clinical observations; however, the nature of the subject matter limits testing of hypotheses in ways open to workers in other fields.

The scope of psychiatric study ranges from the smallest cells of the body to large, intricate social systems. Human beings are influenced in their emotions, thoughts, and behavior by their genetic inheritance, the conditions of their birth and development, and the stresses and supports of the environment. Although it is clearly easier to study the structure, function, and pathologic disorders of discrete organ systems than the workings of the human personality, psychiatry, through systematic observation, experimentation, and rational thought, has continued to generate concepts and hypotheses that effectively aid in the diagnosis and treatment of mental disorders.

This chapter will summarize and discuss some of the major issues in the history of psychiatry, tracing the development of its most important concepts. Psychiatrists have supported the somewhat inconsistent concepts that mental disorders are medical illnesses and that each patient must be understood as a unique individual. Indeed, physicians in all medical specialties must sooner or later confront the challenge of the mind-body problem. How medicine has dealt with that issue has been a barometer of its fortunes during various epochs since Greek medicine raised the study of illness from the sleep of superstition.

THE MIND-BODY PROBLEM

For centuries, philosophers and physicians have been asking whether a valid distinction could be made between mind and body. Once a conclusion was reached that such a distinction might be possible, the next logical questions were about the nature of each and how each influenced the other. These questions have been at the center of psychiatric concern for many years and are now vital issues in other areas of medicine as well. Workers in behavioral medicine are now asking how thoughts and feelings can affect the immune system, cardiovascular function, and the operation of the digestive tract—and, conversely, how alterations in somatic function can affect cognition, emotion, and behavior.

The **integrationist** point of view implicit in these questions is a recent development in psychiatry and medicine. Historically, the **idealists** have accorded primacy to the psyche, holding the body to be merely a temporary vessel containing the immortal soul; while the **materialists** have regarded physicochemical processes as the basis of all reality and have posited the mind as an epiphenomenon of those processes.

Those who take the mind to be a special attribute of human beings apart from the physical have been mainly theologians and philosophers. Particularly since Descartes, they have tended to divide the essential unity of man into body and psyche. All that was corporeal could be relegated to the scientist, but the human psyche as a gift from God could not be subjected to the same detached scrutiny as the circulatory and skeletal systems. Aberrant behavior or modes of thinking were variously regarded theologically as signs of "divine madness," possession by demonic agents, or a loss of the soul. Men and women "gone mad" were sometimes elevated to the status of prophets or shamans, sometimes burned as sorcerers or witches. Treatment might include exorcism, prayer, immolation, or forced confession. Disorders of the mind were the province of priests and inquisitors, and the content of madness was not interpreted in light of the individual's personal history but from the perspective of prevailing religious dogma. Although the positive contributions religious experience can make to mental health must be recognized, it must also be acknowledged that medicine struggled for centuries before the study and treatment of disturbed individuals were freed from the constraints of revealed religion.

The dominance of theology over the study of the mind produced a counterreaction as early as the days of Greek medicine. For centuries since that time, rigid empiricists skeptical of philosophic or theologic interpretations of madness have regarded insanity neither as a divine gift nor as a curse of Satan but as a form of illness due to organic causes. Whether those causes were deemed to be a wandering uterus (**hysteria**) or an excess of black bile (**melancholia**) is less important than the idea that mental symptoms were regarded as manifestations of bodily processes and not divine or demonic influences. The neurophysiologist Ralph Gerard (1959) said, "No twisted thought without a twisted molecule." Significant triumphs of this approach include the finding of *Treponema pallidum* in the brains of patients suffering from "general paresis of the insane" (tertiary neurosyphilis) and the identification of nicotinic acid deficiency in patients with pellagra.

Neglected by this tradition, however, was the significant range of problems that might have reflected psychic conflict or maladaptive social behavior. Furthermore, the *meanings* of the individual patient's communication have always been of less importance to the organicists than those pathophysiologic findings that can be observed and measured in the laboratory. This tradition viewed human behavior as determined principally by organic processes—analogous to Pasteur's concept of illness from invasion of microorganisms. The strict organicist could not conceive how the mind could influence the body or behavior.

By contrast, the contents of human thought and the motivations of behavior were very much a concern of theologian idealists. The *Malleus Maleficarum* is a rich store of clinical observations on human sexual fantasies, paranoid ideas, and anxiety as well as speculation concerning their meaning. According to the idealist view, human beings were responsible for their mental diseases precisely because they were free, which implied voluntary consortium with the Devil. It is in this context that the materialism of the 17th and 18th centuries was advanced as a liberating doctrine, counteracting the fanaticism of the demon-fighters. Paradoxically, human dignity was restored by "reducing" human beings to intricate machines.

HISTORICAL CONSIDERATIONS OF THE MIND-BODY PROBLEM

For most of history, societies have held neither to a radical materialist position nor to one of extreme idealism. Most cultures have been **dualistic,** conceding a place to both mind and body, though often regarding them at odds rather than forming a psychophysical unity. In ancient religions, the body was regarded as frail and of minor importance. It was vulnerable, became diseased, and perished. This perception of the impermanence of the flesh led ancient thinkers to perceive the soul as separable from the flesh at death and capable of leading an immortal extracorporeal existence.

In the writings of the ancient Hebrews, the mind-body dualism was part of the West's earliest philosophic heritage. The Hebrews regarded the soul as the seat of feeling and intelligence as well as of personality. At death, the soul was thought to leave the body and pass to Sheol, the abode of the dead. Prophetic tradition later regarded resurrection of the body as essential to life beyond death, since it was impossible to conceive of continuance of the personality apart from the body. The prophets saw humans as complex beings with lower and higher parts, one linked to the life of Nature and the other to the Spirit of God. Interestingly, there was no proper term for "body," because the Hebrew concept of personality did not call for a special word to denote the bodily organism. In the Old Testament, "flesh" was the prevailing term for humanity's earthly part and "spirit" for the heavenly part, while the "soul" was the union of flesh and spirit in the living organism.

This notion of mind-body integration had no parallel in other pre-Christian cultures. Indian tradition (particularly Buddhism) perceived a clear division between body and psyche. Buddha taught that the body can never be the greatest of blessings. The Greek Orphic and Pythagorean schools felt also that all suffering proceeds from the body. Observing the rapid transition from life to death, from dream to waking, and noting states of possession and fainting, they developed the idea of an essential separation of body and psyche.

In *Phaedo,* Plato wrote of the soul as of divine origin and thus imperishable. Sensuality was seen as the worst of plagues, impeding the soul's efforts to return to its celestial home. Though Plato contended that mind and body were fundamentally different in character, he held that the body could exert a damaging influence upon the psyche, impairing its capacity for rational thought and good judgment. Emotions were deemed to be the product of the body and continually in a state of war with "higher thoughts." This implacably dualist theory demanded that the soul strive to keep the senses and all appetites strictly subjugated. Though both the Platonic and Buddhist doctrines held the mind to be the more lasting of the 2 entities, in neither system was it deemed capable of favorably influencing physical health; all it could do was curtail the body's excesses and attempt to escape from its demands.

We can find echoes of Plato's ideas in Freud's concept of drives and their impact upon ego functioning. Freud contended that the drives—and emotions produced by their frustration—could disrupt rational thinking and distort the proper testing of reality. Just as Plato expressed the wish that humankind could be free from the demands of the body to contemplate the true and the beautiful, so too did Freud value the state in which body tensions were abated or sublimated, freeing us to establish healthy object relations and a mature ego.

Not all Greek thinkers perceived a clear division between mind and body. Heraclitus saw body and soul as existing in a state of constant interchange. Aristotle went further in abandoning most of Plato's dualism in putting forth the idea of the organic: An object was organic when its parts functioned together in an attempt to achieve the ends for which the object as a whole was designed. Body and soul, then, were distinguished as concepts but not separable as facts; the soul was thought to form with the body a single life process. In addressing the question whether body and soul are identical, Aristotle stated that the question was analogous to asking whether wax and the shape imprinted on it were identical. Soul, or psyche, was thought to be the essential nature of the body, providing it with its *telos,* or purpose.

The mind-body issue puzzled over by Greek, Hebrew, and Indian cultures came under scrutiny in Christian theology. Nowhere is Christianity's basic ambivalence about the mind-body question expressed with such tension and power as in the writings of Saint Paul, who used the words "soul" and "spirit" to express the inward, godly nature of man, while body had come to be practically synonymous with "flesh." The strong organic unity of the Old Testament was seemingly severed. Yet the notion of the incarnation (*Fleischwerdung,* "made flesh") in the New Testament links it with the earlier Hebraic idea that "flesh is dignified as being brought into a living unit with spirit, the dust of the earth with the breath of life" (Abraham, 1909). Paul ultimately saw in man not an irreconcilable antithesis between matter and spirit but a psychophysical unity of soul and body. The body as the part of being that links man to nature takes a lower position than the soul through which man comes into relationship with God. In Paulist theory, the psyche of man is no mere epiphenomenon of matter, a phantom of molecular processes; the body can affect the soul, but it can in turn be transformed by the spiritual. Thus Paul introduces an **interactionist** concept of the mutual impact of spirit and matter upon each other. Later in the Middle Ages, Thomas Aquinas also affirmed the indissoluble bond between matter and spirit.

This notion of integration of mind and body became a dominant theme in the Renaissance, when artists like Leonardo da Vinci and Michelangelo set out with renewed vigor to study the human form and through painting and sculpture effect a genuine reconciliation of material and spiritual experience. As Leonardo wrote, "It is through substance that spiritual life must be communicated; and this life must be expressed in a concordant vital motion of the body."

With the rise of the scientific revolution, philosophers shifted their concern with soul and spirit to the mind as the seat of cognition and will. The questions that were to interest them the most did not focus on the influence of a corrupting body on an immortal soul but instead on how extensionless substance (mind) could move or change solid matter. Most philosophers fell into one of 2 camps: the **monistic** theorists, who denied that there are 2 things to be related; and the **dualistic** theorists, who admitted that there are 2 things and offered a variety of explanations for their relationship. Some monists took the materialist position that everything that exists is ultimately dependent on objectifiable physical processes. An alternative monist viewpoint, extreme idealism, as espoused by Bishop Berkeley, held that minds and their perceptions were the only things that really exist: "To be" implied either "to be perceived" or "to be a perceiver"; consequently, one could never be certain of the reality of physical objects, since all we know of them is simply how they appear in our minds as categories of perception. Berkeley thus contended that we could perceive only images and never raw reality. Kant was a critic of Berkeley, claiming that he had degraded bodies to the state of mere illusion (a position very close to the Buddhist doctrine). Kant was concerned that idealism obliterated any valid distinction between what existed in bodies and what lay outside them.

Dissatisfaction with the extreme monistic theories of both materialism and idealism spurred the rise of **double-aspect models.** To Spinoza, a proponent of this view, mind and body were but different aspects of an underlying unity (neither mind nor body) that admits of varying representations. This is analogous to modern theories of light, which is viewed as a wave from one scientific perspective and a bundle of particles from another. The nature of light permits it to be perceived in 2 entirely different forms of some (as yet unknown) underlying unity. The "self" has been described by the philosopher P.F. Strawson as a type of entity such that *both* mental and corporeal characteristics are equally applicable to a single individual.

The double-aspect theory has been applied by René Dubos (1960) to the nature of medicine itself from ideas that have been promoted with differing emphasis from antiquity to the present day. Dubos talks about health being preserved by a way of life and health restored by treatment of disease. Both of these models were found in the Greek medical tradition.

The myths of Hygieia and Asclepius symbolise the never-ending oscillation between two different points of view in medicine. For the worshippers of Hygieia, health is the natural order of things, a positive attribute to which men are entitled if they govern their lives wisely. According to them, the most important function of medicine is to discover and teach the natural laws which will ensure a man a healthy mind in a healthy body. More sceptical, or wiser in the ways of the world, the followers of Asclepius believe that the chief role of the physician is to treat disease, to restore health by correcting any imperfections caused by the accidents of birth or life.

The double-aspect model is developed further in the current **biopsychosocial model,** championed recently by George Engel (1977), which stresses that an understanding of physical and mental health is incomplete if based solely on an understanding of chemical or molecular processes. What happens to a woman when she first looks at her new baby can perhaps be correlated with ion-exchange processes, enzymatic release, and neuronal action potentials, but it can never be completely reduced to them. The biopsychosocial model offers an **integrationist** vision of the traditional division between mind and body. It regards such a cleavage as a false dichotomy obscuring man's inextricable organic unity. Any monist theory that denies either the reality of our bodies and their processes or the mind and its meanings and psychologic associations is equally unhelpful in our attempt to understand health and illness.

The mind-body issue is not some remote province of dead philosophers. A recent book by Karl Popper, a philosopher, and Sir John Eccles, a Nobel laureate neurophysiologist, deals imaginatively with the issues presented here. Eccles proposes a theory of the **"self-conscious" mind** based upon his survey of recent neuroanatomic and neurophysiologic research. It is conceived of as an independent entity that is actively engaged in reading out information from the multitude of active centers in the modules of the liaison areas of the dominant cerebral hemisphere. The model suggests that the self-conscious mind selects from the cerebral centers information in accord with its attention and interests and integrates its selection to give unity to conscious experience from moment to moment.

The self-conscious mind also has the ability to act on neural machinery. Popper reminds us that it is an error of current biomedical theory to think in reductionistic terms in which there is a tendency to explain events on one level in terms of the mechanisms of a lower plane. He asserts that there is also another concept, which he terms **downward causation,** in which the macrostructure as a whole may act on and alter the more elementary subsystems or constituent particles. This idea is relevant to the attempt of psychosomatic medicine to comprehend how symbols, meanings, psychologic associations, and emotions can affect cellular behavior in the body. Popper believes that we have become confused in thinking about mind-body issues because of biology's emphasis on seeing organisms as interlocking hierarchies of different "things" rather than processes. He contrasts this to modern physics, which does not see matter as substance but as dense energy transformable into other forms of energy: "The universe appears to be not a collection of things, but an interacting set of events or processes." Popper contends that the correlation of mental events with brain events does not mean a dependency on them. A true interactionist, he writes: "Besides the physical objects and states, I conjecture that there are mental states and these states are real since they interact with our bodies."

It is the recognition of the validity of mental states as having rules, processes, and structures of their own that is embodied in the revolution of psychiatric thought in our century. It permits us to move beyond the classic reductionistic agenda and talk about an integrative **biopsychosocial model.**

HISTORICAL SURVEY OF THE GROWTH OF PSYCHIATRY

Psychiatry has fought to gain acceptance as a medical specialty and claim the treatment of mentally ill patients as a domain for physicians. As a medical specialty, it has attempted both to understand the origin of mental disorders and to discover treatment methods that are effective and safe.

PREHISTORIC & BIBLICAL TIMES

From ancient times, medicine has had difficulty in asserting the right and power to care for the mentally ill. According to Zilboorg and Henry (1941), most primitive and ancient societies regarded mentally disturbed individuals as either "too sacred and good, or too powerful for anyone to venture to reduce them to the unblessed state of normalcy." Early medicine was not clearly demarcated from religion, and priests often served as physicians. The distinction between physical and mental illness did not exist in the ancient world. All sickness was perceived as mental in the sense that it reflected some spiritual problem. For example, a totem may have been violated, an angry spirit may have possessed a person's body, or a vindictive enemy may have cast a dangerous spell.

In early Eastern and Western theology, mental phenomena were not regarded as natural events that could be studied with objectivity. In Deuteronomy (28:28) we read, "The Lord shall smite you with madness and blindness and confusion of mind." Whenever mental processes were seen to reflect theologic issues, science and medicine were prohibited from intervening. Yet even centuries before Christ, the Hindu physician Susruta advanced the idea that passions and strong emotions might cause not only mental disease but physical illness as well. Such ideas were not elaborated until the 19th and 20th centuries.

THE GRECO-ROMAN ERA

The Greeks were the first to study mental diseases scientifically and separate the study of the mind from religion. Greek medicine was influenced by Ionian natural philosophy, which sought "natural" explanations for events. The Ionian philosophers attempted to trace every effect back to its cause and show how the sum of all causes and effects made up a universal order. Most importantly, they believed that the secrets of the world could be unlocked by unbiased observations of things and by the power of reason. Greek medicine sought universal laws that could form the basis of a real science of illness. It searched for insights into the laws that governed illness, seeking the connection between part and whole, cause and effect.

Greek medicine fought also to free itself from the influence of natural philosophy, which had earlier helped in throwing off the mantle of theology. Hippocratic thought did not isolate a disease and examine it solely as a special problem in itself. In *On Airs, Waters, and Places,* the physician is advised to look steadily and clearly at the *person* who has the disease and see that individual against all of the natural surroundings with their universal laws and special characteristics. In *On the Divine Disease* (epilepsy), the author makes the critical claim that this disease is no more or less divine than any other and arises from the same natural causes as others do.

The Greek physician began to insist upon detailed observation of the needs of each patient without recourse to the theories of natural philosophy. The Greek medical ideal was based on the idea of the **organic.** The medical approach was to comprehend the function of the part within the whole and provide the appropriate treatment of the part. The Greek physician was concerned with health and not only with disease. There was an *arete,* an excellence in the symmetry of the parts of forces in which normal health consisted. The ideals of Greek medicine focused on how those balances of nature that supported and maintained health could be restored and assisted. Their ideas are evocative of current ideas of "behavioral medicine," where the notions of how people eat, sleep, exercise, and handle stress are related to vulnerability to illness.

The Hippocratic tradition had most influence on Greek thought on the nature and viability of the mind. Hippocratic writing always emphasized the natural origins of mental illness: Depending upon the case being discussed, Hippocrates advanced either an anatomic theory of madness (disease or injury of the brain), a physiologic theory (the various body fluids are responsible for mental illness), or a psychologic theory (that emotional states may produce significant mental or physical changes). Hippocrates located the human capacity to feel, think, or dream in the brain. He was the first to propose what Freud later emphasized, that dreams are the expression of our wishes given access to consciousness when the demands of reality are removed. The Hippocratic tradition attempted to synthesize the contemporary philosophic, anatomic, physiologic, and psychologic information and theories to give a picture of the human being functioning as a whole.

Later Greek philosophy, whether reflected in Stoicism or Epicureanism, gave greater emphasis to human beings' relationships to their fellow human beings and society rather than the cosmos. It stressed the importance of feelings and sensations. These schools regarded the individual as a *tabula rasa,* influenced only by the experiences of the environment. The themes of individualism, environmentalism, and the influence of anatomy and physiology on thinking were introduced by the Greeks, but their development into a coherent theory of body and mind did not take place until over 2 millennia later.

Many of these themes influenced Roman philosophy and medicine. **Cicero** acknowledged the role of emotions in mental disorders, while **Plutarch** wrote a clinically accurate and compassionate description of a depressed individual. We find in the Roman writer **Celsus** a concern with the treatment of the mentally ill. He wrote that it was proper to confine or restrain persons who behave violently in order to prevent them from injuring themselves or others. He advocated sudden fright as therapy for mental disease. The notion that restraint, coercion, and fright might bring mentally ill individuals to their senses persisted in medicine until recently.

Perhaps the last of the great classical physicians was **Galen,** who held that mental diseases could be caused by direct affliction of the brain or by "consensus," a sympathetic response of the brain to an illness in another part of the body. He postulated that the seat of the soul is inseparable from the nerve centers. He attempted a descriptive psychology that divided the "rational soul" into 2 parts: external and internal. The external functions are those of the 5 senses; the internal functions are imagination, judgment, memory, apperception, and movement. The concept of separate psychologic functions would receive more detailed attention in the 20th century with the rise of **ego psychology.**

EARLY CHRISTIAN & MEDIEVAL PERIODS

The end of the classical era and the coming of the Dark Ages ushered in an epoch of political chaos and war and a decline of humanistic and scientific learning. The world of barbarian invasions, the destruction of the Roman Empire, and the influx of Eastern mystery cults as well as the rise of Christianity did not provide an environment favorable to dispassionate research concerning the mind and body. Throughout the West and Middle East, religious thought turned to faith, salvation, and ecstatic experience. Not only in medicine but also in mathematics, history, and philosophy, the dogma of revealed truth preempted scholarship and research. The Edict of Milan, whereby Constantine established Christianity as the religion of the Roman Empire in 313 AD, specifically interdicted the study of Plato and Aristotle. In order to establish the authority of the Church, remnants of pagan culture were stamped out. The Codex Theodosianus of 438 AD condemned magic and endorsed the prosecution of the "possessed" as well as of witches and sorcerers. Thus, the study and treatment of the mentally ill became an issue for religion, not for medicine. Hippocrates' view that mental disorders were not punishments or gifts of the gods was forgotten. Study of anatomy was hindered by Church strictures against dissection of human cadavers. Zilboorg and Henry (1941) note that mental diseases, which were apparently increasing in incidence, were excluded from medicine and became a part of general superstition. The Church, frightened and puzzled by mental illness, began to regard study of such illness as work of the Devil. Study of the symptoms of mental illness and the content of thought of those afflicted continued, but under the auspices of demonology. The so-called *stigmata diaboli*—anesthetic spots and nevi that were the signs of possession—were clearly identified by clerical observers. These "manifestations of the devil" were later observed in hysterics by Charcot in the 19th century.

The Arabs, who achieved political power in the Middle East in the 7th century, were able to keep some of the spirit of classicism alive and, by rejecting demonologic ideas, continued to make sound observations about the mentally ill. The great Arab physicians and philosophers preserved and transmitted the scientific observations of Aristotle, along with the concept that what may be true in theology did not necessarily apply to philosophy or science.

Despite prevailing superstition, a few Western European religious leaders taught an enlightened and humane psychology. The Abbot of Stella even came close to asserting the existence of the unconscious when he stated that not everything now present is continuously present, nor does all that a person knows remain always directly present in the eye of the mind. During the Middle Ages, a considerate and kind attitude toward the possessed began to find expression. The powers of the saints were invoked for their cure. Some of the great spiritual leaders of the age, like John of Salisbury and Peter Abelard, denied the power of the Devil to produce mental aberrations.

Yet the number of mentally ill persons increased, and with it the uneasiness of clerical and secular authorities. Torture and immolation soon became weapons in the fight against disorders of the mind. The idea took root that physical illnesses were due to natural causes and mental illnesses to supernatural ones.

Conditions of war, epidemic, and superstition in the Middle Ages led to outbursts of mass hysteria. The flagellants during the 13th century spawned a variety of imitative self-punitive groups all over Europe. There was all manner of ecstatic outbreaks, ascetic flagellants, and wandering eccentrics. In the late Middle Ages, when the authority of the Roman Catholic Church began to be threatened, heterodoxy came to be equated with sorcery, and the mentally ill became innocent victims of theologic anxiety and cultural change. Just as the Renaissance was offering promise of a new spirit of humanism and learning, the saddest chapter in the history of psychiatry began. When the physician to Pope Innocent X said, *Gaudet humore melancholico daemon* ("the devil rejoices in a bath of melancholy humor"), he summed up the belief that moral transgression and mental illness were regarded as one and the same.

The form of moral transgression that preoccupied the Renaissance was sexuality. It was believed that demons entered into carnal relations with the possessed. The witch—a woman who was tainted by devils and snared men into mortal sin through her sexuality—became a fearful figure. The battle against demonic agencies was spearheaded by 2 Dominican monks, Johann Sprenger and Heinrich Kraemer, who wrote the *Malleus Maleficarum,* in which the "treatment" prescribed for mental illness was torture even to the extreme of death. The authors denied that mental aberrations were the result of natural causes and attributed hallucinations, delusions, and sexual anxiety to Satan. In one paragraph, they destroyed the entire classical heritage of scientific observation and concern about the mentally disturbed:

> Those err who say that there is no such thing as witchcraft, but that it is purely imaginary, even although they do not believe that devils exist except in the imagination of the ignorant and vulgar, and the natural accidents which happen to a man he wrongly attributes to some supposed devil. For the imagination of some men is so vivid that they think they see actual figures and appearances which are but the reflections of their thoughts, and then these are believed to be apparitions of evil spirits or even the spectres of witches. But this is contrary to true faith which teaches us that certain angels fell from heaven and are now devils, and we are bound to acknowledge that by their nature they can do many things which we cannot do, and those who try to induce others to perform such evil wonders are called witches. And because infidelity in a person who has been baptized is technically called heresy, therefore such persons are plainly heretics.

The implications of this statement are that even if people fall ill and the disease alters their thoughts and perceptions, creating illusions, this is done solely of their own free will. Those who accept Satan must be punished, and the immortal soul imprisoned in the sinful body must be set free. Thus was established the rationale for the *auto-da-fé;* the burning of the witch or sorcerer was justified as an act of mercy and religious devotion. The *Malleus* held that stories of sexual activity with demons were literal recountings of actual events and not the products of disturbed minds. It was never considered that sexual frustration and restraint resulting in erotic fantasies could account for these lurid confessions. The era was antierotic and misogynistic as well as anxious to preserve the authority of the Church against heresy.

THE RENAISSANCE & THE RISE OF SCIENCE

What followed publication of the *Malleus* in 1487 was an epoch of cruelty, yet simultaneously one of creativity and a renewed sense of discovery of nature and of human beings. The 16th century was the time of Luther, Leonardo da Vinci, Copernicus, Erasmus, Francis Bacon, Montaigne, and Shakespeare. These were times that permitted the most terrible burning of witches but also supported the rise of humanism, creativity in the arts, the return to secular learning, and the scientific assertion that evidence rather than dogma was the cornerstone of knowledge.

Gradually, some medical authorities such as Levinus Lemnius asserted, again, that mental diseases, including epilepsy, were not supernaturally inspired. Montaigne wrote: "Is it not far more natural to think that our mind is deranged by the vulnerability of our crazed spirits than to believe that a mere mortal with the help of strange spirits could in person fly out through the chimney on a broomstick?" Despite the humanism of the Renaissance and the rediscovery of Greek and Roman medicine, the burning of witches continued well into the so-called Enlightenment. In Switzerland in 1782, the last "witch" to die in Europe was executed by decapitation.

The great scholars of the 16th century such as Erasmus, Thomas More, Juan Luis Vives, and Francis Bacon turned their attentions to the mind as something apart from the soul. The properties of the mind came to be associated with the body and with social circumstances rather than with the soul. The emphasis began to shift away from metaphysics and toward description and empirical experimentation. Human motivation—the drives, wishes, and impulses that lead to action—was considered apart from divine or satanic influences. This led to an interest in the role of human emotions in mental illness and to further study as well of treatment of the mentally ill.

Though scientists became bolder in studying natural phenomena in the 17th and 18th centuries, there was still a reluctance to consider the mind itself as a suitable object for empirical study. What progress was made during that time in the study of human behavior was from the perspective of physiologic and physical organization. **Johann Weyer** proposed that careful attention be paid in all cases to the ideational content of each patient's illness, but this revolutionary concept was abandoned almost at the moment it was proclaimed. As scientists turned their attention toward hu-

man behavior, medicine gradually returned to the view that mental disease was the direct product of untoward conditions in the brain.

This transition did not immediately signify the advent of more humane treatment for the mentally ill or the end of belief in demonic possession and satanic influences. Even the neuroanatomist **Thomas Willis** (1621–1675) believed in devils and in the efficacy of harsh treatment of the mentally ill—ie, the use of threats, fetters, and blows as adjuncts to medical treatment. Such methods were thought to act by inducing the mind to give up its arrogance and wild ideas. The American **Benjamin Rush** (1745–1813) similarly believed in the intimidation of difficult patients as well as in the salutary effects of emetics, purgatives, and bloodletting for mental illness.

It seems hardly possible nowadays that these scientists should have harbored punitive and abusive attitudes toward mentally ill people. They may have shared the widespread fear of these persons historically inspired by theologic doctrine, but the absence of an internally consistent model that could be used to understand the mind and mental illness was probably a more important reason. The mind considered as an entity apart from the body or soul had yet to emerge as an object of scientific study, though it was of interest to the philosophers Hobbes, Spinoza, Descartes, and Locke. The materialist tradition became even stronger during the 18th century, and while it ultimately superseded demonology, it seemed at the same time to make no place for the psychologic understanding of humankind. The doctors who took a humane approach to the mentally ill had only their intuitive habit of sympathy for suffering people to guide them. There was no systematic study of the roles of drives, developmental disorders, and psychic conflict in the origin of mental disorders. It was the hope of Descartes and others that the relationship between thoughts and organs could be clarified by a process of reasoning. This search for a synthetic understanding became a project that contemporary psychiatry was to pursue with vigor and imagination if not always with success.

THE ENLIGHTENMENT & THE RISE OF HUMANISM

The philosophers of the Enlightenment celebrated human reason as perhaps the most valuable aspect of human existence and continued to resist the authority of religious dogma. The idea that each individual possessed a rational faculty had political ramifications that were expounded in the writings of Rousseau, Paine, and others who stressed the doctrine of "inalienable rights." As we have already noted, the triumph of human reason led to the dominance in Western thought of materialistic attitudes which, somewhat paradoxically, regarded human beings as essentially machines despite their newfound freedoms.

The Enlightenment introduced reform in the care of mentally ill persons, including the establishment of mental hospitals and the development of better clinical observations, nosologies of mental disorders, and theories about the causes of mental disorders.

Two men who strove to create humane conditions for the mentally ill were **William Tuke,** who founded the York Retreat in England to serve as a model for a humane setting for treatment of mentally ill patients; and **Philippe Pinel,** who, as physician-in-chief at Bicêtre in Paris, lived with his patients, studying their habits and individual personalities. He advocated not only physical treatment but also "moral treatment," a purely psychologic approach.

In the early years of the 19th century, psychiatry became the first medical specialty separately organized as such. Great hospitals were built, and complex systems were designed for classification of mental disease. As the interest in nosology increased, interest in the patient as an individual diminished. Yet the 19th century was also a time when a broader range of mental phenomena came to be examined. Interest focused not only on the severely mentally ill, who needed confinement in hospitals, but also on the common "neuroses" that afflicted courtiers and bankers as well as ordinary people. Psychiatrists began to study not only their patients' brains but their individual experiences as well, along with interplay of conflicting psychologic forces. Full comprehension of the role of these dynamics in the production of symptoms awaited the discovery of the unconscious.

THEORIES OF THE UNCONSCIOUS

One of psychiatry's most important scientific contributions has been the concept that human thoughts and feelings have patterns and structures that can be investigated. Much of what constituted the scientific revolution dealt with the "primary" qualities of matter and descriptions of the size, shape, and movement of spatially discrete bodies. Basic laws and principles of behavior have not, in the past, been accorded the same scientific respect as the study of primary properties of physical objects. Within medical science, psychiatry has been in the vanguard of concern about the meanings of human thought and behavior, regarding them as important biologic as well as psychologic events and central to the evaluation of symptoms.

Meanings, however, are often difficult to discern. Communication of ideas and feelings is essential to human survival, yet people have the ability to distort, dissociate, and disguise their intentions not only from others but also from themselves.

The concept that ideas and mental processes exist outside of awareness and indeed are inaccessible to conscious perception has been a provocative notion in Western thought. How can one become aware of mental activity that is by definition not consciously perceptible? For the clinician, the significance of the unconscious lies in its presumed effect on motivation and behavior. Patients seek help from psychiatrists and other mental health practitioners in order to gain a clearer understanding of dysfunctional patterns of behavior that have eluded their awareness and comprehension.

The work of **Sigmund Freud** is so well known to the general public that the idea of the unconscious is sometimes believed to have sprung fully formed from his brow. Yet the idea of unconscious processes was part of the tradition of 19th century Romantic German philosophy and literature and before that of 18th century French thought.

ANIMAL MAGNETISM & HYPNOSIS

Franz Anton Mesmer (1734–1815), a physician who exerted great influence among the aristocrats and intelligentsia of Europe, posited the existence of a fluid that filled the universe and was the means through which humans were connected to nature and to one another. According to his theory, the origin of disease could be traced to disturbances of this fluid in the body; health depended upon reestablishment of the proper balance of this fluid. The "magnetizer" (therapist) cured patients by utilizing his own fluid—his own "animal magnetism"—to correct their imbalances.

Mesmer claimed that he was able to effect cures by instigating **crises,** ie, by repeatedly provoking the symptoms from which patients suffered, in order to exhaust the symptoms to the point of disappearance. Mesmer felt that success in this effort depended on rapport between the magnetizer and the patient. He observed that after emergence from their crises, patients generally remembered nothing of what had occurred. He understood intuitively that some elements in our lives are too painful, threatening, or dissonant to be remembered and examined by conscious observation. Yet Mesmer also understood the therapeutic necessity of somehow coming to terms with one's past because of the tremendous power it could exert over one's present circumstances.

The concept and practice of **hypnosis** (Gk *hypnos* "sleep") gradually supplanted magnetism and began, through the efforts of **James Braid** (1795–1869), to find its place in received science. Hypnosis provided a means of examining the unconscious content and processes of mental life. By the mid 19th century, the principle that the unconscious existed as a separate entity alongside ordinary waking consciousness was well accepted. It was deemed to be a repository for forgotten ideas and sense impressions that were not amenable to easy access by the conscious mind. The unconscious was believed to exert some undefined influence over conscious thought and to play a role in the pathogenesis of somatic symptoms. Conversely, it was believed that access to the unconscious permitted greater control over otherwise involuntary somatic processes, leading to cures of a variety of disorders. What emerged was a model of the bicameral mind, divided into conscious and unconscious chambers with a dynamic interaction between the two. Problems in this interaction were thought to result in various degrees of somatic and psychologic distress.

Hippolyte-Marie Bernheim (1840–1919), a professor of internal medicine, wrote a textbook that highlighted the importance of suggestion in hypnosis and demonstrated that commands issued to a subject in a hypnotic state could be carried out in a waking condition, without the subject's knowledge. Bernheim came to believe that subjects were amenable to therapeutic suggestion in an unhypnotized state, calling this procedure **psychotherapy** and himself the "father of psychotherapy." Thus, the ground was being prepared for the procedure that Freud was later to develop into the instrument of psychoanalysis: **free association.**

THE SALPÊTRIÈRE SCHOOL: CHARCOT & L'HYSTERIE

In 1870, **Jean-Martin Charcot** (1825–1893) had established himself as the foremost neurologist of his day and the Salpêtrière as a center of medical learning. Charcot became fascinated with the investigation of hysteria through the use of hypnosis. His emphasis was on the clinical distinction between patients who suffered from organic lesions and those whose symptoms were produced "hysterically." While Charcot was ultimately able to distinguish between the two, he was not able to ascertain how psychologic factors could generate somatic symptoms. Charcot took a step toward answering that question in 1884 when he turned his attention to posttraumatic paralysis in 3 men admitted to the Salpêtrière with paralysis involving one arm following a psychologically traumatic incident. He demonstrated not only that the nature of the symptoms was exactly the same as in hysterical paralysis but also that they could be made to disappear *or could be reproduced* under the influence of hypnosis. Furthermore, the symptoms could also be reproduced by posthypnotic suggestion.

Charcot, then, was the first to study the role of psychologic trauma in production of symptoms. Drawing upon his studies of patients under hypnosis, he hypothesized that a hypnoid state is induced following trauma such that these symptoms can be provoked by suggestion even though it is not possible to relieve the symptoms in the waking state. Charcot cleaved to the notion of the unconscious, perceiving it as a storehouse of memories and events sequestered from ordinary consciousness, acquired in a hypnoid state, and resulting in physical symptoms. For this formulation and for his explication of the pathogenic mechanisms of trauma, Charcot is rightly honored as one of the founders of modern psychodynamic theory.

SIGMUND FREUD & PSYCHOANALYSIS

Sigmund Freud (1856–1939) was born in Moravia, moved to Vienna with his family when he was 4, and made his home there until he fled to England the year before his death. His route to fame as founder of psychoanalysis was somewhat circuitous. As a student, Freud did research in histopathology. He then turned his attentions to the new field of neuropathology and wrote an important paper on the structure of the nervous system. He later became a clinical neurologist and wrote respected treatises on cerebral palsy and aphasia.

In 1895, Freud wrote *A Project for Scientific Psychology,* in which he attempted to link various psychologic processes with areas of neuronal discharge. This is noteworthy for the development of the concept of **ego.** In this work, which was not published during his lifetime, Freud hypothesized that the ego was actually a collection of neurons whose main function was inhibition of cerebral excitation in the service of maintaining a grasp on reality.

The Exploration of Neurosis & the Origin of Psychoanalysis

Just as was true of Charcot, Freud's study of neurotic patients formed the basis of his theories of the unconscious. Freud's interest in the problems of hysteria, first aroused by watching Charcot's demonstrations of posttraumatic paralysis, was later intensified by his colleague Josef Breuer's famous patient, Anna O, whose hysterical symptoms reportedly disappeared when Breuer made her aware of their precipitating events through the use of hypnosis. In the *Preliminary Communication* (1893), Breuer and Freud highlight the effect of psychic trauma on the pathogenesis of hysterical symptoms. Freud went on to develop the concept that the dynamic tension preserving symptom formation in this manner was a **defense** against conscious knowledge of the traumatic event. Freud noted also that the mental material being defended against was the representation of current or past sexual trauma.

Freud soon abandoned the notion that trauma was necessary for the generation of neurotic symptoms; he concluded that neurotic symptoms could represent a defense against unconscious **fantasies.** Freud's conception of the unconscious, then, expanded to include not only suppressed memories but fantasies as well.

Freud's idea of the aim of therapy was not to unearth traumatic episodes but to ferret out unconscious fantasies. In his *Introductory Lectures,* Freud defined these fantasies as representing the desire for wish fulfillment, ie, the gratification of sexual impulses. The pathogenesis of neurotic symptoms, then, is the process of compromise between the impulse toward sexual gratification (the energy for which was called **libido**) and the defenses of the ego. Freud wrote that no neurosis could occur without such a conflict. In view of the opposition from the ego defenses, the libido **regresses** to a psychic state that was relatively atraumatic and **fixates** its energy at this stage. As a result, the symptom becomes "a derivative, distorted in manifold ways of the unconscious libidinal wish fulfillment" securing an "exceedingly restricted . . . hardly recognizable" gratification of this wish. As we shall see, the nature of the defense mechanisms will determine the outward form of the symptom.

Freud did more than change the aim of therapy in his investigation of the neuroses; he also changed the technique. In *Studies on Hysteria,* Freud tells how a patient, Elizabeth von R, suggested to him that she be allowed to use the method of **free association** that is now a mainstay of psychoanalytic technique. This development was crucial in that it provided the clinician with an alternative to hypnosis as a means of gaining access to the unconscious. Freud in this way formulated the **fundamental rule** of psychoanalysis, which was for the patient to say whatever came to mind, no matter how embarrassing or seemingly irrelevant the material. As with magnetizers and hypnotists, Freud noted that subjects would often experience **resistance** to compliance with the rule. Freud also noted inappropriate feelings of love or hatred of the clinician during psychoanalysis and called the phenomenon **transference,** claiming that it represented emotions directed toward significant figures in early development that were "transferred" onto the therapist. Transference material served as a valuable source of important inferences about unconscious processes. Before Freud, the clinical significance of the relationship between the therapist and the patient was not recognized, particularly its usefulness as a means of identifying unconscious themes.

In his studies of neurosis, Freud extended our knowledge of the unconscious and further characterized the dynamic nature of its interaction with conscious thought. Psychoanalysis, as a means of identifying and working through unconscious mental material, represented a revolutionary development in the history of psychiatry insofar as it (1) provided a technique other than hypnosis that could lead to the exploration of unconscious material; (2) broadened the subject matter of analytic work to include exploration of unconscious wishes and fantasies; and (3) defined a therapeutic relationship that itself was thought to recapitulate important unconscious dynamics in the life of the patient.

Dreams & the Evolution of the Topographic Model

Freud wrote that the "interpretation of dreams is the *via regia* to a knowledge of the unconscious in psychic life." He posited that the usual defenses which keep unconscious contents from emerging into awareness are slackened; consequently, the dream manifests unconscious ideation albeit in disguised form.

Freud's theory of dreams can be summarized as follows:

Underlying the **manifest content** of a dream is the **latent dream content,** which is essentially the uncon-

scious wish that would otherwise awaken the dreamer from sleep. The central premise of the **dream work,** the process whereby the latent dream content is transformed into its manifest form, is that the unconscious wish is unacceptable to the dreamer. In order to avoid the consequence of a more blatant display of this wish, Freud assigns to a **censor** the function of keeping the wish within the bounds of consciousness. Yet the dream work consists of the unconscious mental operations by which the latent content becomes sufficiently disguised to bypass the censor to appear in the manifest dream. These mechanisms include (1) **condensation,** wherein a single element of the manifest dream may come to represent several unacceptable ideas; (2) **displacement,** wherein an important unconscious idea can be represented by a seemingly trivial detail in the dream; (3) **symbolization,** wherein a particular element of the manifest dream represents an element in the latent content; and (4) **dramatization,** wherein thoughts otherwise not amenable to visual representation receive just such a representation. Having been transformed by these 4 processes, the latent content undergoes a **secondary elaboration** that serves the function of synthesizing these distorted fragments into the manifest dream content. The process of interpreting the dream, then, involves essentially the reverse of the process by which the manifest content of the dream was formed. Like the untangling (so it can be discarded) of a hysterical symptom, this could be accomplished by psychoanalysis using free association.

From this theory of dreaming, Freud was to generate a new conceptualization of the mind involving the dynamic interaction of 2 systems "of which one constitutes the wish expressed by the dream, while the other acts as censorship upon this dream wish, and so forces a distortion of its expression." The former Freud labeled "the system **unconscious**"; the latter was called "the system **conscious**." Inherent in the idea of the system conscious was that of "the system **preconscious**," which contains ideas that are not in active consciousness at a given time but could become manifest without further distortion. This **topographic model** represents further developments in characterizing the unconscious as opposed to the conscious. Going beyond the formulation of the cases presented in *Studies on Hysteria,* Freud described in greater detail the contents of the unconscious and the processes by which unconscious material can reach consciousness. In later elaborations of this model, 2 different modes of thinking are deemed to be characteristic of each. Specifically, **primary process,** or a more primitive, irrational, and pictorial mode of representation, was said to predominate in the unconscious; whereas **secondary process,** or verbal, linear, rational thought, was deemed to be more characteristic of the system conscious. At this point, the dream itself could become a focus for therapy.

The Structural Model & the Redefinition of the Ego

Ultimately, Freud's observations led him to conclude that his earlier concept of the **pleasure principle** was insufficient to explain the myriad clinical phenomena he encountered. He discovered that not all human behavior served the pursuit of pleasure. He increasingly focused on the tendency of the organism to protect itself from overstimulation, serving the end of maintaining psychologic equilibrium. Freud corroborated this idea with the observation of the **repetition compulsion,** observing that even in play, children tend to repeat emotionally traumatic life events. He thus postulated that there was a set of "life instincts" **(eros)** which included the sexual instincts; and the "death instinct" **(thanatos),** both of which were consigned to the unconscious.

Freud realized that positing these 2 competing instincts in the unconscious deprived the topographic model of its usefulness. The mind could not be described simply in terms of the conscious and unconscious. With the publication of *The Ego and the Id* in 1923, he discarded this model in favor of the **structural** model, wherein mental phenomena were deemed to manifest the dynamic interaction of 3 intrapsychic agents. The **id** comprised the drives, fantasies, and repressed ideas and emotions that could not find representation in consciousness in unmodified form. The **superego,** hypothesized to be an independent, unconscious psychic structure only after splitting off from the ego, contained both the **ego ideal**—that which the individual would most like to emulate—and the social and religious sanctions of a given culture. The **ego,** then, was the "coordinated organization of mental processes." The nature of this "coordination" was such that while one part of the ego was responsible for successful navigation in the world, utilizing processes of perception and motor action, the other part was involved in the process of defense, both in waking life and in dreaming. Consequently, the ego was said to be part conscious and part unconscious. It is depicted as serving 3 masters and arbitrating between 3 kinds of anxiety in attempting to balance the demands of reality, the id, and the superego or otherwise face "reality anxiety," "drive anxiety," or "guilt anxiety," respectively.

The transition to the structural model represented a shift in emphasis from exclusive concern with the conscious and unconscious mind to the study of ego functions. The subject matter of analysis changed from unconscious wishes to defenses against them. Examination of these defenses in the context of the analytic relationship would strengthen the ego and help the patient deal more effectively with the demands of life. (See Chapters 3 and 5 for details on psychoanalytic theory and the mechanisms of defense.)

Freud in Perspective

Although Freud has been popularly regarded as a champion of the role of early environmental influences on behavior, he in fact searched all his professional life for the expression of biologic factors in the human psyche. He was made uncomfortable by his inability to ground his theories of mental function in human biology. He believed that his use of purely psychologic concepts to explain human motivation and behavior would be superseded one day by models from the neurosciences and biochemistry. Early in his psychoanalytic career, he made an attempt to correlate mental functions with hypothesized neuronal circuits. However, he realized that despite the ingenuity of many of the ideas expressed in *A Project for Scientific Psychology,* there was a weakness in this attempt to "neurologize" psychology. The prevailing techniques of psychoanalysis and those of the neurosciences did not permit a meaningful correlation between complex psychologic events and neural pathways. Freud never published this work and repeatedly cautioned his followers against a premature synthesis of biology and psychology.

According to Freud, the historical role of psychoanalysis would be to study in depth mental phenomena that had never before been examined. The instruments of such study were free association and dream interpretation. The scientific ethos of his day was reflected in Freud's firm belief in the empirical clinical method. Freud's speculative mind never hesitated to put forth new theories; through his "metapsychology" as well as by his clinical work, he made many contributions to our understanding of how the mind functions and psychopathologic disorders develop. Among his many important contributions can be listed the following:

(1) Identifying the etiologic role of **intrapsychic conflict** in the neuroses.

(2) Emphasizing the influence of **early maturational factors** (particularly childhood sexuality) on later adult development.

(3) Delineating the existence of **defense mechanisms** in warding off conflictual thoughts or feelings and their impact on neurotic symptoms, dreams, character structure, and slips of the tongue.

(4) Discovering the role of **transference** (unconscious attitudes toward the therapist that were earlier directed to parental figures) in the psychotherapeutic situation.

(5) Clarifying the role of **anxiety** as a sign of unconscious conflict.

(6) Identifying the 2 major modes of thought mechanisms: **primary** and **secondary processes.** The latter is linear, logical thought; the former is a process of analogic thinking in which time sequences become confused and their emotional similarities rather than conceptual logic determine associative processes.

(7) Investigating **regressive behavior,** whereby earlier, more infantile choices become the objects of desire and the modes of thought and communication become more primitive.

(8) Elaborating the phenomenon of **fixation**—a state of maturational arrest, so that the individual cannot advance to the next stage of development because of conflict or frustration.

(9) Identifying unconscious moral precepts **(the**

superego) derived from identification with the parents and the role of cultural values in shaping conscience and feelings of guilt.

(10) Observing **repetition compulsion,** the tendency of patients to repeat painful or frustrating earlier experiences.

(11) Observing the phenomenon of **narcissism,** where individuals take themselves rather than others as their prime object of love and interest.

Freud was a bold thinker, mixing clinical observations with theoretical speculations. He tried to understand the workings of the mind from a developmental perspective, through observing the impact of family and society on the growing individual while studying the impact of genetic and constitutional factors on the psychologic growth of the individual. Freud discovered that just as biologic influences can alter the functioning of the mind, so too (as revealed in his early studies on hysteria) could cognitive and emotional factors change the working of the body. Freud's clinical observations were a powerful impetus for the development of psychosomatic medicine. He helped bridge the conceptual gap between the psychologic and the organic by pointing out that the *meanings* of individual experience were in themselves *biologic* events. Later, he and many of his followers became more interested in the adaptational components of the mind—the so-called **ego functions.**

THE FOLLOWERS OF FREUD

The Ego Psychologists

Anna Freud (Sigmund Freud's daughter), **Heinz Hartmann, Ernst Kris,** and **Rudolf Loewenstein** were concerned with the role of psychic conflict and its effects on neurotic illness and the development of conflict-free mental functions. This idea served to emphasize the autonomy of the ego beyond what was envisioned by Freud. The end result, then, would be to assert that the mind could transcend a life of seemingly endless compromises between psychic agencies. This led to the consideration of maturational stages beyond those addressed in classic psychoanalytic theory by clinicians such as **Erik Erikson.** For Erikson, it was important not only that maturing individuals should develop the capacity for sexual bonding but that they should be capable of forming stable **identities** and living their adult lives with **integrity.**

Considerations of Personality & Society: Horney & Sullivan

The observations and ideas of Freud stimulated interest in the concept of **personality.** This construct has been defined in various ways. Gordon Allport (1937) has called it "the dynamic organization within the individual of those psychophysical systems that determine his characteristic behavior and thought." Most authors think of personality as a fairly stable complex of individual traits, styles, needs, habits, or motives. There has been an abiding interest in the relationship of certain personality traits to the development of psychiatric disorders (eg, schizophrenia, depression) and somatic illnesses (eg, peptic ulcer, coronary artery disease). The issues of biologic (genetic, constitutional) causation of personality as contrasted to sociocultural environmental influences determining these traits have continued into the 20th century, with much debate and disagreement. Certain clinician-theorists take the view that experiences in the family and society shape the individual personality, while others stress internal biologic processes.

Two influential psychiatrists who emphasized the environmental and social aspects of personality and disease were Horney and Sullivan. **Karen Horney** wished to go beyond what she considered the "mechanistic" and "biological" theories of Freud. She described 10 basic **neurotic needs** an individual acquired in the search for resolution of disturbed human relationships:

(1) The need for affection and approval.

(2) The need to restrict one's life within narrow borders.

(3) The need for a partner who will take over one's life.

(4) The need for power.

(5) The need to exploit others.

(6) The need for prestige.

(7) The need for personal admiration.

(8) The need for ambition for personal achievement.

(9) The need for self-sufficiency and independence.

(10) The need for perfection and unassailability.

Horney felt that conflicts over these needs are avoidable or resolvable if the child is reared in a home where there is **security, trust,** and **warmth.** Unlike Freud and Jung, she felt that conflict is an outgrowth of social conditions and not part of human nature.

Harry Stack Sullivan believed that personality is the relatively stable pattern of interaction with other people that characterizes each individual. Thus, for Sullivan, personality cannot be divorced from its interpersonal context. Anxiety, which is the main component of neurotic distress, arises as a consequence of interpersonal situations. Interpersonal relations mediate the basic human needs, which Sullivan believes are (1) tenderness, (2) security, (3) intimacy, and (4) peers. He refers to the **self-system,** by which he means all of the behaviors the child acquires in the course of interpersonal relationships that serve the function of avoiding or minimizing anxiety. Some of these behaviors crystallize into specific **security operations**—disordered responses which are inappropriate to the purpose of avoiding anxiety-producing events and which conflict with other sequences of responses that would lead to satisfaction.

Both Horney and Sullivan were greatly influenced by concepts of **learning theory** (see Chapter 3).

Learning has been defined by Hilgard and Bower (1966) as "the process by which an activity originates or is changed through reacting to an encountered situation." There have been many approaches to learning in our century, particularly **classical conditioning** (Pavlov), **trial and error** (Thorndike), and learning through observational activity and **identification** (Bandura). Specific therapies based on learning theory have taken their place along with psychoanalysis as approaches to treating patients with phobias and anxiety reactions, and they have also been used for habit abatement (eg, to stop smoking and drug abuse). (See Chapters 46 and 51.)

Jung & the Collective Unconscious

Carl Gustav Jung (1875–1961) was an early disciple of Freud who later broke with him over Freud's emphasis on infantile sexuality as the dominant factor in neurotic illness. Jung believed sexuality was but one of many influences that shaped personality and made one susceptible to mental illness. He believed that both ontogenetic factors (those arising during the course of the individual's lifetime) and phylogenetic factors (those derived from the individual's biologic and cultural ancestry) shaped the contents of the unconscious. Just as the neurotic individual must somehow bring to consciousness repressed wishes, feelings, and conflicts, so too must the influence of phylogenetic remnants in the unconscious be understood. Jung thus distinguishes the **personal unconscious,** which contains repressed or forgotten experiences of the individual's past; and the **collective unconscious,** which contains memories of the individual's ancestral and racial history. Memories in the collective unconscious are organized around images called **archetypes.** These memories and images may intrude into consciousness and must be integrated and understood during maturation.

Jung developed many other ideas, particularly the compensatory nature of the unconscious, which was derived from clinical practice. He believed that dreams were not always expressions of repressed childhood wishes but might also represent images of more general aspects of the personality that had been denied conscious expression. He believed also that dreams might be more than mere representations of past conflicts and might, in fact, suggest future solutions to problems. Jung was greatly concerned with the issue of integration of the personality—the blending of capacities for feeling, intuition, sensation, and thought. He felt that each of us developed one or 2 of these basic traits and subordinated the others. Treatment could help the individual not only resolve past conflicts but live a richer and more integrated life.

BEYOND FREUD

While Freud was boldly exploring the role of the unconscious in the development and expression of mental disorders, other psychiatrists continued the phenomenologic tradition of careful observation of the mentally ill. **Emil Kraepelin** (1855–1926) studied mental illnesses by recording their signs, course, and final outcome. On the basis of his data, he was able to differentiate manic-depressive psychosis from dementia praecox, which he regarded as an incurable affliction. **Eugen Bleuler** (1857–1939), working at the Burghölzli hospital in Switzerland, reorganized Kraepelin's classification of dementia praecox and introduced the term **schizophrenia,** which he believed was characterized by dissociation of thoughts and emotions. He was far more sanguine about its outcome than was Kraepelin.

In the first half of the 20th century, a number of organic therapies were introduced to treat the major psychoses. Examples are **malaria therapy,** introduced by Julius von Wagner-Jauregg in 1917 (for which he received the Nobel Prize); **insulin coma therapy,** discovered by Manfred Sakel; **electric shock** treatment, pioneered by Ugo Cerletti and Lucio Bini; and **psychosurgery,** introduced by Egas Moniz.

Study of the psychoses led to a better understanding of the role of family dynamics and social stress in the origin and expression of mental illness. New therapeutic approaches in working with severely disturbed patients included supportive psychotherapy, milieu therapy, family therapy, and the development of protective alternative environments.

The study of the psychoses also stimulated investigations of the anatomy, physiology, and chemistry of the brain. These studies have resulted in a better understanding of the circuitry and chemical constituents of the central nervous system and their possible roles in disorders of thought, perception, and emotion (see Chapters 10 and 11).

Exciting new biologic approaches in psychiatry have been introduced during the past 30 years. Advances in the study of electrophysiology of the brain; the discovery of the neurotransmitters and their possible role in mental illness; twin studies in the investigation of genetic factors in affective disorders and schizophrenia; the development of pharmacologic agents to deal with anxiety, depression, mania, and agitation; and the realization that the brain functions as a neuroendocrine organ—all have added greatly to the scientific basis of psychiatry. Many of them are discussed in the chapters that follow (eg, Chapters 10, 11, and 52–54).

During this century, various schools of therapy have claimed success for some particular mode of treatment while excluding or even ridiculing others. The modern trend is to combine biologic, psychologic, and social interventions in a tailored approach to a particular patient with a specific disorder. Research studies now in progress may well lead to recommendations for specific treatment in certain clinical situations and more information about which psychiatric disorders respond best to "single-agent" therapy or combinations of treatments. Psychiatrists of the future, like internists of today, will be aware of the wide range of interventions available and their indications and cost. Like internists also, they will be qualified to administer some forms of treatment themselves and in other instances will refer patients to specialists in biofeedback therapy, behavior therapy, psychoanalysis, and other special fields.

Studies in Human Development

Our understanding of psychopathology will increase as we acquire more knowledge about the normative stages and crises of human development (see Chapters 6–8). Observational studies of mothers and infants over the past few years have provided data about the importance of attachment, emotional communication, and physical comforting to affective and cognitive growth. Sophisticated longitudinal studies are being conducted that will add to our knowledge of all phases of human development. They will indicate what kinds of social, educational, and family support are necessary to help children master the major tasks of succeeding stages and develop appropriate and flexible responses to maturational and environmental stresses. As we understand more about development, we will be better able to plan strategies for prevention and early detection of mental disorders.

Neurochemistry & Neuroendocrinology

Great advances in this area of research have been made over the past decade. Our understanding of the role of chemical brain mechanisms in the etiology of the psychoses, anxiety reactions, and psychosomatic conditions is advancing rapidly. New drugs with more specific behavioral impact and minor side effects will emerge from further studies of neurotransmitters and their receptors. The roles of the neural peptides in physiologic processes, learning and memory processes, and the response to stress are just beginning to be clarified. The discovery of the endorphins and the possibility that the body may manufacture its own ataraxic drugs (through the discovery of benzodiazepine receptors) suggest that the brain may possess its own pharmacopeia for reducing pain and dysphoric affects. Speculation that humans may engage in certain stressful activities because of the reinforcing effects of the secretion of body chemicals may lead to insights into the reasons for repetitive harmful or maladaptive behavior.

Advances in Information Processing

Psychiatrists who use the **biopsychosocial model** are often inundated with information about the patient's childhood, family and cultural background, health history, unconscious processes, cognitive capacities, and social relationships. It is a difficult task to organize, synthesize, and reason from this abundance of data in making diagnoses and planning treatment. Computers and video technology will make data processing available to the clinician. Emphasis will be placed on how psychiatrists collect, collate, and rea-

son from their information pool. Such techniques will help students and residents identify new ways of understanding the doctor-patient interaction and the inferences and decisions that can be drawn from it.

Advances in Behavioral Medicine

Psychiatrists and other physicians, in cooperation with behavioral scientists, are working toward an integration of the behavioral and biomedical sciences in the search for ways to understand and treat mental and physical illness. As Schwartz and Weiss (1978) note, the aim of behavioral medicine is to study those basic mechanisms "whereby behavioral phenomena influence the epidemiology, etiology, pathogenesis, prevention, diagnosis, treatment and rehabilitation of physical disorders."

Behavioral medicine is helping to develop sophisticated techniques that may be effective in changing pathophysiologic processes either directly or by stress-reducing mechanisms. Such modes of treatment may include (among others) psychotherapy, relaxation techniques, behavior modification, biofeedback, hypnosis, and controlled imagery (see Chapter 51).

Psychiatry is a medical specialty. Though many components must come together to assist a student to develop psychiatric skills, the profession has always believed that a psychiatrist is first a physician. Professional identity is centered on a scientific and compassionate concern for individuals in distress. Psychiatric clinicians must be aware of their patients' medical disorders and of the variety of social stresses and supports that affect their lives. The psychiatrist is expected to combine scientific rigor in making clinical observations with a humanistic appreciation of issues of sex, age, culture, and socioeconomic status as they affect patients and their families. Psychiatrists must be at ease in understanding the brain and its complex network of neuronal centers, neurotransmitters, and the drugs that act upon them. But they must also be sensitive to the uniqueness of each patient's personality, with an individual balance of cognitive and emotional styles, patterns of adaptation and defense, internal conflicts, and fantasies. The psychiatrist should also become aware of how social and cultural factors may contribute to the development of mental disorders. As this review has indicated, it is the blending of scientific knowledge, psychologic intuition, and social responsibility that has marked the best epochs of psychiatric history.

What emerges from this brief look backward at some of the historical issues of psychiatry is the conviction that a new science of human behavior is emerging, one that combines the study of the brain and its connections to the body with investigations of the problems of developing interpersonal bonds, the effects of social organization, and the disorders of communication. The new science is learning how to apply the theories that deal with open systems (cybernetics and information theory) to the observations of ethology, neurophysiology, psychoanalysis, endocrinology, and developmental psychology. It studies the mutual influences of both heredity and learning on the plasticity of human behavior. Psychiatry today mixes science and intuition while using powerful and increasingly more specific medications as well as the art of therapeutic communication. It is a growing, lively field, sometimes uncertain of itself but creatively grappling with that most complex problem, the psychologic development of human beings and the afflictions of the mind.

REFERENCES

Abraham I: Page 722 in: *Encyclopedia of Religion and Ethics*. Vol 2. Hastings J (editor). Clark, 1909.

Ackernecht E: *Short History of Psychiatry*. Hafner, 1968.

Allport GW: *Personality: A Psychological Interpretation*. Holt, Rinehart, & Winston, 1937.

Ayala FJ: Biology as an autonomous science. *Am Sci* 1968;**56:**207.

Bernheim H-M: *Hypnosis and Suggestion in Psychotherapy*. University Books, 1963.

Charcot J-M: *Lectures on the Diseases of the Nervous System*. New Sydenham Society (London), 1877–1889.

Dubos R: *Mirage of Health*. Allen & Unwin, 1960.

Ellenberger H: *The Discovery of the Unconscious: The History and Evolution of Dynamic Psychiatry*. Basic Books, 1970.

Engel GL: The need for a new medical model: A challenge for biomedicine. *Science* 1977;**196:**129.

Erikson E: *Childhood and Society*. Norton, 1963.

Fine R: *A History of Psychoanalysis*. Columbia Univ Press, 1979.

Foucault M: *Madness and Civilization: A History of Insanity in the Age of Reason*. Pantheon Books, 1965.

Freud S: *Standard Edition of the Complete Psychological Works of Sigmund Freud*. Hogarth Press, 1953–1966.

Gerard R: Neurophysiology: Brain and behavior. Pages 1620–1638 in: *American Handbook of Psychiatry*. Vol 1. Arieti S (editor). Basic Books, 1959.

Horney K: *The Neurotic Personality of Our Time*. Norton, 1937.

Jung CG: *Memories, Dreams, and Reflections*. Pantheon Books, 1961.

Jung CG: *The Structure and Dynamics of the Psyche*. Vol 8 of: *The Collected Works of C.G. Jung*. Pantheon Books, 1960.

Kolata GB: New drugs and the brain. *Science* 1979;**205:**774.

Kuhn T: *The Structure of Scientific Revolutions*. Univ of Chicago Press, 1970.

Mora G: The history of psychiatry: Its relevance for the psychiatrist. *Am J Psychiatry* 1970;**126:**957.

Schwartz G, Weiss S (editors): *Proceedings of the Yale Conference on Behavioral Medicine*. US Department of Health, Education, and Welfare Publication No. (NIH) 78–1424, 1978.

Sullivan HS: *Conception of Modern Psychiatry*. Norton, 1947.

Yoshida H, Yamamura HI: *Pharmacologic and Biochemical Aspects of Neurotransmitter Receptors*. Wiley, 1983.

Zilboorg GA, Henry GW: *A History of Medical Psychology*. Norton, 1941.

3

Models of the Mind

Frances Cohen, PhD, & Dennis Farrell, MD

Various theories have been developed to explain how personality and behavior in humans develop and change and what factors interfere with normal growth or lead to pathologic states. This chapter will outline 4 main approaches to understanding human behavior: psychoanalytic theory, behaviorist (learning) theory, humanistic-existential theory, and general systems theory. No one of the 4 approaches offers a "best" way to understand patients. Taken together, the different perspectives help us understand the complexities of human behavior and how best to treat patients with emotional and behavioral problems.

PSYCHOANALYTIC APPROACH

Dennis Farrell, MD

Chapter 2 recounts how Freud's earliest ideas about how the mind works were stimulated by clinical work with patients. At first these were mainly patients suffering from functional organic complaints—cases of "hysteria" that comprised a significant part of the caseload of neurologists in late 19th-century Europe. Experiments with hypnosis had shown that the unconscious meanings of symptoms could be brought to consciousness in such patients; and the same memories and fantasies determining these symptoms could be made to disappear from consciousness by the process of posthypnotic suggestion. But hypnosis and its successor, the "pressure technique," utilizing strong positive suggestion in the waking subject, both proved unreliable forms of therapy. Freud then made a discovery that proved crucial for the development of psychoanalysis—that hypnosis and direct suggestion were not necessary if the patient could be encouraged to say whatever spontaneously came to mind and could voluntarily suspend critical control over thoughts, feelings, and fantasies. This method of **free association** has remained the patient's and analyst's principal route of access to the unconscious. A technique that solicits the random thoughts of sick people might seem the antithesis of the deliberate and systematic technique of "scientific inquiry," which focuses sharply on a specific area of concern. Yet having the

patient pursue the process of free association, with or at times without the analyst's encouragement and help, consistently uncovered the origins and meanings of symptoms and often led to their remission.

Generalizing from his work with patients as well as from his study of dreams and such phenomena as slips of the tongue, Freud adopted a **psychodynamic theory** of analysis which holds that the workings of the mind are best understood as the result of an interplay of forces. Freud found that when these forces were in opposition, one side or the other was often repressed, or withheld, from consciousness. **Repression** was a force that emanated from the more conscious part of the mind and was called into service to avoid pain aroused by feelings stirred up when disturbing (usually sexual) impulses threatened to dominate conscious awareness.

Freud's notion of **intrapsychic conflict** as a source of repressed thoughts or impulses accounted for a host of phenomena, including "the psychopathology of everyday life"—slips of the tongue and the tendency to forget names or dates that have painful associations. Freud's study of this phenomenon led him to the conclusion that the unconscious was a vastly more significant part even of normal mental life than people generally understand, since by its very nature it eludes conscious awareness.

In patients with neuroses, however, the unconscious is manifested in disturbances of thought, feelings, and behavior that arise chiefly in the mind though perhaps secondarily induced by external events and stimuli. Symptoms may include involuntary movements, interference with motor function, or odd sensations, as in hysteria; strong and seemingly inappropriate emotions or moods, as in anxiety attacks or depressions; or uncontrollable and repetitive thoughts and actions, as in obsessions and compulsions. Irrational fears characterize the phobic disorders. These symptoms are experienced by the patient as strange, uncontrollable, and disruptive of normal function. If evidence of unconscious processes were demonstrable only in mental patients, the claims of psychoanalysis might have been rejected, but Freud demonstrated in *The Interpretation of Dreams* (1900) that in our dreams we display samples from our vast inventories of unconscious thoughts, impulses, and fantasies.

BASIC PRINCIPLES OF DYNAMIC PSYCHIATRY

From the beginning, perhaps the most fundamental postulate of psychoanalysis had been the doctrine of **psychic determinism**—the idea that all psychic events and processes follow certain strict laws of causality, as in the universe of physical events and processes, and that all psychologic events can be traced back to one or more antecedents. A given psychic event is usually *over*determined—*multiply* determined—by a series of various antecedents. A familiar figure in a dream, for example, may be a reflection of the dreamer's conscious waking thoughts as well as an expression of unconscious impulses or fantasies about that person.

Freud's central idea of a **dynamic unconscious,** together with his conviction about psychic determinism and his discovery of the tool of free association, led to the first systematic psychologic exploration of mental life in depth. In his attempt to discover the way the mind works, he pursued the idea that a dynamic unconscious implies forces at work within some sort of structure; Freud further thought that the whole had to be governed by some basic principle.

From his background in the physics, physiology, and neuroanatomy of his day, Freud arrived at a physicalistic conception of the mind as a structure—the **psychic apparatus**—energized by **drives**—the psychologic manifestations of basic biologic processes. These instinctual drives could not be directly observed but had to be inferred from their derivatives of wish, impulse, and fantasy. Their intensity reflected their force or pressure toward discharge; the obvious and most important example was the sexual drive. The counterforce, as we have seen, was designated **repression.** Thus far, Freud had developed a concept of a structure within which mental forces interact.

Two principles of mental functioning governed the operation of these forces: the pleasure principle and the reality principle. The **pleasure principle** asserts that human beings seek satisfaction of their wishes and needs—equated with pleasure—and that where possible they avoid pain. The pleasure principle dominates the beginning of life, as shown by the infant's imperious demand for gratification; it is modified only gradually through interaction with the external world—the world of physical objects and those all-important "objects" of the child's interests and needs, the parents. The **reality principle** asserts the need to accommodate reality, with all of its constraints, conditions, and frustrations. The pleasure principle is modified only insofar as experience requires it to be: The child learns to postpone immediate gratification in the interest of more lasting satisfactions, including the need to maintain a sense of being loved and admired by its parents. The reality principle, then, joins and ultimately moderates the pleasure principle with a resulting series of complex accommodations between basic needs and wishes and the external reality we encounter in life.

THE STRUCTURE & DEVELOPMENT OF THE MIND

The Topographic Model

Freud's first attempt at understanding the structure of the mind is called the topographic model. This scheme conceptualizes a stratification of the mental apparatus from conscious to preconscious to unconscious levels of mental functioning. At the **preconscious** level are those mental contents not in conscious awareness but capable of being brought to conscious awareness by an effort of will. The **unconscious,** as we have seen, contains mental material not accessible to conscious awareness but accessible by inference from noting discontinuities in the train of conscious thought and by examining such phenomena as emotional conflicts, symptoms, hypnotic suggestion, and dreaming.

Because of the relaxation of conscious control during sleep, the study of dreams became for Freud the "royal road to the unconscious." In concluding that "a dream is but the [disguised] fulfillment of a wish," Freud accomplished 2 things: (1) He offered support for his notion that the unconscious consisted of drives pressing for discharge; and (2) he offered evidence that the unconscious mind was capable of an entirely different kind of thinking.

This special mode of thought, termed **primary process,** differed from ordinary, conscious **secondary-process** thinking in its dependence on wishful, emotional instinctual matters and by its disregard of realistic considerations of which the unconscious, by definition, has no direct knowledge. Primary-process thinking relates to drives seeking discharge or, if they are blocked, to the creation in **unconscious fantasy** of the desired thing or person.

Negation and contradiction do not exist in the unconscious; memories are organized around wishes rather than concepts. Ideas are readily **condensed** (eg, the person in the dream who is at once one's mother and one's sister), or **displaced** from one thing or person to another (eg, a tyrannical boss becomes in a dream a Nazi SS officer), or **symbolized** (eg, a young girl dreams of a snake in her bed). Accordingly, the unconscious can accommodate diverse and "perverse" sexual impulses (primitive or not) and destructive impulses, so long as quantitative limits are not exceeded. However, each individual has a unique limit to the quantity of impulses that may be accommodated. This conception—derived from studies of the way dreams are formed—was of course strikingly different from the way our rational thought processes proceed under the aegis of the conscious self, aware of external reality and seeking to integrate and preserve a sense of a coherent and consistent personality. The **ego,** at this stage in the development of Freud's thinking, denoted person, or self. The next major revision of Freud's theory radically changed the use of this term.

The Structural Model

In 1923, Freud presented his structural theory of the mind, which supplanted the former topographic theory with an overall concept of the mind as an apparatus composed of 3 distinct "agencies": id, ego, and superego. These constructs refer to collections of related functions: The **id** was the successor to the unconscious of the old topographic scheme. It contained the drives and their derivatives—repressed wishes and fantasies—as well as psychic contents that never had been conscious. The pleasure principle ruled in the id, and primary process was the mode of thought.

The **ego** was now conceived of as a *system* of functions, in contrast to the person-ego of the earlier theory. This new ego system went beyond the self to include much that remains unconscious. Defenses against internal conflict are a function of the ego and operate for the most part as unconsciously and automatically as do the impulses of the id. For example, we are not normally aware of repressing all of the primitive sexual and aggressive impulses that could find outlets in action if the "veneer" of civilization and responsible maturity were suddenly stripped away—impulses that in fact do occasionally appear more or less undisguised in our dreams.

The **superego** was a theoretical construct for the critical, judging, and admonishing functions within the mind. It arose from a psychologic **introjection** ("taking in") of the child's perception of parental authority. This process most often occurs when the child begins to turn away from its intense love and hate relationships with its parents to devote its attention to learning about the world and growing up. A subagency of the superego, more conscious and deriving more from the child's wish to identify with the parent—mostly with the parent of the same sex—was named the **ego ideal.**

Psychosexual Development

In addition to the theoretical constructs of the mind as a complex structure having dynamic forces in interaction, psychoanalysis took into account the genetic, or developmental, aspect of the mental apparatus. The emphasis was at first very much on the earlier, more basic dimensions of human experience. These are most subject to repression in later development, as evidenced by the universality of **infantile (childhood) amnesia** for perhaps our most significant life experiences, those of early childhood. Freud and other early analysts only gradually came to appreciate the importance of **infantile sexuality,** an appreciation derived mainly from clinical work with patients and from the analysis of dreams.

While dreams and the "psychopathology of everyday life" pointed to an endless train of minor disturbances of psychic equilibrium in every human being and upheld the validity of the dynamic point of view, it was in the study of patients suffering from overt symptoms of intrapsychic conflict that Freud was able to reconstruct the sexual life of the child. Working with adult patients, he found that emotional symptoms reflected conflicts of a sexual nature—conflicts arising often in adolescence or adult life from situations in which thoughts and feelings unacceptable to the personality as a whole had been stimulated; but these conflicts in turn had their origins in sexual feelings and impulses in early childhood and prohibitions against them. It was clear that infantile sexual material persisted in unconscious fantasy form in these patients and accounted for certain aspects of their adult behavior as well as much of their overt symptoms.

Clinical theory soon came to include a sequence of **psychosexual stages** in the development of the sexual drive, or **libido;** in the maturation of the body and nervous system; and in interaction with the objects of the child's interests, wishes, and needs (see Chapter 6). First, the **oral phase** of infancy was defined, one in which the libido is concentrated in the pursuit of satisfaction through feeding and sucking at the breast, the source of all satisfaction and frustration. Beginning at about the second year and overlapping with the oral phase, the **anal phase** becomes dominant, when urges, wishes, and fantasies center around toilet training and the anal erogenous zone becomes the focus of the child's interest and holding back or expelling stool the overriding issue in the relationship with the primary caregiver. During the **phallic phase (genital phase),** from about age 3 to age 5, the genitals become the focus of the child's interest, with masturbation the means of releasing tension and with other "component" manifestations of the sexual drive, such as the urge to peep and to exhibit oneself, expressing themselves. This latter phase includes the psychologic drama of the **Oedipus complex,** the culmination of childhood sexuality.

The **oedipal situation** was named for Sophocles' play *Oedipus Rex* to underscore Freud's belief in the universality of the oedipal experience despite countless variations shaped by the personality, the behavior of parents, the family constellation, and the culture. In its most typical form in Western culture, the child 3–5 years of age falls in love in a new and recognizably sexual way with the parent of the opposite sex; desires exclusive possession of that parent; and wants to be rid of the other (rival) parent. Fantasies connected with masturbation arouse great sexual tension and feelings of anxiety and guilt. The little boy's anxiety typically takes the form of fear of retaliation by the powerful father and a fantasied threat by the father to cut off the boy's penis. This **castration anxiety,** combined with normal love for the father, compels repression both of sexual yearnings for the mother and of hostile death wishes toward the father. Freud acknowledged his difficulty in understanding female sexual development during this phase; on the whole, he considered it to be analogous to male development—here, love for father, hatred and rivalry toward mother as the oversimplified formula (as in Euripides' play *Electra*). However, he called the girl's reaction to the discovery of the difference in anatomy between the sexes **penis envy,** a counterpart to the boy's castration anxiety. Penis envy is expressed in a young girl's curiosity about the penis and a wish to have one. In a similar vein, some boys envy the woman's ability to bear children. What was previously largely conscious in the child—and usually quite evident in the child's behavior and overt expressions of feeling—now becomes unconscious; with resolution of the Oedipus complex, the child identifies with the parent of the same sex and turns its interest away from the family toward peers of the same sex, toward school experiences, and toward the problems and delights of growing up as a boy or girl. The child's sexuality becomes relatively quiescent during this **latency period** until the resurgence of **genital sexuality** in puberty.

Subsequently challenged—and to some extent modified and expanded—Freud's scheme of female psychosexual development, together with the more definite body of data pertaining to the male, became an accepted part of psychoanalytic **libido theory.** In early psychoanalytic theory, the years of adolescence and adulthood had been relatively ignored, since the attainment of genital sexuality in adolescence was thought either to proceed normally, with incorporation of pregenital drives into personality traits and within sexual play, or else to give rise later to inhibitions or neurotic symptoms.

Clinical Phenomena

Freud's early studies of hysterical neurotic symptoms showed that a compromise was formed between an **impulse** and a counterforce, or **defense:** By repression, the idea accompanying the impulse was withheld from conscious awareness, but if this equilibrium was disturbed, the impulse proved strong enough to force its way in disguised form into awareness. The symptom (phobia, obsession, a functional paralysis, etc) resulted both from the impulse seeking gratification and from the force opposing its expression. The purpose of psychotherapy was to help the patient resolve this conflict in a more favorable way by acknowledging and eventually abandoning the infantile wishes so harshly condemned by the child's superego. This process allows the ego to adapt and modify the libidinal strivings so they can seek appropriate satisfaction in reality.

The process of psychoanalysis (see Chapter 43), however, was complicated by several factors. The pathogenic forces did not subside with the patient's decision to enter therapy. In an important revision of an earlier theory, Freud realized that the ego uses anxiety as a signal of internal danger, such as the threatened emergence into consciousness of a painful idea. This **signal anxiety,** operating automatically and unconsciously, activates habitual **defenses** (see Chapter 5).

Two other seemingly destructive phenomena occurring during treatment—resistance and transference—could then be understood as manifestations of the continuing interplay of forces within the patient extended to include the person and aims of the analyst in the intrapsychic conflict. **Resistance** could be thought of as that part of the patient committed to the status quo and fearful of awareness of bad and dangerous repressed impulses. **Transference** was a reliving of the most dynamically important aspects of childhood experience and occurred because of the patient's need to reexperience rather than remember a relationship that had been lost or missed in childhood and was therefore deeply longed for. Many aspects of transference could also appear as resistance: A hostile transference to the analyst obviously could pit the patient against the analyst's wish to understand, and a positive transference might initially encourage the patient to work in analysis but could also (for instance) ward off "negative" feelings that needed to be understood. In any case, once these 2 phenomena were recognized, the basics of psychoanalytic technique could be defined: to help the patient identify and deal with the inevitable resistance to greater awareness and change and to uncover the past—especially the dynamically important repressed aspects of past experience—by interpreting the transference. The patient's reliving of basic conflicts was essential, and the ever-changing transference situation was the thread followed throughout treatment by the analyst in an attempt to reconstruct the patient's childhood experience. Both phenomena—the many complex patterns that could be identified either as "resistance" or as "transference" phenomena—were almost always seen in every case; and it was exploration of these seeming complications of the therapeutic process that led to major conceptual advances and to the most distinctive features of psychoanalytic technique.

Countertransference is a phenomenon that includes not only the analyst's personal neurotic tendencies to develop transference reactions to the patient but also those blind spots and limiting factors that could interfere with understanding of the patient's problems.

These concepts of repression, resistance, transference, and countertransference have remained indispensable to therapists for the conduct of psychodynamic therapy.

LATER DEVELOPMENTS

Basic Principles

Developments in psychoanalysis after Freud's introduction of libido theory and id psychology included basic revisions of the theory of instinctual drives. From the early libido theory, Freud took up the question of the psychology of self-love, or **narcissism,** and its relationship to the degree and quality of outwardly directed erotic investments **(object libido).** Later, observing many manifestations of aggression directed both outwardly, in destructiveness, and inwardly, as in masochistic or self-punitive behavior and in unconscious guilt, Freud constructed the idea of a **life instinct (eros)** and a **death instinct (thanatos)** in opposition. While such a theoretical elaboration has been considered too speculative for clinical relevance by most psychoanalysts, aggression has been recognized as an important force within the personality. Most psychoanalysts today think in terms of basic forces—conceptualized as libidinal and aggressive drives in inter-action within the personality—that are uniquely expressed in the mental life of each individual.

Structure & Development

Since Freud's death in 1939, leading psychoana-lytic theoreticians such as Anna Freud (1946) (his daughter), Heinz Hartmann (1958), and David Rapa-port (1959) inaugurated a shift of emphasis to the newer **ego psychology,** complementing but not re-placing the older **id psychology.** Psychoanalysts now take the view that the ego represents the part of the per-sonality most attuned to the outer world, in significant part through **inborn, primarily autonomous func-tions** such as perception, the control of movement, memory, and a growing capacity for thought, speech, and communication through language. The ego has the task of maintaining a relationship to reality, accu-rately perceiving and assessing external reality, and regulating the individual's behavior accordingly. Dominating specific lower-level processes is the **syn-thetic function** of the ego, through which conflicting tendencies are reconciled in the best way possible. This self-regulation includes the ability, only gradu-ally developed, to resist impulses, postpone gratification, and tolerate unpleasant mental states such as anxiety, tension, and disappointment while substitutes are sought for the needs of the personality in an increasingly complex interaction between the ex-ternal world and the self. Piaget's work on the normal maturation of cognition in the child is an essential complement to this dynamic point of view (see Chap-ter 6).

This new interest in the ego included but was not limited to those aspects of ego functioning that are more or less conscious or preconscious. Unconscious aspects of ego functioning, especially the elaboration of defenses and their influence upon character forma-tion, were also extensively studied. Anna Freud's work in particular illuminated the variety of defenses used by the ego to deal with the unwelcome thought, impulse, or feeling by removing it from awareness **(repression);** rejecting its significance or importance **(denial);** expelling it entirely from oneself **(projec-tion);** asserting the opposite attitude or feeling in con-sciousness **(reaction formation);** or, at a more ad-vanced level of defense, dealing with the threatening mental content by means of intellectualization, ratio-nalization, or transformation, as in humor or artistic productions **(sublimation).** The whole subject of "defense" has been approached by psychoanalysts mainly from the perspective of the study of conflictual and unconscious aspects of mental functioning (see Chapter 5).

Erik Erikson (1950, 1959) (see Chapter 7) added a new dimension to the classic scheme of psychosexual development through his concept of the **psychosocial stages of development.** Erikson demonstrated through cross-cultural as well as analytic study the in-dividual's dependence for psychologic growth and de-velopment not only on the primary objects of child-

hood but on the social environment as well, ie, the institutions and mores of the culture into which one is born. Erikson's concepts do not end with consider-ation of the conflicts and resolutions of childhood but include an examination of the entire course of normal development, the typical crises and tasks and resolu-tions at various stages of the life cycle. His treatment of the crisis of adolescence and the process of identity formation is particularly noteworthy. More recently, Vaillant (1977) and others have studied the process of change throughout the adult life cycle by means of lon-gitudinal studies of normal (nonpatient) populations.

While psychoanalysis has come to devote attention to adolescence and adulthood, more interest has been focused on the earliest years of life—on infancy and the pre-oedipal phases of development. Clinical study of this early period has been directed toward (1) deeper understanding of transference phenomena in the treat-ment of more disturbed patients—those with develop-mental arrests, or **fixations,** at the pre-oedipal level of development; and (2) direct infant and child observa-tion, as in the work of Fraiberg (1959) and Mahler and coworkers (1975). Clinical observations growing out of the earlier focus on the ego as a system with various functions and attributes have recently stressed how the internalization of experience partly entails the building up of internal images of the self in interaction with oth-ers. These internal images, conscious and uncon-scious, are considered by the **"object relations"** theo-rists to be the basic units of experience. According to this theory, the way individuals relate to each other is determined largely by the way they view themselves and feel about themselves in unconscious fantasy (eg, as "good" or "bad" in relation to the other person). Most object relations theory subordinates the drives, libido, and aggression to what is postulated as a pri-mary need of the self to relate to other people, over and above satisfaction of particular instinctual needs.

Clinical Phenomena

Three major perspectives within modern psycho-analysis—ego psychology, object relations theory, and the recent work of Kohut (1971) focusing on dis-orders of the "self experience"—share an interest in extending psychoanalytically oriented therapy to an increasingly broad range of patients, ie, to include pa-tients with more serious personality and behavior dis-orders (see Chapter 36). In all of these cases, a psycho-analytically oriented clinical approach provides an in-depth view of the workings of the mind.

BEHAVIORIST (LEARNING THEORY) APPROACH

Frances Cohen, PhD

The behaviorist approach began to take form around the turn of the 20th century in protest against psychoanalytic theories. Behaviorally oriented theorists argued that subjective experience and unconscious forces were not public events accessible to verification by others and thus were not appropriate data for science.

The roots of this perspective can be traced to the Russian physiologist Ivan Pavlov (1849–1936), who described and studied the phenomenon of the conditioned reflex. Pavlov found that if a stimulus (eg, food) that automatically elicits a response (eg, salivation) is presented immediately after a tone is sounded, after several repetitions the tone alone will elicit the response. The intial stimulus is called the unconditioned stimulus (UCS), and the one it is paired with is called the conditioned stimulus (CS). This principle is known as **classical conditioning** and is diagrammed below.

Before conditioning: USC (food) ⟶ **Salivation**
Conditioning: CS (tone) + UCS (food) ⟶ **Salivation**
After conditioning: CS (tone) ⟶ **Salivation**

Through the process of classical conditioning, a stimulus that did not previously elicit a response came to elicit it.

Pavlov's principle of conditioning was taken up by the American psychologist John B. Watson (1878–1958) as a procedure that could be used to study human behavior more objectively. Watson formulated a point of view called **behaviorism.** Watson used the principle of classical conditioning in a now famous experiment with an 11-month-old boy named Albert ("Little Albert") to demonstrate the role of learning in abnormal behavior. To establish a conditioned association, the experimenter stood behind Little Albert and made a loud noise whenever he reached for a white rat. The loud noise elicited a fear response in Little Albert. After several repetitions, Albert became disturbed at the sight of the rat even when no noise was present. His fear also became generalized to other furry animals and objects. Thus, an irrational fear had been learned through conditioning.

E.L. Thorndike and B.F. Skinner expanded the behavioral approach by developing a second basic concept of learning. Thorndike (1913) noted that responses that have rewarding consequences are strengthened or learned, whereas those with negative consequences are weakened or extinguished, the so-called "law of effect." The same principle applies in the control of people's behavior through reward and punishment. Skinner (1953) elaborated on this view and emphasized the importance of external, not internal, events in determining an individual's behavior.

UNDERLYING ASSUMPTIONS OF LEARNING THEORY

The behaviorists view personality as a collection of *acquired* behavior patterns that are governed by principles of learning and subject to environmental influences. According to this view, since all behavior is learned, recourse to unconscious motives to explain behavior is unnecessary. Causes of behavior are sought in the environment rather than in the psyche. Behavior is thought to be acquired, maintained, changed, or extinguished according to basic laws of learning and is consequently subject to prediction and control. Maladaptive behavior is based on faulty learning, inappropriate associations, or failure to learn certain types of behavior, such as how to express aggression.

Behaviorists reject the "disease model" of neurotic disorders—the idea that maladaptive behaviors are caused by some underlying illness or disorder. Central to the psychoanalytic view is the idea that behavior is determined and that neurotic symptoms represent the surface manifestations of underlying intrapsychic conflicts. Psychoanalysis searches for the basic cause in its approach to a neurotic condition. To behaviorists, however, the symptom is the problem—remove the symptom and the "disease" is cured. Behaviorists find support for their view in the fact that there is little evidence of symptom substitution after behavioral treatments. To reiterate: To a behaviorist, the origins of symptoms are not of interest; of importance are the circumstances that maintain maladaptive behavior.

CONCEPTS & PRINCIPLES OF LEARNING THEORY

The basic principles of learning theory focus on environmental conditions related to the acquisition, modification, and elimination of response patterns. Behaviorists distinguish between 2 main types of learning: classical conditioning and operant conditioning. As described above, in **classical conditioning,** a stimulus that did not previously elicit a given response has come to elicit it after pairing of an unconditioned stimulus (eg, food) with a new stimulus (eg, tone). The process can also work in reverse: If a conditioned stimulus (eg, the tone) is repeatedly presented without the unconditioned stimulus (eg, food), this will lead to **extinction** (ie, the elimination of the learned response).

Dollard and Miller (1950) described how principles of learning theory explain the phenomenon of conditioned anxiety. If a child is frightened upon falling into a swimming pool, a conditioned response may be learned (water → anxiety), and the child may become anxious when near any swimming pool or large body of water (stimulus generalization). This conditioned anxiety may have important long-lasting effects. If people avoid a situation to avoid the anxiety, they may never discover the reason for the anxiety and may never know that one can learn to swim and enjoy the water. Thus to avoid anxiety, people may continue to engage in seemingly useless patterns that remove anxiety but prevent the individual from discovering that the original reason for the fear is gone.

Conditioned reactions may also occur in medical treatment. Cancer patients often develop conditioned reactions to the medical procedures they must undergo and may, for example, become nauseated and vomit upon entering the x-ray department for radiation treatment or when handed a pill in chemotherapy treatment.

The classical conditioning paradigm was used by Mowrer and Mowrer (1938) to develop a treatment for enuresis during sleep in children. The researchers employed a fine mesh bedsheet so that the first drop of urine closed a circuit that set off a loud bell (an unconditioned stimulus that will wake a sleeping child). After a few nights of this treatment, most children woke up in response to the full bladder (conditioned stimulus) before they wet the bed.

In **operant conditioning,** the subject (person or animal) is put into a situation in which he or she learns to make a response that satisfies a need or achieves a desired goal. A hungry rat may be placed in a cage with a lever. When the rat accidentally activates the lever, a pellet of food drops from a reservoir. After a while, the rat will activate the lever whenever it is hungry. Learning to press the lever is operant conditioning. Being rewarded for working hard, playing the piano well, and getting good grades are all examples of operant conditioning. Reinforcement is sometimes given unknowingly. For example, teachers may fall into the error of reinforcing acting-out behavior by singling the child out for attention—a "reward" that may strengthen rather than weaken the behavior pattern. Ignoring the child's acting-out behavior may be the best way to extinguish the pattern. **Extinction** of a previously learned response occurs when reinforcement is withheld.

The principle of **reinforcement** holds that an association will be established between a stimulus and a response when a drive has been gratified. There are 2 types of reinforcers: Primary reinforcers are factors that satisfy innate needs such as for food, water, or sex; secondary reinforcers are learned through association with primary reinforcers, eg, social approval, money, and clothes. If a parent who provides food also gives a child an expensive toy after a good performance, the toy and similar objects serve as secondary reinforcers.

Reinforcement schedules. The way reinforcement is presented—whether it is given after every response (continuous reinforcement), after every other response (fixed ratio schedule), or on a random basis (variable intermittent)—influences how strong a learned response will be. Not using reinforcement every time actually produces a stronger learned response (the Las Vegas slot machine is an example). Hundreds of experiments have shown that a continuously reinforced response will be extinguished faster than one reinforced on a variable intermittent schedule. Thus, to extinguish a response, one must be careful to avoid *any* reinforcement of that response. If parents want to break a 4-year-old of the habit of crying every night at bedtime in order to be picked up, they should *consistently* adopt a new strategy. If they ignore the crying, the habit will eventually be eliminated; if after a few nights they relent and pick up the child, the partial reinforcement of the habit will make it harder than ever to extinguish. This principle has important implications for our understanding of the persistence of certain kinds of human behavior.

Punishment is an aversive event or the withholding of a positive event, contingent on a behavior, that decreases the frequency of that behavior. Punishment (like reward) is defined as such solely by the effect it has on the behavior. Thus, spanking a child, which a parent might consider "punishment," may not decrease the frequency of the undesirable behavior but may instead serve as a positive reinforcer by providing attention.

Although punishment may teach one what he or she is doing wrong, it does not teach how to behave in an acceptable manner. Thus, if punishment is used, it must be accompanied by reinforcement of other more adaptive behaviors. Another problem with punishment procedures is that punishment may only suppress rather than eliminate the undesirable behavior, so that the behavior may reemerge later. An individual may learn to avoid the punishment situation altogether and thus have no opportunity for reinforcement of desirable behaviors. Punishment might also result in the modeling of an undesirable behavior (eg, a child frequently struck by the parents may learn to be aggressive when frustrated). In general, except in the case of self-injurious or highly dangerous behaviors, it is best to try other intervention strategies besides punishment first.

Stimulus generalization is the tendency of a response that has been conditioned to one stimulus to become associated with other similar stimuli. For example, if one is afraid of a white rat, one may more easily become afraid of other furry animals.

Shaping is a process of reinforcing successive approximations of a desired behavior. (Its use in therapy is discussed below.) Animal trainers used this technique long before Skinner wrote about it. For example, to train a dog to roll over on command, one cannot initially reinforce rolling over, because dogs normally do not roll over except occasionally in play. The trainer must first reinforce sitting down, then lying down, then lying on one side, and finally rolling over. After one response is learned (eg, sitting down on command), reinforcement is given only for the next successive approximation. Circus animals' feats are a clear demonstration of how operant conditioning can be used to shape responses.

Social learning theory. In recent years, the behaviorist approach has been augmented by theorists taking a social learning approach. These latter theories emphasize the importance of cognition—thoughts, values, expectations—in influencing human behavior. To social learning theorists such as Bandura and Walters (1963), Rotter (1966), and Mischel (1968), an individual can learn without eliciting a response or receiving any positive or negative reinforcement.

For example, Bandura discusses **observational learning,** the process resulting from watching how another person behaves in a particular situation. Later, in the same situation, the observer may act as the model did. This may be how people learn to drive a car. It is thought that many children learn aggression through watching it on television. Modeling is an important way to help children prepare for dental work or unpleasant medical procedures. Many hospitals use films that show children coping with hospital procedures as a way of preparing children before their admission to the hospital. Factors such as the sex, power, and personal attributes of the model influence the extent to which a model is imitated.

Rotter (1966) emphasized the importance of the expectations people have and the values they place on particular types of reinforcement. One's **locus of control** is the generalized feeling that one does or does not control what happens to him or her. "Internals" feel they can control what happens to them; people with an external locus of control feel they cannot—that the environment or "fate" determines what will be. This attitude can have important ramifications for health-related behavior. "Externals" may feel there is no reason to take preventive health measures or to alter diet or other personal habits, since "what will be, will be." Internals are more likely to seek information in health settings and to follow preventive health measures.

Therapy and behavior change. (See Chapter 46.) Proponents of the behavioral approaches view abnormal behavior as the result of (1) the failure to learn important adaptive behaviors, (2) learning of maladaptive behavior, or (3) conflicts that require the individual to make difficult discriminations between similar stimuli. According to learning theory, any complex pattern of responses, including neurotic symptoms such as phobias and hysterical paralyses, can be learned. Behaviorists see all behavior as malleable, whether it is normal or abnormal. What is learned can be unlearned, and what has not been learned can be. Behavior therapists apply the principles of learning theory to alter or eliminate undesirable behaviors. A direct attack is made on symptoms, with no attempt to help the patient gain insight. The goal is to discover what maintains the undesirable behavior and determine how to change it. Two types of behavior therapy will be described: operant techniques and systematic desensitization.

Basic **operant techniques** can be used in mental hospital settings. For example, Ayllon (1963) used these principles with a schizophrenic woman who insisted on wearing several layers of clothing—dresses, shawls, sheets, towels—weighing about 25 lb. Ayllon used a shaping technique, with food as the reinforcer. He told the patient that in order to enter the hospital dining room she would have to be weighed and must weigh less than a specified target weight. At first, she had to reduce the weight of clothing to 23 lb. After she met this requirement, a stricter one was imposed. The patient did miss a few meals during the process, but after a few months she was wearing only 3 lb of clothing. This conditioning treatment did not cure the schizophrenia, but it did affect her relationship with her family and other patients, since more people were willing to talk to her after she stopped looking so bizarre.

Systematic desensitization, developed by Wolpe (1961), is a technique based on the principle of counterconditioning, in which a person substitutes for the undesired response one that is incompatible with it. Anxiety responses are extinguished by gradually associating the anxiety-producing stimulus with an incompatible response, namely, relaxation. Systematic desensitization is most effective in treating phobias and anxieties that can be broken down in concrete elements.

In systematic desensitization, a person sets up a hierarchy of stimuli ranked according to the amount of anxiety they produce. For someone with a snake phobia, thinking about a picture of a snake might produce mild anxiety, looking at a picture of a snake moderate anxiety, and letting a snake crawl over one's neck extremely high anxiety. The person is also trained in deep muscle relaxation. The therapy consists of starting at the low end of the hierarchy, asking the person to relax, and then asking the patient to imagine the lowest-level anxiety-causing image. When the person is able to maintain deep relaxation while imagining the low-level stimulus, the same procedure is followed with the next one in the hierarchy, until the person is able to approach the once-dreaded object without becoming anxious.

●　　　●　　　●

This discussion of the behaviorist approach illustrates the development of this perspective from a strict behaviorism that denied the importance of inner thoughts to a form that emphasizes a person's expectations, values, attitudes, and general beliefs. Behaviorist therapies do not involve only the application of learning principles; many elements of the psychotherapeutic process—such as empathy, caring, listening, catharsis, cognitive structuring—also operate in behavioral change therapies. Behavioral change techniques can be used in conjunction with more psychodynamic approaches, and Arnold Lazarus (1981) suggests that using both dynamic and behaviorist approaches as applicable may result in better treatment outcomes.

HUMANISTIC-EXISTENTIAL APPROACHES

Frances Cohen, PhD

The humanistic and existential approaches to the understanding of human nature emerged in the 1940s–1960s in reaction to world events (such as the atrocities of World War II) and to the perceived inadequacies of the behaviorist and psychoanalytic approaches. To the humanist and existentialist, the behaviorist approach is oversimplified, since it professes no concern with internal processes and individual experience; and the psychoanalytic approach is overly pessimistic and mechanistic with its emphasis on pathologic processes. The humanistic and existential approaches emphasize individual uniqueness, the importance of a quest for values and meaning, and freedom to choose. Both approaches place great emphasis on the phenomenal field of the individual—experience known only to that person. Where they differ is that the existentialists take a more pessimistic view of people and of the difficulties in achieving a fulfilled life than do the humanists.

HUMANISTIC PERSPECTIVES

Abraham Maslow (1968) and Carl Rogers (1961) are the major humanistic theorists. Maslow objected to personality theories developed from the study of maladjusted or neurotic people and developed his approach to personality from the study of healthy, creative people. He felt that theories of personality based on the study of mental illness underemphasized the positive features of the personality. He believed that in every person "there is an active will toward health, an impulse toward growth, or toward the actualization of human potentialities" (Maslow, 1968:153).

Maslow arranged needs into a hierarchy, as shown in Fig 3–1. Basic needs must be satisfied first before higher needs can begin to be met. For example, a starving person is concerned with finding food, not with self-actualization. Failure to gratify needs at a lower level blocks personal growth and prevents attainment of higher needs.

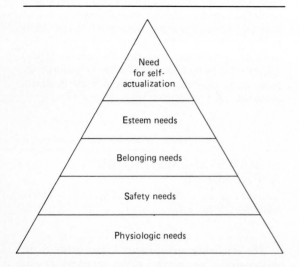

Figure 3–1. Maslow's hierarchy of needs.

The basic **physiologic needs** include oxygen, food, water, and sex. **Safety needs** include security, stability, and shelter. Needs for **love and belonging** include the need to give and receive affection and to feel that one belongs to a group or society. Once the needs for love and belonging are not pressing, then needs for **esteem** (self-respect and the respect of others) press for satisfaction.

When all of the other needs are satisfied, the need for **self-actualization** becomes dominant. The concept of self-actualization was first expounded by Kurt Goldstein (1939), a neuropsychiatrist. Self-actualization is the realization of our potentials, the exercise of all of our talents. Most people do not reach the self-actualization level, according to Maslow, because they never really satisfy their needs for love and esteem or because the environment blocks them. The environment can block or threaten the need for self-actualization if it prevents the individual from satisfying lower-level needs.

To understand personality better, Maslow decided to study people who were achieving a full life rather than those seeking therapy because of problems in living. He informally collected information about a group of people he considered to be self-actualized, ie, fulfilling their potentials. Among the people in his sampler were historical figures such as Abraham Lincoln, Henry David Thoreau, Eleanor Roosevelt, and Albert Einstein as well as some of his contemporary friends. Maslow found that these self-actualized people had certain characteristics in common, which he listed as follows:

(1) Accurate perception of reality.
(2) Acceptance of reality.
(3) Spontaneity.
(4) Ability to focus on problems to be solved rather than on the self.
(5) Need for privacy.
(6) Self-sufficiency.
(7) Capacity for fresh, nonstereotyped appreciation of people and objects.
(8) Capacity for peak experiences and ability to attain transcendence.
(9) Identification with humanity.
(10) Capacity for feelings of intimacy with a few others.
(11) A democratic attitude.
(12) Ability to distinguish means and ends.
(13) A broad sense of humor.
(14) Creativity.
(15) A nonconformist personal style.
(16) Ability to transcend dichotomies (eg, ability to see things other than in black and white, good and bad terms).

Maslow was one of the first psychologists to discuss the importance of "peak experiences"—those ecstatic moments one feels when in love or while listening to music, after accomplishing some great creative achievement or undergoing a mystical or religious experience. Everyone can have peak experiences, though they are more common among self-actualized people. A person living a peak experience can become so absorbed in the aesthetic experience that the self disappears; the experience is pure delight, with disorientation as to time and space; the person reacts to the perception as if it were something "out there," a perception of a reality independent of humankind and persisting beyond one's own life.

The humanist sees the most basic striving of the individual as that toward the maintenance, enhancement, and actualization of the self. According to Rogers, people usually behave in rational ways and choose pathways leading toward personal growth. (Maslow takes a slightly more complex view.) Rogers (1961:177–178) described this perspective in a passage that likens humans to the lion:

> Sometimes people express this concern by saying that if an individual were to be what he truly is, he would be releasing the beast in himself. I feel somewhat amused by this, because I think we might take a closer look at the beasts. The lion is often a symbol of the "ravening beast." But what about him? Unless he has been very much warped by contact with humans, he has a number of the qualities I have been describing. To be sure, he kills when he is hungry, but he does not go on a wild rampage of killing, nor does he overfeed himself . . . . He is helpless and dependent in his puppyhood, but he moves from that to independence . . . . He is selfish and self-centered in infancy, but in adulthood he shows a reasonable degree of cooperativeness, and feeds, cares for, and protects his young. He satisfies his sexual desires, but this does not mean that he goes on wild and lustful orgies. His various tendencies and urges have a harmony within him. He is, in some basic sense, a constructive and trustworthy member of the species *felis* [sic] *leo* . . . . Fully to be one's own uniqueness as a human being, is not, in my experience, a process which would be labeled bad. More appropriate words might be that it is a positive, or a constructive, or a realistic, or a trustworthy process.

Because these approaches place great emphasis on the role of values and self-fulfillment, their proponents insist that values be based on each individual's own considered choices rather than on blind acceptance of the values of society. Rogers and others stress the need for each person to develop a clear sense of self-identity.

Humanists—in contrast to psychoanalytic and behaviorist opinion—see human behavior as basically good and rational and determined by the individual interacting with the environment. The psychoanalytic view is that conflict is inherent in the human condition, with unconscious factors playing a major role in the development of personality. Irrational behavior is seen largely as arising from the influence of the unconscious. Behaviorists take a nonjudgmental, neutral view, finding that individuals may be good or evil, rational or irrational, depending on early conditioning, though behavior is determined by environmental conditioning.

Humanistic theorists regard aggression and cruelty as pathologic behavior resulting from frustration by a corrupting environment, so that faulty learning and maladaptive defense mechanisms cause mental illness and block personal growth and fulfillment. That is, one may learn faulty values or modes of coping or may be forced to concentrate on meeting basic needs rather than higher ones. If feelings or thoughts incongruent with the individual's self-concept are repressed, the result may be less personality integration and signs of maladaptive behavior. Thus, abnormal behavior results from a failure to strive toward one's potential.

Humanistic Therapy

Humanist-oriented therapists try to release the individual's potential by encouraging self-acceptance "as is," with both strengths and weaknesses. This is done (1) by creating a nonthreatening environment for open self-examination; (2) by empathetically understanding the patient's unique worldview; and (3) by encouraging full self-acceptance and confidence in one's ability to act on choices. The therapy is viewed as an "authentic" encounter between 2 individuals, and the client plays a major role in directing the course of therapy. The assumption is that people have within themselves the resources to understand and alter their view of the self and to direct their own behavior. Much of the therapist's role consists of showing empathic understanding and unconditional positive regard (showing genuine care about the individual as a human being, without placing conditions on the therapist's acceptance).

EXISTENTIAL PERSPECTIVES

Existential theories also emphasize the uniqueness of the individual but place more emphasis on irrationality and the difficulties of self-fulfillment. Their central concern is with the challenge of human existence—the need to establish a personal identity and sense of meaning. The basic concepts of these theories stem from European existential philosophers such as Heidegger, Kierkegaard, and Sartre. In the USA, Paul Tillich (1952) and Rollo May (1958) have been influential proponents of this view. The psychiatrists Jaspers, Binswanger, and Boss developed an existential approach to psychotherapy.

Existentialist opinion holds that the basic motivation of human behavior is to find the best way of life and to actualize potentials. This does not occur as a natural unfolding, as the humanists believe, but involves a painful process of soul-searching and decision making. Modern society imposes a heavy burden of spiritual strain and confusion with the breakdown of traditional mores and beliefs. People can resolve this dilemma either by giving up the search and submerging themselves in the group or by striving to define themselves and their existence. The first way is seen as inauthentic and leading to anxiety and despair.

Existential Anxiety

A central theme of existentialism is the encounter with nonbeing, or nothingness. Existential anxiety is the state in which one is aware of the possibility of nonbeing. Nonbeing—the opposite of being—in its ultimate form is death. Awareness of the inevitability of death produces anxieties regarding the unpredictability of life and concerns about whether one is living a meaningful life. Tillich (1952:45), a theologian, describes the process as follows:

> Nonbeing is omnipresent and produces anxiety even where an immediate threat of death is absent . . . . It stands behind the insecurity and homelessness of our social and individual existence. It stands behind the attacks on our power of being in body and soul by weakness, disease, and accidents. In all these forms fate actualizes itself, and through them the anxiety of nonbeing takes hold of us. We try to transform the anxiety into fear and to meet courageously the objects in which the threat is embodied. We succeed partly, but somehow we are aware of the fact that it is not these objects with which we struggle that produce the anxiety but the human situation as such.

If people lack the courage to confront this existential anxiety, they may choose "secure" paths and deny themselves directions that might offer greater self-fulfillment. Neurosis is seen as a way of avoiding nonbeing by avoiding being, of surrendering part of one's potentialities in order to save the rest. Thus, failure to reach one's full potential is due to an inability to confront existential anxiety and to give life a sense of meaning by taking responsibility for one's life.

Tenets of Existentialism

The existentialists emphasize that people are what they make of themselves. Sartre's proposition—that the essence of a person is his or her existence ("J'existe, donc je suis" ["I exist, therefore I am"])—suggests that there is no essential nature of humankind except what is self-created. Tillich (1952:149–150) describes this as "the most despairing and the most courageous sentence in all existentialist literature." Creating the right kind of life and accepting responsibility for who one is can be agonizing. One's essence is shaped by the value choices one makes and the meaning one creates. Viktor Frankl's (1962) experiences in the Nazi concentration camps led him to focus on the **will-to-meaning,** the way individuals find meaning in life even in the midst of a cruel and seemingly irrational world.

More than other approaches, existentialism emphasizes the importance of the spiritual aspect of the person, something ignored by most modern 20th-century psychology and by medicine. Through confrontation with the threat of nonbeing, people are required to answer to themselves for what they have made of themselves.

Existential Therapy

In its application to psychotherapy, the existential approach—more a point of view than a system—combines the existential philosopher's concerns and attitudes toward the human condition with the approach of depth psychology, ie, attempting to understand the patient's subjective experience in all its depth and complexity. The existential approach is seen as a necessary complement to psychoanalysis rather than as an alternative. The existential therapists use some techniques common to psychoanalysis, such as free association and dream analysis.

The existential viewpoint emphasizes the ways in which people are unique rather than alike. More important than the freudian defense mechanisms and characterologic reactions are the modes of **being-in-the-world,** not only taking care of biologic needs or sharing experiences with others but of developing through life and through constant change a feeling of self-identity. People are conceived of as never static but always in transition, coming into being, becoming, evolving. They are seen as going through constant changes—constantly giving up the old, constantly trying to create a unique self and a unique world.

The aims of existential therapies are to help patients confront their total subjective experiences in all of their ramifications, including the anxiety of nonbeing; to recognize what their values are; and to decide on a meaningful way of being. Through therapy, individuals are confronted with questions about the meaning of existence. The encounter with the therapist is an important component of the process—it must be based on trust, openness, and respect for the other person's subjective experience (see Chapter 45).

GENERAL SYSTEMS THEORY APPROACH

Dennis Farrell, MD

The 3 models presented so far represent theories of personality—detailed schemes that explain how behavior and internal psychologic structures develop and change. The fourth model is not an elaborate theory of personality but rather a grand unifying theory providing a perspective on how to understand people in all their complexity and in their interactions with the world around them. General systems theory forms the basis of the biopsychosocial model discussed in Chapters 1 and 2.

General systems theory was first proposed by the biologist Bertalanffy (1968a, 1968b) to account for a wide range of phenomena in the physical world and in nature that seem capable of explanation only on the basis of the concept of **system.** It came to be applied to such seemingly diverse fields as mathematics, engineering, physics, biology, and the social sciences. It has appealed to workers in diverse fields, as if in response—in Bertalanffy's words—to a "secret trend in various disciplines, the striving for unification of the scientific outlook." From a historical perspective, it can be viewed as a counterbalance to what has been the prevailing trend in Western science toward ever-increasing specialization—with the inevitable narrowing and compartmentalization of knowledge as specialists learn more and more about less and less. Through its formulations, which bridge the gap between diverse disciplines, systems theory has attempted what Bertalanffy (1968a:14) has described as "scientific interpretation in theory where previously there was none."

General systems theory holds that the most significant aspect of nature is organization. Living creatures are organized sets of systems, with "system" defined as a complex of interrelated elements. Living systems are **complex systems,** or sets of hierarchically organized systems composed of different levels. Miller (1978), for example, postulates the following hierarchy of levels: cell, organ, organism, group, organization, society, supranational system. Each higher-level system typically contains new characteristics that emerge only at that level. A corollary to this proposition is that such new "emergent properties" cannot be completely understood simply by adding up the parts of which the property seems to be composed; the whole property is greater than the sum of its component parts.

Systems are characterized by organization, interrelatedness and interaction of parts, control mechanisms, and tendencies toward both stability (homeostasis)) and change (heterostasis). The "leading part" of a system at each level regulates the balance between stability and change and maintains the boundary of the system. Wiener (1948) showed that information in a system is mathematically equivalent to energy in physics. Information may be defined as "the amount of complexity, patterning, or organization in a signal or message" (Kaplan and Sadock, 1981). Information and controlling and self-steering mechanisms (which involve a feedback of information) are built into the functioning of living organisms (and sophisticated machines). Living organisms are, however, open systems engaged with the environment in a continuous exchange of matter and energy and information. They are not passive but intrinsically active, even without external stimuli. "The stimulus (ie, a change in the external conditions) does not *cause* a process in an otherwise inert system; it only *modifies* processes in an autonomously active system" (Bertalanffy, 1968a: 209–219).

General systems theory follows the organismic school of biology in holding as a basic tenet the fundamental inseparability of the apparatus and mechanisms determining the activity of a living being (Goldstein, 1939). Since general systems theory originates in biology, it can embrace both mind and body, the experiential and behavioral, and the individual and the social in its overall scheme of different levels and aspects of systems operating according to the same basic principles—the need for organization, interaction of parts, control mechanisms, and maintenance of boundaries.

For example, cybernetics, developed by Norbert Wiener in 1948, helped clarify the way in which the feedback mechanism is fundamental to a host of regulatory processes in both humans and machines. Studies in this field—eg, in biofeedback, one's ability to warm or cool a hand or to raise or lower blood pressure given feedback on the effects one is producing—have demonstrated the intimate link between psychologic and physiologic events. A general systems approach encourages a holistic picture of the individual. To think of people as energy machines, as stimulus-response robots, or as sophisticated walking computers has increasingly come to be seen as a hopelessly narrow view of living beings. Roger Sperry (1981), a neuroscientist whose important contributions include work on mutual isolation of the cerebral hemispheres (split-brain research), offers the following analogy: "Just as the programming variables of a TV monitor have to be included in order to account for the electron flow pattern of the system, so also in the brain the subjective, mental variables of cerebral function have to be included to give a full account of the flow patterns of neural excitation."

Growth and development, the evolution of species, even the rise and fall of civilizations and cultures all illustrate that along with the tendency toward stability and homeostasis, there is in living matter and particularly in human life the tendency toward increasingly higher levels of organization. This point of view incorporates the total range of activity not only of the individual but also of family and group and cultural levels. Processes emerging at higher levels of hierarchically organized systems acquire the power to dominate those operating at lower levels. For example, the value system of an individual, a group, or an entire culture can become a major causal determinant of behavior, at times superseding even the most basic instincts such as self-preservation (eg, the Japanese kamikaze pilots in World War II who sacrificed themselves for their emperor and country). Such a phenomenon cannot be understood on the basis of a model which postulates that behavior is strictly a set response to a stimulus or a way of reducing tension. Nonetheless, families or groups do obey certain natural laws embodied in the concepts making up general systems theory.

General systems theory can also help us comprehend certain aspects of individual or group psychopathology, ie, system malfunctioning or breakdown. The effects of information input overload have been studied at levels of living systems ranging from the single cell to military and industrial organizations. Processes by which systems adjust tend to be **isomorphic,** ie, similar in form between levels. The overworked medical student, after an initial increase in the rate of assimilation of information, may resort to **omission** and **error,** 2 typical adjustment processes to the stress of input overload; the individual neuron behaves in much the same way in response to excessive stimuli.

Alvin Toffler's term "future shock" (1970) vividly conveys the reaction of a society overwhelmed by the rapidity of environmental change. This concept explains much about the typical life-styles and attitudes of inhabitants of the contemporary metropolis in highly technologic societies. As an extreme example, just as an overloaded telephone network can break down *as a system* without any dysfunction in any of its component parts, so a person can succumb to the sheer accumulation of stresses without necessarily having organ failure.

Just as machines cease to function adequately when signal transmission is interrupted, so do individuals or groups where there is some interference with information transmission from one part of the system to another. In systems terms, people are active systems determining their own reactions to their human environment on several levels simultaneously by means of an archaic "decider subsystem" (based on primitive childhood perceptions of self and others) as well as a more mature, reality-attuned "decider subsystem" of the conscious ego. Mental health requires good communication between these subsystems—another way of talking about the need to integrate past and present in coping with life.

General systems theory appeals to many students of the life sciences because of the broad scope of its conceptualization. It is of greatest use when one attempts to study different levels of organization in interaction with one another within a system, eg, mind-body interactions or the interplay of individual and family or group dynamics. It has played an important part in unifying a number of trends that have moved toward a more holistic view of the human being—one that embraces not only the person's biology or psychology but also his or her unique subjective and objective reality, created by certain biologic givens and the social and cultural milieu into which the person was born and moves through life. A systems approach departs radically from the study of the individual in isolation. Physicians, more than most persons, need to keep a systems perspective in mind. An apprehensive adolescent patient presenting in a frantic, keyed-up state with symptoms of rapid pulse and insomnia may be manifesting primary disturbance at the **cellular** or **organ** level (eg, amphetamine toxicity, thyrotoxicosis); at the **organismic** level (anxiety over threatened breakthrough of forbidden sexual impulses); at the **group** level (intolerable family pressures, scapegoating by peers at school); at the **societal** level (unemployment, racial discrimination); or even at the **supranational system** level (threat of war, mobilization for military service).

Disturbance at one level affects functioning at other (usually adjacent) levels. The physician needs to keep all levels in mind in searching for the primary disturbance, as opposed to secondary effects of superficial manifestations, in order to know how to intervene effectively and intelligently. A systems approach is the basis for a truly biopsychosocial approach in psychiatry. It reminds physicians of the complexity of human nature and demonstrates that all "models of the mind" are essentially complementary.

SUMMARY

The models discussed in this chapter offer different vantage points from which to gain a better understanding of the individual. No one theory offers the best perspective. Rather, each emphasizes a different aspect of the person and different intrapsychic mechanisms involved, as shown in the illustrative case below.

Illustrative Case

A 60-year-old black woman with little formal schooling and a history of stomach problems was seen in the surgery clinic because of a breast lump. The surgeon performed needle biopsy to rule out the possibility of a cyst and then ordered a mammogram, which showed a probability of cancer. The surgeon, a white man, recommended a surgical biopsy to remove the lump and confirm the presence of cancer. The patient refused the biopsy despite the surgeon's repeated efforts to explain why it was needed.

A nurse who spoke with the patient and used the different models outlined in this chapter discovered the many reasons for the patient's refusal. From a psychoanalytic perspective, the nurse explored the unconscious meaning the woman's breasts had for the patient and the way she felt about white men in positions of authority. Although the patient was not aware of her feelings, her breasts were clearly a badge of femininity to be protected at all costs, especially from the hands of white authority figures who could not be trusted to be anything other than exploitive. Cancer symbolized death and evoked negative depressive images.

From the behaviorist approach, the nurse realized that because of her lack of formal education, the patient could not understand how the human body worked. Since her stomach had hurt after she had the needle biopsy, the patient decided that the "roots of cancer" had spread to her stomach, signifying that the cancer was so far advanced nothing could be done about it. Why go through surgery, pondered the woman, when it had already spread so far? She wondered why she should go through all that pain and discomfort if she was going to die soon in any case. The nurse also discovered that white male authority figures had several times tried to take advantage of the patient, who had therefore established a conditioned reaction to such men.

From a humanistic-existential point of view, the nurse explored the patient's ideas about the meaning of life, her fears of a protracted illness ending in death, and her desire to maintain as much control over her life as possible. The patient was preoccupied with fulfilling survival needs and became anxious whenever she had to think about the possibility of death before her time.

From a general systems theory perspective, the nurse asked how the patient's family was functioning and how her family members felt. The patient reported that her teenaged son kept telling her, "Don't let them take anything from you." Her daughter, on the other hand, was a nurse who urged her to undergo the biopsy procedure as soon as possible. These differing viewpoints imposed further stress. The nurse also discovered that the patient's "stomach problems" were being treated by an internist and that at times the stomach pain was so severe that it affected the patient's thought processes. The patient felt her internist had never properly explained the stomach problems and was therefore trying to conceal the severity of her condition.

The patient refused the biopsy. She returned to the clinic 6 months later complaining of pain in the breast. This time the patient sought out a black surgeon on the staff, recommended by her internist, who was able to convince the patient to have the biopsy that same afternoon. He also referred her to a health educator who taught her more about the anatomy of the body and what to expect from a mastectomy.

The illustrative case presented above shows the many factors influencing the patient's attitude toward the biopsy and refusal to allow it and how some changes had to occur (increased severity of symptoms; a surgeon who was a nonthreatening authority figure; more information) before change could be effected in the situation. It is useful to apply these different perspectives sequentially in pondering difficult cases such as the one presented. Treatment plans that incorporate a variety of techniques also increase the likelihood of achieving significant change.

REFERENCES

Ayllon T: Intensive treatment of psychotic behavior by stimulus satiation and food reinforcement. *Behav Res Ther* 1963;**1**:53.

Bandura A, Ross D, Ross S: Imitation of film-mediated aggressive models. *J Abnorm Soc Psychol* 1963;**66**:3.

Bandura A, Walters RH: *Social Learning Theory and Personality Development*. Holt, Rinehart, & Winston, 1963.

Bertalanffy L von: *General System Theory*. George Braziller, 1968a.

Bertalanffy L von: General system theory: A critical review. Pages 11–30 in: *Modern Systems Research for the Behavioral Scientist*. Buckley W (editor). Aldine, 1968b.

Dollard J, Miller NE: *Personality and Psychotherapy*. McGraw-Hill, 1950.

Erikson EH: *Childhood and Society*. Norton, 1950.

Erikson EH: *Identity and the Life Cycle*. Internat Univ Press, 1959.

Fraiberg S: *The Magic Years*. Scribner, 1959.

Frankl VE: *Man's Search for Meaning*. Beacon, 1962.

Freud A: *The Ego and the Mechanisms of Defense*. Internat Univ Press, 1946.

Freud S: The interpretation of dreams (1900). In: *Standard Edition of the Complete Psychological Works of Sigmund Freud*. Vols 4 and 5. Hogarth Press, 1959.

Freud S: The question of lay analysis (1926). In: *Standard Edition of the Complete Psychological Works of Sigmund Freud*. Vol 20. Hogarth Press, 1959.

Goldstein K: *The Organism*. American Book, 1939.

Hartmann H: *Ego Psychology and the Problem of Adaptation*. Internat Univ Press, 1958.

Kaplan HI, Sadock BJ (editors): *Modern Synopsis of Comprehensive Textbook of Psychiatry/IV*, 4th ed. Williams & Wilkins, 1985.

Kohut H: *The Analysis of the Self*. Internat Univ Press, 1971.

Lazarus AA: *The Practice of Multimodal Therapy*. McGraw-Hill, 1981.

Mahler MS, Pine F, Bergman A: *The Psychological Birth of the Human Infant*. Basic Books, 1975.

Maslow AH: *Toward a Psychology of Being*, 2nd ed. Van Nostrand, 1968.

May R: Contributions of existential psychotherapy. In: *Existence: A New Dimension in Psychiatry and Psychology*. May R, Angel E, Ellenberger HF (editors). Basic Books, 1958.

Miller JG: *Living Systems*. McGraw-Hill, 1978.

Mischel W: *Personality and Assessment*. Wiley, 1968.

Mowrer DH, Mowrer WM: Enuresis: A method for its study and treatment. *Am J Orthopsychiatry* 1938;**8**:436.

Pavlov IP: *Conditioned Reflexes*. Oxford Univ Press, 1927.

Rapaport D: The structure of psychoanalytic theory: A systematizing attempt. In: *Psychological Issues*. Vol 6. Internat Univ Press, 1959.

Rogers C: *On Becoming a Person*. Houghton Mifflin, 1961.

Rotter JB: Generalized expectancies for internal versus external locus of reinforcement. *Psychol Monographs* 1966;**80**:609.

Skinner BF: *Science and Human Behavior*. Macmillan, 1953.

Sperry RW: Changing priorities. *Annu Rev Neurosci* 1981;**4**:12.

Thorndike EL: *The Psychology of Learning*. Teachers College, 1913.

Tillich P: *The Courage to Be*. Yale Univ Press, 1952.

Toffler A: *Future Shock*. Random House, 1970.

Vaillant G: *Adaptation to Life*. Little, Brown, 1977.

Watson JB: *Behaviorism*. Norton, 1924.

Watson JB, Raynor R: Conditioned emotional reactions. *J Exp Psychol* 1920;**3**:1.

Wiener N: *Cybernetics*. Wiley, 1948.

Wolpe J: The systematic desensitization treatment of neuroses. *J Nerv Ment Dis* 1961;**132**:189.

4

The Mind & Somatic Illness: Psychologic Factors Affecting Physical Illness

Stuart J. Eisendrath, MD

Example: A 60-year-old woman entered a hospital emergency room complaining of light-headedness and chest palpitations. Shortly thereafter, she suffered a cardiac arrest that was successfully treated, and she was transferred to the coronary care unit. When she was examined, she was not only anxious but also depressed. On questioning, she revealed that the date of her cardiac arrest was the 1-year anniversary of her husband's death from cardiac arrest.

Example: A 40-year-old businessman underwent a traumatic divorce and became seriously depressed. The wife to whom he had been devoted had left him for a 25-year-old tennis teacher. Two months later, the businessman was found to have an aggressive lymphoma, and he died 3 months later after several unsuccessful trials of chemotherapy.

Example: A 4-year-old boy had always had excellent health. Two weeks after his only sibling was born, however, he developed persistent cough and fever. He eventually required hospitalization for treatment of pneumonia.

The above are examples of typical clinical situations in which attentive and alert clinicians may see the influence of psychosocial factors on physical health. Physicians have been aware of this relationship since ancient times. The study of this relationship, usually termed **psychosomatic medicine,** has undergone marked conceptual shifts in the past decade. Today, theorists believe that there are no "psychosomatic" diseases per se and that all physical diseases have psychosocial components. These components may predispose to illness, initiate it, or maintain it. This chapter focuses on the development of theories of psychosomatic medicine in the 20th century.

Mind/Body & Stress

Before the 1900s, the philosophy of Cartesian dualism viewed the mind and the body as separate entities. Organized religions claimed the mind and spirit as their domain, while physicians were ceded the body. This dichotomy was heightened by scientific progress in the late 1800s. The discovery that bacteria were causative agents of disease emphasized the physical aspects of medicine and also led to the concept of linear causality: one type of bacterium directly causes one disease. This oversimplified concept of a unitary cause of disease—one factor directly causes one specific disease—influenced the development of psychosomatic theory for several decades.

Cannon was one of the pioneers working in psychosomatic medicine. He performed intricate laboratory experiments that studied the effects of fear and rage on animals. Cannon saw that animals responded to emergencies with adaptive changes in physiology that prepared them for "fight or flight." Cannon theorized that the mechanism involved in inhibition of anabolic (parasympathetic; cholinergic) functions and an activation of catabolic (sympathetic; adrenergic) functions. This combination of processes supplied the animals with energy needed to meet the emergency.

Selye (1974) extended the work of Cannon. He postulated that the entire organism responded to stress; eg, blood flow might be shunted from the gastrointestinal tract to the heart, brain, and musculature during stress. Such an adaptation would help the organism deal with stress over the short term, but if the stress was prolonged, the adaptation might result in increased friability of the gastrointestinal mucosa and eventual ulceration. Selye proposed that responses to stress could be triggered in inappropriate situations if the organism had been accustomed to react in that way. Later research in autonomic conditioning suggests that such inappropriate reactions may be difficult to extinguish.

Other workers also built upon Cannon's efforts. Wolff and coworkers (1950) investigated the human response to stress. They perceived stress-induced diseases as a protective human response to threatening situations, and they believed that the organ system affected by such stress played a specific and symbolic role in the overall response; eg, an individual who wished to be rid of a troublesome person might develop hyperactivity of the colon and resulting diarrhea. One of the noteworthy aspects of Wolff's work was the ingenuity of his experimental methods, which made use of emotionally charged interviews or movies in order to provoke measurable responses in his experimental subjects.

Personality & Medical Illness

In the 1940s, Dunbar (1942, 1946) began developing her "personality profiles" of specific diseases. She felt that each disease was associated with a specific cluster of symptoms, and she therefore reviewed psychologic data about patients with diseases such as hypertension, diabetes, rheumatoid arthritis, and myocardial infarction and from these formulated typical behavior patterns, family histories, and patterns of onset of illness that seemed to be associated. She suggested, for example, that people with myocardial infarction tend to be compulsive and to overwork and that the infarction tends to follow exposure to shock, particularly at work.

The idea that a specific personality may be associated with a certain disease is most evident in current research into the behavior of people thought to be likely candidates for heart attacks. Friedman and Rosenman (1974) labeled the behavior of these patients type A. Further work has suggested that these patients chronically feel the pressure of time and that they harbor feelings of hostile competitiveness.

A major deficit in the "specific personality" approach to understanding the relationship between psychologic makeup and disease is that almost all of the data rely on retrospective analysis. People who already have a certain disease are studied psychologically in an attempt to discern whether certain personality traits caused the disease. But specific psychologic profiles are of limited value. Researchers following the model of direct linear causation derived from Koch's postulates tended to adopt the approach in the 1930s and 1940s that personality might "cause" disease. Treatment techniques (chiefly psychoanalysis) that tried to eradicate the precipitating psychologic factor were notably unsuccessful, however.

It therefore became clear that direct, unitary causation did not operate in the development of diseases. Dunbar herself was careful to avoid implications of cause and effect in her work. Alternative explanations of the behavior associated with certain diseases were formulated. Perhaps the behavior resulted from the disease, or perhaps the behavior and the physical illness were both phenotypic expressions of some common gene. These theories suggested that psychologic treatments that attempted to change behavior might not "cure" disease. Current research is evaluating how changes in type A behavior traits affect a person's chances of incurring myocardial infarction. Prospective studies in progress can avoid the deficits of earlier work. Current studies of the effects of behavioral intervention on myocardial infarction recurrence are inconclusive. The hypothesis that psychologic factors cause disease will still not be proved, however, even if behavioral treatments are shown to be effective in preventing disease.

In contrast to Dunbar's personality-specific research, Alexander (1950) explored the relationship between specific psychologic conflicts and disease states. He investigated 7 diseases regarded as classic psychosomatic disorders: peptic ulcers, bronchial asthma, rheumatoid arthritis, ulcerative colitis, essential hypertension, thyrotoxicosis, and neurodermatitis. His work attempted to answer the main question in psychosomatic medicine in the 1930s and 1940s—why does the individual have these specific symptoms?

Alexander believed that psychosomatic diseases developed out of "visceral neurosis." Physiologic changes accompanied unresolved emotional conflicts and eventually resulted in pathologic derangements in the organ system. For example, Alexander hypothesized that individuals with peptic ulcer disease suffered from infantile desires for others to supply love, support, advice, and money. When frustrated, these desires intensified but then produced guilt and shame in these patients, who wanted to appear as capable, independent adults. The desire to be cared for was equivalent to the infantile wish to be fed, and the conflicting drives for independence and dependence were expressed as increased gastric secretions. The secretions in turn led to formation of ulcers.

Alexander advanced the theory of psychosomatic medicine significantly by abandoning a model of disease based on unitary, direct causation. He postulated a 3-part constellation of factors necessary to produce disease: (1) The individual must have a specific set of psychologic conflicts; (2) a specific situation that triggers the onset of disease must occur; in ulcer disease, this might be the loss of a person on whom the patient depended; and (3) the individual must have a constitutional vulnerability, an "X factor," that biologically predisposes the patient to that specific illness.

Alexander's work suffered because it was based on retrospective analysis. Mirsky (1958) investigated Alexander's ideas in an ingenious prospective study that used army recruits who were entering basic training. The recruits were divided into 2 groups on the basis of high or low levels of serum pepsinogen, a genetically determined trait that correlates with some types of ulcer formation. Those recruits with high levels of serum pepsinogen were found to have the infantile features suggested by Alexander; moreover, they could be identified from their responses to psychologic testing by independent raters who did not know their serum pepsinogen levels. The recruits who subsequently developed ulcers associated with the stress of basic training proved to be from the group who had high levels of serum pepsinogen.

Further Development of Theories of Psychosomatic Medicine

The Mirsky study tended to confirm many of Alexander's ideas but left many questions unanswered. How did stress lead to formation of ulcers? Why did the psychotherapeutic approaches have such variable success in treatment of psychosomatic disorders such as ulcers?

Mirsky's study opened a new area of inquiry in psychosomatic medicine. Could an inherited biologic tendency toward gastric hypersecretion lead to psychologic sequelae? For example, a newborn with high rates of gastric secretion might biologically require hourly feedings to diminish gastric acidity. If the mother fed the newborn at "average" intervals of once every 3 hours, conflict concerning dependence on others for attention and nurturance might be created in the newborn's personality. The genetic predisposition to gastric hypersecretion could lead to somatopsychic effects. Personality development could therefore be a result of physiologic events, rather than the reverse.

Grinker and colleagues (1973) began integrating such possibilities into a unified field theory of psychosomatic medicine. This approach was basically a general systems model of illness. This theory emphasized that each element of the human "system" (eg, personality or genetic constitution) had multiple reverberating connections throughout the system. Biologic and psychosocial forces could interact with each other to produce disease. The effect of this theory was to clearly point out the inadequacy of the unitary, direct causation model of disease.

At the same time, the work of Engel directed psychosomatic theory toward less specific but broader concepts of the production of illness. Engel (1975) noted that loss of an important person in the patient's life frequently preceded the onset or exacerbation of illness. Engel himself described how he suffered a myocardial infarction on the last day of a mourning period for his twin brother.

Engel (1967) believed that loss led to several phases of response. At first, the individual was aroused to search for the lost object. If the search failed, the person entered a state of "conservation-withdrawal" and ceased to search; physiologic processes (eg, gastric secretion) became hypoactive. Engel believed that such a sequence could lead to a "giving up-given up" state, in which the individual felt helpless to change his or her situation and hopeless about receiving aid from others. Such a condition predisposed a person to development of illness. Engel did not believe that this condition was in itself sufficient to cause illness, nor did he feel that this condition had to exist before illness occurred. Such a condition could make the person vulnerable to illness, however.

Animal experiments lent support to Engel's position. Kaufman and Rosenblum (1969) used different species of monkeys to study the physiologic response of an infant who was separated from its mother. The infant's patterns of behavior tended to follow the series of responses outlined by Engel, and the incidence of illness increased. Among certain species, however, the pattern was moderated if the deprived young monkey was provided with social support.

Epidemiologic studies have also supported Engel's work. Holmes and Rahe (1967) evaluated the effects of stressful events on the occurrence of physical illness. In both retrospective and prospective studies, they found that the number and magnitude of life changes (eg, bereavements, new jobs, moving to another place) correlated with the onset and severity of disease. Their work suggests that changes in life may encourage the development of disease, but in a nonspecific way.

Other researchers have evaluated bereavement as one specific and powerful type of life change. Rees and Lutkins (1967) noted that the number of deaths among relatives of patients who had died was 7 times higher than in the general population. Parkes and Brown (1972) found similarly elevated mortality rates in another population of bereaved individuals. These findings have been reproduced in many countries. It is clear that loss of an emotionally important person is associated with increased incidence of both illness and death, particularly in young widowers.

Reiser (1975) believed that there are 3 phases related to illness. During the period before illness develops, the patient is shaped by genetic constitution and early psychosocial experiences. When the illness appears, the prior "programming" is activated by nonspecific psychosocial stresses, such as bereavement. Other factors, such as environmental exposure to viruses or malignant transformation in cells, may then challenge the stressed individual and produce disease. In the third phase, after the onset of disease, psychosocial forces operate to modulate the course of the disease.

Biopsychosocial Model of Disease

Engel (1977) synthesized the advances in psychosomatic medicine by developing the biopsychosocial model of disease, which recognizes that *all* diseases have biologic, psychologic, and social components. Engel's model emphasizes the view that each individual is composed of systems and is in turn part of larger outside systems. Each person is composed of molecules, cells, and organs; each person is also a member of a family, community, culture, nation, and world. Every individual has a biologic, psychologic, and social structure that may affect other levels of the system and vice versa. As an example, Engel (1980) described a patient undergoing cardiac arrest, an account paraphrased here and used to illustrate how Engel's theory may be applied:

A patient suffers chest pain and goes to a hospital emergency room. Because he has had one previous myocardial infarction, he suspects that he is having another. He is examined by a new intern, who also suspects an infarction and who attempts to insert an intravenous line. After several unsuccessful attempts, the intern leaves the patient alone in his cubicle and goes to get assistance. While unattended, the patient continues to feel pain and also feels alone and worried about the competence of his caretakers. He suffers a cardiac arrest and is immediately resuscitated successfully by the emergency team.

If the viewpoint adopted by the clinician is a biomedical model based on linear causality, the successful resuscitation of the patient is a laudable event. If psychosocial factors are taken into account, however, important information is revealed about the patient and the incident; namely, that the patient's pain, fear, and doubts most likely affected the physical disease process, possibly through direct vagal effects, increased levels of circulating catecholamines, or other physiologic responses. If medical personnel had considered psychosocial factors and started appropriate treatment—eg, ensuring constant attention by the nursing staff or using anxiolytic medications—the cardiac arrest might not have occurred at all. The biopsychosocial model does not simplistically assert that the myocardial infarction was a direct result of the patient's psychology. It does provide a broader understanding of disease processes, and it encourages physicians to think about truly comprehensive treatment that considers both the physical and the psychosocial elements of disease.

The model also includes sociocultural factors in its conception of disease. It has been widely demonstrated, for example, that pain as a presenting symptom is affected by sex, race, and ethnic origin. The biopsychosocial model holds that a stoic New England Yankee may be experiencing as much pain as an expressive Italian patient with the same disease.

Psychoimmunology

The biopsychosocial model provides one approach to describing the relationship between disease and psychosocial factors. Research in psychosomatic medicine has shifted from the "why" questions so common in the 1930s and 1950s to "how" questions; eg, how does the bereavement experience become translated into physical illness? Or, as Weiner and coworkers (1957) ask, how is psychologic experience transformed to bodily change?

Psychoimmunology is one area of research that is trying to explain the relationship mentioned above. Since immunocompetence protects an individual against infections as well as cancer, alterations in immune status may be expected to have serious effects. Many of the clincial studies that would clarify the effects of psychologic stress on immune function are only now getting under way. Preliminary work does suggest, however, that stress can have powerful effects on immune function.

Bartrop and associates (1977) studied the spouses of survivors of an Australian train wreck and found that at 5 weeks after bereavement, these individuals had depressed lymphocyte function (T cell response to mitogens). This T cell response was 10-fold less than that of controls.

Greene and colleagues (1978) evaluated patients for life change factors along the lines of the work of Holmes and Rahe. In those individuals who had undergone stressful life changes, they found evidence of decreased lymphocyte cytotoxicity. Locke (1982) investigated college students coping poorly with stress and found decreased natural killer cell activity (part of the body's immunologic defense system). Both studies suggest that individuals under stress, particularly those not coping well, may be at increased risk for infection and malignant changes in cells. Although studies using humans are at an early stage, substantial animal experimentation exists that supports the findings of Greene and Locke and their colleagues. Work studying the effect of stress on animals has shown increased susceptibility to illness caused by many types of infectious agents. Other work suggests that stress may also predispose animals to cancer.

Riley (1975) exposed 2 groups of mice to the Bittner virus, which usually causes mammary tumors. One experimental group was kept in a stress-free setting. The other group was placed in a high-stress, crowded environment. At the end of the experiment, the incidence of tumor was 7% in the first group and 92% in the second group.

In exploring the alteration of immune function, Ader and Cohen (1975) induced immunosuppression in rats as a conditioned response. They exposed rats to saccharin, together with cyclophosphamide, an immunosuppressant. Subsequent reexposure of the rats to saccharin alone produced immunosuppression, which although not as great as that associated with cyclophosphamide, was nonetheless significant and demonstrated that immunosuppression may be a learned behavior. The results of these experiments have been duplicated by other researchers.

Results from animal experimentation studies suggest that psychosocial forces may have a powerful effect on physical health. The question of how the effects are mediated remains. Rogers and coworkers (1979) suggested 3 possibilities. One mechanism may involve the hypothalamic-pituitary-adrenal axis. It has been known for years that stress can cause an acute increase in cortisol production. This increase, in turn, may lead to impaired cell-mediated immunity. The issue is complicated, however, because prolonged stress may not have the same effects as short-term stress and may actually be associated with enhanced cell-mediated immunity.

A second possible mediator of stress is the autonomic nervous system. For example, since lymphocytes are known to have beta-adrenergic receptors, release of catecholamines by the sympathetic nervous system would affect lymphocyte function.

A third possible mechanism is that the nervous system may be directly linked to the immune system. The conditioned response in the experiment of Ader and Cohen (1975) might be explained by such a mechanism, since the increased amounts of cortisol alone cannot fully explain their findings of immunosuppression. In addition, Besedovsky (1977) has immunized rats and found increased electrical activity occurring immediately afterward in the ventromedial hypothalamic nuclei. Workers speculate that there must be some afferent link between antigen stimulation and hypothalamic function, and the idea is supported by experimental studies showing that anaphylactic reactions may be prevented by experimentally inducing hypothalamic lesions.

Research in fields such as endocrinology and cardiology will extend the knowledge of psychophysiology already gained from the psychoimmunologic studies described above.

SUMMARY

The field of psychosomatic medicine is no longer restricted to the study of the 7 classic psychosomatic diseases (peptic ulcer, bronchial asthma, rheumatoid arthritis, ulcerative colitis, essential hypertension, thyrotoxicosis, and neurodermatitis). The focus of study has shifted from theories of unitary psychogenic causes of disease to an approach that integrates psychosocial and biologic factors.

The biopsychosocial model may be applied to all diseases and is especially useful in helping to decide which treatments to use; eg, the clinician who realizes that peptic ulcer disease has psychologic and social components as well as physical elements will consider not only cimetidine but also psychotherapy as possible treatments. Treatment based only on biologic considerations may be useless in coronary artery disease unless the patient's psychosocial characteristics are taken into account. Even if type A behavior is discounted as an influence on disease, the patient's compliance with medication requirements and changes in exercise, smoking, and diet may all affect progression and disease.

As Lipowski (1977) noted, the cause of disease remains a focus of interest in psychosomatic medicine. Another major interest is the investigation of how psychologic processes are mediated in the production of disease. As this relationship is elucidated, new types of treatment are sure to follow.

REFERENCES

Ader R, Cohen N: Behaviorally conditioned immunosuppression. *Psychosom Med* 1975;**37**:333.

Alexander F: *Psychosomatic Medicine: Its Principles and Applications.* Norton, 1950.

Bartrop RW et al: Depressed lymphocyte function after bereavement. *Lancet* 1977;**1**:834.

Besedovsky H et al: Hypothalamic changes during the immune response. *Eur J Immunol* 1977;**7**:323.

Dembroski TM et al: Stress, emotions, behavior, and cardiovascular disease. In: *Emotions in Health and Illness: Theoretical and Research Foundations.* Temoshok L, Van Dyke C, Zegans L (editors). Grune & Stratton, 1983.

Dunbar HF: *Emotions and Bodily Change,* 3rd ed. Columbia Univ Press, 1946.

Dunbar HF: The relationship between anxiety states and organic disease. *Clinics* 1942;**1**:879.

Engel GL: The clincial application of the biopsychosocial model. *Am J Psychiatry* 1980;**137**:535.

Engel GL: The death of a twin: Mourning and anniversary reactions. Fragments of 10 years of self-analysis. *Int J Psychoanal* 1975;**56**:23.

Engel GL: The need for a new medical model: A challenge for biomedicine. *Science* 1977;**196**:129.

Engel GL: A psychological setting of somatic disease: The giving up-given up complex. *Proc Roy Soc Med* 1967;**60**:553.

Friedman M, Rosenman RH: *Type A Behavior and Your Heart.* Knopf, 1974.

Greene WA et al: Psychosocial factors and immunity: Preliminary report of the annual meeting. American Psychosomatic Society, March 31, 1978.

Grinker RR: *Psychosomatic Concepts,* 3rd ed. Jason Aronson, 1973.

Holmes TH, Rahe RH: The social readjustment rating scale. *J Psychosom Res* 1967;**11**:213.

Kaufman IC, Rosenblum L: Effects of separation from mother on the emotional behavior of infant monkeys. *Ann NY Acad Sci* 1969;**159**:601.

Lipowski, ZJ: Psychosomatic medicine in the seventies: An overview. *Am J Psychiatry* 1977;**134**:233.

Locke SE: Stress adaptation and immunity. *Gen Hosp Psychiatry* 1982;**4**:49.

Locke SE et al: The influence of stress on the immune response: Preliminary report of the annual meeting. American Psychosomatic Society, March 31, 1978.

Mirsky IA: Physiologic, psychologic, and social determinants in the etiology of duodenal ulcer. *Am J Dig Dis* 1958;**3**:285.

Parkes CM, Brown RJ: Health after bereavement: A controlled study of young Boston widows and widowers. *Psychosom Med* 1972;**34**:449.

Rees WD, Lutkins SG: Mortality or bereavement. *Br Med J* 1967;**4**:13.

Reiser MF: Changing theoretical concepts in psychosomatic medicine. Pages 477–500 in: *American Handbook of Psychiatry,* 2nd ed. Vol 4. Basic Books, 1975.

Riley V: Mouse mammary tumors: Alteration of incidence as apparent function of stress. *Science* 1975;**189**:465.

Rogers MP, Dubey D, Reich P: The influence of the psyche and the brain on immunity and disease susceptibility: A critical review. *Psychosom Med* 1979;**41**:147.

Rose RM: Endocrine responses to stressful psychological events: Advances in psychoneuroendocrinology. *Psychiatr Clin North Am* 1980;**3**:251.

Selye H: *Stress Without Distress.* Lippincott, 1974.

Weiner H et al: Etiology of duodenal ulcer. *Psychosom Med* 1957;**19**:1.

Wolff HG, Wolf S, Hare CE (editors): *Life Stress and Bodily Disease.* Williams & Wilkins, 1950.

Stress & the Mechanisms of Defense

5

Mardi J. Horowitz, MD

Stress reactions provide a model for the integration of biologic, psychologic, and sociologic perspectives in medicine. The word "stress" itself implies an overloading of systems that will break down if sufficient strain is exerted on them. Increasing activity in the effort to cope with stress in a system that is about to fail may interfere with the function of other systems.

The biologic, psychologic, and social systems are interrelated, so that an overload in one will have an impact on the others. Physiologic responses to psychologic stressors include arousal of the nervous, musculoskeletal, cardiovascular, and endocrine systems. Psychologic responses include heightened activity of cognitive and emotional processes, especially those that assess the outside world in relation to inner perceptions of how things "should be." Social stress involves people impinging on one another via conflicting activities, plans, values, and priorities for the use of resources.

In each system, the overload may be handled by reactive processes. These are often called mechanisms of coping and defense.

PHYSICAL RESPONSES TO PSYCHOSOCIAL STRESSORS

A threat to the physical integrity of the body from the environment is a universal stressor. The body mobilizes to defend itself by fighting or fleeing. In most mammals, perceived threats produce increased cardiovascular activity to prepare the tissues for increased oxygen consumption, with constriction of peripheral blood vessels, reduction in digestive functions, dilatation of the pupils, increased sweat gland activity, and piloerection. Underlying these physiologic responses are metabolic changes based on hormone secretions, biochemical shifts, and alterations in the clotting mechanisms of the blood.

These changes result in fear, manifested by trembling, pounding pulse, sweaty palms, "butterflies" in the stomach, pharyngeal constriction, a staring countenance, and a dry mouth.

Mental Response

In civilized societies, the fear response is less common, because challenging circumstances are more often met by revised mental strategies and plans than by physical responses. As a result, the well-organized physical readiness for fight or flight deteriorates, and the body's response itself may become a psychologic stimulus to which the individual must then react.

Emotional Response

The fight or flight response is dramatic. A less dramatic psychophysiologic response is one that Selye (1976) calls the "general adaptation syndrome." It consists of 3 phases: an alarm reaction, followed by a stage of adaptation, and finally a stage of exhaustion, because the resources for arousal are not replenished as fast as they are expended. Passage through these phases of the general adaptation syndrome involves adjustments in the brain, the autonomic nervous system, and the endocrine system (especially the pituitary).

Endocrine Response

The initial phase of the general adaptation syndrome is characterized by increased secretion of pituitary and adrenocortical hormones that have both inflammatory and anti-inflammatory effects. With repeated presentation of the stressor over many days or weeks, there is enlargement of the adrenal cortex, atrophy of the thymus gland, and bleeding gastric ulcers due to the preponderance of anti-inflammatory hormones.

Physical Illnesses of Stress

Following the work of Claude Bernard, Walter Cannon, Hans Selye, and others on such biologic features as the fight or flight response, the disruption of internal equilibriums or homeostasis, and the general adaptation syndrome, investigations have continued on the relationship between serious life events, reactive human stress, and a variety of potentially related psychologic and physical illnesses. Holmes and Rahe (1967) showed an increase in morbidity from all types of illness in relation to life events such as loss of job or promotion in rank, death of a loved one, and divorce. (The works by Dohrenwend and Dohrenwend [1974], Goldberg and Breznitz [1982], and Gunderson and Rahe [1974] listed in the references examine the relationship between stressful life events and the onset of psychologic and physical illnesses.)

STRESSFUL LIFE EVENTS & STRESS-RELATED STATES OF MIND

Stressful events are defined here as those which are quite serious for the average person and which require some form of defense or adaptational behavior. Examples are deaths, separations, accidents, a diagnosis of serious illness, impending danger or pain (eg, a scheduled operation), and even vague symptoms that might be due to heart disease or cancer. For medical students, the first experience with a cadaver, the first operation, and the first patient death can also be quite stressful. A stressful event confronts the individual with new, disturbing information—eg, seeing oneself bleed, or being told by a physician that x-ray study has disclosed an area that might be cancer.

The word "stress" also denotes the state of the individual during and after stressful life events. To some extent, everyone receives, interprets, and reacts to stressful events in peculiar ways depending upon special meanings from developmental sources, special meanings and associations from current life experiences, and special ways that have become habitual and predictable at a personal or cultural level. A person in a state of stress typically shows a variation from some established pattern of behavior. For example, one who is usually only mildly tense and able to sleep without hypnotics may, following an automobile accident, exhibit a "stress reaction" characterized by anxiety, insomnia, and intrusive images. Patients told they have serious illnesses such as heart disease may have similar reactions.

The psychologic responses commonly seen after stressful events are described below.

PSYCHOLOGIC STRESS RESPONSE SYNDROMES

Fearful or Anxious States of Mind

The perception of fear and of being threatened, associated with a sense of vulnerability and preparations for responding, characterizes either a fearful or an anxious state of mind. The sensations are identical in many persons. Whether the state is called fear or anxiety depends upon the circumstances. If the response is justified by the situation, we say it is fear. If not, we call it anxiety. It may be "an anxiety attack" if it is sudden, or just an anxious mood if it emerges slowly and continues for some time.

Fear or anxiety may be a conditioned emotional response; may be based on unconscious mental processes; or may be based on conscious and rational assessment of stimuli.

Conditioned Emotional Responses

An important principle of learning theory is that conditioned associations can be established between ideas and feelings. A dangerous stimulus provokes fear. Later, there may be recurrent fear with a repetition of the stimulus. Because of stimulus generalization, there may be similar emotional responses to stimuli that are in some way similar but not rationally associated with a potential danger. A typical example is the child scratched by a cat. It is natural and adaptive for the child to be frightened when it sees the same cat the next day. It is a phobic response if that child 10 years later, after suitable experiences with harmless cats, is terrified of being near cats because the fear response has not been unlearned.

The equivalent term in psychodynamic psychology is **traumatic anxiety.** A dangerous situation appears to overwhelm the individual's coping capacity and may result in panic. Repetition of the situation—or anything symbolic of it—again generates fear even though the repetition is not itself dangerous. For example, after a severe automobile accident, one may feel dread when asked to ride in a car the next day.

Signal Anxiety

Because thought proceeds both consciously and unconsciously, one is able to experience internal threats as well as external ones. Signal anxiety is the process by which one "recognizes" the presence of some kind of threat. Recognition need not be conscious, since much information processing occurs without conscious awareness.

The following example illustrates anxiety signaling the presence of a conflict: A superior orders a worker to do something the latter perceives as wrong. The worker realizes at once that refusal or argument could lead to an unfavorable annual performance assessment. Speaking out thus creates a situation of personal danger (a withheld raise or promotion). Remaining silent is also dangerous if it violates the worker's self-image as an honest and courageous person. If the worker doesn't know what to do or feels that speaking out would be right but risky, the result might be signal anxiety—a red flag that says "watch out."

An affect, whether as a signal or as an expressive response, can be threatening. Anxiety, guilt feelings, shame, remorse, disgust, and sadness can be extremely painful. The mind can avoid routes of awareness that lead to such extremes of pain. The way of avoiding awareness, or of avoiding certain impulses to act, is often called a **defense.** The "forces" behind expressions (of sexual desire, for example) are called **impulses.** The counterforce is called a **defense,** and the complex is called an **impulse-defense configuration.** Some impulses are also called **drives,** or **instinctual drives.**

Anxiety is not the only signal affect, but it is emphasized in the psychiatric literature. Guilt, shame, disgust, pride, joy, and other feelings also have signal properties, since they feed back a "state of things" message into the psychic system. In a way, all signal affects are small samples of what may lie ahead if contemplated actions become actual ones. Guilt reactions to "bad thoughts" warn the individual about how he or

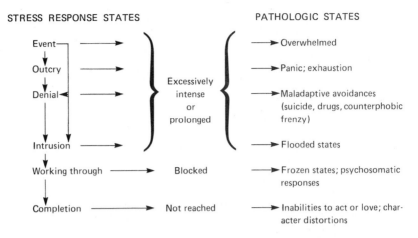

STRESS RESPONSE STATES   PATHOLOGIC STATES

Figure 5–1. Stress response states and psychologic intensification.

she might feel if contemplated behavior is not modified to conform with the demands of good conscience.

PHASES OF THE PSYCHOLOGIC RESPONSE TO STRESS

General stress response tendencies proceed in phases. The degree of stress and the time for anticipation before an external stress event will alter the nature of responses after the event. Individual history and character patterns will affect the order of entry into phases, the time in each phase, and the clinical manifestations within a phase. The usual pattern, in spite of these variations, is an initial response of outcry, followed by denial, then intrusion, then working through and, finally, completion. As shown in Fig 5–1, the initial outcry may not occur, and one may enter directly into the denial or intrusion phase. Responsiveness to stress is not abnormal; however, excessive re-

Table 5–1. Some signs and symptoms of denial phase of stress response syndromes.

Perception and attention	Daze. Selective inattention. Inability to appreciate significance of stimuli.
Consciousness	Amnesia (complete or partial). Nonexperience.
Ideational processing	Disavowal of meanings of stimuli. Loss of reality appropriateness of thought by use of disavowal. Inflexibility of organization of thought. Fantasies to counteract reality.
Emotional manifestations	Numbness.
Somatic manifestations	Tension-inhibition-type symptoms.
Actions	Frantic overactivity to withdrawal.

Table 5–2. Operational definitions of some important signs and symptoms of denial.

Avoidance of associational connections: Inhibiting expectable and fairly obvious personal or general continuations of meaning, implications, contingencies.

Numbness: A present subjective sense of not having feelings or of feeling "benumbed."

Reduced level of feeling responses to outer stimuli: Include flatness of expectable emotional responses, constriction.

Rigidly role-adherent or stereotyped: Carrying on by playing a part, socially automatic response sets.

Loss of reality appropriateness of thought by switching attitudes: Going from strong to weak, good to bad, active to passive, liking to disliking, or other changes to the degree that thought about any one meaning or implication is blunted and confused.

Unrealistic narrowing of attention, vagueness, or disavowal of stimuli: Include inflexibility of attention deployment, lack of centering on a focus, and avoidance of certain otherwise likely perceptual information. Include insensitivity to changes in body.

Inattention or daze: Include staring off into space, failure to determine significance of stimuli, clouding of alertness.

Inflexibility or constriction of thought: Failure to explore relatively obvious or likely avenues of meaning other than the given theme under contemplation.

Loss of train of thought: Temporary or micromomentary lapses in continuation of a communicative experience, or reports of similar inability to concentrate on a line of inner processing of information.

Loss of reality appropriateness of thought by sliding meanings: Distorting, minimizing, or exaggerating to the point where real meanings are clouded over.

Memory failure: Inability to recall expectable details or sequences of events; amnestic areas; inability to remember in usually expectable manner.

Loss of reality appropriateness of thought by use of disavowal: Saying to oneself or others that some meanings that are obvious or would be fairly obvious are not so.

Warding off trains of reality-oriented thought by use of fantasy: Excessive focus on what might have been, what could be, or imaginative stories as a way of not facing realistic consequences or implications.

Table 5–3. Some signs and symptoms of intrusion phase of stress response syndromes.

Perception and attention	Hypervigilance and startle reactions. Sleep and dream disturbance.
Consciousness	Intrusive-repetitive thoughts and behaviors (illusions, pseudohallucinations, nightmares, ruminations, and repetitions).
Ideational processing	Overgeneralization. Inability to concentrate on other topics; preoccupation. Confusion and disorganization.
Emotional manifestations	Emotional attacks or "pangs."
Somatic manifestations	Symptomatic sequelae of chronic "fight or flight" readiness (or of exhaustion).
Actions	Search for lost persons and situations; compulsive repetitions.

Table 5–4. Operational definitions of some important signs and symptoms of intrusion.

Pangs of emotion: A "spell" or episode or wave of feeling that has a quality of increasing and then decreasing rather than being a prevailing mood or subjective tone.

Rumination or preoccupation: Continuous conscious awareness about the event and associations to the event beyond that involved in ordinary thinking through of a problem or situation to a point of decision or completion. It has a sense of uncontrolled repetition to it.

Fear of losing bodily control, or hyperactivity in any bodily system: Include subjective sensations of urinating or defecating involuntarily; fears of being unable to control vocalization; arm movements; hiding; running: obvious somatic responses such as excessive sweating, diarrhea, tachycardia.

Intrusive ideas in word form: Appearance of sudden and unbidden thoughts.

Difficulty in dispelling ideas: Once an idea has come to mind, even if thinking about it were deliberate, the person cannot stop awareness of the idea or topic. Emotions and moods that cannot be stopped are included.

Hypervigilance: The person is excessively alert, overly scanning the surrounding environment, too aroused in the sense of perceptual search, tensely expectant, or more driven toward obtaining stimuli than normal.

Reenactments: Any behavior that repeats any aspect of the serious life event from minor ticlike movements and gestures to acting out in major movements and sequences. Include enactments of personal responses to the life event, whether or not they were part of the real action surrounding the event.

Bad dreams: Any dream with unpleasant subjective experience, not just the classic nightmare with anxious awakenings.

Intrusive thoughts or images while trying to sleep: See Intrusive ideas and Intrusive images.

Intrusive images: Unbidden sensations in any modality, including any hallucination or pseudohallucination that comes to mind in a nonvolitional manner. The emphasis here is on sensory quality, which, however similar to that of ordinary thought images, may be more intense and may occur as a sudden, unwanted entry into awareness.

Startle reactions: Flinching after noises, unusual orienting reactions, blanching or otherwise reacting to stimuli that usually do not warrant such responses.

Illusions: A misperception in which a person, object, or scene is misappraised as something else; for example, a bush is seen for a moment as a person, or a person is misrecognized as someone else.

Hallucinations or pseudohallucinations: An imaginary or fantasy-based emotional reaction as if it were real, whether or not the person intellectually thinks it is real. Include "felt presences" of others in the room. Smell, taste, touch, movement, auditory, and visual sensations, as well as "out of the body" experiences are included.

sponses may be pathologic, as shown below in Fig 5–1. Outcry is the almost reflex emotional response to the sudden impact of unexpected new information. The expression may take the form of weeping, panic, moaning, screaming, or fainting. For example, a woman told that her husband has just died in a mine disaster may sob in anguish. Clinically, it is useful to keep in mind certain characteristics of the phases of denial and intrusion.

Denial

Denial is the phase in which there is some combination of emotional numbing, ideational avoidance, and behavioral constriction. The signs and symptoms of denial are listed in Table 5–1 and defined in Table 5–2. Emotional numbing is a positive sensation; ie, the individual is often aware that he or she is not having a normal reaction to stimuli, as might occur in other circumstances. One may even have a sense of being insulated, in a cocoon, "not quite myself"—or that reality is "not real." Ideational avoidance may also be consciously recognized by the individual and obvious to companions. Ideational avoidance includes not having a train of thought directly implied by a stress or a stimulus.

Behavioral constriction is another pattern that may be subjectively experienced and, whether or not it is subjectively experienced, may be noted by observers. It consists of a focus of activities that is narrower than would otherwise be the case for the individual. It can reach extreme forms, as when a person faced with some personal tragedy repetitively cleans up a room rather than taking necessary adaptive action.

The widow in the mine disaster example might enter the denial phase after a day or so of feeling very emotional (in the outcry phase). Relatives might come to the house, both to help out and to attend funeral services. Since they are probably not as deeply affected by the loss, they may already have entered the intrusion phase (see below). They would have many thoughts about the deceased, cry episodically, and experience feelings of sadness and painful loss.

The widow, in contrast, might be numb, fearless, and even busily involved in planning for the immediate future and "entertaining" the relatives. If the relatives are charitable but ignorant of stress response tendencies, they may say that "she is very strong" and "doing very well." If they are less charitable, they may say that "she didn't really care for him."

Intrusion

Intrusion is the period of unbidden ideas and pangs of feeling and of direct or symbolic behavioral reenactments of the stressful event. Intrusions include nightmares about the stress event, recurrent unbidden images, and startle reactions to perceptual or associational reminders. This variety of intrusive signs and symptoms is listed in Table 5–3 and defined in Table 5–4.

The widow might enter an intrusion phase after a period of denial, but this phase might not begin until after the relatives have left. Weeks or months later, she might then begin to alternate between periods of denial and numbing and waves of searing grief, despair over the emptiness of her life, and even a hallucinatory sense of the "presence" of the dead husband.

Order of Phases

One may enter the sequence of phases (as in Fig 5–1) at any point and go through the phases in any order. For example, a couple in a car suddenly veers off a mountain road and descends a steep slope strewn with boulders and trees. The driver remains calm, skillfully maneuvering the car past obstructions, while the passenger thinks of the destructive possibilities, is terribly frightened, and faints. As the car comes to rest, the driver relaxes, thinks of the same shattering possibilities, and only then experiences fear. When remedial or evasive action is possible, alert perception, planning, and execution have first claim on cognition; fearsome images of possible injury are warded off. Later, recognition of possibly disastrous outcomes and emotional flooding may occur.

CONTENTS OF CONCERN

In the preceding sections, common signs and symptoms of stress were summarized. Here, we consider briefly the constellations of ideas and emotions that are aroused by serious life events.

Any event is appraised and assimilated in relation to the past as well as the current cognitive and emotional set of the person experiencing it, so that idiosyncratic responses result. But human beings are as similar as they are different, and certain conflicts between wishes and realities seem fairly universal after stress events such as accidental injury, illness, and loss. Clinical studies reveal the following themes as common, though often unconscious, problems for the working-through process initiated by stressful life events. Such thematic contents are manifested as intrusive ideas, as ideas that are warded off, and as ideas that are deliberately contemplated.

Fear of Repetition

Anticipation of repetition of stressful events conflicts with the wish to avoid unpleasantness. People fear actual repetitions yet cannot avoid thinking about stressful events. They also become fearful just thinking repeatedly about the event. For example, a person who has had one heart attack fears another. The individual may think often about the illness and reexperience the stress with anxiety and discomfort.

Shame Over Helplessness or Emptiness

Fantasies of omnipotence express the universal wish for control over one's life. The opposite is the fear of helplessness.

The delusion of omnipotence—having an invulnerable body or being able to prevent disease in others—is a universal hope and sometimes a deeply held belief. Failure to prevent accidents and the breakdown that may result from illness are perceived as weakness or loss of control. Patients with heart disease or back injuries, for example, may apologize profusely because they cannot perform heavy household chores, or they may do heavy work to avoid "shirking" or being "useless." After a fire has burned down the family home, parents may feel diminished in the eyes of their children because the family situation is not as comfortable as before. Magical thinking (that fantasy is reality) often extends the boundaries of such irrational attitudes, so that inability to master a stressful event is unconsciously regarded as equivalent to a loss of bowel or bladder control or a regression to infantile helplessness.

Rage at "the Source"

Rage is a natural response to frustration. As strange as it sounds, an important theme after stress events is anger at any symbolic figure who can, however irrationally, be considered responsible. A woman who cuts her finger while slicing meat may feel an impulse to say to a nearby child, "See what you made me do!" Asking, "Why did it happen?" after a stress event is usually associated with a need to find out who is to blame and who should be punished. Rage may come in conflict with a sense of social morality. A common example is rage at a person who has fallen ill, a feeling that conflicts with the recognition that it is not the sick person's fault and that compassion and not blame is the appropriate emotional response.

Guilt or Shame Over Aggressive Impulses

When violence is part of the stressful event, this in itself seems to stimulate internal aggressiveness. Aggression conflicts with a sense of conscience and leads to feelings of guilt or shame. Negative feelings toward a person who has died and consequent reactive guilt or shame are common manifestations of this type of conflict.

Another impulse that may evoke guilt feelings or shame is the urgent need to look at a potential threat. This virtually instinctive impulse would seem to be conflict-free, but that is not the case when other persons are victims. For example, there may be severe injury to others in an accident. Because social convention and natural revulsion dictate looking away from or covering up the bodies, staring at the bodies is unwarranted aggression, and having done so may lead to subsequent feelings of anxiety and guilt. Such self-accusation is overly harsh. Individuals feel a strong need to examine potential threats as an attempt to master their fear and avoid the discomfort associated with the fearful state.

Fear of Aggressiveness

Conflict also occurs between destructive fantasies and the wish to remain in control. For example, a soldier traumatized by repeated combat experiences may fear that on return to civilian life he will physically attack people who frustrate him only slightly.

Survivor Guilt

When others have been injured or killed, one is relieved to realize that he or she has been spared. At the level of magical thinking, the irrational belief may emerge that destiny chooses one possible victim and spares another, as if to placate primitive gods, and that if one has avoided serious injury it is at the expense of those not spared. The wish to be a survivor thus leads to self-castigation for selfishness.

Fear of Identification or Merger with Victims

An emotion related to survivor guilt is the fear of not being separate from the victim. At a primitive level of thinking, persons are not conceptualized as separate. If something has hurt another, there is a primitive fear that it may hurt oneself. This may set in motion a train of thought assuming the self as victim, even when this conflicts with reality.

Sadness in Relation to Loss

Any painful stressful event has an element of loss and conflicts with the universal wish for permanence, safety, and satisfaction. The loss may be another person, an external resource, or an aspect of the self. Naturally, some losses are more symbolic than real, but they are no less important. A person who has been laid off from work because a plant has closed may suffer a loss of self-esteem from deprivation of the work role even though economic forces and not personal inadequacy or misbehavior are responsible.

The common forms and contents of psychologic reactions to stress have been summarized above. One should learn to look for these patterns in patients who have experienced serious stressful events or have received bad news about their health status. It is especially important to know the signs and symptoms of the denial and intrusion phases and to realize how pervasive the stage of denial can be. The physician often has to repeat information at various times and in various doses before it is truly "heard."

As for intrusive experiences, such as unwelcome fantasy images related to the stressful event, it is helpful to ask directly about such experiences, since patients often do not report such matters spontaneously. The common concerns of patients are often surprising, because some of them seem "irrational." Physicians are most often surprised by the angry response of some patients and make the mistake of being hurt by it rather than understanding it as a stress response and main-

taining rapport with patients as they attempt to master the stressful situation.

COPING & DEFENSE

Following serious life events or threats, emotional excitation increases, and the individual may feel disorganized or out of control. To avoid excessively painful or helpless states of mind, various self-regulatory processes are called into service. Coping mechanisms may be conscious or unconscious.

The ideal coping mechanism is to solve the problem and thus survive the threat, but the operational goal is often to maintain a sense of equilibrium without being flooded with unwanted levels of emotion.

Operations aimed at achieving coping or defensive goals are motivated by anticipation of the physical or emotional pain that will occur if nothing is done. This itself is a thought process that may proceed unconsciously, ie, the anticipation of consequences.

Once control mechanisms are set in motion, they have their own consequences. Stopping thought to reduce emotion may offer temporary relief but may also interfere with effective planning. Denial may lead a patient to postpone treatment; eg, the patient who denies the presence of gangrene may refuse to authorize an amputation that would increase the chances for survival.

Defense, like anxiety, is a broad, multidimensional term. A defense is a process used to respond to a dangerous or threatening situation. Defenses are mechanisms for avoidance of anxiety (primary gain), and anxiety is a motive for the use of defenses. Many defenses are ways of avoiding awareness of inner urges, ideas, and feelings. These specific methods for warding off mental experience are called defense mechanisms. The person remains unaware both of what is warded off and of the defense mechanism that accomplishes the maneuver.

When defenses alone are insufficient to prevent anxiety, symptoms may occur. The psychologic symptom is sometimes a compromise between the warded-off urges and the defensive process. The symptoms may also provide secondary gain, as through suffering (relieving guilt), attention getting, or avoidance of onerous responsibilities.

COMMON DEFENSE MECHANISMS

Denial

The most frequently encountered defense in general medical practice is denial: avoidance of awareness of some painful reality. It is accomplished by withholding conscious understanding of the meaning and implications of what is perceived—especially by refusing to take in the extended significance of new information. Magical thinking ("Pay no attention and it will go away") also plays a powerful role in denial. Within limits, denial is a normal process used to slow down the response to bad news. Persons with myocardial infarctions treated in coronary care units persist in telling themselves and others that their pain was due to "indigestion." Physicians may ignore the early warning signs of cancer in themselves on the grounds that "it means nothing." While denial is considered a "normal" defense, since it may allow a graded acceptance of bad news, it is maladaptive if it interferes with rational action.

Repression & Suppression

Repression consists of withholding from conscious awareness an idea or feeling. Conscious expulsion of thoughts from the mind is called suppression. Repression differs from suppression in that it is an involuntary rather than a voluntary process. It may operate to exclude from awareness what was once experienced as inability to remember an important but traumatic event (eg, amnesia) or to curb ideas and feelings that have not yet reached consciousness but would emerge were it not for the defensive process. For example, one may repress the awareness of erotic arousal by an inappropriate love object or may repress hatred for someone he or she "ought to love."

Displacement

In displacement, the avoided ideas and feelings are transferred to some other person, situation, or object. For example, hypochondriac patients may displace worry and ward off a concern that their minds are failing and will focus concern instead on a body part.

Reaction Formation

In reaction formation, a warded-off idea or feeling is replaced by an unconsciously derived but consciously felt emphasis on its opposite. For example, an older boy is jealous of a baby brother and has a fantasy that if the baby were to die, he would again be the center of his parents' attention. Having such a fantasy, he realizes, is "bad," because he has been "ordered" to love the baby. Reaction formation consists of replacing the wish to be rid of the brother with an exaggerated concern for the baby's welfare. If the defense works adaptively, he cares for his brother even though he wishes, occasionally, for the restoration of his only-child status. If the conflict is intense, the reaction formation may lead to symptoms. For instance, such a boy might have a compulsion to check up on the baby to make sure it is all right, not suffocated, or kidnapped.

Projection

In projection, a warded-off impulse or idea is attributed to the external world. For example, people who struggle with their own hatred may develop a delusion that others are out to get them. This both gives them an acceptable rationale for hating and allows them to avoid recognition of their own destructive impulses.

Regression

Regression consists of turning back the maturational clock and going back to earlier modes of dealing with the world. Some persons confronted with the stress and environmental cues of hospitalization become, for example, "regressively" childlike in terms of demands, demeanor, and dependence on others.

Turning Against the Self

In this defense, an inappropriate impulse directed outward is redirected at the self. The guilt that would follow from aggression against an object of hatred can be avoided by hurting oneself (as by self-mutilation).

Isolation

The process of isolation consists of splitting of ideas and feelings, as in having the obsessive idea or image of "killing" without feeling anger or hostility toward the object. This defense leads to flatness of affect or seeming indifference.

Undoing

Undoing expresses both the impulse and its opposite, as in being very domineering one minute and then offering obsequiously to defer to another. In rapid repetition, undoing may lead to indecisiveness.

Rationalization

Rationalization consists of proclaiming logical reasons for actions actually performed for other reasons, usually to avoid stress or self-blame. Rationalization is also used to justify avoiding unpleasant duties.

Sublimation

Sublimation is the process whereby one replaces an unacceptable wish with a course of action that is similar to the wish but does not conflict with one's value system. For example, aggressive wishes may be sublimated into working hard to solve social problems.

Acting Out

Acting out consists of engaging in activities in a different arena from the one in which the basic impulses came into conflict with values. In acting out, feelings are displaced from one arena to another. A patient angry with the doctor may, for example, pick a fight with someone else but still hope the fight will nonetheless affect the physician.

COPING

The term "coping" usually suggests that the subject is reacting as adaptively as possible to a difficult situation. The term "defense" sometimes suggests a maladaptive type of response. Here, however, no clear distinction is made between coping and defense mechanisms; they are regarded as different aspects of essentially the same processes. Defense often occurs at an unconscious level of information processing and adds components to consciously mediated choices of action in response to threats.

Defensive Denial

It is always important to assess whether a process of psychologic defense or strategy for coping is adaptive or maladaptive. Denial can be adaptive when it prevents one from being overwhelmed with panic; it can be maladaptive in that it tends to interfere with realistic planning. To make matters more complex, the average person processes information at various levels of awareness and in the context of a variety of belief systems. Take as an example a man who has had a heart attack and is being cared for in the hospital. He may be aware of the risk to his life and at the same time behave as if the illness were only a minor one. He may show different degrees of awareness of his health status at different times. When the chief resident comes by on ward rounds, the patient may converse with the doctor as if he fully understands his present situation. Moments later, in the presence of a nurse, he may insist on getting out of bed, loudly asserting that he is not seriously ill. A conversation with the doctor on Tuesday may show a realistic appreciation of the changes in life-style that will be necessary after discharge. On Wednesday the patient may still, at some level, deny the implications of his illness. The denial can be said to be adaptive in reducing fear and allowing pacing of decisions, helping the patient to feel less troubled; but postponing awareness of what must be faced may also lead to hazardous choices of action.

Coping Strategies

Strategies for coping with threats involve choices about what to think about and what to do.

A. Changing the Mental Focus: For example, one common reaction to serious news is to think intensively about it—another is to avoid thinking about it. By switching between "thinking about it" and "not thinking about it," people can adjust the input of information and in that way modulate their emotional responses. Relatives of a patient undergoing major surgery must wait in the hospital to learn the outcome. During this time they may contemplate a successful result as well as the possibility of death. Thinking about the impending surgery and the possibility of death will cause fear and anxiety. Talking, reading, or thinking about other topics will temporarily take their minds off the threatening situation and restore emotional stability. Another type of coping is to restrict or extend the interval of time that must be dealt with. For example, a patient facing a procedure such as bronchoscopy may focus on an extremely short interval, such as 2 or 3 seconds, or may contemplate the present moment in terms of long stretches of time so that it pales in significance. Another common coping or defensive strategy is to switch back and forth between reality and fantasy. For example, after the death of a loved one, the survivor may cope with grief by musing on happy memories of the relationship or by fantasizing some future reunion. Another way of coping would be to think realistically about all of the changes that must now take place.

B. Altering Modalities of Thought: Another coping strategy involves using different modalities of thought. A person who usually thinks in words may, in very stressful situations, use more visual imagery. For example, a person in the hospital unable to eat and maintained with intravenous fluids may placate the sensation of hunger by imagining the sight and odors of a favorite meal. At the other extreme, a person who has been in an automobile accident and has seen the carnage may attempt to avoid all mental images and to process the accident only in verbal terms.

C. Shifting Roles: Another common coping strategy is to change one's activity status, as in changing states of consciousness. One may become more aroused, which can be maladaptive if it leads to hypervigilance, or may escape into long periods of sleep or a state of reduced activity. Shifts in roles of oneself and others also provide opportunities for both coping behavior and defensive behavior. A hospitalized patient lying in bed and being attended in various ways has a tendency to regress. This is not necessarily maladaptive, although regression is one mechanism of defense. The patient in this example returns to a state in which it is all right to depend on others for feeding, bathing, and toilet care. Group attachments and opportunities for increased interpersonal relationships also help one cope with stress. One advantage of having several patients in the same room is that they form bonds that help all of them cope with their situations.

People seem to have some control over which of several available self-images is dominant at a given moment. Some persons under the stress of illness become more aloof and withdrawn instead of forming increasing attachments to others. This may be their way of focusing energy on the internal situation in order to deal with it. Others assume greater than usual competency, behaving more courageously, wisely, or altruistically than before.

D. Seeking New or Additional Information: This is an important way of coping with a stressful event. The physician gives the patient expert advice and information on topics the patient is unfamiliar with. It is the physician's responsibility to interpret this information and help the patient appraise its implications. Other members of the health team often are involved in helping the patient practice new behavior, just as a physical therapist establishes a supportive relationship with a patient learning to walk on crutches or learning to use a prosthesis.

The above are examples of common coping strategies. The achievement of humor and wisdom, the use of philosophic or religious perspectives during stressful situations, and the creation of new identities and capacities are creative methods of coping and achieving personal growth in the face of crisis.

Different individuals favor different defenses and coping strategies. The physician who provides help through a period of illness will understand the patient's habitual styles of coping and interact appropriately with that patient.

Helping a patient endure a period of stress involves activities or interventions at the biologic, psychologic, and social levels. At the biologic level, support to various strained organ systems is indicated in addition to whatever can be done to combat pathogenic influences. At the psychologic level, an understanding of the stress response syndrome itself is useful to the person experiencing it and to that person's immediate caretakers, whether they are members of the health team or of the family. Social activities to increase support may also be useful. Counteracting feelings of helplessness by pointing out what companions or relatives can realistically do for a suffering person will often provide the relationship so necessary to maintaining a sense of well-being.

REFERENCES

Cannon WB: *The Wisdom of the Body*. Norton, 1939.

Dohrenwend BS, Dohrenwend BP (editors): *Stressful Life Events: Their Nature and Effects*. Wiley, 1974.

Freud A: *The Ego and the Mechanisms of Defense*. Internat Univ Press, 1946.

Goldberg L, Breznitz S: *Handbook of Stress*. Free Press, 1982.

Gunderson E, Rahe RH (editors): *Life Stress and Illness*. Thomas, 1974.

Holmes TH, Rahe RH: The social readjustment rating scale. *J Psychosom Res* 1967;**11:**213.

Horowitz MJ: *Stress Response Syndrome,* 2nd ed. Jason Aronson, 1986.

Janis IL, Mann L: *Decision Making*. Free Press, 1977.

McLaughlin P: *The Mechanisms of Defense*. Appleton-Century-Crofts, 1969.

Selye HA: *Stress in Health and Disease*. Butterworth, 1976.

Selye HA (editor): *Selye's Guide to Stress Research*. Vol 1. Van Nostrand Reinhold, 1980.

White R, Oviliand RM: *Elements of Psychopathology: The Mechanisms of Defense*. Grune & Stratton, 1975.

Child & Adolescent Development

Aubrey W. Metcalf, MD

CONCEPTS OF CHILD DEVELOPMENT

An understanding of the processes of growth and development has become indispensable for the study of human biology and behavior; the field is now a basic science in all clinical curricula. Advances in knowledge during the last 2 centuries have revealed a striking orderliness and continuity in the immensely complicated, mysterious, and beautiful transformations that occur from conception to old age. These advances provide clues to how we come to be the way we are. Much detailed study has yet to be done, but the main mechanisms of biologic development are well understood in animals and young humans, and their links to behavioral development are rapidly being clarified. As research on personality in later life accumulates, it becomes apparent that changing phases and developmental tasks are characteristic not only of the early years but of the entire life cycle. For the clinician, an understanding of this lawfulness of development serves as a framework within which each individual patient can be assessed and understood.

Originally, the scientific study of humans, while thought of as describing a whole individual, was mostly focused on how the various subsystems (the individual organ complexes) work within any one person. In the late 19th century, academic psychologists began to explore such isolated human capacities as sensory discrimination, consciousness, and intelligence. Early in the 20th century, practitioners of the new science of psychoanalysis evolved a theory of the structure of the mind and called its subsystems id, ego, and superego. More recently, human behavioral development has been viewed from the standpoint of supersystems: the mother-infant dyad, the conjugal relationship, the family, and larger social groups.

THE HISTORY OF INQUIRY INTO GROWTH & DEVELOPMENT

Phylogeny & Ontogeny

Phylogeny is the study of the successive forms of life that have evolved on the earth. Although humans

originally saw themselves as the center and purpose of creation, the painful reappraisal started by Wallace, Darwin, and Huxley 130 years ago has assessed the place of humankind in nature more modestly but more correctly, and we now begin our study of human beings with what we know about the ascent of phyla and the biology and behavior of other living things. Ethologists and anthropologists have described many homologies between human beings and animals in form, physiology, and even feelings. In common with other primates, humans are social, curious, aggressive, sensual, and intelligent beings. These similarities are not surprising in view of what we have learned about speciation. We assume that many of the behaviors that evolved to ensure the survival of young mammals for 60 million years are directly carried over into human life—especially the first few months and years of it. This mammalian heritage appears to control development, with decreasing influence, throughout the life cycle.

Ontogeny is the study of the succession of forms each individual passes through in a lifetime. Even before the connection between animals and humans was established, and quite apart from all speculation about the ascent of phyla, there was conjecture about the mechanism of physical development in any one individual. The ancients were aware of the continuous and progressive changes in the organism from earliest life through maturity, but their concept was not "developmental" as the word is used today. Their theory of embryology was founded on the homunculus theory of "preformationism," first proposed by a Greek philosopher in the fifth century BC. This was a linear model of development—what we now call growth, ie, increase in the number and size of cells (technically, hyperplasia and hypertrophy). Since this notion did no violence to the myths of the time or to the later Judeo-Christian doctrine of divine creation, it was unchallenged for more than 2000 years until microscopic study revealed that older embryos had organs and tissues not present in younger ones of the same species. This showed that development was not simple linear enlargement but a progression through successive stages. The theory of "predeterminism" was invoked to explain the origin of these changes in physical form; such changes constituted a puzzle that persisted unsolved until the development of the scientific method and specialized experimental techniques in modern times.

Physical Epigenesis

As microscopes improved and experimental embryology replaced predeterminism, the modern theory of epigenesis arose (epigenetic = after genes). This theory holds that the genes cause early formation of certain cells that act as organizers of surrounding undifferentiated cells, inducing them to form the various organs. Experiments performed during embryogenesis revealed that many of these organizers function according to a biologic timetable. In such systems, there is a critical stage before or after which contiguous cells do not change in form under the influence of the organizer cells. Either they receive proper stimulation from the organizer and develop normally, or they do not develop their proper organ system at all. The timetables for physical development in the growing embryo are more or less fixed genomically* in most species and are well along toward completion by the time of birth. After birth, further development depends increasingly on the environment, with experience and practice assuming a larger role the higher the organism is on the phylogenetic scale.

Behavioral Epigenesis

In behavioral epigenesis, the genes are responsible for certain primitive reflex responses that in turn act as organizers of further responses. These combinations (stimulus plus response) alter the organism in specific ways in accordance with natural laws. As a result, the organism learns and develops different behaviors.

For some functions, there are **critical periods** in time after which behavioral differentiation is incomplete or impossible. For example, cats blindfolded from birth lose the ability to see if their eyes are not uncovered before the end of the critical period. These timetables are more or less fixed genomically, depending on the species and the age of the organism.

THE CAUSES OF DEVELOPMENT: "INSTINCTS" & "LEARNING"

The Development of Individuals: Ontogeny

When we consider the forces that drive individual development, it is obvious that ontogeny does not rely entirely on chance conditioning. Examples are numerous of animals acting in ways they have had no opportunity to learn. We ordinarily call such behavior instinctive (unlearned) and conclude that it represents some internal system fixed by inheritance.

If we follow the analogy of the ascent of phyla, we might imagine that the needs and frustrations of the individual organism force (cause) the next step in maturation, just as we see the exigencies of the environ-

ment shaping new species through mutation and natural selection. A version of this has appeared in theories that try to explain behavior as simply stimulus-response learning or efforts to avoid pain and maximize pleasure. But a closer look reveals that the need for food, drink, and protection from predators is alone insufficient for development. For both the one-celled animal and the infant human, the *causes* of individual development are those stimuli to which the young organism is sensitive at each level of its developmental cycle.† The natural environment of plankton is water, and they divide faster in warmer water. The natural element of infant humans is the **caregiving situation** within which development and learning occur, so long as the experiences are not too discrepant from the environment of evolutionary adaptedness. The infant's delight at seeing the mother is not at first connected to the conscious experience of needing her physical or nutritional support but a response to specific stimuli for which the infant is primed. This appears to be an instinctive mechanism for achieving attachment in infants and caregivers.

Imprinting & Social Bonding

The concept of imprinting (*"Prägung"*) was popularized by Konrad Lorenz (1957), who presented himself to newly hatched goslings before they had an opportunity to experience nurturing by their own mother and found that the newly hatched birds perceived him—but not other geese—as a member of their species. Scott (1963) showed that there was a sensitive period in the life of puppies in reference to fear responses. So long as a puppy was no older than 5 weeks when first exposed to a human, it approached at once. If over 7 weeks elapsed before first exposure to humans, the puppies kept away for several days. If not exposed until 15 weeks of age, the animal kept away permanently unless special training was provided. Concepts such as "imprinting" and "sensitive periods" of learning have demonstrated how intrinsic inclinations and epigenetic timetables may limit the extent to which many species can adapt to changes in the environment. Although of primary importance for some animals, their presence in humans is not convincing, with the striking exception of the attachment behaviors of the first year of life. This topic is discussed in the next section of this chapter.

Two important discoveries derive from these studies. First, behavioral development after birth, especially in primates, does not proceed spontaneously or simply as the result of genomically fixed unfoldings but only through experience in the "environment of evolutionary adaptedness." Second, the great importance of social bonding for the normality of subse-

---

*The word "genomic" is used here to refer to the direct action of genes—in contrast to the term "genetic," which is used more broadly to refer to the original or developmental source of a behavior or symptom.

†For every organism, there is an environment within which its physiologic and behavioral systems operate best at any one point in its ontogeny. This has been given the somewhat cumbersome name "environment of evolutionary adaptedness" by John Bowlby (1983).

quent development has been clarified. The young must have the expectable interactions with their parents and peers. Attachment behaviors are thus formed by social experience, and without such experience animals are unable to subsist in the wild and in some cases unable to mate and rear young. The higher the species on the phylogenetic scale, the more severe the impairment if infants are isolated. What is true of animals is also true of human infants, as shown many times by unfortunate examples of abandonment or abuse.

Human Behavior: Instinctual & Noninstinctual

"Behavior" in the human fetus begins with characteristic simple reflex responses to sensory input. After birth, and within the environment of evolutionary adaptedness, these constitutional tendencies extend to form the first-step behaviors of normal development— in newborns, eye and head orientation, rooting, sucking, grasping, and swallowing. First-step success clears the way for the next one, and so it goes. The new behaviors become the epigenetic substrates for the next step in development. The infant's actions may themselves evoke the environmental response necessary for a succeeding developmental step. The baby's smile, for example, provokes and sustains the positive social responses the infant needs to develop normally.

Behavioral maldevelopment may of course result from heritable defects, noxious intrauterine influences, maternal illnesses, or birth trauma; but the chief cause of behavior disorders with onset in early infancy is interference with the interpersonal processes necessary for normal behavior. Social interaction is as essential as physical development in the making of an intact human individual. (Rutter has recently reviewed the role of life experience in development.)

In higher animals of the class Mammalia, instinctive behavior is not ready at birth as it is in insects. What is inherited is the *potential* for developing certain sorts of behavior systems, given the anticipated experiences of that species in its environment of evolutionary adaptedness. This capacity permits greater individual adaptability than other animals possess, but it also imposes a risk of distorted or destructive behavior if the environment during development and the environment to which the species is adapted are vastly different. The current concern with the importance to bonding of interaction between mother and infant immediately after birth reflects awareness that there may be limits to the capacity of human infants to adapt to variations in the caregiving environment. Social experiences of humans in their natural environment are linked in infancy with nurturing by the caregivers. Indeed, for humans, the social behaviors are now held to be more important than the more "primary" motivators of behavior such as pain, hunger, or response to physical danger. From the first bond with the caregiver, interpersonal relationships are major factors in the growth of personality, and disturbed or inadequate relationships underlie much unhappiness and mental illness in humans.

THE DEVELOPMENTAL PERSPECTIVE

The usefulness of these epigenetic theories in answering difficult questions about human conduct has convinced most students of normal and abnormal behavior that to understand, treat, and predict the outcome of any individual, the stage of development must be known. Almost all modern theories of personality and psychopathology thus have what could be called a developmental perspective, whose main characteristics have been well described by Breger (1974): (1) The progression of behavioral maturation is from the less complex to the more complex; (2) what emerges in the immediate (and even the distant) future is relatively dependent upon what has already arisen; and (3) above all, the effect of any experience will often depend upon the stage at which it occurs in the development of the individual.

The third characteristic is of the greatest importance in our understanding of the ontogeny of personality and mental function. Environmental stresses may lead to very different results in a growing child depending upon the child's stage of development. Imagine the consequences for a daughter of her mother's death if the daughter is a 4-month-old baby, a 4-year-old child, or a 40-year-old adult. The birth of a sibling has different consequences for a 1-year-old or 6-year-old than for a 2-year-old. Understanding the normal progression of the individual's ability to cope with and understand the environment helps the clinician differentiate pathologic social maturation from normal variations and will help the therapist decide what treatment is likely to be beneficial.

The most important aspect for medical practice of any theory of psychology or psychopathology is its usefulness in the prediction of future development and in suggesting means of altering the course of existing maldevelopment in the direction of health. Unfortunately, no single theory is adequate to explain the diversity of human individuals and cultures, although neurophysiologic, behavioral, and ethologic research is beginning to merge with more sophisticated observations of human feelings and behavior.

It should be emphasized that most research in developmental psychology has been done within narrow cultural parameters—namely, with middle-class white subjects. This does not necessarily invalidate the findings for other cultural groups, but caution should be used in the application of these findings. The pertinence of generalizations varies according to the age of the subject. The behavior of unborn and newly born infants is affected very little by culture beyond the influence of the physical environment. Infant humans are strikingly similar to each other across all societies and are, for that matter, very similar to other young primates when it comes to behaviors observed in the first few weeks and months of life. Yet from the middle of the first year onward the young of differing cultural groups become so increasingly like that group and different from other groups that more and more elaborate explanations are required to account for any deviations from behavior considered normal for that group. It remains to be seen to what extent theories of psychology and psychopathology in Western middle-class culture will apply to others.

Although the theories of development described here and in Chapters 3 and 7 are most familiar to health professionals, not all theories of learning are based on developmental concepts, and much of what we know about how we learn has been without reference to the learner's age or stage of development. Classic conditioning research led to the discovery of operant, or instrumental, learning, in which behavior is modified by positive or negative reinforcement at any age. Skinner (1953) and Sears and coworkers (1957) applied these learning theories to the study of how children change during development, and Bandura and Walters (1963) demonstrated how offering models for observation is an effective way of teaching new behavior even without reinforcement. There need be no conflict among different theories, because learning can occur by multiple mechanisms.

Development and learning can be profitably viewed as sequential or progressive from one stage to the next, with the types of learning that are dominant in each stage being somewhat different from those that are dominant in other stages. In all stages, the learner's role is usually not simply passive but quite active.

THEORIES OF DEVELOPMENT

A number of theories of human development are derived from clinical experience and experiment. Many of them contribute useful perspectives, and several aspire to the status of general theories of behavior. The 2 best-known systems used by clinicians today are those derived from classic psychoanalysis and Piagetian developmental psychology. The former has been criticized as being excessively intrapsychic and unyielding to systematic validation; the latter because it takes no account of emotions or the biologic mechanisms of development. Both are closed systems and products of Western culture, but they have long histories of clinical usefulness and serve as appropriate instruments for further research and validation in other cultures. Recently, general systems theory and research in animal ethology have provided tools that are improving and expanding the study of infancy and early childhood.

Psychoanalytic theories of development, classic and Eriksonian, are introduced in Chapter 3. Erikson's view of the life cycle will be further elaborated in Chapter 7. Two other influential theories are discussed here because of their special relevance to child development. These are Piaget's theory of cognitive development and Bowlby's attachment theory.

JEAN PIAGET
(1896–1980)

Piaget is the best-known child psychologist in the world, and his theory of cognitive development has been the most influential. His hypotheses have formed the basis of an entire discipline (he called it "genetic epistemology") and have provided a formal philosophic stimulus for clinical research in a number of other fields in psychology. For Piaget, the *intellectual* functions are the core of personality formation and serve to coordinate development in all spheres. He did not offer a theory of development of emotional life in childhood, though he acknowledged its importance.

Piaget was the first modern theorist to emphasize that the infant is active from the beginning in exploring the world and striving for a more gratifying mastery of it. The process is genomically inherited and proceeds in all children through a series of fixed developmental phases and subphases. It is epigenetic in that mastery of each phase is dependent on success in mastering the elements of the preceding one and forms the basis for future refinement.

Piaget holds that there are 2 fundamental processes by which the organism adapts: assimilation and accommodation. **Assimilation** is the absorption ("taking in") of an experience as a whole, insofar as the individual understands it. It consists of fitting an experience into an existing cognitive structure. An analogy is assimilation of food by the digestive tract, which is limited by the extent to which the organism is able to digest it. **Accommodation** is the process of changing the existing cognitive structure in order to adjust to new experiences. The digestive tract of a species may evolve so that individuals of the species can digest new foods, or a theory may be modified to explain contradictory data. Learning proceeds by assimilating new perceptions in terms of the existing cognitive capacity and refinement of the cognitive structure to accommodate new perceptions.

Piaget describes 4 stages of development of cognition (Table 6–1): the **sensorimotor stage** and **stage of preoperational thought,** in early childhood; the **stage of concrete operations,** roughly the grammar school years; and the **stage of formal operations,** the teenage years. Some children reach and master the oncoming stage a bit sooner than others, but this is not a function of intelligence. Very intelligent children in the preoperational stage are unable to perform ordinary tasks of the concrete stage even though they may be able to read, write, and speak far in advance of their peers. Each stage reinterprets previous understanding and experience according to new ways of thinking and organizing information.

Sensorimotor Stage
(Age 0–16/24 Months)

During the sensorimotor stage, the biologic apparatus determines the experience of the child. The senses receive stimuli, and the motor apparatus responds in a stereotyped or reflex way: stimulus in, response out.

Table 6–1. Summary of human development from multiple perspectives.

	DEVELOPMENTAL LANDMARKS Performance Levels (A. Gesell, etc)	PSYCHODYNAMIC DEVELOPMENT			INTELLECTUAL DEVELOPMENT Cognitive Stages (J. Piaget)
		PSYCHOSEXUAL STAGES (S. FREUD) Ego Defense Mechanisms (G. Vaillant)	PSYCHOSEXUAL STAGES Psychosocial Modes Psychologic Tasks and VALUES (E. Erikson)	ATTACHMENT THEORY (J. BOWLBY) Psychologic Characteristics (A. Freud)	
INFANCY					
Birth	Reflex smile/grimace. Develops eye/head control.	ORAL _"Narcissistic" defenses_ Projection (delusional in older persons) Denial (psychotic in older persons) Distortion	ORAL-RESPIRATORY-SENSORY-KINESTHETIC Incorporative mode _Trust versus mistrust_ HOPE		SENSORIMOTOR STAGE I. Reflex (0–2 months)
2 mo	Social smile. 180-degree visual pursuit.			1. PREATTACHMENT: (0 TO 8–10 WEEKS) Orientation to signals without discrimination of a figure	II. Primary circular reaction (2–6 months)
3 mo	Reaches for objects; rolls over.			II. ATTACHMENT-IN-THE-MAKING: (8–10 WEEKS TO 6 MONTHS) Orientation and signals directed toward one (or more) discriminated figures	III. Secondary circular reaction (2–8 months)
6 mo	Transfers objects; raking grasp.				IV. Secondary schemes (8–12 months)
9 mo	Sits up well; purposeful release; prehension deft; cruises at rail.			III. CLEAR-CUT ATTACHMENT: (6 MONTHS TO END OF LIFE) Maintenance of proximity to a discriminated figure by means of local motion as signals	V. Tertiary circular reaction (12–16 months)
1 yr	Walks unassisted; uses 3–4 words; builds towers of 2 cubes.	ANAL _"Immature" defenses_ Projection Schizoid fantasy Hypochondriasis Passive-aggressive behavior Acting out	ANAL-URETHRAL-MUSCULAR Retentive-eliminative mode _Autonomy versus shame and doubt_ WILL		VI. Invention of new means through mental combinations (16 months on)
18 mo	Scribbles with crayon; uses 10–20 words; builds towers of 5–6 cubes; names a few pictures.			_Exuberant exploration_ _Realizes omnipotence is limited, becomes conservative_ Oppositional behavior Messiness	
2 yr	Runs and falls; uses 3-word sentences; names several body parts; uses appropriate personal pronouns.			Parallel play Pleasure in looking and being looked at	
PRESCHOOL					
3 yr	Rides tricycle; copies a circle; can stand on one foot; talks of self and others.	PHALLIC/INFANTILE GENITAL _"Neurotic" defenses_ Intellectualization Repression Displacement Reaction formation Dissociation	GENITAL/OEDIPAL Intrusive-inclusive mode _Initiative versus guilt_ PURPOSE	IV. GOAL-CORRECTED PARTNERSHIP: Disgust Orderliness possible Fantasy play Masturbation begins Curiosity heightened	STAGE OF PREOPERATIONAL THOUGHT (PRELOGICAL) (1) Development of symbolic functions (2) Differentiation between signs and symbols (3) Use of language (4) Observational learning, representation versus direct action
4 yr	Buttons clothes; throws ball overhand; copies square; draws a person; says ABCs.			Cooperative play Imaginary companion Task perseverance Rivalry with parent of same sex Problem solving Games with rules begin	(5) Egocentrism (6) Thinking by intuition

SCHOOL AGE / ADOLESCENCE	Defenses	Psychosocial / Psychosexual	Latency / Adolescence	Cognitive
SCHOOL AGE				**STAGE OF CONCRETE OPERATIONS**
5 yr — Copies triangle and diamond; ties knots in string; complete toilet self-help.	**LATENCY** — *Continues "neurotic" defenses (see Preschool) and begins "mature" defenses (see Adolescence)*	**PSYCHOSEXUAL MORATORIUM** — *Industry versus inferiority* — SKILL	**LATENCY** — *Hobbies / Ritualistic play / Rational attitudes about foods / Enjoys friends and "best friends" / Invests self in teachers and older leaders*	Child begins to be rational and more stable in thought. An orderly conceptual framework is applied in understanding the world. Physical quantities such as weight and volume are now viewed as constants despite changes in shape and size.
6 yr — Can roller-skate; prints name; ties shoelaces.				
7 yr — Knows seasons of year; rides 2-wheeled bike.				
8 yr — Shares ideas; names days of week; repeats 5 digits forward.				
9 yr — Can define such words as sympathy and foolish.				
10 yr — Able to rhyme; repeats 4 digits in reverse.				
11 yr — Understands pity, grief, surprise; knows where sun sets.	— PREADOLESCENCE —			
ADOLESCENCE	EARLY ADOLESCENCE	**PSYCHOSOCIAL MORATORIUM** — *Identity versus role confusion* — FIDELITY	**ADOLESCENCE** — *Rebelliousness / Loosens family ties / Runs in cliques / Responsible independence emerges in fragments / Work habits solidify / Obvious heterosexual interests (girls usually before boys)*	**STAGE OF FORMAL OPERATIONS**
12 yr — Can comprehend definitions of scientific words of great complexity such as entropy.	"Mature" defenses: Altruism / Humor / Suppression / Anticipation / Sublimation			Child can now deal deductively not only with the reality the child sees but also with abstractions and propositional statements. The adolescent uses deductive reasoning and can evaluate the logic and quality of his or her own thinking. Increased powers of abstraction enable him or her to deal with laws and principles. Although egocentrism is still evident, balanced idealistic attitudes emerge in late adolescence. Some "normal" people do not advance this far in intellectual development; many do not lose their essential egocentrism at all. Egocentrism returns at senescence.
13 yr				
14 yr — Can divide small number in head.				
15 yr — Can repeat 6 digits forward and 5 digits backward.	MIDDLE ADOLESCENCE			
16 yr				
17 yr	LATE ADOLESCENCE			
18 yr				

*In each of the 3 center columns on psychodynamic development, the different styles of printing are vertically matched to the names and systems of the theorists in the heading box.

At first, the child experiences this process somewhat as a spectator. A feedback loop is formed, and the result is the first cognitive structure beyond the reflexes. Piaget calls this structure (stimulus-response-awareness) a **schema.** The schema is a cognitive behavioral unit that can be used, together with other **schemas,** as a building block to construct more complex structures that he called **schemata**—through circular reactions, first accidental and then purposeful. For example, as the reflex grasp becomes purposeful, what is grasped finds new uses beyond simply being mouthed. As development proceeds in this manner, children become aware that they can influence the environment and begin to see that they are in some vague way a cause of interesting actions that can be repeated in useful or amusing ways.

Between 8 and 12 months, the exploring and experimenting infant begins to distinguish objects as separate from the activity they were once associated with. Thus, a rattle that was originally only shaken, sucked at, and dropped is also thrown and sought, used for banging and poking, and otherwise employed as a tool. This is quite an "intellectual" leap from the discovery that the rattle could be mouthed or made to make a noise.

At the end of the sensorimotor stage (during the second year), children begin to become aware that material objects have an existence apart from the uses to which they are put. They can, for a time, maintain a mental image of the object. Piaget calls this **object permanency.*** This ability will lead children to look for a lost toy in the place where they saw it disappear. In the latter part of this stage, which corresponds to the beginning of language use (symbolization), children are able to imagine a familiar object in a context of new action or a familiar action involving a new object—without having to discover everything by trial and error. Piaget holds that when symbolization starts to occur with some frequency, the child leaves the sensorimotor stage and begins to function intelligently.

Stage of Preoperational Thought (Age 2–6)

The child begins to use symbols and language during the preoperational stage. This is the time of greatest active exploration of the surrounding world. Increasingly, language and thought processes replace solely physical sensations and activities. Children in this stage are **egocentric** and perceive themselves as the center of the universe. There is little objectivity or perception of the self as a separate entity. Events are

judged by their superficial impact without regard for logic or hidden possibilities. Early in this period, children may believe that everything that moves is alive and may impute magical powers to parents and other adults. They do not employ logical processes in arriving at conclusions and are confused by being asked how they know what they know. They are unable to reverse a thought process. Shown a picture of a result, they cannot reconstruct the starting point. They do not rank things relatively except in terms of opposites, eg, "bad" or "good. " Moral laws exist as indivisible parts of certain types of behavior. To obey adults is to be "good"; to disobey is to be "bad," even if doing so is accidental or unavoidable.

Stage of Concrete Operations (Age 6–12)

The name Piaget gave to this stage (concrete operations) exemplifies the manner of functioning now possible; the child employs **operational thinking.** Impressionistic intuition is replaced by small, logical steps in reasoning, and the data used are **concrete;** that is, they are constant, reproducible, and communicable. Concrete operations still depend on perception, but the perceptions are no longer egocentric. Rather, they are external and susceptible to validation by thinking through or acting through. Children of this age are able to organize data as parts of a whole and to keep the whole and the parts in mind at the same time. Even the brightest preoperational 5-year-old is unable to say whether there are more crows in the world or more birds, whereas the 8-year-old has no difficulty with the question. Still, both children will be unable to distinguish moral judgments from physical processes. The concept of infection can be understood but will also be connected with morality. Thus, being "bad" may be seen to be the cause of illness.

Although children in this stage of development are limited in what they can achieve intellectually by the literal quality of their understanding, they are able to order their lives according to rules and do so with enthusiasm. There is a general decrease in egocentrism, and the moral authority of the parents begins to be less magical and absolute. The child occasionally can see things from someone else's point of view.

Stage of Formal Operations (From Age 12 Onward)

At some time between age 12 and 15, some (not all) children acquire a capacity for abstract reasoning. When in the concrete stage, children live in the present, doing what they know best and reacting to the world in an immediate, superficial way without much thought about the past or future. During adolescence, children become able to think ahead and hypothesize from here and now to a number of different outcomes elsewhere and in the future. They also learn to think backward to analyse why a present situation exists, and they develop the capacity to "think about thinking." Fantasy, which in earlier developmental periods focused on wish fulfillment, now becomes a powerful

---

*Not the same as **object constancy,** a phrase introduced by Mahler and coworkers (1975) to characterize that stage of life (usually reached by 36 months) when a child can retain the relatively unambivalent concept of a loving mother in its mind even when she is absent for some time. In psychoanalysis, the word "object" denotes the libidinal object, the loved person in the infant's life. Piaget uses the word only to denote inanimate "things."

instrument for experimental manipulation of ideas and essences. As summarized by Maier (1969), cognitive activity evolves in 3 steps: from doing, to doing knowingly, and finally to concept formation. During the stage of formal operations, the individual can invent propositions based on no real life experience. According to Piaget, when these propositions can be organized into systems that can be used as a way of looking at life, cognitive development is complete.

Regression During Stress & Illness

Physicians and others caring for sick or injured people have noted that stress is often accompanied by regression of cognitive functioning. An adult is apt to become as "concrete" and egocentric as a child of 8 when health is threatened. Even well adolescents and adults may have ideas about illness that fall short of their cognitive mastery of other nonstressful subject matter. Piaget's special importance has been that he emphasized clinical *developmental* psychology. For decades before it became popular to do so, he was insisting that the child understands the world differently from adults and learns in a different way. Everyone who works with children (and with adults under stress) is in Piaget's debt for these insights. Comments on how children's cognitive powers affect their responses to illness are included in the descriptions of the developmental phases in the next section of this chapter.

JOHN BOWLBY (1907–)

The body of thought that has come to be called **attachment theory** begins with the 1958 publication of "The Nature of a Child's Tie to His Mother," by British psychoanalyst John Bowlby. In this and in subsequent major works, Bowlby reinterprets his original psychoanalytic understanding of early development in terms of animal ethology and modern evolutionary theory. In addition, he takes into account the newer ideas of control systems and the model of information processing.

Bowlby emphasizes Darwin's explicit view that every feature of anatomy, physiology, and behavior in an animal species contributes—or once contributed—to the survival of that species in its natural environment. The behaviors underlying mating, the care of infants, and the attachment of young to their caregivers*

---

*In this chapter, the word "caregiver" (and the feminine third-person pronoun) are used to denote the primary person to whom the child becomes emotionally attached or bonded. In most families and most societies, this person is the biologic mother. But such bonds form with others also; not all "mothering" is done by mothers, or by women for that matter. Although certain kinds of "caregiving" can of course be done by others than the attachment figures (such as the professional child attendant in kibbutzim), the word here is meant to denote the object of primary emotional attachment.

are obviously of the greatest importance to survival and are so stable across human cultures that they have come to be numbered among the few instinctual systems of the species. Survival through years of helpless dependency is not left to chance or to the dedication of caregivers alone. A behavioral system evolved to make certain that the infant itself would be motivated to remain with its caregivers. Protection from predators, Bowlby maintains, is the evolutionary purpose of attachment behaviors. In general, attachment behaviors are those observable actions of a child that promote an appropriate nearness to the attachment figure so that dangers may be avoided.

Bowlby's basic assumption is that humans are born with fragmentary skills that enable them to survive in the environment of evolutionary adaptedness. For any individual human, this environment is represented by a caregiver (usually the biologic mother) in an established social unit. The main behaviors that serve the attachment system are, at first, signals—crying and looking, then smiling and cooing. Later, verbalizing predominates, but nonverbal signaling remains a powerful part of attachment behavior throughout life.

The stages of attachment are shown in Table 6–1. At birth, before attachment occurs, the infant is distressed by pain, hunger, and cold. Crying alerts the caregiver to the infant's needs. Later, when the infant has become attached to a specific person, it will cry not only in response to physical discomfort but also whenever the caregiver goes away or when frightening or unusual things happen, such as the approach of a stranger or a large dog. Cessation of crying and other attachment behaviors depends on the degree of alarm or distress. Just seeing the caregiver approaching may be enough, or in some cases nothing short of a clinging embrace will terminate the attachment behavior. As long as the child is comfortable and the caregiver is in sight, the child may wander a good distance before the proximity limit for that situation is exceeded and attachment behavior is stimulated in child or caregiver. If there is some threat to continued proximity—especially if the caregiver appears about to move away—the child may spontaneously move nearer to the caregiver.

Attachment behavior must be distinguished from the **attachment bond** implied by the behavior. The strength of the bond may be correlated with the passion of the behavior when the bond is severed, but it is not necessarily true that the absence of attachment behavior implies an absence of the attachment bond. Once formed, the attachment bond persists and is manifested by the emotional consequences of long separations. Anger, apparent indifference, or cold behavior in a child separated from its attachment figure by death or desertion is the child's emotional and cognitive reaction to the trauma of separation and not a sign of absence of attachment.

Bowlby's control systems theory of emotion explains how basic feelings (such as fear) help the infant adapt and survive: fear is innate, not learned behavior. From the first, sudden strong stimuli are frightening.

Shortly after birth, looming figures or a sensation of dropping from a safe (held) position causes distress. By age 2 or 3 months, being alone or in strange surroundings elicits obvious fear. By the time attachment to caregivers begins (between 3 and 6 months), fearful behavior and attachment behavior are aroused by the same stimuli; the child is alarmed by the danger, and this alarm precipitates action to increase proximity to the caregiver. If adequate proximity cannot be achieved quickly, the child will then feel distress that is both more severe and qualitatively different from the original sense of alarm. Bowlby called this different kind of distress **anxiety**.

The infant experiences minor degrees of anxiety (awareness of not being close enough to the attachment figure) repeatedly and learns to master anxiety if ready access to the attachment figure is maintained. After about 6 months, the infant will anticipate the discomfort of anxiety on seeing its caregiver preparing to leave and will activate its attachment behaviors and protests in an attempt to prevent departure. The more consistent the caregiver's behavior is in the mind of the child, the more separation the child is likely to tolerate. In the presence of the attachment figure, the child is likely to feel the opposite of anxiety—**security**—unless fearful that the attachment figure will unexpectedly leave or become unresponsive. The very young baby explores the body of the attachment figure, so that the attachment and exploration systems coincide; this favors the development of a strong bond. Later, the caregiver serves as a secure base from which to explore at some distance, so that exploration behavior is balanced by attachment behavior. A child who feels secure is able to explore; when security is threatened by alarm or separation, attachment behavior predominates. If security is threatened much of the time, the child's capacity for learning and for developing social relationships is impaired.

Bowlby's approach to the dawn of social relations has clarified the essentially social origins of the child's tie to its caregiver. Earlier theories from psychology and psychoanalysis held that infants become attached to their caregivers only secondarily, out of a primary need for nourishment. If, as it seems, attachment is served by a separate behavioral system (although overlapping with the nutritional system), then a host of findings from animal research and observations of human maldevelopment are easier to comprehend. The following sections of this chapter have been greatly influenced by these considerations, and examples demonstrating their usefulness are offered there.

SUMMARY OF THEORIES OF CHILD DEVELOPMENT

Table 6–1 summarizes 5 perspectives on human development. They are, of course, not the only views on the subject. The psychodynamic approaches of the psychoanalytic schools are heavily represented in this table because they are most used in clinical psychiatric practice. Theories of personality and psychopathology derived from nonanalytic psychology and philosophy, especially the modern humanistic theories, are mentioned in other chapters in this text.

CHILD DEVELOPMENT FROM BEFORE BIRTH TO ADOLESCENCE

THE PREPSYCHOLOGIC PERIOD: CONCEPTION THROUGH AGE 2 MONTHS

Prenatal Life

Cerebral processes and responses can be demonstrated in utero (such as conditioning of the fetal electroencephalogram to a sound), but it is not known whether the gestating infant must have any specific sensory experiences in order to develop properly, nor do we know what (if any) noxious sensory input distorts or impedes that development. Excess or deficiency of maternal circulating hormones (eg, thyroid, pituitary, adrenocortical, and sex hormones) are known to adversely affect physical development, especially of the central nervous system; but damage to the fetus occurs only as a result of physical and chemical agents—directly through trauma and disease, and indirectly through ill health of the mother. There is no evidence that the mother's emotional state, attitudes, thoughts, or conflicts have any effect on the fetus. Aside from obstetric complications, the chief dangers to the fetal nervous system are maternal viral infections and severe protein malnutrition. Chronic alcoholism in the mother during pregnancy results in several types of abnormality. Central nervous system metaplasia (increases in number and complexity of cells) is maximal during the first 3 months of pregnancy, and protein starvation during this period is devastating for future intellectual development. Unlike most of the rest of the body, if brain tissue fails to receive adequate nourishment in this period, repair cannot be achieved by proper feeding later. This vulnerability continues, but to a lesser extent, throughout gestation and the first few years of life.

Birth & the Neonatal Period

Much creative energy has been expended in contemplating the physical act of obstetric delivery as a possible factor in emotional development. Despite the most eloquent conjectures, however, current evidence indicates that birth is an experience of negligible psychologic importance to the infant. However, it is of major psychologic importance to the mother and her supporters, which means that even if it is never shown that favorable conditions at delivery are crucial to the *child's* psychologic future, they certainly may be to the mother and others and thus indirectly to the child. A satisfied mother and father and a smiling baby are more likely to form early and strong bonds with each other. This common sense assumption has led some progressive obstetric units to provide a more homelike atmosphere in labor and delivery rooms and to allot a more active role to the parents, including the presence of the father (or other supporting adult) during the birth process and afterward.

One thing that is certain is that the infant even at the moment of delivery is not a "tabula rasa" on which experience writes all. In the delivery room, some infants are observed tracking with their eyes certain colors and shapes of light while ignoring others. Within a few days, and without much experience, this skill improves markedly. What appears to be happening is that the infant is already seeking a pattern. At this point, it is a relatively nonspecific pattern, but it is definitely not indiscriminate. With time, what infants seek becomes shaped by what they actually get and how satisfying it is; but from the first there are inclinations to react in predictable ways to certain patterns of sight, sound, and touch.

Mutually satisfying caregiver-child interactions consolidate the rhythms of the baby's life and lead to more awake-alert times within which learning takes place before physical tensions such as hunger or other discomforts stimulate the child to cry. The act of being satisfied serves as an early prototype of a future feeling of trust or security. If needs are satisfied efficiently and empathetically, a sense of trust and security begins to take form; if not, the result is mistrust and distress, the forerunners of insecurity, anxiety, and psychic conflict in later life. These are, of course, concepts inferred from appearances and an adult's perspective.

The Dawn of Psychologic Awareness

The prenatal and early neonatal period appears to be dominated by biologic needs and responses. The mother or other caregiver is the "auxiliary ego" who makes life not only bearable but possible, and it is mostly through her—the rhythms of her body during gestation and her physical interventions and social stimulations after birth—that the child experiences the world. The caregiver's physical ministrations bridge the physiologic gaps that delivery creates in the systems of breathing, feeding, elimination, regulation of body temperature, etc. Up to this point, it is doubtful if any experience is appreciated in a psychologic way by the child. For an event to have psychologic meaning for an infant, one must assume the existence of rather sophisticated innate mental processes and the ability to discriminate between external and internal stimuli. These hypotheses are tempting because the normal infant behaves so naturally within its environment of evolutionary adaptedness, but there is no evidence that physically difficult labor or discomfort—or even cruelty or neglect in the first several weeks—limits the

child's potential for future development unless tissue damage is sustained. In fact, the gravest congenital abnormalities requiring multiple surgical procedures and other painful methods of treatment ordinarily do not result in psychologic maldevelopment. It is only later, when the child's psyche is organized by the quality and frequency of the caregiver's social responses, that we can speak of a truly psychologic life in a child. Nevertheless, future research may reveal that certain early stimuli have epigenetic importance for optimal development later in life, and this possibility should be borne in mind in our handling of the youngest of infants (see Stern reference).

Coalescence of Ego Fragments: The Experience of Infancy

We assume that "awareness" in neonates consists only of being comfortable or not and that infants differentiate only vaguely, if at all, between the outer and inner environments. The fixed-action patterns present at birth—rooting, sucking, postural adjustment, looking and listening, grasping and crying—stimulate the caregiver to provide what is needed to relieve discomfort. This process is experienced by the infant as a sensorimotor cycle as described by Piaget: sensory input and motor output, with not much evidence of the "throughput," or mental functions, that will make such a difference later, as cognition develops.

We infer that during the first months of life, infants gradually begin to perceive a difference between the "central self" and what they experience as more peripheral. Although they seek to escape from unpleasant stimulation, the usual salient experience consists of repeated exposure, in a decidedly social context, to pleasurable and tension-relieving stimuli. (This "coming inside" of the external world, chiefly through the mouth in feeding but through other sensory modalities as well, has given rise to the concept of **orality** in psychoanalytic theory.) Because the early organismic and attachment needs cannot be met by the child, it may be that they are particularly distressing when relief must be even briefly postponed. This is perhaps why symptoms and fantasies from this early "oral" phase of life are so persistent in serious mental disorders assumed to have their origin in very early life.

Constitutional Givens & Environmental Responses

In the first weeks or months of life, infants begin to show characteristic styles of behavior that develop into consistent patterns. The constancy tends to persist until about 2 years of age, after which time traits of individual diversity start to appear. Caregivers react to the infant's style of behavior for better or worse according to their expectations and tolerance, and their responses tend to shape the child's behavior.

There is no question that "difficult babies" are a great trial to their caregivers, and this should be kept in mind in evaluating later behavior problems. The family's ability to provide a good emotional environment may be limited, and these deficiencies begin immediately to influence genomic potential so that a child's competence at age 2 or age 6 may fall far short of its potential at birth.

Of all the characteristics of newborns that stimulate parental responses and affect what the child learns, the most striking is gender. Whether the infant is a girl or a boy elicits responses from the parents congruent with their hopes, fears, identifications, and preconceptions. These parental responses feed back into the child's developing self in a way that shapes the direction of the child's responses and, later, the child's feelings about himself or herself. Those who deal with newborns and infants often hear parents attribute qualities to their children that are not obvious to others. Boys, for example, are commonly seen by their fathers as tough, aggressive, and destined for success in sports, while girls are often described as sweet, shy, and in need of daddy's protection even though the 2 children may appear to an objective observer to be indistinguishable in behavior.

The Role of the Father

The role of the father may be as important to the infant as that of the mother. If the mother is the primary caregiver, the father can be the first alternative caregiver. The relationship between fathers and infants is only now being examined closely, but it appears that fathers can serve as primary caregivers just as well as mothers. It is an advantage for infants if there is more than one attachment figure in the home, but the commonly held conviction that infants develop best in a home with both a father and a mother is based on convention and tradition rather than research data.

The Deviant Child/Pathogenic Caregiver Issue

Aberrations of infant development that result from physical defects, extremes of constitutional style, etc, may be noted at or soon after birth. If dealt with skillfully by the caregiver, they may resolve, but such aberrations may persist despite ideal nurturing. If the caregiver continues to function without guilt, rage, or rejection and there is no further insult, the child will develop to the limits of its constitutional potential— which still may be defective. However, ideal nurturing in needy cases is not as common as might be wished. Caregivers are human and have their own problems stemming at times from their own suboptimal rearing. Considering the variations in environments, certain behavioral extremes of "deficiencies" may result even though not predetermined by any genomic predispositions. Such situations contribute to the diversity of humankind and, although unfortunate, cannot be considered pathologic. An example would be a passive infant born to a very dependent woman with little formal education and low self-esteem. In the absence of contrary influences, it would be no surprise if this infant developed in a borderline retarded way, even though there were no indications of subnormal intellectual potential early in life.

Precursors of Attachment: The "Prepsychologic" Phase of Attachment (Table 6–2)

Although from the start the infants orient themselves toward external signals emanating from human beings, they do not at first discriminate between one person and another but seem to be scanning for patterns and for things that move. Very young infants respond preferentially to soft, high-pitched voices and soothing, cooing sounds, and as early as the fourth week of life the infant will turn toward its primary caregiver's voice while ignoring others. The social smile becomes distinguishable from the reflex grimace between the fourth and eighth weeks. The infant's smile and its first gurgles and coos are powerful "social releasers" that elicit attention and affectionate behavior from the caregivers. As yet, however, the smile, vocalization, and general excitement at the appearance of a human face and the sound of a human voice are still fixed-action responses similar to the palmar grasp reflex.

The infant makes a ready and positive response to strangers up to about the 18th week. The infant's pleasure in these interactions is not simply related to anticipated relief of hunger or physical discomfort but is a **primary social drive** that is additionally reinforced as the child associates the caregiver with gratifying experiences. The close child-caregiver bond provides protection and physical sustenance and is a necessary preparation for socialization in later life. What brings children and caregiving persons together for these protective and nurturing ends is **attachment behavior.** The appearance of the promiscuous social smile and the beginning of discrimination between the primary attachment figure and others signal the end of the prepsychologic period of life.

THE PERIOD OF ATTACHMENT: THE INFANT AT 2–9 MONTHS

The Positive Phase of Attachment (Table 6–2)

During the third month, an infant recognizes the primary caregiver and soon begins to reserve its most vivacious smiles and kicks for that person. Mothers will say, "He sees me now" or "She knows it's me." By 6 months, infants are alert, attentive to the environment, and eager to move out into it, and they grasp purposefully at whatever comes into view as long as they can see their own hands in the field. They try to sit up and to watch or follow anything that moves, as long as it does not approach too fast or make too much noise. They are especially eager to get at and stay close to mother, hold onto her, and climb on her. They lose awareness of objects out of sight and quickly lose interest, after a brief moment of perplexity, if a toy they have been playing with suddenly disappears under a blanket. By this time, they have begun to associate

Table 6–2. The development of attachment.

I. **"Prepsychologic" phase of attachment (conception to 2 months of age)**
   Follows moving objects with eyes. Listens.
   Searches for and enjoys the patterns of the human face but does not discriminate between faces.
   Prefers mother's voice by 1 month.
   Entrains gross body movement with human speech.
   Demonstrates reflex grimace without eye crinkling.
   (Eye crinkling combined with "reflex" grimacing signals the social smile, which marks the end of the "prepsychologic" phase.)
II. **Positive phase of attachment (2–7 months)**
   Definitely recognizes attachment figures.
   Reserves the most vivacious smiles for them.
   Most home-reared children focus attachment on one figure.
   Indiscriminate smiling peaks between 14th and 18th weeks.
   Sobering and staring at strangers begins between the 18th and 24th weeks and signals the end of the positive phase of attachment.
III. **Limiting phase of attachment (6–10 months)**
   Unmistakable fear of strangers appears at about 26 weeks of age in home-reared infants. This is not separation anxiety. The appearance of fear of strangers ends the positive phase of attachment.

certain objects with activities that have provided gratification, such as holding a bottle.

Between 4 and $6\frac{1}{2}$ months, most home-reared children narrow their attachment behavior to focus on the figure of their primary emotional caregiver and, to a lesser extent, the several other social respondents in the home, especially the father. Weakly attached infants are more likely to confine their social behavior to a single person. Social interaction with one or a few constant people is essential for formation of secure attachments. It is not known how much social interaction is necessary, and it probably varies. Between the fifth and seventh months, the tendency to focus on a particular figure is strongest, and when this attachment has been achieved, the tendency to seek other figures for attachment declines dramatically. This change is reminiscent of the critical periods for imprinting in animals. The sensitive phase within which attachment can be formed normally ends as early as the sixth month or as late as the eighth month. If the infant has not had consistent access to a figure on which to focus, the ability to form attachments seems to wane after about the 18th month, and thereafter it is extremely difficult to accomplish.

Investigations designed to determine whether multiple or changing caregivers might provide adequate infant care have not established conclusively that such arrangements would be suitable substitutes for the traditional main-caregiver/subsidiary-caregivers system that characterizes the human family unit. Data from natural experiments and from scientific projects are not comparable, and what constitutes a "good" outcome is difficult to agree upon. Most children reared in kibbutzim, communes, and other multiple-caregiver situations natural to the culture grow up to be indistinguishable, as a group, from the general population, but there is evidence that children reared primarily with peers rather than in traditional families have different personality structures.

While the complexity and richness of relations with attachment figures continue to grow, the endearing positive response to strangers, which is maximal at 14–18 weeks, gives way to sobering and staring at 18–24 weeks. This shift in attitude about strangers signals completion of the positive phase of attachment.

The Limiting Phase of Attachment (Table 6–2)

After 6 months, conditions for the development of attachment in home-reared children are complicated by the emergence of fear responses. As noted above, sobering and staring at strangers begin around the 18th week. Frank **fear of strangers** is manifest at variable times, beginning at about 26 weeks in home-reared infants, but is usually not well established until the eighth month. This response is fear of the stranger and not merely **separation anxiety,** because it occurs while infants are securely in the arms of their primary caregivers. It is important to note that these 2 types of behavior, although interrelated, are differentiable and may appear independently (either one before the other).

Separation anxiety, which prompts what has been described here as attachment behavior, is the sense of discomfort a child feels when being threatened by or experiencing an unpleasant separation from the attachment figure. Naturally, stranger fear and separation anxiety often function together; the child tries *to move away from* a frightening situation and *go toward* the person or place that offers protection and safety. Since fear of the stranger reinforces attachment behavior, it functions to enhance the already well-developed attachment drives, thus bringing to a close the positive phase of primary attachment. Thereafter, the infant may go to others and be friendly but will not develop the same emotional attachments accorded to his or her own emotional caregivers. This focus on the immediate family provides an apprenticeship in human relations that must be mastered before the child can move comfortably outside the family circle.

Screening for Attachment Adequacy

Since the most important achievement of the first year is a secure attachment to one or more caregivers, pediatricians and others caring for children must watch for normal development of that phenomenon or for its absence. Attachment behavior can be roughly assessed early in the first year primarily by noting the infant's response to the human face peering down. During the third and fourth month, the **social smile** is fully developed. Anyone can elicit such a smile in a well-attached baby of this age by approaching slowly and presenting one's face for inspection. Soft vocalizing helps. If the infant is well and not distracted, it will smile when the observer smiles. Although the infant may smile in response to other cues as well, the human face, smiling, nodding, and cooing, is the strongest stimulus. Absence of this characteristic response at this age warrants investigation for some physical or psychologic abnormality.

Beginning in the seventh month, attachment to the primary caregiver can be easily tested in the clinic or elsewhere. The following is an example: As the pediatrician approaches the child and its mother, the child shows concern at the intrusion of a strange face. While safely on its mother's lap, a child not otherwise distressed will continue to smile broadly at her, reaching for her and playing with her hair—but will immediately become sober when looking at the pediatrician and will not return a smile but will turn back to the mother instead. This is the beginning of active discrimination between familiars and strangers that a fully attached infant will normally show. At 7 or 8 months, the child may cry when put on the examining table and protest vigorously when handled off the mother's lap. The child's distress at separation from the mother and the strange face of the examiner is an indication that the attachment system is in good order;

it is not an occasion for disapproval or reproach of the child (Main, 1985).

Cognitive Advances

At 6–9 months, when fear of strangers is developing, the first cognitively intentional acts are observed. In Piaget's charming phrase, the child learns to initiate "procedures calculated to make interesting spectacles last." Deliberate action begins. Since some kinds of behavior produce results, such as the noise of a rattle or the movement of a toy puppy pulled by a string, interest shifts from the action itself to its repeatable consequences. Still, the infant is inclined to equate the movement or gesture with the result, an essentially magical procedure.

THE INFANT AT 9–12 MONTHS

Physical & Cognitive Abilities

Near the end of the first year, the child can sit, crawl toward attractive objects and away from repugnant or fearsome ones, cruise at the rail, walk a few steps, fixate and track with the eyes, grasp with either hand, and convey what is grasped to the mouth. It has command over its motor systems, mental representations of familiar people and objects in the environment, and rudimentary devices for securing and retaining things and people that are wanted or needed. Objects now have an existence that survives loss of visual or tactile contact with them, so that the child may search for a toy that has somehow disappeared. If a ball is placed under a blanket where the child can see a bulge, it will reach under the blanket and retrieve the ball. However, if the ball is taken from under the first blanket and put under another one, even though the child sees this happen, it will not search at the second site. This illustrates Piaget's assertion that infants do not distinguish a "thing" from the motor action with which the "thing" is associated.

Attachment & Stranger Fear Responses

By 12 months, the infant is well attached to its primary caregiver and to others in the household to a lesser extent. The ability to discriminate between people and the fear of strangers bind the child to the nuclear family and serve to protect the child from predators and other dangers. Sustained by the active social relationships formed, the young child is now equipped to venture into the world of experience beyond the caregiver's embrace.

Negative Effects of Overlong Separation

Since attachment is necessary for healthy physical and emotional development, and since separation is tolerable only in moderation, overlong separation in early life can be expected to have morbid consequences. Bowlby and coworkers have described how young, well-attached children respond to long separation from their parents without adequate substitutes—as happens, for example, when a child is left in a residential nursery because its mother has been hospitalized—with protest, despair, and detachment. The **protest phase** begins after about 3 days of separation, with crying, calling, and searching for the attachment figure. The child clamors for the attention of caretaking adults but knows they are only substitutes. Anger leads to ambivalence when the mother does return, so that the child may avert its face, reject the mother's offers of affectionate hugging, and cling to an attendant instead. In the **despair phase,** the child is still attached to the absent mother but communicates an air of hopelessness. Finally, if the separation continues, the child becomes **detached,** progressively more interested in the environment but more so in the material objects there than in people. If the mother returns before detachment occurs, the child may *appear* to be quite indifferent to her. All this has put a great strain on the child's ability to trust the caregiving environment. If the primary caregiver responds to the child's apparent indifference by rejection, disastrous disaffection and estrangement may be the result.

Children placed for adoption can move from a foster home to the adoptive home with little difficulty until they are about 6 months of age; after that time, many children become visibly upset, and by the eighth month, all children show serious upset when moved from a foster home to the adoptive home—especially if the foster home was a socially stimulating one in which the child had developed strong affiliations. The distress is due to rupture of the attachment bond that begins to strengthen during the sixth month, and the sequence of protest, despair, and detachment occurs as just described. Some forms of such distress, especially protest and despair, continue to occur on long separations up to the third year or even later, regardless of the circumstances necessitating the separation and despite loving attentions from multiple and changing nonattachment figures. The presence of a sibling, grandparent, or other secondary attachment figure can greatly reduce the stress of separation, and special attention by a trained substitute caregiver who does not rotate with others on a workshift schedule will minimize the potential damage.

All this is not to say that there can be no repair or recovery if a child makes unsatisfactory primary attachments in infancy or must endure painful separations later. Initiation or resumption of affectionate care at any stage of development may reverse the process and limit developmental damage.

The Security/Exploration Balance

As mobility skills and hand control begin to develop at about age 1 year, exploration of the environment tests the child's ability to tolerate short separation from the caregiver. Easy access to the caregivers is an essential precondition to exploratory freedom. Secure children explore the world, learning as they go; less secure ones are less eager to do so, and cognitive development is correspondingly affected. Securely attached youngsters have no trouble breaking off briefly to seek comfort in proximity to caregivers when fearsome events stifle exploratory impulses.

THE SECOND YEAR: MASTERY OF THE BODY

Physical & Social Advances

The child's second year is characterized by increasingly vigorous autonomous behavior but a corresponding ready distress upon unexpected separation from attachment figures. To be with someone who is familiar is of the utmost importance at this age. The fear of separation, however, is not the only fear experienced. Sudden sounds, the appearance of strange objects and unfamiliar people, and the rapid approach or looming presence of large objects initiate the fear response and stimulate attachment behavior. There is little indication that imagination or fantasy plays any part in the fear response; children are innately fearful of these things, and they learn to fear other things that have been associated with pain or frightening experiences, such as large animals or noisy machinery. They learn also to be aware of fear in their parents and siblings and express it as their own.

This year of life has been called the period of mastery of the body, since exploration of the child's own body, especially the erogenous sites, is a primary preoccupation. As new motor skills are acquired, the child takes great pleasure in using them, especially if the parents' praise and pleasure are forthcoming. Because motor development outruns the emergence of rationality and discretion, conflicts with what the parents consider appropriate behavior inevitably arise. When the child's demands are thwarted, frustration and rage may result, and the child sets out to test the limits of the parents' indulgence and tolerance. Since the child is small, the parents usually are successful in removal or restraint except in areas of physiologic function where they cannot exert control—eating, drinking, and excretion of urine and feces.

By the 18th month, the child is able to use spoons, cups, and other simple household items in appropriate ways. By age 2, small toys, cars, dolls, and playhouse furniture are beginning to be used in imaginative play.

At this point in life, both boys and girls are likely to have established an exuberant relationship with the world. Shyness with strangers lessens, and children resume the search for social relationships. This imposes new demands on the primary caregivers to keep up with their children and protect them from harm.

Parental Example & Intervention

During the child's second year, 2 major influences begin to exert their effect on behavior and personality: parental example (modeling) and parental intervention (positive and negative reinforcement). Even before this time, children are eager to imitate and identify with one or both parents; the peek-a-boo, patty-cake, and baby-talk games of the first 6 months are common examples. Later, toddlers will delight in imitating complex parental behaviors based on observation without having grasped the purpose of the behavior. "Shifting gears" in the car seat is an example. This phenomenon illustrates not only increasing mastery of the body but also the process of internalization of the child's perception of the parents' motivations and thought processes. The cat is petted or its tail pulled, teddy bears punished or rewarded, and all manner of familiar adult behaviors are acted out. This propensity to imitate adults and to absorb their emotions reinforces the child's inclination to respond with fear, anxiety, or distress to the same stimuli that evoke these responses in the parents.

The shaping effect of parental intervention becomes more important as language becomes the chief means of interaction between parents and children. Although this influence may start to have some effect as early as the third month, it becomes maximal after age 1, when the child becomes able to divine the parents' intentions, "see through" their plans, and accurately assess their emotions. This awareness makes for conflict and the internalization of conflict. The child wants to do something, and the parents object. Their opposition is "internalized" as the child modifies its behavior in order to please them and avoid losing their love and kind ministrations. A common example is the internalization of the concept "No!" Toddlers often act as if "no" were still external. A child may reach for the television knobs and then, hand poised in the air, say "No!" firmly and pull away. Once internalized, the powerful concept of "No!" can be turned against the parents as the child realizes they can be opposed in some ways. The well-known oppositionism of this age group has been dubbed "the terrible twos."

During this period, toilet training depends partly on maturation of the nervous system. Bowel and bladder control is important to the extent the parents think it is. Overconcern about "accidents" focuses the child's attention on these physiologic activities and confers an unwarranted importance on struggles between parent and child about matters over which neither has good control.

The child's interest in his or her body at this time emphasizes the parts that give pleasure and are under some kind of control. Excretory products are not repulsive at first. A little boy enjoys directing his stream of urine, and fecal play is a transient phenomenon in some children. A general tendency to "make a mess" is often noted, as are all physical activities that have some semblance of mastery of the environment. Since fine motor control is not yet achieved and judgment is immature, household items are at risk of destruction. Since this is also the time when the child has the power to expel or retain feces—and perhaps is engaged in a contest with the caregiver over who is to control that pleasurable activity—it has been called the **anal-sadistic stage** in psychoanalytic descriptions of development.

Cognitive Advances

During the second year, the child can be observed studying situations and devising experiments in order to create new experiences. As new skills are acquired, they are perfected by repetition and practice. Consolidation by repetition is a recognized feature of mentation and shows that the function itself is a source of pleasure apart from any need to relieve boredom or tension or derive erotic pleasure. During this period, the child does with the body what it will later do with language, which eventually supersedes action as the chief means of dealing with the world and conforming to its social requirements. It is for this reason that Piaget calls the first 2 years of life the "sensorimotor" stage and considers it preintelligent (ie, prior to verbal conceptual thinking).

By about 16 months, as cognition matures, sensorimotor activity is slowly replaced by increasingly conceptual processes. Objects have acquired some permanency in memory and an existence independent from the actions with which they are associated. It is now common to imagine displacements of objects and logical to search for them in places where they might be lying hidden. Studies have shown that the primary caregiver is usually the first "object" to acquire such permanency in the child's mind and that children whose attachments are strong and positive are better able to develop mental images of other things.

The child's experiences in communicating with its parents serve as inner directives about which cognitive impulses can be freely entertained and which must be kept from consciousness because of their forbidden content. By this process, the "unconscious mind" begins to take form. Szurek (1969) argues that the parents' own unconscious sanctions are sensed by the child and received as authoritative along with their overt and conscious directives. As long as the parents are relatively free of conflict about their values, the child can tolerate rather strict "instructions" about what may or may not be thought. The developmental processes are strong, however, and their force will sometimes be exerted against the parents' opposition.

Parents should tactfully help children gratify as many of their mental impulses as reasonably possible in the social and cultural context. When necessary frustration produces rage and tantrum behavior, children should be given a firm explanation of where, when, how, and with whom the sought-for gratification can be achieved rather than an angry or anxious negative or positive response. Parents should cultivate a habit of nonretaliatory acceptance of their children's anger but should not hesitate to use gentle physical restraint if the children try to hurt the parents or themselves.

THE CHILD AT AGE 2–4

Physical & Social Advances

The third and fourth years are those during which the expansion of mental life is most striking. There is an enormous increase in the ability to use words and symbols (pictures and gestures) and to combine them in new ways to enrich the inner life with fantasy and to explore and control the outside world. Although there is great variation in the age at which children master language, most children by age 2 have a speaking vocabulary of 100–300 words and are able to understand several hundred more. If their attachments are secure, they begin to spend less time with the parents and look outward for amusement, especially in the company of other children. **Parallel play** comes first, in which young children are observed playing "together" but not yet "with each other." Between ages 2½ and 3, **associative play** evolves with elements of peer interaction and cooperation, and during the fourth year **cooperative play** with one other child is possible. It is not until the fifth year that cooperative play in a group becomes a regular feature of childhood behavior.

Fantasy

Fantasy play is the means by which children aged 2–4 master the world. In fantasy, they can manipulate, reverse, modify, and improve their lot in ways that are beyond their control in real life. After unpleasant or frightening incidents, the child can relive those experiences in fantasy and play and often revise and master them. This is the rationale of play psychotherapy. (See Chapters 41 and 57.)

Sibling Rivalry

Age 2–4 is the time when a child is most likely to be presented with a baby brother or sister. Next to long separation from the primary attachment figure or other catastrophe in early life, the advent of a sibling is the most impressive psychologic event in childhood, and its effects continue to be felt throughout life in attitudes about competitors and dependents. It provides a special opportunity for the development of important social skills but is also the nidus around which neurotic distortion may collect.

Most commonly, there is threatened or actual diversion of the mother's love and attention from the child who has enjoyed it undiluted for 2 or 3 years. The child may respond with babyish activity and demands for attention and may regress in behavior to an earlier stage of development. The parents' response to regression will determine whether adaptation with few residual effects will occur or whether it will remain a focus of anxious concern and bitterness for the child. Even the busiest new mother can find time to respond by allowing a bit of regression in her 2-year-old and to express her understanding of why it is happening. The birth of a sibling is a time when the father or other family adult not directly involved with the new baby should spend more time with the older child.

Transitional Objects

Many parents are annoyed when their children—even up to the school-age years—have some object they like to hold and carry about with them, usually a blanket, stuffed animal, or other article of soft material that they seek out in times of disappointment, fatigue, or pain. The psychodynamic explanation of this phenomenon remains a subject of debate, but there is no evidence that the practice has any pernicious effect so long as the child does not *prefer* the transitional object to the attachment figure.

Gender Identity

Children during the third and fourth years (if not earlier) discover the difference betwen boys and girls and have a natural curiosity about it. Starting in the second year, but mostly in the third and fourth, there is an increasing interest in bathroom matters and in the genitals and genital play, although this is usually forbidden by the adults in the family, who do not tolerate genital exhibitionism as they may have tolerated and encouraged other types of showing off. The restriction does not lead to conflict if the parents accept the impulse as natural but indicate that social tradition calls for privacy in these matters.

It is also at this age that awareness of being male or female occurs. How the parents act in their gender roles and what they demand from their sons and daughters determine how children internalize their gender.

Cognitive Advances

Age 2–4 is the time when children, having mastered the sensorimotor mechanisms of their bodies, begin to use symbols and syntax in dealing with the world. They "reason" by intuition rather than by logic. All things are judged by surface appearance and interpreted by post hoc reasoning. Children at this age are confused by causality, attributing effects to the loudest, most recent, or most impressive preceding event. For example, a 3½-year-old boy might assume that a thunderstorm has caused him to have a sore throat and that the doctor's examination cured it.

During this period, children are relatively egocentric; they personalize their observations and experiences. Although many children show a spontaneous empathy for the distress of others even at as young an age as 1 year, they cannot be objective about why they feel that way, and they either do not comprehend at all or, at best, repeat without understanding what they are told.

THE CHILD AT AGE 4–6

Childhood Sexual Experience

During the years from age 4 to age 6, overt sexual behavior becomes differentiated from attachment behavior. Most adults cannot remember their own sexual preoccupations during this time, and many prefer to believe that children are "innocent" of such thoughts.

Whether this new, overtly sexual behavior constitutes the emergence of a new instinctual system or is an outgrowth of the old attachment system is still being debated. It is clear, however, that the forms taken by new sexual initiatives will be affected by what is acceptable in the family and will reflect parental attitudes, especially unconscious ones. Commonly, a father will be pleased by his daughter's coquettishly "feminine" behavior and will respond positively to it, and the mother responds in the same way to her son's "manly" behavior. Their positive responses to the sexual content of the children's behavior will be limited, however, so that in the long run, the child must endure disappointment. But the need for parental nonsexual love, attention, and direction—the attachment needs—continues for many years.

Sexual behavior adds a complex emotional dimension to the child's relationship with the parents. The child's understanding of this behavior is determined largely by the sophistication of its cognitive processes. Parental disapproval of sexual behavior by a small boy may arouse concern about potential harm to the penis, which he perceives as central to his sexual feelings. When he learns that females do not have penises, the immature little boy—and the little girl also—may wonder where the missing penis might be and how it came to be lost or hidden. Children of this age are not far removed from the phase of development when they dealt with the world only through their bodies, and they are greatly concerned about bodily integrity and any possible threats to it.

The little girl at age 2 or 3 may become concerned when she discovers she lacks a penis and may not be fully satisfied by reassurances that she has not lost hers, that she has something of equivalent value inside her body, and that she will someday be able to produce a baby. Despite the fear and doubts resulting from sexual thoughts and fantasies at this age, the child's self-respect still rests on how the parents behave toward her and how they behave toward each other. The mother's security as a female adult, as demonstrated by the respect she receives from her husband, is the daughter's best source of reassurance that she is a worthy and fully equal member of the family despite the absence of a penis. Although a girl of 4 or 5 can easily grasp the idea that she has *internal* organs of comparable value, for many youngsters at age 2 and 3, appearances are all-important even in the face of adult assurances to the contrary. At this age, both boys and girls are very impressed with the penis. Later, when the mystery of procreation becomes comprehensible, both girls and boys are fascinated by that process. Some of the aggressive behavior boys direct toward girls—and their bragging and self-aggrandizing—can be traced to a wish that they could have the female's procreative abilities.

Boys at about age 4 focus a good deal of attention on the penis, and this leads naturally to use of the penis, especially when erect, as something to thrust against or into objects or people in a sensual or aggressive way.

The experience in Western culture is that between ages 4 and 6 years, both little boys and little girls go through a phase of immaturely perceived sexual love for the parent of the opposite sex, followed by the inevitable disappointment when it becomes clear that competition with the father (or mother) for exclusive possession of the other parent is a lost cause. The child must relinquish the parent as sex object without losing the parent's support and love and yet retain an interest in the opposite sex. How well the 3 parties handle the renunciation will determine to a great extent the child's emotional stability and maturity in later life. If the parents are themselves free of conflicts about the child's sexual impulses and careful to avoid any semblance of participation in sexual behavior with the child, the child will eventually learn to select appropriate sexual objects outside the family. The result will be increased self-respect and even pride in having taken a step toward growing up.

The differences between sexual behavior in developing boys and girls may depend in part on the fact that, although the first love object for both is a woman, the boy must renounce the sexual elements of this love while preserving the possibility of such sexual love with another woman later. The girl does not have to experience this painful separation of loves so acutely, since her attachment to her mother can continue along with the development of her heterosexual interest in her father and other males.* It seems certain now that girls may achieve femininity without going through an acute phase of envying boys, although many girls go through a phase of wishing they had a penis (not necessarily wishing they were boys), and some girls experience a sense of deficiency about this, especially in families where boys are more highly valued by the parents. Girls may dress like boys and engage in activities traditionally associated more with boys than with girls, such as rough competitive play. Such behavior may be a repudiation of femininity. It is common in Western society for alternations of sex identification to continue for several years until a sense of self as female becomes established. Aside from this, girls who otherwise identify completely with their mothers and have no problems about accepting their own femininity may seek assertive goals much as boys do simply because of the physical mastery and competitive gratifications that can be achieved in that way. If the child's sexual feelings during this early period of sexual discovery and experimentation are accepted by the parents as natural and dealt with by means of simple explanations and reassurance, the child will turn its attentions to things in which success is possible while quietly continuing to explore sexuality in secrecy or with other children.

If this period of life is disrupted by separation or by illness or injury of the child or parents or if there are covert seductions, sexualization of the child/parent relationship, reversals of the child/parent roles, vicarious encouragements of sibling sexual play, etc, anxi-

---

*Controversy over the psychology of female sexual development has continued ever since Freud advanced his first tentative conclusions 80 years ago. At present, opinion is widely diverse even among psychoanalysts.

ety will be experienced in the context of the child's sexual preoccupations and may leave psychic stains that will persist as dominant themes in psychologic treatment later.

Guilt

The rudimentary moral sense developing in the child during this period engenders feelings of guilt that can be relieved by punishment and forgiveness. Guilt may arise over secret behavior or secret thoughts and fantasies. Provocative behavior toward the parents may be unconsciously calculated to elicit punishment for relief of guilt about sexual, hostile, or destructive fantasies of which the child feels the parents would disapprove. This inclination to punish oneself continues to some degree throughout life, in proportion to the dominance of an unconscious talion principle of wrongdoing and its deserved consequences ("an eye for an eye," etc).

The Role of Fantasy

One of the most remarkable human traits is the capacity for fantasy and the use of words and symbols and directed memories to enhance fantasy. Children try to make sense out of experiences; they hypothesize, engage in research, and reach conclusions—as their elder counterparts must do also—on the basis of imperfect understanding, and attempt to control and change what they find unsatisfactory. When humans fail, they have recourse to imagination and verbal ratiocination where problems yield to magical solutions and defects can be relived as victories. All this is explicit in children's games, the stories they invent, and the fairy tales they love. Some of the fantasies of childhood survive in the unconscious and reappear in adult life in the form of dreams, in the free association of patients in psychiatric treatment, and in the waking lives of psychotic patients. The ability to fantasize increases as the cognitive skills gain sophistication. At each succeeding level of development, earlier conscious preoccupations are reworked. Through this process, some unconscious distortions, formed in childhood and resurfacing in psychotherapy, can be examined and corrected.

The Effects of Illness in Childhood

A child's reaction to illness or injury is conditioned by 3 factors: (1) the specifics of the disorder (severity, duration, signs and symptoms); (2) the stage of psychologic development already achieved, and its stability; and (3) the response of parents and siblings. The most obvious reaction is regression, eg, clinging, whining, thumb-sucking, and bed-wetting in a child who has outgrown such "babyish" behavior. The younger child is most fearful of separation; an older preschooler may also fear mutilation (if surgery is necessary) or may perceive the illness as punishment for misdemeanors committed or contemplated.

Children also tend to take cues from their parents. If the parents are horrified, paralyzed with fear, dis-

gusted, or angered by the child's misfortune, and if they withdraw, they will compound the psychologic and physical damage. Psychologic trauma can be minimized if the parents maintain a compassionate and supportive attitude and are especially attentive during the most stressful phase without being overindulgent.

Cognitive Advances

During the preschool years, the child's thinking is largely egocentric, as it was during the sensorimotor period. It is still impossible at this age to hold in mind both the concept of a thing in its entirety and the individuality of its parts. Appearance dominates judgment, so that something very long and thin may be considered "larger" than something with much more bulk but not so long. Most things are seen in terms of absolutes: best/worst, bad/good, etc. The 5-year-old is not adept at comparisons or basic mathematical concepts. When they are spread out in front of her, a little girl may know there are 10 pieces of candy. After they are lumped into a mound or put into a paper sack, she is no longer sure and must count them again.

Words are especially important in this very egocentric stage. Children are often deeply hurt by being called names, because words are perceived as concrete things and have a magical capacity to stand as accomplished facts, as if the name-caller were actually making them into the derogated thing.

Children of this age have only a vague concept of time. Today, yesterday, and tomorrow may be clear enough, but the child 4–5 years old has difficulty envisioning how long it will be from now until 2 or 3 days from now, and the distant past and recent past may be lumped together as "day before yesterday." A physical illness may be described as the result of some aspect of the child's personal experience, usually a single sensory experience. "How did you get sick?" "It was the night, at night," or "I played with John." Toward the end of this period, a grasp of impersonal causality begins to dawn and egocentrism weakens.

THE SCHOOL-AGE YEARS: AGE 6–12

During the sixth or seventh year, most children have matured enough so that they can spend part of each day in some kind of educational experience and apart from their attachment figures. They have all the cognitive abilities and controls that are needed to conduct themselves well away from home. By this time, children have renounced incestuous love and have turned toward relationships with peers and interests in how the world works.

However, what may appear to be independent functioning at this age still depends on reliable adult backing for its consolidation and continuance. Under conditions of social deprivation, when children of this age are left to their own devices, a premature and pathologic spirit of independence and self-reliance may develop. Although perhaps permitting survival in abnormal circumstances such as war or mass disasters, too much independence too early prevents the full development of the individual.

Sexual Latency, or Moratorium

The disappearance of observable sexual behavior in most children in Western society at this age (and the disinclination of adults to acknowledge such behavior in children of any age) first suggested that this period was one of sexual latency and diminished sex drive. What seems more likely is that the energies formerly expended on sexual competition within the family are now turned outward (**sublimated**). Internally, eroticism continues in clandestine forms.

Despite frequent regression in the face of disappointment and frustration, school-age children are resourceful in their own behalf and are beginning to be less rigid in their moral judgments. It is natural at this time to conform to the mores and "dress code" of schoolmates, and there is often also a general disillusionment—at least overtly—with the parental image. If the parents continue to offer loving support and guidance, the child will continue to identify with the general characteristics of the parent of the same sex. During elementary school years and adolescence, when issues of self-esteem are so important, the child needs the help of parents, older siblings, and teachers in gradually acquiring skills that call for patience and practice.

During this period, there is an obvious voluntary separation of the sexes. Protestations of contempt by each group for the other may be an attempt to control uncomfortable interests in sexuality. Preference for playmates of the same sex appears to be a cultural phenomenon, since overt heterosexual behavior is evident and encouraged in some cultures during the preteen years.

Cognitive Advances

During this phase, maturation of the central nervous system and cumulative life experiences enable children to relate the parts of an object to its whole and to retain a concept of the whole while considering the parts. Children learn not only to conceive a course of events from the beginning to the end but also to understand it back from the end to the beginning. Piaget calls this **operational thought.** In the early (concrete) stage of operational thinking, the operations still depend on the child's perception of how things appear to be. Later, during adolescence, "formal" (abstract) thinking begins: thinking about thought.

In this concrete stage, children begin to understand systems of classification. For example, "nesting" is descriptive of all classes that are additive; each larger category sums up all of the previous parts. It is only now that they can understand the question, "Are there more birds or more crows in the world?" With this ability, children can conceptualize experiences individually and then organize them as parts of a larger whole. The change is from an inductive to a deductive way of understanding the world and from magical thinking to a more scientific approach. This knowledge precedes the ability to apply the knowledge very well or to put it into words—a 7-year-old has difficulty explaining *why* there are more birds than crows—and the new skills are used mostly in the service of the social and gratification aims characteristic of earlier phases of development, such as defeating others in competition or getting more treats.

Because the child at this age is better able to perceive cause and effect, there is a shift from categorical judgments learned by rote toward cognitive manipulation of rules and reasons. As the ability to understand and manipulate the environment increases, the environment becomes more stimulating, a better place to be. Cooperative play in groups occurs, since intrafamilial competitiveness can now be expressed through games and fantasies. As the child proceeds through the elementary school years, rules become more reasonable and ideas of punishment less strict. Right and wrong begin to lose their absolute qualities.

School

Going to school is the single most significant developmental event of childhood. When children leave their families and even their neighborhood groups to go to school for a significant part of most days, all of the deficiencies of social and behavioral interaction that have been tolerated or gone unnoticed in the home environment come to light. Although there are many causes of school difficulties and suboptimal achievement in class, the most prevalent ones are cultural or economic deprivation resulting in ego development inadequate to the task of schooling.

ADOLESCENCE

The task of describing the extraordinarily complex and variable normal adolescent experience is not undertaken here, but the following can act as an outline and summary of adolescent development.

Despite the time that has elapsed since Freud first began to write about it, the major developmental concerns of adolescence remain the same 2 he considered: (1) establishment of a firm individuality (a sense of self or ego identity) and (2) integration of the pubertal surge of sexual and aggressive impulses. Both of these, familiar from childhood, are the psychologic concomitants of the physical developments of puberty: The maturing motor system of the body approaches adult strength and adeptness; the hormonal shift and spurt announce the capacity for fertilization; and the increase in neuronal complexity in the brain makes adult thinking and judgment possible. Social skills developed in relationships with family members, playmates, and others determine whether the transition to adulthood will be turbulent or smooth over a short or long course of time. Studies of other societies and of different social classes within Western society indicate vast differences in the degrees of difficulty experienced during this period.

Adolescence begins with the recognizable physical changes of puberty. The subsequent stages of psychologic advance, regression and regrouping, partial fixation, and further advance are diverse and may occur simultaneously or alternatingly in any one young person. The end point of adolescence is defined by social rather than physical criteria and is the subject of much dispute between the generations. Eventually, however, the press of physical maturation carries the young person out of adolescence and into adulthood.

For our purposes here, the end of adolescence is defined as that point in young life when the major social investiture for the given social class is complete—so that the obligations and privileges of adulthood are assumed. The duration of this process will be short or long in direct relation to local conditions of survival, ie, the need to augment the procreative, work, or fighting forces. In many societies it is quite short; in some classes of Western society, it is an extended period complicated by irresolution or enhanced by refinements of education, travel, or pleasure-seeking activity.

An Outline of Adolescence

Those who have studied and written about normal adolescence in North America commonly perceive 3 stages: early, middle, and late. Some add preadolescent and postadolescent ("youth") phases, which helps to emphasize that this period is inextricable from what went before and what follows. In most instances, it is clear that in the year or so before the onset of puberty there begins a restless increase in motor and psychologic needs typical of the same individual during ages 2–4. The young person is harder to get along with; the activities of the school years are no longer so satisfying; and parental control becomes difficult to sustain. A characteristic of this period is that children of both sexes turn away from their mothers, the boy to his "gang" and the girl to her circle of close friends. These changes intensify as physical development proceeds.

Early adolescence. Adolescence begins with the advent of pubertal change, when new ways of self-expression (sexual and social) and new skills emerge. These new interests are noticeable because people outside the family become the objects of further attachment. The relationships available within the family are no longer sufficient to gratify the new aspirations of a progressively more vigorous and sexual person. Early adolescents usually make an effort to contain their drives within the bounds of family life, but the result may severely test the parental relationship. If demands for growing space and sexual expression can be recognized and progressive emancipation allowed, the family will remain a source of support and guidance during these experimental sallies into a widening world.

Much has been written of the "turbulence" of adolescence in Western society. However, it is only when behavior is primarily antiself, antifamilial, or antisocial that one must suspect pathogenic forces at work, especially within the family. These potentially destructive forces sometimes lead young people to seek support and remedial experiences elsewhere. If a benevolent outside environment meets the need, the troubled youngster may be able to continue normal development and make a successful adult adjustment. More often, however, such conflicts lead to fixation at an immature stage, premature rupture of family relationships, or partial regression to earlier stages.

Despite the risks, most young people are irresistibly drawn toward the satisfactions and prerogatives older people seem to enjoy, especially in the area of sexual experience. Even in what is perceived to be a permissive modern society, young people continue to experience conflict over sexual impulses and their expression. Childhood fantasies about sexual anatomy and function may persist into these years in spite of free access to accurate information about sex and procreation.

In most socioeconomic classes, overt sexual behavior during early and middle adolescence is suppressed, deflected, or repressed, despite the exploitation of sexuality in our culture. Premature sexual experience is eluded through the escape channels of masturbation and verbalization of fantasies with peers of the same sex.

Early adolescence is characterized by increased introspection and self-absorption, exciting but unspeakable new sensations (including masturbation to orgasm), and changes in physical proportions such that the body image established through the school years is destabilized. Since much of what is happening cannot even be discussed with the parents, young people at this age form intense personal relationships with one or 2 "best friends" of the same age and sex. Transient identification with adolescent or adult groups provides opportunities for young people to try various roles. The first contact with drugs usually occurs at this time—mostly marihuana and the inexpensive hallucinogens as well as "uppers" and "downers." The influence of respected peers is of great importance in avoiding or pursuing destructive drug use. Constructive friendships, sexual fantasy, and growing pleasure in physical and intellectual activity are in most cases preferred alternatives to drug abuse or hazardous sexual escapades.

The attention of adolescents fluctuates back and forth from friend to self, to idealized heroes and back again to self. Bursts of activity alternate with almost interminable periods of passive absorption in music, reading, video games, and television. A wish to be different is paradoxically combined with a passionate insistence on sameness, so that having the same designer brand of jeans or jacket or the same earrings as their special friends becomes an urgent necessity. Adolescents seem to form a subculture—a world apart to which only the young can belong.

It was once assumed that a turbulent adolescence was essential to full development. However, research by Offer (1969) and others has demonstrated that only about one-fifth of normal adolescents have a stormy time; about the same proportion proceed smoothly to normal adulthood; and the remainder show turmoil and anxiety in surges, with spurts of development and periods of stress and stalled progress.

Middle adolescence. Eventually, after consolidation through relationships with peers has occurred and experience with fantasy loses its appeal, boys and girls become overtly interested in each other as the objects of sexual behavior, and middle adolescence holds sway. The boy has commonly focused until now on male identification models, whereas the girl has in most cases maintained an active interest in boys and in both male and female idols. Such interest is usually free of conscious sexual content. With the beginning of focused heterosexual interest, the preoccupation with intimate friendship, masturbation, and sexual play with members of the same sex are replaced by identifications with *groups* of people. The demanding, argumentative, dependent relationship with the father or (most often) mother often suddenly resolves. School clubs, athletics, and social activities of all kinds now provide opportunities to add a physical dimension to relationships with young people of the opposite sex. Access to cars, later hours, more money, and less adult supervision have the same effect.

During this period of increasing sexual expression, it continues to be obvious how private conversations ("woman talk", "man talk") with peers of the same sex protect against premature heterosexual activity. Excessive modesty (or its equivalent, nervous flirting) reflects the strength of the sexual impulses and the energy being expended on their suppression. Undoubtedly, some adolescents accelerate their development during this phase, while others, feeling hopelessly outclassed and frightened, falter and stop in some fixated state. Still a third group, inconsistently guided or ignored by their parents at earlier stages, take license for freedom and attempt by extreme behavior to provoke parents and other authority figures to set needed minimum limits.

In early mid adolescence, as the search for self-mastery and satisfying heterosexual relationships reaches its apex, we see all the forward, backward, and lateral movement that characterizes the adolescent in our society. The object of "first love" usually resembles in some way the parent of the opposite sex, or—if the conflict over renouncing the parent as a sexual goal was too intense—he or she may have diametrically opposite physical traits. The young person usually identifies with the parent of the same sex at this time, often in open imitation of dress and mannerisms. The boy becomes suddenly more integrated, genuinely manly, as compared with earlier strutting and posing. The girl becomes more womanly, as compared with her former vanities and affectations. This accomplishment marks the end of the middle adolescent period.

Late adolescence. In late adolescence, a consolidation of personality occurs, with relative stability and consonance of feelings and behavior. There is often a decrease in introspection and creative imagination characteristic of earlier adolescence. By the end of this period, one can recognize in young people's styles of behavior striking similarities to those they formerly repudiated in their parents. The admired and respected parental values have been made their own, and in this way the generations are linked. The gender and libidinal struggles of mid adolescence yield center stage to the search for vocational choice and a satisfying position in the social group. Students who have done poorly in grades 8–11 suddenly, with the close of the major developmental press of the first 2 adolescent phases, may take up their studies with dedication and qualify for college.

For some young people in middle-class society, late adolescence means that school is finished and work and spousal choices are made or imminent. They pass immediately into adulthood. For others, late adolescence marks the beginning of long years of further schooling and professional training—a phase of adulthood beyond adolescence but short of the full investments of adulthood. In this "youth" phase, some of the hallmarks of adolescent student status persist.

Psychologically speaking, however, normal adolescence comes to a close in the college years (at about age 20) for those continuing in school. Adolescent-type conflicts may linger, but adolescence is over. A 24-year-old graduate student with identity diffusion or antisocial behavior, which might be normal for some 16-year-olds, is not a person with prolonged adolescence but an adult with problems.

Along with the maturing cognitive abilities, people in late adolescence usually become less preoccupied with themselves and more concerned with cultural values and ideologies. They become seriously interested in theology, ethics, or politics, but usually still in a tentative, reversible way, expecting that bad outcomes can be expunged, amnesty granted, and records sealed. Commitment to a "cause" may also represent some of the energy loosened from family ties and is an outlet for energies not yet invested in love and other adult preoccupations.

Cognitive Advances

During the elementary school-age years, problem-solving activity is mostly limited to actual situations in the real or fantasy world. At some time between ages 12 and 15—usually in the stage described here as early adolescence—some young people develop the ability to deal with abstractions, to think also about possibilities. Piaget calls this the **stage of formal operations** to emphasize that the form of the proposition is what is important, not the content, as in the formulas of mathematics. In formal-stage thinking, the individual abstracts the key elements and then is able, through mental processes, to combine, reverse, and recombine them into possibilities that perhaps never were or may never become actualized. This capacity contributes to the adolescent's propensity toward moral abstraction, grandiosity, idealism, and dedication to things that "could be but are not." Although Piaget described this development as the final stage in normal cognitive growth, it should be regarded as a special achievement rather than a universal expectation. As Dulit (1972) and others have demonstrated, only about one-third of adults function to a large extent in the formal stage; another third do so some of the time but have no need for it in their daily lives; and the rest never achieve it at all. Although the capacity for formal thought is correlated with normal intelligence, it is not directly related to it. Failure to progress to the concrete stage from preoperational thinking is evidence of mental deficiency or disorder; this is not necessarily the case with failure to achieve the formal stage in adolescence. Most people move on from the concrete stage to learn workaday techniques for solving life's problems and have no practical use for the skills of the formal stage.

Attachment

The second decade of life is the time when people learn how to care for themselves in the world. The dependence on the primary attachment figures characteristic of the first decade—being cared for—gives way gradually to a measured independence. Physical and emotional separation from the parents occurs, sexual identity is consolidated, and sexual interest is directed toward peers. By the close of adolescence, love rela-tionships are reflecting the quality of the old attachments, this time including tender and satisfying genital sexuality with an emotionally valued partner.

When this process is accomplished, usually early in the third decade, the young adult is prepared to begin to care for others. The attachment cycle completes itself in the quality of care provided to a new generation. At this point, young adults can return to their parents on a basis of equality. Old attachments continue to express themselves in attenuated form in letters, telephone calls, and visits, and attachment figures are sought out in times of sadness or adversity, giving structure and continuity to personal relationships over a lifetime.

Most writers in this field of study agree that psychologic development can continue throughout life, and understanding later life phases is important in medical treatment. Since so many clinicians have found Erik Erikson's work on the entire life cycle helpful, the next chapter will describe Erikson's view of each phase in detail. A summary of it is included in Table 6–1.

REFERENCES

Bandura A, Walters R: *Social Learning and Personality Development*. Holt, Rinehart, & Winston, 1963.

Bowlby J: *Attachment*, 2nd ed. Vol 1 of: *Attachment and Loss*. Basic Books, 1983.

Bowlby J: The nature of the child's tie to his mother. *Int J Psychoanal* 1958;**39**:350.

Breger L: *From Instinct to Identity: The Development of Personality*. Prentice-Hall, 1974.

Dulit E: Adolescent thinking à la Piaget: The formal stage. *J Youth Adolesc* 1972;**4**:281.

Engel G: *Psychological Development in Health and Disease*. Saunders, 1962.

Erikson E: *Identity and the Life Cycle*. Internat Univ Press, 1959.

Gesell A: *Gesell and Amatrude's Developmental Diagnosis*, 3rd ed. Knoblock H, Pasamanick B (editors). Harper & Row, 1974.

Lewis M: *Clinical Aspects of Child Development*, 2nd ed. Lea & Febiger, 1982.

Lorenz K: Der Kumpan in der Umwelt des Vogels. English translation in: *Instinctive Behavior*. Shiller C (editor). Internat Univ Press, 1957.

Maccoby E: *Social Development: Psychological Growth and the Parent-Child Relationship*. Harcourt Brace Jovanovich, 1980.

Mahler M, Pine F, Bergman A: *The Psychological Birth of the Human Infant*. Basic Books, 1975.

Maier H: *Three Theories of Child Development*, rev ed. Harper & Row, 1969.

Main M, Kaplan K, Cassidy J: Security in infancy, childhood and adulthood: A move to the level of representation. Growing points in attachment theory. *Monogr Soc Res Child Dev* 1985;**50**:1.

Mussen P, Conger J, Kagan J: *Child Development and Personality*, 5th ed. Harper & Row, 1979.

Offer D: *The Psychological World of the Teenager*. Basic Books, 1969.

Piaget J, Inhelder B: *The Psychology of the Child*. Basic Books, 1969.

Rutter M: Meyerian psychobiology, personality development, and the role of life experiences. *Am J Psychiatry* 1986;**143**:9.

Scott J: The process of primary socialization in canine and human infants. *Monogr Soc Res Child Dev* 1963;**28**:1.

Sears R, Maccoby E, Levin H: *Patterns of Child Rearing*. Harper & Row, 1957.

Skinner B: *Science and Human Behavior*. Macmillan, 1953.

Stern D: *The Interpersonal World of the Infant*. Basic Books, 1985.

Szurek S: The needs of adolescents for emotional health. Page 157 in: *Modern Perspectives in Adolescent Psychiatry*. Howells J (editor). Oliver & Boyd, 1969.

Thomas A, Chess S: *The Dynamics of Psychological Development*. Brunner/Mazel, 1980.

Vaillant G: Theoretical hierarchy of adaptive ego mechanisms. *Arch Gen Psychiatry* 1971;**24**:107.

Winnicott D: Transitional objects and transitional phenomena. *Int J Psychoanal* 1953;**34**:1.

7

Normal Psychologic Development

Nancy B. Kaltreider, MD

This chapter will set out a broad framework of normal developmental patterns as currently understood in Western society, relying principally on Erik Erikson's model of psychosocial stages. Particularly in childhood, additional models stressing cognition and learning theory are a useful supplement to this broadly based approach. (See Chapter 6.) A complex of biologic, constitutional, cultural, and environmental factors influence each phase of development. Thus, behavior of any individual at any given stage cannot be attributed to any single factor, and of course it would not be possible to specify perfect conditions for rearing all children. However, children arrive in the world with inborn needs and propensities, and they must progress through fairly distinct developmental stages each of which involves certain hazards along with the potential for growth. The use of a systematic framework for describing psychologic development is helpful in understanding the life stresses of patients in all types of medical practice.

ERIK ERIKSON
(1902–   )

Erik Erikson was born in Germany and began his professional training in Vienna, where he was analyzed by Anna Freud and was the first man trained as a Montessori teacher. He ventured to the USA in 1933 and continued his studies of the meaning of children's play. He lived with a number of Native American tribes to observe how child-rearing practices prepared young people to assume the social roles expected of them as adults. He participated in the Berkeley longitudinal multiracial study of normal child development. Out of these cross-cultural experiences came his first book, *Childhood and Society* (1959), which summarized his interests in the synthesis of developmental and social tasks. He has always been somewhat ahead of his time, writing in the 1950s about black identity, the changing role of women, and the alienation of young people in Western culture.

Erikson developed one of many approaches to understanding the psychosocial developmental sequence. It has the advantage of covering the total life span and interweaving concepts of psychodynamics, family structure, social setting, and individual historical-cultural factors. The information in Chapter 6 on cognitive and behavioral development in the early years should be integrated with what is said in this chapter in order to provide a more comprehensive view.

Erikson's view of psychologic development (Table 7–1) is analogous to that of embryogenesis: Anything that grows has a basic plan; and out of this plan the elements of the personality arise, each having its time of special ascendancy, until all parts of the psyche form a functioning whole.

On the continuum of development, the individual is confronted by major "tasks" that must be accomplished in a series of stages. Each stage is dominated by one main task, though elements of others may have to be dealt with also, and each stage is related to the others as parts of a sequential developmental whole. Grappling with the major and minor tasks is the developing individual's way of achieving the "success" of normality manifest in a healthy personality—a hazy concept defined as follows by Jahoda (1958): "A healthy personality *actively* masters his or her environment, shows a certain unity of personality and is able to perceive the world and him [self] or herself correctly." Normality is much more than just the absence of maladjustment. Failure to master the major task of any developmental period leaves an area of vulnerability that may become manifest later as impaired adult function.

Table 7–1. Erikson's conception of developmental sequence.

Psychosocial Stage	Age (years)	Polarity
I. Oral-sensory	0–1	Trust versus mistrust
II. Muscular-anal	1–3	Autonomy versus shame and doubt
III. Locomotor-genital	3–6	Initiative versus guilt
IV. Latency	6–12	Industry versus inferiority
V. Puberty and adolescence	12–20	Identity versus role confusion
VI. Young adulthood	20–30	Intimacy versus isolation
VII. Adulthood	30–65	Generativity versus self-absorption or stagnation
VIII. Maturity and death	65 and older	Ego integrity versus despair

Erikson's Stage I. Trust Versus Mistrust: Birth to 1 Year

The first component of a healthy personality that must be developed is a sense of basic trust, a conviction that oneself and the world are both worthy of trust. What is needed for the essential forming of human attachment is consistent parenting and stimulation. Without it, even if adequate food, clothing, and shelter are provided, the infant will fail to sit, stand, or speak and may even die before its first birthday. With appropriate stimulation, reflexive behavior is slowly replaced by voluntary movements. Because the ability to take in by mouth corresponds to the parent's intention to feed and welcome the new baby, the mouth is the focus of the first approach to life (the "oral stage"). But the baby is receptive to the environment in many other ways, so that visual and other (nonoral) tactile stimuli are eagerly received.

The need for parenting. By 6–9 months, interaction with the environment becomes more active. Teeth can now bite into and through; eyes can focus so that the hands can grasp objects; hands not only grasp but hold; and ears can localize the source of sounds. Taking now extends to holding onto, and biting encourages weaning.

The critical role of the primary caregiver has been demonstrated using an animal model. Harlow and Harlow (1971) separated infant monkeys from their mothers at birth and put them in cages with so-called surrogate mothers. The infant monkeys preferred cuddling with a terry cloth mother doll to receiving milk from a wire doll. To Harlow's greater surprise, the monkeys raised without mothering or peer interaction for 6 months were later found to be sexually inept and completely uninterested in mothering their own offspring. In humans, when the reinforcing interaction with the parent fails, the situation falls apart and the infant tries to restore control by random activity; it may activate itself to exhaustion or find its thumb and damn the world. Severe early social deprivation or gross inconsistencies in parenting may set the pattern for major adult mental disorder.

The first stage of development, which takes place during the first year of life, should result in a feeling of basic trust in the world derived from the parents' consistent care. The danger in this period is a sense of mistrust leading to feelings of emptiness and to withdrawal from a nonloving world.

Erikson's Stage II. Autonomy Versus Shame & Doubt: 1–3 Years

A review of the chapter headings in Spock's (1957) baby book suggests that some major changes are occurring around age 1 year: "feeling his oats"; "the passion to explore"; "getting more dependent and more independent at the same time"; "biting humans"; "the small child who won't stay in bed at night."

As children discover themselves, they are increasingly delighted with the idea of autonomy. However, it is the sense of basic trust and love that has freed them to explore, and they must frequently return to home base for reassurance. As muscles mature, the infant begins to experiment with 2 different modalities: holding on and letting go. Psychoanalytic theorists have called this the anal period, because sphincter control is a model of the crisis faced. External controls at this stage must be reassuring enough to allow children to trust themselves, yet firm enough to protect them from a feeling of anarchy ruled by poorly controlled drives. With too much shaming, children seek to produce only repetitive controlled situations in the model of the adult obsessive compulsive. They may develop a permanent sense of being "too little" and may respond with a secret determination to get away with things unseen. Much of the struggle is apt to focus on sphincter control, since control of elimination is of great importance in most human societies. Erikson calls this preoccupation "the ideal of a mechanically trained, faultlessly functioning, and always clean, punctual, and deodorized body." Language development begins to help in the evolution of control systems. The ideal is to say, "Look at the pretty flower"—and thus divert the child from eating it.

So the second stage is based on a sense of mastery—that the child can feel in control of its drives and able to separate briefly from the parent without feeling unable to deal with the world. Even at this early age, signs of severely disordered behavior can appear with an unclear level of contribution from both developmental and genetic factors. Such children may seem unable to relate from birth or may show initial adaptation followed by regression. They are generally indifferent to others, unable to use language for communication, and show an obsessive desire for sameness.

Erikson's Stage III. Initiative Versus Guilt: 3–6 Years

Erikson wrote as follows: "Having found a firm solution of his problem of autonomy, the child of 4 or 5 is faced with the next step—and with the next crisis. Being firmly convinced that he is a person, the child must now find out what kind of person he is going to be. And here he hitches his wagon to nothing less than a star; he wants to be like his parents, who to him appear very powerful and very beautiful, although quite unreasonably dangerous." The child "identifies with them" and plays with the idea of how it would be to be them. No matter what the cultural background, almost every child seems to have some variety of the daydream, "When I grow up I will marry Mommy [or Daddy]." Although first formally recognized by Freud in the analysis of neurotic patients, the so-called Oedipus complex is a recurrent theme in world literature. The child attaches considerable significance to the fantasy of replacing the parent of the same sex. In the case of both sexes, the wish is strong enough to create a period of conflict in the child, since the very nature of the wish implies rivalry with the parent of the same sex and aggressive fantasies directed against that parent.

But this period creates the impossible situation in which the rival parent is also the object of love. Guilt over the aggressive wishes can be discerned in the content of the frequently appearing "night terrors" in which the young dreamer is punished by monsters. The increased mastery and pride in being big now receives its severest setback in the clear fact that in the sexual and reproductive sphere the child is vastly inferior to the same-sexed parent.

Rivalry with parent. Resolution of this crisis seems tied to a strengthened identification with the parent who has so recently been the rival. For the boy, it is as if he reasons as follows: "Since I cannot take my father's place, I will be like him." If because of death, divorce, or any other reason the parent of the same sex is unavailable during this period, delinquent behavior in later childhood and adolescence is more apt to occur. The new sense of initiative spreads to enjoyment of competition, pursuit of goals, and pleasure in conquest.

The stage is thus set for the entrance into "real life"—except that school must come first. Thus, at ages 4 and 5, the child toys with the fantasy of "becoming" the parent, then renounces that idea, then develop a stronger sense of identification with the parent of the same sex, and finally marshals new energies for dealing with peers and school.

Erikson's Stage IV. Industry Versus Inferiority: 6–12 Years

In most cultures, children begin to receive some type of systematic instruction at about age 6. Energies previously expended in dealing with oedipal matters are now freed for full involvement in learning and doing. In contrast to earlier autonomous play, the object now is "being the best" in comparison with peers rather than adults. The child's abundant resources are turned toward mastery of the new social environment of school. Physical maturation slows, and social sex roles begin to be more clearly defined.

The success for which a child strives is a sense of accomplishment for having done well—failure is avoided at all costs. Most of a child's energy is poured into the effort to develop mastery and control. Piaget stresses that children build their mental capacities to order and relate experience to an organized whole. They may become preoccupied with establishing systems of classification. Collecting things and arranging them in order is a popular hobby. Life proceeds smoothly in a carefully structured world, but when that structure is threatened, children quickly fall back upon earlier intuitive methods of functioning. A major cause of vulnerability during this period is that they are still children, incomplete adults, and apt to feel inferior. Unsuccessful resolution of earlier phases leaves ongoing conflicts that may siphon off needed energy. Freudians refer to this interval as the latency period, which refers to lack of striving toward involvement with a partner of the opposite sex. More recently, it has been argued that the prolonged "latency" of sexu-

ality is more of a middle-class cultural phenomenon than an inborn suspension of drive.

Society enlarges. Children begin to see their parents as representatives of a larger society and to measure them against other representatives. The mother may find her view of the world held in less esteem than one offered by an admired grade-school teacher. The base of identification broadens, as does the child's awareness that there are many authorities besides the parents.

Erikson notes that many of the individual's later attitudes toward work can be traced to the sense of industry fostered during this period. In taking a quick developmental history, the latency period is a profitable one to inquire about, because clear successes suggest that healthy resolution of previous crisis periods has occurred.

One could say that personality at the first stage ("basic trust") crystallizes around the conviction, "I am what I am given"; that of the second ("autonomy"), "I am what I will." A third ("initiative") can be characterized by "I am what I imagine I will be"; and latency ("competence") by "I am what I learn." With the establishment of a good relationship to the world of skills, childhood as such comes to an end.

Erikson's Stage V. Identity Versus Role Confusion: 12–20 Years

Anna Freud (1958) wrote, "Adolescence is by its nature an interruption of peaceful growth, and the upholding of a steady equilibrium during the adolescent process is in itself abnormal." In other words, it seems almost impossible to sever parental ties and develop a firm self-concept without experimentation and some crisis—for both the adolescent and the parents. Offer's recent work suggests that many individuals progress through this period of transition without major upheaval.

Assessment of adolescent changes must be very cautious, since the normative crises produce inconsistent and unpredictable behavior. Adolescents are faced with physiologic revolution from within and a society structured by previous generations from without; somehow, they must evolve a sense of who they are in their own eyes and in the eyes of others. Erikson's phrase "identity crisis" is now widely used, but it is important to remember that Erikson sees adolescence as a developmental phase and not an affliction.

Physical changes. Physical changes are prominent and dramatic in adolescence, and preoccupation with these changes is inevitable. There is a wide variation in the onset and tempo of puberty, so that the adolescent lives through a period of being different from peers in both physical development and interests. Often there is a particular concern with sexual characteristics—body hair, the breasts, the penis—with frequent shower room comparisons. The body is subjected to such careful scrutiny that the slightest perceived defect—a cowlick or a pimple—is submitted to anxious inspection and study. Early adolescents may transiently develop physical features associated with the opposite sex—prepubertal mammary fat in boys or a lanky "tomboy" look in girls. Adolescents often undergo medical examinations with self-conscious reluctance, fearing perhaps that the doctor will discover something abnormal or see evidence of masturbation.

The adolescent who comes to a physician for a checkup or with some minor physical complaint may be motivated by unspoken fears. The physical act of masturbation is more acceptable in our current society than was formerly the case, but the fantasies associated with the act are still a rich source of guilt feelings; reaction to these feelings may bring teenagers in for reassurance that their bodies are intact and sexually normal. Young patients seeking help for overweight may really be wondering if their late-developing bodies will ever achieve the desired physical configuration. Fears of venereal disease or pregnancy and a need for contraceptive advice are probably the most common reasons teenagers seek out physicians, yet they may be strangely silent on these subjects in the office. Sympathetic questioning and an offer of factual sexual information are most useful, but the doctor must detect the underlying concern rather than present a prepared speech. The fact that a teenager is sexually active does not guarantee an adequate knowledge of the "facts of life."

Tension and anxiety. Adolescents have brought with them from the latency period an increased tolerance for tension that makes the organized pursuit of learning possible. They now have an opportunity to rework childhood problems. Suddenly the young person's struggle for individualism is pitted against society's dictum about his or her appropriate role. Youth is characteristically a period of social ferment, and Goodman (1962), in *Growing Up Absurd,* suggests that nonconformity is often an imaginative response to an adult world that fails to provide decent jobs, homes, and values into which young people may grow. In contrast to earlier agricultural cultures, our society is not prepared to grant full entry into adult life until after the second decade, and postgraduate education and professional apprenticeships may postpone full adult status into the thirties. Adolescents develop new defenses to deal with intensified drives. They may develop interests in abstruse subjects, convening for hours to discuss erudite problems and taking uncompromising stands on both practical and idealistic grounds. This rigidity may be intensified when young people find their parents disappointing models and fear that circumstances will cause them to "end up in the same way." Group sanctions play a major role in the development and internalization of standards.

Sexual changes. On the threshold of puberty, both sexes go through a stage of having one "best" friend of the same sex, frequent crushes on idealized figures, and a comfortable attraction to members of both sexes. Szurek (1971) observes that the chum becomes the object of intense interest and absorption. Even a short separation must be quickly ended by a phone call. "The need to validate his or her own reactions, feelings, thoughts with another undergoing similar experience appears insatiable." Fashions and fads are used to emphasize the adolescents' unique identity as a group. Girls mature 1–2 years earlier than boys and develop heterosexual interests more in the form of a yearning for tender love than relief from erotic tensions. In early puberty, boys are still oriented mostly toward peer groups, and the stirrings of sexuality are manifested in homosexual play, dirty language, exhibitionistic bragging about physical prowess, and general restlessness. Adolescence involves experimentation with a wide variety of roles. The adolescent must abandon the familiar love objects of childhood and often seems driven to create conflict in order to achieve separation from the parents. Open hostility and disenchantment, particularly with the parent of the same sex, accompanies a shift in family dynamics and reappraisal of the power structure. Independence from parents—so assiduously sought and so necessary—may be followed by feelings of emptiness (almost of mourning) on the part of both the adolescent and the parents.

Role confusion. The danger of this stage is role confusion. When this is based on a strong previous doubt about one's true sexual identity, delinquent and outright psychotic episodes are not uncommon. "Falling in love" is often used as a validation of one's own identity. If marriage occurs when the partners are young, still seeking their own identities, disappointment is frequent. When precipitated or followed soon by pregnancy, the necessary role adjustments may force premature settling into a life-style inappropriate either to parenting or to the couple's own needs. All too often, a young girl's wish for a child is really a wish to be mothered.

Experimentation with roles may lead to a feeling of being "phony" or even to a perverse choice of identity most abhorrent to the parents—as if it is better to be known as a "pothead" or an "easy lay" than to be not quite anybody. The considerate, submissive adolescent who remains tied to the family may achieve tranquility at the cost of not "growing up."

Consolidation. Late adolescence is a period of consolidation. It is a decisive turning point and may mark the onset of mental disorder. As the last vestige of childhood is given up, choices must be made about a basic philosophy of life, acceptance of authority, and orientation toward achievement. Not everyone is prepared to make commitments to a life role at the same time. An adolescent may choose to put off the decision until a broader range of life experiences has accumulated—to "take a moratorium" in Erikson's phrase. The common phenomenon of dropping out of school for a year of "bumming around" may be a healthy adaptive mechanism. In Erikson's words, "By free role experimentation [he] may find a niche in some section of society, a niche which is firmly defined and yet seems to be uniquely made for him." Young women are now struggling to realize a broader range of role possibilities that represent serious commitments and not just something to do "until the right man comes along."

Psychodynamic theories of adolescence have been colored by the fact that investigators have derived their data chiefly from observation of turbulent adolescent boys. More commonly, however, the progressive phases of adolescence include substantial periods of mastery and pleasure for those who have successfully weathered earlier developmental stages. The reworking of the past is seen in the merged issues of autonomy, sexuality, and identity; the cauldron within which these ingredients are stirred is the family, so that an interactive system is involved. Along with profound physical changes, maturation of cognitive skills and defensive flexibility are reflected in the need to build an independent value system. Friendships, peers, and adult mentors ease the transition from home to the adult world.

In summary, adolescence is a time of crisis with enormous potential for growth. At no other phase of life are the promise of finding oneself and the threat of losing oneself so intertwined. Upheaval is the external indication that internal adjustments are in progress as adult sexuality is integrated and identity choices are made. *It may be quite difficult to distinguish adolescent chaos from serious mental disorder.*

Erikson's Stage VI. Intimacy Versus Isolation: 20–30 Years

Continuing work by developmental theorists has underlined Erikson's premise that psychologic change is continuous throughout life; adulthood cannot be understood just by projecting forward salient issues of childhood. The popularity of *Passages* by Sheehy (1977) suggests the reader's recognition of patterns, so that although each individual's life is unique, there are anticipated steps though perhaps unequal in outward impact or varying in chronologic order. In their study of adult development, *The Seasons of a Man's Life,* Levinson and his colleagues (1978) describe these as "eras," periods of adult life that have distinct unifying qualities. Work published by Vaillant and Milofsky (1980) on the natural history of male psychologic health supported the major hypotheses of Erikson's writing: "First, the stages of men's life cycle must be passed through sequentially; failure to master one stage usually precludes mastery of subsequent stages. Second, the age at which a given stage is mastered varies enormously. Third, the stage attained by middle life appears quite independent of childhood social class or education, although adult maturation is correlated with whether childhood was conducive to basic trust, autonomy, and initiative."

Position of women. Most published developmental studies follow the time-honored tradition of studying men and extrapolating the results to women. Currently the issues are harder to define, because we are in a period of such rapid societal change. In less than a generation, the number of women holding jobs has more than doubled, mostly as a result of entry of married women into the work force. The chief impetus for this change is financial need, but the increased level of education achieved by women has not resulted in significantly higher economic status. For women, the issues of identity and autonomy may be only partially resolved when they enter the developmental phase of motherhood and then reenter the job market in later adult life. The stairstep pattern of developmental tasks is overlaid by more awareness of the biologic timetable; choices about pregnancy can only be made during the fertile years. The impact of the range of choices—to marry or stay single; whether or not to have children; to stay at home or to combine career and family; to be gay or bisexual; to be a single parent or to raise children in a communal setting—will require careful study to be integrated with our current understanding of normative adult development.

Early adulthood is a period of abundant possibilities—biologic, social, and otherwise—in which the individual must find some balance between settling down and moving forward. The task is to create a new life, apart from the parents but with a goal structure and openness to reattachment with new close ties.

Intimacy. Erikson writes, "It is only after a reasonable sense of identity has been established that real intimacy with the other sex—or, for that matter, with any other person or even oneself—is possible." This is the period of establishment of a stable love relationship in contrast to the more transitory ties of adolescence. The adult consolidation of the self as able to love helps in the resolution of earlier ambivalent relations with parental figures. The step toward intimacy is a frightening and decisive one—as perceptively viewed by Cleaver (1968) in a letter to Beverly in *Soul on Ice:*

> The reason two people are reluctant to really strip themselves naked in front of each other is because in so doing they make themselves vulnerable and give enormous power over themselves one to the other. . . . You beautifully spoke in your letter of "What an awesome thing it is to feel oneself on the verge of the possibility of really knowing another person. . ."

The fear of the commitment involved with intimacy can lead to a choice of isolation or of highly stereotyped interpersonal relations. It may seem safer to choose self-absorption than to seek an elusive closeness that seems potentially dangerous to one's own identity. There are other factors that interfere with intimacy. Young adulthood is a period of vigor and activity, with the establishment of a variety of different roles that are important in achieving identity and status.

When Freud was once asked what a normal person should be able to do, he replied simply, "To love and to work." In young adulthood, the balance of these—with love seen as the expansiveness of generosity as well as genital love and with work seen as a general productiveness that would not so preoccupy the individual that his or her capacity to be a loving, sexual being would be lost—may be a difficult goal to achieve.

The critical task of young adulthood, then, is the development of intimacy built on a strong sense of personal identity. The newly mature individual recognizes the essential loneliness of human existence and the vulnerability of closeness and yet chooses this special relatedness over protective self-absorption. The sense of self includes choices of vocation and life-style that are extensions of individual identity.

Such thoughts naturally lead to the next and major period of adulthood.

Erikson's Stage VII. Generativity Versus Self-Absorption or Stagnation: 30-65 Years

Generativity is primarily the interest in establishing and guiding the next generation, although this same impetus may be applied to other altruistic concerns or to creative activity. Attitudes toward one's own children seem to derive largely from the quality of one's own early parental ties. The birth of each child necessitates further adjustments and shifts in the marital relationship and family constellation. Family size has a direct bearing on the individualization of care for each child. Particular developmental periods in children may be harder for each parent to handle. There is a new sense of time. One woman put it like this: "It is as if there are two mirrors before me, each held at an angle. I see part of myself in my mother, who is growing old, and part of her in me. In the other mirror, I see part of myself in my daughter."

Possible life-styles. Many different possible lifestyles are now open to most people. There may be a retreat from the demands of generativity to pseudointimacy, often with a pervading sense of stagnation and interpersonal impoverishment; or the children may be clung to, since their departure will mean loss of identity. Perhaps as the cultural emphasis slowly shifts away from the worship of motherhood, a woman's sense of identity will be broader-based and not restricted to her reproductive function. For both parents, the maturation of children may provoke feelings of envy or unrealistic identification. The child's ultimate independence can leave the parent feeling rejected or deserted, a potential candidate for psychosomatic illness or depression.

Abandoning illusions. Mid life can be characterized as a period of surrendering illusions. Review of the road taken and reflection on the future make it clear that the world is no longer one of infinite possibilities. There are often discrepancies between what one had hoped to become and what one did become, uneasily expressed in the question, "Of what value is my life?" Preparation for the second half of life may be a time for perceiving creative new directions, with a sense of continuing growth and the interconnectedness of generations. It may also be a period of awareness of vague physiologic changes, a growing sense of time limitation, with death no longer an abstraction and time now measured in years left to live rather than time since birth. The neglected parts of the self urgently seek expression during a complex time when one may be responsible both for the care and education of the young

and the care and retirement of the aged. Jung (1933) emphasized the concept of individuation: "The serious problems of life. . . are never fully solved. If it should for once appear that they are, this is the sign that something has been lost. The meaning and design of a problem seem not to lie in its resolution but in our working at it incessantly. This alone preserves us from stultification and petrification." Thus, the second developmental stage of adulthood is marked by a concern for the next generation—a caring about the future rather than unsatisfying preoccupation with oneself.

The final stage of adulthood, with awareness of approaching death, is still the least well understood.

Erikson's Stage VIII. Ego Integrity Versus Despair: 65 Years & Older

Biologic aging. This is a period of biologic decline. The process is perhaps best characterized by its tremendous individual variation, but there are some common experiences. Engel and coworkers (1956) observe that people over 60 generally note a decrease in energy and strength. Tolerance to stress is impaired, and the potential loss of loved ones by death or loss of status by economic adversity and retirement are common sources of anxiety and depression. The fantasy of immortality is undermined by illness and death among contemporaries. Increased concern with minor symptoms is common. There may be noticeable impairment of recent memory, difficulty in learning new skills, and an apparent sharpening of remote memory.

Older people seeking medical care have many understandable concerns: What will be found? Will I still be seen as a worthwhile person? Will the advice seem merely palliative for one so close to the end of the race?

Increase of aged population. The number of old people in the population is increasing rapidly. Many of course are widowed, perhaps living alone or left behind in a declining central city or impoverished rural area. The chronic debilitating changes of physical decline are frequent reminders of passing time. A retired physician has said, "If I wake up in the morning and feel no pain, I'll know that my nervous system has worn out, too." It may be easier for the elderly patient to adapt to disability and decline than it is for the younger, cure-oriented physician. It is important for physicians caring for old people to continue to investigate the possibility of reversible changes, often secondary to depression, nutritional deficiency, or drug imbalance. Medical evaluation offers an excellent opportunity to help the elderly patient maximize independence and gain an increased sense of well-being. Even very old people have great potential reserves of creativity and physical and emotional energy. With environmental enrichment and exercise programs, significant improvements can continue to be achieved both in cognitive and in physical functioning.

Erikson speaks of an ideal old age as the fruit of the 7 earlier stages: a sense of integrity. "It means a different love of one's parents and an acceptance of the fact that one's life is one's own responsibility." It is a sense of history, of comradeship with the "ordering ways of distant times and different pursuits." A sense of integrity provides a successful solution to the fear of death as the end of an unfulfilled life. Older people may have a sense of pride in their past performances and in the achievements of their offspring or others whose lives they have influenced. They may show a sense of mellowness, a tolerance for self and others. A social worker once commented, "If you want to be a dear little old lady at 70, you must begin early, say at 17."

Losses during old age. Unfortunately, our society seems to assume that the chronologically old must inevitably suffer losses of social and economic resources and that they can only apprehensively anticipate physical and mental decline. With retirement and reduced income, self-regard and a sense of purpose may deteriorate. There is an increase in alcoholism, accidents, invalidism, and—in men—a striking increase in the suicide rate. In *Poorhouse Fair,* Updike (1977) catches the mood of confused rage the aged occupants of the county poor farm feel toward the world that has in the end discarded them.

The goal to be sought in this final stage of life is a sense of wisdom and a readiness to accept the totality of the life cycle. This sense of adult integrity comes close to the earliest period of infantile trust. Erikson suggests that healthy children will not fear life if their elders have integrity enough not to fear death. Weisman (1972), in a study of the attitudes toward death of a large number of aging patients, comments that death is not always construed as a bitter blow of fate but may be welcomed as an appropriate and timely culmination of the events that make up a life. Death with open awareness may be more harmonious than death cloaked in a conspiracy of silence and depression.

The crisis of life ends with an echo of the original theme of basic trust, and the circle is complete. The patterns discussed here are but one way of representing the major pathways of growth and development in current Western civilization. Each stage bears the imprint of previous stages as well as the human ability to adapt. In the turbulence of developmental crises, it often seems that little has gone before or lies ahead. However, when life is viewed as a continuum of challenge and potential for growth, the perspective gained may help the individual deal with the developmental tasks of each period.

REFERENCES

Adelson J (editor): *Handbook of Adolescent Psychology.* Wiley, 1980.

Blos P: *On Adolescence: A Psychoanalytic Interpretation.* Free Press, 1962.

Butler R: Psychiatry and the elderly: An overview. *Am J Psychiatry* 1975;**132:**893.

Cleaver E: *Soul on Ice.* McGraw-Hill, 1968

Colarusso CA, Nemiroff RL: *Adult Development.* Plenum, 1981.

Engel GL, Reichsman F, Segal H: A study of an infant with a gastric fistula. *Psychosom Med* 1956;**18:**374.

Erikson E: *Childhood and Society.* Norton, 1959.

Feinstein SC: Identity and adjustment disorders of adolescence. Chapter 39.8 in: *Comprehensive Textbook of Psychiatry/IV.* Kaplan HI, Sadock BJ (editors). Williams & Wilkins, 1985.

Fraiberg S: *The Magic Years.* Scribner, 1959.

Freud A: Adolescence. *Psychoanal Study Child* 1958;**13:**255.

Gilligan C: *In a Different Voice.* Harvard Univ Press, 1982.

Goodman P: *Growing Up Absurd.* Random House, 1962

Greenspan S: Normal child development. Chapter 32.1 in: *Comprehensive Textbook of Psychiatry/IV.* Kaplan HI, Sadock BJ (editors). Williams & Wilkins, 1985.

Harlow H, Harlow M: Psychopathology in monkeys. In: *Experimental Psychopathology: Recent Research and Theory.* Kimmel HO (editor). Academic Press, 1971.

Jahoda M: *Current Concepts of Positive Mental Health.* Basic Books, 1958.

Jung C: *Modern Man in Search of a Soul.* Harcourt Brace Jovanovich, 1933.

Keniston K: *The Uncommitted: Alienated Youth in American Society.* Harcourt Brace, 1965.

Levinson DJ et al: *The Seasons of a Man's Life.* Knopf, 1978.

Maier HW: *Three Theories of Child Development.* Harper & Row, 1969.

Neugarten BL: Time, age, and the life cycle. *Am J Psychiatry* 1979;**136:**887.

Offer D, Sabshin N: *Normality and the Life Cycle.* Basic Books, 1984.

Sheehy G: *Passages.* Bantam, 1977.

Spock B: *Baby and Child Care.* Pocket Books, 1957.

Szurek S: The child's needs for his emotional health. In: *Modern Perspectives in Child Psychiatry.* Howells J (editor). Brunner-Mazel, 1971.

Updike J: *Poorhouse Fair.* Knopf, 1977.

Vaillant GE: *Adaptation to Life.* Little, Brown, 1977.

Vaillant GE, Milofsky E: Empirical evidence for Erikson's model of the life cycle. *Am J Psychiatry* 1980;**137:**1348.

Weinberg J: Geriatric psychiatry. Chapter 53 in: *Comprehensive Textbook of Psychiatry/III.* Freedman AM, Kaplan HI, Sadock BJ (editors). Williams & Wilkins, 1980.

Weisman A: *On Dying and Denying.* Behavioral Publications, 1972.

Aging

8

Leon J. Epstein, MD, PhD

Definition of Old Age

Disagreement exists about the definition of old age: Does it begin at 60, 65, or 70 years of age? In this chapter, 65 years of age has been chosen with the awareness that the psychologic phenomena associated with aging and its organic and psychosocial consequences may vary widely in their impact on specific individuals. Aging proceeds at different rates in different individuals and at different rates within specific organ systems. Many persons seem old in body or spirit at age 50 years and others scarcely so at age 65.

A Public Health & Social Perspective on Aging

Mandatory retirement at a specific age has a varied impact on how people maintain their health after retirement, and in the USA it is currently the subject of conflicting legislation at both the state and the national level. Many persons, perhaps most, eagerly look forward to retirement. Many retire with great satisfaction, especially those who did not enjoy their occupation or those whose self-esteem was not strongly associated with their work role. It is therefore to be expected that workers retiring from more prestigious occupations or jobs associated with power and socially esteemed perquisites may face greater difficulties in adjusting to retirement. The frequency of occurrence of sudden death as a supposed consequence of retirement has been grossly exaggerated, however, since it is known that many who retire do so because of illness.

The delivery of health services to the elderly is an important social issue that is certain to gain increasing attention. Services to persons over 60 years of age account for half of all health care expenditures despite the fact that this group currently represents only about 20% of the total population of the USA. Five percent of these individuals are in custodial settings of some kind, and the chances of living in such a setting increase to about 20% at age 85 years and older. These figures represent more than 1 million people, a number of great importance in terms of economic cost, human suffering, and family disruption.

With respect to mental health services in the USA, although persons over age 65 years represent only 11% of the general population, they constitute almost 30% of first admissions to psychiatric inpatient units, and 1 out of every 16 persons in this age group has psychiatric symptoms severe enough to require hospitalization for treatment. Furthermore, it is estimated that this age group will grow to nearly one-fourth the population of the USA within 40 years. It should be noted, however, that the late years are for many a time of grateful rest, satisfaction, continuing growth, exercise of wisdom, contentment, and reasonably good health. During these years, many older people may effectively exercise the same techniques of coping with life that served them well in former years, and they may feel relief rather than loss at their release from former responsibilities. In this respect, retirement may be an event to be anticipated with pleasure and characterized by enjoyable interaction and personal fulfillment.

It is important to emphasize that the aged cannot be viewed as a homogeneous segment of society. There are vast physical, physiologic, emotional, cultural, and socioeconomic differences among aged individuals. In clinical practice, it is therefore impossible to generalize about delivery of comprehensive health care for a given individual, although it is difficult to avoid some generalities and stereotypes in a discussion as brief as this.

Old age is undeniably a time of loss, both psychologic and physiologic, including loss of familiar environment, loss of social relationships, loss of significant persons, and the anticipation of death.

Biology of Aging

Many of the changes in the aging process may not be "abnormalities," and the goal of a "cure" is therefore questionable. It is often difficult to distinguish between changes due to aging and those due to disease, and patients often seek treatment because of a combination of these factors. Authors who have described some of the changes in the aging process generally agree to the following:

A. Skin and Hair: Aging skin becomes dry, wrinkled, inelastic, and thinner. As a result of increased vascular fragility, small hemorrhages occur with little or no trauma. Keratoses develop on the face, arms, and trunk. Hair is progressively lost, and sweating is diminished.

B. Muscles: There is a gradual loss of muscle mass and strength in the aged. The lessened activity often associated with retirement accelerates this loss. There is an actual loss of muscle cells and subsequent replacement by fibrous tissue.

C. Nervous System: Reflexes generally are slower (though not always), and reactions to stimuli are slower and less efficient. There is often some impairment in recent memory, and there may be a narrowing of interests, loss of adaptability, difficulty in accepting new ideas, and marked possessiveness. With additional pathologic changes there may be senile dementia (marked confusion, loss of orientation, memory, reasoning ability, and appropriateness of response). The nervous system demonstrates (possibly more clearly than any other system) the poorly defined borderline between normal, expected, and tolerable changes due to aging and pathologic changes due to disease.

D. Special Senses: There may be some loss of the senses of taste and smell, which may alter a person's appreciation of food. Farsightedness usually occurs earlier than the other changes listed here and often occurs before age 65 years. There is also some reduction in visual fields, slowing of dark adaptation, and increased threshold for light stimulation, which results in difficulty in seeing in dim light. These changes in vision may limit activity and further increase existing difficulties in adapting. Hearing generally decreases with increasing age, usually most markedly in the higher frequencies, and at times progressing to involve speech frequencies. Hearing loss may also limit social relationships and increase the isolation that is a serious problem for many older persons.

E. Cardiovascular System: There is a decrease in cardiac output at rest, a loss of ability to respond to the stress of exertion, an increase in peripheral resistance, and a tendency toward increased systolic blood pressure. It is often difficult to separate expected cardiovascular changes due to aging from those due to disease.

F. Respiratory System: A decrease in total lung capacity, a decrease in vital capacity, and an increase in residual volume occur. Maximal breathing capacity decreases, at times markedly. Diminished resiliency of the lungs, slowing of the rate of diffusion and gas exchange, and loss of vascular pathways occur. Shortness of breath—which these changes produce to a greater or lesser degree—may hamper activity.

G. Gastrointestinal Tract: The gastrointestinal tract shows some loss of motility and decreased peristalsis. Decrease in gastric acid and decreased absorption of iron may occur, resulting in anemia. The intake and enjoyment of food may be reduced by bad teeth or poorly fitting dentures.

H. Urinary Tract: Renal blood flow and the glomerular filtration rate are usually markedly diminished. In women, loss of abdominal and pelvic muscle tone and stretching of pelvic ligaments may result in stress incontinence, incomplete emptying of the bladder, and chronic bladder infections. In men, prostatic enlargement may produce incomplete emptying of the bladder, nocturia, and persistent infection. Polyuria and incontinence are other common problems that may profoundly affect social adaptation.

It is evident that many of the organic changes described above affect psychosocial adjustment. Changes involving the senses—especially losses in vision and hearing—interfere with interaction and communication with others and may lead to emotional difficulties and virtual exclusion from certain impor-

tant individual and group relationships. The exclusion resulting from physical impairment has been observed to be a precursor of paranoid ideation; the individual imagines (projects) what others may be saying or doing in the absence of more meaningful involvement or communication with them. Debilitating illness and the older person's response to a loss of strength, attractiveness, vigor, and self-concept as an energetic and healthy person may preclude even the already lessened interaction and involvement with others that may be present.

There is some confusion about the decrement in mental functioning with aging. It is true that there is a loss in speed of response, but measures of intellectual functioning may be obscured by diminished attention span or decreased motivation in the testing situation as well as by a slowing of response. For most persons, nevertheless, there is some decrement in intellectual functioning, and decrease in brain weight by as much as 50% is recognized by age 75 years, although intellectual functioning is reduced to a far lesser extent.

One must distinguish between "normal" senescence and senility. **Senescence** involves slowing, varying from scarcely noticeable to moderate changes in function. These losses are not severe enough to interfere with the maintenance of relationships with others. **Senility** is a serious illness and pathologic process in which there is severe memory loss, disorientation, deterioration in personal habits, extreme decline in intellectual functioning, and often death within several years (see Chapters 10 and 24). Worldwide, about 10% of persons over age 65 years suffer this serious decline, and the incidence increases, so that about 20% of persons 85 years of age or older have undergone these changes. It is not known how a significant increase in life expectancy would affect the incidence of senility.

Illustrative case. An 86-year-old widow had been living in a modest 1-bedroom apartment since the death of her husband about 20 years previously. A neighbor had been purchasing her groceries and supplies for her about once a week and had been repaid by the patient's daughter, who used the patient's Social Security income. Her apartment was fairly neatly maintained, mainly because of the help of the daughter who visited her mother several times a week. The patient had few friends in the community, because most of her former companions had already died. She spent most of the day watching television, looking out the window, and preparing rather simple meals. Her health had been good, and it had not been necessary for her to seek medical care for several years.

Two months prior to presentation, the patient fell while getting out of bed to void in the middle of the night, and she suffered a fractured right femur. Although an open reduction was necessary, the healing process seemed uneventful. During hospitalization, she appeared confused and bewildered. She was unable to state her age or her date of birth, the name of her daughter, or the names of her grandchildren. She did not know her telephone number or her address. She was totally unable to describe the state of her finances. There was no evidence of hallucinatory experiences or delusional thinking.

The patient's mental condition did not improve during a month of hospitalization. The results of an extensive battery of laboratory and radiologic studies were within normal limits for her age. It was obvious that she would not be able to return to living alone in her apartment, nor would she be able to live with her daughter, who was unable to provide suitable attention. Upon her discharge from the hospital, she entered a nursing home.

A common assumption in the situation outlined above is that the onset of the patient's confusion was acute and brought about by the fracture. The more probable explanation is that the low demands of her living situation enabled her to function despite moderately severe senile brain disease of the Alzheimer type. Had there been a history of prolonged hypertension or stroke, the alternative diagnosis of multi-infarct dementia would have been more appropriate.

In elderly persons living in undemanding situations, moderately severe dementia may often go unrecognized until some event breaks the tenuous equilibrium in their lives.

Developmental Tasks

A number of authors have described developmental tasks, or tasks for mastery in later years. Erikson (1982) describes old age as ushering in the culmination of the life cycle, when it is to be hoped that the individual accumulates mature judgment and knowledge "freed of temporal relativity" and feels a sense of satisfaction with the life that has been lived (see Chapter 7). In Erikson's terminology, the individual achieves a state of **ego integrity.** The opposite, the state of **despair,** is characterized by fear of death and relative dissatisfaction with the only life one has lived. Others have viewed the task of old age as survival through the extension of previously successful habits of mastery; the integration of the past, leading from maturity to wisdom; the acceptance of the altered condition of later maturity; the acknowledgment of the finitude of life, albeit with humor and the attainment of modified ideals; or the finding of protectors and providers, as in childhood.

Although differences exist in the emphases listed above, most observers of elderly people agree that the later years ordinarily present most people with major changes in socioeconomic style of life, outlets for achievement, and roles within the family. Some of these changes relate to the task of preparing for (or denying) death. Studies of old people also share a common emphasis on changes in the psyche, eg, heightened egocentricity and weakening of repression as a mental mechanism, with the subsequent development of anxiety at a time of diminished potential for dealing with it.

Many observers point to the old person's work of confronting late developmental tasks not only with an altered psychic apparatus but also with a profoundly altered cerebral capacity to manipulate and store percepts and maintain cognition. These changes may usher in a state of relative inattention to the world and lead to increasing introversion and preoccupation with a simplified past.

A task important to the emotional well-being of the older individual is modification of the goals the aging person had hoped to realize and acceptance of ideals that are more appropriate for a person with increasing limitations in intellectual functioning, social and economic achievement, and ability to master the environment by using the adaptive techniques successfully applied in the past. The individual must be able to accept without shame the limitations of diminishing assertiveness, increasing passivity and dependency, and increasing spectatorship rather than leadership or participation. Related to the reassessment of ideals is the need to accept and integrate changes in one's self-image, with successful mastery leading to continued self-respect.

An additional task to be mastered in later years is the acceptance of changes in the strength of drives. A frequent complaint in the elderly is that "there is no drive left." Older people must also learn to accept some deterioration of the central nervous system, manifested as increasing slowness in manipulating memories for thinking; difficulty in making, storing, and retrieving new information; and the limitation imposed on incoming information by sensory deficits such as impaired vision or hearing. Prevalent social attitudes that are not based on scientific fact also affect older people's perception of drives; eg, many older people decrease their sexual activity out of proportion to the change in their actual desires and physical capabilities because society dictates that "old folks just don't do that kind of thing." Few nursing homes provide the privacy adequate for intimate emotional and physical caring.

Sometimes individuals resist facing the developmental tasks of this phase. They may refuse to modify their demands in the light of decreased physical and mental abilities, deny their increasing limitations, and use many defense mechanisms to deny their decline, all of which may result in a variety of psychopathologic manifestations (eg, paranoid blaming, obsessive stubbornness, hostile aggressiveness). The converse—with equal potential for pathologic consequences—is premature resignation and capitulation to an exaggerated view of the physical and mental decline associated with aging. Two lifelong male friends in their late 70s died within a short time of each other, seemingly the victims of opposite maladjustments to aging. One refused to cut back in his vigorous physical activity, frequent trips, and excessive smoking, despite a recent heart attack and failing lungs. The other responded to his friend's death by stopping almost all of his activities, involvements, and indulgences out of fear; he died of nonspecific causes several months later.

The 2 most important developmental tasks of old age must be given the same degree of attention as the tasks of earlier phases. These critical tasks are (1) acceptance of changes in ideals and self-concept resulting specifically from advancing age and (2) acceptance of changes in the physiologic processes of the body. The first task includes the ability to accept the loss of significant people in one's life and to accept the idea of one's own approaching death.

Psychologic Mechanisms of Adaptation & Coping Strategies

The elderly may respond in a variety of ways, both organic and psychologic, to pressures from organic or psychosocial loss or stress. The coping strategies used are by no means unique to this age group but reflect coping styles developed earlier in life (in late life they may be less subtly employed, however). Frequent responses are somatization as an unconscious attention-seeking maneuver, withdrawal, projection in the form of blaming others, denial, and depression. For example, people whose physical attractiveness was a source of attention in earlier years may continue to command attention to their bodies through the unconscious elaboration of bodily concerns and psychosomatically induced somatic change. Depression is manifested as anorexia and weight loss, leading to electrolyte imbalance, nutritional deficiency states, and the potential for irreversible physical damage. The potential for suicide is great in depressed elderly people.

An accurate history is required to help determine the significance of the current organic and psychosocial clinical picture in view of the patient's previous adjustments to changes in life. It is crucial to assess the extent of loss suffered by the patient, especially that associated with isolation, since such isolation is often linked to ill health. Two-thirds of aged mental hospital residents are divorced, have survived the death of a spouse, or have never been married. This number is higher than the percentage in the general population of old people who are not hospitalized. This fact may simply reflect the personality traits of these people and social factors that may have contributed to their being divorced or remaining unmarried.

A number of hypotheses have been expressed about the behavior of elderly people. Although the dependency of infants and elderly people is often compared, infants are developing from helplessness to self-sufficiency, whereas older people are losing self-sufficiency and becoming increasingly more helpless. Some have seen old age as an overlapping of the waning powers of maturity and the increasing helplessness of a second childhood. The response to anxiety in the elderly is described by one writer in musical terms as the "da capo effect"—playing through a passage (the earlier problems or their solutions) again. Much of the behavior of elderly people has also been viewed as different strategies of coping; eg, the reminiscence characteristic of old age enables older people to relive the satisfactions of previous years and experience gratification when opportunities for gratification from present endeavors have decreased.

The paranoid thinking so often observed in elderly persons may result when aging individuals in increasing decline project feelings of insecurity associated with their many losses. For example, old people may feel less anxious if they choose to believe that others are deliberately withholding important information from them rather than admitting that they themselves are losing their hearing or suffering a decline in memory. The price paid for this coping mechanism is fewer interpersonal relationships and decreased ability to assess reality.

In this same vein, some clinicians regard rigidity as a normal coping device that enables the elderly to deal with change. Rigidity may enable people to remain in those settings to which they had previously adapted successfully. Memory loss may produce a distortion or displacement of events that is used as a defense mechanism to deny reality. Other symptoms associated with organic brain disease are also psychologic defense mechanisms. Certain individuals who feel uncertain about the future may become stingy with what remains of their lives and transfer this feeling to their material possessions by adopting a hoarding or miserly attitude. As insecurity increases, the elderly person may exaggerate genuine economic problems: "I'm afraid that I'm going to be old and poor because I can't take care of myself anymore, and the government is out to get us old people [because of cuts in federally funded health care]. What they don't take away, my children will." Furthermore, with the elderly, aggressiveness may emerge as controls diminish, especially when a situation is aggravated by the use of alcohol. The aggression may in turn lead to disturbing behavior toward others. Also, since behavior that once served a person well becomes fixed, the conservatism of the elderly may be seen as a reiteration of behavior that maintained self-esteem during earlier periods of higher capacity and security.

One of the most common characteristics of old age is increasing dependence. Many elderly people, fearful of isolation and loneliness, may attach themselves to a "protective other," whether this be spouse, relative, or friend, and they seek constant reassurance that this person will not forsake them. Almost any absence may be viewed as abandonment. A loss of status with age also occurs in a culture that emphasizes youth, beauty, power, and success; for many old people, the result is lowered self-esteem and increasing dependence on the help of others to achieve gratification of needs. The more unwilling a person is to accept a dependent attitude, the more disguised may be the search for help, eg, as manifested in invalidism or depression.

Other factors, such as the sociocultural setting, unquestionably contribute to difficulties of adjustment in the aged. In fact, elderly people in the USA are often seen as a disadvantaged minority group. In an increasingly urban social setting that emphasizes technologic productivity, the role of the elderly undergoes drastic change. Although retirement benefits may provide an income (though limited, for many), the altered role in society may cause serious problems, especially when loss of a role contributes to an overall self-concept of uselessness. Less affluent people may have an advantage in this respect in that these families tend to be less mobile, and the elderly are therefore better able to maintain continuing contact with their children as well as with other family members and may thus suffer fewer losses. The absence of some such links with others has resulted in a decreased network of communication and interaction for many elderly, which can promote withdrawal and progressively decreasing personal interaction, so that isolation and loss of self-esteem may occur.

The Physician & Elderly Patients—Special Problems

Depression may be cited as a prime example of the difficulties associated with elucidation of any disease in the aged that has a complex etiology involving interrelated organic, interpersonal, and social factors.

Depression has been viewed almost as a characteristic of senescence despite the fact that many old people are cheerful, wise, and content. However, depressive symptoms are well known to physicians who care for older patients, and in recent years, depression in the elderly has received increasing attention. Despite this, depressive illness in the elderly is easily and frequently overlooked. Depressive symptoms may be regarded as consistent with the process of senescence or may be confused with symptoms of various organic diseases. **Pseudodementia** is a constellation of signs and symptoms often associated with an organic process (eg, poor memory, decreased reasoning ability, confusion); these symptoms also occur in major depressive disorders. Symptoms and signs of depression may also be dismissed as being "just natural for an old person." The degree of hopelessness may be out of proportion to circumstances and may be an unrealistic response to an illness or other stresses.

Illustrative case. A 67-year-old man recently retired as president of a sizable corporation which he had started as a young man and which had gradually grown under his leadership. He was a vigorous, active man at the time of his retirement, regularly played golf and tennis, and enjoyed a rather active social life. He had 2 sons who seemed to effectively assume the managerial role that he had had for so many years.

About 6 months after his retirement, the man requested an appointment with the physician who had been treating him for many years. He complained of fatigue, which was certainly out of keeping with his prior history. There were also numerous physical complaints referable to many organ systems. He also expressed a disinterest in golf, tennis, and the social activities that he had previously enjoyed. He stated, "I just feel played out." He was waking up several times during the night. He noted that his appetite was fair, although his zest for food was somewhat diminished.

There was no expression of guilt or self-depreciation, and he did not express feelings of depression or undue sadness. Results on physical examination and an extensive battery of laboratory studies were unrevealing.

The clinical picture of depression described above is not unsusual in an elderly person who suffers a loss—in this case, the loss of position and power which the man had formerly enjoyed and which meant a great deal to him. Failure to express feelings of melancholy, guilt, self-depreciation, or other signs of depression frequently seen in younger patients is not unusual and often results in a failure to diagnose depression in the elderly. This oversight is particularly unfortunate in elderly patients, since depression is often reversible, but should it become more severe, poor hydration and inadequate nutritional status may result, as well as a worsening of any preexisting organic conditions, even to the extent of irreversible damage in an older person with less stable physiologic equilibrium.

The older attitude that the mental symptoms of old age are largely the result of organic deterioration has been tempered in recent years by a greater emphasis on the importance of psychogenic factors, and this is particularly true of depression. However, many questions remain unanswered—eg, whether depressive disorders with mental symptoms are age-linked and specific to old age; whether they are recurrences of an affective disorder from earlier life; or whether these disorders are similar to the depressive episodes that occur in earlier life but for some reason are delayed until later life. Perhaps many individuals with depression in old age also suffered similar depression in early life but managed to avoid hospitalization because of better means of coping (eg, better physical health, economic supports, family protection, or special skills).

Although it is generally acknowledged that considerable interaction occurs between the experiences of an individual, the current environment, the person's changing physical condition, and mental health, it is not clear what the precipitating factors really are that lead to depression in the elderly. Investigators have emphasized **age-related stresses** (eg, physical illness, bereavement, economic deprivation, poor living conditions, social isolation, deafness or blindness, rejection by children); **hereditary factors;** and **personality before onset of illness.**

The clinician should not forget the positive aspects of social relationships in maintaining the quality of life; there is evidence that those who have someone to confide in during their later years have better morale than those lacking such a confidant. Social interaction and activities are much related to morale, and limitations in these areas may serve to promote withdrawal or demoralization. Successful social programs for the elderly incorporate such factors as providing a sense of usefulness, involving older people in planning, and structuring the environment to help make it easier to establish social relationships with others. A creative approach is required to stimulate the interests of aging individuals, particularly those who are isolated or who have had limited opportunities for social interaction.

The relationship between elderly people and their physicians is different from that between doctors and younger people. For many older people, a visit to their physician constitutes far more than a search for diagnosis and treatment. It often represents a significant social interaction, perhaps one of the increasingly few such relationships for the elderly patient. The care with which older patients may prepare for a visit to a physician is well known and may include careful attention to dress or grooming. Hypochondriasis may often unconsciously represent both a search for a significant relationship and a socially acceptable pathway for formation of a dependent attachment to the doctor. In caring for elderly patients, the physician confronts chronic illness and end-stage disease, which may frustrate all attempts at cure and may contradict the image of the physician as the all-conquering healer.

The problems of the elderly are complex, since older people often have physical disabilities in addition to changes resulting from the "normal" aging process. They undergo comparable changes in psychologic functions that may be sources of support or stress (more often both). The person's response to these closely related factors and the ability to pursue the developmental task of integrating a lifetime of experiences into a meaningful whole determine the kind of adjustment achieved during this period of life.

REFERENCES

Binstock R, Shanas E (editors): *Handbook of Aging and the Social Sciences*. Van Nostrand Reinhold, 1976.

Birren JE, Schaie KW (eidtors): *Handbook of the Psychology of Aging*. Van Nostrand Reinhold, 1977.

Birren JE, Sloan RB (editors): *Handbook of Mental Health and Aging*. Prentice-Hall, 1980.

Breslau LD, Haug MK (editors): *Depression and Aging: Causes, Care and Consequences*. Springer, 1982.

Butler RN: *Why Survive? Being Older in America*. Harper & Row, 1975.

Comfort A: *The Biology of Senescence*. Elsevier, 1979.

Erikson EH: *The Life Cycle Completed*. Norton, 1982.

Miller NE, Cohen GD (editors): *Clinical Aspects of Alzheimer's Disease and Senile Dementia*. Raven Press, 1981.

Death & Bereavement

9

Charles M. Binger, MD, & Dennis P. Malinak, MD

The certainty of death is universal to human experience and is one of the mysteries at the core of the world's religious and philosophic systems. Some postulate that the fear of death is the prototype of human anxiety. Many maintain that paying attention to death is morbid; this is not only untrue and defensive but also not helpful, especially for physicians, who must be actively concerned with the dying process, its psychologic aspects, and its effect on patients, their loved ones, and not least of all those who care for the dying.

In modern Western society, death is generally considered an unacceptable topic for attention or conversation, and it perhaps occupies the same position that sex did in the Victorian era. Death from chronic illness has increased in recent times, especially in older age groups. Consequently, death more often occurs in settings outside the home and among people who have already been substantially separated from family and from economically productive roles in society. Until fairly recently, most people died at home, and the family was responsible for laying out the corpse. Increasingly, it is hospitals and custodial institutions that care for the terminally ill, and it is the funeral industry that prepares the body for burial and arranges the funeral. (Interestingly, mortuary institutions are called "homes," a remnant of the past.) Fewer and fewer children and young adults have participated in the death of another person. As an individual's connection with the process of dying becomes increasingly remote, the opportunity to contend adequately with one's own death and to mourn appropriately the death of others seems to diminish.

A profound contradiction exists in thinking about death: On the one hand, death is considered a termination; on the other, for some people it is an entry to another realm. Society must push the dead away so that both those closest to the dead and the larger group of mourners can recommence their participation in the normal affairs of the community, yet simply disposing of the dead and excluding them provoke too much anxiety in the living, who are left behind with the knowledge of their own ultimate fate. Recognition of the need to allay this anxiety accounts for the existence of funerals, which are one of the primary rites of passage and which are found in almost all societies. The funeral provides a way of combining disposal of the body with its transmutation to the spiritual realm. The funeral also provides an opportunity for the collective and ritualized expression of grief; the chance to summarize and recognize the achievements and personal-

ity of the deceased; the chance to participate in a concrete demonstration of the finality of that person's life; and the opportunity to perform various special religious, philosophic, or personal rites to ensure the appropriate passage of the deceased.

Studies have demonstrated that as a group, physicians have significantly stronger anxieties about death than do most other people. This anxiety may play a significant role in the choice of profession, since becoming a doctor may be a way of confronting conflicts and fears concerning death. Physicians are trained as healers and as the enemy of illness and death; in one sense, death is an unacceptable outcome that is tantamount to failure. Physicians are also trained to assume an active therapeutic role, whereas chronically or terminally ill patients often require a restrained and supportive approach. Physicians may need to reconsider or reformulate these assumptions and training practices in order to be at their most effective; at the very least, they can try to understand their attitudes and those of their patients toward death and dying.

The Meaning of Death

What is the great fear that death holds? Pattison (1974) described the fears faced by a dying person as fear of the unknown, fear of loneliness, fear of loss of family and friends, fear of loss of the physical body, fear of loss of self-control (ie, control of bodily functions), fear of pain, fear of loss of identity, and fear of regression. Physicians can attend to several of these fears. Effective analgesics preclude the need for patients to suffer excessive physical pain. The fear of an actual experience of loneliness may be lessened by ensuring a continued human presence around the patients, encouraging the support of family and friends, and not relegating the dying patient to a remote room at the end of the hall. The patient's sense of self-control may be maximized by including the patient in treatment decisions and by providing dignified assistance with failing bodily functions. Informed consent and thorough but easily understood explanations of the disease and its treatment may lessen fears of the unknown.

On a somewhat more philosophic level, Kastenbaum and Aisenberg (1972) described 3 aspects of the fear of death: dying, in which the individual fears personal suffering and indignity; afterlife, in which the person fears punishment or rejection; and extinction, or ceasing to be, which many consider to be the most basic fear of death.

Although the fear of death and anxiety about death have received the most attention in the literature, sadness seems to constitute an equally important and deep response to impending death in many individuals: sadness over the loss of family, friends, and future hopes and plans. The dying person has much to grieve for; everything is being lost.

The human need for symbolic immortality and a sense of historical connection beyond the individual's lifetime is related to and in a sense overcomes the fear of death. Lifton and Olson (1974) feel that the sense of immortality is expressed in 5 modes: biologic, creative, theologic, natural, and experiential. **Biologic immortality** involves living through one's offspring, a demonstration of the continuity of germ plasm. **Creative immortality** allows people to live on through works of art, writing, or the heritage of the deeds performed during their lifetimes. **Theologic immortality** involves religious or philosophic symbols of life after death or life beyond death. **Natural immortality** is that achieved through the continuity of nature: "From dust you came and to dust you must return." **Experiential immortality** is a feeling of intense well-being and joy in being alive that transcends the fear of death; the person focuses on living more completely in the present and participating fully in all that life has to offer.

These modes of symbolic immortality provide a sense of relatedness to that which has preceded and that which follows, and they are a means of mastering the anxiety about death. To the degree that physicians can help patients to achieve some form of the symbolic immortality described above or at least deal with their fear of mortality, they can extend their range of care beyond simply making a dying patient's last days more comfortable. For example, bedside conversations with a patient about major and minor life accomplishments, which may range from paintings to business dealings to rearing children, may promote a sense of contribution and significance. The physician may offer religious consultation with hospital religious advisers or outside clergy and encourage the formal and informal sharing among patients of philosophies, attitudes, and coping strategies. All but the most gravely ill patients should be encouraged to participate as fully as possible in their remaining days of life: Some people may read all the books they never had time for; others may review their accumulating slide collection or spend another summer in the mountains.

Types of Death

In the Western world, it is the responsibility of the physician to complete the death certificate. According to Shneidman (1976), the signing of the death certificate gives death its operational meaning (ie, the cause of death is not "known," and the person is not dead until the certificate is signed) and its administrative meaning (ie, the signing process starts the legal machinery that settles the dead person's affairs). The first section of the US Standard Certificate of Death identifies the deceased; the second section states the cause of death (eg, pneumonia, meningitis). The bottom third of the form includes miscellaneous items such as place of burial and the name of the funeral director, but the most important section is that with the words "accidental," "suicide," and "homicide." If none of these items is checked off, the death is assumed to be due to natural causes (it is from these categories that Shneidman derives the NASH classification of death: *N*atural, *A*ccidental, *S*uicidal, *H*omicidal). With the exception of suicide, this classification scheme carries an assumption that people are passive agents with regard to their own deaths. Shneidman has proposed several changes in the standard death certificate, including a requirement that the decedent's intentions be specified, ie, that deaths be classified as *intended, unintended,* or *subintended.*

In an **intended death,** the individual plays a direct and conscious role in effecting his or her own death (eg, suicide).

An **unintended death** is one in which the deceased has played no significant role; death is therefore essentially due to trauma from without or biologic failure from within due to age or disease.

Subintended deaths are those in which the decedent has played a covert, usually subconscious role in hastening his or her own demise. This category of death is an important one, and more deaths may be assigned to it than most people care to believe. Many people involved in automobile accidents have subconscious suicidal impulses, for example. Hastening death through poor health care (eg, smoking and alcohol abuse) is another example of subintended death.

As medical experience with death and dying grows and as more people come to believe in the interaction of the body and the mind, the number of deaths assigned to the subintended category may increase. Every experienced and perceptive physician has known patients who successfully survive an operation or medical crisis only to succumb because they seem to lack the will to recover or because they fail to comply with treatment. (Conversely, many physicians have cared for patients with seemingly terminal illness who survived, apparently because of a conscious or unconscious desire to live.)

Death & the Life Cycle

Our concept of death continues to evolve both cognitively and emotionally throughout life. It is helpful in dealing with children to know how they think about death, and to achieve that requires some understanding of the timing of their cognitive development. Younger children often indulge in animistic thinking (everything is alive) as well as magical thinking (the equation of wishes and thoughts with action). An example of the latter is a case in which a little girl wishes for a pony and feels guilty when her cat runs away and dies, because she thinks it was her desire to have the pony that led to the cat's death.

Development is discussed in Chapters 6 and 7, but it is worthwhile here to describe how children's conceptions of death fall into 3 broad stages. The first stage, up to about age 5 years, is one in which death is not recognized as final but rather is regarded as separation or something like sleep. During the second stage, between the ages of 5 and 9 years, the child tends to personify death. Death is still external and can be personally avoided: One can outrun "the death man" or lock the door against the bogeyman. By age 9 years, the child enters the third stage and begins to form an adult idea of death, including its finality and inevitability. In cognitive terms, the simple statement "I will die" implies self-awareness, logical thought processes, and understanding of probability, necessity, causation, personal time (the length of a person's life span) and physical time (time that exists independently of the individual), finality, and separation.

It is important for the physician to realize that even very young children may experience considerable anxiety about death, although their concept of it differs significantly from that of the adult. It is also important to realize the futility and frustration involved in trying to explain a concept that is beyond the child's level of comprehension.

Emotional development continues throughout life, with a series of broadly defined stages and developmental tasks, as described in Chapters 6, 7, and 8. The meaning of death for a given individual must be related to that person's stage of development as well as to details of the personal life, circumstances, and social system. For example, the adolescent's typical concerns about body image and control will influence concerns and conceptualization about death (eg, adolescents may worry about never having had sex, or they may feel that they disappointed their parents by not going to a "good" college). Young adults may be more concerned about never having married or never having had children or about unrealized professional goals. People facing death who are new parents will be riddled with anxieties about the care of their young children and will be filled with regret about not being able to see the children grow. Middle-aged adults whose lives have achieved a degree of financial and social stability may be filled with resentment over the lost chance to enjoy the fruits of earlier labors. Elderly persons are confronted with the harsh inevitability of death as more and more of their friends and colleagues die; they must also look back upon their lives with the knowledge that there is little chance for major modification. As Erikson (1950) pointed out, people may approach death with a sense of contentment and satisfaction with past accomplishments or with regret and despair.

The Process of Dying

People have a stable set of adaptive and defensive mechanisms that are developed early and carried through life. Thus, in general, people die as they have lived; they react to the stress of impending death in a way similar to the way they have reacted to various stresses in life—though perhaps in an exaggerated fashion.

Illustrative case No. 1. A bank president in the last stages of terminal gastrointestinal cancer inexplicably disallowed visits from any of his colleagues. In conversation with the patient, an astute medical student detected the man's great unspoken fear (in a man who highly valued dignity and decorum) that he would vomit during one of these visits because of the potent anticancer drugs he was receiving. Simple rearrangement of the medication schedule enabled the patient to feel comfortable about having visits again, and a significant lifting in mood followed.

Another important principle to remember has been called the primary paradox: Although people recognize that death is universal, they (their unconscious minds) cannot imagine their own. As Tolstoy wrote in *The Death of Ivan Ilyich:* "Ivan Ilyich saw that he was dying. In the depth of his heart he knew he was dying, but not only was he not accustomed to the thought, he simply did not and could not grasp it. The syllogism he had learnt from Kiezewetter's logic: 'Caius is a man; men are mortal; therefore Caius is mortal,' had always seemed correct as applied to Caius, but certainly not as applied to himself. That Caius—man in abstract—was mortal, was perfectly correct, but he was not Caius, not an abstract man, but a creature quite separate from all others. He had been little Vanya, with a mamma and a papa . . . with toys, a coachman and a nurse. . . . Caius really was mortal and it was right for him to die; but for me, little Vanya, Ivan Ilyich, with all my thoughts and emotions, it's altogether a different matter."

Other investigators, most notably Kübler-Ross (1969), have proposed a series of psychologic stages through which the dying patient progresses. The Kübler-Ross stages need not be viewed as inevitable occurrences but rather as representative samples of the emotional reactions experienced by terminally ill patients. She speaks of 5 reactions:

(1) Denial and isolation. The patient's initial reaction is one of brief shock followed by the feeling that "it cannot be true." Denial occurs in all patients to some degree throughout illness and serves to protect the organism from emotional overload.

(2) Anger. The patient asks, "Why me?" The anger is displaced and projected in all directions, so that family and medical staff should be prepared to receive hostility that is not really meant for them.

(3) Bargaining. The patient attempts to bargain for time or reduced pain, and the bargain usually represents a pact with God or the fates. It represents an extension of the childhood attitude that being good may earn the patient special favors.

(4) Depression. Depression takes 2 forms: **reactive depression,** or mourning for things already lost (eg, depletion of finances, loss of job, loss of function); and **preparatory depression** (ie, the patient is going to lose everything and everybody held dear).

(5) Acceptance. When the patient accepts the inevitability of death, the patient's sphere of interest diminishes, and the patient draws inward. This attitude is not to be confused with hopeless giving up, which is perhaps a more common and more unfortunate reaction.

These stages share certain similarities with aspects of bereavement that are discussed below and also with the general reactions of the stress syndrome considered in Chapter 5.

In caring for a terminally ill patient, the physician must decide whether and how to tell the patient that the illness is terminal. It is a very rare patient who is unaware of a terminal prognosis. Some patients may unconsciously be aware of the wish of the family and caretakers to deny the inevitable. It is usually a great relief to the patient if the information is out in the open so that feelings can be discussed and plans made. "What tormented Ivan Ilyich most was the deception, the lie, which for some reason they all accepted, that he was not dying but was simply ill . . . and wishing and forcing him to participate in that lie."

Illustrative case No. 2. A blustery truck driver denied the implications of his terminal illness until one evening when he shared with his physician the previous night's dream of driving an unknown cargo down a dark and lonely road. The sensitive physician was able to gently broach the subject of death with this indirect permission from the patient.

Glaser and Strauss (1974) described 4 patterns of awareness found in hospital settings: (1) **closed awareness,** in which patients do not know of their terminal illness but everyone else does; (2) **suspected awareness,** in which the patient suspects what others know; (3) **mutual pretense awareness,** in which everyone, including the patient, knows the terminal prognosis but all pretend otherwise; and (4) **open awareness,** in which personnel, patient, and family know the prognosis and act on the knowledge openly and appropriately. Physicians should be alert to indications from patients (usually indirect) that they are ready to talk about certain issues. They should also allow patients the degree of denial they need, but without contributing to the denial system.

In dealing with dying children, it is a serious mistake to think that children older than age 4–5 years do not realize the seriousness and probable fatal outcome of their condition. It is a pathetic situation if a fatally ill child must suffer the loneliness and isolation of having no one with whom to share concerns because parents and physicians are attempting to shield the child from a prognosis that is usually sensed. As with adults, children must know that their concerns are shared, that they will not be deserted or lied to, that everything possible is being done, and that they will not undergo unnecessary discomfort.

Illustrative case No. 3. A 7-year-old girl with rapidly progressive acute leukemia was told that she had a minor blood abnormality and that she would be well enough to resume school in the fall. This bright youngster could not understand the look of sadness in the eyes of her adult visitors, or why relatives were flying in from distant states, or why the other children seemed so ill on the ward (a pediatric cancer ward). The pediatric resident felt trapped between the family's wish to shelter the patient and the bewilderment, anger, and loneliness of the child, whose life was numbered in days. With considerable effort, a social worker convinced the parents that it would be appropriate to share the prognosis with the patient. The girl's initial sadness and fear were followed by relief, increased family sharing and support, and significant calm acceptance, and the patient spent much time comforting younger children on the ward.

At some early point in training and frequently thereafter, prospective physicians must come to terms with their own anxieties and attitudes about death and dying. This process can be facilitated if they review their own experiences with serious illnesses, accidents, or deaths of family members and friends and if they follow a patient and family through the process of dying and bereavement and stay with them. *Perhaps the most important service a physician can perform is to let the patient know that the doctor will be there and that the patient will not be abandoned,* in effect saying, "You do have a terminal illness, but we will go through it together." It is important to allow the patient room for hope, which does not mean the physician can lie or exaggerate. Implicit in the doctrine of informed consent is the patient's right to know what is being done in treatment and to have some choice in the matter. With appropriate help, patients can exercise the necessary bodily and mental functions as much as they are able in the face of diminished control and can thereby preserve their self-esteem and maximal independence for as long as possible. Confused patients may be respectfully reoriented by a greeting such as, "How are you on this 12th morning of August?" or they can be tactfully reminded of the day's visitors. Excretory functions represent an important real and symbolic area of control for many patients. The dignity maintained by using a wheelchair or walker to go to the bathroom instead of requesting a bedpan may be well worth the effort involved and the risk of a fall. Adequate and anticipatory pain relief should be provided and discomfort minimized. Physicians can assist family members and friends in working through the grief they will soon experience and at the same time can keep open the channels of communication with the dying. By their example, physicians can impart the courage to accept what cannot be changed and can provide for as dignified and appropriate a passing as the situation allows.

The Impact of Death on Loved Ones

Terminal illness exacts a heavy toll from all those involved with the dying person. The importance of defining the family as a unit of treatment is becoming increasingly evident. The task of the physician extends beyond caring for the dying patient to feeling concern for family and friends and assisting them in achieving an adequate adjustment to the loss. On one hand, family members are an integral part of the experience of death for the terminally ill patient; on the other hand, terminal illness causes major changes in family structure. The person accustomed to being the prime financial supporter may need to assume major responsibility for the children; conversely, the person responsible for most of the child care may suddenly be forced into the job market. Loneliness, resentment, guilt, and fear must be faced. Major decisions about children, home, and finances have to be made rapidly at a time of confusion and stunned preoccupation. The survivors need to reassess the meaning and direction of their own lives; in a real sense the patient's problems have ended, whereas those of the family have escalated.

Freud (1917) identified the characteristics of mourning as painful dejection, loss of interest in the outside world, loss of capacity to adopt any new object of love, and inhibition of activity. Lindemann (1944) published the first field study of acute grief and described what he thought were its 5 major characteristics: somatic distress, preoccupation with the image of the deceased, guilt, hostile reactions, and loss of previous patterns of conduct. He defined the task of working through grief as emancipation from bondage to the deceased.

The essential task of mourning or grieving is the withdrawal of emotional concern and attachment from a lost object (person) and the preparation for relationships with new objects.

Stages of Mourning

Various authors have described the phases of mourning. Physicians should be familiar with these phases as well as with signs that indicate an unsuccessful or pathologic outcome of the mourning process. Parkes (1972) listed 5 stages of bereavement: alarm, numbness, pining (searching), depression, and recovery. These stages share certain similarities with the reactions of the dying patient discussed above and with the characteristics of the stress syndrome discussed in Chapter 5. These stages and phenomena vary in sequence, duration, intensity, and even occurrence in any given individual.

The initial reaction of alarm is essentially a reflex and physiologic alteration (increased heart rate and blood pressure) that occurs when acute stress exceeds the person's threshold of tolerance. Alarm is followed by numbness, which, if not excessive, is an adaptive defense mechanism that regulates the inflow of painful information so that it is not overwhelming. The third stage is essentially one of pining and searching for the lost object; it may be characterized by frequent hallucinations and pseudohallucinations of the deceased and by comments such as "I can't help looking for him even though I know he is dead." Parkes lists the components of this stage as a high state of alertness and sensitivity to stimuli, restless movement, preoccupation with thoughts of the deceased, development of a perceptual set of the deceased (ie, fixing in the mind of a set of images and reminders of the dead person), loss of interest in the outside world, calling for the person, and direction of attention to the environment where the person might be.

Illustrative case. A middle-aged widow spoke of her experience in the supermarket 3 weeks after the unexpected death of her husband: "I've actually always enjoyed grocery shopping, and that day everything seemed so normal and even carefree. My greatest concern of the moment was what to prepare for dinner. Then I suddenly realized that my husband would not be at dinner. I became shaky and for some reason walked over to the magazine and book rack; that was where he often browsed when we came to the market together. I kept seeing his favorite foods as I wandered along the aisles and for an instant thought that 2 men in the store might be him. I left the supermarket without my groceries."

Gradually, the loss becomes more real, and despair sets in as searching for the object decreases. This is the stage of depression and disorganization. As Freud stated, "Each single one of the memories and situations of expectancy is met by the verdict of reality that the object no longer exists." In the terminology of learning theory, patterns of previous behavior and assumptions are extinguished; ie, when behavior fails to result in previously obtained rewards (reinforcement), that behavior decreases in frequency.

The final stage of grief and mourning is that of recovery and reorganization, with a turning toward new goals and new persons.

Illustrative case (cont'd). Several months later the same woman as in the illustrative case above again talked about her experience in the supermarket: "For some reason, grocery shopping was a major focus of my grieving. I guess it represented a concrete way of caring for my husband, and I couldn't pretend to be buying food for 2. For weeks I needed a friend or one of the children to take me shopping because I got shaky and confused. After that I just got mostly sad. I must have been quite a sight standing in the checkout line with tears in my eyes. But my husband never came home to dinner, and now I only get a little sad at the store."

Several important phenomena occur during the mourning process. Characteristically, this process is not a period of continual depression but rather of episodic pangs of acute, intermittent grief. Symptoms include sleep difficulties, loss of appetite, and activation of the autonomic nervous system (eg, dryness of the mouth, tachycardia). Anger, guilt, and fear are common, in addition to sadness and a sense of loss. Anger has many facets and includes resentment toward the deceased for leaving and toward fate or God for dealing such a cruel blow; anger is also a reaction to the inevitable frustration occurring in the search for the deceased. Medical staff, friends, and relatives should be aware that the hostility often directed toward them is usually neither personal nor rational; to turn away from the bereaved as a result only compounds the pain.

Guilt is also present and stems from several sources. On a more conscious level, there is almost always the question, "Could I have somehow done more?" The empathic physician will often find it helpful to respond to this inquiry, even if it remains unasked. On a more unconscious level, guilt results from those ambivalent and hostile feelings harbored for the deceased. Relief that the death is someone else's and not one's own results in **survivor guilt** (see Chapter 5). Fear arises from the need to face a drastically changed reality without the support of the deceased, from the forced realization of one's own mortality, and often from the sheer intensity of the emotions and reactions experienced (eg, "Am I going mad?"). The bereaved person may adopt traits and mannerisms of the lost person, a normal process termed **identification.**

The time course of the mourning process is lifelong; in fact, one of the ways in which the deceased continues to live is in the memories of others. With time, however, memories become less painful and less intrusive. The pangs of acute grief usually peak during the second week following the death of the loved one. The major mourning period lasts between 6 and 18 months, with most people able to resume work and relatively normal functioning in less than half a year.

Bereavement in Children

Children are particularly susceptible to the stress of a death in the family, and they are vulnerable to the heightened danger of development of psychopathologic symptoms. Children's concepts of death vary with their developmental level. Children are also particularly affected by the alteration in family dynamics caused by death, which also activates numerous anxieties. Because of their tendency toward magical thinking, children often have feelings of being responsible for the death of the loved one, and they frequently harbor fears that they will be the next to die. They often resent the parent or parents who spend so much time with the dying family member, and they have fears of abandonment as well as anger toward the parents for allowing death to happen.

Unfortunately, the surviving parent or parents are often so overwhelmed with their own grief that they cannot offer sufficient support to the child. People cannot and should not attempt the impossible task of sparing the child the pain of loss but should instead help the child or adolescent grieve in a way that is appropriate to that individual's developmental level. The child's ability to mourn is greatly facilitated when surviving family members accept and support the child's reactions and allow the child to mourn with them. Young children in particular need the assistance of adults in expressing feelings of ambivalence, pain, and loss. Adults should provide names for the feelings the child may be experiencing but cannot verbalize. The child should also be reassured of the continuity of relationships with other people both within and outside the home.

Determinants of Grief & Pathologic Grief

Among the major factors that determine the course and outcome of the mourning process are (1) the developmental level of the bereaved individual; (2) the history of prior losses and stresses and how these have been dealt with; (3) the nature of the relationship with the deceased, especially the degree of conscious and unconscious ambivalence and hostility felt toward the dead person; (4) the current social support system of the bereaved; (5) the bereaved person's preparedness for the death (ie, whether the death was expected or unexpected); (6) the degree of economic disruption occasioned by the loss; and (7) the sociocultural setting of the bereaved and its provisions for facilitating the mourning process through rituals.

The mourning process is essential for the mental health of the bereaved individual. Unsuccessful or pathologic mourning is of 2 general types: (1) prolonged and unresolved grief and (2) delayed or denied grief. Symptoms include exaggerated guilt or self-reproach, extreme or abnormal identification with the deceased, phobias, hypochondriasis, psychosis, significant drug or alcohol use, prolonged immobilization (such as the inability to resume relatively normal functioning by the end of 1 year), or delay of the onset of grieving for more than a few weeks after death has occurred.

Illustrative case. A young man became incapacitated for months after his father died of stomach cancer. He developed physical symptoms of abdominal pain and vomiting, became fearful of crowds, and began heavy use of alcohol. A psychiatric consultation revealed the following factors: The father had been a harsh and punitive man for whom the son harbored significant resentment but upon whom he had been somewhat dependent financially; at age 5 the son had witnessed the accidental death of an older, and perhaps favored, brother; and the son had recently moved to a new city, where he had no close acquaintances. A brief course of psychotherapy resulted in a decrease in alcohol abuse and gastrointestinal symptoms, along with increased expression of feelings of anger, guilt, and loss. The young man subsequently moved back to the city where his family lived.

The Role of the Physician

Because of their closeness to the dead person during the last stages of illness, physicians have a special relationship with the deceased's survivors. Work with the family starts well before the terminally ill person's death, if possible, and includes the building of a trustful, empathic relationship founded on honest and appropriate communication. The physician should offer a realistic appraisal of the situation but at the same time allow for hope. The concept of anticipatory grief encourages family members to verbalize their thoughts and feelings and to begin to contemplate what life will be like without the dying person. Channels of open communication should be established with the dying person, so that important final personal communications between persons who have shared their lives may take place. Physicians should help facilitate this sharing process by letting patients and their families know that they are available and willing to talk about issues of mutual concern, whether it be directly and openly or through some metaphor or allegory that is comfortable to patients and their families. Anticipation of practical arrangements regarding the funeral, a will, housing arrangements, and so on should be encouraged.

During acute grief, physicians must first come to terms with their own thoughts and feelings about the patient's death; if the physician communicates a sense of acceptance of the outcome as opposed to a feeling of personal defeat, the bereaved will stand a greater chance of accepting the death. During the initial period of numbness and grief, financial, household, funeral, and other arrangements must be made. The physician may enlist the aid of friends for these tasks, educate them about what to expect (eg, irrational periods of anger), and correct possible misconceptions (eg, that dwelling on the deceased is morbid, when in fact working through grief requires recurrent review of many aspects of the lost person). Friends may also be called upon to provide for emotional support of any children involved.

Many bereaved people are perplexed or frightened by the nature and intensity of their reactions. The physician can reassure the mourner that guilt, anger, numbness, and even hallucinations are normal parts of the mourning process. At the same time, the physician should be alert to the possible manifestations of pathologic grief described above. Should such manifestations appear, careful monitoring by family and friends and possible consultation with the physician may be required.

The question whether medication should be prescribed for bereaved individuals arises frequently. Mourning is a necessary though painful process. Drugs stifle the emotions and inhibit the work of grief, and they should be prescribed only in rare instances. In the words of one patient, "I was furious when they offered me Valium; I wanted and needed to feel the pain of my father's death." It is important, however, that bereaved persons have enough sleep; hence, should severe insomnia persist, a sleep medication may be required.

SUMMARY

In medicine, physicians dedicate themselves to relieving pain, promoting health, and helping their fellow human beings. Nowhere else is there a greater opportunity to realize these ideals than in dealing with the dying patient and the bereaved family. In a sense, the quantity of life is less important than the quality of life, and the latter includes the quality of dying. To help someone die with dignity, with the benefit of companionship, minimal pain, and the knowledge that those left behind are in caring hands, is a great service.

REFERENCES

Anthony EJ, Koupernick C: *The Child and His Family: The Impact of Disease and Death*. Wiley, 1973.

Binger CM et al: Childhood leukemia: Emotional impact on patient and family. *N Engl J Med* 1969;**280:**414.

Bowlby J: *Attachment and Loss*. Vol 3: *Loss, Sadness, and Depression*. Basic Books, 1980.

Easson WM: *The Dying Child*. Thomas, 1970.

Erikson EH: *Childhood and Society*. Norton, 1950.

Feifel H: *The Meaning of Death*. McGraw-Hill, 1965.

Feifel H: *New Meanings of Death*. McGraw-Hill, 1977.

Freud S: Mourning and melancholia (1917). In: *Standard Edition of the Complete Psychological Works of Sigmund Freud*. Vol. 14. Hogarth Press, 1957.

Furman E: *A Child's Parent Dies*. Yale Univ Press, 1974.

Glaser B, Strauss A: *Awareness of Dying*. Yale Univ Press, 1974.

Hinton J: *Dying*. Penguin Books, 1967.

Kastenbaum R, Aisenberg R: *The Psychology of Death*. Springer, 1972.

Kübler-Ross E: *On Death and Dying*. Macmillan, 1969.

Lifton R, Olson E: *Living and Dying*. Bantam Books, 1974.

Lindemann E: Symptomatology and management of acute grief. *Am J Psychol* 1944;**101:**141.

Parkes CM: *Bereavement*. Internat Univ Press, 1972.

Pattison EM: Help in the dying process. Chapter 34 in: *American Handbook of Psychiatry*. Vol 1. Arieti S (editor). Basic Books, 1974.

Shneidman ES: *Death: Current Perspectives*. Mayfield, 1976.

Shneidman ES: *Deaths of Man*. Penguin Books, 1974.

Spinetta JJ: The dying child's awareness of death: A review. Pages 430–436 in: *Annals of Progress in Child Psychiatry and Child Development*. Chess S, Thomas A (editors). Brunner/Mazel, 1975.

Tolstoy L: *The Death of Ivan Ilyich and Other Stories*. Signet, 1960.

Waechter E: The response of children to fatal illness. In: *Current Concepts of Clinical Nursing*. Duffy M et al (editors). Mosby, 1971.

Weisman AD: Thanatology. Chap 27.2 in: *Comprehensive Textbook of Psychiatry/IV*, 4th ed. Kaplan HI, Freedman AM, Sadock BJ (editors). Williams & Wilkins, 1985.

10

Brain & Behavior

Jonathan Mueller, MD, & Howard Fields, MD, PhD

The practice of psychiatry requires a working knowledge of brain structure and function as well as of individual psychology. Knowledge about psychodynamic concepts complements and strengthens the clinician's understanding of behavioral and intrapsychic changes associated with alterations in the structure and function of the central nervous system. In this chapter, a review of the gross anatomy of the brain is followed by descriptions of disorders of the central nervous system that illustrate the role of the brain in human behavior.

Until recently, psychiatric education has emphasized the diagnosis and management of schizophrenia, depression, and anxiety disorders. To a surprising extent, the study and management of memory disorders, aphasias, head trauma, epilepsies, and dementia syndromes have been neglected.

In evaluating and managing patients with brain lesions, several factors must be taken into account: Personalities, intellectual gifts, and cognitive processes prior to brain injury are highly individual; lesions that produce changes in behavior and cognition are themselves never exactly the same; and social support networks and the motivation to improve following brain damage vary tremendously. Nevertheless, many characteristics are shared by brain-injured patients, and a knowledge of common syndromes aids the clinician in developing an individualized approach. The psychiatrist who is unaware of neurobehavioral syndromes will miss those diagnoses, to the detriment of the patient's care. For example, altered behavior due to organic causes (eg, inattention or diminished language comprehension) may be mistakenly interpreted as a problem in psychodynamic motivation. The clinician must distinguish behavioral and cognitive changes due to brain lesions from psychologic reactions due to the awareness of acquired deficits in mental and motor abilities. Since intact portions of the brain compensate for damaged portions, this task may be difficult.

GROSS ANATOMY OF THE BRAIN

An appreciation of neuroanatomy requires a knowledge of 3 different levels of the brain and the manner in which they are connected. MacLean (1969) used the term "triune" to describe 3 brains (Fig 10–1) essentially working as one: (1) a **neomammalian brain** (the neocortical mantle); (2) a **paleomam-**malian brain** (limbic or visceral brain); and (3) an ancient **reptilian brain** ("R complex"). These 3 levels will be discussed below under the headings of neocortical surface anatomy, limbic system anatomy, and brain stem anatomy.

Neocortical Surface Anatomy
(See Figs 10–2 and 10–3)

The adult human brain weighs about 1350 g and contains over 10 billion nerve cells. The surface of the 4 cerebral lobes (Fig 10–2) is irrigated by 3 major blood vessels: the anterior, middle, and posterior cerebral arteries. Major boundaries are formed by the **longitudinal cerebral fissure,** which separates the left from the right hemisphere at the midline; the **central sulcus** (fissure of Rolando), which separates the frontal from the parietal lobe; and the **lateral cerebral sulcus** (fissure of Sylvius), which forms the superior margin of the temporal lobe.

Many classification schemes have been devised to describe the structure and function of the brain. In 1909, Brodmann identified 47 different areas of the

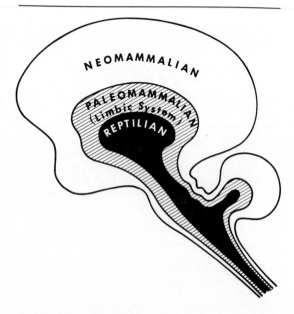

Figure 10–1. MacLean's "triune" brain. (Reproduced, with permission, from MacLean PD: The brain, empathy and medical education. *J Nerv Ment Dis* 1967;144:374. Copyright © 1967 by Williams & Wilkins.)

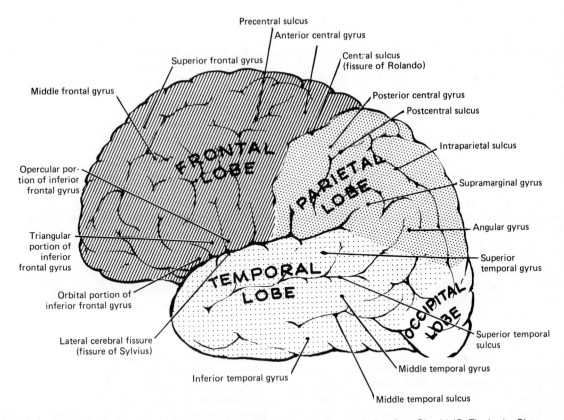

Figure 10–2. Lateral view of left cerebral hemisphere. (Reproduced, with permission, from Chusid JG: The brain. Chapter 3 in: *Correlative Neuroanatomy & Functional Neurology,* 19th ed. Lange, 1985.)

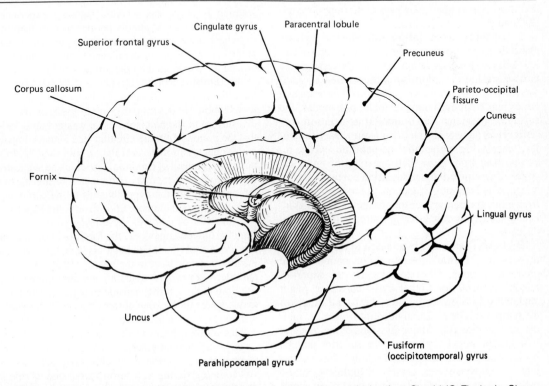

Figure 10–3. Medial view of right cerebral hemisphere. (Reproduced, with permission, from Chusid JG: The brain. Chapter 3 in: *Correlative Neuroanatomy & Functional Neurology,* 19th ed. Lange, 1985.)

cerebral cortex (Fig 10–4) on the basis of cytoarchitecture; this classification is still the most widely used.

A. Organization of the Cortex: The cortex consists of motor, sensory, and association areas.

1. Motor cortex–The motor cortex lies anterior to the central sulcus and may be subdivided into motor, premotor, supplemental motor, and frontal eye field areas (see also p 119).

2. Sensory cortex–The primary sensory cortex consists of regions that receive projections from thalamic relay nuclei. (Note that olfactory stimuli have no thalamic relay stations.) **Auditory impulses** stimulate the eighth cranial nerve, traverse brain stem pathways, and are conveyed by auditory fibers from the medial geniculate body of the thalamus to Heschl's gyrus (the primary auditory cortex) in the superior temporal plane. Surrounding Heschl's gyrus is the auditory association cortex known as Wernicke's area, located in the posterior third of the superior temporal gyrus. **Visual impulses** travel from the retina in the optic nerve and tract to reach the lateral geniculate body of the thalamus; they are then conveyed by fibers that sweep backward after a slight forward loop to reach the banks of the calcarine fissure (the primary visual cortex) on the medial aspect of the occipital lobe. Surrounding this primary visual cortex are the parastriate and peristriate visual association areas. **Tactile impulses** are mediated by fibers arising in the trunk and limbs and traveling up the spinal cord and by fibers arising from the face; these fibers converge in the ventral basal complex of the thalamus and then are projected to the postcentral gyrus (the primary sensory projection cortex). Association fibers then pass to the superior parietal lobule.

3. Sensory association cortex–The sensory association cortex of the temporal, parietal, and occipital lobes is the foundation for the processing and cross-correlation of information transmitted by auditory, visual, and tactile fibers. The sensory association cortex may be divided into unimodal, polymodal, and supramodal regions. The **unimodal association cortex** receives input exclusively from one sensory stimulus, whereas the **polymodal association cortex** receives input from more than one type of unimodal cortex. The **supramodal association cortex** performs a high-level integratory function. It receives no input from either the primary sensory or the unimodal association cortex; its only afferent source is the polymodal cortex.

B. Lobe Divisions: In addition to the functional division of the **frontal lobe** into motor, premotor, and prefrontal regions, 3 horizontal gyri—the superior, middle, and inferior frontal gyri—constitute major landmarks. In a similar fashion, the lateral aspect of the **temporal lobe** is also divided into superior, middle, and inferior gyri. Major divisions of the **parietal lobe** are the postcentral gyrus, the superior parietal lobule, and the inferior parietal lobule. This last region, which consists exclusively of high-level (polymodal and supramodal) association cortex, is subdivided into supramarginal and angular gyri. The

occipital lobe, also divided into superior and inferior gyri, contains the cuneus and lingual gyrus.

C. Sensory Cortex-Limbic System Connections: Through the sensory cortex-limbic system connections, the sensory information reflecting experience in the "outer world" is communicated to the "inner world" of emotions and drives, which are presumed to be governed by the limbic system.

Since the 1960s, it has been recognized that visual association fibers travel forward from the occipital region through the inferior and middle temporal gyri to reach the temporal pole. Fibers then sweep backward and medially to impinge on the amygdala, a component of the limbic system. The amygdala has been conceptualized as a gate, bridge, or way station between the sensory cortex and the hypothalamus.

D. Frontal Lobe-Limbic System Connections: Pathways that arise in the orbitomedial and dorsolateral prefrontal regions impinge on the hypothalamus and brain stem directly. Since these fiber systems are bidirectional, they offer a pathway whereby the frontal lobes not only can monitor but could also actually modulate core brain or autonomic system activity.

Limbic System Anatomy

The term "limbic system" refers to a group of structures anatomically situated between the diencephalon and telencephalon. Functionally, these structures mediate transactions between the extracorporeal world (as elaborated in the sensory association cortex) and primitive internal or visceral drives and responses "represented" in the hypothalamus. To the extent that learning is a process whereby sensory experience achieves meaning or attains permanence in memory by being paired with the experience of pleasure or pain at the core brain or "visceral" level, all learning may be said to be mediated by the limbic system.

A. Limbic Circuits: Despite the fact that Willis in the 17th century and Broca in the 19th century used the term "limbic" to describe the ring of tissue on the medial surface of the hemispheres, it was not until 1937 that the notion of limbic circuitry had a major impact on psychiatry. In that year, Papez published "A Proposed Mechanism of Emotion," in which he suggested that a group of structures participated in transferring information from the hypothalamus to the cortex and back to the hypothalamus. Specifically, the Papez circuit (Fig 10 – 5) involves the transfer of information from the hippocampus over the fornices to the mamillary bodies of the hypothalamus and then via the mamillothalamic tract to the anterior thalamus. From the anterior thalamus, fibers ascend through the anterior limb of the internal capsule to reach the cingulate gyrus, where they sweep posteriorly via the retrosplenial cortex to once again reach the hippocampus. Today the fornix is known to be a bidirectional pathway largely involving cholinergic pathways. It is believed to be part of an intrinsic or obligatory pathway involved in registering new information, and its role in emotional experience continues to be examined (Gray, 1983).

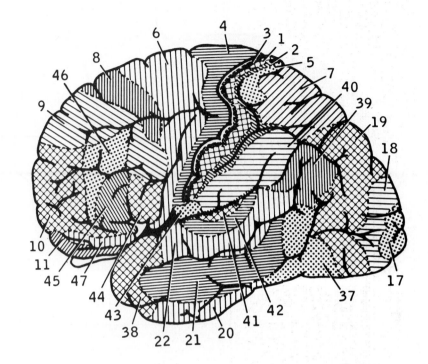

A

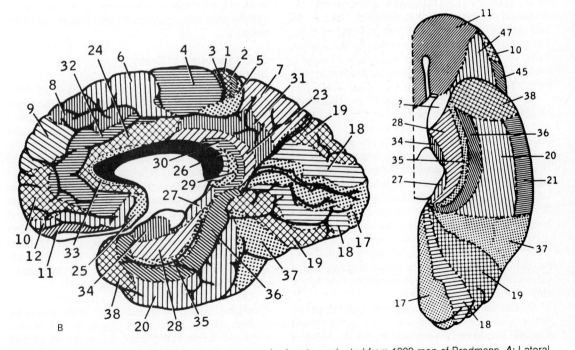

B

Figure 10–4. Cytoarchitectural zones of the human cerebral cortex, adapted from 1909 map of Brodmann. *A:* Lateral surface. *B:* Medial surface. **At right:** Basal surface. (Reproduced, with permission, from Adams RD, Victor M: *Principles of Neurology,* 2nd ed. McGraw-Hill, 1981.)

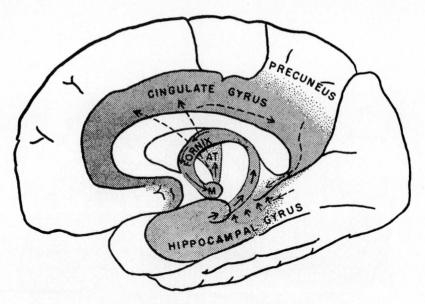

Figure 10–5. The Papez circuit, as described by MacLean. AT = anterior thalamus; M = mamillary bodies of the hypothalamus. (Reproduced, with permission of Elsevier Science Publishing Co., Inc., from MacLean PD: Psychosomatic disease and the "visceral brain." *Psychosom Med* 1949;11:340. Copyright © 1949 by The American Psychosomatic Society, Inc.)

Eleven years after Papez published his now famous paper, Yakovlev (1948) suggested that in addition to the medial structures described by Papez, 3 lateral cortical regions (the orbitofrontal cortex, temporal pole, and insula) played an important role in motivation. Yakovlev also highlighted the strategic position of 2 subcortical structures that Papez had not included in his circuit, the amygdala and dorsomedial thalamus.

In 1952, MacLean explicitly linked the medial limbic circuit of Papez with the basolateral limbic circuit of Yakovlev, referring to them as the limbic system, or visceral brain (Fig 10–6). The following is a brief summary of the major limbic system connections: (1) Both circuits exert powerful downward and presumably regulatory effects on the brain stem. (2) Both circuits have intrinsic connections, and the Papez circuitry has been described as "reverberating." (3) The basolateral limbic circuit has particularly strong upward connections to the sensory and frontal cortex, while the hippocampus (medial limbic circuit) receives sensory and frontal lobe input via multisynaptic pathways that converge on the entorhinal area before entering the hippocampus itself.

B. Limbic System-Neocortex Connections: Fibers arising from limbic structures in the medial temporal lobes travel to prefrontal regions by 2 distinct routes: a direct pathway via the uncinate fasciculus and an indirect pathway via the dorsomedial nucleus of the thalamus. Another example of limbic system-neocortex connections is the diffuse projection system that arises from the nucleus basalis of Meynert in the basal forebrain and travels to widespread areas of the neocortex, as well as to the hippocampus and amyg-

dala. Recent evidence suggests that degeneration of neurons in this limbic forebrain region may be responsible for the cholinergic deficit seen in Alzheimer's dementia.

Some Features of Brain Stem Anatomy

The reptilian brain consists essentially of brain stem and basal ganglia. Coursing through the upper brain stem is a dense network of interneurons known as the **reticular activating system.** From the reticular formation in the midbrain, fibers ascend both to the ventral forebrain and to the intralaminar and reticular nuclei of the thalamus. Thalamic fibers in turn project to diffuse areas of the cortex. Nauta (1958) coined the term **septo-hypothalamo-mesencephalic continuum** to describe a central core containing multiple neural tracts that connect (1) the septal region (the most anterior portion of the reticular activating system), (2) the hypothalamus, and (3) the midbrain. This continuum (Fig 10–7) is roughly synonymous with MacLean's reptilian brain ("R complex") (Fig 10–1).

The **septal region** consists of a group of nuclei located beneath, in front of, and medial to the head of the caudate nucleus. In the 1960s, it was found that electrical stimulation of the septal region in both animals and humans resulted in a strong sensation of pleasure, and the septal area thus was labeled a "pleasure center" (see p 104).

The **hypothalamus** consists of multiple nuclei located behind and above the optic chiasm, beneath the thalamus, and above the pituitary. The hypothalamus forms the floor and part of the lateral wall of the third

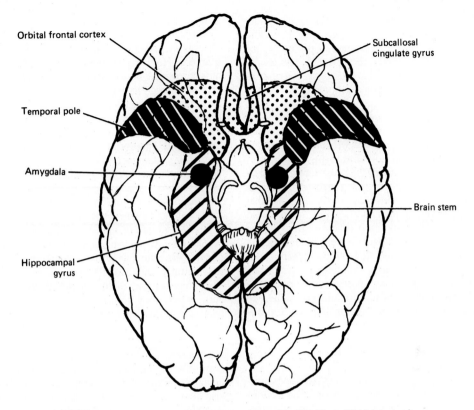

Figure 10–6. Orbital view of the limbic system. (Modified from KE Livingston.)

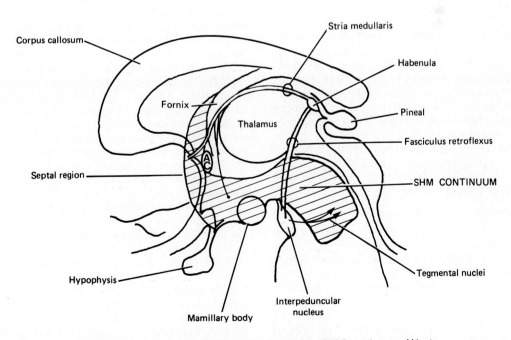

Figure 10–7. Septo-hypothalamo-mesencephalic (SHM) continuum of Nauta.

ventricle and has as its posterior border the mamillary bodies. The hypothalamus functions as a final common outflow pathway for autonomic discharge and plays a major role in regulation of pituitary function. It also contains regions central to the expression of drive states and appears to function as a homeostatic control device for maintenance of the internal milieu.

The **midbrain (mesencephalon),** a region of the upper brain stem, is of special importance to psychiatrists, since it is the site of origin of 2 major ascending **dopaminergic pathways.** Fibers arising from the substantia nigra and traveling to the neostriatum (caudate nucleus and putamen) form the **nigrostriatal pathway.** The **mesolimbic pathway** consists of fibers that arise from the ventral tegmental area of the midbrain and ascend to the frontal and limbic regions of the forebrain. (The antipsychotic effects of neuroleptic agents appear to be mediated by postsynaptic dopamine blockade in the mesolimbic pathways, while parkinsonian symptoms are produced by dopamine blockade at the level of the neostriatum.) In addition to these dopaminergic pathways, **noradrenergic pathways** and **serotoninergic pathways** arise from the more posterior regions of the brain stem and, together with dopaminergic pathways, constitute the **medial forebrain bundle.**

In summary, the septo-hypothalamo-mesencephalic continuum has extensive intrinsic connections and exerts a powerful upward influence on the cortex via the ascending reticular network and the numerous pathways of the medial forebrain bundle. In addition, the continuum is itself subject to downward influences from the medial and basolateral limbic circuits.

ANATOMY & PHYSIOLOGY OF PAIN

Both perception of pain and response to pain vary greatly among individuals. These behaviors range from the reflex withdrawal of a burned finger from a hot stove to the experience of pain in a limb amputated long ago, and from the anesthesia of conversion disorders ("hysterical anesthesia") to the analgesia produced by placebos. Knowledge of the neuroanatomy and physiology of pain is critical to understanding behavior in response to pain. This brief discussion will focus on peripheral receptors and transmitters, spinal reflexes, a system for central transmission of pain, and a system for modulation of pain.

Pain Transmission Systems

Pain sensation is triggered by stimuli that are potentially damaging to tissue. Nociceptors ("pain" receptors) in the periphery are probably free nerve endings. In peripheral nerve, the pain message is carried by 2 classes of small-diameter primary afferent fibers, the unmyelinated fibers and the myelinated fibers. In conscious patients, it is possible to electrically stimulate peripheral nerves and correlate fiber types with the sensations they produce. When the small myelinated

primary afferent fibers are activated, subjects begin to report pain. When the threshold for unmyelinated fibers is exceeded, the pain becomes burning and unbearable. Human peripheral nerve studies in which tungsten microelectrodes were used to stimulate single nerve fibers confirmed that pain is only elicited by activity in small-diameter myelinated and unmyelinated fibers. Although large-diameter fibers do not respond selectively to noxious stimuli, they are necessary for the "normal" quality of pain perception. When input from large-diameter primary afferent fibers is blocked, noxious stimuli produce an abnormal burning sensation. The activity in these large-diameter fibers is known to inhibit spinal pain transmission neurons, and this may account for the excessive response to noxious stimuli in subjects with large-fiber block.

The pain-transmitting small-diameter primary afferent fibers bifurcate as they enter the spinal cord and run rostrally and caudally for several millimeters. They enter the gray matter and terminate in the dorsal horn, where they contact neurons of the projecting pain pathways such as the spinothalamic and spinoreticular tracts. The primary afferent fibers contact projection cells both directly and via small relay interneurons in the superficial layers of the dorsal horn. In addition to the primary afferent terminals, relay interneurons, and projection cells, the dorsal horn also contains inhibitory interneurons that function in pain modulation circuits (described below).

The present working knowledge of the central pathways transmitting pain is based on observations in the 1850s by Brown-Séquard, who demonstrated that "pain" involves crossed pathways in the spinal cord and that hemisection of the cord results in contralateral analgesia below the lesion. Gowers studied patients with discrete spinal lesions and reported in 1886 that the anterolateral column of the spinal cord was the important spinal pathway for pain. In 1911, Spiller, on the basis of studies of lesions in monkeys, encouraged the neurosurgeon Martin to cut the anterolateral column of the spinal cord in patients with severe pain, predicting that this would produce lasting pain relief. In fact, it did. Although the spinothalamic tract is in the anterolateral column, it is not clear that this tract is the only major pathway for pain sensation. Cutting the anterolateral quadrant of the cord also results in interruption of fibers that project to parts of the brain stem reticular formation, which in turn projects to the thalamus. This projection is called the spinoreticulothalamic pathway.

Fig 10-8 illustrates that phylogenetic development is accompanied by increasing size of the spinothalamic tract. To a certain extent, the spinoreticulothalamic tract also grows, and this pathway is phylogenetically the oldest. If we accept the hypothesis that subhuman animals feel pain, then we have to seriously consider the medial spinoreticulothalamic tract an important pathway of pain. Since lesions in the spinal cord and lower medulla must destroy *both* pathways, this does not resolve the question of which is the major pain pathway. In the rostral medulla, the direct spino-

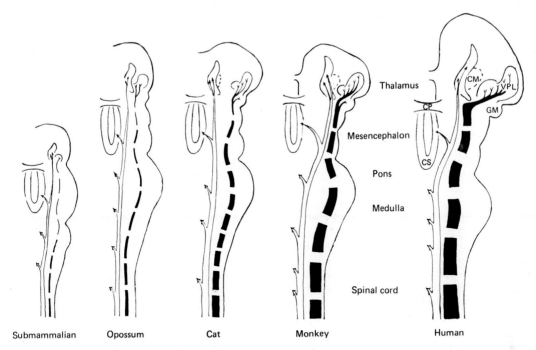

Figure 10–8. Phylogenetic tree of the spinothalamic tract. Schematic representation of the course and distribution of rostral projections from the spinal cord in the frog, opossum, cat, monkey, and human. Neospinothalamic system (interrupted black lines) versus paleospinothalamic system (uninterrupted outline). CP = commissura posterior; CS = central gray substance; CM = nucleus centromedianus; GM = nucleus corporis geniculati medialis; VPL = nucleus ventralis posterolateralis. Note the progressive increase in size of the neospinothalamic pathway. (Reproduced, with permission, from Mehler W: Some observations on secondary ascending afferent systems in the central nervous sytem. Chapter 2 in: *Pain: Henry Ford Hospital International Symposium.* Knighton RS, Dumke PR [editors]. Little, Brown, 1966. Copyright © 1966 by Little, Brown and Co.)

thalamic fibers take a more lateral course, which is separate from the medial spinoreticular system. Although stimulation of either of these tracts produces pain, there is a qualitative difference in the experience the patients report. Stimulation of the lateral (direct) spinothalamic tract produces a sensation of *sharp* localized burning, numbness, or cold. Stimulation of the medial spinothalamic tract, presumably activating the spinoreticulothalamic system, produces a *severe* burning pain that evokes strong emotional responses (anxiety, fear).

In summary, there are at least 2 pain pathways. It appears that the lateral spinothalamic tract is more concerned with discrete, localized, acute pains, eg, pinprick. The medial spinothalamic and spinoreticulothalamic pathway probably mediates more diffuse, chronic "clinical" types of pain. The clinical and behavioral significance of each one may be different. Cordotomy is an effective operation for pain relief probably because *both* pathways occupy the same region in the spinal cord and thus are simultaneously cut.

At present, cortical involvement in pain sensation is a subject of controversy. The thalamic regions receiving fibers directly from the spinal cord project to the parietal lobe and are probably reciprocally connected. The connections of the other thalamic regions involved in pain sensation are more diffuse and may include cortical and subcortical limbic structures.

Central Pain Syndromes

Isolated lesions in the lateral spinothalamic tract at the level of the rostral medulla result in pain in a high percentage of cases. A similar pain syndrome can be produced by chemical lesions of the lateral spinothalamic tract in the medulla, mesencephalon, or thalamus (the pain of thalamic syndrome). These central pain syndromes may result from lesions that interrupt the lateral (direct) spinothalamic tract while more or less sparing the medial spinoreticulothalamic tract.

Pain Modulation Systems

There is good evidence to support the concept of a neural network that selectively inhibits pain transmission. Stimulation of certain brain stem sites near the midbrain periaqueductal gray matter has been shown to produce analgesia in humans and laboratory animals. This modulating action is exerted at the level of the spinal cord dorsal horn. Stimulation of the periaqueductal gray matter inhibits spinal cord dorsal horn neurons that transmit pain. This action is mediated in part by a descending pathway that projects from the nucleus raphe magnus of the medulla to those regions of the dorsal horn where nociceptive projection cells are located.

The periaqueductal gray matter and the spinal cord dorsal horn contain high concentrations of opiate receptors, ie, membrane-bound proteins that stereospecifically bind opiate agonists (eg, morphine) and antagonists (eg, naloxone). Injecting small quantities of opiates at either site will produce analgesia. Furthermore, endogenous opioid peptides (endorphins) released by nerve cells can also produce analgesia by binding to opiate receptors. Examples of 2 such endorphins are leu-enkephalin and met-enkephalin. These enkephalins are found in very high concentration in the periaqueductal gray matter, nucleus raphe magnus, and spinal cord dorsal horn, and there is evidence that they are released in the presence of stress or pain and contribute to the action of the pain modulation system. Furthermore, there is evidence that morphine and other narcotic analgesics inhibit pain by activating cells in the periaqueductal gray matter and nucleus raphe magnus, which then project to and inhibit spinal cord pain transmission cells.

In addition to explaining how opiate analgesics relieve pain, knowledge of this pain modulation system has resulted in improved understanding of the variability of the pain experienced by different patients with similar tissue damage. One expression of this variability is the analgesic response of some patients to placebo. Placebo administration results in significant pain relief in about one-third of patients with severe pain (eg, postoperative or cancer pain). Recent studies have shown that this effect can be reduced by the opiate antagonist naloxone. This suggests that placebo analgesia results in part from activation of the endorphin-mediated analgesia system.

In summary, it is now clear that a full understanding of pain requires knowledge not only of the transmission system but of the modulation system as well. A more rational approach to the diagnosis and management of clinical pain problems can be expected to follow increased information about both systems.

EPILEPSY

Epilepsy and all seizure disorders illustrate the most basic relationship between the brain and behavior. These disorders result in intermittent paroxysmal dysfunction of the brain, which is manifested by synchronous high-voltage electrical discharges and by a variety of motor, sensory, and behavioral phenomena. Once called "the sacred disease," epilepsy has served as a scientific model for understanding the role of the brain in human behavior.

Classification of Epilepsy

There have been many attempts to classify the epilepsies. Difficulties are encountered because a single underlying pathologic process can produce various manifestations in different patients and because a variety of different processes (eg, tumor, infarct, vascular

malformation) can result in clinically indistinguishable seizures. There are a variety of diseases whose sole manifestation is a seizure disorder. Each of these diseases has a somewhat different clinical and electroencephalographic manifestation. Thus, the epilepsies have 2 distinct aspects: First, epilepsy can be a general (nonspecific) response of the brain to a variety of metabolic and structural insults. Second, the epilepsies include a group of clinically distinct nervous system diseases.

Table 10–1 represents one clinically useful empirical classification scheme. The 2 major divisions are **primary epilepsies,** in which there is no known brain abnormality other than the clinical paroxysmal dysfunction; and **secondary epilepsies,** in which there is a known structural or metabolic abnormality of the brain.

Table 10–1. Classification of epilepsies.*

Primary generalized epilepsies
Absence seizures:
  Classic absence seizures of childhood, with diffuse 3-Hz spike-and-wave complexes.
  Absence seizures of juvenile myoclonic epilepsy, characterized by staring and diffuse 3- to 6-Hz multi-spike-and-wave complexes during adolescence.
  Juvenile absence seizures with diffuse 8- to 12-Hz rhythms.
  Myoclonic absence seizures, with diffuse 3- to 6-Hz multi-spike-and-wave complexes.
  Myoclonic absence seizures, characterized by staring, fragmentary myoclonus, automatisms, and diffuse 12-Hz rhythms.
Myoclonic seizures:
  Myoclonic seizures of early childhood, with 3- to 6-Hz multi-spike-and-wave complexes without mental retardation (Doose's syndrome).
  Juvenile myoclonic seizures of Janz or benign myoclonic seizures of adolescence and late childhood, with diffuse 4- to 6-Hz multi-spike-and-wave complexes.
Clonic-tonic-clonic (grand mal) seizures.
Tonic-clonic (grand mal) seizures.
Partial epilepsies
Simple partial.
Complex partial:
  Simple partial at onset followed by impairment of consciousness and automatisms.
  Impairment of consciousness at onset:
    Motionless stare and impaired consciousness followed by automatisms (temporal lobe epilepsy).
    Complex motor automatisms at start of impaired consciousness (frontal lobe, somatosensory, or occipital lobe epilepsy).
    Drop attack with impaired consciousness and automatisms (temporal lobe syncope).
Secondary generalized epilepsies
Simple partial evolving to tonic-clonic (secondary tonic-clonic).
Infantile spasms (propulsive petit mal, infantile myoclonic encephalopathy with hypsarrhythmia, or West's syndrome).
Myoclonic astatic or atonic epilepsies (epileptic drop attacks of Lennox-Gastaut in children with mental retardation).
Progressive myoclonic epilepsies in adolescents and adults with dementia (myoclonic epilepsies of Lafora, Lundborg, Hartung, Hunt, or Kuf).
Unclassified epilepsies

*Modified from the classification of the International League Against Epilepsy and the World Health Organization.

Most (not all) primary epilepsies are generalized at onset—ie, there are electroencephalographic and clinical signs of widespread bilateral involvement of brain areas—with no preceding focal discharge. There is impairment of consciousness, and symmetric motor manifestations are seen. The **primary generalized epilepsies** usually appear before adolescence, are associated with normal intelligence, respond well to medical management, and may resolve, so that medication can be withdrawn. Seizures that are generalized at onset and have an obvious cause (eg, birth trauma, lipidoses) are termed **secondary generalized epilepsies** (previously called symptomatic epilepsies). If the underlying disease can be treated, the seizures will stop; if not, seizure control may be difficult or impossible.

Partial epilepsies are those in which the seizure discharge is limited to part of the brain, usually one hemisphere. If there is any impairment of consciousness during the seizure, it is referred to as a **complex partial seizure.** Partial seizures may spread and become generalized. They are then classified as secondary generalized epilepsy. Partial epilepsies are usually produced by structural lesions involving the limbic cortex, often the temporal lobe. Partial epilepsy includes temporal lobe or psychomotor seizures.

Complex partial seizures are of importance in psychiatry because the manifestations during seizures may resemble those seen in psychiatric illness. For example, visual and auditory hallucinations (including hearing voices) are not rare. Objects in the environment may appear to shrink or move. Of particular interest are subjective changes such as a feeling of familiarity *(déjà vu),* of strangeness *(jamais vu),* or of unprovoked fear or anxiety. Other manifestations include automatisms such as lip smacking or chewing movements; more complex behavior including incoherent speech, driving, or walking may occur during the seizure, and the patient will have no memory of these acts. Strange smells, tastes, visceral sensations, or vertigo may occur and should raise the suspicion of complex partial seizures. In addition to these seizure phenomena, patients with complex partial seizures involving the temporal lobe may have an increased incidence of psychopathologic manifestations between seizures. The 2 most frequent are aggressive behavior and a lasting schizophrenialike illness that occurs after repeated seizures.

Newer monitoring techniques that simultaneously videotape the patient's behavior and electroencephalographic changes have permitted more accurate localization of the seizure focus. In cases of complex partial epilepsy that are refractory to anticonvulsant medication, excision of the seizure focus can lead to complete seizure control and some amelioration of the behavioral disturbance.

Mechanisms of Epilepsy

Partial epilepsies have been studied in a variety of animal species in which focal cortical lesions lead to paroxysmal discharge. In patients with partial epilepsy, the origin of the seizure can often be located between seizures by recording intermittent focal spikes on the electroencephalogram. In animals, such spikes can be produced by certain experimental focal cortical lesions. It is now clear that these surface spikes are generated by synchronous activity in cortical neurons. Intracellular recording has demonstrated that individual cortical neurons generate massive depolarizations that are synchronous with the spikes recorded at the cortical surface. These massive depolarizations are called paroxysmal depolarization shifts and are thought to represent a failure of normal synaptic inhibitory mechanisms. A variety of insults could produce this, including a reduction in the amount or efficacy of the inhibitory transmitter gamma-aminobutyric acid or an inadequate glial uptake of potassium.

In animals with induced focal cortical lesions, these intermittent focal spikes may increase in frequency until they produce a prolonged depolarization with continuous repetitive firing of cortical neurons. Under these circumstances, the seizure activity may spread to adjacent cortex or across the corpus callosum to become generalized.

Whether results in animal models are relevant to human partial epilepsy is uncertain; however, paroxysmal depolarization shifts have been recorded in human cortical tissue taken from a seizure focus. At present, there are no well-studied experimental models for the generalized epilepsies. In addition, brain tissues from patients with generalized epilepsy show no consistent pathologic changes.

DRIVES & DRIVE DISORDERS

At its most elemental level the human organism, like crawling life, has a mouth, digestive tract, and anus, a skin to keep intact, and appendages with which to acquire food. Existence, for all organisms, is a constant struggle to feed—a struggle to incorporate whatever other organisms they can fit into their mouths and press down their gullets without choking . . . . If at the end of each person's life he were to be presented with the living spectacle of all that he had organismically incorporated in order to stay alive, he might well feel horrified by the living energy he had ingested. The horizon of a gourmet, or even the average person, would be taken up with *hundreds* of chickens, flocks of lambs and sheep, a small herd of steers, sties full of pigs, and rivers of fish. The din alone would be deafening.

This quotation from Becker (1975) illustrates the pivotal role of drives—in this case, the drive to eat. Philosophers have long debated the meaning of universal and innate biologic forces or drives manifested in all forms of life. Scientists have tried to translate these concepts into considerations of matter and energy, brain tissue and nerve transmission.

Freud's (1895) *Project for a Scientific Psychology* represented an attempt to consider how energy manifests itself and is transmitted in the brain and how objects in the external world begin to assume a particular charge or meaning for the observer. After hypothesizing the transfer of electrical energy (cathexis) from one neuron to another, Freud extended his model to include objects invested with or deprived of cathexis. For example, he spoke of infants as extending libidinal pseudopodia toward objects in the world.

While reflex behavior is fully *predictable,* other more complex forms of behavior exist that do not correlate as precisely with external stimulus conditions but are still far from voluntary. Students of behavior have invoked as hypothetical mechanisms the concept of motivational states that determine the intensity and direction of complex behaviors. Reflexes, drive behaviors, and fully voluntary behaviors thus seem to exist not as sharply demarcated features but along a continuum.

Theories of Drive

Various approaches to understanding drives can be seen in the work of ethologists, developmental psychologists, and anatomists.

A. Innate Capacities: Ethologists such as Lorenz and Tinbergen have made important discoveries about what they term "innate capacities." Turning away from the complexity of human behavior, ethologists have studied instinct or drive by working with animals such as fish, birds, and insects.

Tinbergen's work with the male stickleback fish is a good example of this approach. While the presence of male fish with bright red bellies during mating season provokes fighting or attack behavior in other males, it provokes approach or mating behavior in females. Colorless models resembling stickleback fish fail to elicit this behavior in either males or females. On the other hand, crude pieces of wood painted with a patch of red elicit only male approach. From this sort of work arose the notion of a "sign stimulus" or "releaser"—a particular configuration or feature embedded in a complex stimulus—that triggers instinctual behavior such as eating, mating, or attack. Since these stereotyped response behaviors occur in animals raised in total isolation, ethologists speak of them as operating through "innate releasing mechanisms."

The following is an example of the types of behavior arising from triggered innate release mechanisms: When parent thrushes alight on the nest of newborns and shake the nest, the mouths of the newborn chicks gape upward. A few days later, touching the side of the young thrush's mouth produces the same response. Shortly thereafter, the sight of the parent bird (or even of a human finger) elicits gaping behavior that is still vertically oriented. Still later, gaping behavior is directed toward the visual stimulus. Two distinct types of behavior are seen: (1) a response initially elicited and controlled by proximal (vestibular or tactile) stimuli and (2) a response gradually recruited by more distal stimuli such as visual stimuli.

B. Human Reflexes: Early reflex behaviors such as sucking, grasping, and turning the head toward a stimulus (eg, a nipple or a finger touching the infant's cheek) occur not only in awake infants but also in infants who are asleep or in coma. Sucking behavior also

occurs in anencephalic infants. Although the extensor plantar response may persist for a year, most of these primitive reflexes disappear by the age of 4–6 months. However, they often reemerge in human adults with frontal lobe disorders (eg, tumor or advanced Alzheimer's dementia). Thus, these primitive behaviors appear to have been held in check by the frontal neocortex.

C. Anatomy of Specific Drive Behaviors:
1. Rage–In the 1890s, it was noted that cerebral decortication in dogs caused them to respond to trivial stimuli (pinching of the tail, being removed from the cage, or even having a fly land on the animal's nose) with disinhibited rage.

In the 1920s, Cannon studied adrenal medullary sympathetic discharge in decorticated cats and described their massive reaction to trivial stimuli (eg, touching the cat's back) as "sham rage," consisting of the following behavior: (1) pupils dilating and hair standing on end, (2) hissing and growling, (3) baring the teeth and fangs, and (4) arching the back and lashing the tail. In 1928, Bard pointed out that this entire sequence depended on the integrity of the posterior hypothalamus.

2. Eating–Feeding and eating have been studied in rather fine detail. Following initial observations that destructive lesions in the ventromedial hypothalamus resulted in hyperphagia and obesity, other reports began to document profound anorexia and weight loss following destruction of the lateral hypothalamus. Thus, there arose the concepts of a ventromedial "satiety center" and a lateral "feeding center," or "appetite center." Reports of stereotactic surgery of the hypothalamus in animals, along with a few dramatic case reports of humans with lesions in these areas, have supported these initial observations. However, several lines of inquiry—as shown in the examples below—suggest that it may be inappropriate to conceptualize hypothalamic areas as "centers" for eating or satiety.

Lesions in the hypothalamus interrupt ascending dopaminergic pathways of the medial forebrain bundle. Severing these fibers outside the hypothalamus also produces the diminished arousal and aphagia seen with lateral hypothalamic lesions. In fact, animals with lesions in the hypothalamus do not have an isolated or selective loss of interest in food. Rather, they appear to manifest syndromes of multimodal sensory inattention—ie, reduced responsiveness to visual, auditory, tacticle, and olfactory stimuli presented to the side opposite the lesion.

Although animals with ventromedial hypothalamic lesions usually eat more food than animals without lesions, if the food is adulterated (eg, made bitter with quinine), they actually eat less than normal animals do. Thus, they seem to show an exaggerated response to both noxious and pleasant stimuli.

Animals starved prior to destruction of the lateral hypothalamus will eat and gain weight immediately after the lesion is produced—apparently in an attempt to bring their weight to a "set point."

These observations point to the difficulties in conceptualizing "centers" for activities as complex as eating.

A hierarchical network approach to eating behavior recognizes contributions to this behavior from 3 levels of control: (1) The hypothalamus, with its "hard-wired circuitry," regulates glucose levels, monitors fullness of the stomach (satiety versus hunger), and determines the "set point," ie, *how much to eat.* (2) The limbic system, in concert with the sensory systems, governs the selection of foods appropriate to appease the appetite, ie, *what to eat.* (3) The prefrontal regions are involved in decisions about table manners, ie, *when, where, and how to eat.*

Disturbances at each of these levels can be seen: (1) Tumors of the diencephalic region may disrupt carbohydrate metabolism and lead to hyperphagia, rage, and obesity. Patients with dysfunction of appetite regulation may even tear doors off refrigerators in order to satisfy the carbohydrate drive. This is termed "appropriate megaphagia," since the items ingested are not qualitatively different from what is normally eaten. (2) Patients with medial temporal lobe disorders (eg, Klüver-Bucy syndrome) may ingest items such as tea bags or cigarette butts. This "inappropriate hyperphagia" has been interpreted as reflecting sensory-limbic disconnection with consequent visual agnosia, manifested in this case by the inability to recognize and discriminate between the edible and inedible items. (3) Dementia or frontal lobotomy may lead to disruption of social behavior with loss of table manners.

3. Pleasure–Animal experiments begun in the 1960s have shed light on the neural substrates for "pleasure." After electrodes were implanted in certain regions of the medial forebrain bundle, the animal could press a bar to receive an electric current to the brain (pleasure stimulus). Animals were observed to press the bar repeatedly—even to the point of neglecting water and food or to the point of exhaustion—and to cross an electric grid to receive further pleasure stimulation.

Modulation of Drives

Drives depend on neural circuits whose developmental maturation is vulnerable to chemical and structural insults. Structurally intact circuits are themselves subject to modification and modulation by numerous forces. Examples of factors that shape and modulate the circuitry from which drives arise include the following:

A. Genetics: Individuals with Down's syndrome (trisomy 21) appear to have a biologic disinclination to violent behavior.

B. Circadian Rhythms: Cortisol secretion, motor activity, and body temperature are all subject to 24-hour cycles. A pathway from the retina to the supraoptic nucleus of the hypothalamus plays a major role in adjustment to changes in the light-dark cycle.

C. Hormones: Castration and antiandrogens are used to treat sex offenders in Europe. The human brain

itself may have a "sexual identity": A region of the anterior hypothalamus (preoptic nucleus) has been termed "dimorphic" in rats, since its gross anatomy is shaped by exposure to circulating estrogens. Alpha-fetoprotein produced by the fetal liver protects the developing human fetal brain of both sexes from masculinization by circulating maternal estrogens. The third or fourth month of human gestation appears to be a "critical period" for the development of sexuality.

Drive Disorders

Psychiatrists and neurologists seldom see isolated drive disorders. Constellations of drive disorders, however, are seen frequently in the context of neuropsychiatric disorders. The following are examples of human drive disorders:

A. Anorexia Nervosa: This disorder is characterized by loss of 25% of baseline ideal weight; altered body perception and fear of obesity; amenorrhea; lanugo; hypotension; bradycardia; and peculiar behavior associated with eating and weight control, such as hoarding food, abusing laxatives, binge eating (bulimia), and vomiting. Anorexia occurs more frequently in females than in males (20:1) and is most common in the age group from 15 to 25 years. The role of psychodynamic factors in this disorder is unclear. Behavioral regimens (eg, confinement to bed until satisfactory weight gain occurs) in conjunction with psychotherapy appear to be the only successful approach to treatment (see Chapter 3).

B. Kleine-Levin Syndrome: Episodic hypersomnia (up to 20 hours) alternates with hyperphagia, gorging of food, and hypersexuality (masturbation and aggressive sexual behavior) in this syndrome in adolescent boys. Patients are amnesic for these episodes, which recur at intervals of 3–6 months, last 1–3 weeks, and remit spontaneously.

C. Depression: Major depression is associated with the following neurovegetative signs:

1. Sleep–The amount of sleep is classically diminished in depression. Early morning awakening and rumination are prominent manifestations, but prolonged sleep with frequent arousals can also characterize major affective disorders. Hypersomnia is well recognized in "atypical depressions."

2. Eating–Anorexia with weight loss is common, but overeating is often seen in "atypical depressions."

3. Sex drive–Diminished interest in sex is often seen as one manifestation of anhedonia (inability to find pleasure in events that previously afforded enjoyment).

4. Motor activity–Psychomotor retardation is common in depression.

D. Mania: Diminished need for sleep, hyperactivity, pressure of speech, and hypersexuality are common in manic states.

E. Klüver-Bucy Syndrome: Manifestations include placidity (tameness), visual agnosia, lack of sexual inhibitions, and a tendency to place objects in the mouth.

F. Complex Partial Seizures: Hyposexuality

and increased preoccupation with abstract intellectual interests (eg, philosophy, religion, and morals) are seen in patients with complex partial seizures. It is as if these intellectual interests had preempted biologic drives.

G. Wernicke-Korsakoff Syndrome: Korsakoff's amnestic syndrome is preceded by the characteristic triad of Wernicke's encephalopathy, ie, confusion, ataxia, and eye movement disorders (nystagmus or ophthalmoplegia). As part of Korsakoff's syndrome, one may see profound apathy in which neither sex nor alcohol interests the patient. Korsakoff's syndrome is a useful model for a drive disorder, with lesions distributed in strategic midline structures: (1) mamillary bodies in the posterior hypothalamus (part of Papez circuit); (2) the periaqueductal region (from the third to fourth ventricles), with lesions interrupting the ascending fibers of the medial forebrain bundle and the reticular activating system; and (3) the dorsomedial nucleus of the thalamus, which is a crucial bridge between multiple limbic regions and the frontal lobes.

SLEEP & SLEEP DISORDERS

Sleep has many of the attributes of a drive. Sleep deprivation leads to an increased "urge" to sleep and to extended periods of sleep immediately following the deprivation. After several days of sleep deprivation, a confusional state may occur with disordered attention, emotional lability, reduced memory, delusions, and even hallucinations. The physiologic function of sleep is unknown. Current knowledge suggests that people follow the urge to sleep to avoid the consequences of sleep deprivation. To date, no one has proposed a better explanation for the function of sleep than Freud, who believed it provided a time for dreaming and discharging unconscious wishes and expressing unconscious fantasies that were unacceptable to conscious thought and expression.

Physiology of Sleep

Most animals experience a daily cycle of changes in levels of alertness and arousal as well as sleep and waking. Sleep was originally thought to be a passive process (ie, essentially a functional deafferentation), based on observations of animals falling into continual sleep or coma if the forebrain is deafferented by transection of the brain stem at the mesencephalic level. However, the observation that lesions of the pons just in front of the trigeminal nerve cause animals to be hyperalert and sleep much less than normal indicates that normal sleep is an active process that requires activity of neurons in the brain stem. In fact, neurophysiologic studies have demonstrated that nerve cells in the pontine reticular formation begin to discharge minutes prior to the onset of certain stages of sleep.

The sleep cycle consists of several distinct stages defined by the appearance of certain wave patterns on the electroencephalogram. The time required to pass through the complete sequence of sleep stages is about 90 minutes, and the cycle is repeated 3–5 times each night. There are 2 distinct states of sleep: **slow-wave sleep** and **rapid eye movement (REM) sleep.**

Slow-wave sleep—also called non-rapid eye movement (NREM) sleep—is divided into 4 stages (Fig 10–9): Stage 1 is characterized by an electroencephalogram in which the alpha rhythm has disappeared and the electroencephalographic background consists of low-voltage fast activity. In stages 2–4, the electroencephalogram becomes more synchronized (lower frequency, higher amplitude) and the subject more difficult to arouse. The longest and deepest period of slow-wave sleep each night is the first period of stage 3 and 4 sleep, usually within 2 hours after falling asleep. During this period, subjects are aroused with great difficulty and frequently demonstrate a transient confusional state. Stage 4 sleep, the deepest stage of slow-wave sleep, resembles hibernation in that blood pressure, pulse, respiratory rate, and body temperature all drop and the brain oxygen consumption is very low. It is not known where in the brain slow-wave sleep is initiated, but its electrical manifestations can still be observed in cortex that is disconnected from the brain stem.

After the intial slow-wave sleep stages, the electroencephalographic pattern usually shifts abruptly to the desynchronized (higher frequency, lower amplitude) pattern seen in stage 1 sleep. Despite some similarity with the "waking" electroencephalographic pattern, it is difficult to waken subjects in this stage of sleep. This is sometimes referred to as "paradoxic sleep." One of the most striking features of this stage is intermittent rapid eye movements. Because of these eye movements, this stage is termed rapid eye movement (REM) sleep. During REM sleep, there is also a striking loss of limb muscle tone, which resembles paralysis. In normal subjects, REM sleep only occurs after a preceding period of deeper (stages 2–4) sleep. Studies indicate that dreaming occurs mainly during REM sleep. More than 80% of subjects aroused during REM sleep report vivid and colorful visual imagery. Subjects aroused 10 minutes after the REM period has terminated seldom report complete dream imagery. Since subjects usually have several REM episodes each night, they probably have several dreams, although they rarely remember more than one. If REM sleep is selectively blocked by wakening the subject at the beginning of REM sleep, a specific "REM debt" builds up, and the subject does not feel adequately rested. REM sleep is apparently triggered by neurons in the dorsolateral midbrain and pontine reticular formation.

Sleep Disorders*

Several of the drive disorders described previously are characterized by abnormalities of sleep. Hypersomnia is a key feature of the Kleine-Levin syndrome, and disorders of sleep are seen frequently in patients

---

*This section is contributed by James J. Brophy, MD.

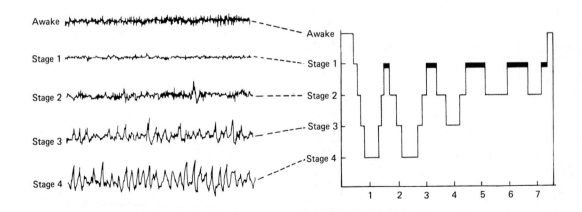

Figure 10–9. *Left:* Electroencephalographic recordings during different stages of wakefulness and sleep. Each line represents 30 seconds. The top recording of low-voltage fast activity is that of an awake brain. The next 4 tracings represent successively deeper stages of NREM (slow-wave) sleep, characterized by lower-frequency, higher-amplitude waves. *Right:* A typical night's pattern of sleep staging in a young adult. The time spent in REM sleep is represented by a **dark bar.** The first REM period is usually short (5–10 minutes), but periods tend to lengthen in successive cycles. Conversely, stages 3 and 4 dominate the NREM periods in the first third of the night, but they are often completely absent later. (Reproduced, with permission, from Kelly DD: Physiology of sleep and dreaming. Chapter 40 in: *Principles of Neural Science.* Kandel ER, Schwartz JH [editors]. Elsevier, 1981. Copyright © 1981 by Elsevier Science Publishing Co., Inc.)

with depression and mania. Insomnia (ie, trouble falling asleep, waking up during the night, or awakening too early without a rested feeling) is one of the most common complaints in general medical practice and occurs in about 30% of the normal population.

A. Insomnia: Insomnia is usually considered to be sleep deprivation or a marked change in the perceived sleep pattern. Factors contributing to insomnia include (1) situational problems such as transient stress, job pressures, and marital discord; (2) aging; (3) medical disorders that inevitably include pain and physical discomfort; (4) drug-related episodes, including withdrawal from alcohol or sedatives; and (5) psychologic conditions, particularly the major mental illnesses such as schizophrenia and affective disorders.

Schizophrenic patients vary markedly in the degree of sleep disturbance they endure. In acute episodes, the disruption is severe, even to the point of total insomnia. The chronic schizophrenic or the patient in remission often has no complaints, and an electroencephalographic pattern is not remarkably abnormal.

Sleep disturbance is one of the most common symptoms of affective disorders. Some patients with bipolar disorder sleep more when they are depressed and less when they are manic, but there is much variation. Primary depressions usually show sleep continuity disturbances, shortened REM stage latency, more REM sleep at the beginning of the night than in early morning hours, and a marked reduction in sleep stages 3 and 4. In the manic phase, REM sleep is decreased, but there are varying reports on slow-wave sleep. In both unipolar and bipolar disorders, patients in the depressed phase usually have a decreased total sleep time. The incidence of excess sleep in depression is low—about 8%. There is no correlation of particular types of depression with specific types of sleep problems.

B. Hypersomnia: Hypersomnia is seen in narcolepsy, Kleine-Levin syndrome, and sleep apnea.

1. Narcolepsy–This sleep disturbance usually occurs before age 40 and includes one or more of the following 4 conditions: sleep attacks, cataplexy, sleep paralysis, and hallucinations. **Sleep attacks** are sudden, reversible, short (lasting about 15 minutes) episodes occurring during any type of activity. Electroencephalographic recordings usually show a direct progression to REM sleep. The patient awakens refreshed, and there may be a refractory period of 1–5 hours before another attack occurs. **Cataplexy** is a sudden loss of muscle tone, with effects ranging from weakness of specific small muscle groups to general muscle weakness that causes the person to slump to the floor, unable to move. Cataplexy is often initiated by an emotional outburst (laughing, crying, anger) and lasts from several seconds to 30 minutes. **Sleep paralysis** involves acquisition of flaccid muscle tone with full consciousness, either during awakening or while falling asleep. There is usually intense fear, which is occasionally accompanied by auditory hallucinations. The attack is terminated by touching or calling the patient. **Hypnagogic hallucinations,** either visual or auditory, may precede sleep or occur during the sleep attack. If the hallucinations occur during awakening, they are called **hypnopompic hallucinations.** The occurrence of the symptoms of the narcoleptic tetrad are as follows: sleep attacks, almost 100%; sleep attacks and cataplexy, about 70%; sleep paralysis alone, about 5%.

2. Kleine-Levin syndrome–Hypersomnic attacks may last up to 20 hours and occur infrequently (3–4 times per year). There is confusion upon awakening. This syndrome is a separate entity from narcolepsy.

3. Sleep apnea–Apneic episodes occur in both REM and NREM sleep. Noisy, stertorous snoring and hypersomnolence the next day are common. Intellectual and personality changes include decreased attention span, decreased memory, and hyperirritability. There are 2 types of sleep apnea: **central apnea,** in which there is a cessation of respiratory movement with loss of airflow; and **obstructive apnea,** in which there is persistent respiratory effort but upper airway blockage.

C. Stage 4 Sleep Disorders: The most common of these disorders is **enuresis,** which is usually seen with variable nightly occurrence in children. While it often seems that the wetting occurred during dream sleep, it is actually seen most frequently in stage 4 sleep, with some preponderance in the first third of the night. **Somnambulism** also is reported mostly in children, usually during stage 3 and 4 sleep. **Pavor nocturnus** (night terrors) usually occurs in young children, predominantly in stage 4 sleep. As in somnambulism, amnesia for the episode occurs.

SYNDROMES OF DENIAL, NEGLECT, & INATTENTION

The parietal lobe receives and integrates tactile, visual, and auditory information. As it has grown through evolution, it has (1) pushed the motor area anteriorly, (2) pushed the visual cortex backward and downward, and (3) led to the development of an operculum (flap) composed of temporal, parietal, and frontal cortex.

The right parietal lobe region and the prefrontal region have been referred to as "silent areas," since lesions in these regions may not produce gross disturbances of motor or sensory function. On the other hand, it is definitely not the case that the surgeon can remove these areas with impunity.

Assessment of Parietal Lobe Disorders

Several factors complicate assessment of parietal lobe disorders. Patients with lesions of the left parietal lobe frequently have receptive aphasia and, therefore, may be unable to understand the examiner's statements and questions. Patients with lesions of the right parietal lobe have problems sustaining and directing attention and may be only marginally cooperative. Since patients with parietal lobe disorders may be either unaware of their deficits or unable to communicate with the examiner, the history obtained from friends and family becomes invaluable.

During the mental status examination, extreme care must be taken to avoid overlooking any of the following: (1) language problems (see Language Disorders, below); (2) problems with the distribution of attention; (3) visual, spatial, or constructional deficits (see Apraxia and the Callosal Syndromes, below); (4)

body image distortions; (5) tactile problems; (6) motility disturbances; and (7) other neuropsychiatric disturbances.

Denial of, Neglect of, & Inattention to Illness

In 1914, Babinski coined the term **anosognosia** to denote neglect of left hemiplegia following right cerebral infarction. He observed that his patients either were unaware of or seemed to ignore their deficits. His first patient was a woman who, despite an otherwise excellent recovery, never once over a period of years complained of or even alluded to her hemiplegia. When asked to move her arm, she behaved as if the examiner were talking to someone else. A second patient not only failed to move her paralyzed arm when asked to do so but would sometimes say, "There, it's done" without having moved at all. Babinski noted that each of these patients had left-sided weakness with sensory deficits in the affected limb. He speculated that anosognosia might be peculiar to patients with lesions of the right hemisphere. It is important to note that "denial of illness" is a somewhat clumsy translation of Babinski's original term, since it implies that patients have some level of awareness of their deficit but either repress or suppress this knowledge. Because most cases of anosognosia occur in association with right parietal lobe disorders and because neglect or inattention can also be produced in animals by surgically manipulating the parietal lobes, it seems unlikely that psychodynamic factors play a primary causative role in most neglect syndromes.

Right hemispheric lesions in at least 5 different areas can each produce striking neglect syndromes both in animals and in humans. These areas include the inferior parietal lobule, the prefrontal convexity, the cingulate gyrus, the thalamus, and the hypothalamus. It has been postulated that each of these areas is part of an anatomic loop connecting cortical, limbic, and reticular structures. Lesions at any level of this loop might thus produce attentional deficits. It is of particular interest that structures in the left parietal lobe play a role in the distribution of attention to objects and events in the right hemispace, while homologous structures in the right parietal lobe appear to play a role in the distribution of attention not only to the contralateral but also to the ipsilateral hemispace.

Body Image Distortions

Patients with lesions of the parietal lobe may deny the existence of a paralyzed limb or may admit its existence but repudiate ownership, claiming that it belongs to someone else. One male patient with left hemiplegia constantly lay on his right side, protesting that he had a paralyzed brother beside him. He explained that because this situation was offensive to him, he preferred to turn his back on his brother. On one occasion, without being aware that he was being observed, the patient was overheard addressing his brother: "How are you?" "Do you want a cigarette?" In another case, a physician observed a male patient searching under the bed for his left arm, which he felt was missing. A patient whose limb is paralyzed secondary to parietal lobe disorder may adopt a facetious or condescending attitude toward the compromised limb, referring to it as a "piece of meat" or "dumb slob" or giving the offending body part a pet name. (Critchley [1979] used the term "misoplegia" to describe a violent dislike for the paralyzed limb.)

Tactile Sensory Disturbances

Patients with parietal lobe disorders may have tactile sensory disturbances despite the absence of gross sensory deficits. Their response to a tactile stimulus may be delayed, or they may have a distorted perception of the stimulus. Patients may experience **tactile (haptic) hallucinations,** such as the hallucination of a 3-dimensional object in the hand or of a "phantom limb." Persistence of tactile experience or displacement of sensory experiences from one side of the body to the other may also occur. More commonly, however, careful examination discloses striking deficits in the synthesis, interpretation, and differentiation of primitive sensory experiences. **Astereognosis** (tactile agnosia) refers to the inability to recognize a 3-dimensional object by palpation. Disorders of tactile discrimination are not limited to the appreciation of shape and may occur with reference to texture **(hylognosis),** size **(macro- or microstereognosis),** or pattern **(graphanesthesia).** Finally, impaired ability to recognize the posture of an extremity **(statagnosis)** tends to be associated with bizarre subjective experiences and may play a major role in determining a patient's mental attitude toward the disability.

Motility Disturbances

Patients with parietal lobe disorders manifest greater unilateral incapacity than would be expected on the basis of their motor weakness. Unilateral diminution in spontaneous movements and wasting of the hand muscles and shoulder girdle muscles suggest the importance of intact sensory pathways to motor activity and to the maintenance of muscle mass.

LANGUAGE DISORDERS

Aphasia usually suggests pathologic changes in the left hemisphere. Aphasic patients with posterior lesions may present with acutely disorganized and incoherent speech that is sometimes mistaken for schizophrenic "word salad," while patients with anterior lesions are often noted to be severely depressed, frustrated, or irritable. Aphasialike disorders may be induced by medications; lithium toxicity, for instance, may produce **dysnomia** (word-finding difficulty). Management of patients with organic brain disease and especially those with language disorders requires an appreciation of both the functional deficits and preserved skills of the patient. Without assessing a patient's ability to comprehend, name, repeat, read, or write, the clinician's ability to help either the patient or the patient's family is severely limited.

Language Versus Speech Disorders

Although combinations of speech and language disorders may be seen, it is important to distinguish these 2 types of disorders. **Dysarthrias** (disorders of speech) are due to pathologic changes in the neuromuscular apparatus responsible for the mechanical production of speech. Dysarthria may be seen either with lower brain stem lesions affecting the cranial nerves subserving motor speech outflow or with disruption of corticobulbar fibers traveling from the cortex to the brain stem. In speech disorders, articulation is characterized as spastic, flaccid, ataxic, or hypo- or hyperkinetic. In contrast, **aphasias** (disorders of language) are due to disruption of the neural machinery responsible for the reception, processing, and production of language-dependent ideas. Aphasic patients demonstrate abnormalities not only in spoken but also in written communication.

Language Circuitry of the Left Hemisphere

Since the 1860s—based on the work of Pierre Paul Broca, a French surgeon and anthropologist—it has been known that the vast majority of language disorders occur following damage to the left hemisphere. Ninety-seven percent of right-handers have left hemispheric dominance for **propositional language** (the ability to use semantics and syntax to convey an idea or proposition). Ten percent of the population are left-handed, and over two-thirds of left-handed individuals have left hemispheric dominance for language skills.

The language circuitry of the left hemisphere (Fig 10–10) involves regions of the temporal, parietal, and frontal cortex surrounding the lateral cerebral (sylvian) fissure. Damage to the perisylvian* region produces major aphasic syndromes whose features depend on the size, extent, and location of the lesion. Auditory fibers travel from the medial geniculate body of the thalamus to Heschl's gyrus in the superior temporal plane. Surrounding Heschl's gyrus is the auditory association cortex known as **Wernicke's area.** From Wernicke's area, fibers sweep backward and upward in the arcuate fasciculus, traveling through the inferior parietal lobule to reach the foot of the third (inferior) frontal gyrus. This frontal region, known as **Broca's area,** can be thought of as motor association cortex. As an extension of premotor cortex, it serves as an auditory encoder that generates articulatory programs for the region of the motor cortex subserving the mouth, tongue, and larynx.

Since the entire perisylvian area is supplied by the middle cerebral artery, varieties of aphasia reflect which branch or branches of this artery are occluded.

---

*By "perisylvian" is meant the area surrounding the lateral sulcus, also known as the sylvian fissure or sulcus.

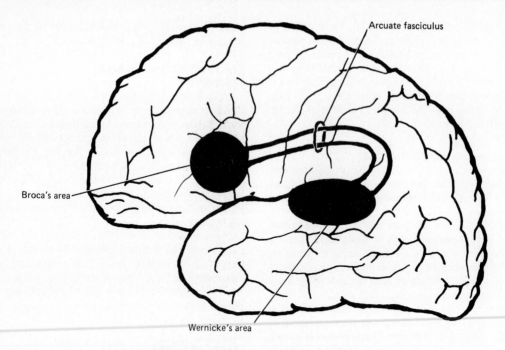

Figure 10–10. Perisylvian language circuitry.

Aphasias Due to Lesions in the Perisylvian Area (Table 10–2)

The 3 major aphasias discussed below all result from pathologic changes in the perisylvian area of the left hemisphere, and all 3 are characterized by inability to repeat spoken language. Patients with **Wernicke's aphasia** cannot repeat because they are unable to decode auditory messages. Those with **Broca's aphasia** fail to repeat because they cannot encode messages that have been understood. Patients with **conduction aphasia** cannot repeat because they are unable to transfer information from an intact auditory decoding apparatus to an intact auditory encoding apparatus. If the entire perisylvian area is destroyed, patients lose both spontaneous speech and auditory com-

prehension. These unfortunate individuals, whose lesions lie either in the internal carotid artery itself or near the organ of the middle cerebral artery, are said to have **global aphasia**.

A. Broca's Aphasia: Broca's aphasia ("motor" aphasia) is characterized by poor articulation and severe impairment of verbal fluency (the ability to produce spontaneous, effortless speech) and is often accompanied by paralysis of the right face and arm. Comprehension is relatively unimpaired, and following recovery, patients often report that they knew precisely what they wanted to say but were unable to say it.

Because the speech of these patients consists mainly of noun and adjective phrases or clichés, with

Table 10–2. Classification of aphasic syndromes.

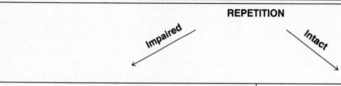

Perisylvian Syndromes			Nonperisylvian Syndromes
	Fluency	Comprehension	
1. Broca's aphasia	−	+	1. Anomic aphasias
2. Wernicke's aphasia	+	−	2. Transcortical aphasias
3. Conduction aphasia	+	+	Motor
4. Global aphasia	−	−	Sensory
			Mixed ("isolation of the speech area")
			3. Subcortical aphasias
			Basal ganglia/internal capsule
			Thalamus
			Marie's quadrilateral space

omission of connecting words such as conjunctions and prepositions, it is often described as "telegraphic" and "agrammatical." Despite severe impairment in fluency, patients are sometimes capable of serial speech such as counting or reciting. Cursing and singing may also be preserved. Patients with Broca's aphasia tend to be angry, depressed, and frustrated. Surprisingly, however, suicide attempts in this population are extremely rare.

B. Wernicke's Aphasia: Wernicke's aphasia often occurs in the absence of motor impairment. Speech is fluent and effortless but devoid of meaning, and comprehension is grossly impaired. Lesions producing this "fluent" aphasia are located in or near Wernicke's area. Since the auditory association cortex functions as an auditory decoder or phonetic analyzer for spoken language, destruction of this area leads to inability to extract meaning from spoken language.

The affective behavior of patients with Wernicke's aphasia ranges from euphoric indifference to paranoid agitation. Management is complicated by the patients' lack of insight into their illness, and rehabilitation therapy cannot be initiated until they become aware of their deficits. Individuals with Wernicke's aphasia are at risk for sucide at 2 points in the course of their illness: (1) following sudden onset of a comprehension deficit, when their lack of insight and misinterpretation of others' actions may lead to chaotic paranoid behavior; and (2) as they begin to become aware of their impairment.

C. Conduction Aphasia: In conduction aphasia, spontaneous speech and comprehension are both preserved, but the patient has almost complete inability to repeat spoken language. This condition results from lesions that spare both Broca's area and Wernicke's area while disrupting the fibers of the arcuate fasciculus that connect these 2 regions.

Aphasias Due to Lesions Affecting Nonperisylvian Language Areas

The following language disorders result from lesions in the nonperisylvian area of the left hemisphere. Patients with these disorders are able to repeat spoken language.

A. Anomic Aphasias: Anomic aphasias are characterized by severe impairment of word-finding ability. (As a general rule, all aphasias are accompanied by some difficulty with word finding.) Patients with anterior lesions appear to have problems with word **production,** while patients with posterior lesions have difficulty either with **selection** of the correct word or with **access** to their "central word lexicon." The most severe anomic aphasia is that associated with lesions in the region of the dominant inferior parietal lobule. Damage to either the angular or supramarginal gyrus can produce anomia of such severity that patients not only fail to benefit from phonemic or semantic cues but may also be unable to recognize the name of a common item when presented with a list containing the word.

Word-finding difficulty may occur in the absence of a structural lesion, eg, with physical exhaustion, dehydration, fever, or metabolic encephalopathy. Thus, care should be taken to differentiate true anomic aphasia from transient language disorders that merely reflect physiologic disequilibrium.

B. Transcortical Aphasias: These aphasias are characterized by impairment of either fluency or comprehension, depending on whether the lesion is anterior or posterior. The aphasias are termed transcortical because they typically result from infarctions at the border zone between the middle cerebral artery and either the anterior or the posterior cerebral artery (Fig 10–11).

1. Transcortical motor aphasia–This form of aphasia results either from a medial frontal lobe lesion of the left hemisphere secondary to occlusion of the anterior cerebral artery or from damage to the prefrontal convexity following infarction at the border zone between the anterior and middle cerebral arteries. It has been argued that the language disturbance resulting from anterior cerebral artery infarction reflects "limbic akinesia," or difficulty with the initiation of motor speech, rather than true aphasia.

2. Transcortical sensory aphasia–This condition, which results from watershed infarctions between the middle and posterior cerebral arteries, is often misdiagnosed until it is systematically assessed. Because patients with the disorder have fluent speech and are capable of repeating spoken language, it is often mistakenly assumed that comprehension is also intact. These patients should serve as important reminders that language skills (eg, repetition and comprehension) may be dissociated. Unless a comprehension deficit is recognized, these patients may be misdiagnosed as confused, uncooperative, or amnestic.

3. Mixed transcortical aphasia–Near drowning, carbon monoxide poisoning, or sustained anoxia secondary to hanging may result in infarction of the entire ribbon of cortex stretching along the border between the middle cerebral artery and both the anterior and posterior cerebral arteries—a condition known as mixed transcortical aphasia or "isolation of the speech area." Patients with this disorder produce no spontaneous speech and are incapable of comprehension. However, since, perisylvian speech areas are preserved, they are able to respond in parrotlike fashion, even repeating long and complex phrases.

C. Subcortical Aphasias: The third group of language disorders in which repetition is preserved is referred to as the subcortical aphasias. Three types have been described: The anterior type results from vascular disorders in the basal ganglia or anterior limb of the internal capsule. The posterior type results from vascular disorders in the thalamus. Both of these are characterized by an initial period of mutism. While the first evolves into transcortical *motor* aphasia, the second evolves into a transcortical *sensory* aphasia with prominent paraphasias. The third type of subcortical aphasia arises from pathologic changes in the area

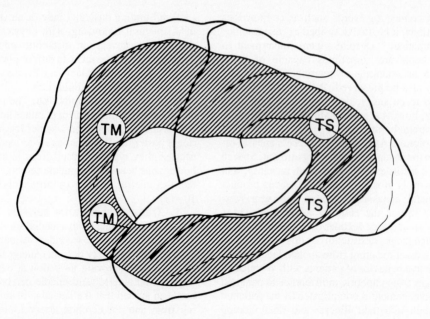

Figure 10–11. Diagram of approximate boundaries of borderzone area. Pathologic changes are present in the lined area but not in the inner language area in most instances of borderzone aphasia. TM = possible sites of transcortical motor aphasia; TS = possible sites of transcortical sensory aphasia. Involvement of borderzone area both anteriorly and posteriorly underlies the mixed transcortical aphasia picture. (Reproduced, with permission, from Benson DF: *Aphasia, Alexia and Agraphia.* Churchill Livingstone, 1979.)

known as Marie's quadrilateral space (Fig 10–12), and in this type, initial mutism persists as global aphasia. The importance of the subcortical aphasias is 2-fold. First, they demonstrate that language circuitry is not limited to neocortex. Second, the subcortical syndromes may represent an exception to the general rule that word-finding difficulty accompanies all aphasic disorders.

Disturbances of Prosody

The "expressive" ability to modulate pitch, melody, and rhythm to impart emotional coloring (prosody) to one's own speech and the receptive ability to detect prosody in the speech of others are important "nonpropositional" aspects of language. Patients with Broca's aphasia, Parkinson's disease, and moderately advanced dementia have difficulty with the inflection, rhythm, and melody of their speech. Recent evidence suggests that patients with damage to the right frontal region homologous to Broca's area may lose the ability to impart prosody to their speech, while patients with posterior right hemispheric lesions in areas homologous to Wernicke's area may lose the ability to decode or perceive affective coloring in the speech of others. Although aprosody and dysprosody are only now beginning to be studied, the possibility of dissociations between felt inner emotion and affective expression is clearly of significance to psychiatrists, since it confounds the diagnosis of depression in patients with organic brain disease and may also represent an underrecognized complication of neuroleptic drug administration.

APRAXIA & THE CALLOSAL SYNDROMES

The term "apraxia" has been used in a confusingly large number of ways. In fact, many clinicians still use

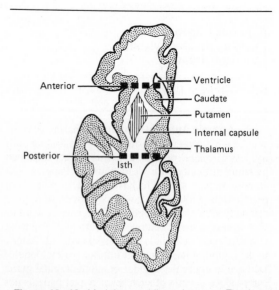

Figure 10–12. Marie's quadrilateral space. The heavy broken lines indicate the anterior and posterior boundaries of the space. Isth = isthmus or temporal stem. (Reproduced, with permission, from Benson DF: *Aphasia, Alexia and Agraphia.* Churchill Livingstone, 1979.)

the term to describe disorders of movement they are unable or unwilling to characterize in some other way. The clinician who accepts another's diagnosis of apraxia without personally examining the patient adopts the ambiguity and uncertainty of the previous examiner. Thus, clinicians are advised to ask the previous examiner to specify what has been observed and then to examine the patient personally.

Constructional Apraxia

The term "constructional apraxia" is a somewhat awkward means of denoting difficulty with "constructions," eg, copying a simple drawing or reproducing a pattern. Constructional ability may be assessed in several ways (see Chapter 18). Since the earliest reports of constructional difficulty appeared, debate has continued about whether the deficit reflects (1) a perceptual problem with the spatial aspects of visual and tactile experience or (2) a motor disorder of programming complex movements in space. It now seems that the right and left hemispheres make separate and distinct contributions to performing complex constructional tasks. The right hemisphere appears to play a largely perceptual role, while the left hemisphere is instrumental at the executive or planning level of motor constructions. Thus, differences in constructional deficits are based on whether lesions are right-sided or left-sided.

Patients with right-sided lesions draw energetically and often add extra strokes. Their productions tend to be scattered and fragmented; boundaries are not observed, and virtually all aspects of spatial relations appear to be lost. These patients may also have difficulty dressing themselves and show hemispatial neglect (for the left side of space).

Patients with left-sided lesions draw slowly and seem to benefit from having a model to copy (this does not help patients with right-sided lesions). Their drawings tend to be somewhat more coherent but are simplified and lack inner detail. The coexistence of language disturbances and elements of Gerstmann's syndrome—alexia, agraphia, right-left confusion, and finger agnosia—may be seen.

Apraxia for Dressing

Difficulty in orienting articles of clothing with reference to the body can be seen in patients with dementia or right parietal lobe disorders but is probably most common in confusional states.

Apraxia of Gait

Patients with expanding frontal lobe lesions or lesions in the region of the supplemental motor area and patients with normal-pressure hydrocephalus may have great difficulty in initiating gait. Because they look as if their feet are glued to the floor, they are sometimes said to have a "magnetic gait." Patients with apraxia of gait are unable to use their limbs properly despite unimpaired strength and intact sensation. Their deficits are not limited to walking and appear to reflect a diffuse problem with the initiation of movements in the lower extremities. These patients may, for example, be unable to perform on command such acts as kicking an imaginary ball or drawing a circle with their feet while lying supine.

Apraxia of Speech

Apraxia of speech is a communication disorder intermediate between true aphasia and dysarthria. It is characterized by prolongation and segregation of syllables. Apraxia of speech, along with dysarthria, is often a component of Broca's aphasia. Apraxic "groping for articulatory postures" lends a plaintive quality to patients with Broca's aphasia. For the speech pathologist, however, it suggests that a particular therapeutic strategy (melodic intonation therapy) may be helpful.

Ideational Apraxia

Ideational apraxia denotes disturbance in the planning of a complex gesture or act even though each of its component parts can be executed singly without difficulty. The problem is one of the sequencing and integration of motor behavior over time.

Ideomotor Apraxia

Ideomotor apraxia denotes a disconnection syndrome wherein certain skilled movements cannot be performed in response to verbal commands, although they can be performed spontaneously. Behavioral neurologists in the USA use the term ideomotor apraxia only if the following criteria can be met: (1) Motor systems are intact, ie, no paralysis, paresis, slowing of movements, incoordination, or other movement disorder; (2) there is no sensory loss in the limbs; and (3) the disorder is not the result of inattention, lack of cooperation, poor comprehension, or intellectual deterioration.

Ideomotor apraxia is caused by interruption of the pathways between the perisylvian area involved with language and the motor association areas involved with voluntary (willed) behavior. A review of these pathways may be helpful. When one is asked to perform a particular act with the right hand, comprehension and performance involve the circuitry from Wernicke's area via the arcuate fasciculus to Broca's area and thence to the left motor cortex. If one is asked to perform the same act with the left hand, the command must be relayed from Wernicke's area in the dominant hemisphere to the right motor cortex. Two possible pathways might be imagined: (1) from Wernicke's area in the left hemisphere via the posterior commissure to the Wernicke's area homolog in the right hemisphere, and then to the right motor cortex; or (2) from Wernicke's area via the arcuate fasciculus to Broca's area, from Broca's area via the anterior corpus callosum to the Broca area homolog in the right hemisphere, and then to the right motor cortex (Fig 10–13). Since there is no clinical evidence that patients with lesions of the posterior corpus callosum (infarction of the posterior cerebral artery) have difficulty using the left hand to follow complex commands, the anterior route appears to be the actual pathway.

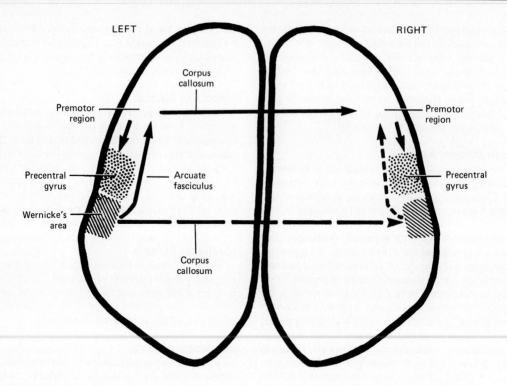

Figure 10–13. Diagram of human brain (viewed from above) shows hypothesized pathways for intra- and interhemispheric information transfer following verbal command to perform limb movements. (Reproduced, with permission, from Geschwind N: The apraxias: Neural mechanisms of disorders of learned movements. *Am Sci* 1975;**63**:188.)

Apraxia may occur with damage to the pathway from Wernicke's area to the right motor cortex at any of 3 sites: (1) If the anterior portion of the corpus callosum is damaged (due to commissurotomy or infarction of the territory irrigated by the anterior cerebral artery), the pathway from Wernicke's area to Broca's area and then to the left motor cortex is intact, and patients can perform tasks on command with the right hand. However, since the left hemisphere cannot communicate with the right hemisphere homolog of Broca's area, these patients are unable to carry out commands with their left hand despite fully intact strength, coordination, and sensation in the left hand. (2) Lesions producing Broca's aphasia are usually large enough to produce paralysis of the right arm. Even though comprehension is intact, the patient is unable to perform the task with the paralyzed limb. Since the command cannot travel from the left hemisphere to the right motor cortex, the patient will also be unable to use the left hand. (3) Apraxia can result from left middle cerebral artery infarctions that spare Broca's and Wernicke's areas as well as the pathways that cross the corpus callosum but disrupt fibers traveling from Wernicke's area to Broca's area (ie, as in conduction aphasia).

Since left middle cerebral artery infarctions are not rare, one might expect ideomotor apraxia to be common. In fact, it is infrequently reported. There appear to be several reasons for this: (1) Apraxia may be a transient phenomenon that disappears as edema diminishes or as alternative pathways are recruited. (2) Patients themselves are usually unaware of ideomotor apraxia, since they can perform volitional acts spontaneously. (3) Patients with apraxia are sometimes considered to be simply confused or to have comprehension problems. (4) Those testing for apraxia may fail to utilize strict criteria.

Patients should be tested for ideomotor apraxia by requesting them to pantomime certain learned movements involving facial muscles (cough, suck, blow out a match) or the limbs (wave good-bye, flip a coin, salute the flag, comb the hair). If the patient is unable to perform either type of task on command, the tasks are restructured in one of the following 3 ways to determine whether performance improves: (1) imitation of the act (visual cuing); (2) handling the object (tactile cuing); and (3) spontaneous manipulation of the object (visual and tactile cuing). If the patient is unable to perform the act on verbal command but can perform the act following one of these 3 maneuvers, ideomotor apraxia has been demonstrated.

It is important to remember that one of the criteria for apraxia is intact comprehension. Comprehension can be tested in aphasic patients (1) by asking them questions of graded difficulty that require head nodding, head shaking, or yes and no responses; and (2) by asking them to perform movements involving use of the axial muscles (movements that can be executed with extrapyramidal motor systems whose origins appear to arise from diffuse areas of the cortex) or eye movements. Intact comprehension is demonstrated if the patient can perform these tasks.

Callosal Syndromes

The corpus callosum, composed of 200 million fibers, is the largest of several nerve fiber bundles connecting the hemispheres. It consists of the rostrum, genu, trunk, and splenium (Fig 10–14). Three other telencephalic interhemispheric pathways are the anterior commissure, hippocampal commissure, and massa intermedia. In addition, there are 2 midbrain commissures: the posterior and habenular commissures.

When surgical section of the corpus callosum was first performed in patients with intractable convulsions, behavior did not appear to be affected by the procedure. Large-scale studies in the 1940s led researchers to comment jokingly that the corpus callosum served only to transmit seizures from one hemisphere to the other or to keep the hemispheres from collapsing onto themselves. After Sperry's pioneering work on animals whose interhemispheric pathways had been surgically sectioned, Geschwind and his coworkers (1962) were able to document symptoms of

callosal syndrome in a patient whose corpus callosum had been severed to control seizures. Since that time, a uniform clinical picture has been described in patients whose corpus callosum has been surgically transected or damaged by disease. These patients behave as if their 2 hemispheres were functioning autonomously. For example, the patient may open a drawer with one hand and immediately close it with the other or may button a shirt with the left hand and then unbutton it with the right hand (the "alien hand syndrome"). From observations that patients who wrote in a normal fashion with the right hand were unable to write with the left and were unable to name (although they could demonstrate recognition of) pictures of items that had been seen exclusively by the right hemisphere, researchers have gained insight into hemispheric specialization. Particularly important was the recognition that even though the right hemisphere was essentially mute, it was still able to process things in complicated ways. Geschwind's research on disconnection syndromes in animals and humans, published in 1965, has become a cornerstone of behavioral neurology in the USA. Even though the apraxias were not the first disorders of higher cortical dysfunction to be conceptualized as disconnection syndromes, they have served as a prototype for the study of mind-brain relations.

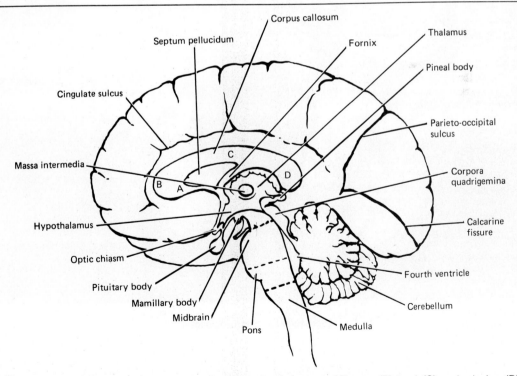

Figure 10–14. *Above:* Medial view of the left hemisphere, showing rostrum (A), genu (B), trunk (C), and splenium (D) of the corpus callosum. *Right:* Corpus callosum, its radiation, and indusium griseum (E), displayed from above. (Figure at right reproduced, with permission, from Gluhbegovic N, Williams TH: *The Human Brain: A Photographic Guide.* Harper & Row, 1980.)

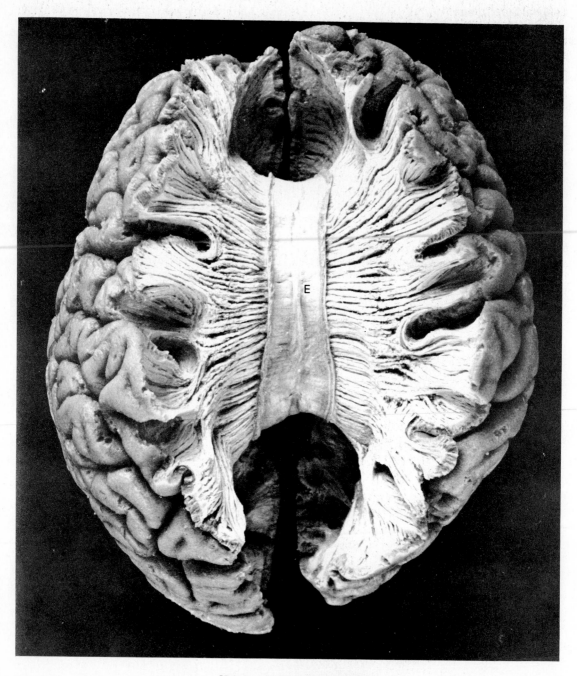

[See legend on preceding page.]

MEMORY DISORDERS

The following case report demonstrates the importance of differential diagnosis of amnestic behavior. This section will present some of the major categories of memory disorders of organic origin that should be considered when confronting such a case.

Illustrative Case

A carpenter was in good health until the age of 51, when he had an episode of depression characterized by crying spells, withdrawal, insomnia, anorexia, and diminished libido. These symptoms responded to a 2-month course of amitriptyline. Two years later, he had a single seizure, attributed to alcohol withdrawal.

At age 53, the carpenter had an argument with his wife at their home in rural New England. The next day he appeared at the emergency room of a San Francisco hospital, where he told a physician that he had "come to" lying in a doorway, not knowing who he was or how he came to be there. He described having hallucinated the presence of a woman who held his hand and who laughed gently at his predicament. A veteran's identity card was found on his person, and further questioning was not done. The patient was transferred to the San Francisco Veterans Administration Medical Center, where he was admitted with the complaint of loss of memory for all events of his past life and loss of personal identity.

A Minnesota Multiphasic Personality Inventory done shortly after admission was interpreted as revealing "a lack of normal defensiveness, a plea-for-help configuration, highest scores on Pd, Hy, and D scales, with no evidence of thought or affect disorder." IQ scores for verbal and performance tasks were in the bright normal to superior range. Neurologic examination, CT scan of the head, isotope brain scan, and electroencephalogram with nasopharyngeal leads disclosed no abnormalities.

Under hypnosis, the patient related the following: As a naval corpsman, he had grown attached to a woman who was a nurse commander. They enjoyed an intense affair and became drinking partners. At age 25, he had seen this friend taken up for a pleasure ride in a small aircraft by a physician at an East Coast naval base. The plane exploded in midair, killing both passengers, and the patient gathered the remains in body bags. He took no time off from work, but shortly thereafter he requested and was granted a transfer to the West Coast. Hypnosis was terminated by vocalization of anger toward his wife, accompanied by the sudden onset of "migraine headache."

On another occasion during this hospitalization, the patient's family telephoned cross-country to speak with him. Although he spoke for some time with his daughter, he claimed that a loud buzzing and sudden headache made him unable to hear his wife's voice. Recall of his past life returned over the period of a week. After repeated episodes of drinking on passes and on the ward, the patient was asked to leave the hospital.

The patient reportedly returned home and later suffered a sudden onset of weakness in the right face, arm, and leg, 3 days of confusion, and transient slurring of speech. He was told by his local physician that he had had a "stroke." The patient recovered completely over 6 months. Alcohol abuse continued, and he was convicted twice of charges of driving while intoxicated.

Eighteen months later, at the age of 54, the patient was brought to the San Francisco Veterans Administration Medical Center for the second time with complaints of memory loss. He was found to have pneumonia and was admitted to the medical service, where he was unable to recall his name, age, residence, prior occupation, or any events of the recent or remote past. Examination of his personal effects revealed his driver's license and a receipt for $17,000 deposited in a San Francisco bank 2 days before admission. The patient consistently denied any knowledge of how he came to be 3000 miles from home. Several hours after admission, he was shown his wallet and regained knowledge of his name but continued to complain of inability to recall his past.

Examination on the medical ward 24 hours after admission revealed an engaging and articulate man who expressed pain, puzzlement, and embarrassment over recent events. He was fully oriented, had an 8-digit memory span, and retained 2 of 4 objects at 5 minutes (the other 2 were retrieved with category cues). He was able to recite the names of 6 presidents backward without difficulty, and he had no memory loss for events following his admission. The patient's initial affect was one of bewilderment and concern over his loss of memory, but his face contorted suddenly and he broke into sobbing. In response to questioning, he again related the story of his deceased friend, referring to his hallucination 18 months previously as "obviously not real, but more compelling than life." The patient volunteered that he had not thought of this episode or of the woman for over a year. He then abruptly began to speak in a pressured way of his anger toward his wife, who had recently asked him to give $5000 of his inheritance to her daughter by a former marriage so that the daughter could build a house. The patient's $17,000 deposit represented the total amount of his paternal inheritance.

The patient was transferred to the inpatient psychiatry ward but left after 2 days against medical advice, traveled to southern California to visit relatives, and returned to San Francisco within the week. He drank heavily for 3 weeks, had a seizure in a downtown bar, and was returned to the San Francisco Veterans Administration Medical Center at his request. He again claimed loss of recent and remote memory as well as loss of personal identity. On the third day of hospitalization, after accidentally dropping some coins onto the floor and bending over to pick them up, he reported the sensation of a "curtain lifting," with all the events up to the time of his falling off the barstool prior to admission returning "in a flood."

One month later, following a minor head contusion

and scalp laceration, the patient was admitted to the hospital for the fourth time in 2 years. He complained of tremulousness, right-sided weakness and paresthesia, and loss of identity with inability to recall anything from the past. He was treated medically for alcohol withdrawal syndrome. A neurologic examination was remarkable only for a positive Hoover sign (failure while supine to push down with the "good leg" while attempting to elevate the "bad leg"), and his neurologic complaints were ascribed to a psychogenic origin. The patient refused psychiatric care and left the hospital when informed that further hospitalization would need to involve a treatment contract in which his alcoholism would be addressed.

Korsakoff's (Amnestic) Syndrome

Wernicke's encephalopathy constitutes the acute phase of 2 distinct disorders—Wernicke's syndrome and Korsakoff's syndrome—both of which are caused by thiamine deficiency. Confusion, ataxia, and eye signs (nystagmus or ophthalmoplegia) comprise the traditional triad of symptoms in patients with Wernicke's encephalopathy. Because these patients are profoundly inattentive, it is inappropriate to characterize them as having a memory disorder (see Chapter 18). In the chronic stages of thiamine deficiency, however, apathy and memory disorder are the 2 most salient features. The hallmark and sine qua non of Korsakoff's syndrome is a dissociation between immediate recall and recent recall (the latter sometimes referred to as recent memory or short-term memory). In addition to significant problems registering new information, these patients demonstrate long-term memory problems (retrograde amnesia). One can think of this long-term memory deficit as a reflection of the difficulty these patients had registering new information at earlier times (anterograde amnesia). Thus, the extent of retrograde amnesia probably reflects the period of time over which the patient has suffered anterograde amnesia.

Unless formal testing of memory is performed routinely (see Chapter 18), the memory deficits associated with thiamine deficiency are easily mixed, since these patients often converse in what appears to be a normal or even glib fashion. Moreover, their performance on tests of intellectual functioning is not significantly impaired by their amnestic state. Confabulation (the filling-in of memory blanks with what may appear to be fanciful information) is not an invariable part of the syndrome but tends to occur in the earlier stages and during recovery. While confabulation has been construed as intentional misleading of the examiner, it is probably best viewed as an attempt by the patient either to make sense of the world or to cooperate with the examiner despite depleted information stores.

Since lesions in Korsakoff's syndrome are localized to specific anatomic sites, the syndrome provides a model for the study of amnesia and brain localization. Petechial hemorrhagic lesions stretch from the third to the fourth ventricle in the midline along the cerebral aqueduct. Lesions in the mamillary bodies and in the dorsomedial nucleus of the thalamus are also predictable findings. While the periventricular lesions lie in the ascending reticular network, lesions in the mamillary bodies lie in the medial limbic circuit described by Papez. The dorsomedial thalamus is a prominent way station for fibers passing from medial limbic structures such as the amygdala to the prefrontal cortex.

Alcoholic Memory Blackouts

In contrast to Korsakoff's syndrome, in which both the anatomy and pathophysiology are reasonably well understood, alcoholic blackouts represent a common occurrence whose pathogenesis is poorly understood. Two types of blackouts have been described: en bloc and fragmentary.

The onset of **en bloc blackouts** is abrupt, and the duration is from minutes to days. During blackouts, patients are incapable of registering new information and may ask the same question or tell the same story repeatedly. Despite their anterograde amnesia, these patients may have unimpaired ability to move about, drive an automobile, and perform routine tasks. The hallmark of the en bloc blackout is that forgetting is complete and memory cannot be recovered for a period of time despite attempts to "jog the memory" with cues, hypnosis, or amobarbital interviews.

Fragmentary blackouts are more common than en block blackouts. Patients with fragmentary blackouts have "spotty" recall for events that happened during the blackout and sometimes report that events happened "as in a dream" or "a picture out of focus." During recovery, islands of recall seem to coalesce, and retrieval of information is facilitated by "jogging the memory." Casual observers cannot distinguish behavior of patients during alcoholic blackouts from their behavior during mild states of inebriation.

Transient Global Amnesia

The typical picture of transient global amnesia is that of a 50- or 60-year-old man who experiences a sudden onset of confusion with loss of ability to learn new information. Attacks last hours to days, and during this period patients tend (in contrast to patients having an alcoholic blackout) to be agitated and aware of their problem. They may, for example, repeatedly ask questions such as "Where am I?" or "What is happening?" An attack rarely (if ever) occurs more than once in any individual. Seizure activity, vasospasm, and occlusive transient ischemia of medial temporal lobe structures have been suggested as possible causes of transient global amnesia.

Traumatic Amnesia

Following nontrivial head injury, memory problems are common. Traumatic amnesia refers to loss of memory both for a period of time preceding the head injury (retrograde amnesia) and for events following the injury (posttraumatic [anterograde] amnesia). Posttraumatic amnesia prevents the patient from registering new information. For example, a hospitalized patient may recognize visitors and talk with them but the next day have no recollection of the visit. In general, posttraumatic amnesia lasts minutes to hours following return of consciousness; if it exceeds 24 hours, the patient usually has sustained severe and permanent neurologic deficits such as those associated with prolonged coma. Termination of posttraumatic amnesia tends to be abrupt and often occurs after a period of sleep or following some emotionally meaningful event such as the visit of a close friend. Because the extent of retrograde amnesia immediately following injury may initially encompass years of the patient's life but later shrinks to a minute or less in all but the severest cases of head injury, the term "shrinking retrograde amnesia" is appropriate. Phenomenologic studies of traumatic amnesia reveal that shrinkage of retrograde amnesia follows and depends on resolution of the anterograde amnestic deficit. Following head injury or confusional states, a remarkable phenomenon known as "reduplicative paramnesia" involving bizarre distortions of memory is sometimes observed. For example, a patient with paramnesia who is asked, "Where are you?" may admit being in a hospital but inisist that the hospital itself is across the street from his or her home or that the hospital room is even in a wing of the home.

Amnesia Following Seizures

Following major motor seizures, patients are invariably amnestic for the seizure itself as well as for a variable period after the seizure. In general, the same is true of complex partial seizures, although some patients have such seizures during which they remain conscious. During the confusional period that follows seizures, patients may respond to gentle attempts to assist them with agitation or aggression but will later be amnestic for this period of abnormal behavior. Continuous absence ("petit mal") is a rare condition in which patients lose touch with the environment for prolonged periods and thus are amnestic for events.

Acute Confusion

Although acute confusion of toxic, metabolic, or infectious origin is not considered a true amnestic state, patients with acute confusion may be unable to register new information over prolonged periods. If examined following resolution of their confusion, they may appear "amnestic" for the confusional period. Toxic states for which a person has no recall can occur with phencyclidine (PCP) abuse. This drug is a known "dissociative/amnestic" agent, and a person under its influence may commit crimes of violence for which he or she later has no recall.

Memory Impairment

Memory impairment unaccompanied by other evidence of intellectual deterioration is termed an amnestic syndrome. Early problems with memory become increasingly more severe in presenile and senile dementia of the Alzheimer type. The term "benign senescent forgetfulness" has been used to designate the almost universal memory problems that occur with increasing frequency in the seventh, eighth, and ninth decades. This "benign" variant of forgetfulness is in all likelihood related to the memory deficits seen in dementia syndromes, differing only in degree of impairment.

Patients with moderately advanced dementia are usually unaware of their memory dysfunction and therefore not concerned about it. Depressed patients with complaints of cognitive deficits (depressive pseudodementia) are preoccupied with what they take to be memory deterioration and may seek help for this complaint. Thus, even though some patients in the earliest stages of dementia may be aware of and upset by their memory problems, patients who present with complaints of memory problems are more likely to have an affective illness.

Differential Diagnosis of Organic & Functional Amnestic Disorders

Among the nonorganic (psychogenic) memory disorders are the following: dissociative episode (fugue state), feigned amnesia (malingering), factitious amnesia (a variant of Ganser's syndrome), and conditions in which thought processes are disrupted by intrusive thoughts or images (major affective illness, schizophrenia, posttraumatic stress disorder). Although the latter are psychiatric conditions, their "biologic" features suggest that the term "psychogenic" is used here in a somewhat strained sense.

In differentiating organic from functional amnestic disorders, the clinician should consider the following factors: age; medical history (especially history of neurologic disorders); psychiatric history; the presence or absence of psychosocial precipitants (in what environment or under what circumstances the amnestic episodes occur); affective behavior during the episode; the patient's desire for recovery; what type of information is forgotten (loss of personal identity implies functional illness); evidence that the patient is registering some types of information while selectively ignoring others; the patient's response to cuing techniques (eg, hypnosis, use of amobarbital); and where the patient is when memory function is recovered.

FRONTAL LOBE SYNDROMES

Understanding the behavioral manifestations of frontal lobe disease requires a knowledge of frontal lobe functions and of frontal connections to the rest of the central nervous system.

Frontal Lobe Connections

A. Sensory Input: Sensory input to the prefrontal region does not arise from primary sensory regions but rather from the high-level (polymodal and supramodal) association cortices of the temporal, parietal, and occipital lobes. Sensory information presented to the frontal lobes is therefore already highly processed. Input to the frontal convexities from the inferior parietal lobule serves as one example of such highly processed sensory input.

B. Motor Output: The frontal lobe cortex contains 4 motors areas: (1) the motor strip containing giant pyramidal (Betz) cells, (2) the premotor region, (3) the frontal eye fields, and (4) the supplemental motor area. The frontal cortex, along with much of the neocortex, projects to the basal ganglia. Projections to the head of the caudate nucleus (which are not bidirectional) are particularly prominent. The importance of these frontostriatal ("psychomotor") pathways is suggested by the fact that the head of the caudate nucleus also receives limbic system input from such regions as the hippocampus and the amygdala. Thus, the basal ganglia can be seen as a point of convergence for frontal lobe and limbic system information.

C. Limbic System Input: As mentioned in the earlier discussion of limbic system anatomy in this chapter, there are numerous links between prefrontal and limbic areas. These may conveniently be subdivided into 3 categories: (1) direct pathways from the medial temporal lobe structures to frontal cortex via the uncinate fasciculus; (2) indirect fibers connecting frontal and limbic system regions via the dorsomedial nucleus of the thalamus; and (3) indirect fibers passing from the hippocampus to prefrontal regions via the cingulate gyrus.

D. Septo-Hypothalamo-Mesencephalic Continuum Input: There are direct pathways from the dorsolateral convexities and orbitomedial portions of the prefrontal area to the septo-hypothalamo-mesencephalic continuum.

Behavioral Changes in Frontal Lobe Syndromes

Behavioral changes following frontal lobe damage may be grouped into 3 broad categories: personality, intellect, and motor function disturbances.

A. Personality Disturbances: The case of Phineas P. Gage, a 25-year-old construction foreman working on a railroad bed in Vermont, is perhaps the most famous example of personality disturbance associated with frontal lobe syndromes. According to the case report of Harlow (1868), Gage was using a tamping iron to pack blasting powder into a hole when the powder exploded. The explosion drove the tamping iron through his face and out the top of his skull, transecting his frontal lobes. After the accident, he became, in the words of his physician, ". . . fitful, irreverent, indulging at times in the grossest profanity (which was not previously his custom), manifesting but little deference to his fellows, impatient of restraint or advice when it conflicts with his desires, at times pertinaciously obstinate yet capricious and vacillating, devising many plans for future operation which are no sooner arranged than they are abandoned in turn for others appearing more feasible . . . . His

mind was radically changed, so that his friends and acquaintances said he was no longer Gage."

Studies of individuals who suffered penetrating head injuries during World War I showed personality disturbances of 2 distinct types. Individuals with orbitomedial disorders appeared puerile, disinhibited, and euphoric ("pseudopsychopathic"). Those with brain injury limited to the dorsolateral convexities appeared apathetic and indifferent ("pseudodepressed"). Since patients rarely have lesions limited to either of these regions, it is more common to see admixtures of these 2 personality types. Geschwind has described these patients with irritability, apathy, and euphoria as manifesting "the impossible triad of frontal lobe pathology."

B. Intellectual Disturbances: Characterization of intellectual deficits following frontal lobe damage has been a vexing problem. In the late 1940s (10 years after psychosurgery had come into use), essentially no neuropsychologic changes had been consistently noted in postsurgical patients even though psychologists searched diligently for intellectual deterioration in these patients. Failure to correlate intellectual deficits with prefrontal lobe damage called into question the established view that the frontal lobes were the highest seat of human intelligence and suggested that they might even be superfluous structures, since they could apparently be removed with relative impunity. Since that time, the consequences of frontal lobe damage have been somewhat clarified, largely as a result of the work of Luria, a Russian neurologist and neuropsychologist (see Luria, 1980). After seeing thousands of patients personally, Luria concluded that the frontal lobes have 4 functions: (1) generating plans for action; (2) programming the components, or subroutines, of actions; (3) monitoring ongoing activity with reference both to the goal and to environmental shifts; and (4) correcting the course of activity already in progress.

Obviously, the frontal lobes do not act independently. They depend on high-level sensory input from the temporal, parietal, and occipital lobes. Patients with frontal lobe damage may have the following problems: (1) difficulty suppressing irrelevant associations, or intrusions; (2) inability to anticipate the consequences of their actions, ie, physical damage to property, self, or others and emotional consequences for self and others; (3) inability to formulate an approach to complex problems that extend over time; (4) remarkable dissociation of speech from action (eg, a patient told to "squeeze a ball when the light goes on" may say "I must squeeze the ball" when he or she sees the light but will fail to carry out the action); and (5) difficulty understanding metaphors, similes, and parables (the "inability to assume the abstract attitude" described by Goldstein in the 1940s as the hallmark of organic disease).

Patients with frontal lobe damage have been said to manifest "frontal amnesia." In actuality, these patients do not have amnestic problems similar to those of patients with Korsakoff's psychosis. However, they are sometimes unable to hold in conscious awareness the various pieces of information required for a specific action. It has been speculated that these individuals fail to generate mnemonic associations; thus, their forgetting may reflect not so much a retrieval blockade as a disinclination to remember or a failure to generate "limbic tags" for events.

Intelligence tests do not appear to measure well the type of deficits seen following frontal lobe damage. The Wisconsin Card-Sorting Test (in which patients are asked to infer from the examiner's responses whether they are shifting cards by the appropriate criterion) and various maze-learning tasks have proved helpful in neuropsychologic assessment of frontal lobe damage. Tests that measure the ability to sustain, shift, or direct attention might be expected to be most sensitive to frontal lobe lesions.

C. Motor Function Disturbances: The motor changes following frontal lobe damage may include the appearance of primitive reflexes such as grasping, sucking, and snouting reflexes. However, in many patients with significant prefrontal lobe damage (eg, lobotomized psychiatric patients), these reflexes cannot be elicited. The grasp reflex is most frequently observed in patients over age 60, but its presence does not correlate well either with gross brain damage or with intellectual deterioration.

Disturbances associated with difficulty in overcoming motor inertia are seen in patients with frontal lobe damage. These include apraxia of gait, characterized by difficulty initiating gait; decreased "ocular palpation of the environment," which may contribute to the patient's tendency to make judgments on the basis of incomplete information; and palilalia, characterized by repetition of the last elements of an utterance (either the entire last word or the last syllable). Difficulty "changing sets" has long been recognized as a problem following frontal lobe damage. Patients asked to draw a series of geometric shapes such as a circle, triangle, and square may perseverate the production of one of these 3 elements. Luria has recommended the use of a simple bedside test in which patients are asked to perform a 3-step command—striking the top of a table with the edge of an open hand ("cut"), then striking the table with a closed fist ("pound"), and finally striking the table with an open palm ("slap")—as one index of frontal lobe function.

Many of these problems with inertia and perseveration resemble symptoms that arise from disorders of the basal ganglia. Since there are strong frontostriatal connections, it becomes difficult and even somewhat meaningless to attempt to separate frontal (cortical) from striatal (subcortical) symptoms.

MOVEMENT DISORDERS

Although virtually all neurologic diseases have psychologic correlates, the movement disorders serve as striking prototypes of neuropsychiatric disorders. The connections between neurology and psychiatry are particularly strong in Parkinson's disease, Huntington's disease, tardive dyskinesia, Gilles de la Tourette's syndrome, and Wilson's disease. Therefore, each of these disorders will be considered here.

Parkinson's Disease & Other Extrapyramidal Motor Disorders

A. Pathologic Physiology: Tremor, muscular rigidity, and bradykinesia (the parkinsonian triad) are due to pathologic changes in the posterior portion of the septo-hypothalamo-mesencephalic continuum—specifically, in the substantia nigra of the midbrain. This darkly pigmented area lies at the junction between the cerebral peduncles and the tegmentum of the midbrain. Dorsal and medial to the substantia nigra lies the ventral tegmental area of Tsai, which is the origin of the mesolimbic dopaminergic pathways projecting to the limbic and frontal cortices. Destruction of the dopaminergic neurons in the substantia nigra leads to a decrease in the dopamine content of the neostriatum (caudate nucleus and putamen) and alters the cholinergic-dopaminergic balance. This imbalance of acetylcholine and dopamine may be treated with either dopamine agonists or anticholinergic drugs.

B. Dementia in Parkinson's Disease: For many years, it was thought that intellectual deterioration was not an intrinsic feature of Parkinson's disease. It now appears that parkinsonian patients are at high risk (10 times that of age-matched controls) of developing dementia. The incidence of neuropathologic changes of the Alzheimer type is higher in patients with Parkinson's disease than in age-matched controls. Because so many symptoms of dementia in parkinsonian patients seem to involve a *slowing* of both mentation and motor activity, it has been suggested that the basal ganglia may play an important role in cognitive activity. Since dopaminergic pathways that ascend from the ventral tegmental region of the midbrain also travel to the frontal lobe cortex, damage to these mesolimbic and mesofrontal pathways may play a role in the dementia of Parkinson's disease.

C. Drug-Induced Parkinsonism: Drug-induced parkinsonism may occur within 5–30 days after starting neuroleptic treatment. Although the parkinsonian triad of symptoms is present, the severity of symptoms in drug-induced parkinsonism differs from that in Parkinson's disease in that bradykinesia is often the most prominent feature, muscular rigidity is less pronounced, and tremor may be insignificant.

Acute **dystonia,** if present, usually appears in the first 5 days of neuroleptic treatment and is very painful. Dystonic reactions may be seen in the eyes, neck, tongue, jaw, or trunk and are frequently misdiagnosed as hysteria, malingering, or seizures. A drug such as benztropine mesylate, diphenhydramine, or diazepam should be administered intravenously. If dystonic reactions recur or persist, a neuroleptic agent or lower potency such as thioridazine or chlorpromazine may be indicated. Serum calcium levels should be measured to rule out hypocalcemia.

Akathisia, an inner sense of restlessness that may or may not be accompanied by gross motor restlessness, may occur 5–60 days after initiating treatment with dopamine blockers. Antihistamines and propranolol are more efficacious than purely atropinic substances in treating akathisia.

"Rabbit syndrome," a fine perioral tremor, may appear months after starting an antipsychotic agent. It is frequently misdiagnosed as tardive dyskinesia but is actually a parkinsonian phenomenon that responds to treatment with anticholinergic agents.

Huntington's Disease

Movement disorder and dementia are the 2 major features of Huntington's disease. The age at onset of this autosomal dominant disorder ranges roughly from 25 to 50 years, with peak onset in the fourth decade. Recent work on localization of the gene for Huntington's disease raises hope that early detection and possibly even treatment may be forthcoming. It is impossible to distinguish tardive dyskinesia from Huntington's disease, except on the basis of a family history of Huntington's disease.

George Huntington's (1872) description of the disorder deserves to be repeated here:

> The *hereditary* chorea, as I shall call it, is confined to certain and fortunately a *few* families, and has been transmitted to them, an heirloom from generations away back in the dim past. It is spoken of by those in whose veins the seeds of the disease are known to exist, with a kind of horror, and not at all alluded to except through dire necessity when it is mentioned as *"that disorder."* It is attended generally by all the symptoms of common chorea, only in an aggravated degree, hardly ever manifesting itself until *adult* or *middle* life, and then coming on gradually but surely, increasing by degrees, and often occupying years in its development, until the hapless sufferer is but a quivering wreck of his former self . . . . There are three marked peculiarities in this disease: 1, its hereditary nature; 2, a tendency to insanity and suicide; 3, its manifesting itself as a grave disease only in adult life.
>
> (1) Of its hereditary nature. When either or both the parents have shown manifestations of the disease, and more especially when these manifestations have been of a *serious* nature, one or more of the offspring almost invariably suffer from the disease, if they live to adult age. But if by any chance these children go throughout life *without* it, the thread is broken and the grandchildren and great-grandchildren of the original shakers may rest assured that they are free from the disease. . . . Unstable and whimsical as the disease may be in *other* respects, in *this* it is firm, it never skips a generation to again manifest itself in another; once having yielded its claims, it never regains them. In all the families, or nearly all in which the choreic taint exists, the nervous temperament greatly preponderates. . . .

Although patients may present with either motor or psychiatric symptoms, the former are more likely to bring the patient to medical attention. Initially, patients may fidget, twitch, grimace, and speak in a slurred fashion. As the disorder progresses, movements become conspicuously clumsy, of greater amplitude, and assume a bizarre and grotesque quality.

Personality disorder, thought or affective disorder, and dementia may occur. Violence and hypersexuality (often of a bizarre nature) are among the striking behavioral abnormalities that Huntington noted:

> (2)The tendency to insanity, and sometimes that form of insanity which leads to suicide, is marked. I know of several instances of suicide of people suffering from this form of chorea, or who belonged to families in which the disease existed. As the disease progresses the mind becomes more or less impaired, in many amounting to insanity, while in others mind and body both gradually fail until death relieves them of their sufferings. At present I know of two married men, whose wives are living, and who are constantly making love to some young lady, not seeming to be aware that there is any impropriety in it. They are suffering from chorea to such an extent that they can hardly walk, and would be thought by a stranger, to be intoxicated. They are men of about 50 years of age, but never let an opportunity to flirt with a girl go past unimproved. The effect is ridiculous in the extreme.

In patients with Huntington's disease, atrophy of the caudate nucleus leads to ballooning of the lateral ventricles, which can be seen on CT scan in the late stages of illness. Metabolic changes in the head of the caudate nucleus can be demonstrated early with positron emission tomography.

Since the mean life expectancy of patients with Huntington's disease is 16 years following diagnosis, it is important to realize that symptomatic relief is available. The movement disorder, the agitation, and the violent behavior described above can be treated with dopamine blockers such as haloperidol. For disturbances of affective behavior, which may reflect either depression due to a biochemical imbalance or reactive depression, treatment with lithium or tricyclic antidepressants should be considered.

Tardive Dyskinesia

Chlorpromazine was approved as an antipsychotic agent by the FDA in March, 1954. Two years later, the first cases of persistent abnormal movements following discontinuation of antipsychotic drugs were reported.

A. Pharmacologic Factors Affecting Onset and Treatment: Tardive dyskinesia is a late-onset disorder that occurs months to years after initiation of treatment with dopaminergic blocking agents. Suggested mechanisms for a functional dopaminergic excess have included (1) increased circulating blood levels of dopamine, (2) increased dopamine release by dopaminergic neurons, and (3) increased responsiveness to dopamine at the postsynaptic receptor sites. The precise pharmacologic basis remains unclear. In all likelihood, tardive dyskinesia involves an imbalance of neurotransmitters (eg, dopamine, acetylcholine, and gamma-aminobutyric acid) and perhaps neuropeptides such as cholecystokinin and somatostatin as well.

Discontinuing dopamine-blocking agents is desirable but may not always be possible if psychosis is poorly controlled. Temporary worsening of the movement disorder is to be expected following cessation of administration of these agents. Drug holidays (weeks or months) are indicated to determine whether patients continue to require antipsychotic medications.

Increasing the dose of dopamine-blocking agents is not suitable treatment for tardive dyskinesia, since it will only mask the symptoms while pathophysiologic changes continue.

If patients are being treated with anticholinergic agents such as tricyclic antidepressants or with antihistamines, discontinuing these agents may produce dramatic alleviation of the movement disorder.

Although lecithin and choline have been used for treatment of dyskinesia, these agents do not appear efficacious. Lecithin causes a fishy odor, and choline must be given in massive doses.

B. Types of Tardive Dyskinesia: Patients may present with one or more of the types of tardive dyskinesia described below. Older patients tend to have the buccolingual-masticatory and orofacial syndromes, whereas adolescents and young adults are more likely to develop choreiform movements primarily of the extremities.

1. Buccolingual-masticatory dyskinesia– The movements for this type include twisting, turning, protruding, and smacking the tongue and lips.

2. Orofacial dyskinesia–This form is characterized by facial tics, grimacing, and blinking.

3. Axial dyskinesia–Truncal movements such as shoulder shrugging, lordotic posturing, and pelvic thrusting may all be seen in patients with axial dyskinesia.

4. Appendicular chorea–Choreiform movements of the fingers, hands, arms, or legs have a rapid, dancelike quality. Since these choreiform movements are usually accompanied by some degree of athetosis (slow, writhing movements), the term choreoathetosis is often employed. Ballistic movements, eg, a throwing movement of the arm, are occasionally seen.

C. Differential Diagnosis: It is impossible to distinguish tardive dyskinesia from Huntington's disease clinically. This leads to a particular problem: If a patient with a psychotic behavioral disturbance is treated with antipsychotic agents and years later develops a movement disorder, the clinician seeing the patient for the first time is likely to attribute the movement disorder to prior neuroleptic drug treatment. Thus, Huntington's disease can be masked unless a family history is determined.

Gilles de la Tourette's Syndrome

This syndrome is characterized by chronic multiple motor and vocal tics. The age at onset is 2–15 years. Motor tics frequently consist of sniffing, snorting, or blinking; vocal tics consist of clicks, grunts, barks, coughs, or yelps. Coprolalia (the compulsive uttering of obscenities) is said to occur eventually in 60% of cases. Although mental and mood changes are not an intrinsic part of the syndrome, suicide may occur secondary to profound social disruption produced by the disorder. Tourette's disease may exist for many years before the diagnosis is made. The cause and pathogenesis are unknown, but administration of central nervous system stimulants such as methylphenidate may precipitate the disorder. Dopamine-blocking neuroleptic agents usually afford some symptomatic relief (see also Chapter 52).

Wilson's Disease (Hepatolenticular Degeneration)

Wilson's disease is an autosomal recessive disorder in which copper is deposited in the liver and lenticular nucleus (putamen and globus pallidus) of the basal ganglia. The defect in copper metabolism consists of diminished levels of ceruloplasmin, which may be documented by serum assay. The neurologic manifestations of the disease reflect progressive extrapyramidal dysfunction accompanied by deterioration of personality (eg, irritability, depression, psychosis) and intellect. Early signs include tremor, bradykinesia, dysarthria, and dysphagia. Eventually, the patient develops a characteristic picture—a "vacuous smile," great difficulty chewing and swallowing, constant drooling, and a coarse "wing-flapping" tremor when the arms are outstretched. Deposition of copper in the cornea (Kayser-Fleischer ring) may be seen with a slit lamp in advanced stages. Treatment consists of reduction in dietary copper, use of sulfurated potash to prevent absorption of copper, and administration of the copper-chelating agent penicillamine.

Family members should be screened once the diagnosis is made.

REFERENCES

Babinski MJ: [Article without title.] *Rev Neurol (Paris)* 1918;**34:**365.

Babinski MJ: Contribution à l'étude des troubles mentaux dans l'hémiplégie organique (anosognosie). *Rev Neurol (Paris)* 1914;**27:**175.

Bard P: A diencephalic mechanism for the expression of rage with special reference to the sympathetic nervous system. *Am J Physiol* 1928;**84:**490.

Becker E: *Escape From Evil.* Free Press, 1975.

Benson DF: *Aphasia, Alexia and Agraphia*. Churchill Livingstone, 1979.

Benson DF: *Psychiatric Aspects of Neurologic Disease*. Vol 2. Grune & Stratton, 1982.

Broca P: Anatomie comparée des circonvolutions cérébrales: Le grand lobe limbique et la scissure limbique dans la série des mammifères. *Rev Anthropol [Series 2]* 1878;**1**:385.

Broca P: Perte de la parole: Ramollissement chronique et déstruction partielle du lobe antérieur gauche du cerveau. *Paris Bull Soc Anthropol* 1861;**2**:219.

Brodal A: *Neurological Anatomy*, 3rd ed. Oxford Univ Press, 1981.

Brophy JJ: Psychiatric disorders. Chap 18, p 658, in: *Current Medical Diagnosis & Treatment 1984*. Krupp MA, Chatton MJ (editors). Lange, 1984.

Critchley M: Misoplegia, or hatred of hemiplegia. Pages 115–120 in: *The Divine Banquet of the Brain*. Raven Press, 1979.

Critchley M: *The Parietal Lobes*. Hafner, 1953.

Freud S: Project for a scientific psychology (1895). In: *Standard Edition of the Complete Psychological Works of Sigmund Freud*. Vol. 1. Hogarth Press, 1966.

Geschwind N: The apraxias: Neural mechanisms of disorders of learned movements. *Am Sci* 1975;**63**:188.

Geschwind N: Disconnexion syndromes in animals and man. (2 parts.) *Brain* 1965;**88**:237, 585.

Geschwind N, Kaplan E: A human cerebral disconnection syndrome. *Neurology* 1962;**12**:675.

Goldstein K: The effects of brain damage on personality. *Psychiatry* 1962;**15**:245.

Gray JA: *The Neuropsychology of Anxiety*. Oxford Univ Press, 1982.

Harlow JM: Recovery from the passage of an iron bar through the head. *Mass Med Soc Publications* 1868;**2**:329.

Huntington G: On chorea. *Med Surg Reporter* 1872;**26**:320.

Lorenz K: *The Foundations of Ethology*. Springer-Verlag, 1981.

Luria AR: *Higher Cortical Functions in Man*, 2nd ed. Basic Books, 1980.

MacLean PD: The brain, empathy and medical education. *J Nerv Ment Dis* 1967;**144**:374.

MacLean PD: Some psychiatric implications of physiological studies on the frontotemporal portion of the limbic system (visceral brain). *Electroencephalogr Clin Neurophysiol* 1952;**4**:407.

MacLean PD: *A Triune Concept of Brain and Behavior*. Univ of Toronto Press, 1969.

Marsden CD, Fahn S: *Movement Disorders*. Butterworth, 1981.

Mountcastle VB: *Medical Physiology*, 14th ed. Mosby, 1980.

Mueller J: Neuroanatomic correlates of emotion. Chap 10, pp 95–121, in: *Emotions in Health and Illness*. Temoshok L, Van Dyke C, Zegans LS (editors). Grune & Stratton, 1983.

Nauta WJH: Hippocampal projections and related neural pathways to the midbrain in the cat. *Brain* 1958;**81**:319.

Papez JW: A proposed mechanism of emotion. *Arch Neurol Psychiatry* 1937;**38**:725.

Pfaf DW: *The Physiologic Mechanisms of Motivation*. Springer-Verlag, 1982.

Plum F, Posner J: *The Diagnosis of Stupor and Coma*, 2nd ed. Davis, 1972.

Sperry R: Some effects of disconnecting the cerebral hemispheres. *Science* 1982;**217**:1223.

Willis T: *Cerebri Anatome*. Martzer and Alleftry (London), 1664.

Yakovlev PI: Motility, behavior and the brain: Organization and neural coordinates of behavior. *J Nerv Ment Dis* 1948;**107**:313.

Neurobehavioral Chemistry & Physiology

11

Jack A. Grebb, MD, Victor I. Reus, MD, & Nelson B. Freimer, MD

Modern psychiatry seeks to correlate the vast amount of new research in basic neurosciences with observations of normal and abnormal human behavior. Research has focused on the identification of specific neurochemical pathways in the brain, the classification of receptor subtypes for each neurotransmitter, and the continued elucidation of the physiology and behavioral role of the neuroactive peptides (eg, endogenous opioids).

The virtual explosion of information in the basic neurosciences has resulted from the expanded application of existing research tools as well as new technologic advances, including such important techniques as radioimmunoassay, radioreceptor assay, recombinant DNA techniques, high-performance liquid chromatography, gas chromatography-mass spectrometry, electron microscopy, regional cerebral blood flow measurement, computerized tomography, computer-analyzed electrophysiology, and magnetic resonance imaging. Positron emission tomography is particularly useful because it permits in vivo determination and measurement of metabolic and neurochemical processes in human brain. Positron emission tomographic scans are generated by labeling test substances with a radioactive compound, which produces positron-emitting isotopes (commonly fluorine 18) that can be localized in tomographic brain sections. Early studies focused on mapping brain metabolism with 2-deoxyglucose. Recently, scanning techniques have been adapted to the study of neurotransmitters and their receptors. For example, the functional activity of dopamine receptors has been visualized using binding with labeled spiperone, a neuroleptic agent with presumed high affinity for D_2 receptors. Other studies with different ligands have identified dopamine receptor changes in Huntington's disease, Parkinson's syndrome, and normal aging. Development of a quantitative means for evaluating positron emission tomographic findings and specific assessment of other neurotransmitter receptor systems are the main foci of current research. Additional in vivo imaging techniques (eg, topographic magnetic resonance spectroscopy) promise similar focal metabolic assessment with considerably less invasive risk to the patient. Psychiatrists must now be familiar with at least the basic concepts of these techniques in order to fully understand and critically evaluate much of the recent literature.

TRANSMISSION OF NERVE IMPULSES IN THE CENTRAL NERVOUS SYSTEM

The most important fundamental unit of transmission of nerve impulses in the central nervous system is the synapse, which is a specialized area of contact between nerve cells that enables interneuronal communication to occur. There are 3 types of synapses. First and most important, there are **chemical synapses,** which use a chemical messenger that is released by the presynaptic neuron when it is stimulated. Once in the synaptic cleft, this chemical can act on receptors located either on presynaptic cell membranes (autoreceptors) or on postsynaptic cell membranes. The effects of this receptor interaction may be either stimulatory or inhibitory; however, in the central nervous system, it is the combined effects of multiple inputs to a single neuron that determine its actual functioning. Second, there exist **electrical synapses,** whose role remains poorly understood. Third, there are **conjoint synapses** that operate via both chemical and electrical transmission of nerve impulses. In addition to facilitating synaptic communication, nonsynaptic areas of neuronal membranes may contain receptors for chemical signals floating freely in the brain extracellular fluid. Neurons may be further affected by changes in pH, electrolyte concentrations, and other chemical constituents of the surrounding extracellular fluid and cerebrospinal fluid. For example, cerebrospinal fluid prostaglandins and especially calcium have major regulatory functions in transmission of nerve impulses.

Chemical transmission has been the focus of most of the recent research in neurobehavioral sciences, and 3 general categories of **neuroregulators** have been described: neurotransmitters, neuromodulators, and neurohormones. Although the differentiation of these messengers is clear in theory, they often have overlapping roles in vivo. **Neurotransmitters** are the "classic" chemical signals. They are released into the synaptic cleft quickly (1–2 ms) by the presynaptic neuron when it is stimulated. They then bind to receptors on either the postsynaptic or presynaptic cell membranes. The physiology and chemistry of neuro-modulators are not yet clearly understood. It is known, however, that **neuromodulators** also bind specifically to receptors, although their function is to modify the response of the receptor to the neurotransmitter by tempering or adjusting transfer of the message rather than to actually transmit the message. Neuromodula-tors may be released by presynaptic nerve cells and may exercise their effects on a single synapse. It is also possible that neuromodulators may come from non-neuronal tissue and be distributed in cerebrospinal or extracellular fluid, thereby affecting large numbers of neurons. In addition, it appears that neuromodulators have a longer duration of effect (perhaps minutes) than do neurotransmitters. The distinguishing feature of **neurohormones** is their release by nerve cells directly into the systemic circulation rather than into the synap-tic cleft, extracellular fluid, or cerebrospinal fluid. Neurohormones may then be transported throughout the body to affect peripheral organs as well as the cen-tral nervous system.

Discovery of the **coexistence of neuroregula-tors**—the presence of more than one neuroregulator (neurotransmitter, neuromodulator, or neurohor-mone) with a single neuron—is one of the most impor-tant recent developments in neuroscience. It now ap-pears that many neurons in the central nervous system demonstrate coexistence. The number of coexisting neuroregulators released upon stimulation apparently varies; however, the basic physiology of these coexist-ing neuroregulators is largely unknown. Coexistence has significant implications for understanding regula-tory mechanisms in normal and disease states. It is possible, for example, that a nerve cell might contain both a neurotransmitter and a neuromodulator. If the neuromodulator decreases the response of the postsyn-aptic neuron to the neurotransmitter and if an apparent overactivity of the neurotransmitter is noted in disease states, the cause may be an excess of neurotransmitter, a deficiency of neuromodulator, or both.

Steps in Synaptic Transmission

The first 3 steps in synaptic transmission are the synthesis, transport, and storage of the chemical mes-senger. The actual release of the chemical messenger usually involves a calcium-dependent process that causes a synaptic vesicle containing the neuroregula-tor to fuse with the postsynaptic membrane and release its contents through exocytosis.

The principal site of action of neuroregulators is the synapse. Synapses are not only axodendritic but also axoaxonic, axosomatic, and dendrodendritic. Synap-tic receptors are complexes of one or more proteins floating in the lipid portion of the nerve cell mem-brane. Current knowledge suggests that synaptic re-ceptors may have as many as 3 basic components: a recognition site, a modulator, and an effector. Each component and its corresponding functions may be represented by one or more proteins existing in a com-mon area of the membrane and interacting when the receptor is stimulated.

The **recognition site** of the receptor exists on the external membrane and is responsible for the speci-ficity of receptor response by preferentially binding only certain neuroregulators. The modulator compo-nent may exist as a separate protein that connects the activated recognition site to the effector. The **modula-tor protein** may itself have binding sites located on the external membrane, where neuromodulators or neurohormones bind to modulate receptor function. For example, a neuromodulator may bind to a modula-tor protein and change the latter's conformation. This change in conformation may affect the conformation of receptor proteins and inhibit binding of the neuro-transmitter.

The **effector protein** is usually either a nucleotide cyclase or an ion channel. The effector protein is often adenylate cyclase, which catalyzes the conversion of adenosine triphosphate to cyclic adenosine $3',5$-monophosphate, which is often called the "second messenger" because it links extracellular chemical messengers and the physiologic response. The cyclic adenosine $3',5$-monophosphate can then activate cyto-plasmic enzymes, phosphorylate membrane proteins, induce synthesis of messenger RNA, or affect micro-tubular assembly at the cellular level. An ion channel (the other common type of effector protein), when ac-tivated, changes its conformation to increase or de-crease passage of specific ions into the neuron.

Termination of neuroregulator activity may occur through 4 mechanisms. First, the neuroregulator or products of its degradation may be brought back into the neuron through active, energy-dependent reup-take. Second, the neuroregulator may be degraded by enzymes either extraneuronally or intraneuronally. Third, the released neuroregulator may diffuse away from the postsynaptic cell into the brain extracellular fluid.

It is necessary to think of the steps in synaptic trans-mission as a dynamic flow, with change in one step af-fecting all other steps. Most drugs currently used in psychiatry initially exert their specific action on a sin-gle component of the synaptic receptor; however, the specific acute change may have complex effects on other components, and acute effects may differ markedly from chronic effects once the central ner-vous system has attained a state of equilibrium with the drug.

Regulation of Synaptic Transmission

Because recent research about the biology of be-havioral disorders has centered on abnormalities of the regulation of chemical transmission, it is therefore critical to understand the normal regulation of this pro-cess. The amount of neuroregulator that is synthesized may be controlled by varying the amount of necessary precursors and by altering the activity of the synthetic enzymes for specific neuroregulators, particularly en-zymes controlling rate-limiting steps. The transport and storage of neuroregulators are also subject to regu-lation by changes in microtubule, microfilament, and vesicle assembly and function at the cellular level.

The actual release and action of neuroregulators have received most of the emphasis in research on regulatory processes. Presynaptic inhibition may occur through a variety of mechanisms; eg, with repeated stimulation, a presynaptic neuron eventually releases smaller amounts of neuroregulator. Presynaptic neurons with autoreceptors may respond to the released neuroregulators to decrease (or possibly increase) synthesis and release of neuroregulators. The amount of neuroregulator released may also be reduced either by an independent inhibitory presynaptic neuron with an axoaxonic connection or by an inhibitory presynaptic neuron stimulated by a collateral fiber of the presynaptic neuron itself. Postsynaptic inhibition may be either direct or indirect. Direct inhibition occurs when an inhibitory postsynaptic potential is generated in the cell by an inhibitory neurotransmitter. Indirect inhibition occurs during the refractory period after the development of an action potential in a postsynaptic cell.

The sensitivity of the receptor is also subject to regulation, and the concepts of supersensitivity and subsensitivity are widely accepted. **Sensitivity** denotes the degree of neuronal response to a particular agonist. Changes in sensitivity may occur through a change in the absolute number of available receptors or through a change in the actual function of the receptor complex. The modulation of receptor sensitivity is thought to be involved in the development of tolerance and dependence. In **tolerance,** the chronic administration of a drug results in the need for an increasing amount of the drug to achieve the same effects originally produced by a smaller amount. In **dependence,** a state of homeostasis occurs in an organism as a result of the presence of an active drug in the system. If the drug is stopped, the system is no long in homeostasis, and withdrawal phenomena occur.

The proteins of the receptor complex exist in the fluid matrix of the bilayer lipid membrane, which itself is a site of regulation of neuronal homeostasis and activity. There is an increasing awareness that localized areas of the membrane may rapidly become more or less fluid (viscous), primarily as a function of phospholipid methylation. Such changes in membrane viscosity may hypothetically affect the function of receptors in various ways. For example, a more viscous membrane might force more receptor recognition sites out into the synapse, thereby increasing sensitivity. Conversely, a more fluid membrane might allow the various proteins of the receptor complex to become more widely separated and result in decreased sensitivity.

A new concept in neuroregulation is **chronobiology** (study of the effect of time on living systems), based on the observation that most biologic systems in the central nervous system—including neuroregulator production, neuroendocrine function, receptor sensitivity, and behavioral attributes such as rest and activity—follow a regular temporal cycle in their occurrence. **Circadian rhythms** are variations in biologic activity occurring during the course of a day (ie, 24 hours). Other important rhythms occur at the same time each month or each year. Rhythms may be regulated either by endogenous mechanisms or by exogenous (environmental) cycles (eg, the light-dark cycle of day and night or the varying daylight hours at different times of year). The various rhythms in normal controls are said to be synchronous. In disease states these rhythms may become asynchronous, and daily patterns of sleep or appetite may be disrupted.

The biologic basis of the pacemaker for circadian rhythms in humans is poorly understood, though the suprachiasmatic nucleus and pineal gland are thought to play important roles. Circadian rhythms have many implications for neurobehavioral physiology. The time of measurement of any central nervous system function must be noted, since activity may vary dramatically during the course of a day. Furthermore, the concept of biologic rhythm implies that the response of the central nervous system to environmental stimulation and to drugs changes over a period of time. Some have postulated that asynchronous biologic rhythms contribute to some mental illnesses, eg, abnormalities in sleep rhythms and in diurnal mood variations as well as the tendency for recurrence and seasonal occurrence of depression. In support of this hypothesis, antidepressant agents have been shown to affect circadian rhythms, and these effects may be the mechanisms of the drugs' therapeutic actions in some patients.

Recent study of the role of ion complexes in regulating cell function is important in psychopharmacology and in understanding the mechanisms of pathologic behavior. The calcium messenger system is the focus of particularly intense investigation. Calcium ions (Ca^{2+}), acting as both extracellular and intracellular messengers, regulate neurotransmitter and hormone secretion. Gross changes in extracellular Ca^{2+} concentration have been implicated in mood state changes in patients with bipolar affective disorder. It is likely, however, that disequilibration of the tightly controlled system regulating intracellular Ca^{2+} concentration is of greater significance. A complicated pump system maintains a large Ca^{2+} concentration differential across the cell membrane by regulating Ca^{2+} entry into the cell. The process depends upon control of the activity of specific Ca^{2+}-binding proteins, with calmodulin probably the most important in brain. Stimulation of the Ca^{2+}-binding system by hormones, neurotransmitters, or depolarization results in alteration of intracellular Ca^{2+} concentration through either intracellular Ca^{2+} release or opening of membrane Ca^{2+} channels. Small changes in Ca^{2+} flux can result in significant disequilibrium; whether such disequilibrium results in behavioral change is unclear. However, evidence for mood-stabilizing effects of Ca^{2+} antagonists active at voltage-dependent Ca^{2+} channels suggests that depolarization abnormalities may be important. These agents do not seem to block Ca^{2+} channels directly; they act by binding to nearby receptors.

There appear to be marked variation and heterogeneity in the concentration of Ca^{2+} antagonist receptors in brain. The functional significance of such variation is still unclear; however, mood-stabilizing effects have been described for different classes of Ca^{2+}-blocking agents with varying receptor specificities. Most of these reports have focused on the effects of verapamil and nifedipine. It is likely that other classes of Ca^{2+}-blocker not yet available for clinical use may show greater specificity for central nervous system receptors. Diphenylbutylpiperidine neuroleptic agents (represented by pimozide) are unique in their potent antagonism of Ca^{2+} channel receptors. These agents have been reported to be particularly effective in treating the "negative" symptoms of schizophrenia (eg, emotional withdrawal and poverty of speech and affect).

NEUROTRANSMITTERS

The 3 classes of neurotransmitter substances are the monoamines (biogenic amines), amino acids, and peptides. The monoamines include the catecholamines (dopamine, norepinephrine, epinephrine), an indoleamine (serotonin), a quaternary amine (acetylcholine), and an ethylamine (histamine). (See Table 11–1 for a summary of major precursors, enzymes, and metabolites of these substances.)

Neurotransmitter Research

The synthesis and metabolism of individual neurotransmitters are discussed below for 2 reasons. First, many of the synthetic enzymes as well as the products of metabolism serve as markers in research for the presence and activity of these neurotransmitter systems. Second, both synthesis and metabolism may be affected by drugs. It is unlikely that individual pathways specifically related to complex behaviors will be found; however, it may be that small groups of major pathways will be shown to be essential for proper expression of certain emotions or behaviors.

One focus of investigation is receptor subtypes for specific neurotransmitters. It seems that for most neurotransmitters, there is more than one type of receptor

that will respond specifically to that neurotransmitter. These different receptor types vary in their sensitivities, structural characteristics, and responses to the neurotransmitter. Research is therefore being directed toward the development of drugs that affect specific receptor subtypes but not others. Ideally, new drugs will affect the receptors involved with the abnormal behavior and not cause the adverse effects associated with some currently used drugs.

Research in most neurotransmitter systems also includes neurotransmitter challenge tests. **Challenge tests** involve in vivo testing of the biologic state of a specific neurotransmitter or neuroendocrine system by means of baseline measurement of a biologic or behavioral variable, followed by the administration of a specific biologically active agent affecting a neuroregulator system. The effects on the original variable are then measured over time. For example, it has been thought that some depressed patients might have abnormally sensitive receptors for acetylcholine. Physostigmine is a potent inhibitor of acetylcholinesterase, which is the major mechanism of termination of acetylcholine neurotransmission. Challenge testing in this case would involve measurement of baseline mood and pupillary size, administration of physostigmine, and assessment of its effects on those measurements. Eventually, a battery of such challenge tests could be used in the baseline assessment of patients with mental disorders, thereby providing specific measurement of crucial neuroregulatory systems. Rational pharmacotherapy would then be based on the results of such a test battery.

It now appears that neurotransmitter synthesis and release are partially controlled by the concentration of their precursors in dietary intake. High-carbohydrate, low-protein meals elevate brain tryptophan levels and accelerate serotonin synthesis. Brain concentrations of tyrosine and its catecholamine products may be elevated by consumption of protein and, as shown in preliminary studies, by consumption of the artificial sweetener aspartame. The behavioral effects of caffeine appear to depend upon its regulation of release of adenosine, a nucleic acid that may have neuroregulatory properties.

Table 11–1. Monoamine neurotransmitters and related compounds.

Neurotransmitter	Principal Synthetic Enzymes	Primary Precursors	Primary Brain Metabolites
Dopamine	Tyrosine hydroxylase*	Tyrosine L-Dopa	Homovanillic acid
Norepinephrine	Tyrosine hydroxylase* Dopamine β-hydroxylase	Tyrosine L-Dopa	Methoxyhydroxyphenylglycol
Epinephrine	Tyrosine hydroxylase* Dopamine β-hydroxylase Phenylethanolamine-N-methyltransferase	Tyrosine L-Dopa	Methoxyhydroxyphenylglycol
Serotonin	Tryptophan hydroxylase*	Tryptophan	5-Hydroxyindoleacetic acid
Acetylcholine	Choline acetyltransferase*	Choline	No specific metabolite
Histamine	Histidine decarboxylase*	Histidine	No specific metabolite

*Rate-limiting enzyme, or enzyme associated with rate-limiting step in synthesis.

Dopamine

Dopamine is synthesized through a number of enzymatic steps from the amino acid tyrosine. The rate-limiting enzyme is tyrosine hydroxylase, which requires pteridine cofactor for activity. The principal degradative path is through the action of monoamine oxidase to 3,4-dihydroxyphenylacetic acid and then through catechol-O-methyltransferase to homovanillic acid, the major metabolite of dopamine. It has been demonstrated that there are 2 types of monoamine oxidases (MAO-A and MAO-B) in the central nervous system that differ in their substrate affinity, with MAO-B more selectively metabolizing dopamine and MAO-A more selectively metabolizing norepinephrine and serotonin.

The importance of MAO in dopamine metabolism has been highlighted by serendipitous observations of the effects of 1-methyl-4-phenyl-1,2,3,6-tetrahydropyridine (MPTP), a central nervous system toxin. An epidemic of parkinsonism among users of a synthetic heroin containing MPTP suggested a model for studying dopamine depletion in the substantia nigra. It is now known that the dopamine-depleting effects of MPTP depend upon its conversion to 1-methyl-4-phenylpyridinium iodide (MPP+), a reaction that is catalyzed by MAO-B and blocked by MAO-B-selective inhibitors. These findings have led to the hypothesis that parkinsonian syndromes may result from environmental toxins that aggravate the diminution in dopaminergic function associated with aging. The MPTP-MAO model of dopamine depletion may be important in quantifying dopamine activity in mood and thought disorder and in understanding movement disorder in long-term recipients of neuroleptics.

Together with norepinephrine, dopamine regulates motivational arousal and the reward-reinforcement system; however, these functions have not been localized to a specific pathway. Dopamine is also thought to be involved in temperature regulation, which may be relevant in neuroleptic malignant syndrome, a disorder associated with administration of some antipsychotics (eg, phenothiazines). (See Chapters 24 and 52.)

A. Dopaminergic Pathways: There are 5 recognized dopaminergic neuronal pathways in the central nervous system:

1. The nigrostriatal pathway has cell bodies of dopaminergic neurons in the substantia nigra. These neurons project to the caudate nucleus and putamen of the corpus striatum. Normally, this pathway is involved in the initiation and coordination of muscle movement. Dopamine shares a dynamic balance with acetylcholine in this pathway. It is thought that there is a dopamine excess and an acetylcholine deficiency in Huntington's chorea and Gilles de la Tourette's syndrome. The reverse imbalance exists in Parkinson's disease. An excess of both dopamine and acetylcholine may possibly lead to idiopathic orofacial dyskinesia (Meige's dystonia, or Brueghel's syndrome). This pathway is involved in neuroleptic-induced extrapyramidal syndromes and probably in the development of tardive dyskinesia as well (see Chapter 10).

2. In the mesolimbic-mesocortical pathway, cell bodies of dopaminergic neurons exist in an area medial and superior to the substantia nigra. These neurons project to the limbic system and neocortex. This pathway is thought to be involved in the control of normal emotions and behaviors and is conceivably the site of pathologic changes in schizophrenia and other psychotic illnesses.

3. The tuberoinfundibular (tuberohypophyseal, hypothalamic-hypophyseal) pathway has cell bodies of dopaminergic neurons in the arcuate nuclei and periventricular area; these neurons project to the median eminence of the hypothalamus and to the posterior pituitary. This pathway regulates release of prolactin from the pituitary. Dopamine itself is thought to act as a prolactin-inhibiting hormone.

4. The medullary periventricular pathway has cell bodies of dopaminergic neurons in the motor nucleus of the vagus nerve and the nucleus tractus solitarii. The projections are not well defined, but this group of cells is thought to be involved in the control of food intake and perhaps in the physiologic derangements causing eating disorders (see Chapters 10 and 39).

5. A group of incertohypothalamic neurons project from the dorsal and posterior hypothalamus to the dorsal anterior hypothalamus and the lateral septal nuclei. The role of these neurons is unknown.

B. Dopaminergic Receptors: Three types of dopamine receptors have been characterized. The existence of D_1 and D_2 receptors has been firmly established; the existence of D_3 receptors remains controversial.

1. D_1 receptors are located on postsynaptic cells and activate dopamine-sensitive adenylate cyclase. They are essentially absent in the tuberoinfundibular pathway.

2. D_2 receptors are located on postsynaptic cells and either do not affect or may actually inhibit dopamine-sensitive adenylate cyclase. Guanosine triphosphate further regulates the effects produced by stimulating these receptors. This is the only type of dopamine receptor in the pituitary.

3. D_3 receptors are located on presynaptic neurons and are also called autoreceptors. Their activation decreases the amount of dopamine synthesized in the presynaptic cell. These receptors are found in the nigrostriatal and mesolimbic pathways but not in the tuberoinfundibular and mesocortical pathways.

C. Dopamine Hypothesis of Schizophrenia: (See also Chapter 27.) The dopamine hypothesis of schizophrenia proposes that hyperactivity of the dopamine system (possibly the D_2 receptors in the mesolimbic-mesocortical pathway) may exercise a causative role in schizophrenia. The major support for this hypothesis is that the clinical potency of the neuroleptics is well correlated with their ability to block D_2 receptors. Postmortem examination of the brains of schizophrenic patients has revealed an increased number of D_2 binding sites; however, this may be partially attributed to the effects of neuroleptic medication.

There appear to be some schizophrenic patients with low monoamine oxidase activity, which would reduce the rate of degradation of dopamine. There may also be a subgroup of people with low dopamine β-hydroxylase activity. This enzyme converts dopamine to norepinephrine; therefore, low dopamine β-hydroxylase causes a relative dopamine excess and norepinephrine deficiency. Since the various aspects of this hypothesis are still the focus of current research, it is more important to understand the concepts of dopamine regulation than it is to comprehend any of the currently hypothesized specific dysfunctions.

There is an increasing awareness of the role dopamine plays in the affective disorders. The hypothesis is that dopamine levels are low in depressed patients, particularly those with significant motor retardation. Conversely, dopamine levels are thought to be high in mania and may be particularly important in the shift from depression to mania. The biologic correlates at the time of major clinical change in patients (eg, shift from depression to mania or from nonpsychotic to psychotic states) are of major interest for researchers. Dopamine challenge tests with measurement of growth hormone or prolactin response are being used to assess the functional status of a patient's dopaminergic system.

D. Neuroleptics: (See also Chapters 27 and 52.) Neuroleptics are the major drugs used to treat psychotic conditions, including schizophrenia. The antipsychotic effects of neuroleptics may not become apparent for 3 weeks, whereas their dopamine receptor-blocking effects occur immediately. Many neuroleptics also significantly block alpha-adrenergic, serotoninergic, histaminergic, and cholinergic receptors; therefore, not all of the actions of neuroleptics can be directly ascribed to their immediate dopamine-blocking effects.

The major adverse side effects associated with neuroleptics are parkinsonlike symptoms and the potential development of tardive dyskinesia. The traditional explanation of this disorder is that chronic dopamine blockade by neuroleptics causes the equivalent of denervation and postsynaptic dopamine hypersensitivity. Although this theory may explain withdrawal dyskinesias, more recent research indicates that presynaptic oversecretion of dopamine coupled with noradrenergic hyperactivity is the cause of tardive dyskinesia in at least some patients with this disorder. This theory fits in with the observation that the most effective drugs for tardive dyskinesia involve beta-adrenergic blockers and gamma-aminobutyric acid-containing drugs, which may decrease dopamine activity. The use of cholinergic drugs to help correct a hypothesized dopamine-acetylcholine imbalance has not been of much clinical benefit. Also, recent reports have noted that in some patients with bipolar affective disorders who have been treated with neuroleptics, tardive dyskinesia is active during depression and absent during mania. This observation supports the hypothesis of dopamine overactivity in mania.

E. Amphetamines: Amphetamines cause the release of both dopamine and norepinephrine from synapses and also significantly block their reuptake. Both chronic and acute amphetamine use in humans may produce a psychosis indistinguishable from paranoid schizophrenia that may serve as a model for schizophrenia. (See Chapter 25.) Amphetamines have been used successfully to treat some depressed patients, particularly older ones with medical illnesses. Sympathomimetics have also been used to treat childhood hyperactivity; traditionally, this has been called a "paradoxical effect." Studies have shown that amphetamines do increase vigilance and response time in both normal and hyperactive children.

Norepinephrine & Epinephrine

Norepinephrine shares the synthetic pathway of dopamine. Dopamine is converted to norepinephrine by dopamine β-hydroxylase, a copper-containing enzyme. Norepinephrine is metabolized by monoamine oxidase (more selectively by MAO-A) and catechol-O-methyltransferase to methoxyhydroxyphenylglycol. Epinephrine is currently considered to play only a minor role in central nervous system function. It is produced when phenylethanolamine-N-methyltransferase converts norepinephrine to epinephrine.

The noradrenergic pathways are thought to play a role in regulation of mood, learning, memory, reinforcement, anxiety, and the sleep-wakefulness cycle. Beta receptors—specifically, those located in the hippocampus and septal nuclei—seem to be involved in the sensation of anxiety. Alpha receptors may regulate the initiation of feeding, and beta receptors may participate in the induction of satiety.

A. Noradrenergic Pathways: There are 2 large groups of noradrenergic neurons:

1. The locus ceruleus in the upper pons is the site of most noradrenergic neurons. These neurons project to the cerebral cortex, hypothalamic and thalamic nuclei, and limbic system.

2. The lateral tegmental neurons are loosely scattered within the lateral ventral tegmental fields and may be an important source of noradrenergic fibers to the basal forebrain, hypothalamus, and amygdala.

B. Adrenergic Pathways: Epinephrine-containing neurons are intermingled with the noradrenergic neurons of the lateral tegmental area and are found also in the dorsal medulla. They are believed to project to the locus ceruleus, mesencephalon, and hypothalamus. Epinephrine-containing neurons in the nucleus tractus solitarii may play a role in the control of blood pressure.

C. Noradrenergic Receptors: There are 4 types of noradrenergic receptors:

1. Alpha$_1$ receptors are postsynaptic and do not activate adenylate cyclase when stimulated.

2. Most α_2 receptors are presynaptic, activate adenylate cyclase when stimulated, and are more sensitive to alpha-adrenergic agonists than are postsynaptic adrenergic receptors. They function to reduce norepinephrine synthesis in the presynaptic neuron. Some α_2 receptors are postsynaptic.

3. Beta$_1$ receptors are postsynaptic and may be presynaptic. They activate adenylate cyclase when stimulated.

4. Beta$_2$ receptors are postsynaptic and activate adenylate cyclase when stimulated. There is some evidence for presynaptic β_2 receptors that function to increase presynaptic function. Both types of beta receptors predominate at the ends of the locus ceruleus tracts, and there may be beta regulation of α_2 receptors in the mammalian central nervous system.

D. Monoamine Hypothesis of Affective Illness: (See Chapter 30.) The monoamine hypothesis of affective illness states that a functional underactivity of norepinephrine or serotonin may cause depression and that increased activity in the noradrenergic and serotoninergic pathways may result in mania. The basis for this hypothesis rose from 2 major observations. First, researchers noted that reserpine not only depleted central stores of catecholamines and indoleamines but also inhibited their storage. It also caused depression. Second, antidepressant drugs (see Chapter 53) either blocked reuptake of catecholamines and serotonin or effectively blocked their degradation. The major problem with this hypothesis and the supporting evidence is that although the acute changes associated with antidepressant drug therapy seem to increase noradrenergic and serotoninergic activity, the chronic changes appear to be significantly different. Studies of patients undergoing chronic (1–3 weeks) treatment with antidepressant drugs have indicated the following changes: decreased postsynaptic β receptor and presynaptic α_2 receptor sensitivity or activity; increased α_1 receptor sensitivity; and increased norepinephrine release (possibly due to decreased α_2 receptor sensitivity). These studies seem to support a different hypothesis—namely, that noradrenergic *over*activity is involved in depression and that treatment with antidepressant drugs reduces overall noradrenergic activity. Research on the monoamine hypothesis of affective illness continues.

Recent models of mood disorders have highlighted the importance of disequilibrium of the noradrenergic system. There is evidence to support the following criteria for disequilibrium: impairment of feedback control, erratic basal output, disruption of normal circadian rhythms, decreased selectivity in response to environmental stimuli, and restoration of efficient regulation by mood-stabilizing drugs. The postsynaptic α_2 receptor system, which normally provides negative feedback inhibition to norepinephrine release, appears to be desensitized in some depressed patients. A singular change has been hypothesized in patients with panic disorder. Yohimbine, a selective α_2 receptor antagonist, reproduces panic symptoms in susceptible individuals. Alprazolam, a benzodiazepine, appears to attenuate the noradrenergic effects of yohimbine in patients with panic disorder but not in control subjects. The action of other antipanic agents at the α_2 receptor remains unclear.

Investigators have pursued 2 additional lines of study in their research into the role of the noradrenergic pathway in depression. First, it has been noted that urinary excretion of methoxyhydroxyphenylglycol in depressed patients follows 2 patterns. Patients with low urinary methoxyhydroxyphenylglycol levels have a norepinephrine deficiency, whereas those with normal or high levels may not. Second, noradrenergic challenge tests with clonidine (a specific α_2 agonist) or amphetamine followed by measurement of their effects on the neuroendocrine system have been used to assess central noradrenergic function. These challenge tests may enable clinicians to differentiate subtypes of depressed patients on a biologic basis and may eventually have implications for treatment.

Although much research in schizophrenia has focused on the role of dopamine, there is evidence to support overactivity of norepinephrine as a causative factor in some schizophrenic patients. Both clonidine and propranolol (a beta-adrenergic blocker) have been successful in the treatment of a few psychotic patients.

E. Drugs Commonly Used in Affective Disorders: (See Chapters 53 and 54.) Many commonly used psychotropic drugs have major effects on the adrenergic system. The tricyclic antidepressants and the monoamine oxidase inhibitors have strong noradrenergic effects as well as a broad range of actions affecting the serotoninergic, cholinergic (mostly muscarinic), and histaminergic ($H_1 \gg H_2$) systems.

The antiadrenergic antihypertensive drug clonidine has been used to treat opiate withdrawal. Presumably, clonidine binds to presynaptic α_2 receptors and reduces the amount of norepinephrine synthesized and released during the withdrawal period. Clonidine has also been reported to be effective in the treatment of some cases of depression, mania, anxiety, and tardive dyskinesia. The beta-adrenergic blocking drugs, of which propranolol is the best known, either are nonselective in their blockade effects or have some selectivity for β_1 blockade. No specific blockers of β_2 receptors are in clinical use. Lithium inhibits stress-induced release of norepinephrine as well as norepinephrine reuptake. Chronic lithium treatment may decrease beta receptor function and increase alpha receptor function.

The major adverse adrenergic side effects of monoamine oxidase inhibitors and tricyclic antidepressants are mediated primarily by α_1 receptors and consist of postural hypotension, dizziness, and reflex tachycardia. Tyramine-induced hypertensive crises in patients taking drugs also inhibit liver and intestinal monoamine oxidase activity. A surge of adrenergic activity occurs when tyramine-rich foods such as cheese, beer, or wine are consumed.

Serotonin

Serotonin is synthesized through a number of enzymatic steps from the amino acid tryptophan. The first enzyme in this pathway is tryptophan hydroxylase, which requires oxygen and pteridine cofactor for activity. The concentration of tryptophan appears to be a primary regulatory factor. Serotonin is metabolized by monoamine oxidase (preferentially by MAO-A) to 5-hydroxyindoleacetic acid. It is not known how much cerebrospinal fluid 5-hydroxyindoleacetic acid is derived from the spinal cord and how much comes from brain.

Serotonin is thought to play a role in circadian rhythms, the perception of pain, the sleep-wakefulness cycle, and mood. It is also involved in control of feeding, motor activity, and temperature. It affects the prolactin, cortisol, growth hormone, and possibly the β-endorphin neuroendocrine systems.

A. Serotoninergic Pathways: Serotoninergic neurons are concentrated in the area of the median and the dorsal raphe nuclei, caudal locus ceruleus, area postrema, and interpeduncular area. Both the medial and dorsal neurons project to the thalamus, hypothalamus, and basal ganglia. The medial neurons also project to the amygdala, piriform cortex, and cerebral cortex. Descending fibers from this group of serotoninergic neurons innervate the spinal cord, modulate the sensitivity to pain input, and therefore probably play a key role in mediating the analgesic actions of morphine and related opioid compounds. Antidepressants that affect the serotoninergic system have been widely used clinically to control chronic pain.

B. Serotoninergic Receptors: Two types of serotoninergic receptors have been identified. S_1 receptors preferentially bind serotonin, require guanosine triphosphate for activity, and activate adenylate cyclase. S_2 receptors preferentially bind spiperone (a neuroleptic not available for clinical use in the USA), do not require guanosine triphosphate for activity, and do not activate adenylate cyclase. There is some evidence that S_2 receptors are the primary mediators of serotoninergic behavioral effects. There is also evidence for the existence of presynaptic serotoninergic receptors of an unknown type.

C. Role of Serotonin in Affective Illness and Schizophrenia: (See Chapter 30.) Serotonin is implicated as part of the cause of affective illness. Traditional psychiatric theory has claimed that low serotonin levels are associated with depression and high serotonin levels with mania. Some depressed patients have been shown to have decreased levels of 5-hydroxyindoleacetic acid in cerebrospinal fluid, and these patients seem to show greater anxiety and to be at greater risk for suicide than other patients.

The "permissive serotonin hypothesis" states that low levels of serotonin "permit" low levels of catecholamines to cause depression, whereas high levels induce mania. Somewhat in conflict with these theories is the observation that chronic treatment with antidepressant drugs reduces the number of S_2 receptors, which might imply an *over*activity of serotonin in at least some types of depression.

The transmethylation hypothesis of schizophrenia postulates that metabolic errors in the serotoninergic system might produce psychotomimetic indoleamine derivatives (see Chapter 27). Major support for this hypothesis has come from research into the actions and effects of LSD, which has extraordinarily specific effects on the serotonin system as a receptor blocker and as a partial agonist even though it affects both the serotoninergic and dopaminergic pathways.

D. Psychotropic Drugs: The main psychotropic drugs affecting the serotoninergic system are the tricyclic antidepressants and monoamine oxidase inhibitors, which were discussed in the previous section on norepinephrine. Loading with L-tryptophan (a precursor of serotonin) has been shown to increase central nervous system levels of serotonin; this amino acid has been used both as a hypnotic and as an adjuvant chemotherapeutic agent for antidepressant treatment.

At the onset of therapy, lithium likewise increases serotonin levels; however, after 2–3 weeks, lithium appears to reduce stimulant-induced release of serotonin.

Acetylcholine

Acetylcholine is synthesized from choline and acetyl-CoA by the enzyme choline acetyltransferase. Acetylcholine is rapidly metabolized in the synaptic cleft by acetylcholinesterase. About half of the choline produced by this degradation is taken back into the presynaptic neuron. Acetylcholine synthesis is regulated mostly by the availability of choline and somewhat by the feedback of acetylcholine in the choline acetyltransferase enzyme.

In the normal central nervous system, the cholinergic neurons are thought to modulate arousal, rapid eye movement sleep, pain perception, learning, memory, and thirst. Perhaps the most significant role of the cholinergic system in disease occurs in Alzheimer's dementia. A specific destruction of the neurons of the nucleus basalis of Meynert has been observed in at least a subgroup of patients with this disorder. (See Chapters 10 and 24.) Dementia in general is associated with a decrease in acetylcholine concentrations in the temporal neocortex, hippocampus, and amygdala. Attempts to facilitate cholinergic function with increased amounts of choline precursors such as lecithin in the diet have been disappointing, although this approach may prove useful in a subgroup of patients with dementia.

A. Cholinergic Pathways: Cholinergic neurons are found in the corpus striatum, nucleus accumbens septi, motor cortex, and thalamus. A large ascending system of cholinergic neurons originates in the reticular formation and projects to the hypothalamus, thalamus, hippocampus, and neocortex. A specific concentration of cholinergic cells in the nucleus basalis of Meynert projects to the cerebral cortex.

B. Cholinergic Receptors: Cholinergic receptors are subdivided into muscarinic and nicotinic types. Many psychotropic drugs, including tricyclic antidepressants, monoamine oxidase inhibitors, and neuroleptics, lead to the common anticholinergic adverse side effects of blurred vision, dry mouth, sinus tachycardia, constipation, and urinary retention. Trazodone is reported to have fewer anticholinergic side effects than the other antidepressants. Nicotinic receptors are much less common than muscarinic receptors in the central nervous system; however, they do exist and are responsible for the stimulating effects of tobacco. A third type of presynaptic cholinergic receptor may also exist.

C. Role of Acetylcholine in Affective Illness:
There is an increasing appreciation of the possible role of acetylcholine in the genesis of affective disorders. A homeostatic balance of acetylcholine with norepinephrine has been hypothesized. Depression is thought to be associated with cholinergic overactivity and mania with adrenergic overactivity. It has been suggested that the shortened interval between initial onset of sleep and onset of rapid eye movement sleep seen in depression may reflect cholinergic hypersensitivity in the central nervous system; furthermore, response to early correction of this disturbance with antidepressant therapy may predict the eventual therapeutic outcome. It has been further suggested that the derangement of the cortisol axis seen in depression is also due in part to cholinergic overactivity in the central nervous system. Cholinergic challenge tests with cholinomimetic agents may prove to be useful markers of cholinergic function in the central nervous system.

D. Psychotropic Drugs: Drugs with anticholinergic activity (benztropine, trihexyphenidyl) are frequently used to treat neuroleptic-induced extrapyramidal symptoms. (See Chapter 52.) They function by decreasing the dopamine-acetylcholine imbalance caused by dopamine blockade. Although they are usually effective in this role, there is contrary epidemiologic evidence that use of anticholinergic drugs increases the likelihood of tardive dyskinesia; therefore, these drugs should be used with caution.

Histamine

Histamine is synthesized from histidine by the enzyme histidine decarboxylase.

A. Histaminergic Pathways: Histamine is found in the highest concentrations in the hypothalamus and is believed to be a neurotransmitter in projections to the cerebral cortex, thalamus, corpus striatum, nucleus accumbens septi, and hippocampus.

B. Histaminergic Receptors: There are 2 types of histaminergic receptors: H_1 and H_2. H_1 receptors are therapeutically blocked by antihistamine medications used to control allergic symptoms. H_1 blockade may lead to sedation, weight gain, and hypotension. H_2 receptors activate adenylate cyclase and are found in the neocortex and hippocampus.

C. Psychotropic Drugs: Cyproheptadine is a potent H_2 antagonist that also has complex effects on the dopamine, acetylcholine, serotonin, and norepinephrine pathways. It has been used successfully in the treatment of Cushing's disease and anorexia nervosa. Doxepin, a tricyclic antidepressant, is a potent blocker of H_1 and H_2 receptors, being about 6 times more powerful than cimetidine as an H_2 blocker and about 1000 times more powerful than diphenhydramine as an H_1 blocker. Doxepin has been useful in the treatment of peptic ulcer disease, particularly in patients whose disease has a significant affective component and in those who have developed adverse psy-

chiatric reactions to cimetidine (eg, depression or psychosis).

Amino Acids (Including Gamma-aminobutyric Acid)

Gamma-aminobutyric acid is an inhibitory amino acid neurotransmitter present in 60% of synapses in the human central nervous system. Other possible inhibitory amino acid neurotransmitters include glycine, taurine, and β-alanine. Glutamic acid appears to act as an excitatory amino acid neurotransmitter at many sites in the human central nervous system. Other probable excitatory amino acid neurotransmitters include aspartic acid, cysteic acid, and homocysteic acid. Elucidation of the action of amino acid neurotransmitters is complicated by the fact that they play common metabolic roles as well as perform neurotransmitter functions. Neurons containing gamma-aminobutyric acid appear to affect anxiety, emotions, and the control of eating. Disease or derangement of the neuronal system containing gamma-aminobutyric acid may lead to disorders in these functions as well as to overt seizure disorders.

Gamma-aminobutyric acid is synthesized from glutamic acid by the enzyme glutamic acid decarboxylase and is metabolized eventually to succinic acid by gamma-aminobutyric acid transaminase. Both of these enzymes require pyridoxal phosphate as a cofactor for activity. Gamma-aminobutyric acid acts by increasing cell membrane permeability to chloride ions.

A. Gamma-aminobutyric Acid-Containing Neuronal Pathways: Gamma-aminobutyric acid is widely distributed in inhibitory interneurons but is concentrated in the substantia nigra, globus pallidus, hypothalamus, and cerebellar and cerebral cortices. It is the neurotransmitter for the cerebellar Purkinje cells, which project to the vestibular and cerebellar nuclei. There is also a tract of cells containing gamma-aminobutyric acid running from the corpus striatum to the substantia nigra that may interact in a complex relationship with the endogenous opioid system.

B. Gamma-aminobutyric Acid Receptors: There are probably at least 2 different types of gamma-aminobutyric acid receptors in the central nervous system; however, they have not yet been well differentiated.

C. Psychotropic Drugs: The gamma-aminobutyric acid receptor complex contains a modulating protein that has a binding site for benzodiazepines. The action of benzodiazepines is thought to be due to their binding to the benzodiazepine recognition site and facilitating the inhibitory effects of gamma-aminobutyric acid transmission. Barbiturates also may act by facilitating neurotransmission involving gamma-aminobutyric acid. Both anxiolytic and anxiogenic endogenous ligands for this binding site have been identified.

PSYCHOENDOCRINOLOGY

Psychoendocrinology (more specifically, psycho-neuroendocrinology) is a subspecialty of endocrinology that takes into account the fundamental relationships between central nervous system biology, behavior, and the endocrine system. The classic chemical messengers of the endocrine system are the hormones, which are chemical signals released into the systemic circulation that may exert either local effects close to their site of release or effects far distant in the body. The 3 major structural classes of hormones are the steroids, peptides, and amino acids. It is the peptide class that has attracted the most interest in psychoendocrinology.

As mentioned above, the peptides coexist with the biogenic amines in presynaptic terminals—ie, are cotransmitters—and are apparently released along with the biogenic amines when the neurons containing them are stimulated. Table 11–2 contains a list of some currently known coexisting biogenic amines (specifically, monoamines) and peptide neuroregulators. Until recently, it was thought that only one neuroregulator existed in any one type of cell. Given the importance of the biogenic amines in both normal and abnormal human behavior, the relationship between the 2 classes of compounds is thought to be important, although it is not completely understood at this time. There is evidence that peptides not only act as neuromodulators and neurohormones at distant sites but also may have local effects similar to those of classic neurotransmitters. Many of these peptides (eg, corticotropin-releasing factor, adrenocorticotropic hormone) are also involved in regulation of the traditional hormonal axes (eg, the cortisol axis).

An important quality distinguishing peptides from classic neurotransmitters is their polymorphism; there are now known to be at least 9 endogenous opiates and 5 forms of cholecystokinin, each of which may be localized to different neurons. The identification and isolation of new peptides have been revolutionized by DNA technology. Molecular cloning has permitted the exact sequencing of a number of peptides and their precursors. Through examination of precursor sequences predicted by cloned mRNA, it is now possible to postulate the existence of previously undetected peptides. Such sequencing techniques are likely to identify and localize enzymes required for the formation of peptides from precursors, as well as for the inactivation of peptides. This information will help clarify the functional significance of specific peptide systems.

The synthesis of neuropeptides involves transcription of DNA in the cell nucleus to form RNA, which through the process of translation, guides the production of proteins in cytoplasm. Both of these steps are under multiple regulatory controls. The product of translation is a precursor protein that is metabolized into active components by peptidases. This system allows many peptides to be derived from a single gene product and involves yet another step that can be regulated. The peptides are transported, stored, and released in a manner basically similar to that described for conventional neurotransmitters.

It is hypothesized that in contrast to monoamines and amino acids, peptide neuroregulators can act at sites more distant from their site of release; can affect neuronal function over a longer period of time; can modulate rather than directly transmit messages; and can coordinate complex behaviors rather than simply activate single cells. The action of the peptides is terminated by the action of peptidases.

The basic role of neuroendocrine systems and the peptides in particular in mental disorders is still largely unknown; however, abnormalities in these systems have been identified in some mental disorders. These abnormalities of regulation may represent markers of dysfunction or may themselves be directly responsible for pathophysiologic changes. Major depression is the illness with the most clearly defined neuroendocrine abnormalities, including (1) increased cortisol secretion with loss of the usual dirunal variation, (2) blunted growth hormone response to insulin-induced hypoglycemia, and (3) blunted thyrotropin response to infusion of thyroid-releasing hormone. Anorexia nervosa is a syndrome that also has multiple neuroendocrine abnormalities; however, it has been difficult to determine which of these are secondary to the malnutrition. Neuroendocrine function in schizophrenia and mania has also been extensively investigated, with inconsistent results.

Table 11–3 sets forth the major central nervous system neuroactive peptides and their relationship, if any, to commonly described endocrinologic axes. Clinicians should note that the name given to a component of the neuroendocrine system may represent only the first recognized function and not other functions or even the chief function. Many hormones are also structurally similar and may have potentially overlapping effects on receptors. Although anatomic localizations are given for many of the neuroactive peptides, much of this information was obtained from nonhuman animals, and there may well be large interspecies differences.

Table 11–2. Examples of monoamines and peptides that are found in the same neurons.

Monoamines	Coexisting Peptides
Dopamine	Cholecystokinin Enkephalins
Norepinephrine	Enkephalins Neurotensin Somatostatin
Serotonin	Substance P Thyrotropin-releasing hormone
Acetylcholine	Enkephalins Vasoactive intestinal peptide
Epinephrine	Enkephalins

Table 11–3. Central nervous system neuroactive peptides and the psychoendocrine system.

Traditional central nervous system-hypothalamic-anterior pituitary axis
  Cortisol: corticotropin-releasing hormone, adrenocorticotropic hormone, cortisol
  Gonadal regulatory steroids: gonadotropin-releasing hormone, luteinizing hormone, follicle-stimulating hormone, estrogens, progesterone, androgens
  Thyroid: thyrotropin-releasing hormone, thyroid-stimulating hormone, thyroid hormones
  Growth hormone: growth hormone-releasing hormone, somatostatin, growth hormone
  Prolactin: prolactin-inhibiting hormone, prolactin-releasing hormone, prolactin
  Melanocyte-stimulating hormone
Central nervous system-N hypothalamic-posterior pituitary axis
  Vasopressin
  Oxytocin
Central nervous
  Melatonin
Other central nervous system peptides
  Endogenous opioids
  Substance P
  Cholecystokinin
  Vasoactive intestinal peptide
  Angiotensin I, II, and III
  Neurotensin
Other central nervous system peptides (not discussed in text)
  Bombesin
  Bradykinin
  Calcitonin
  Cardioexcitatory peptide
  Carnosine
  Gastrin
  Gastrin inhibitory peptide
  Glucagon
  Insulin
  Motilin
  Neuronal growth factor
  Neuronal polypeptide
  Secretin
  Sleep-inducing peptide

Central Nervous System-Hypothalamic-Anterior Pituitary Axis

The basic organization of the central nervous system-hypothalamic-anterior pituitary axis involves input from the limbic system and cortex to the hypothalamus, which in turn releases releasing and inhibitory factors affecting the pituitary. The pituitary releases trophic hormones that may stimulate the peripheral glands to release hormones. All of the released products have the potential to provide feedback regulation to previous components of the axis. Although the following sections discuss the hypothalamic factors and pituitary trophic hormones under the heading of the final hormone of their systems, many of the substances have been found to exist elsewhere than in the hypothalamus, and many may have direct effects unrelated to their hormonal action.

A. Cortisol: The regulatory controls in the levels of cortisol are corticotropin-releasing hormone and arenocorticotropic hormone. A diurnal variation in adrenocorticotropic hormone and cortisol occurs in humans, with peak cortisol levels occurring around 6–7 AM. Hypercortisolism (Cushing's syndrome) may cause depression, mania, confusion, and psychosis. Apathy, fatigue, and depression are common symptoms in hypocortisolism (Addison's disease). The entire axis is important in the physiologic response to stress and may be involved in the control of mood and behavior. In addition to its direct hormonal actions, cortisol also induces protein synthesis and modulates production of synthetic enzymes in the central nervous system. Both corticotropin-releasing hormone and adrenocorticotropic hormone have been shown to exist in the central nervous system outside the hypothalamus. Extrahypothalamic adrenocorticotropic hormone is found in the brain stem, thalamus, and limbic system, where it may play a modulating role in attention, memory, and learning. High cortisol levels with loss of the usual diurnal variation in levels have been reported mainly in patients with depression but may also be found in some patients with mania, obsessive compulsive disorders, schizoaffective disorders, or eating disorders. The role of extrahypothalamic corticotropin-releasing hormone is not known.

There is a good deal of interest in the possible direct effect on behavior of corticotropin-releasing hormone. When administered centrally in animals, it causes behavioral effects similar to those observed in animal models of anxiety and depression. A subgroup of depressed patients has also demonstrated an attenuated adrenocorticotropic hormone response to corticotropin-releasing hormone stimulation. This response contrasts with that of control subjects and with the adrenocorticotropic hormone hyperresponsivity of most patients with Cushing's disease. The relationship between corticotropin-releasing hormone and brain noradrenergic, serotoninergic, and cholinergic systems enables clinicians to consider corticotropin-releasing hormone hypersecretion and hypothalamic-pituitary-adrenal disequilibrium in terms of traditional neurotransmitter models of mood disorder.

B. Gonadal Regulatory Steroids: The peptides involved in the regulation of production of estrogens, progesterone, and androgens are gonadotropin-releasing hormone, luteinizing hormone, and follicle-stimulating hormone. The primary role of the gonadal regulatory system is regulation of gonadal function and control of gonadal steroid hormone production, with specific reference to puberty, the menstrual cycle, and menopause. Disturbances in regulation are undoubtedly involved in premenstrual tension syndrome.

Gonadotropin-releasing hormone is structurally similar to thyrotropin-releasing hormone and exists chiefly in the hypothalamus but is also found in the amygdala and midbrain. There is evidence that gonadotropin-releasing hormone functions as a neuromodulator and that it has both inhibitory and excitatory effects on postsynaptic cells. Its primary effect is presumably on sexual behavior; however, it may also be involved in the general control of alertness and anxiety as well as in early development of the central nervous system.

Anorexia nervosa is characterized by pathologic changes in the gonadal regulatory system—specifically, by reversion to prepubertal patterns of secretion of the hormones of this system, with low levels of gonadotropin-releasing hormone and no circadian or monthly variation in hormone levels. In psychologic terms, anorexia nervosa is seen as a retreat from adult responsibility and sexuality; in physiologic terms, the patient with anorexia nervosa has a sexually immature gonadal regulatory system. The common theme of sexual immaturity is an interesting connection between biologic and psychoanalytic approaches to this syndrome (see Chapter 39).

There is evidence that estrogens have an antidepressant effect in some women, and antiandrogens have been reported to be of use in the treatment of male sexual offenders. The observation that many serious mental illnesses have their onset at puberty may be related to the dramatic changes in the gonadal regulatory system that occur at that time.

C. Thyroid: The peptides involved in the regulation of triiodothyronine (T_3) and thyroxine (T_4) production are thyrotropin-releasing hormone and thyrotropin. The thyroid regulatory system is known to play a critical role in central nervous system development, as shown by the profound neurologic and other abnormalities seen in perinatal hypothyroid states. In adults, gross hyperthyroidism may cause anxiety, restlessness, and irritability. "Apathetic" hyperthyroidism, characterized by depression and withdrawal, may also occur, especially in geriatric patients. Hypothyroid states are characterized by depression, cognitive impairment, confusion, and psychosis. Thyrotropin-releasing hormone is widely distributed outside the hypothalamus in the cerebral cortex, brain stem, spinal cord, periventricular area, amygdala, and basal ganglia. Thyrotropin-releasing hormone is released from neurons upon stimulation (and therefore has neurotransmitterlike properties). It generally has an inhibitory effect on postsynaptic cells. It is thought that thyrotropin-releasing hormone is involved in the regulation of mood and behavior in addition to and independently of its traditional endocrine role. Infusion of thyrotropin-releasing hormone produces a transient improvement in mood in some depressed patients—an effect also observed, however, in other psychiatric patients and in normal volunteers.

A blunted thyrotropin response to infusions of thyrotropin-releasing hormone has been noted in about one-third of patients with major depression (see Chapter 30), and abnormal augmented responses have been observed in one-fourth of all depressed women. The latter finding is frequently associated with increased antithyroid antibody titers. Triiodothyronine as a supplement to tricyclic antidepressant has been shown to accelerate response to antidepressants in some individuals, particularly women. Supplementing tricyclic antidepressant therapy with triiodothyronine also has been effective in treating depressed patients who have

failed to respond to tricyclic antidepressants alone (see Chapter 53). These effects may be related to the observation that the regulatory peptides and hormones of the thyroid system are able to regulate the number of available central nervous system beta-adrenergic receptors. It should be noted that many patients with acute psychiatric illness have transient elevations of thyroid hormone levels at the time of admission to the hospital, although the interpretation of this finding is unclear.

D. Growth Hormone: The peptides regulating the release of growth hormone are growth hormone-releasing factor and somatostatin (growth hormone-inhibiting factor). Gross disorders of growth hormone regulation result in acromegaly or dwarfism. Release of growth hormone increases with exercise and stress. Somatostatin is found in high concentrations outside the hypothalamus, especially in the cerebral cortex and amygdala, but it is also found in the brain stem, basal ganglia, and hippocampus. It has been demonstrated that somatostatin is released from neurons upon stimulation and serves as a potential neurotransmitter or neuromodulator; it may also have an inhibitory effect on postsynaptic neurons. The behavioral effect of somatostatin is to decrease activity and increase sedation. A significant alteration in somatostatin regulation may account for many of the neuroendocrine changes noted in major depressive illness, and the role of somatostatin as a possible neuromodulator of acetylcholine may be important in the mechanism of Alzheimer's disease.

E. Prolactin: The controls regulating the release of prolactin are prolactin-inhibiting hormone and prolactin-releasing hormone. Prolactin bears certain structural similarities to growth hormone. It is found in increased levels during sleep, exercise, pregnancy, and nursing. Neuroleptics cause a marked increase in circulating prolactin, because they block the tuberoinfundibular receptors for dopamine, which may function physiologically as prolactin-inhibiting hormone. Hyperactivity of the prolactin regulatory system may lead to lethargy, irritability, and increased thirst.

F. Melanocyte-Stimulating Hormone: The regulatory peptides for melanocyte-stimulating hormone are melanocyte-stimulating hormone release-inhibiting hormone and melanocyte-releasing hormone. Little is known about the role of these substances in the central nervous system; however, melanocyte-stimulating hormone may be involved in learning and memory, and there have been a few reports that melanocyte-stimulating hormone and melanocyte-stimulating hormone-inhibiting hormone have an antidepressant effect.

Central Nervous System-Hypothalamic-Posterior Pituitary Axis: Vasopressin & Oxytocin

Vasopressin (antidiuretic hormone) and oxytocin are both synthesized in the supraoptic nuclei and paraventricular nuclei of the hypothalamus. These nuclei send projections to the posterior pituitary, whence the hormones are released into the circulation. The 2 hormones are derived from 2 different precursors. These 2 precursors also produce the 2 specific neurophysins, or carrier proteins. These carrier proteins may also have independent effects on the central nervous system. The paraventricular nuclei also project to the amygdala, locus ceruleus, thalamus, nucleus tractus solitarii, hippocampus, and septal nuclei.

Neurons containing vasopressin project to the anterior pituitary and into the cerebrospinal fluid through cells ending in the third ventricle. Release of vasopressin is increased by pain, stress, exercise, morphine, nicotine, and barbiturates and is decreased by alcohol. Vasopressin is thought to play a role in attention, memory, and learning and may also have an antidepressant effect. A number of specific agonists and antagonists of vasopressin have recently been developed, and their use in experimental animal models will help clarify the role of vasopressin in the central nervous system.

Oxytocin has been shown to be released by neurons and may function as a neurotransmitter; it appears to have an inhibitory effect on postsynaptic cells. The fact that suckling causes release of maternal oxytocin is an excellent example of a neural afferent-endocrine efferent reflex arc.

Central Nervous System-Pineal Gland Axis: Melatonin

Melatonin is synthesized from serotonin in the pineal gland by the action of serotonin-N-acetylase and 5-hydroxyindole-O-methyltransferase. The pineal gland also contains many other peptides, including vasopressin and luteinizing hormone-releasing hormone. The major regulator of melatonin synthesis is the light-dark cycle, with synthesis being increased during darkness. Regular fluctuations in the production of melatonin occur even without light-dark cues but create a longer cycle. The pineal gland is thought to be regulated by a major beta-adrenergic mechanism, and propranolol decreases melatonin synthesis. Melatonin itself seems central to the regulation of circadian rhythms and sexual maturation.

Other Central Nervous System Peptides

A. Endogenous Opioids: The endogenous opioids consist of a large number of naturally occurring morphinelike compounds. The 2 major enkephalins are met-enkephalin and leu-enkephalin. The enkephalins are found in high concentrations in the brain stem, amygdala, cerebral cortex, corpus striatum, thalamus, and periaqueductal gray regions.

The α-, β-, and γ-endorphins are derived from a large, nonopioid precursor protein. Beta-endorphin is found in high concentrations in the pituitary, anterior hypothalamus, septal region, and periaqueductal gray regions.

Mu receptors bind morphine preferentially and may be involved in the mediation of the analgesic effects of the endogenous opioid system. Delta receptors bind enkephalins preferentially and may be the opioid receptors primarily affecting behavior and seizure threshold. Kappa receptors bind dynorphan preferentially. They are located deep in the cerebral cortex and are thought to influence sensory integration. This function is manifested clinically by sedation and analgesia. Other types of receptors include σ and ϵ; however, these have not yet been clearly characterized.

Beta-endorphin release is increased by stress, and the general role of the endogenous opioids would appear to include regulation of pain, anxiety, and memory. Other likely effects include regulation of sexual activity, feeding, temperature, and blood pressure. A variety of endogenous opioid abnormalities have been reported in schizophrenia, affective illnesses, and eating disorders. Treatment of mental disorders with both opioid agonists and antagonists (eg, naloxone) has thus far yielded conflicting results.

B. Substance P: Substance P may be the principal neurotransmitter for the primary afferent sensory fibers from the dorsal root ganglion to the substantia gelatinosa of the spinal cord. Substance P is found in particularly high concentrations in the hypothalamus, median eminence, and basal ganglia; it is also found in the brain stem, amygdala, hippocampus, and cerebral cortex. It has been demonstrated that substance P is released from neurons upon stimulation and serves as a possible neurotransmitter. It often has an excitatory effect on postsynaptic cells. Substance P appears to modulate pain perception and possible motor control. Levels of substance P have been reported to be markedly reduced in patients with Huntington's chorea.

C. Cholecystokinin: Cholecystokinin has also been shown to be released from central nervous system neurons and may therefore be a neurotransmitter. It is found in high concentrations in the hippocampus and cerebral cortex as well as in the brain stem, basal ganglia, hypothalamus, and amygdala. It is thought that cholecystokinin may partially mediate the sensation of satiety, and its coexistence with dopamine in the nucleus accumbens septi argues for a prominent role in the pathophysiology of schizophrenia.

D. Vasoactive Intestinal Peptide: Vasoactive intestinal peptide is structurally similar to glucagon and is released from central nervous system neurons upon stimulation (thereby indicating a possible role as a neurotransmitter). It is found in especially high concentrations in the hippocampus and the cerebral cortex, where it appears to be organized within single cortical columns. It is also found in the brain stem, basal ganglia, hypothalamus, and amygdala. The role of vasoactive intestinal peptide is not known.

E. Angiotensin II: Angiotensinogen is converted by renin into angiotensins II and III. Although angiotensin II has received the most attention, all 3 compounds may be active in the central nervous system as neuroregulators. Angiotensin II is concentrated in the periventricular region; its major behavioral effect thus far discovered appears to be stimulation of water drinking.

F. Neurotensin: Neurotensin may be an excitatory regulator and is found in the highest concentrations in the hypothalamus and substantia nigra as well as in the nucleus accumbens septi, septal area, spinal cord, brain stem, interneurons of the substantia gelatinosa, and the motor trigeminal nucleus. It has been thought to regulate pain, sensitivity, arousal, and body temperature.

FUTURE DIRECTIONS

Three new areas of research in biologic psychiatry and the related basic neurosciences are psychoimmunology (properly psychoneuroimmunology), developmental psychobiology, and molecular genetic neuroscience.

Psychoimmunology is analogous to psychoendocrinology in that it expands the study of immunology to include the relationships between central nervous system biology, behavior, and the immune system. In reference to the biopsychosocial model of disease, 2 lines of research demonstrate how environmental influences may affect immune function. First, animal models have demonstrated that environmental stress may affect the immune system and the immune function may, in fact, be a conditioned response. Second, it is known in clinical medicine that both the onset and course of illnesses involving the immune system (eg, rheumatoid arthritis, systemic lupus erythematosus, and cancer) may be altered by psychosocial stresses.

The immune system is reciprocally linked with the nervous and endocrine systems, centrally and peripherally. In animal studies, hypothalamic and limbic system lesions may either impair or amplify suppressor T cell activity. In addition, various peptide and catecholamine receptors are found on the surface of circulating lymphocytes.

Although glucocorticoids were thought to suppress immune function, it is now apparent that they can either amplify or depress immune response under different physiologic conditions. Various immune products, eg, thymosin (the thymic hormone) or lymphokines, influence the secretion of corticotropin-releasing hormone and adrenocorticotropic hormone. Preliminary evidence indicates that lymphocyte receptors for glucocorticoids and catecholamines are altered in subsets of depressed patients. The plethora of opiate receptors on lymphocytes suggests an additional mechanism for hormone-immune system interactions. Studies of stress response may elucidate these interactions; acute exposure to stressors tends to suppress humoral immunity, whereas repeated exposure often leads to enhanced antibody response.

The linked evolution of the nervous, endocrine, and immune systems may be thought of in terms of a progressive sophistication in the process of distinguishing "self" from "nonself" in complex organisms. Aberrations in the recognition of self and nonself are thought to be the basis of autoimmune disease; an ever increasing number of diseases with behavioral manifestations are now known or suspected to be of autoimmune origin, including Graves' disease, Hashimoto's thyroiditis, multiple sclerosis, lupus erythematosus, and myasthenia gravis. It now appears likely that the development of lithium-induced thyroid disease is related to prior susceptibility to autoimmunity. There is also preliminary evidence that in some families and populations, psychiatric disorders are associated with particular haplotypes of the major histocompatibility complex known as the HLA system. Although it is possible that HLA is merely a marker for the inheritance of these syndromes, its role in regulating immune responses suggests that autoimmunity may be implicated in the pathogenesis of the illnesses themselves.

Developmental psychobiology is the study of the influence of the external environment on the development, maintenance, and natural degeneration of the central nervous system. It is a common misconception that brain development is unaffected by the environment until puberty, after which functioning then slowly degenerates with age. Experiments in which animals were exposed to enviromental stresses, specific patterns of learning, dietary changes, and varying degrees of sensory input have clearly demonstrated that such fundamental central nervous system properties as receptor number, cell division and migration, branching of dendrites, formation of synapses, and protein synthesis may all be affected by environmental factors. Recognition of these forces has resulted in increased research in behavioral teratology and has led to evidence that any significant environmental stimulus (eg, drugs; psychologic or physical stress) occurring during a critical period of neural development may have subtle but permanent effects on neural regulation and behavior.

Workers in **molecular genetic neuroscience** are exploring central nervous system function and dysfunction through the application of molecular genetic principles. The importance of protein synthesis in central nervous system development and function is already clear, and modern techniques in genetic research make it conceivable that genetic markers and genetic manipulations may become critical in the understanding of the molecular basis of mental disorders.

REFERENCES

Alexander P (editor): *Electrolytes and Neuropsychiatric Disorders*. S P Medical & Scientific Books, 1981.

Black I et al: Biochemistry of information storage in the nervous system. *Science* 1987;**236:**1263.

Burns SR et al: The clinical syndrome of striatal dopamine deficiency. *N Engl J Med* 1985;**312:**1418.

Charney D, Heninger G: Noradrenergic function and the mechanism of action of antianxiety treatment. *Arch Gen Psychiatry* 1985;**42:**458.

Cooper J, Bloom F, Roth R: *The Biochemical Basis of Neuropharmacology*, 5th ed. Oxford Univ Press, 1986.

Costa E, Racagni G (editors): *Typical and Atypical Antidepressants: Molecular Mechanisms*. Vol 31 of: *Advances in Biochemical Psychopharmacology*. Costa E, Greengard P (editors). Raven Press, 1982.

Costa E, Trabucchi M (editors): *Regulatory Peptides: From Molecular Biology to Function*. Vol 33 of: *Advances in Biochemical Psychopharmacology*. Costa E, Greengard P (editors). Raven Press, 1982.

DeFeudis F, Mandel P (editors): *Amino Acid Neurotransmitters*. Vol 29 of: *Advances in Biochemical Psychopharmacology*. Costa E, Greengard P (editors). Raven Press, 1981.

Fauman M: The central nervous system and the immune system. *Biol Psychiatry* 1982;**17:**1459.

Frost JJ: Imaging neuronal biochemistry by emission computed tomography: Focus on neuroreceptors. *Trends Pharmacol Sci* 1987;**7:**490.

Guillemin R, Cohn M, Melnechuk T (editors): *Neural Modulation of Immunity*. Raven Press, 1985.

Hanan I, Koslow SH (editors): *Physico-chemical Methodologies in Psychiatric Research*. Raven Press, 1980.

Hirata F, Axelrod J: Phospholipid methylation and biological signal transmission. *Science* 1980;**209:**1082.

Hofer M: *The Roots of Human Behavior*. Freeman, 1981.

Holbreich U (editor): *Hormones and Depression*. Raven Press, 1987.

Iversen SD, Iversen LI: *Behavioral Pharmacology*, 2nd ed. Oxford Univ Press, 1981.

Krieger D: Brain peptides: What, where, and why? *Science* 1983;**222:**975.

Krieger D, Martin J: Brain peptides. (2 parts.) *N Engl J Med* 1981;**304:**876.

Lynch DR, Snyder SH: Neuropeptides: Multiple molecular forms, metabolic pathways, and receptors. *Annu Rev Biochem* 1986;**55:**773.

Motulsky H, Insel P: Adrenergic receptors in man. *N Engl J Med* 1982;**307:**18.

Sachar EJ (editor): Advances in psychoneuroendocrinology. *Psychiatr Clin North Am* 1980;**3:**2. [Entire issue.]

Schmitt F, Bird S, Bloom F: *Molecular Genetic Neurosciences*. Raven Press, 1982.

Schwartz JH, Costa E: Neuropeptide synthesis and function. *Annu Rev Neurosci* 1986;**9:**277.

Shepard G: *The Synaptic Organization of the Brain*, 2nd ed. Oxford Univ Press, 1979.

Sibley DR, Lefkowitz RJ: Molecular mechanisms of desensitization using the beta-adrenergic receptor coupled adenylate cyclase system as a model. *Nature* 1985;**317:**124.

Snyder SH: Neuronal receptors. *Annu Rev Physiol* 1986;**48:**461.

Snyder SH, Reynolds IJ: Calcium antagonist drugs. *N Engl J Med* 1985;**313:**995.

Stahl SM, Leendees KL, Bowery NG: Imaging neurotransmitters in living human brain by positron emission tomography. *Trends Neurosci* 1986;**9:**241.

Takahashi J, Zatz M: Regulation of circadian rhythm. *Science* 1982;**217:**1104.

Williams RH (editor): *Textbook of Endocrinology*, 7th ed. Saunders, 1985.

Wurtman, RJ: Behavioral effects of nutrients. *Lancet* 1983; **1:**1145.

12

Psychiatric Diagnosis & Psychosocial Formulation

Howard H. Goldman, MD, PhD, & Steven A. Foreman, MD

Diagnosis is the process of matching a patient with observed or reported or reasonably presumed symptoms and signs with a known pathologic entity or syndrome. What makes diagnosis the starting point of medical care rather than its intellectual terminus is the process of **psychosocial formulation,** whereby each patient is managed individually according to his or her special needs and resources.

Clinical psychiatry is thus concerned with 2 related processes: (1) diagnosing mental disorder and (2) assessing psychiatric factors in health and illness. The former is a specialized domain, defined by concern for particular disorders (eg, schizophrenia, depression). The latter is a generic process common in evaluating all patients regardless of diagnosis and may extend beyond the traditional boundaries of medicine to include assessment of "problems in living" and normal human behavior. Clinical psychiatry shares this 2-dimensional approach with other medical specialties. Cardiologists, for example, are concerned not only with diagnosing cardiac disease but also with assessing cardiovascular function in all patients. Although they share important similarities in the objectives of patient assessment, psychiatry and other medical specialties have some important differences as well.

The basic processes of diagnosis are quite similar in the various branches of clinical medicine. The clinician observes patterns of signs and symptoms characteristic of a syndrome or specific disorder and decides on a name, or diagnosis. The diagnostic label implies that *this* patient's pattern of signs and symptoms is similar to the pattern observed in other patients with the same diagnosis. The pattern of signs and symptoms may have the same cause (etiology) or may develop in the same way (pathogenesis) or may be associated with the same abnormalities (pathology). The diagnostician observes the patient and tries to answer 2 questions: (1) Does the patient have frank . . . [mental, cardiac, etc] disease? (2) Does the patient have signs or symptoms of . . . [mental, cardiac, etc] dysfunction that suggest the onset of disease or suggest that the patient's clinical status would be compromised or deteriorate under stress such as an intercurrent illness, surgery, or death of a loved one? The clinician may also look for evidence of special skills or strengths or signs of abundant health that may enable the patient to adapt well to a particular situation or stress.

For most purposes of clinical assessment, it is sufficient to say that there *is* or *is not* evidence of disease. In some cases, however, the diagnostician may want to speculate about the circumstances (tolerance limits) under which the patient can be expected to function within "normal limits." In clinical psychiatry, the diagnostician first determines whether mental disorder is present or absent (**diagnosis**) and then goes on to assess the patient's mental function, behavior, social circumstances, and personality—a process called **psychosocial formulation.** Each patient is described uniquely, and the description is expanded to include personal information useful in patient care. To conclude only that a patient's psychiatric status is "within normal limits" generally is unsatisfactory. **Psychodynamic formulation** is one type of psychosocial formulation based on psychoanalytic theories of mental function and dysfunction. It is the most common formulation encountered in clinical psychiatry and is discussed later in this chapter.

Before undertaking to outline current theories of mental function and disorder, let us explain why psychiatric evaluation should go beyond assessment of the presence or absence of disease to an evaluation of individual psychic function.

There is a growing body of knowledge about the significance of behavior, emotion, personality, social circumstances, life-style, and stressful life events on health and illness. Clinical evaluation is incomplete without an assessment of these factors (psychosocial formulation). Unlike the diagnostic process, which tells us how one patient is similar to others, the process of psychosocial formulation tells us how each patient is unique. It attempts to explain why a patient presents at a particular time with a specific set of complaints. For example, a man with hemoptysis who waited 2 months before seeking treatment presented with vague complaints of chest pain. The physician found the chest pain to be benign, and hemoptysis proved to be the clue to malignant disease. Questioning the patient revealed that he presented with complaints on the anniversary of his child's death following cardiac surgery; and because his mother had died of lung cancer, he had denied the significance of the cough out of fear. The psychosocial formulation made on each patient can help the physician understand the patient's psychologic defenses and personality, so that an individualized approach to treatment can be planned.

How can the physician help the patient understand the illness and cooperate in making informed decisions about treatment? What psychosocial factors will affect compliance with treatment? What are the patient's social and family resources in coping with the illness? Is special assistance needed at times of stress? The process of psychosocial formulation parallels the diagnostic process both in medicine and in psychiatry. Its goal is to enable the therapist to understand each patient individually.

THEORIES OF MENTAL DISORDER

It would greatly simplify both psychiatric teaching and patient care if mental disorders could be explained by reference to basic principles that would also explain behavior, thoughts, and emotions, ie, by a "unitary theory" that would combine diagnosis and psychosocial formulation in one process of clinical evaluation. In this section, we will describe some unitary theories that have been offered for that purpose; discuss briefly their limitations; and then go on to recommend in their stead a biopsychosocial model made up of useful elements derived from biomedical as well as psychosocial observations. The biopsychosocial model encourages us to go beyond diagnosis and include psychosocial formulation as an essential part of the evaluation of every patient. The result is a pluralistic model that can be used as a guide to the clinical approach to the patient.

UNITARY THEORIES

In psychiatry, it is often assumed that an understanding of mental disorders confers understanding of normal behavior as well. The relationship is perceived as transitive: the study of one aspect of psychiatry informs the other. Although generally valid, this assumption has given rise to some overly simplified theories of psychopathology. Some theories assume that *all* mental disorders can be understood by reference to a *particular* model of how the mind works. To oversimplify for the sake of example—behaviorist theories explain mental disorders as maladaptive learning; psychodynamic theories (such as psychoanalysis) hold that mental disorders represent dysfunctional attempts to resolve psychologic conflicts derived from unconscious drives and wishes; and psychobiologic theories hold that all psychopathology results from defects in neurophysiologic processes.

These unitary theories provide the clinician with a single framework in which to search for the diagnosis of all mental disorders as well as for the understanding of human behavior in health and illness. Unitary theories have a kind of elegant economy, so that we can use the same basic principles for the purposes of diagnosis and for understanding every patient's thoughts, feelings, and behavior.

The unitary psychobiologic theory of mental disorder holds that all psychopathology can be understood as expressions of specific abnormalities in neurophysiologic function. In the narrowest of unitary theories, all disorders are claimed to result from deficiencies of a vitamin or mineral essential to neurotransmission or from an excess or lack of some endogenous compound. More sophisticated unitary psychobiologic theories may view specific mental disorders as the result of a diversity of influences on a central neurophysiologic abnormality responsible for all mental disorders (eg, a defect in a particular mental mechanism, such as selective attention). The diverse manifestations of mental disorders can be viewed as highly individual expressions of the basic pathophysiologic process, as epiphenomena unrelated to etiology. For example, if selective attention is the core defect in mental disorder, depression may represent an inability to harbor positive feelings about oneself and the future, and a phobia may represent an inability to undergo particular experiences without feeling anxious or panicky.

For the clinician working in the context of a unitary theory, diagnosing specific disorders is less important than identifying the fundamental abnormality and noting its effect on the individual. The goal is to correct the defect by vitamin supplementation, specialized training, etc, depending upon the physician's "school" of therapy.

In a unitary psychodynamic theory of mental disorder, all forms of psychopathology are viewed as examples of developmental arrest or regression along a chronologic plane of psychologic maturation. Symptoms and signs are viewed as responses (adaptive or maladaptive "defenses") characteristic of a particular level of development. General principles explain psychologic maturation, the conflicts that emerge along the developmental sequence, and the patterns of response. The general principles may be applied to each person's life experience to produce a unique understanding of an individual. Obeying basic laws of behavior, otherwise unique individuals may have common patterns of behavior and exhibit the same signs and symptoms of maladaptive responses. These common expressions of psychopathology may be grouped into syndromes or disorders. According to psychodynamic theories, disorders are clusters of signs and symptoms typical of a particular developmental level.

According to a unitary psychodynamic theory of mental disorder, diagnosing a specific disorder is less important than assessing individual psychologic maturity and appreciating the symbolic significance of individual symptoms. This process of psychosocial formulation is often called "psychodynamic formulation."

Theories of psychopathology that look to a single cause of mental disorder tend to hold that treatment should also be a unitary concept, as in the case of psychotherapy—individually tailored, of course, to each patient's signs and symptoms. A general theory of treatment emerges from the dominant basic theory of psychopathology. The concept of "panacea" is derived from such unitary theories. The challenge of this approach is to develop a *unique* treatment with a *unitary* therapy.

The word "panacea" now carries a pejorative connotation, because the unitary theories of etiology and treatment upon which the panaceas were based were overly simplistic and failed to explain the diverse pathologic manifestations of mental disorder encountered in clinical medicine. Similarly, unitary theories of mental disorder have fallen out of favor as a basis for understanding *all* forms of psychopathology.

BIOPSYCHOSOCIAL MODEL

Current thinking in clinical psychiatry holds that no *single* theory of psychopathology is adequate to explain all that needs to be explained about mental disorders. Instead, psychiatry has embraced a biopsychosocial model, recommended by George Engel and others before him, that attempts to integrate 3 perspectives into a comprehensive view of human behavior in health and illness. Drawing upon biomedical, psychologic, and social theories of psychopathology, the biopsychosocial model permits us to distinguish the 2 major patient assessment processes in clinical psychiatry and, for that matter, in general medicine: (1) diagnosis and (2) individual psychosocial formulation. In the absence of a widely accepted theory of psychopathology to explain the pathogenesis of mental disorder, diagnosis becomes a process of categorizing signs and symptoms that occur together in recognizable patterns. This descriptive (phenomenologic) process seeks to define disease entities carefully enough so that similarities of underlying pathogenesis or etiology can be discerned.

Criteria for inclusion or exclusion from a diagnostic category consist of verifiable signs and symptoms with a specified duration and intensity and a common natural history, prognosis, and response to treatment. Once a diagnosis has been made and the patient placed in a particular diagnostic category, the process of individual psychosocial assessment can begin. As noted in the introductory paragraphs, whether the diagnosis is psychiatric or somatic, individual psychosocial assessment is essential for evaluating patients comprehensively. As Francis Scott Smyth, former Dean of the School of Medicine, University of California (San Francisco), once noted, "To know what kind of a person has a disease is as essential as to know what kind of disease a patient has" (Smyth, 1962:499).

For the present at least, the search for a unitary theory of psychopathology can be said to have intellectual appeal but no urgent utility. We do not need a theory linking diagnosis and pathogenesis in order to arrive at a correct diagnosis, a realistic individual psychosocial assessment, and an effective plan of treatment. It is not essential to associate psychologic development or personality in a causal relationship with a diagnosis of depression, schizophrenia, or ulcerative colitis. As a practical matter, it is sufficient to diagnose mental illness in a biomedical mode and to assess our patients individually in a psychosocial mode. The diagnostic process enables us to select a known category of dysfunction or disorder that fits the patient's symptoms and signs—ie, to define how the patient is similar to other patients. The more difficult process of psychosocial assessment helps us to understand the meaning and expression of this disorder in a unique individual.

CLINICAL USE OF THE BIOPSYCHOSOCIAL MODEL

Ordinary People was a popular novel and successful movie in which Conrad Jarrett, the young protagonist, is portrayed as being depressed. The character will serve as a clinical example to illustrate 2 important points: (1) the utility of the biopsychosocial model to guide clinical assessment and (2) the benefit of both diagnosis and psychosocial (in this case, "psychodynamic" formulation for patient evaluation and treatment. We have selected this example because the young man has a disorder—a major depressive episode—that may be explained and treated both biomedically and psychosocially. The case demonstrates the need to diagnose a disorder for its biomedical benefits and to formulate the individual psychodynamics for its psychosocial benefits. Occasionally, patients can be treated successfully from only one perspective. Generally, a biopsychosocial perspective encouraging both diagnosis and formulation is optimal.

Conrad Jarrett was hospitalized and treated with electroconvulsive therapy after a suicide attempt following an extended period of depressed mood with guilt feelings marked by self-reproach, hopelessness, and thoughts of death. He was socially withdrawn and seemed to have lost all sense of pleasure. He also experienced difficulty sleeping, agitation, and poor appetite. He had nightmares in which he reexperienced a boating accident that cost his older brother his life. With the help of a psychiatrist, he eventually came to realize that his guilt over having survived the accident might explain his depression.

Conrad had always resented his brother and felt he was neglected by his mother, who favored the dead brother. He suspected that some part of him wanted the brother to die and that he did not try hard enough to rescue the drowning boy. The feelings left him despondent and angry. The suicide attempt represented an unconscious wish both to be punished and to punish his mother.

It is useful to examine these events from both a biomedical-diagnostic and a psychosocial perspective. Our understanding of Conrad and our approach to his treatment will be influenced by both points of view: He is suffering from a major depressive episode, characterized by depressed mood and a pattern of behavior including withdrawal from pleasurable activities, guilt and self-reproach, hopelessness, and suicidal thoughts. He is also suffering from a sleep and appetite disturbance. A major depressive episode is often characterized by abnormal laboratory findings (eg, in the dexamethasone suppression test) and a favorable response to antidepressant medication or electroconvulsive therapy. The psychodynamic formulation, developed during psychotherapy, provides an individualized understanding of the psychosocial forces contributing to this patient's depression. The formulation helps us understand the unique presentation of *this* young man undergoing a major depressive episode.

As is often the case in practice, we do not know whether the biomedical-diagnostic or the psychosocial perspective contributes more to our understanding of the cause and pathogenetic mechanism of Conrad's illness. We do not know if some still unidentified constitutional predisposition must be present for major depressive disorder to occur. We do not know if the physiologic findings (such as abnormalities in dexamethasone suppression or a depletion of catecholamines in the brain) are the cause of the depressive episode or the result of psychodynamics. We do know that not all patients with major depressive episodes have the same psychodynamic formulation and that not all individuals with the same personality structure and similar life experiences suffer major depressive episodes.

Since we have agreed not to seek unitary explanations for this and other types of mental disorder, we need not restrict ourselves to any one therapeutic resource. Controlled clinical trials have demonstrated that antidepressant medication is usually necessary for optimal control of depressive symptoms in major depressive episodes and that psychotherapy (especially focused on social adaptation) is essential for maximal recovery of social function. Insight psychotherapy is intellectually satisfying for some patients and may help prevent the painful repetition of depressive episodes by enabling patients to recognize their mixed feelings toward loved ones, even after the death of loved ones or their loss through divorce, separation, etc. Medication has also been shown to prevent recurrences of depressive symptoms, even without psychodynamic understanding of the disorder.

Continuing research may someday clarify the connection between the psychodynamics of depression and the psychobiology of major depressive episodes. Meanwhile, a dual perspective—biomedical and psychosocial, diagnostic and individualized—is essential to comprehensive patient care.

DIAGNOSIS & PSYCHOPATHOLOGY

Diagnosis in psychiatry is a complex and challenging process even though it may require less experience than psychodynamic or psychosocial formulation. Diagnosis serves several purposes, some of which benefit the patient, while others benefit the provider of care, the patient's family, or society. We diagnose mental disorders in an attempt to communicate more reliably and effectively with one another about a certain class of problems. A diagnosis is a type of "shorthand" for defining an individual's problems in a way that will be recognized by patients, doctors, and society. In addition, the act of diagnosis confers the "sick role" on the patient, granting exemption from certain responsibilities as well as giving permission to engage in certain types of behavior and to expect certain types of behavior from others.

A diagnosis also implies a degree of understanding of a pattern of illness, suggesting a **specific treatment** and an expected outcome, or **prognosis.** Establishing a diagnosis may also make the physician or other care provider feel better about dealing with the uncertainties of illness, human suffering, and death. Sometimes the process of diagnosis is all the physician can offer, but it should be offered even so. The danger that a psychiatric diagnosis may function as a social label or stigma is a risk that must be accepted. The benefits of specific treatment may depend on specificity and precision in diagnosis. Leprosy, syphilis, lung cancer, tuberculosis, and mania are all stigmatizing diagnoses. Failure to make the diagnosis could deprive a patient both of specific treatment and of the general supportive care called for in such cases.

Precision in diagnosis is important also for **research.** If we are to understand illness, we must be able to describe it reliably enough to achieve a degree of homogeneity in a study population and perhaps in that way discover a common cause of a pattern of illness or dysfunction. Communication, research, and treatment are 3 important reasons why phenomenologic descriptions and classification into specific disorders are important even without a full understanding of underlying causes and pathophysiologic mechanisms.

Diagnosis involves 3 processes that will be discussed in turn in the following sections. The diagnostician begins by organizing a set of **symptoms and signs** elicited from the history and from the physical and mental status examinations. These observations are then grouped into **syndromes.** Further specification produces diagnoses of **mental disorders.** Mental disorders are characterized by deviations from a socially defined norm in thoughts, perceptions, mood, and behavior that impair social functioning. As noted above, psychopathology is the study of these deviations, the symptoms and signs of mental disorders, and their etiology and pathogenesis.

Symptoms are subjective complaints; signs are objective evidence of a pathologic state. A symptom could be a headache, a fear, or a report of auditory hallucinations; a sign may be nystagmus, tachycardia, or loosening of associations. Symptoms frequently occur in characteristic clusters called syndromes. A syndrome is a set of symptoms and signs that occur together in a recognizable pattern.

A disorder is more specific than a syndrome. A disorder is also a set of symptoms and signs but with a specified course of the illness, premorbid history, and pattern of familial occurrence. It is assumed that every disorder has a specific pathogenesis, although the pathogenesis may be unclear. The same syndrome can occur in many different disorders or diseases. In psychiatry, the term "disorder" is occasionally distinguished from "disease." A disease is even more specific than a disorder in that a known cause *and* a specific pathogenesis are implied.

The goal of medicine is to understand pathologic processes so they can be prevented or treated effectively. Most medical treatment is symptomatic or syndromic in nature. We would prefer to base all treatment on an etiologic diagnosis, as we do with antibiotic drugs or vitamin therapy for specific infectious diseases or vitamin deficiencies, but in most cases we treat symptoms (pain), signs (fever, inflammation), or syndromes (congestive heart failure, hypercortisolism [Cushing's syndrome], dementia, depression). Therapy differs with the level of diagnostic specificity. For example, fever can be treated with aspirin, but it is important to know whether the fever is part of a syndrome along with productive cough that might respond to antibiotic therapy, in contrast to a syndrome of fever, joint pain, and rash, which might suggest a different therapy.

A syndrome consisting of fever and productive cough, without more, might represent a bacterial or fungal disorder. Further historical details, physical examination, x-ray studies, and laboratory procedures will help make the distinction. If the sputum cultures grow *Streptococcus pneumoniae* and the chest x-ray shows a patchy density in the right lower lobe, we can make the diagnosis of a specific disease: pneumococcal pneumonia. For the patient with this diagnosis, specific antibiotic treatment is indicated.

In psychiatric disorders the pathologic features are rarely shown on x-ray films. No bacillus or enzymatic defect has been shown to cause schizophrenia or bipolar affective disorder. For this reason, we rarely speak of **diseases** with known causes and pathophysiologic mechanisms. Instead, we speak of **disorders** we think represent particular underlying but as yet unknown disease processes. In some cases, the disorders are little more than **syndromes**—clusters of observable symptoms and signs.

The third edition of *Diagnostic and Statistical Manual of Mental Disorders (DSM-III)* together with its revision *(DSM-III-R)*, now the standard diagnostic text in psychiatry, attempts to formalize the nomenclature by organizing psychopathology into a series of disorders (see Chapter 23 for details). In most instances, *DSM-III* makes no assumptions about the causes or the pathophysiologic mechanism underlying the disorders. It recognizes limitations to our understanding of psychopathology. *DSM-III* defines disorders by means of **inclusion and exclusion criteria.** The criteria consist chiefly of the clinical manifestations (symptoms and signs) along with a statement about duration of the pathologic state, the course of illness, the premorbid history, impairment of function, and whether the patient meets the criteria for a different disorder. Defining disorders by inclusion and exclusion criteria is a process of phenomenologic description.

Diagnostic Criteria

The diagnostic criteria for psychiatric disorders are organized into a standardized format and nosology in *DSM-III*. The standard format includes the cardinal features, associated features, and exclusionary criteria. The depression of Conrad Jarrett, the protagonist in *Ordinary People,* can be used to illustrate the use of *DSM-III-R*.

The diagnostic criteria for major depressive episode are listed below:

A. "At least five of the following symptoms have been present during the same two-week period and represent a change from previous functioning; at least one of the symptoms is either (1) depressed mood, or (2) loss of interest or pleasure. (Do not include symptoms that are clearly due to a physical condition, mood-incongruent delusions or hallucinations, incoherence, or marked loosening of associations.) (1) Depressed mood (or can be irritable mood in children and adolescents) most of the day, nearly every day, as indicated either by subjective account or observation by others. (2) Markedly diminished interest or pleasure in all, or almost all, activities most of the day, nearly every day (as indicated either by subjective account or observation by others of apathy most of the time). (3) Significant weight loss or weight gain when not dieting (eg, more than 5% of body weight in a month), or decrease or increase in appetite nearly every day (in children, consider failure to make expected weight gains). (4) Insomnia or hypersomnia nearly every day. (5) Psychomotor agitation or retardation nearly every day (observable by others, not merely subjective feelings of restlessness or being slowed down). (6) Fatigue or loss of energy nearly every day. (7) Feelings of worthlessness or excessive or inappropriate guilt (which may be delusional) nearly every day (not merely self-reproach or guilt about being sick). (8) Diminished ability to think or concentrate, or indecisiveness, nearly every day (either by subjective account or as observed by others). (9) Recurrent thoughts about death (not just fear of dying), recurrent suicidal ideation without a specific plan, or a suicide attempt or a specific plan for committing suicide.

B. "(1) It cannot be established that an organic factor initiated and maintained the disturbance. (2) The disturbance is not a normal reaction to the death of a loved one (uncomplicated bereavement). *Note:* Morbid preoccupation with worthlessness, suicidal ideation, marked functional impairment or psychomotor retardation, or prolonged duration suggest bereavement complicated by Major Depression.

C. "At no time during the disturbance have there been delusions or hallucinations for as long as two weeks in the absence of prominent mood symptoms (i.e., before the mood symptoms developed or after they have remitted).

D. "Not superimposed on Schizophrenia, Schizophreniform Disorder, Delusional Disorder, or Psychotic Disorder not otherwise specified."

Conrad Jarrett meets the criteria for major depressive episode by virtue of an extended period of depressed mood (more than 6 months after the death of his brother), associated with anorexia, insomnia, social withdrawal, and loss of interest in all activities (anhedonia). He awakened from sleep terrified by dreams of the boating accident, unable to go back to sleep. His primary problem, leading to hospitalization, was a suicide attempt, presumed to be secondary to feelings of despair, hopelessness, and guilt. He was otherwise healthy and had no other history of emotional disturbance.

Multiaxial Diagnosis

According to *DSM-III-R,* Conrad suffered a major depressive episode. This diagnosis is considered an axis I disorder. Axis I is used to record the majority of disorders we will consider in this book. However, our current approach to diagnosis is multiaxial, made up of 5 axes or dimensions:

Axis I	Principal mental disorders.
Axis II	Personality disorders (adults) or developmental disorders (children).
Axis III	Physical disorders relevant to patient management.
Axis IV	Severity of psychosocial stressors within past year (rating of 0–7).
Axis V	Global assessment of functioning (rating of 1–9).

As noted, axis I is reserved for all mental disorders other than personality disorders or developmental disorders, which are recorded on axis II. The axis II disorders are considered predisposing conditions for certain axis I disorders—or even for nonpsychiatric disorders. For example, dependent and obsessive compulsive personalities seem to be at greater risk for depression. Perhaps a more careful examination of Conrad Jarrett's personality might reveal evidence of compulsive traits. In addition, certain personality styles are thought to predispose to physical illness as well.

Physical disorders, recorded on axis III, may complicate the course of mental disorders, precipitating an acute decompensation reaction, exacerbating symptoms, and interfering with specific kinds of treatment. In *Ordinary People,* we are given no information about physical disorders. Conrad might have been a diabetic. If his diabetes had been out of control, he might have felt more depressed. Increased feelings of depression might have caused him to ignore his personal care, thus interfering with control of his diabetes. In later life, his diabetes might have led to heart disease, making it more difficult to treat future depressive episodes with tricyclic antidepressants.

Clearly, a psychosocial stressor, the accidental death of his brother, figured prominently in the pathogenesis of Conrad's major depressive episode. This kind of stressful life event would be rated as severe ("6"), or perhaps even catastrophic ("7") because of the circumstances of the accident. Although we are given limited information in *Ordinary People,* Conrad probably had functioned at a very good ("8") or good ("7") level in the year preceding the depressive episode. Apparently, he was reasonably well adjusted, performing adequately in school and with friends. It is not made clear in the movie, but his relationships with his brother and mother seem not to have been strong and supportive.

These multiple axes help us to understand and describe many aspects of our patients. In addition to providing a multidimensional description of patients, a multiaxial approach to diagnosis offers practical advantages. Each axis represents a different perspective on treatment: A specific psychotropic medication or psychotherapeutic technique may be chosen on the basis of axis I. Axis II tells us what to expect from a patient in response to the stress of illness. It also suggests the risk of further illness. (See discussion of personality styles in medical management in Chapter 36.) Physical disorders (axis III) may complicate treatment. Identifying psychosocial stressors (axis IV) suggests interventions designed to ease environmental stress or improve coping mechanisms. Stressful life events that cannot be changed may become the focus of psychotherapy. Information on the previous level of adaptation tells the health care provider what to expect from a patient. Axis V tells us about the patient's "baseline," or "premorbid," functioning. A patient with very good premorbid functioning may be expected to resume good functioning following treatment. The prognosis is usually less hopeful for a patient with poor premorbid functioning.

In this book, we will focus primarily on axis I and axis II disorders. In general, we do not discuss details of patient assessment on axes III–V. Chapter 41 (Mental Disorders of Childhood and Adolescence) does use the multiaxial approach to diagnosis to illustrate its application. Mastery of multiaxial diagnosis takes considerable practice and experience. *DSM-III* and *DSM-III-R* are discussed in more detail in Chapter 23. A glossary of terms describing the signs and symptoms of mental disorders is provided as an appendix to this text. The student should review the material in the glossary before proceeding with the remainder of the text.

REFERENCES

Campbell RJ: *Psychiatric Dictionary,* 5th ed. Oxford Univ Press, 1981.

Diagnostic and Statistical Manual of Mental Disorders (DSM-III), 3rd ed. American Psychiatric Association, 1980.

Diagnostic and Statistical Manual of Mental Disorders (DSM-III-R), 3rd ed, revised. American Psychiatric Association, 1987.

Engel G: The need for a new medical model: A challenge for biomedicine. *Science* 1977;**196:**129.

Goldman HH: Nonunitary disease hypotheses. *Schizophrenia Bull* (Jan) 1977;**3:**3.

Guest J: *Ordinary People.* Viking, 1976.

Holmes OW Sr: *Medical Essays.* Houghton Mifflin, 1895.

Kaplan HI, Freedman AM, Sadock BJ (editors): *Comprehensive Textbook of Psychiatry/IV,* 4th ed. Williams & Wilkins, 1985.

Kolb LC, Brodie HKH: *Modern Clinical Psychiatry,* 10th ed. Saunders, 1982.

Schneider K: Primäre und sekundäre Symptome bei Schizophrenie. *Fortschr Neurol Psychiatr* 1957;**25:**457.

Smyth FS: The place of the humanities and social sciences in the education of physicians. *J Med Educ* 1962;**37:**495.

Spitzer RL, Skodol AE, Gibbon M: *Psychopathology: A Case Book.* McGraw-Hill, 1983.

Psychiatric Epidemiology & Mental Health Services Research

13

Howard H. Goldman, MD, PhD

Acronyms Used in This Chapter

CMHC	Community mental health center
DIS	Diagnostic Interview Schedule
ECA	Epidemiologic Catchment Area
FTE	Full-time equivalents of employees
GHQ	General Health Questionnaire
NIMH	National Institute of Mental Health
RDC	Research Diagnostic Criteria
SADS	Schedule for Affective Disorders and Schizophrenia
SADS-C	SADS-current disorders
SADS-L	SADS-lifetime disorders
SCID	Structured Clinical Interview for *DSM-III*
VA	Veterans Administration

The role of the psychiatric epidemiologist is to gather data on the frequency and distribution of mental disorders in the population and determine patterns of occurrence with respect to age, sex, race, geographic location, socioeconomic status, life-style, diet, health status, and other factors affecting the presence and severity—or the absence—of mental disorders. These data provide clues to the etiology and pathogenesis of mental illness, help identify individuals at increased risk for specific disorders, and aid in assessing the needs of the population for mental health services.

Mental health services investigators add to this epidemiologic data base the information on distribution of health care providers (various treatment and support facilities, agencies, etc); patterns and trends of services used; costs of care; and projections of services needed in the future. They also evaluate the processes and outcomes of patient care.

Psychiatric epidemiology and mental health services research are multidisciplinary fields, involving physicians, demographers, statisticians, economists, sociologists, psychologists, and anthropologists in the attempt to devise improved methods of identifying and caring for the mentally ill.

DEFINITIONS

Measurements of Frequency & Risk

Frequency is measured in terms of **incidence** (number of new cases) or **prevalence** (number of existing cases) and is calculated as follows:

$$\text{Incidence rate} = \frac{\text{Number of persons developing a disease}}{\text{Total number at risk}} = \text{Per unit of time}$$

$$\text{Point prevalence} = \frac{\text{Number of persons with a disease at a certain point in time}}{\text{Total number in group}}$$

$$\text{Period prevalence} = \frac{\text{Number of persons with a disease during a period time}}{\text{Total number in group}}$$

As shown above, incidence is a measure of **risk** (ie, the probability or chance of a particular illness or injury occurring). **Individual risk** is generally considered to be equal to the incidence rate; eg, if the incidence of a disorder is 5000/100,000 people per year (annual incidence), the individual risk is considered to be 5% per year. The **population at risk** for an illness is in part defined by the nature of the illness. For a broad category such as physical or mental illness, the only individuals excluded from risk are those already ill. However, risk may be **factor-specific** (eg, functional vaginismus is sex-specific; sudden infant death syndrome is age-specific; occupational injuries are exposure-specific, ie, occur only in those exposed to the workplace environment), or it may be **factor-related** (eg, the risk of dementia is near zero before 60 years of age and rises to 3% at age 70 and 17% at age 80).

Data on the distribution of a specific illness in the population provide the basis for determining what factors (eg, age, sex, exposure to certain agents) constitute **risk factors,** ie, factors that increase the probability or chance of the particular illness or injury. Relative risk and attributable risk are both measures of *how much* risk is associated with a specific factor. **Relative risk** is expressed as the ratio of the incidence in one group to the incidence in another (eg, 12,000/100,000 versus 3000/100,000 = relative risk of 4:1). The difference in incidence (ie, 9000/100,000, or 9%, in this example) is considered the **attributable risk.** Obviously, the nature of the factor and the nature of the groups being compared must be taken into account in determining relative risk and how much risk can be attributed to a specific factor. For example, some groups are better-defined (male/female, exposed/unexposed), while some are less well defined (races are mixed; age groups and geographic breakdowns are arbitrarily chosen); the relationship of cause and effect for factor and disease may be direct, indirect, or unknown; and in cases of exposure, the degree, number, and timing of exposures must be considered, etc. In some cases, even though a specific factor is known to increase the risk, the amount of increased risk cannot be quantified.

As shown in the formulas for calculating prevalence, **point prevalence** is a measure of the number of existing cases at a specific point in time. The "point" may be in calendar time (eg, first day of the year; midpoint of the period of study), or it may be defined by a specific event (eg, at the time of examination or survey of the subjects studied; on the third day of treatment).

Period prevalence is the number of existing cases during a defined period of time. For **annual prevalence** (an example of period prevalence), the numerator of the formula may be calculated as follows: point prevalence on the first day of the year plus annual incidence (new cases during the year). **Lifetime prevalence** (also a form of period prevalence) reflects the number of individuals affected by a disorder at some time during their lives.

Depending on the nature and duration of the disorder being studied, prevalence figures may have to be adjusted to take into account the number of individuals who have died or recovered spontaneously or through treatment. Thus, for an acute disorder whose average duration is 6 months and whose annual incidence is 5%, the rate (5% per year) would be multiplied by the duration (½ year), yielding a point prevalence of 2.5%.

Some general conclusions can be drawn regarding incidence and prevalence: Prevalence rates for chronic disorders are often greater than incidence rates; for acute disorders, the reverse is usually true. Effective treatment of a disorder will not affect incidence (since it is a measurement of new cases only) but will affect prevalence (since cured cases no longer "exist"). Prevention will affect both incidence and prevalence.

True incidence and prevalence reflect the numbers of people who have a disorder, whether or not they are being treated for the disorder. **Treated incidence and prevalence** reflect only the numbers of people receiving treatment in specified settings.

Mental health services researchers analyze the following statistics to calculate treated incidence and prevalence in inpatient facilities: the **resident census,** number of inpatients on a specific day; number of **admissions,** new patients; **readmissions,** patients returning for treatment of a new bout of illness; **additions,** admissions plus readmissions; **discharges,** patients with authorization to leave the facility; and **terminations,** patients who died or discontinued involvement with the facility.

In outpatient facilities, patients are classified as new, continuing, or terminated, and statistics are recorded in the **caseload,** a census reflecting the number of patients in continuing treatment ("on the books").

Treated point prevalence, the resident census or caseload, is the number of patients on a specific day.

Treated period prevalence is usually measured in terms of **episodes of care** rather than numbers of patients. For example, annual episodes of inpatient care is the sum of the resident census (point prevalence) and annual additions (period incidence). Community surveys, however, may provide data on the proportion of individuals with mental disorders who were "under care" (ie, treated prevalence) in the past year.

The volume of services may be calculated in terms of the number of **outpatient visits** or **inpatient days.** The service capacity may be measured on the basis of **FTEs** (full-time equivalents of employees; 2 half-times equal one full-time), **examining room capacity** (outpatients), or **bed capacity** (inpatients).

Some estimates on utilization of health care in a system of facilities do not take into account whether a patient has been treated in one facility several times or has been treated in several different facilities (eg, hospital emergency room, alcohol residential treatment center, and alcohol outpatient clinic) during the period of the study; these estimates are termed **duplicated counts.** In contrast, **unduplicated counts** identify each individual in treatment in the system, assuring that each person is counted only one time.

Assessment of Diagnostic Accuracy

The **reliability** of a process or instrument of measurement is the extent to which it yields reproducible results (see Chapter 21 for details). In psychiatric epidemiology, identification of cases of mental illness (by recognition of signs, symptoms, or traits) is reliable if the process is consistent (ie, with agreement among epidemiologists in a specific case) and is repeatable (ie, with agreement on successive occasions).

A process or instrument of measurement has **validity** if it measures what is intended to be measured. Reliability is a prerequisite for validity. **Bias,** a systematic error encouraging one outcome or answer over others, may be introduced into epidemiologic assessments if the process or instrument of assessment lacks content validity, predictive validity, or construct validity (see Chapter 21) or if the results are inaccurately interpreted.

The value of a diagnostic test is related to its sensitivity and specificity. A test has **sensitivity** if it accurately detects the *presence* of a disorder in individuals who *have* the disorder; it has **specificity** if it accurately detects the *absence* of a disorder in individuals who *do not have* the disorder. The results of a given test may be **true-positive** (disease present and results positive), **false-positive** (disease absent and results positive), **true-negative** (disease absent and results negative), or **false-negative** (disease present and results negative).

Sensitivity and specificity are reported as percentages, calculated as follows:

$$\text{Sensitivity} = \frac{\text{True-positive}}{\text{True-positive} + \text{false-negative}} \times 100$$

$$\text{Specificity} = \frac{\text{True-negative}}{\text{True-negative} + \text{false-positive}} \times 100$$

The **predictive value** of a diagnostic test is also expressed as a percentage, with the percentage reflecting how often the test outcome is expected to agree with the actual diagnosis. Predictive value is calculated as follows:

Positive predictive value =
$$\frac{\text{True-positive}}{\text{True-positive + false-positive}} \times 100$$

Negative predictive value =
$$\frac{\text{True-negative}}{\text{True-negative + false-negative}} \times 100$$

PSYCHIATRIC EPIDEMIOLOGY

The discussion of psychiatric epidemiology in this chapter* focuses on the question, How many people in any defined population (but the United States population in particular) have a mental disorder? The methods and findings are shaped by prevailing **theories of psychopathology.** As described in Chapter 12, **unitary theories** hold that all mental illness is derived from a single process, whereas **nonunitary theories** hold that mental illness comprises a heterogeneous group of distinct mental disorders that result from various processes. Proponents of a unitary theory of psychopathology identify cases of mental illness on the basis of the presence or absence of a wide variety of nonspecific symptoms and signs indicative of mental illness (eg, hallucinations, recurring headaches, palpitations, depressed mood, sleep disturbances). Differences in the severity, number, or pattern of occurrence of these symptoms and signs are usually viewed as variations in the expression of a single disease process (eg, inadequate psychosocial development or adaptation, social stress, neurotransmitter deficiency). In contrast, proponents of a nonunitary theory focus on identifying cases of specific mental disorders, each of which is presumed to have a different cause or causes and each of which is defined by a different set of diagnostic criteria (specific symptoms, signs, and natural history).

Because of the breadth of the definition of mental illness in prevailing unitary theories of psychopathology, epidemiologic studies conducted according to a unitary theory find a higher rate of mental illness than do studies conducted on the basis of a nonunitary theory (25% versus 10–16%). These findings are discussed in more detail below.

---

*The *DSM-III-R* classification of mental disorders is discussed in detail in Chapter 23, and epidemiologic findings for specific mental disorders are reviewed in Chapters 24–41. Social and cultural factors influencing the epidemiology of mental disorders are described in Chapters 14 and 15.

HISTORY OF PSYCHIATRIC EPIDEMIOLOGY IN THE USA & CANADA

The earliest epidemiologic data on mental illness were treated prevalence statistics. Superintendents of mental asylums counted and recorded descriptions of admitted and discharged patients and speculated on the relationships between their disorders and their sex, age, race, country of birth, moral upbringing, alcohol use, and social class. In the 19th century, asylum superintendents examined patterns of occurrence and discovered that many patients were from areas close to an asylum, which led to the recognition that the true prevalence of mental illness was higher than their data (treated prevalence) suggested. By 1850, they had succeeded in increasing the number of asylums, treating more patients, improving the methods of documenting cases, and developing a census of the institutionalized mentally ill and mentally retarded; however, methods were not yet developed to study the true prevalence of mental illness.

During World Wars I and II, statistics were compiled in the USA on young men rejected for military service, servicemen receiving medical discharges, and war casualties. These statistics, which provided the basis for analysis of both the physical and mental status of this defined population, revealed that a large number of men were disqualified for military service because of mental illness or retardation, and nearly one-third of all medical casualties in World War II were due to "combat fatigue," "war neurosis," and other neuropsychiatric disorders.

Between the wars, the mental hygiene movement sponsored several efforts to assess the nature and scope of mental illness in the USA. Malzberg in New York, Faris and Dunham in Chicago, and Hollingshead and Redlich in New Haven began to look at the correlates of mental illness (eg, criminality, race, ethnic background, and social class), and the modern era of psychiatric epidemiology was initiated (see also Chapters 14 and 15).

Post-World War II epidemiologists focused their attention on studies of the true prevalence of mental illness. Many investigators followed the dominant unitary theories of psychopathology, influenced strongly by psychoanalytic thinking. The diagnostic nomenclature of this era lacked specificity and reliability. The pioneers in these efforts were Srole, Rennie, and Langner in the USA and the Leightons in rural Canada.

In the 1950s in Baltimore, Pasamanick and his colleagues adopted a nonunitary (disorder-specific) approach to studying the true prevalence of mental illness. This approach gained momentum with the increase in biomedical knowledge of mental disorders and the development of more specific and effective treatments for psychiatric states and syndromes (eg, psychosis and depression) and specific disorders (eg, lithium-sensitive bipolar affective disorder). Since the late 1960s, psychiatric epidemiology has moved in the direction of the disorder-specific approach, and advances in research methods have facilitated efforts to determine rates of specific mental disorders. Recently, the National Institute of Mental Health (NIMH) published data from the Epidemiologic Catchment Area (ECA) program designed to study the incidence and prevalence of more than 20 mental disorders in 5 communities in the USA (Table 13–1).

EPIDEMIOLOGIC FINDINGS

The earliest studies of the true prevalence of mental illness in the general population found lifetime and point prevalence rates ranging from 18 to 24%. When nonspecific symptoms related to mental disorders were assessed, much higher rates were discovered.

The first important United States community survey based on a disorder-specific approach was conducted in Baltimore in 1954 by Pasamanick and his associates (1956). They found a 10% point prevalence rate of specifiable mental disorders (defined according to the World Health Organization's International Classification of Disease). In a New Haven, Connecticut, survey that was originally done in 1967 and updated in 1975, Weissman and her colleagues (1978) reported a point prevalence rate of approximately 16% in the population over age 19.

The Monroe County (New York) case register—a detailed record of all individuals in treatment in all medical and mental health settings (including private office practice) in the county surrounding Rochester, New York—provides a valuable data base for many epidemiologic studies. On the basis of this source of unduplicated counts of mentally disabled patients, the annual incidence rate of mental illness in the USA is estimated to be 5%.

In 1978, Regier and his associates at NIMH reviewed the epidemiology of mental illness in the USA for the President's Commission on Mental Health. Favoring the disorder-specific approach, they synthesized the findings of many studies and concluded that the point prevalence rate of all "diagnosable" (ie, specific) mental disorders in the USA was 10% and that the annual incidence rate was 5%, yielding an annual prevalence rate of 15%. The more recent NIMH-ECA survey found 6-month prevalence rates of approximately 19%, indicating earlier estimates were conservative.

EPIDEMIOLOGIC RESEARCH METHODS

Epidemiologic findings are determined by the criteria and methods used to define and identify cases of mental illness.

Table 13–1. Six-month prevalence of DIS/*DSM-III* disorders for estimated number and percent of US civilian population, based on 1980 US census and three ECA sites.*†

Disorder	Estimated US Population (Aged 18 or Older)	
	Number (in millions)	Percent
Any DIS disorder	29.4	18.7
Any DIS disorder except phobia	22.6	14.4
Any DIS disorder except substance abuse	22.1	14.0
Substance abuse disorders	10.0	6.4
Alcohol abuse/dependence	7.9	5.0
Alcohol abuse	7.2	4.6
Alcohol dependence	4.6	2.9
Drug abuse/dependence	3.1	2.0
Drug abuse	2.1	1.3
Drug dependence	1.7	1.1
Schizophrenic/schizophreniform	1.5	1.0
Schizophrenia	1.4	0.9
Schizophreniform	0.1	0.1
Affective disorders	9.4	6.0
Manic episode	1.0	0.7
Major depressive episode	4.9	3.1
Dysthymia	5.1	3.2
Anxiety/somatoform disorders	13.1	8.3
Phobia	11.1	7.0
Panic	1.2	0.8
Obsessive compulsive	2.4	1.5
Somatization	0.1	0.1
Antisocial personality	1.4	0.9
Cognitive impairment (severe)	1.6	1.0

*Source: Taube CA, Barrett S (editors): *Mental Health, United States-1985.* Alcohol, Drug Abuse, and Mental Health Administration, US Department of Health and Human Services, 1985.
†The 3 ECA sites were not chosen to be a representative sample of the USA, so the study results cannot be used to estimate precisely the number of Americans afflicted. However, by projecting the data and standardizing the rates to the 1980 census on the basis of age, sex, and race, an approach is provided for those who wish to make projections to the total population.

Criteria

Psychiatric research was limited by the low reliability of diagnostic procedures, due largely to the lack of formal inclusion or exclusion criteria. To correct this problem, Feighner and his colleagues (1972) proposed a set of criteria outlining symptoms and signs for specific mental disorders. Building on this work, Spitzer and coworkers (1978) added criteria regarding the severity, duration, and course of specific disorders, with all terms defined operationally for more than 20 diagnoses. Their criteria, called the Research Diagnostic Criteria (RDC), were found to have diagnostic reliability between raters on concurrent assessments (reliability of 0.75–1.00, indicating significant agreement) and when used in succession by 2 raters. The RDC influenced the development of the *DSM-III* criteria in current wide-scale use (see Chapter 23).

Survey Methods

In community studies, some information is gathered from the population through survey, while other data are extrapolated from existing sources (census data, hospital records, etc). Contacting subjects by mail or telephone ("self-report" questionnaire) is an **indirect method** of survey. **Direct methods,** which typically involve the subject in face-to-face interview with a trained professional, may be **structured** (prescribed format followed for all subjects) or **unstructured** (format varies as judged appropriate by the professional). While unstructured interviews are usually conducted by clinicians who can make clinical judgments about the presence or absence of mental illness, structured interviews may be conducted by either clinicians or nonclinicians trained as interviewers. Nonclinicians can only be trained to make a limited number of clinical observations; on the other hand, interviews conducted by clinicians are more expensive and thus are usually reserved for studies in which clinical judgment is essential.

Survey Instruments

Several of the better known diagnostic instruments, representing different approaches to case identification, are discussed below.

The **General Health Questionnaire (GHQ)** is a 60-item self-report diagnostic screening instrument developed by Goldberg (1972) to detect psychiatric illness in community settings, particularly among medical outpatients in primary care. (Briefer, 28- and 30-item versions have also been developed.) It is focused on psychologic components of illness, ie, symptoms and signs suggestive of emotional disorder, especially anxiety and depression. For example, the GHQ asks, "Have you recently been getting a feeling of tightness or pressure in your head?" or " . . . felt that life is hopeless?" The respondent selects one of the following response categories: "Not at all," "No more than usual," "Rather more than usual," "Much more than usual." The first 2 responses are scored as "negative"; the latter 2 are "positive."

As a screening instrument, the GHQ does not identify specific mental disorders. Instead, it searches for common symptoms and signs of emotional distress found in most individuals with mental illness and not commonly reported by emotionally well people. It attempts to distinguish between "cases" and "normals"; although there is no sharp dividing line, the probability is great that an individual who exceeds the "case threshold" (ie, scores positive on 11 or 12 of the 60 items) has a mental disorder. In this sense, the GHQ is a nonspecific diagnostic measure compatible with a unitary theory of psychopathology—similar to the Cornell Medical Index used in the Midtown Manhattan study.

The GHQ is brief and easy to administer and has proved understandable and generally acceptable to patients. It is objective, reliable, sensitive (0.91), and specific (0.95). It is useful for screening primary-care populations for patients undergoing emotional distress. Research has shown that patients identified by the GHQ as emotionally distressed and subsequently treated have improved markedly.

The **Schedule for Affective Disorders and Schizophrenia (SADS)** is a clinician-administered diagnostic interview schedule designed by Spitzer and Endicott (1979) to identify patients in over 20 RDC diagnostic categories. The exact number of RDC categories varies with the 3 versions of the SADS: current disorders (SADS-C), lifetime disorders (SADS-L), and combined SADS. The interview schedule covers over 200 items and takes 1½–2 hours to complete. The interview is structured, but clinical judgments are required. The SADS not only identifies the features of various diagnostic categories but also assesses the severity of illness in 8 summary scales of psychopathology (eg, depressed mood and ideation, anxiety, delusions-hallucinations). It may be used in case identification for present or past illnesses and in evaluating clinical change when used at 2 points in time. The SADS is reliable and valid (when compared with other measures of mental disorder) and is in widespread use in research employing RDC diagnoses. Because it requires a lengthy complex interview by an experienced clinician, the SADS is expensive and is thus practical to use only when RDC precision is demanded.

The **Diagnostic Interview Schedule (DIS)** was developed by Robins and her coworkers (1981) in cooperation with the NIMH for use in its ECA surveys in 5 population areas in the USA. It is a nonclinician-administered interview schedule developed to make nearly 30 diagnoses according to *DSM-III* and Feighner criteria as well as RDC criteria. The DIS also expands the list of SADS diagnoses, although it is less sensitive in identifying schizophrenia in acutely disturbed paranoid patients. It is not designed for use in assessing changes in the severity of symptoms and signs. Like the SADS, it provides current and lifetime diagnoses, relies on complex questions with branching logic, and takes a long time to complete. Using nonclinician interviewers narrows the range of clinical judgments that can be made and thus limits its value in identifying serious illness in suspicious or uncooperative patients with severe disorders such as schizophrenia. Nonclinicians, however, are not as expensive to train and use as interviewers and can be equally well trained to use the DIS reliably. As a result, the DIS is the best available instrument for large-scale disorder-specific community surveys. Examples of DIS questions and assessments are presented in Fig 13–1.

Although most diagnostic interview schedules are used for research or clinical screening, they may be used in some routine clinical practice and in clinical training as well. Simple standardized interviews can become a regular part of evaluation of patients, or they can be used for teaching diagnostic interviewing to students and clinical trainees. The **Structured Clinical Interview for** *DSM-III* **(SCID),** developed by Spitzer and Williams (1983) under contract with the NIMH, is being used in this way.

After inquiring about any periods of depressed mood lasting 2 weeks or longer and discovering that during at least one period the person had not been physically ill and had not been taking any medicines, street drugs, or alcohol (that might have accounted for the depressed mood), the interviewer says, "I am going to ask about other problems that you might have had during any period of being depressed or having no interest in things." The interviewer then asks 16 questions grouped into the 8 categories related to the diagnostic criteria for major depressive episode (see Chapters 12 and 30), including the 5 questions listed below:

	I Worst Period	II Ever in Lifetime	
Have you ever had a period of a week or more when you had (Did you have) trouble falling asleep, (PAUSE) staying asleep, (PAUSE) or waking up too early? STOP AFTER FIRST "YES"	1 345 _____	1 345 _____	S L E E P
Have you ever had a period of a week or longer when you were (Were you) sleeping too much?	1 345 _____	1 345 _____	
Has there ever been a period lasting a week or more when you felt (Did you feel) tired out all the time?	1 345 _____	1 345 _____	T I R E D
Has there ever been a period of a week or more when you talked or moved (Did you talk or move) more slowly than is normal for you?	1 345 _____	1 345 _____	S L O W
Has there ever been a period of a week or more when you felt (Did you feel that) you had to be moving all the time—that you couldn't sit still and paced up and down?	1 345 _____	1 345 _____	R E S T L E S S

If the person being interviewed has been using drugs or alcohol or has been physically ill during any period of depressed mood, the examiner must inquire about the association of substance use or illness with the symptoms and signs in each question. If the person describes symptoms or signs (unassociated with substance use or illness) in at least 4 of the 8 categories, the examiner asks the person about the "worst spell of depression . . . when you had these symptoms all together. . . ." Each question is asked again to determine if symptoms and signs in at least 4 of the 8 categories occurred together during the worst period of depressed mood lasting 2 weeks or longer. If so, the person meets the diagnostic criteria for major depressive episode. Further questioning determines current status, in addition to lifetime history of major depressive episodes.

Figure 13–1. Use of the Diagnostic Interview Schedule (DIS), questions on major depressive disorder. The 2 sets of numbers to the right of each question are for coding responses, one for occurrence during the "worst period" and the other for occurrence "ever in lifetime." 1 = no; 3 = yes, but associated with drug or alcohol use; 4 = yes, but associated with a physical illness; 5 = yes.

SPECIAL AREAS OF EPIDEMIOLOGIC RESEARCH

The clinical goal of psychiatric epidemiology is better treatment or prevention of mental disorders. Epidemiologic data can identify the risk factors contributing to illness or even the pathogenesis and causes of specific mental disorders. The search for social and cultural causes and risk factors in mental illness has involved sociologists and anthropologists in the study of psychiatric epidemiology. Social class, social stress, cultural conflict, migration, racism, sexism, ageism, and unemployment all have been implicated by epidemiologic research in the pathogenesis of mental illness (see Chapters 14 and 15 for discussion). Genetic factors, too, have been considered in psychiatric epidemiology. Studies of monozygotic twins with family histories of mental disorder who are reared apart (see Chapter 27) and pedigree analysis of families and isolated communities with high rates of consanguinity have revealed clues to the hereditary component of several mental disorders. Epidemiologic investigation of dietary practices, toxic exposures, and contagion have all contributed to our ability to treat and prevent mental disorders (see below).

Epidemiology has helped shape the classification of mental disorders, especially through studies of the natural history of mental illness. Emil Kraepelin first distinguished the manic-depressive psychoses (bipolar affective disorder) from dementia praecox ("premature dementia" indicating schizophrenia) on the basis of serious mental disturbance. The manic-depressive disorders were marked by episodes of severe disturbance separated by intervals of relative health and return to premorbid (preillness) functioning. Dementia praecox was marked by a deteriorating course with episodes of severe illness but no return to premorbid functioning. Although Kraepelin's observations are basically correct, more recent longitudinal studies of schizophrenia have demonstrated that **continuing** deterioration is not an essential feature of the disorder even though there is rarely a return to premorbid status.

Accurate identification and classification of specific mental disorders have contributed to research on more specific treatments. Epidemiologists often assist clinical researchers in selecting homogeneous study populations for further investigation. Active research in epidemiology, joining neuroscientists, geneticists, and other biologic scientists with sociologists, anthropologists, and other behavioral scientists, holds promise for better understanding of the causes and pathogenesis of mental disorders.

PREVENTION & EPIDEMIOLOGY

Prevention of mental illness has been an important goal of epidemiologists in public health. Preventive psychiatry is characterized by 3 types of prevention (Caplan, 1964): **Primary prevention** reduces or elim-inates the incidence of symptoms and signs of mental disorders; it stops illness (morbidity and perhaps mortality) before it occurs. **Secondary prevention** reduces the prevalence of mental illness without directly altering its incidence by early treatment of acute cases, reducing the duration of illness and its associated morbidity and mortality. **Tertiary prevention** reduces the morbidity and mortality rates associated with mental disorders by rehabilitation; the incidence and prevalence of the disorders are not affected, although pain and suffering may be relieved. Effective prevention requires specifying the disorder or problem to be prevented, demonstrating risk factors, and identifying and evaluating proposed interventions. Psychiatric epidemiology provides the specific basis of preventive psychiatry, as illustrated in the following examples of each type of prevention.

Primary Prevention

Pellagra is a potentially fatal disorder characterized by dementia, diarrhea, and dermatitis. The dementia, occasionally associated with psychotic symptoms, may bring patients with pellagra to the attention of psychiatrists and mental hospital personnel. Before the cause of pellagra was identified, clinical epidemiologists noted the seasonal nature of the illness and its association with poverty. In the USA, pellagra was a serious problem in the southeastern states in the early 1900s, accounting for as many as 10% of admissions to mental hospitals and occurring in outbreaks in all types of institutions. In the early 1920s, Joseph Goldberger, a Public Health Service epidemiologist, showed that a dietary deficiency was associated with pellagra. In particular, Goldberger and his colleagues (1925) demonstrated that the typical diet of the poor farm worker—cornmeal, meat, and molasses—lacked a nutritional element contained in yeast and green vegetables that could prevent pellagra. Only later was nicotinic acid (niacin) identified as the specific dietary deficiency. An improved standard of living and diet, as well as vitamin enrichment of grain products, has led to the virtual elimination of pellagra in the USA; however, it remains a problem in South Africa, Egypt, and India among agricultural workers whose principal source of food is niacin-poor grain.

Primary prevention of organic mental disorders and mental retardation has benefited from epidemiologic data. Data on the association of maternal age and Down's syndrome contributed to an understanding of the cause of this form of mental retardation and provided one mechanism for primary prevention through parental counseling. Data on the association of retardation and behavior disorders in children and the use of lead paint in older housing prompted preventive measures affecting lead content in paint and in other sources of environmental exposure. Other examples of primary prevention in psychiatry include the prevention of measles encephalitis through vaccination and the prevention of problems in emotional development in hospitalized children by permitting parents to stay in the hospital with them.

Some investigators have expanded the concept of primary prevention to include **health promotion** through activities that improve the quality of life and prepare individuals in a general way for adapting to life stresses. In mental health, this area includes general education of parents; counseling in anticipation of death or separation in a family member to reduce pathologic grief; support groups for people and their families with specific medical problems (eg, mastectomies, colostomies, diabetes); support groups for widows; and all sorts of nonspecific support groups. **Mental health education** is sometimes regarded as a form of primary prevention in psychiatry. Critics argue that the problems being prevented are not well specified (if at all) and that the interventions are unproved; proponents point to the obvious benefits expected from such safe, inexpensive, and often enjoyable activities.

Secondary Prevention

Preventing the complications of tertiary neurosyphilis by early treatment of primary and secondary syphilis is an important example of secondary prevention in psychiatry. General paresis of the insane (the paranoid psychosis of neurosyphilis) was at one time a major reason for psychiatric hospitalization. Other examples include the early treatment of stress response syndromes (see Chapter 5) to potentially prevent chronic posttraumatic stress disorder, treating teenage alcoholism to prevent the complications of alcohol-related organic mental disorders, and treating childhood behavioral disorders in an attempt to prevent personality disorders later in life. In a sense, the early treatment of affective disorders (eg, mania and depression) reduces the prevalence of acute symptoms and signs of these disorders, although the incidence of these disorders is not actually affected. As such, the treatment is also a form of secondary prevention.

Tertiary Prevention

Rehabilitation is designed to reduce the severity of symptoms and possibly the number of deaths associated with illness and to restore function lost through disease. In psychiatry, rehabilitation is important in patients with chronic mental disorders (eg, dementia and schizophrenia). It has been shown that stressful life events exacerbate the course of schizophrenia, leading to acute relapses and accelerated decline in social functioning. Intervening with patients and their families (eg, with counseling or psychotherapy) following a stressful life event is both a form of secondary prevention of an acute relapse and tertiary prevention of further deterioration. In chronically institutionalized patients, the decline in social functioning associated with routinized behavior and neglect in some long-term residential settings (called "chronic social breakdown" or "institutionalism") can be reversed by active psychosocial rehabilitation in the form of stimulation, changes in routine, and activities therapy or, occasionally, by release to less restrictive residential settings (Gruenberg, 1980). This form of tertiary prevention so encouraged the field of institutional psychiatry that it stimulated dramatic changes in the delivery of mental health services.

MENTAL HEALTH SERVICES RESEARCH

The treated prevalence of mental illness is the domain of mental health services research. In the work done for the President's Commission on Mental Health, Regier and his coworkers (1978) not only estimated the annual prevalence of mental illness in the USA but also provided a map of the mental health services system, identifying 3 major sectors: (1) the **specialty mental health sector,** comprising all specialized mental health providers (eg, facilities, such as psychiatric hospitals and clinics; and professionals, such as psychiatrists in office practice); (2) the **general medical sector,** which includes the general hospital inpatient/nursing home sector and the primary-care/outpatient medical sector; and (3) the **not-in-treatment/other human services sector.** They estimated that of the 15% of the United States population with mental disorders, one-fifth of patients (3% of the total) were seen in the specialty mental health sector, three-fifths (9% of the total) in the general medical sector, and one-fifth (3% of the total) in other settings or not at all.

The distribution of individuals with mental disorders to treatment settings in the USA, based on NIMH data, is discussed in the following paragraphs.

(1) Three times as many individuals with mental disorders are seen by non-mental health professionals as by mental health professionals. Primary-care visits are shorter and also focus on somatic problems in the general medical sector. This is an important reason for all physicians to be familiar with psychiatric assessment and treatment approaches. Although the most seriously ill patients are referred to the specialty mental health sector, many patients are hesitant to go and will need diagnosis, treatment, and sensitively handled referral by practitioners in the general medical sector.

(2) Office-based private practice psychiatry and psychology, the stereotype of mental health care, accounted for treatment of fewer than 4% of patients with mental disorders, about 0.5% of the United States population, in 1975. Recent estimates indicate that overall use has more than tripled since that time, and psychologists now provide services to about the same number of patients as do private psychiatrists in office practice (Taube and coworkers, 1984).

(3) General hospitals treated nearly 900,000 people with mental disorders in general medical and surgical beds, in addition to almost 1 million mentally ill people who were treated in the beds of all general hospi-

tals *with* specialized psychiatric units. This sector continues to grow in use.

(4) Nursing homes cared for over 100,000 residents (of a total of approximately 1.3 million) with mental disorders (excluding senility or dementia). An additional 550,000 residents have dementia as a primary diagnosis or complicating other disabilities.

(5) Over 2.6 million people were treated in outpatient services in a variety of organized settings. Yet, in spite of the growth of ambulatory services, hospital services also continue to provide intensive care and treatment.

(6) Over 1.5 million people were treated in psychiatric inpatient settings (private and public) and in residential treatment centers (usually for children and adolescents).

MENTAL HEALTH SERVICES

Mental health services include inpatient (hospital), outpatient, partial or part-time hospital (day treatment), residential treatment (24-hour), emergency and crisis intervention, consultation/liaison, and social support services. These services are characterized and be further subcategorized below.

1. INPATIENT SERVICES

Psychiatric hospital care serves many functions unavailable to patients in outpatient settings, especially for seriously ill patients who need specialized diagnostic assessments (eg, close observation of behavior, special neurologic or endocrine tests), treatment (eg, rapid control of psychotic symptoms with parenteral medication, electroconvulsive therapy), and nursing services (eg, because of complex medication regimens or concomitant medical problems). Psychiatric patients also are admitted to hospitals for their own protection and for the protection of others—as in the cases of suicidal or homicidal patients or patients who are so grossly mentally disorganized, apathetic, or cognitively impaired that they cannot care for themselves. Such patients are observed closely, protected, restricted, and confined and usually are treated for a specific mental disorder underlying their self-destructive, neglectful, or otherwise dangerous behavior. In some cases, individuals accused of criminal activity are admitted to a hospital for forensic psychiatric evaluation of competence to stand trial or for assessment of criminal responsibility (see Chapter 58). Psychiatric hospitalization may also be used unnecessarily or inappropriately to provide a home for the homeless, an "asylum" for other dependent individuals, when alternative services (eg, halfway houses, nursing homes, board and care facilities) are not available or when alternative care (eg, intensive outpatient services or part-time hospital care) is not reimbursed by health insurance programs and is otherwise too expensive.

Hospital treatments include medication and other biomedical interventions (see Chapters 42 and 51–54), various psychotherapies (see Chapters 42–50), specialized services (see Chapters 57–60), and social interventions, including occupational, activity, and expressive therapies. All of these treatments and specialized interventions occur within the "healthful environment" or hospital "milieu." The therapeutic use of the hospital enviroment, dating to the original asylum concept, has been termed **milieu therapy.** Although milieu therapy and the "therapeutic community" it seeks to create have been shown to be especially effective for treating drug abusers (Jones, 1953), the benefits of these environmental interventions for all patients remain unproved yet widely accepted as face valid. The critique of long-term institutional care in general (discussed above and in Chapter 14) includes a critique of milieu therapy (Perrow, 1965) and, with it, most forms of psychiatric hospitalization.

Disadvantages of psychiatric hospitalization include the stigma of being a psychiatric patient, diminished self-esteem, and increased dependency and regressed behavior. In addition, psychiatric hospitalizations are expensive. Recent reviews of a variety of clinical trials of brief hospitalization and the use of alternative settings for care indicate that prolonged hospital care (longer than 2 or 3 months) is beneficial for only a small minority of patients, such as patients with schizophrenia who have a healthy premorbid social adjustment (Glick and Hargreaves, 1979; Kirshner, 1982). Although the evidence argues that "less is better," there is no evidence that "none is optimal." Brief hospitalization is essential for many disturbed psychiatric patients; prolonged hospital stays are currently unavoidable for thousands of others.

In 1982, there were approximately 1.9 million episodes of psychiatric inpatient care in the specialty mental health sector and an estimated 1 million or more episodes in the general medical sector. Although the vast majority of hospital stays are for less than 30 days, approximately 75,000–100,000 individuals are long-term residents (1 year or longer) of psychiatric hospitals. Patterns of care vary among the many different hospital facilities that deliver inpatient psychiatric care.

State and county mental hospitals, the descendants of the public asylums founded in the 19th century, have declined in use since 1955, yet they currently provide voluntary and involuntary short- and long-term inpatient care for more total inpatient days than any other type of facility in the specialty mental health sector. Almost 30% of all episodes of inpatient psychiatric care occur and 60% of all inpatient days are spent in these facilities, which serve the poorest and most disturbed of all psychiatric patients. Although the resident census fell to less than 120,000 by 1984, annual additions remained at about 330,000. Approximately 60% of patients in the resident census have been in the hospital for 1 year or longer; approximately 20% have been inpatients for between 90 and 364 days. The remaining 20% of inpatients on a given day are short-term, newly admitted patients. Although state and county hospitals provide the majority of long-term inpatient psychiatric care, of all the additions during the year, 80% are discharged in less than 90 days. Once dominating all psychiatric care, state and county mental hospitals now share the specialty mental health sector with other facilities whose importance has grown since World War II.

Private mental hospitals have experienced relatively stable use since the early 19th century, when they were opened as private asylums and retreats. Growth kept pace with population increases until very recently, when there was a 10% increase in their rate of use, linked probably to increases in insurance coverage for inpatient mental health services. Providing mostly voluntary short-term and some long-term care to paying or insured patients, private psychiatric hospitals have developed under not-for-profit (often university-affiliated) and for-profit management. Recent shifts toward for-profit management (especially by corporate hospital "chains") reflect financial incentives as well as pressures demanding cost-conscious hospital management in a time of increasing fiscal controls.

Psychiatric units in general hospitals, rare before World War II, have expanded their role rapidly, now providing almost exclusively short-term hospital care to voluntary and involuntary patients. Opened under both private nonprofit and public auspices, psychiatric units serve various categories of patients. The public sector units serve poorer, somewhat more disturbed patients, who often require involuntary commitment. In contrast, the private sector units serve insured patients who are typically voluntary and stay in the hospital for a few days longer than patients in public sector units (median: 12 versus 10 days). In some areas, very short stay patients, especially in public sector units, are transferred to state and county hospitals and other facilities.

Veterans Administration (VA) psychiatric inpatient services are provided in psychiatric units in VA general hospitals and in neuropsychiatric hospitals operated by the VA. They provide a mix of inpatient care for alcohol abuse, drug abuse, and general psychiatric problems to armed services veterans and some of their dependents.

Federally assisted CMHCs were created in the 1960s to organize inpatient, outpatient, consultation, and other mental health services into a single, multipurpose organization serving the population of a defined geographic area called a **catchment area.** In the USA, there are approximately 1500 catchment areas and 700 CMHCs. Some of them provide all of the mandated services under one roof; others via affiliated organizations at various locations. When fully federally funded, these CMHCs offered services to the public, regardless of ability to pay. As federal resources declined, CMHCs were forced to eliminate unprofitable services and shift to serving insured or more affluent patients. CMHCs succeeded in providing mental health services to many populations that had never before used mental health services.

2. OUTPATIENT SERVICES

Almost unknown in the 19th and early 20th century, ambulatory psychiatric services expanded dramatically since 1955, when they accounted for 23% of all episodes of psychiatric care. Owing to a 12-fold increase by 1977, more than 4.5 million episodes of outpatient services represent 72% of all organized psychiatric care in the specialty mental health sector. In addition to care provided in outpatient clinics and CMHCs, ambulatory psychiatric services are provided in private offices by psychiatrists, psychologists, clinical social workers, psychiatric nurses, and other licensed mental health counselors. Nearly 10 million people in the USA are estimated to have had one or more outpatient mental health visits during 1980—25% seen by psychiatrists in office practice, 24% seen by psychologists, and the remainder seen by nonpsychiatrist physicians and social workers in office practice and in organized settings (Taube and coworkers, 1984). The median number of visits is 3; the mean is 8 visits, skewed by the 10% of patients who accumulate 25 or more visits each year.

The specific treatments offered to patients in outpatient settings are discussed in detail in Chapters 42–54. Patients with a wide spectrum of problems can be treated in outpatient settings: individuals having "problems in living" and adjustment disorders, medical patients with emotional problems or habits and behaviors that compromise their health status, and almost the whole range of patients with psychotic and other nonpsychotic mental disorders needing psychotherapy, medication management, and social skills training.

3. ALTERNATIVES TO HOSPITAL & TRADITIONAL AMBULATORY CARE

Only the most seriously disturbed or diagnostically complex patients must be hospitalized, although the outpatient management of many others is complicated and demanding of time, commitment, and effort. Because it is often easier for the physician to hospitalize a patient (eg, better supervision of behavior), cheaper for the patient and more remunerative for the doctor (because of better insurance coverage for hospital benefits), and more desirable for the patient's family (to provide relief from concern and, at times, from abuse), hospital care may substitute for outpatient care. This is unnecessary, restrictive, and costly for society. Because insurance coverage is skewed toward hospital care and "standard" practice is difficult to change, alternatives to both hospital and traditional outpatient care are lacking. Alternative facilities would provide more continuous supervision, evaluation, and treatment than outpatient care but would not offer as intensive an array of services as a hospital. Many models of such alternatives have been developed and proved effective. However, too few exist, and where they do exist, they are not well covered by health insurance.

Partial or Part-Time Hospitals

Partial or part-time hospitals offer treatment services in a hospital "milieu" for part of the day—in some cases allowing patients to go home at night and in other cases allowing them to stay at night and work or attend school during the day. Programs offer supervision, observation, individual and group therapy, social and occupational skills training, recreational therapy, and medication management. In spite of documented cost-effectiveness, partial hospitalization has accounted for only 3% of all patient care episodes in the specialty mental health sector since 1965. Insurance benefits are limited; insurers fear that if they were to be insured, partial hospitals would attract a wide range of patients beyond those for whom they serve as a cost-effective alternative to hospital care. Meeting the so-called "latent demand" with a new benefit could result in higher costs rather than savings, unless the partial hospital services could be strictly limited to patients who would otherwise require hospital care.

Residential Treatment Programs*

Residential treatment programs provide 24-hour care in nonhospital settings. **Self-help communities** are usually sponsored by nongovernmental agencies for the purpose of helping people with a particular type of difficulty. The individual lives in the facility full-time for varying periods and usually continues to be affiliated with the group after leaving. Examples of self-help communities include Synanon (originally organized to help people with narcotics problems), residences for alcoholics, Salvation Army, and church-sponsored agencies.

Substitute homes provide shelter and treatment-related programs for longer periods of time. Examples are foster homes, usually for children; board and care homes, primarily for people who are disabled and unlikely to return to productive function; mental hygiene homes, providing special services for the mentally disabled who are unable to live in board and care homes; family care homes, similar to foster homes but taking adults—usually several at one time; residential treatment centers, taking a number of children and offering fairly intensive treatment programs; and "crash pads," a relatively new approach to short-term residence for young people—often in the process of withdrawing from drugs—who need shelter.

Emergency & Crisis Intervention Services

Crisis intervention services are offered by hospital and nonhospital facilities. They provide episodic, acute interventions in life-threatening or extreme circumstances involving patients with mental disorders. They use biomedical and psychosocial interventions; specific treatment methods and techniques are discussed in Chapters 52–54 and 59.

Consultation/Liaison Services

Consultation/liaison services are provided in CMHCs and in general hospitals (see Chapters 55 and 56).

Social Support Services

Social support services are offered by most mental health and community agencies to bolster a patient's natural support system (eg, family, workplace, religious community, neighborhood) or to provide a substitute system of personal and social support. In response to the problems of deinstitutionalized patients with chronic mental illness, networks of community support services (described above) have been established in the USA and in several other countries. These services break with those of earlier reforms by offering services *directly* to chronically ill patients rather than ignoring them while trying to prevent chronicity by the early treatment of acute illness (Tessler and Goldman, 1982).

The following types of social support services are not only designed for patients with chronic mental illness but also for other groups as well:

Nonresidential self-help organizations.* The following are examples of organizations usually administered by people who have survived similar problems and have banded together to help others cope with the same problem: Alcoholics Anonymous (and AlAnon, to help families of alcoholics); Recovery Inc., organized and run by people who have had an emotional problem that required hospitalization; Schizophrenics Anonymous; Gamblers Anonymous; Overeaters Anonymous; colostomy clubs; mastectomy clubs; the Epilepsy Society; the American Heart Association's Stroke Clubs of America; burn recovery groups; the international bypass groups for those who have had surgery for obesity; other groups organized to help people deal with practical and psychologic problems of a particular illness; and friendship centers that assist people in their efforts to find specific kinds of help.

Special professional and paraprofessional organizations.* Examples of special organizations of this type are Homemaker Service, made up of individuals who come into the home to help the partially disabled maintain the household; Visiting Nurse Associations, which usually provide more than medical assistance; adult protective services, oriented toward assisting the elderly; Abortion Counseling and Planned Parenthood Services; genetic counseling services; family service agencies, for marriage counseling and family problems; Travelers Aid, for rendering assistance to new residents and transients; legal aid societies; Big Brothers, Inc., to provide a masculine figure when one is lacking in the family (or Big Sisters for girls); consumer credit organizations, to help the financially naive organize their financial problems; crisis centers, eg, "free clinics" and county-sponsored satellite clinics; and church-sponsored agencies.

---

*This section is contributed by James J. Brophy, MD.

*This section is contributed by James J. Brophy, MD.

MENTAL HEALTH PROFESSIONALS

As noted throughout this chapter, there are many different professional providers in the specialty mental health sector. There is overlap between some of their skills and the services they perform, and there are some areas in which they have specialized professional training.

Psychiatrists are MD or DO physicians who have completed a 4-year residency training program in general psychiatry. Psychiatrists are trained to diagnose and treat patients with physical and mental disorders both biomedically and psychosocially. Usually they are trained in techniques of psychotherapy and are skilled at both diagnosis and psychosocial formulation (psychodynamic, behavioral, or both). They are the only members of the mental health care team licensed to prescribe medication and (along with nurses) to perform complete physical examinations. Subspecialties in psychiatry are discussed in separate chapters (eg, psychoanalysis in Chapter 43, child and adolescent psychiatry in Chapter 57, consultation/liaison psychiatry in Chapters 55 and 56, forensic psychiatry in Chapter 58, and occupational psychiatry in Chapter 60).

Clinical psychologists are doctoral (PhD, EdD, PsyD, DMH) or masters-level mental health professionals who may be licensed as independent practitioners in psychotherapy and psychologic assessment; some masters-level professionals are licensed separately as marriage and family counselors. These professionals attend graduate schools and have clinical placements and internships in which they learn psychotherapy, diagnosis, and psychologic testing under supervision. When licensed, they may diagnose and treat patients with mental disorders. Psychologists often have specialized training in administering psychologic tests and performing behavior and cognitive therapies. They also have more extensive research training than most physicians. Like the services of physicians, those of psychologists are now being reimbursed by insurance. In addition, psychologists are beginning to gain admitting privileges to some hospital inpatient services, permitting them to admit a patient jointly with a physician.

Clinical social workers are doctoral (DSW, PhD) or (more frequently) masters-level (MSW, MSSW) psychotherapists, caseworkers, and marriage, family, and child therapists, trained in accredited schools of social work and social welfare and accredited by the National Association of Social Work as having completed many hours of supervised clinical work. They are licensed by many states as independent practitioners, and increasingly they are being reimbursed by health insurance. Social workers are particularly skilled at psychosocial therapies, are knowledgeable about community and social welfare resources, and have a special interest in families.

Clinical nurse specialists are registered nurses who may take special training in psychiatric nursing. They may be licensed as independent practitioners, but they more often work in organized ambulatory health care settings and in hospitals. Nurses have special skills in the biomedical as well as the psychosocial aspects of mental health care.

Occupational, activities, and recreational/expressive therapists are registered practitioners from a variety of educational backgrounds with specialized training in using art, music, dance, drama, play, and vocational activities to help patients express their feelings and thoughts, learn new behavior, and develop or recover emotionally and socially valuable skills.

Pastoral counselors are clergy with specialized training in counseling patients with emotional disorders.

There are a number of other mental health providers, including **clinical sociologists, clinical pharmacists,** and **clinical specialists** in other related disciplines. They develop clinical skills related to their core academic or professional training and apply them in clinical settings.

Psychoanalysts are graduates of psychoanalytic institutes, including freudian, neo-freudian, and jungian training centers, who have completed a course of study, a personal analysis, and supervised training analyses (see Chapter 43). Although most are psychiatrists, other professionals have been trained as **lay analysts.** Training takes many years following completion of other professional mental health training.

Multidisciplinary teams of mental health professionals function in psychiatric and general hospital and ambulatory settings. The **inpatient team** has a traditional hierarchy and division of labor, with the psychiatrist leading the team, the nurse managing day-to-day ward activities and medication and patient monitoring duties, the psychologist performing psychologic tests, the social worker finding a place for the patient to go to at discharge and arranging the financing of hospital and posthospital care, and the occupational therapist organizing activities for the patient during the hospital stay. This traditional organization is still the mode, although in some settings the inpatient team has evolved with less differentiated functions and roles—and a less hierarchical organization.

The **outpatient team** tends to be less hierarchical, although certain functions are still performed by different disciplines (eg, psychiatrists manage medication and psychologists give tests and conduct behavior treatments). The functions of members of the **consultation/liaison team** are partly differentiated, as described in Chapter 56.

MENTAL HEALTH ECONOMICS

The **direct cost of mental illness** in the USA is conservatively estimated to be approximately $20 billion annually, or nearly 8% of all health care expenditures (Frank and Kamlet, 1984). This figure excludes direct costs associated with drug abuse, alcoholism, mental retardation, and uncomplicated senility; it also excludes the social costs (eg, lost income and productivity) associated with mental illness, estimated to be at least 1.5 times the direct cost. Direct costs associated with alcoholism are estimated to be $9 billion, and drug abuse costs are approximately $1 billion (Cruze and coworkers, 1984). Of the $20 billion in mental health costs, the specialty mental health sector accounts for 53%; the general medical sector accounts for 31%; and the other human services sector accounts for the remainder. (In contrast, the percentages of *individuals* seen in each sector are approximately 20%, 60%, and 20%, respectively.) In the specialty mental health sector, nearly half of the costs go to hospital care—more than in the general medical sector. Physicians' services are about 8% of all direct mental health costs, in contrast to the 18% of direct health costs for all disorders spent on physicians' services. The growth in direct mental health costs was 1.3% per year between 1977 and 1980, compared to 3.6% in growth for all health care costs.

The history of mental health services is also a story of **mental health financing.** The opening of public asylums in the USA in the early 19th century marked the beginning in a shift of fiscal responsibility from families, charity, and other private sources to public sources in state and local government. The movement took another step at the turn of the century with the passage of the State Care Acts, transferring the bulk of fiscal authority and responsibility from local government to state government. The pattern began to reverse somewhat with the introduction of health insurance from 1930 to 1950 and the expansion of private office practice and inpatient psychiatric practice in private nonprofit hospitals.

The federal government became involved in mental health financing in a major way in the 1960s with the Community Mental Health Centers Act, committing federal money for use by local public and private agencies, and the Medicare and Medicaid legislation, committing public resources for health and mental health care in the private sector at public expense. The involvement of the federal government marked a major redirection and set a pattern of hybrid funding for services, mixing federal and state (Medicaid), federal and local (CMHCs), and federal and private (Medicare) resources in a public-private system of care. The revision of the Social Security disability program in the 1970s infused additional federal money into the care and support of the mentally impaired. This level of federal financing allowed states to divest themselves of additional fiscal responsibility for mental health care, shifting public responsibility away from the state for the first time since the turn of the century. The passage of the Mental Health Systems Act in 1980 revised the CMHC legislation and provided the framework for an expanded federal-state-local partnership (Foley and Sharfstein, 1983).

In the 1980s, the pattern of mental health financing is shaped by fiscal austerity, cost containment, and a policy of "new federalism," all of which return fiscal responsibility to the state and local government and the private sector. The repeal of the Mental Health Systems Act before its implementation in 1981 and its replacement with a "block grant" to states at a reduced level of funding, the imposition of Medicaid spending ceilings, and the implementation of a prospective payment system for hospital care in Medicare (limiting payment to a prearranged price based on "diagnosis-related groups") all reflect this new trend in the public sector. In the private sector, mental health benefits in health insurance have been further limited for both inpatient and outpatient care. First restricted in the 1950s in an effort to control costs anticipated for long hospital stays and for open-ended long-term psychotherapy, the "nervous and mental disorder" benefits for *all* patients with mental disorders were limited to fixed dollar amounts per year and in a lifetime; the "out-of-pocket" expenses for each psychiatric care visit were higher than for nonpsychiatric care, and there were limits on the number of visits and on the total days in the hospital per admission, per year, and in a lifetime. Insurance coverage for mental health care does not have "parity" with coverage for other forms of health care. Costs need to be controlled, but cost-containment mechanisms can be designed to minimize their effect on access to needed high-quality mental health care. Investigation in this area of mental health services research is focused on understanding the complex interplay of clinical and economic forces that shape patterns of service use.

The field of mental health economics research is in its infancy. The mental health services system is diverse and highly differentiated into multiple facilities, providers, and financing mechanisms, sometimes cooperating and other times competing for scarce resources. The system is filled with inequities: The poor are still less well served than the rich, and duplication of effort and expense occurs too frequently. The costs increase, and the cherished, expensive treatments (eg, long-term psychiatric hospitalization and psychoanalysis) are more and more difficult to finance and afford. Different professional groups become rivals and competitors as physicians and nonphysicians stake out claims as independent providers of mental health services and eligible recipients of insurance payments. The mental health services system and its financing mechanisms are in flux as the system tries to provide valuable services to the 15–20% of the population with specific mental disorders and to countless others who suffer emotional distress in the course of daily life or physical illness.

SUMMARY

This chapter began by discussing the science of epidemiology and its related discipline, mental health services research, and ended by discussing services, financing, and public health policy. This direction results from following the line of questioning initiated by epidemiologic investigations: Who in the population has a disorder? How and why did they come to have it? What is the risk? How can it be diminished—with what interventions, in what settings, and at what cost? A discussion of rates of incidence and treated prevalence is followed naturally by a consideration of services, programs, insurance policies, and public laws.

Epidemiology is the basic science of public health. The hope is that good science will make better policy and that good policy will improve the public health.

REFERENCES

Baldessarini RJ, Finkelstein S, Arana GW: The predictive power of diagnostic tests and the effect of prevalence of illness. *Arch Gen Psychiatry* 1983;**40:**569.

Brophy JJ: Psychiatric disorders. Chapter 17 in: *Current Medical Diagnosis & Treatment 1988.* Schroeder SA, Krupp MA, Tierney LM Jr (editors). Appleton & Lange, 1988.

Caplan A: *Principles of Preventive Psychiatry.* Basic Books, 1964.

Cruze AM et al: *Economic Costs to Society of Alcoholism, Drug Abuse, and Mental Disorders—1980.* Alcohol, Drug Abuse, and Mental Health Administration, US Department of Health and Human Services, 1984. [Mimeographed data.]

Dohrenwend BP et al: *Mental Illness in the United States.* Praeger, 1980.

Endicott J, Spitzer RL: A diagnostic interview: The Schedule for Affective Disorders and Schizophrenia. *Arch Gen Psychiatry* 1978;**35:**837.

Faris REL, Dunham HW: *Mental Disorders in Urban Areas.* Univ of Chicago Press, 1939.

Feighner JP et al: Diagnostic criteria for use in psychiatric research. *Arch Gen Psychiatry* 1972;**26:**57.

Frank R, Kamlet M: *Direct Costs and Expenditures for Mental Health in the United States—1980.* National Institute of Mental Health, 1984. [Mimeographed data.]

Glick I, Hargreaves WA: *Psychiatric Hospital Treatment for the 1980s.* Lexington Books, 1979.

Goldberg D: *Manual of the General Health Questionnaire.* NFER Publishing Co., 1972.

Goldberger J, Warning CH, Tanner WF: Pellagra prevention by diet among institutional inmates. *Public Health Rep* 1925; **38:**2361.

Goldman HH: Epidemiology. Chapter 2 in: *The Chronic Mental Patient: Five Years Later.* Talbott JA (editor). Grune & Stratton, 1984.

Goldman HH, Adams N, Taube C: Deinstitutionalization: The data demythologized. *Hosp Community Psychiatry* 1983; **34:**129.

Goldman HH et al: The multiple functions of the state mental hospital. *Am J Psychiatry* 1983;**140:**296.

Hollingshead AB, Redlich FC: *Social Class and Mental Illness.* Wiley, 1958.

Jones M: *The Therapeutic Community.* Basic Books, 1953.

Kirshner LA: Length of stay of psychiatric patients. *J Nerv Ment Dis* 1982;**170:**27.

Klerman GL, Weissman MM: Epidemiology of mental disorders. *Arch Gen Psychiatry* 1978;**35:**705.

Kramer M: A discussion of the concepts of incidence and preva-

lence as related to epidemiologic studies of mental disorders. *Am J Public Health* 1957;**47:**826.

Leighton DC et al: *The Character of Danger.* Vol 3 of: *The Stirling County Study of Psychiatric Disorder and Socio-Cultural Environment.* Basic Books, 1963.

McGuire T: *Financing Psychotherapy.* Ballinger, 1981.

Pasamanick B et al: A survey of mental disease in an urban population. *Am J Public Health* 1956;**47:**923.

Perrow C: Hospitals: Technology, structure, and goals. Page 910 in: *Handbook of Organizations.* March JG (editor). Rand McNally, 1965.

Regier DA, Burke JD Jr: Epidemiology. Chapter 6.1 in: *Comprehensive Textbook of Psychiatry/IV,* 4th ed. Kaplan HI, Freedman AM, Sadock BJ (editors). Williams & Wilkins, 1985.

Regier DA, Goldberg ID, Taube CA: The de facto US mental health services system. *Arch Gen Psychiatry* 1978;**35:**685.

Regier DA et al: The NIMH Epidemiologic Catchment Area (ECA) Program. *Arch Gen Psychiatry* 1984;**41:**934.

Robins LN: Psychiatric epidemiology. *Arch Gen Psychiatry* 1978;**35:**697.

Robins LN et al: The NIMH Diagnostic Interview Schedule: Its history, characteristics, and validity. *Arch Gen Psychiatry* 1981;**38:**381.

Spitzer RL, Endicott J: *The Schedule for Affective Disorders and Schizophrenia (SADS),* 3rd ed. New York State Psychiatric Institute, 1979.

Spitzer RL, Endicott J, Robins E: Research diagnostic criteria: Rationale and reliability. *Arch Gen Psychiatry* 1978;**35:**773.

Spitzer RL, Williams JBW: *Instruction Manual for the Structured Clinical Interview for DSM-III (SCID).* New York State Psychiatric Institute, 1983.

Srole L et al: *Mental Health in the Metropolis.* Vol 1 of: *The Midtown Manhattan Study.* McGraw-Hill, 1962.

Taube CA, Barrett S (editors): *Mental Health, United States— 1985.* Alcohol, Drug Abuse, and Mental Health Administration, US Department of Health and Human Services, 1985.

Taube CA, Kessler LA, Feuerberg M: Utilization and expenditures for ambulatory mental health care during 1980. In: *National Medical Care Utilization and Expenditure Survey, Data Report No. 5.* US Department of Health and Human Services Publication No. (PHS) 84-20000, 1984.

Tessler R, Goldman HH: *The Chronically Mentally Ill: Assessing Community Support Programs.* Ballinger, 1982.

Weissman MM, Myers JK, Harding PS: Psychiatric disorders in a US urban population. *Am J Psychiatry* 1978;**135:**459.

Social Psychiatry

14

Joseph P. Morrissey, PhD

The term social psychiatry has not been precisely defined. Broadly speaking, it is a branch of study and research with important clinical applications that is concerned with the etiology, diagnosis, treatment, and prevention of mental disorders.

Despite the ambiguity of the term,* the core research concerns of investigators working in the field are easily identified. The literature addressing the social aspects of the mental disorders is voluminous. In Fig 14–1, the 3 general areas in which workers in this field have busied themselves are shown to be the same as if the subject area were infectious diseases or rheumatology. There has been great interest in the **genesis and distribution of mental disorders** in community populations, with emphasis on social, environmental, and psychologic variables as they affect the incidence and prevalence of mental disorders. Working within an epidemiologic framework, investigators in this area seek to determine how and why differential distributions occur. The assumptions are that mental disorders are not randomly distributed in the population and that by examining their social, environmental, and psychologic concomitants, insights can be gained into their etiology, course, outcome, and prevention.

The second issue concerns the patterns of **recognition of and response to mental disorders**—both the personal responses of the sick individual and the responses of others such as family and friends, psychiatrists, and personnel working in public agencies. Much of the research on personal responses consists of studies of "help-seeking" behavior; studies of public ("other") responses have tended to emphasize the "labeling" function, ie, the criteria and processes involved in identifying symptoms as those of mental illness and the sequestration, excuse from responsibility, or avoidance of the sick individual. Both lines of inquiry have led to the conclusion that social factors play a role in determining the nature, gravity, and outcomes of these recognition and response processes.

The third issue deals with **psychiatric roles and decision making.** Here the focus of attention shifts from the patient to the practitioner. Areas of concern include the ways in which psychiatric practice is shaped by professional ideologies; the structure and dynamics of treatment settings; and social pressures from families, the community, and the legal system. Sociologists have studied the development of schools and movements in psychiatry in relation to both internal and external pressures. Internal pressures are

---

*See Bell and Spiegel (1966), Redlich and Pepper (1968), Srole (1974).

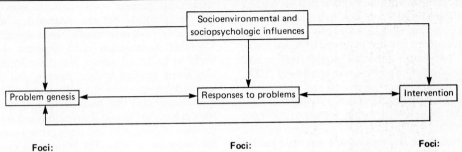

Figure 14–1. Domain and scope of social psychiatry.

created by the ascendancy of different ideologic sub-groups within psychiatry and their patterns of recruitment, socialization, career choices, and preferred practice settings. External pressures are exerted by supportive and competitive relationships with other professions and constituencies as well as by political, economic, and historical forces.

GENESIS & DISTRIBUTION OF MENTAL DISORDERS

The search for social causes of mental disorder has been an important theme in epidemiology and social psychiatry. The epidemiologic studies are discussed in Chapter 13. In this chapter, 2 of the principal social variables—social class and stressful life events—identified as likely to play a role in the onset of mental disorder will be examined.

The Role of Social Class in the Etiology of Mental Disorder

Sociologists have studied the origins, composition, and consequences of social classes or stratification systems in a variety of societies. The number and type of classes in different societies vary, but in modern industrial societies there tends to be a similar social class hierarchy. One of the most widely used frameworks for measuring social class in the USA is Hollings-head's Index of Social Position, which sorts people into 5 classes: I (upper class), II (upper middle), III (lower middle), IV (upper lower), and V (lower lower). One's position on this ladder depends upon the occupation, education, or income of the heads of the family. Since these 3 variables tend to be highly correlated, investigators often rely on only one component. Numerous studies have demonstrated that social position tends to affect life-styles and consumption patterns, political worldviews and values, opportunities for achievement and advancement, and health status and mortality rate.

Indeed, one of the most consistent findings in the psychiatric epidemiology literature is that the highest rates of mental disorder are found in the lowest social class. Dohrenwend and Dohrenwend (1974) documented this pattern in a careful review of 80 studies of the "true" prevalence of mental disorder (both treated and untreated cases) worldwide since the early 1900s. In spite of time and place differences and variations in case-finding procedures, 28 of the 33 studies that measured social class showed that the highest overall rates of functional mental disorder were associated with the lowest social class. This relationship was strongest for urban or mixed urban-rural communities (19 of 20 studies), and it held for schizophrenia (5 of 7 studies) and personality disorder (11 of 14 studies), but not for neuroses or bipolar affective disorder. The latter 2 conditions tend to be more common among the upper and upper middle social classes.

Two competing hypotheses have been offered to account for the high rates of mental disorder in the lowest social class: **social causation** versus **social selection.** The first hypothesis is that environmental and psychologic factors associated with life-styles of the lower social class produce mental disorders; the second holds that preexisting susceptibility to mental disorder leads to low social class position. Implicit in the social selection hypothesis is the notion that genetic or other biologic factors (rather than environmental or psychologic ones) are the primary causes of psychiatric disturbances. Both hypotheses gained prominence from Faris and Dunham's (1939) study of the ecologic distribution of treated mental disorders in Chicago. Since that time, the operative form of each hypothesis has undergone refinement, and a number of variants have been proposed.

On the social causation side, the disproportionate rates of mental disorders in the lowest social class have been explained in terms of social disintegration, value conflicts, blocked aspirations, deprecatory self-concepts, and childhood deprivation. On the selection side, 2 distinct hypotheses have been proposed: **social drift** and **social segregation.** The "drift" hypothesis holds that mental disorder is more common in the lowest class because people from higher classes sink to lower ones as a consequence of their illness. The segregation hypothesis holds that healthy members of the lower class are selected upward in our socially mobile society, leaving behind a "residue" of the ill. Thus, the notion of drift points to *downward* social mobility, whereas the idea of segregation points to *blocked upward* mobility as the most parsimonious explanations for the class-mental disorder relationship.

The evidence in support of these hypotheses is mixed. In 1962, Srole and his colleagues on the Midtown Manhattan epidemiologic study reported data on parental social class as well as the current social class position of their adult respondents. Since the parents' social class was clearly antecedent to the respondents' current (adult) psychiatric status, the investigators reasoned that the direction of causality in any observed relationship would be unambiguous. Their findings did reveal a significant inverse relationship between respondents' parents' social class and rates of psychiatric impairment, but the relationship was much stronger for the respondents' own social position. Moreover, respondents rated impaired were more likely to be found among the downwardly mobile (downward relative to their parents) and less likely among those who were upwardly mobile. The investigators concluded that both social causation (in the form of early childhood deprivation) and selection (in the form of both drift and segregation) contribute to the observed relationship between socioeconomic status and psychiatric impairment.

Other studies have examined the relationships between social mobility and different types of psychiatric disorders, especially schizophrenia and antisocial personality, with equally mixed results. (See Dohrenwend [1975] for a review.) In a rigorous investigation of the class-schizophrenia relationship, however, Turner and Wagenfeld (1967) found convincing evidence for the "residue" as opposed to the "drift" hypothesis. The data base for this study of first admissions for schizophrenic men was drawn from the Monroe County (New York) psychiatric case register. The findings indicated that first admission rates were disproportionately high both for patients of lowest occupational status and for patients whose fathers had lowest occupational status. However, there was little overlap between the 2 groups. Moreover, the amount of downward social mobility among schizophrenic men did not differ significantly from that in the general population. What the data indicated is that the patients tended less than the general population to rise above the parents' social position. Thus, the findings suggest that the accumulation of schizophrenic disorders in the lowest class is not because patients lost positions they had once achieved ("drift") but rather because they failed ever to achieve as high an occupational or social level as did most men of their social class origins ("residue").

All of the studies that have examined the social class-psychiatric disorder nexus suffer from methodologic and research design problems that complicate their interpretation, so that clear support for either explanation has not been forthcoming. Currently, many investigators agree that both factors must be considered, and attention has focused on specific intervening variables linking social class to psychiatric disorder. One of the most closely studied variables is social stress.

The Role of Stressful Life Events in the Etiology of Mental Disorder

The relevance of the stress concept for the understanding of mental disorders comes chiefly from studies of human behavior in extreme situations such as war, natural disasters, and concentration camps and from investigations of the occurrence and response to more ordinary life events. Attention here will be limited to the stressful aspects of everyday life. As Dohrenwend (1975) points out, if social stress plays an important etiologic role in psychiatric disorders (which have been reported to affect as much as 25% of the general population), then the events must be more common in the lives of most people than those occurring in extreme situations (see Chapters 5, 31, and 35).

The Midtown Manhattan study (Srole and coworkers, 1962) established the foundation for much of the current research on psychiatric disorder and life events. Langner and Michael, 2 of the senior investigators on this project, examined the hypothesis that the inverse relationship between mental illness and social class was due to the greater force of life stresses in the lower classes. Their findings (1963) did support this relationship, but the differences in levels of stress were not large enough to account for the observed differences in impairment risk at different social class positions. When the numbers of life stresses were held constant, respondents in lower social class positions still showed greater psychiatric impairment. This im-

plies that the correlation of lower class with higher incidence of mental disorder is not attributable simply to the amount of stress people endure. Langner and Michael suggested that other factors should be examined as intervening variables in the social class-mental disorder relationship, such as personality differences, stress-buffering resources, and differential use of adaptive mechanisms.

The measure of "life stress" used in the Midtown Manhattan studies was based on a 10-item score composed of both childhood factors (eg, parents' poor mental health, economic deprivation, poor physical health, broken homes) and adult factors (eg, poor adult physical health, poor interpersonal affiliations, work worries). More recently, investigators have concentrated on the occurrence of stressful events in adult life as determinants of mental health status. Rabkin (1982) points out that the terms "life events" and "stressors" are used interchangeably in the literature to describe "discrete changes in life conditions that are consensually recognized as entailing some degree of distress, challenge, and/or hazard by the individual and members of his/her social group." These include events such as death of a spouse, divorce, marriage, loss of a job, pregnancy, and a sudden change in financial status. Generally, as Dohrenwend (1975) notes, the assumption is that the *accumulation* of several events rather than one decisive event produces the stressful impact.

Several models of stress and illness have evolved in the social psychiatry literature. According to Rabkin, the most popular current model is the **vulnerability hypothesis,** which holds that chance exposure to stressors triggers psychiatric disturbance in vulnerable people. The reason for vulnerability may vary according to the type of disorder and may include childhood experiences, family relationships, or genetic predisposition. In addition, a variety of resource factors are postulated as potential mediating variables that determine the probability of a person's becoming ill. These may include social supports, financial resources, and personal coping skills.

A number of the studies reviewed by Rabkin provide presumptive evidence that various types of psychiatric disorder—specifically, acute episodes of schizophrenia, depression, and anxiety disorders—may follow the occurrence of life events. For example, Brown and Birley (1968) studied life events of 50 patients suffering acute onset or relapse of schizophrenia and a group of 377 normal controls drawn from the Camberwell district of London. The 2 groups differed in the proportion experiencing at least one major change in their lives in the 3-week period preceding the interview (60% of the patients versus 19% of the controls). The investigators also separated the life events into those over which subjects had control and those over which they had no control, and the relationships still held.

In another study of the same community, Brown and Harris (1978) compared a sample of the depressed women receiving outpatient care with a comparison group of normal controls. Their findings indicated that stressful life events (such as losses of relationships, status, or love) were more common among the women who became depressed than among those who did not. Moreover, the women who were most vulnerable to depression tended to be those who had no intimate relationships, who had 3 or more young children in the home, who did not have an outside job, and who had lost their mothers early in life. All of these conditions were more frequent among women of the lower class.

The relationship between life events and psychiatric disorder has also been investigated in surveys of the general population. Myers and coworkers (1975) studied a community sample of 720 adults in New Haven in 1967 and 1969. Psychiatric symptomatology was measured at each time period by a 22-item index of mental status and life events by 62 items adapted from Holmes and Rahe's Schedule of Recent Life Events and other sources. The findings revealed an inverse relationship between life events and mental status for each time period. Moreover, comparisons of the 2 surveys revealed that a net increase in life events was associated with a worsening of symptoms, while a net decrease was associated with improvement. This pattern held for different types of events and (with statistical controls) did not vary according to age, sex, marital status, religion, or social class.

As noted by Dohrenwend and by Rabkin, however, the "life events" literature still presents a number of methodologic and research design problems. Unresolved issues include the characterization and weighting of events (eg, pleasant versus unpleasant, predictable versus unpredictable, controllable versus uncontrollable), their subjective meaning and timing (eg, rapid versus insidious onset), and their causal direction (eg, consequences versus antecedents of stress). The identification of appropriate population samples and comparison groups has been another methodologic hurdle. Efforts are now under way to develop research designs with longitudinal or prospective measures that can help to resolve these problems. As Dohrenwend points out, only through such designs will we be able to answer the central questions posed by current research: What kinds of life events—over what periods of time and in what combinations and circumstances—are causally implicated in various types of psychiatric disorders?

Current evidence strongly suggests that no simple cause-effect relationship will be forthcoming from life stress and mental illness studies. Rather, as Eisenberg (1977) has noted, a fuller understanding of the mental disorders will require a biopsychosocial model that allows for multiple and interacting causes involving social, environmental, psychologic, and biologic variables.

PATTERNS OF RECOGNITION & RESPONSE TO MENTALLY DISORDERED BEHAVIOR

Regardless of their ultimate causes, the ways in which aberrant behavior or psychiatric symptoms come to be recognized by the individuals affected, their families and friends, or the wider community are all decidedly *social* in nature. Responses of the symptomatic person and others entail a process of social definition that depends upon knowledge and beliefs and the impact of the deviant behavior in the social context. Some research findings about the role of environmental and psychologic variables in the recognition and response process are set forth in the following paragraphs.

Help-Seeking Behavior

Underlying most of the research that has been done on the recognition and response to psychiatric symptoms is an effort to identify the criteria commonly used by the sick individual and others to evaluate the situation. In 1980, Mechanic showed that these appraisals are influenced by a wide range of social factors, including (1) the extent to which symptoms disrupt normal activities and interfere with the performance of social roles; (2) the degree of sophistication about psychiatric matters possessed by the evaluator; (3) the capacity for ignoring or otherwise normalizing symptoms; (4) the subcultural norms pertaining to what kinds of actions are regarded as irrational or inappropriate; and (5) the need to deny a psychiatric condition because of the perceived stigma and embarrassment associated with hospitalization, or because family or other members of the household are dependent on the symptomatic person's continued presence in the household. Mechanic has argued that such criteria are commonly applied by both the sick person and by others in assessing the need to seek help, and that the process is parallel to what occurs in the case of ordinary medical conditions.

Some people seek help for psychiatric problems on their own initiative, as Cockerham (1981) reminds us, whereas others must be cajoled or coerced into obtaining care by threats or deception on the part of the family and friends, or by force. Thus, 2 situations must be distinguished when describing the pathway into treatment. A persistent finding in the literature is that the more bizarre and disruptive the symptoms are, the more likely it is for a person to seek psychiatric care or be required by others to do so. Cockerham's review of current research suggests that social variables, in contrast, appear to exert their strongest influence on *where* to seek help rather than *whether* to seek it.

For psychiatric as well as medical problems, seeking help often proceeds within a "lay referral network" that selectively channels people to helping resources. In a study of why people undertake personal psychotherapy, for example, Kadushin (1969) noted that the decision was traceable to the influence of small "social circles" of friends and supporters of psychotherapy who have sought or received such help themselves. Further support for the importance of lay referral networks is provided by Horwitz (1978) in a study of 120 married lower middle-class and working-class patients at a community mental health center. His findings indicated that help seeking outside the family was chiefly a female pursuit. Women also proved more likely to recognize the existence of mental disturbance in themselves and to enter treatment voluntarily. Men, in contrast, rarely placed themselves in treatment or even discussed their problems with others. Family members attempted to keep the help seeker within the informal network, whereas friends tried to direct the individual to a wider network of professional resources.

In general, persons seeking help on their own initiative differ with respect to a number of sociodemographic and attitudinal variables from other persons in the community not seeking help. Greenley and Mechanic (1976) have reviewed epidemiologic studies in this area suggesting that those who seek out psychiatrists for mental and emotional disturbances tend to be women or Jews living in urban or suburban areas, with high education and income and low religiosity orientations. In a 1979 study comparing national survey data in 1957 and 1976, however, Kulka and his associates found that the general population now is much more likely to define personal problems in psychologic terms and more likely to consult mental helath professionals. Although wealthier and better-educated respondents made greater use of psychiatrists and psychologists in both years, the relationship was much less marked in 1976 than in 1957. These data were interpreted as evidence of the growing availability of services and insurance coverage, which make social class less of a barrier to access. Such findings suggest that the social class-psychiatric treatment relationship so convincingly established by Hollingshead and Redlich in their 1958 study has moderated over the past 2 decades.

There also is an extensive literature on public attitudes and responses to mental disorder measures in terms of hypothetical cases, brief descriptions of behavior, or exposure to a family member who has had a psychiatric episode (see Clausen and Huffine [1975] for an overview). In general, as the behavior described becomes increasingly threatening or bizarre, the more likely it is to be perceived as mental illness. Otherwise, there appears to be a wide tolerance for deviant behavior and a reluctance to conceptualize it in psychiatric ways.

The tendency for members of the public to deny psychiatric symptoms is clearly illustrated in studies of family experiences with recently hospitalized patients. Yarrow and coworkers (1955) analyzed the definitional process on the part of wives whose husbands were hospitalized. The process entailed 5 stages: (1) The wife's first recognition of a problem occurred only after behavior that was not readily understandable or acceptable to her. (2) She then attempted to account for the husband's deviant behavior by applying alter-native explanations such as physical illness, job stress, or character flaws. (3) Her interpretation of the problem vacillated from seeing the situation as normal on some occasions to abnormal on others. (4) She made continual adaptation to her husband's behavior and became defensive about it with others. (5) She finally reached a point where her defenses could no longer cope with the husband's behavior and her definition of normality could no longer be sustained. It was only at stage (5) that mental illness was imputed and intervention by outside authorities was sought. These processes prefigure one dimension of the "family burden" that has become a central concern in current research on the care of chronic mental patients in family and community settings.

One consequence of these normalization and denial processes is the delay in seeking treatment until the situation becomes intolerable and hospitalization inevitable. Although recognition of this tendency has provided a rationale for public education programs about mental illness in the past 2 decades, Mechanic (1980) cautions that there are costs as well as benefits to applying psychiatric labels too readily. He notes that in many cases, early and effective treatment may reduce suffering, minimize disability and family disruptions, and even prevent suicide. Furthermore, effective treatment now exists for the disabling symptoms of schizophrenia, depression, and anxiety. In other areas, however, Mechanic points out that the efficacy of treatment is uncertain, and given the monetary and psychologic costs, limited benefit is derived from encouraging people to go into treatment. While encouragement and support of persons undergoing life crises are necessary, the act of defining people's behavior as mentally disordered may undermine their limited self-confidence and coping abilities. Premature diagnosis may also encourage a stance of dependency that leads to further disability and the acceptance of illness. On the basis of these considerations, Mechanic notes that the major challenge faced by new programs is to provide sustenance and help to those who are going through difficult crises without defining and structuring their problems so as to increase the probability of disability.

Further progress along these lines necessitates advances both in clinical psychiatry and in social psychiatric research. As Clausen and Huffine (1975) point out, "As it becomes increasingly possible to differentiate particular types of disorder responding to particular forms of therapy, . . . the more grossly disrupting behaviors can be limited . . . [and] accorded the status of illness." This would permit reaction patterns to life problems, for which psychiatry can claim no special expertise, to be channeled to other helping resources. Further research on help-seeking processes can also contribute to more appropriate use of psychiatric services. Among the issues in this area that Mechanic identifies as largely unresolved are the social aspects of illness attribution, the social development of different dispositions to seek help, their interactive effects with level of distress and choice of helping resources, and the extent to which help-giving agencies either encourage care among certain groups or impose obstacles to such care.

Social Reaction

The "labeling" of mental disorders as a form of deviant behavior is a major concern of social psychiatric research. In this framework, deviance is not a quality of the act but instead a product of the interaction of the person who performs the act (or manifests the symptom) and those who respond to it. Social groups "create" deviance by making rules whose infraction constitutes deviance and by applying those rules to particular people and labeling them as outsiders. Proponents of this view maintain that persistent rule breaking and labeling initiate a process of social degradation in which individuals are forced to become members of a deviant group. Those so labeled experience a profound and frequently irreversible socialization experience that causes them to accept an inferior status and deviant worldview, with the knowledge and skills that go with it. They thus develop a deviant self-image based upon the reactions of others to their behavior.

The labeling perspective had its origins in the works of Edwin Lemert, Howard Becker, Irving Goffman, and other sociologists, but it has also been supported by psychiatrists such as Thomas Szasz and R. D. Laing. Sedgwick (1982) notes that 2 varieties of labeling theory have been proposed. The weak form allows for a biologic basis of mental illness but maintains that the course of the disorder can be worsened or sharpened by the social handling of the patient in diagnosis and treatment. The strong form, in contrast, attributes mental illness solely to power relationships between the person singled out as being mentally ill and one or more dominant parties (eg, family, psychiatrist, public agencies).

Scheff (1975) has offered an explicit statement of the strong form of labeling, whereby mental illness is seen as "residual rule breaking." The labeling theory of mental illness examines 2 basic questions: (1) Why are some persons labeled as mentally ill while others who behave in similar ways are not so labeled? (2) What are the effects of being so labeled? In Scheff's view, powerless individuals are most apt to be labeled mentally ill, and the effect of labeling is to lock the individual into a "career" in which mental illness becomes a major social role in a life characterized by recurrent hospitalizations.

These contentions have been the subject of controversy for the past 15 years. Scheff's most persistent critic has been Walter Gove, a sociologist who has sought to refute the labeling perspective in a number of studies of mental hospitalization and its stigmatizing effects. Gove's own research (1975) was based on a sample of 258 first admissions to a state mental hospital in Washington from 1961 to 1964. In contrast to Scheff's predictions, Gove found that social resources (ie, high social class and being married) facilitated hospitalization and prompt treatment and that the stigma of hospitalization was negligible. Gove has marshaled a body of secondary evidence to support these findings.

While many investigators believe that the evidence does not support a doctrinaire view of labeling as the primary cause of mental illness, few would deny that labeling has profound consequences for what happens to many persons with psychiatric disturbances. Cockerham (1981) summarizes much empirical research and concludes that people are not randomly or capriciously singled out and labeled mentally ill, even though nonpsychiatric factors influence psychiatric diagnoses and outcomes. He notes that regardless of the theory involved, attributions of mental disorder are based on both verbal and nonverbal behavior in individuals labeled as mentally ill. Furthermore, these behavioral cues indicate the ability of the labeled patient to affect or react to the situation. What seems apparent from Cockerham's assessment is that before labeling occurs, there exists a troubled mind independent of the labeling process. Cockerham notes that when a person with a troubled mind expresses that internal state to others, then labeling occurs. At that point, a variety of social factors are brought into play to influence the responses to—and decisions about—the sick or troubled individual.

That labeling often has serious consequences for persons who are mentally ill can be documented from a number of sources. Goffman's (1961) depiction of mental hospitals as "total institutions," for example, suggests that many of the behaviors attributed to mental patients are social adaptations to the self-mortification and regimentation imposed by the structure and goals of these institutions. The clinical concepts of "institutional neurosis" and "institutionalization" also speak to the consequences of prolonged exposure to debilitating environments in terms of passive compliance, self-neglect, occasional outbursts of aggressive behavior, indifference, and apathy. Gruenberg's (1974) concept of the "chronic social breakdown syndrome" refers to a more severe form of secondary deterioration that has its origins in the social environment rather than the intrinsic features of schizophrenia or other psychotic conditions. Other studies of pathways to treatment, psychiatric diagnostic practices, and hospital discharge criteria also suggest that labeling processes affect the fates of persons with mental disorders.

Thus, although evidence suggests that societal reactions do not "cause" mental disorder, labeling processes do influence the subsequent life experiences of mental patients. Psychiatry, as Sedgwick (1982) notes, has blunted much of the critical edge of the "antipsychiatry" movement by incorporating the weak form of labeling theory in its evolving biopsychosocial model of mental illness. The practice of psychiatry, nonetheless, is still susceptible to critical evaluation for its tendencies toward overdiagnosis, its role in social control, and its assumed dominion over other mental health care providers. An exploration of these issues leads to the third and final domain of social psychiatric research considered in this chapter.

PSYCHIATRIC ROLES & DECISION MAKING

What is the proper role of psychiatry in society? To what extent are its promises kept? Who benefits and who pays for its exercise of autonomy? These are the questions that have prompted critical analyses of the social organization, ideologies, and practices of psychiatry from within as well as outside its ranks. Over the past 3 decades, a sizeable body of literature has developed around such issues. Some highlights of this work will be reviewed here in relation to socialization processes, treatment settings and ideologies, social control, and psychiatric dominance over mental health care.

Professional Socialization

Analysis of the processes whereby medical school graduates are inducted into psychiatry has provided a number of insights into the values, ideologies, and practice orientations of the profession. Two recent contributions in this area are *Training in Ambiguity: Learning by Doing in a Mental Hospital*, by Coser (1979); and *Becoming Psychiatrists: The Professional Transformation of Self*, by Light (1980). The data for these case studies were gathered during the 1960s at university-affiliated teaching hospitals in the urban Northeast. O'Brien Hospital (a fictitious name), the setting for Coser's study, is described as a private mental hospital with 200 patients of the upper and middle class and a staff of 50 psychiatrists. About half of the staff were psychiatric residents. University Psychiatric Center (also fictitious), the setting for Light's study, is described as a small state hospital and community mental health center that had 75 psychiatric residents in training during the time the research was conducted. Both hospitals operated well-known "elite" training centers. O'Brien had primarily a psychoanalytic orientation, whereas University was "analytic-eclectic"—ie, the training program had deep commitments to psychoanalysis but accommodated projects and research in community and social psychiatry, behavior therapy, and psychopharmacology.

Coser's study examines 3 sources of "sociological ambivalence," a condition in which psychiatric residents are expected to live up to contradictory values and expectations: (1) receiving medical training versus engaging in psychodynamic practice; (2) controlling patient behavior (milieu therapy) versus giving treatment (psychotherapy); and (3) having to behave as a professional while learning to become a professional. Coser's analysis suggests that structural arrangements evolved to reduce the contradictions, such as the separation of therapist and management roles and the maintenance of "pluralistic ignorance," or the denial of ambiguity among trainees and senior staff.

In *Becoming Psychiatrists*, Light integrates the literature on psychiatric training with his own fieldwork data, and what emerges is a comprehensive understanding of the resident's worldview. His focus is on the "moral career" of the psychiatric resident, a construct derived from Goffman's (1961) penetrating analysis of the social situation of mental patients. Five stages are identified in the psychiatric resident's socialization process: (1) feeling different and being discredited; (2) moral confusion; (3) numbness and exhaustion; (4) moral transition, or the development of a coherent psychiatric worldview; and (5) self-affirmation, or gaining a sense of mastery over one's work. Light indicates that a major consequence of this socialization is that young psychiatrists move away from being advocates of the patient toward being technicians. The social structural supports for this transformation process are identified, along with the strategies residents employ to cope with the uncertainties of psychiatric knowledge, diagnosis and treatment, and interpersonal relations.

These 2 studies capture much of what is known about the entry-level socialization process in psychiatry. Although generalization from case studies is always suspect, it would appear that the 2 sites described were typical of "elite" residency training programs in the 1960s. Great changes in the practice and orientation of psychiatry have occurred in the past 25 years, and further research is required to update and confirm the relevance of these findings. Furthermore, the profession of psychiatry historically has been composed of multiple ideologic groups, each of which has gone about recruitment and training in its own way. Whether the current trend in psychiatry toward a closer partnership with general medicine will lead to greater homogenization of the profession is an issue that will be studied in the years ahead. Although this convergence of interests may overcome the differences between medical training and psychiatric practice that are highlighted in Coser's and in Light's work, it will also alter psychiatry's relationships with other mental health care providers such as psychologists and social workers. Accordingly, the benefits and costs of these shifting professional alignments must be assessed not only for psychiatry but for its traditional clientele and constituencies as well.

Treatment Settings & Ideologies

Professional socialization, as with its counterpart in everyday affairs, is a lifelong activity. Sociologists have not been content to study residency training but have attempted to explore the ways in which practice settings shape the character and content of psychiatry. Much of our understanding of the role of social, organizational, and ideologic factors in the practice of psychiatry is based upon a number of pioneering case studies of both private and public mental hospitals in the 1950s and early 1960s. Among the more notable studies are works by Stanton and Schwartz (1954), Belknap (1956), and Caudill (1958). These monographs attempted to document the ways in which the formal and informal organization of the hospital affected patients' symptoms and therapy, the "irrationalities" of the social structure, the dislocation of power and communication processes, and, in the case of public institutions, the displacement of treatment goals by custodial functions.

The work of Strauss and his colleagues (1964) stands as one of the most ambitious efforts to uncover the interplay of institutional, ideologic, and professional forces as they affect the practice of psychiatry in hospitals. The study was carried out over a period of several years in one public and one private mental hospital in the Chicago area using quantitative as well as qualitative research procedures. Part of the research involved an effort to establish the content and distinctiveness of 3 ideal-typical psychiatric ideologies: (1) somatotherapeutic, (2) psychotherapeutic, and (3) sociotherapeutic. The results suggested that the first 2 were polar opposites and that the third, at the time, was the least well developed ideologic position. While the investigators had assumed that the sociotherapeutic perspective would be the opposite of the psychoanalytic or psychotherapeutic view, the findings suggested that they were empirically unrelated. Even so, the overall findings demonstrated that the psychoanalytic model was the dominant ideologic perspective for psychiatrists at both hospitals in the early 1960s.

The findings that emerge from all of these studies were generated during a period in American psychiatry that has changed dramatically in the past 25 years. Not only have there been major advances in the scientific basis of psychiatry and psychiatric treatment—there has also been a rapid expansion and differentiation in practice settings. Today, the locus of the profession has shifted away from large public mental hospitals to medical schools, and new practice settings have been created with the advent of community mental health centers, health maintenance organizations, and the expansion of psychiatric units in general hospitals. As the profession attempts to redefine its roles and responsibilities in these new institutional arenas, the challenge for social psychiatric researchers is to update and refine the insights derived from these pioneering studies about psychiatry and its intra- and interprofessional dynamics.

Social Control

In addition to the role of physician-psychiatrist in both office and hospital practice, psychiatrists are called upon to accept bureaucratic responsibilities in the legal, military, and correctional systems. The problem of allegiance to stakeholders rather than to patients in these nonpsychiatric organizations has received considerable attention both within and outside the profession. One area of research has examined the role of psychiatrists in commitment and criminal proceedings, which highlights the social control aspects of psychiatric practice as well as the misplaced confidence in psychiatrists as expert witnesses.

Cocozza and Steadman (1978) report their attempt to assess the 1971 revisions in the New York State Code of Criminal Procedure [Law], in which psychiatrists were called upon to provide evaluations of dangerousness for all indicted felony defendants found incompetent to stand trial. They conducted a longitudinal study of 257 male defendants, representing an entire first-year cohort of cases evaluated under the new procedures. They found that 60% of the defendants were evaluated as dangerous and that nonpsychiatric factors (especially the actual or perceived level of violence associated with the alleged offenses) played a key role in these decisions. The psychiatrists, however, overwhelmingly justified their determinations on clinical and psychiatric grounds (ie, assessed mental illness and antisocial behavior prior to the offense). Furthermore, in 87% of the cases, the psychiatric recommendations pertaining to the defendants' dangerousness were accepted by the courts.

The major contribution of this study was its effort to evaluate the validity of psychiatric assessments. The authors gathered follow-up data over a 3-year period from the hospital records of each defendant and from community arrest reports following their discharge. These data centered around outcome measures of the defendants' actual behavior subsequent to the determination of dangerousness. The findings indicated that psychiatric predictions of dangerousness were not accurate. In fact, defendants evaluated as dangerous proved to be no more dangerous than those evaluated as not dangerous by any of the criteria used.

This study calls attention to the illusion of psychiatric expertise. Psychiatry is seen by the public, the courts, the legal community, and legislators as the professional group rightfully charged with the responsibility to predict potential dangerousness of individuals in conflict with the law. Yet the existence of any such special knowledge or expertise cannot be demonstrated. Indeed, as Cocozza and Steadman observe, "Psychiatrists may . . . be acting more as seers than as scientists in predicting dangerousness." The latent function served by psychiatrists acting in this role may well be to lay a veneer of science and respectability over what in practice is an exercise in social control of disruptive and disturbing behavior.

Similar issues have been raised across the many interfaces between psychiatry and the law. (See Chapter 58.) In whose interest does a psychiatrist act in "forensic" circumstances? To what extent are such actions consistent with the limited knowledge base now possessed by psychiatry? Where does the role of psychiatrist-physician leave off and the role of bureaucratic agent of social control begin? Although mechanisms of social control are necessary to preserve and maintain public order, at what point is more harm than good accomplished when political and correctional actions are justified in the name of "mental medicine"?

The current wave of criticism of Soviet psychiatrists for their role in controlling political dissent illustrates the revulsion some feel over what is perceived as the abuse of a care-giving privilege. Clearly, a profession true to its ideals cannot afford to ignore these issues, which, though they may be perceived differently as the profession changes, are never resolved. All professions must guard against the misuse of their authority and public trust. The changing political and ethical posture of psychiatry warrants close attention from researchers during the current transition and realignment of the profession from a peripheral and isolated specialty to one more central to medical institutions and practices.

Psychiatric Dominance

Psychiatry occupies the dominant position in a hierarchy of occupations concerned with the treatment of patients in the acute phase of illness as well as the long-term care of chronic mental patients. The sources of this dominance flow from psychiatry's license and mandate to treat persons suffering from identifiable mental disorders and from its legal control over hospitals and drug prescription. The position of psychiatry in the mental health care system is legitimized in myriad ways through government regulations and eligibility criteria for third-party reimbursements. The effect of these legal and professional controls is to restrict treatment for most patients to those settings and practitioners that are sanctioned by the profession. As insurance coverage expands, however, nonphysician mental health professionals are being granted status as independent providers eligible for insurance payments.

The Problem of Chronicity

The psychiatric profession has a long-standing bias in favor of acute ("curing") versus chronic ("caring") services and, increasingly, a narrow concern for the medical-psychiatric rather than the broader mental health and social status of its clients. This posture may be consistent with recent advances in the scientific basis of psychiatry and its demonstrated efficacy in the stabilization and control of acute illness, especially in hospital settings.

Although hospitals may still be the preferred setting for the treatment and stabilization of serious acute illness, many would argue that they are counterproductive for the long-term care of chronic patients. Indeed, with changing philosophies of care, the weight of the evidence regarding the overall value of hospitalization has begun to shift; when calculated in terms of psychosocial as well as financial costs, its presumed net benefits are diminished even for many patients with acute conditions.

The aftermath of state hospital deinstitutionalization policies in the USA and other countries, as Morrissey and associates (1980) have noted, has led to the "rediscovery" of chronic mental illness. Changing the locus of care from institutions to the community has not led to a fundamental change in the incidence or prevalence of severe mental disorders. Yet thousands of chronic mental patients now populate local communities, and their treatment and sustenance needs must be met by available resources. The public policy issue that remains unresolved is whether a mental health care system dominated by a medical-psychiatric hierarchy can satisfy the needs of this population.

For many severely disabled mental patients, social supports in the form of housing, vocational, and recreational services become of chief importance once the medical-psychiatric condition is stabilized. Recognition of this has prompted many psychosocial practitioners to seek an alliance with psychiatrists as peers for the joint management of a shared clientele. However, the medical tradition of retaining full clinical responsibility for patients has led psychiatrists to insist on maintaining control over other practitioners involved in mental health service delivery. When current psychiatric practices fail to recognize the psychosocial contributions of nonphysicians, psychiatry falls far short of the biopsychosocial ideal advocated by the profession's academic leaders. The trend toward fuller integration of psychiatry with general medicine may well reinforce this troublesome attitude of mind.

Homelessness

Although deinstitutionalization policies are often cited in the media as the primary cause of urban homelessness, its rapid growth in the 1980s is due more to the shortage of low-income housing, the high rate of unemployment, and other adverse economic conditions. Nonetheless, mentally ill individuals are included among the homeless (Lamb, 1984), and for some, mental illness preceded loss of housing. For others, however, psychiatric symptoms have resulted from the situational crisis of homelessness—if these individuals can be reconnected with stable jobs and affordable housing, their symptoms may subside. Other problems faced by some chronically mentally ill homeless people include, in varying combinations, alcohol and drug abuse, physical illness, entanglements with the law enforcement system, and difficulties in social relationships.

Viewed historically, cycles of reform and neglect in mental health care in the USA often have been stimulated by the transformation of social problems (eg, dependency, senility, criminality, poverty, and racism) into mental health issues (Goldman and Morrissey, 1985). With homelessness, psychiatry and the mental health community must avoid offering once again a mental health solution to a larger social problem. Community care for the chronically mentally ill is still in a fragile and fiscally precarious stage. It could be seriously undermined by false expectations that community support systems will solve the generic problem of homelessness in the USA. Social dependence and homelessness demand social welfare solutions. Disorders need treatment and medical intervention. Mental health professionals must be sensitive to the dual needs of the chronically mentally ill, and adequate resources must be found to deal with their needs.

The elusive goal of a client-centered approach versus a medical-psychiatric-centered system of services for the chronically mentally ill remains a major challenge for public mental health care in the decades ahead. Will psychiatry respond to this challenge in terms of a truly biopsychosocial model of practice? The answer is not known, but it surely will have profound implications for the future of the profession as well as for our ways of thinking about and responding to the social problems posed by mental illness.

REFERENCES

Belknap I: *Human Problems of a State Mental Hospital*. Mc-Graw-Hill, 1956.

Bell NW, Spiegel JP: Social psychiatry: Vagaries of a term. *Arch Gen Psychiatry* 1966;**14**:337.

Brown GW, Birley JLT: Crises and life changes and the onset of schizophrenia. *J Health Soc Behav* 1968;**9**:203.

Brown GW, Harris T: *Social Origins of Depression: A Study of Psychiatric Disorder in Women*. Free Press, 1978.

Caudill W: *The Psychiatric Hospital as a Small Society*. Harvard Univ Press, 1958.

Clausen JA, Huffine CL: Sociocultural and social/psychological factors affecting social responses to mental disorder. *J Health Soc Behav* 1975;**16**:405.

Cockerham W: *Sociology of Mental Disorder*. Prentice-Hall, 1981.

Cocozza JJ, Steadman HJ: Prediction on psychiatry: An example of misplaced confidence in experts. *Soc Probl* 1978; **25**:265.

Coser RL: *Training in Ambiguity: Learning by Doing in a Mental Hospital*. Free Press, 1979.

Dohrenwend BP: Sociocultural and social-psychological factors in the genesis of mental disorders. *J Health Soc Behav* 1975; **16**:365.

Dohrenwend BP, Dohrenwend BS: Social and cultural influences on psychopathology. *Annu Rev Psychol* 1974;**25**:417.

Eisenberg L: Psychiatry and society. *N Engl J Med* 1977; **296**:903.

Faris REL, Dunham HW: *Mental Disorders in Urban Areas*. Univ of Chicago Press, 1939.

Goffman E: *Asylums*. Free Press, 1961.

Goldman HH, Morrissey JP: The alchemy of mental health policy: Homelessness and the fourth cycle of reform. *Am J Public Health* 1985;**75**:727.

Gove W (editor): *The Labeling of Deviance: Evaluating a Perspective*. Halsted, 1975.

Greenley JR, Mechanic D: Patterns of seeking care for psychological problems. In: *The Growth of Bureaucratic Medicine*. Mechanic D (editor). Wiley, 1976.

Gruenberg E: The social breakdown syndrome and its prevention. In: *American Handbook of Psychiatry*, 2nd ed. Arieti S (editor). Basic Books, 1974.

Hollingshead AB, Redlich FC: *Social Class and Mental Illness*. Wiley, 1958.

Holmes TH, Rahe RH: The social readjustment rating scale. *J Psychosom Res* 1967;**11**:213.

Horwitz A: Family, kin, and friend networks in psychiatric help-seeking. *Soc Sci Med* 1978;**12**:297.

Kadushin C: *Why People Go to Psychiatrists*. Atherton, 1969.

Kulka RA, Veroff J, Douvan E: Social class and the use of professional help for personal problems: 1957 and 1976. *J Health Soc Behav* 1979;**20**:2.

Lamb HR (editor): *The Homeless Mentally Ill*. American Psychiatric Press, 1984.

Langner TS, Michael ST: *Life Stress and Mental Health: The Midtown Manhattan Study*. Free Press, 1963.

Light DT: *Becoming Psychiatrists: The Professional Transformation of Self*. Norton, 1980.

Mechanic D: *Mental Health and Social Policy*. Prentice-Hall, 1980.

Morrissey JP, Goldman HH, Klerman LV: *The Enduring Asylum: Cycles of Institutional Reform at Worcester State Hospital*. Grune & Stratton, 1980.

Myers JK, Lindenthal JJ, Pepper MP: Life events, social integration, and psychiatric symptomatology. *J Health Soc Behav* 1975;**16**:421.

Rabkin JG: Stress and psychiatric disorders. In: *Handbook of Stress: Theoretical and Clinical Aspects*. Goldberger L, Breznitz S (editors). Free Press, 1982.

Redlich FC, Pepper MP: Are social psychiatry and community psychiatry subspecialties of psychiatry? *Am J Psychiatry* 1968;**124**:1343.

Scheff T: *Labeling Madness*. Prentice-Hall, 1975.

Sedgwick P: Antipsychiatry from the sixties to the eighties. In: *Deviance and Mental Illness*. Gove W (editor). Sage Publications, 1982.

Srole L: Sociology and psychiatry: Fusions and fissions of identity. In: *Explorations in Psychiatric Sociology*. Roman PM, Trice HM (editors). Davis, 1974.

Srole L et al: *Mental Health in the Metropolis: The Midtown Manhattan Study*. McGraw-Hill, 1962.

Stanton A, Schwartz M: *The Mental Hospital*. Basic Books, 1954.

Strauss A et al: *Psychiatric Institutions and Ideologies*. Free Press, 1964.

Turner RJ, Wagenfeld MD: Occupational mobility and schizophrenia: An assessment of the social causation and social selection hypotheses. *Am Sociol Rev* 1967;**32**:104.

Yarrow MR et al: The psychological meaning of mental illness in the family. *J Soc Issues* 1955;**11**:12.

Contributions of Anthropology to Psychiatry

15

Frank A. Johnson, MD

This chapter will review some of the significant contributions anthropology has made to psychiatry and medicine. Since anthropologists are interested in studying both the similarities and the differences between societies, a variety of health institutions, modes of practice, and manifestations of illness will be presented to illustrate cultural and subcultural diversity. Reference will be made to experience in a number of geographic areas, but this chapter will concentrate mainly on anthropologic factors affecting health care in North American settings. This emphasis is made necessary for reasons of space, but it does introduce some unavoidable bias.

The chapter will be divided into 4 parts: (1) a conceptual and historical overview; (2) a review of the effects of culture on psychiatric disorders and methods of treatment; (3) a review of some cultural features of health care in North American populations; and (4) a discussion of some practical advantages of maintaining a relativistic cultural perspective in the delivery of health care and especially mental health care.

CONCEPTUAL & HISTORICAL OVERVIEW

Definitions

A. Culture: The aggregate of all the beliefs, customs, technologic achievements, language, and history of a people would constitute a culture—although this is only one of many definitions of the word culture. Kroeber and Kluckhohn (1952) apply the term to many different aspects of social organization:

1. Traditional—A culture comprises all of the beliefs, laws, customs, morals, capabilities, and habits of people who cooperatively work and live in an identified social unit (tribes, cities, nations, etc) or in institutions (armed forces, religious orders, hospital staffs, etc). A traditional survey of the culture of physicians would include descriptions of their scientific beliefs, the varieties of medical and surgical subspecialty practices, the work settings, and the economic exchanges and other customs that are features of the delivery of health care.

2. Historical—The term "culture" may be applied to the social heritage—myths of origin, traditions, etc—in a society, transmitted from each generation to the next. A historical resume of the culture of medicine would trace the earliest records of healing procedures, the developments in medical and surgical treatment up to the present time, and the ways in which theories of disease and actual practices have been transmitted through apprenticeships, formal education, and literary records.

3. Normative—Studies of cultures are inevitably concerned with the rules, "norms," standards, ideals, and values that regulate behavior in a society. In the study of medical institutions, such norms would reflect both the implicit and explicit legal and ethical duties owed by physicians and patients to each other.

4. Psychologic—Cultural studies are concerned also with the techniques of adjustment, problem solving, and learning and the ways in which customs, norms, and beliefs are inculcated. In a medical setting, special note might be taken of subjective and motivational factors in health-related interactions, including the patient's fears, expectations, and psychologic defenses against the idea of being ill.

5. Structural—Examination of cultures is concerned with the "anatomy" of the social organizations that bind societies together. In the institution of medicine, the organizational "anatomy" includes agencies of government, accrediting and licensing boards, health-related industries and manufacturers, and, of course, all of the educational institutions and specialty academies and societies that train and certify health care professionals.

6. Genetic—Culture is concerned with the study of products, processes, and artifacts generated by various societies or institutions and with the origin and transmission of ideas and products from the standpoint of their historical significance. The "genetic" aspects of the culture of medicine would include a succession of surgical instruments, pharmacologic substances, and the records of technologic achievements that accompanied their invention and use.

In summary, culture is concerned with the rules concerning communication (language, gestures, rituals); child rearing and training; procurement and preparation of food; family, kinship, and political structures; marital, gender, and leadership roles; beliefs and rituals; ownership of real and personal property; regulation of aggression, sexual behavior, and play; and the use of tools, the exchange of goods, and the designation of services.

B. Cross-Cultural, Transcultural: Before presenting some background information about the field of anthropology, it will be useful to define 2 terms that are commonly confused. The term "cross-cultural" applies specifically to comparisons made between 2 or more distinct social groups to clarify differences or similarities that characterize their group distinctiveness—eg, the differences in child rearing between urban and rural Peruvians. The term "transcultural" is ordinarily applied to characteristics commonly or universally found in all human societies. The distinction between cultural specificity and universal human characteristics is pertinent to the study of medical and psychiatric institutions and to descriptions of patterns of illness.

Two other terms are used in anthropology to distinguish between different modes of communicating and interpreting human experience. Anthropologists use the terms "emic" and "etic" to differentiate between 2 levels of description and explanation. The term "emic," derived from the linguistic expression "phonemic," denotes the vocabulary and explanations of customs and practices used by individuals *within* a particular culture. The term "etic," derived from "phonetic," refers to scientific explanations of cultural practices employed in descriptions made by individuals *outside* the particular culture. Applied to the institution of medicine, "etic" features would be found in the body of accumulated technical data through which diseases are understood, treated, and prevented; practitioners are trained; and health institutions are formed. The "emic" features of medicine would represent the various ways in which people actually experience illness (explain their symptoms; feel pain and fright), clinicians encounter patients (look, feel, and "poke around" for signs and symptoms), and health institutions function in real life (as collections of people with their own attitudes toward their jobs, their health care roles, and the patients they treat). These 2 different ways of looking at human experience are fundamental to an understanding of the cultural aspects of psychiatry and medicine.

C. "Ethno-" Terms: The basic meaning of the combining form "ethno-" is "race, people" (Gk *ethnos*).

1. "Ethnic" (noun) denotes an individual who possesses traits representative of a particular cultural or subcultural group. The adjective "ethnic" refers to the characteristics typical of a specific subculture.

2. "Ethnicity" is an abstract noun denoting qualities recognized by individuals within a given culture as indicative of group identity and by outsiders as attributes that make the group "different" from one's own group and from other ethnic groups.

3. "Ethnography" denotes a written documentary that describes the specific attributes of a given culture. The subjects of ethnographies usually are small, ex-

otic societies. However, an ethnography may focus on a health institution or the peculiar experiences of groups of patients whose distinctive life-styles are mandated by chronic disability (eg, the lives of quadriplegics). Ethnographies may be looked on as "case studies" of particular small societies.

4. "Ethnology" denotes a more comprehensive record of a culture, superseding a written ethnography to include a compendium of the relics, artifacts, literature, myths, beliefs, and cultural practices of a particular society. An ethnology is often organized to go beyond description to present *conclusions* concerning the aggregate patterns of a particular social group. Often this is systematically compared to other cultures or to general categories of social organizations.

5. "Ethnocentrism" denotes 2 separate but related principles: first, the tendency of all cultural groups to accept their own culture as a kind of universal "given"—often without imagining that other human societies might see the world differently; and second, an innate sense of cultural superiority over others on the basis of ethnicity alone. All societies tend to regard nonmembers as potentially barbarous, primitive, and savage and other cultures as not only different but "strange" and even threatening.

6. "Ethos" denotes the collective beliefs, temperaments, and dominant assumptions that influence the formation of "typical" personalities within certain cultures.

Anthropology as a Social Science

Until the late 1800s, the customs and beliefs of exotic societies were reported by explorers and missionaries. In the 17th and 18th centuries, exotic cultures were romanticized as "noble savages," "unspoiled," and closer to nature and God than urban "civilized" folk. In the 19th century, exotic societies were made notorious by their peculiarities and described in pejorative terms as "bestial," "lascivious," "heathen," and "primitive." The customs and languages of these societies were negatively compared with those of Western European industrial societies. European civilization at that time was regarded as the high point in a continuum of progress wrongly thought to be a social form of Darwinian evolution. Slowly and with some difficulty, the science of anthropology was helpful in refuting theories of "racial superiority" spuriously based on political, economic, or historical grounds. Unfortunately, the field has at times created its own biases and stereotypes.

Anthropology has undergone considerable change in the past century. As is true of psychiatry and medicine also, anthropology is concerned with both group and individual behavior. Although the field focuses on the collective behaviors of groups in their distinctive manifestations of living, the method of study often uses information gathered from individual culture bearers ("informants"). To the extent possible, the anthropologist lives among the people and uses "participant-observation" for the purpose of examining as well as seeing the culture being studied. Ethnographers attempt to shed presuppositions and to keep their descriptions of what is seen and heard authentic according to the "emic" terms and explanations provided by the informants. Information must be collected over a period of months or years—preferably during repeated visits. Information relating to medicine and psychiatry is often gathered in the form of prevailing attitudes and beliefs about disease and of descriptions of practices regarding child rearing, health care, and nutrition.

Historically, the fields of medicine and anthropology have been associated in informal and coincidental ways. Physicians commonly went along on expeditions of discovery from continental Europe and England and contributed written accounts of the customs of the people they visited, the occurrence of unusual diseases, or the use of folk remedies to treat disease. With colonization, medical missionaries did informal fieldwork, describing the cultures and languages of the societies they visited. In the earlier years of this century, anthropologists themselves did not accentuate illness variables in their ethnographic work. More recently, anthropology, medicine, and psychiatry have contributed to a specialty called **medical anthropology** that focuses on describing the experience of illness, the institutional characteristics of health care and "patienthood," and the variety of physical and cultural features associated with illness in various societies. Nowadays, this includes the study of these factors in industrial societies as well as developing ones and involves looking at the manifestations of established, traditional, and folk models of care. A subspecialty within the fields of public health and epidemiology called **ethnomedicine** analyzes the rates and characteristics of illness in terms of specific physical, climatologic, and cultural factors affecting particular populations. **Ethnopsychiatry** is a highly specialized field whose practitioners look for explanations of mental and behavioral manifestations in the context of cultural features that may influence the frequency and form of adaptive and maladaptive behaviors.

Since the mid 1800s, the roles of environmental, ecologic, and economic factors in the incidence and prevalence of illness have been studied in an attempt to explain how pathophysiologic processes affect different individuals and groups. In American psychiatry, recognition of the crucial significance of these factors has popularized **biopsychosocial models** of disease (Engel, 1978). The idea is gaining ground that psychiatric disability can only be comprehensively understood through consideration of 4 systems: **biologic systems**—anatomic, cellular, and biochemical factors; **personality systems**—which explain individual behavior in terms of motivations, habit patterns, and cognitive characteristics; **social systems**—in which the characteristics of large groups of people are related to the dynamics of disease or illness behaviors; and **cultural systems**—in which the customs and behavioral inclinations of particular groups are examined to determine their influence on health and disease.

As a science and academic discipline, anthropology is divided into a number of subspecialty areas, 4 of which relate to medicine and psychiatry: physical anthropology, linguistics, cultural anthropology, and psychologic anthropology. **Physical anthropology** involves systematic study of ancient and modern constitutional adaptations of human beings. This specialty is concerned with variations in skeletal growth, body habitus, skin pigmentation, dentition, and muscular development of diverse groups of human beings from prehistoric times to the present. It is concerned with the relationship of dietary factors to physical size and to the development or avoidance of specific diseases (eg, thalassemia, kwashiorkor, sickle cell anemia). Physical anthropologists analyze the genetic factors associated with distributions of blood type, immune reactions, and enzyme deficiencies in their interaction with variables present in pathologic processes within particular cultures.

The contemporary field of **linguistics** developed out of an association with anthropology in the study of exotic and diverse languages. Spoken and written language not only reflects the worldview of a culture but also shapes and limits the way members of a culture express their ideas and perceive the world around them. Study of the diversity of spoken languages and of other cultural differences has reinforced the concept of **cultural relativism.** This principle holds that the language and customs of a people are to be examined in the context of that particular culture and judged primarily in terms of their utility to that culture. Cultural relativism argues against value-laden comparisons between cultures and supports a culture-bound analysis of language and custom.

Cultural anthropology contributes to medicine and psychiatry in 3 principal ways. The first is by providing descriptions of cultures and subcultural groups and their customs, communications, and beliefs. Such understandings have broad implications for the incidence and prevalence of disease, behavior during illness, and the nature of cooperation with health care specialists in preventing or treating disease.

A second major contribution of cultural anthropology to medicine and psychiatry consists of the rich body of information that has increased our understanding of certain universal characteristics of individuals, families, and groups.

The third contribution lies in cross-cultural methods of research that have been applied to clinical studies in medicine and psychiatry. These methods have been fruitful in defining both variations and shared features in the experience of disease among various ethnic and national groups. For example, the incidence of gastric carcinoma, hypertension, and myocardial infarction among some descendants of Japanese immigrants who settled in the USA and Brazil has been compared with the incidence observed in cousin cohorts in Japan. Results showed lower rates of cardiovascular disease among Japanese who did not emigrate but higher rates of gastric carcinoma. Since the hereditary factors are relatively invariant in both groups, some combination of dietary, environmental, and stress factors must be sought in an effort to explain the differences in incidence of these diseases.

Psychologic anthropology focuses on the personality factors and motivational characteristics of individuals that may be correlated with cultural adaptation and maladaptation, adjustment, and disability. Such interests have shed light on the personality characteristics of cultural or national groups (sometimes called "national character"), usually in an attempt to link such characteristics to child-rearing practices, environmental conditions, or distinctive cognitive styles based upon language, physical adaptation, or racial-historical features of these societies. Studies of "national character" have fallen into disrepute, partly because they were politicized and exaggerated into ethnic stereotypes. More recently, studies in psychologic anthropology have stimulated interest in the cognitive aspects of cultural experience. This is investigated through meticulous study of the subjective and introspective lives of individuals within the context of their own cultures. Since these methods look at both self-presentations and cognitive styles within distinctive cultural groups, the potential contributions for psychiatry and medicine are great. If the earlier insights of cultural anthropology are regarded as the "gross anatomy" of social organizations, these newer techniques could be seen as their "histology," through which the microscopic features of clinical transactions can be examined. The outlook for contributions from psychologic anthropology in clarifying illness behavior and disease experience by such techniques is most promising.

CULTURE & PSYCHIATRIC DISORDERS

MEDICAL & PSYCHIATRIC "NORMALITY"

The definition of abnormality and disease in general medical conditions is relatively straightforward, but distinguishing normality and abnormality in psychiatry is a more complex process. Offer and Sabshin (1966) have written about the distinction between disease and health, normality and abnormality, both in general medicine and in psychiatry. They see the process of deciding what is "normal" from 3 perspectives. First, they note that health is often defined in terms of the simple **absence of disease**—ie, regardless of *latent* physical or temperamental abnormality, an asymptomatic nondisabled person is in "normal health." By these criteria, a 42-year-old, slightly overweight American car salesman with narrowed coronary vessels and an aggressive personality style who was experiencing *no* symptoms would be "normal."

Their second perspective uses **statistical frequency** as a criterion for normality. The standard bell-shaped curve would thus define normality in reference to physical or temperamental factors surveyed among large population groups. By these criteria, our 42-year-old car salesman would be "abnormal" in his excessive drive and work orientation and in his vascular changes—irrespective of the absence of symptoms.

A third perspective on normality consists of using **cultural criteria** to establish ranges of "health" and "disease," based upon the idealized beliefs and assumptions held by particular societies and subcultures. For example, at a behavioral level, assertiveness and open competition are positively endorsed by North Americans. Using cultural criteria, then, our salesman now would be considered "normal"—since it is desirable to be eager and aggressive at work.

To understand the confusion inherent in these separate definitions, the distinction between cultural norms and statistical norms is crucial. Cultural norms determine ranges of acceptable behavior based upon idealized criteria that dictate how people *should* dress, how they *may* speak in certain situations, and when and where and how they *may* engage in various behaviors. These idealized standards ("norms") apply to the almost limitless range of human behaviors and actions. These norms are also complex in their variation according to gender, age, and situation. They are not based on any statistical probability that "most people *will or will not* do certain things" but rather on the emotionally compelling, prescriptive basis that "people *should or should not* do certain things." Even though these norms are not substantiated in fact, they act to provide idealized (ie, normative) standards promoted by all societies in their definitions of "right and wrong," or "good and bad," including criteria regarding health and disease.

An integrated perspective described by Offer and Sabshin consists of an **operational blending** of the first three. They conclude that all illness—physical and mental—is best defined from all of the foregoing perspectives. By these criteria, our salesman would be statistically "abnormal," both in his latent myocardial disease and in his overly stressful adaptation to work, even though he is "normal" by symptomatic and cultural criteria. According to an integrated approach, a comprehensive description of this man's health status includes a combination of all 3 perspectives on normality.

CULTURAL INFLUENCES ON CLASSIFICATIONS

The taxonomy of mental and behavioral disorders is derived from combinations of descriptive, etiologic, pathophysiologic, and psychologic criteria. This process has been going on since antiquity in the attempt to "explain" human behavior and misbehavior and continues today in the ongoing effort to apply medical, psychologic, and sociologic criteria to these problems.

Many attempts at systematic classification (including "folk taxonomies") emphasize differences between psychotic and nonpsychotic disorders. Even allowing for cultural variability, Murphy (1976) found that systematic classifications worldwide define the symptom clusters of schizophrenic disorders as psychotic. Most societies classify less socially disruptive disorders as nonpsychotic. From a cross-cultural perspective these nonpsychotic conditions, although they show great variation, can be informally subclassified into (1) **moderate maladaptations and abnormalities** (eg, "dysthymic disorder," "conversion disorder"); (2) **characterologic abnormalities** (eg, "paranoid personality," "narcissistic personality"); or (3) **abnormalities of adjustment** (eg, "conduct disorder," "situational crisis"). Furthermore, many classifications differentiate between behavioral abnormalities due to physical causes (hereditary, toxic, traumatic) and those of obscure origin. In primitive taxonomies, various abnormalities are attributed to magical or telepathic influences—intrusions of "bad spirits," "loss" (or theft) of certain faculties, or the effects of hexes or curses by another person. Both physical and mental disorders may be attributed to deliberate or accidental violation of a ceremonial taboo or failure to observe culturally mandated rituals following deaths, accidents, or quarrels. Scientific explanations of functional disorders are apt to include a combination of hereditary, developmental, social-interactional, and concurrent stress factors. All but the first of these are heavily influenced by cultural differences in the processes of socialization and by differing traditions about what constitutes stress in one society and not in another. Although some sources of stress (eg, puberty, bereavement) are universal, the *meanings* of such stresses and the ceremonial resources for dealing with them vary widely in different cultures. Thus, the processes of diagnosis and treatment may differ in different cultures in 4 ways: (1) in the definitions of what constitute symptoms of disease; (2) in the interpretation and presumed causes of such symptoms; (3) in the classification of symptoms into syndromes; and (4) in perceptions about what constitutes an acceptable method of treatment.

Regardless of their utility and validity, all classifications of psychiatric syndromes are affected by cultural variables. Even refined classifications such as are found in the *Diagnostic and Statistical Manual of Mental Disorders (DSM-III)* or the *Manual of the International Statistical Classification of Diseases, Injuries and Causes of Death (ICD-9)* are composed of verifiable signs and symptoms *and* subjective cultural judgments about what is abnormal. Despite attempts to seek a consensus among specialists in classification (who use statistical frequencies of occurrence and objective criteria), culturally loaded judgments still affect conclusions about the abnormality or normality of these conditions. *DSM-III* explicitly acknowledges this in warning that shared beliefs of religious or cultural groups may be difficult to distinguish from delusions to someone outside the culture. They warn that

such a conclusion is unwarranted, implying that all symptoms must be understood in terms of their meaning within particular cultures and subcultures. This does not mean that classifications of mental abnormality are arbitrary, but it acknowledges that cultural criteria affect the scientific classification of behavioral abnormalities. Many studies show that clinicians vary greatly in their responses when asked to diagnose mental disorders even within a particular national group or culture. Such variability is more prominent in cross-cultural studies or in studies that show differences in diagnostic conclusions about ethnic minorities based either upon communication problems or racially oppressive "pathologizing." Low socioeconomic status is also associated with higher rates of diagnosed illness and may account for some of this variability. (See Chapter 14 for further discussion.)

A simplified way of looking at the effects of culture on the phenomenology, form, and incidence of psychiatric conditions is set forth in Table 15–1. This divides some representative conditions into 2 groups: relatively invariant and relatively variant. Those syndromes described under the *DSM-III* categories as schizophrenic disorders, major affective disorders, organic mental disorders, mental retardation, and substance use disorders have many culturally invariant features. This means that these conditions tend to display similar manifestations, regardless of cultural locale. In contrast, the personality disorders and the syndromes that represent brief or prolonged abnormal reactions to stress (conduct, adjustment, anxiety, somatoform, dissociative, and dysthymic disorders) show a higher degree of cross-cultural variation. Such variation is expressed both in the manifestations of these disorders and in their frequency or infrequency of occurrence.

As might be expected, there is least cross-cultural difference among the "relatively invariant" conditions with respect to their reported incidence and prevalence. Even so, some qualitative differences in their clinical presentations are evident in different cultures, and the meanings and consequences of these condi-

Table 15–1. Relative cross-cultural variance in selected mental and behavioral disorders.*

Relatively invariant
1. Schizophrenic disorders
2. Affective disorders
3. Organic mental disorders
4. Mental retardation
5. Substance use disorders

Relatively variant
1. Conduct disorders
2. Adjustment disorders
3. Anxiety disorders
4. Somatoform disorders
5. Dissociative disorders
6. Dysthymic disorders
7. Personality disorders (axis II)
8. Atypical psychosis

*DSM-III categories.

tions differ according to cultural specification. For example, Japanese schizophrenic patients are more taciturn than North American patients, require less external constraint, and are more adaptive to group conditions in mental hospitals (Caudill and Doi, 1963). Some acute schizophrenic breakdowns in young Japanese men may be accompanied by violence directed toward the mother; this is not characteristic of schizophrenic American men and is believed to be related to the extraordinarily close bond that exists between mothers and sons in Japan. In another cross-national comparison, Townsend (1978) reported that German patients, doctors, and families of patients tend to see schizophrenia primarily as a medical illness whose treatment requires following the advice of doctors and nurses, whereas North Americans, though continuing to seek a medical (ie, biophysical) explanation for schizophrenia, place greater emphasis on the psychologic (ie, personal life history) features of this disorder, with the result that patients are perceived as being partly responsible for their illness and for the success or failure of treatment. One of the commonest qualitative cross-cultural differences in schizophrenia concerns the content of delusions. Delusions characteristically are woven out of the threads which represent the good and evil powers of particular societies (the FBI, Satan, famous personages). Also, some societies favor persecutory themes, while others accentuate religious scenarios.

In the "relatively variant" conditions, broad cultural differences are common and prominent in the manifestations of syndromes. For example, the incidence and symptom patterns of mild to moderate depressive syndromes (dysthymia) show high cross-cultural variation. In Japan and some other Asian communities, depression is more commonly manifested in psychophysiologic symptoms, hypochondriasis, or weakness. In Japan, the cultural suppression of both the cognitive and affective features of depression is in sharp contrast to most Western societies, where it is culturally permissible to manifest some degree of self-contempt, lassitude, and outwardly visible sadness in public interactions. Even if displayed, the meaning of various dysthymic, anxious, phobic, and other "psychoneurotic" symptoms is culturally variable. Since many of these conditions were "discovered" and characterized by Western commentators, cross-cultural comparison is difficult. Although some of these syndromes occur worldwide, specific features are observed most prominently in Western European or Middle Eastern cultures. In other cultures, feelings of sadness, fear, or confusion may be suppressed or redirected into more acceptable forms of expression. Tanaka-Matsumi (1979) has described a common "psychoneurotic" somatoform-type illness among young adults in Japan called **taijin-kyofusho,** characterized by a fear of eye and social contact ("anthrophobia"), concerns about blushing, and obsessions concerning body odor. It is related to the traditional pattern of social interaction in Japan, which places a high premium on the protocol for self-presentation,

something not commonly expected in interactions taking place in most Western societies.

Personality disorders, as defined in current classifications, are even more culturally variable than either the major psychoses or syndromes of dissociative or somatoform symptoms. Although certain aspects of characterologic adaptation are unquestionably universal, in different cultures the manner in which these basic adaptations are blended and stylized by differential socialization makes their cross-cultural standardization very difficult. Moreover, since "disorders of personality" involve a **maladaptive exaggeration** of cultural styles, direct cross-comparison is correspondingly even more complicated.

"Exotic" Psychoses

The most exotic culturally defined symptoms are represented in *DSM-III* by the "atypical psychoses." They are characterized by relatively short duration of illness and are usually brought on by serious psychogenic stress in individuals with mild to moderate difficulties in characterologic adaptation. Pre- and postmorbid status is variable and may include "normal," "hysteroid," eccentric, or violent personality types. These psychotic disorders have a rapid onset, are often exhibitionistic in their symptoms, and are not associated with exposure to toxins, trauma, or metabolic disease. Delusions may be present, but hallucinations are exceptional. Behavioral disorganization and eccentricity are usually more pronounced than are symptoms of disorganization in "thought process." A number of "exotic" syndromes that roughly fit this pattern of atypical psychosis have been described in various societies. The following descriptions of amok, windigo psychosis, and hysterical psychosis are offered as examples.

Amok. This disorder, reported in Malaysia, is characterized by a sudden outburst of destructive violence accompanied by rage and depersonalization, sometimes culminating in violence directed against persons, animals, or inanimate objects. The outbursts often subside into a period of exhaustion or catatonic trance, and the patient is amnesic for the episode following recovery. As Carr (1978) has reported, this exotic syndrome is manifested in varying degrees of severity, some of which are not psychotic. Carr also points out that amok may be factitiously simulated or intentionally induced.

Windigo psychosis. This syndrome is reported among some Native American groups living under harsh environmental conditions in Northern Canada (among some Cree, Ojibwa, and Salteaux communities). The disorder is manifested by obsessive fear of magical transformation into a compulsive cannibal ("windigo") through sorcery. Occurring in hunting societies, the syndrome appears to be related to the mythical belief in possession and transformation brought on by guilt and depression over failure to succeed as a hunter. In vulnerable individuals, this failure may be experienced as the forbidden desire to eat human flesh, which then is unconsciously projected as spirit possession. As with amok, nonpsychotic versions of this syndrome are common.

Hysterical psychosis. (In *DSM-III,* this is called "brief reactive psychosis.") By definition, episodes of hysterical psychosis last less than 2 weeks and are typified by a sudden onset, following stress, of incoherence, depersonalization, and hyperactivity or severe depression, sometimes with looseness of association and disconnectedness from the environment. Agitated, flamboyant, or bizarre behavior occurs in some cases, and the patient is often amnesic for events leading up to and during the psychotic period. Defined as occurring among European and North American populations by Hollender and Hirsch (1964) and others, these syndromes could be considered to be time-limited depressive or agitated psychotic episodes in persons with premorbid histrionic personality disorder (*DSM-III,* axis II). Some authors see these and other related conditions as representing a universal pattern of short-term psychoses that take different forms according to the specific cultures in which they occur. Such a view, however, may obscure the fact that the syndromes may not be homogeneous but may occur along a spectrum of culture-specific reactions to internal conflict or external stress. Carr (1978), for example, has related amok to a sudden breaking away from the strong Malaysian constraints against showing anger. Kleinman (1980), writing about the "culture-bound syndromes," points out that the flamboyance and "exotic" characteristics of these disorders force the observer outside the culture to note their "cultural qualities." This should not obscure the fact that all behavioral conditions are "culture-bound" in the sense that they can only be expressed through the symbolic and communicative processes available within the culture.

Nonpsychotic Disorders

Exotic syndromes that superficially resemble psychoses—especially to clinicians outside the culture—may prove on closer inspection to be acute disorders of brief duration featuring mixtures of what in Western nosology would be considered anxiety, somatoform, and dissociative symptomatology (*DSM-III*). These may include manifestations of panic disorders (eg, hyperventilation, severe anxiety, fear of dying or hurting others), conversion disorders (eg, hysterical seizures, hysterical paralysis), or dissociative disorders (eg, amnesia, derealization, trance, or psychogenic fugue states).

Arctic hysteria (piblokto). This phenomenon occurs chiefly among Inuit (Eskimo) women and is manifested by anxiety and depression (crying, trembling, screaming) and fuguelike states (running naked in the snow, leaping into water), accompanied by confusion, depersonalization, and sometimes violence toward themselves and others. Foulkes (1972) has offered a multifactorial hypothesis explaining the condition as a result of early socialization factors, poor nutrition and vitamin D uptake, abnormal mobilization of plasma calcium, and social isolation.

Susto. Widely reported from Latin America, this syndrome is manifested by states of severe fright (Sp *susto*) and fear of loss of soul (Sp *espanto*), believed to be brought on by magical causes or by real or imagined combinations of interpersonal or physical causes (eg, humiliation, physical injury, curses imposed by other persons or by spirits). In addition to obsessions about who or what is causing such terror, the victims usually show diffuse anxiety, insomnia, anorexia, fatigue, restlessness, and social withdrawal. Susto often includes a fear of "evil eye," the operation of black magic, and spirit possession.

Koro. This syndrome is observed in males in some sections of China and Southeast Asia and is characterized by guilt and obsessions concerning sexual functioning. Victims have the somatic delusion that the penis will retract into the abdomen, potentially causing death. There may be a preoccupation with losing semen, coexisting with increased appetite for sexual encounters and sometimes worries concerning impotence. Diffuse anxiety is usually severe and accompanied by the inability to work and function socially. The syndrome is common in Southeast Asia (Singapore, Thailand) and India and basically resembles what in the West would be termed panic disorder.

CULTURAL ASPECTS OF MENTAL HEALTH PRACTICES

Just as the descriptive and etiologic classifications of mental disorders vary according to cultural factors, the status of practitioners and the range and types of treatments offered are highly variable. In almost all societies, tiers or levels of practitioners are available for the diagnosis and treatment of both somatic and psychiatric conditions. These range from specialists representing the scientific and technical tradition to folk and spiritual healers.

In the USA, psychiatrists, psychologists, psychiatric social workers, and nurse specialists provide psychiatric care either alone or in therapeutic teams. In many areas in the USA and Canada, counseling for psychologic problems is available through licensed practitioners working in agency, institutional, or private settings. Blends of spiritual and counseling procedures are undertaken by some members of the clergy, nowadays usually by persons trained in such techniques. Nonpsychiatric medical practitioners also see and treat many mild to moderately disabled individuals and may prescribe antidepressants or sedatives for depression and anxiety. Treatments for habit disorders are offered in clinics specializing in weight reduction, cessation of smoking, alcoholism, or drug abuse. Group therapies, including self-help groups, are available in some communities. Alcoholics Anonymous offers a widely accessible program for the control of pathologic drinking.

In ethnic subcommunities, folk remedies are available for a variety of behavioral difficulties, psychologic problems, or refractory medical conditions.

Faith healing is claimed by some fundamentalist Protestant denominations. Christian Science readers are specially trained to assist members of that faith in the restoration of physical, mental, and spiritual health. Despite the widespread availability of various spiritual healers in North America, the rational, empirical traditions of medical and psychiatric care offered by medical and psychiatric practitioners represent the prevailing view. Some recent changes in this long-standing trend will be discussed in a following section.

CULTURAL ASPECTS OF HEALTH CARE IN THE USA

This section will discuss cultural aspects of health care in 2 ways: first, by examining the characteristics of the culturally and regionally diverse populations in the USA; and second, by describing some of the cultural features of North American health care institutions and practitioners.

CULTURAL ASPECTS OF THE POPULATION IN THE USA

North American society is one of the most pluralistic ever seen, as witness the striking variations in ethnic background, regional identification, religious affiliation, life-style, and economic and other class-oriented stratifications. Historically, this pluralism is a result of overseas colonization followed by waves of immigration and the tribal diversity of the Native American population. Colonial migration brought British, Dutch, Spanish, and French expeditions financed and encouraged by trading companies that gave rise to agricultural, mining, and shipping industries. Commercial activity brought infusions of the political, legal, religious, and cultural attributes of major European countries. In addition to European colonization and immigration, the importation of African slaves and the later influx of a large Hispanic population in the Southwest have further contributed to American ethnic pluralism. Between 1820 and 1983, about 50 million immigrants entered the USA legally, three-fourths of them from continental Europe and the United Kingdom. Smaller populations emigrated from the Pacific Basin, Asia, the Middle East, and Central and South America. The largest numbers of immigrants arrived on the East Coast during the years 1890–1910. Many of them stayed in the large industrial cities in the Northeast and Midwest; others moved toward the Great Plains, the Northwest, and California.

Despite the striking variety and heterogeneity of both colonization and immigration, the USA has con-

tinued to reflect a modified version of the cultural characteristics of its British antecedents. Although it is difficult and arbitrary to list these characteristics, they cluster around what have been generalized as white Anglo-Saxon Protestant (WASP) values. These fundamental values include a belief in non-Catholic Christianity, freedom, materialism, and individualism. There is a strong investment in productivity and work, sometimes expressed as the American version of the Protestant work ethic. This ethic promotes the idea that those who toil will be rewarded and, conversely, that those who do not toil may well go hungry. A corollary to this belief is acceptance of social stratification (unequal availability of rewards) as natural, because success is ultimately an individual responsibility. There is an explicit commitment to the values of capitalism, ownership of private property, and competition for resources in a laissez-faire marketplace. A respect for civil order and social propriety coexists alongside an attitude of disdain for authoritarian systems of government, religion, or social control. Education is a prized achievement, and the belief persists that technologic and pragmatic solutions exist or can be devised for human problems. Independence, or at least its outward trappings, is highly valued, along with the virtues of self-sufficiency, self-reliance, and, more recently, self-actualization. Protracted states of dependency due to "inferiority," disability, handicap, or unemployment tend to be devalued. Since medical patients often lapse into transient or permanent states of dependency, this causes problems in the relationship between patients, health care providers, and society.

Americans are described as being overly concerned with personal cleanliness and respectability. Compared to European society, they are ambivalent about sexuality, manifesting both a puritanical belief (inherited from both Protestant and Catholic backgrounds) that sex is "bad" and a libertarian attitude that recognizes sexual expression as an individual right that may be enjoyed if not injurious (or scandalous) to others. As a compromise, then, passion and sex in America are "all right" as long as they are not offensive to others or do not seriously interfere with work or family life. Family life itself accentuates the nuclear, one-generation unit, stressing the independence of children after maturity (18–21 years) and the financial autonomy of parents following retirement. Small families are desirable, and there is a normative emphasis on educating them toward independence and upward mobility.

One must remember that these values, derived from the dominant WASP culture, are listed as idealized cultural "norms"—therefore, not necessarily what most of the population actually does but rather what they say they should do. Patients may experience psychologic conflict in their sense of failure to achieve these inflated standards. Persons from minorities also may feel trapped between inflated expectations and diminished opportunities to exemplify the norms.

As in the generalizations about fundamental WASP

values, some statements about American norms for the "sick role" may be made. The conceptual definitions of this role were formulated by Parsons (1951) in idealized terms of institutional expectations. He saw the sick role as outlined by variations among 2 sets of "rights" (ie, exemptions) and "duties" (ie, obligations). Sick people were exempt from responsibility for their condition and from normal social role performance. They were, however, obligated to seek professional assistance and to try to get well. Sick roles are very complex. For example, disabled people often play the part differently on different stages. Their role as performed for their families and friends may differ from what is perceived by health professionals, employers, or insurance company adjusters. Socioeconomic class, occupation, age, or life situation can also affect the way in which the sick role is assumed, depending upon the emotional implications of being disabled and how these affect the working and personal lives of different people. A duodenal ulcer may be a "red badge of courage" for an advertising executive but a sign of physical weakness for a machine shop worker. Sick roles also vary according to the nature of primary gain (eg, unconscious need to be dependent or exempt from blame) and secondary gain (various realistic reinforcements and benefits that accompany the sick role).

Doctors and other health professionals are themselves ambivalent about the sick roles of their patients. They may compassionately treat patients with myocardial infarction but still resent the fact that "these people didn't take proper care of themselves in the first place." Physicians may urge their patients to "take it easy" and recover gradually and at the same time worry that patients may be exaggerating residual symptoms or trying to prolong the special privileges of convalescence. Physicians may openly resent persistence of the sick role in people they seem unable to help or "cure." Worst of all, doctors readily become exasperated with persons who "enjoy bad health" (hypochondriacs) or who are always vaguely, annoyingly, but never seriously sick ("crocks").

However, the most important conclusion about sick roles among Americans compared to people of other nationalities is that they are quite diverse—reflecting wide differences in ethnicity, life-style, forms of health care, socioeconomic status, and geographic region. Furthermore, sick roles change among subcultural groups as their explanations of disease and acceptance of establishment health care take on the characteristics of the dominant society through assimilation.

The overlapping terms "acculturation" and "assimilation" help describe the adaptation of immigrant groups to the culture of the USA. **Acculturation** is defined as a socialization process through which minority groups are gradually incorporated into the dominant culture. It is divided into "internal" and "external" manifestations: internal in the sense of a deep investment in the cultural norms and attitudes of the host society, including acquisition of the language, beliefs, attitudes, and behaviors of the prevailing culture; and external as connoting a superficial accommodation to the practices and protocols of the society. For example, some second-generation Chicanos may be highly Americanized in their consumer orientation, use of health care facilities, and use of English as a second language, while at the same time they may retain and prefer their subcultural identification as Mexican-Americans in the nature of their family roles, their preference for speaking Spanish, and their desire for Latin American foods, living in ethnic neighborhoods, and cultivating social networks primarily within the subculture. **Assimilation** is a term used to denote the eventual disappearance of cultural traits that tend to distinguish individuals from the normative characteristics of the host society. In the USA, assimilation ordinarily means the acquisition of WASP traits, making the latecomers indistinguishable from other assimilated Americans. This includes the use of nondialectal American English and, regardless of ethnic background, the acceptance of American "middle-class" values.

The "melting pot" was an exaggerated assimilation model at the turn of the century, a metaphor that conveyed 2 things: first, that new ethnic groups would be "melted down" and assimilated; and second, that the result would be a new amalgam. Although some immigrant groups (notably those from the United Kingdom, Scandinavia, and Western Europe) were readily assimilated within 2 generations, this was not true in the case of Eastern Europeans, Jews, Asians, Native Americans, Hispanics, and blacks. Furthermore, although the amalgam did change in some ways, many of the suppositions about what Americans ought to be like did not change in response to infusions of immigrant cultures. Such a melting pot ideology also acted to obscure the persistent refusal to admit blacks, Native Americans, and "unmeltable ethnics" (Novak, 1971) to full political, civil, and economic participation in American society.

Some of the earliest improvements in the status of minority and ethnic groups occurred with the unionization of labor early in this century and with the development of coalitions of ethnic groups in big cities. These groups gradually acquired political power, particularly in large midwestern and northeastern American cities beginning in the 1920s. By the 1950s, minority groups began to devise long-term plans for acquiring equivalent civil, educational, and economic opportunities. Basic to their strategy was a recognition that assimilation toward a WASP, American middle-class norm was a process that allowed only small numbers of people to achieve status commensurate with that of nonethnic groups in the larger society. Recognizing this, leaders concentrated on the development of positive ethnic consciousness, political solidarity, and open hostility toward oppressors. Increased opportunities were sought through local, state, and national legislation and in the federal courts. Opportunities first realized in the armed forces and in the federal and state civil service gradually led to greater participation in the open labor market, along with increased access to educational institutions, professions, and the trades. Accompanying these determinative changes in legislation and judicial proceedings, publicity about ethnic and minority experience was influential both in gaining visibility and in making public displays of discriminatory or defamatory attitudes unfashionable.

Affirmative action programs were extended to include women as another legally designated minority, and a series of laws were enacted to equalize opportunities for entry into trades, professions, and educational and training programs. In the past, like other institutions in the USA, the health professions had traditions for training and hiring that discouraged or openly excluded minorities and women. Medical colleges and schools of nursing practiced informal or explicit exclusion of blacks, Jews, and sometimes Catholics, usually with the rationalization that "they have their own schools." Other medical schools, including state institutions, used quota systems that allowed a trickle of ethnics, minorities, and women into the practice of medicine. Similarly, some internships, residencies, and hospital staffs were essentially "closed" to ethnic applicants. Women were of course recruited into nursing and laboratory technology. Blacks and women were abundantly represented among the maintenance, housekeeping, and laundry workers. Since the early 1970s, these trends have been reversed, so that quota systems and exclusion practices are now expressly forbidden by law.

Another important group of Americans who have benefited by affirmative action legislation primarily designed to improve the lot of ethnic minorities and women are the middle-aged and older persons who have used these precedents in protesting discriminatory hiring or firing practices on the basis of age and station in life. Federal medical assistance legislation (Medicare) has extended essential benefits to this needy and illness-prone population, with the result that independent and dignified existence in the later years is now more achievable where that was often not the case before.

AMERICAN MINORITIES & THE EXPERIENCE OF ILLNESS

In any culture, the provision of health care ultimately depends on the client-healer interaction. In some societies, the role of healer may be quite specific; in others, helping relationships may be more temporary or situational. Regardless of the cultural characteristics, the observational skill and empathy present during the communicative interchange determine the quality of information shared by the healer and client regarding the nature of the present illness, the past history, and the interpretation of symptoms and signs. Two factors may complicate the process: **class status** and **ethnic identity.** These factors are particularly prominent in areas of the USA where plu-

ralism and a high degree of class consciousness are accompanied by ethnic and class chauvinism. Either of these can create subtle or sometimes gross differences in worldview, expectations, and communication patterns. A few of these differences are illustrated by examples drawn from some American subcultural groups.

"Latinos"

The largest group of Latinos consists of nearly 10 million Mexican-Americans, sometimes called Chicanos or *La Raza* ("the race"). The ethnic identity is very strong. Culturally, they are of a mixed "Indio" and white Spanish origin and reflect the diversity of population groups in Central America and Mexico prior to colonization. They are a fatalistically religious group, fostering strong mutual support and solidarity, with a high value placed on family and neighborhood. The subculture stresses dignity, manliness, feminine virtue and chastity, the reluctance to accept charity, and a tendency toward strong response to perceived provocation. Anglo-Chicano relations have long been characterized by discrimination and by job and residential segregation, with unequal opportunities for jobs and education. Resurgence of ethnic pride has been conspicuous within the last 20 years, paralleling similar movements in black and other minority communities.

In some surveys, Mexican-Americans have been shown to be relative underusers of health facilities. This may in part reflect the positive and realistic idea that it is natural for people to get sick and that intervention is not always needed. It may also be due to lack of appropriate bilingual services. Cultural beliefs about health care may include simultaneous acceptance of indigenous (folk) and scientific health systems. For some individuals, the *curanderos* offer a complementary alternative to the conventional hospital, clinic, or private office system.

Kay (1981) has described the folk classification of behavioral and mental conditions among Mexican-Americans in the Southwest. An overall category of "emotional illness" (*enfermedad emocional*) is subdivided into "mental illness" (*enfermedad mental*) and "moral illness" (*enfermedad moral*). The first category includes disabilities caused by physical, interpersonal, or spiritual interventions, eg, hex or "evil eye"; the second, abnormalities due chiefly to the (moral) weakness of the individual, eg, alcoholism, drug abuse, pathologic jealousy.

Coalitions of Latino groups have been important in fostering both group identity and political solidarity. However, all Latinos do not share the same culture. The Spanish-speaking population is made up of culturally diverse groups from Central and South America and the Caribbean. These subcultural groups differ from one another in their pronunciation of Spanish, incidence of bilingualism, and educational and economic backgrounds.

Puerto Ricans living in the continental USA presently number almost 2 million. They obtained citizenship following the Spanish-American War and since World War II have demonstrated a high rate of out-migration for the purposes of working on the mainland. Formerly, there was a low literacy rate accompanied by a high birth rate and short life expectancy. Although improvements in both health care and literacy have been made, the unemployment rate continues to be high.

Harwood (1981) has summarized the folk theory of disease among some Puerto Ricans as demonstrating a dualistic division of human nature into a mortal body and an immortal soul. Causes of illness are separated into physical (material) causes, interpersonal causes (from human activities), and spiritual causes (from wandering, disembodied souls or divine, magical sources). Also prominent among Puerto Ricans' thoughts about physical causes of illness is a "hot/cold" theory of disease. According to this theory, arthritis, upset stomach, and respiratory infections are *frio* ("cold" conditions) brought on by drafts of "ill winds" and best treated not with medication but by rest and diet (eating bananas, coconut, white beans). Diarrhea, various skin eruptions, and ulcers are considered *caliente* ("hot" conditions) and may be treated by combinations of medicines (eg, aspirin) and diet (eg, evaporated milk, kidney beans). Conflicts between scientific and folk medicine may lead to inconsistent treatment regimens, since the rationales differ greatly. For example, a Puerto Rican patient with a "cold" illness such as influenza may be unwilling to take a "hot" remedy such as aspirin unless it is combined with a "cold" remedy such as fruit juice.

Pacific Islanders & Asian-Americans (Chinese, Japanese, Korean)

Pacific Islanders and Asian-Americans experienced a special form of immigration, originally coming to the Hawaiian Islands and West Coast as contract laborers in agricultural, mining, or railroad industries. Assimilation has been relatively difficult because of their non-European traditions, distinctive langauges and physical characteristics, and traditional Buddhist and Confucian philosophies. As immigrants, they were originally non-Christian and observed highly different customs and rules of family organization. Oriental Exclusion Acts were passed early in the century to prevent the continued influx of Asians. Municipal, state, and territorial laws were also enacted to discourage opportunities for the purchase of land and other assets. With some exceptions, commercial development was also made difficult. Restrictions on residential and educational opportunities were common. Differences between Chinese and Japanese rates of assimilation have been noted. These partly reflect differences in culture of origin but are attributable also to the greater demographic complexity among Chinese immigrants and to the continuing infusion of newly arriving Chinese from various parts of Southeast Asia. Japanese-Americans, at one time the victims of deprivation of property and civil rights, have nonetheless retained a

positive ethnic identity and generally have prospered in the USA. Earlier in this century, commonalities of Oriental emigrants from various nationalities were more apparent—in terms of reasons for migration, socioeconomic status, and barriers to assimilation and adaptation raised by legal and prejudicial reactions against them. Prejudice has subsided following the war and improvements in civil rights since the 1960s.

Both Chinese- and Japanese-Americans are shown to be relative underusers of the mental health care system. The integrity of the extended family as a support system partly accounts for this, along with a feeling that behavioral problems are in a sense shameful. A sample case illustrates these points.

Illustrative case. A 58-year-old Cantonese man was admitted to a public psychiatric ward after firing a revolver from his apartment window at passing streetcars. His wife and sons described an 8-year history of delusions around the theme that the "Chinese Communists" were about to invade the West Coast and that their advance undercover agents were attempting to contact him. Following the onset of his delusion, he had been unable to work and essentially lived a suspicious, reclusive life at home, preparing his own meals (to avoid being poisoned) and brooding about political conspiracies. His relationships with his wife and sons were poor, but the family continued to support him passively and only intervened when he became threatening. It had not occurred to them that they should consult a psychiatrist. Even after the father was hospitalized, they expressed hope that the doctors might discover a physical cause for his "eccentricities."

Filipinos have a long history of migration to Hawaii and the continental USA. There has also been a new influx of Chinese and Indonesian immigrants during the past 20 years. Some (from Vietnam and Cambodia) are political refugees; others from Hong Kong have immigrated in search of economic and educational opportunities. The need for ethnically and linguistically sensitive health services is particularly evident with these latter groups.

Native Americans

The 1980 USA census lists 900,000 American Indians, nearly one-fifth of them residing in the Southwest, particularly in Arizona and New Mexico. It is estimated that over 700,000 Native Americans were present when the New World was discovered. The population dwindled to 500,000 around the time of the Civil War and was estimated to be 250,000 at the turn of the century. Sovereign status was originally given to tribes and confederations by the British and French governments as a stabilizing gesture during early colonization. After the American Revolution, the United States government followed the same precedent, though continuing to force various tribes beyond the Mississippi River by the time of the Civil War. In 1871, legislation abolished nation status for tribes and thereafter created reservations where Indians lived in the legal status of wards of the federal government. In the 1870s, attempts to encourage Native Americans to emulate the model of independent white small farm operators proved ineffective. Boarding schools created to educate diverse reservation populations have had limited success. The diversity of tribal backgrounds, along with some ancient sources of animosity, has in the past fostered disunity among some of the Native American population. Since the 1960s, there has been more solidarity in presenting concerted multitribal grievances along with demands for improvements in economic, civil, and educational opportunities.

Native American use of health facilities is complex and involves a blending of private, federal, and indigenous services, depending in part upon whether residence and occupation are in urban, rural, or reservation settings. Some groups have sustained a complicated tradition of indigenous caretakers who offer incantations, herbs, and ceremonial practices for physical and behavioral disorders. In some settings, medicine men are preferentially used, and conventional medical treatment is reserved for severe trauma or illness that has not responded to folk methods. In many tribes, medical customs and beliefs are closely intertwined with religious practices.

Statistics have recently shown decreases in maternal and neonatal deaths, tuberculosis, and severe respiratory diseases. However, high rates of alcoholism, accidental deaths, suicide, and homicide are still reported.

Black Americans

Blacks comprise the largest ethnic minority group in the USA, accounting for almost one-tenth of the population. They have been in North America since 1619 and were first brought as indentured servants and then as chattel slaves in response to the economic demands of labor-intensive Southern agriculture. Between the years 1700 and 1860, it is estimated that 500,000–700,000 slaves were imported. Social advantages intended to be conferred by the federal Civil Rights Acts during the Reconstruction period were swiftly nullified by local denials of rights and voting privileges and of equal protection under federal law. In addition to these institutional forms of oppression, antiblack prejudice has continued to be a shameful feature of American society.

Although new civil rights legislation has improved the situation of American blacks during the past 20 years, economic, social, and educational segregation and prejudice are still facts of life for many black citizens. According to Willie (1974), upper- and upper middle-class black Americans enjoy unfettered access to social, commercial, and educational institutions. Middle-class blacks, called "affluent conformists" by Willie, tend to form egalitarian, cooperative marriages in which both partners work and tend to have few children and a high regard for home ownership and education of children. There is a strong identification with church, closeness to relatives, and identification with the place of employment. Despite such identification with WASP cultural norms, a deficiency of capital and prejudicial hiring practices have resulted in fewer jobs for middle-class blacks than for competitive whites.

A third group of working-class blacks are the "innovative marginals" who have stable employment but are characteristically less well educated. Many have dropped out of high school either because of disillusionment or a need to help support the family. The families tend to be large, and the children are not expected to achieve more than blue-collar status. Families tend to maintain continuity in residence and occupation, though the divorce rate is high.

Lower-class blacks are characterized as "the struggling poor." Living at the bare subsistence level, they cluster in large cities and show a high rate of discontinuity in family relationships and employment. The struggle for existence is fierce and is characterized by distrust of one another as well as of the better-off members of the prevailing society.

Generalizations about the health status, attitudes toward illness, and use of professional facilities among blacks in the USA are complicated by class and regional differences and duration of residence (measured in generations) in particular localities. Although there have been many studies of physical conditions, mental illness, and social disabilities among urban and rural blacks, the factors of class, region, and generation-in-locality have often not been taken into account. Jackson (1981) has summarized some deficiencies in research methods and overinterpretation of findings. Compared to white populations, blacks have a higher incidence of hypertension and some cardiovascular diseases. The recently reported higher rates of various neoplasms reflect increased life expectancy and improved case reporting. Overall suicide rates for black men and women are consistently lower than those of the nonblack population, with the exception of young black men. Reported high rates of schizophrenic disorders may be due in part to overreporting and may correlate better with social class than with racial or ethnic factors per se.

Jackson stresses the fact that black Americans constitute an extremely heterogeneous group, so that attempts to reach unified conclusions on the basis of limited research findings are both methodologically inaccurate and racially biased. This of course is true in the case of other ethnic groups also.

Beyond Stereotyping

Ethnicity interacts with other crucial sociodemographic factors (such as gender, age, class, and generation) to influence health attitudes and behavior. Male/female differences, even within a particular culture, are related to distinctions in worldview, assumptions about specific gender roles, and, of course, experiences of health and illness. Age differences also are significant, both within ethnic groups and in cross-cultural comparisons. Similarly, differences in generation determine the degree of subcultural identity, from the extreme of complete immersion in the culture of origin to a high bicultural adaptation or even rejection of "old country" customs and values.

In the past 20 years, many writers have studied the physical and cultural experience of disease among groups with certain ethnic and class characteristics. Anthropologists, social scientists, and clinicians have contributed both to the sophistication of practitioners and health institutions and to the development of services that better serve the needs of medical and psychiatric populations. (For example, see Zborowski's [1969] work on the perception of pain in various American ethnic subcultures.)

Information about ethnicity and the adaptation of medical services to specific populations is now offered in health science education courses and in some medical postgraduate training programs. Since efficient communication is vital to the healer-patient interaction, the need for better understanding of the ethnic, class, and generation characteristics of patients is evident.

INSTITUTIONAL & HISTORICAL ASPECTS OF HEALTH CARE

The cultural characteristics of North American medicine reflect its historical development and particularly the colonization by and immigration of huge numbers of people from all over the world. The earliest practitioners virtually duplicated the prevailing modes of practice in Great Britain and continental Europe. However, indigenous American versions of homeopathic and osteopathic medicine in the 1800s stood in competition with if not opposition to the ascendant school of allopathic medicine. Furthermore, a complex system of folk medicine has always existed alongside professionally trained practitioners and has used nostrums, tonics, purgatives, salves, and poultices for diverse medical conditions. Americans have traditionally been self-medicators. Over-the-counter medications for a broad range of symptoms constitute a kind of "folk medicine" that is so widely practiced that it escapes notice. Herbalists, nutritionists, and proprietors of small apothecaries in Chinese or Latino communities provide medicinals, vitamins, and herbs for a variety of real and imagined illnesses.

Despite cultural diversity and geographic expansion in the USA, the trend has been toward centralization and consolidation rather than regional specialization and diversification. Starr (1983) has summarized some historical, institutional, and cultural factors relating to the growth of American medicine. He perceives the involvement of organized medicine in influencing health policy as a combination of altruistic intentions to elevate standards of practice along with some less noble incentives for limiting the numbers of practitioners and access to hospitals. The upgrading of professional qualifications in county medical societies paralleled the raising of standards for state medical licenses and the development of specialty boards to supervise the quality of postgraduate training and to ex-

amine applicants for specialty certification. The growth in number and variety of American medical periodicals and of the medical textbook industry freed American practitioners from intellectual dependence on European and British centers. Although these developments did not begin to gain momentum until the 1930s, the result has been a virtual preeminence of American medical research on the international scientific scene. These scientific, political, and educational changes in American medicine have sharply divided folk medicine and scientific medicine, with the axis of superiority clearly turning toward allopathic treatment as taught in medical schools and advanced hospital and university centers.

American psychiatry has burgeoned since World War II. Its cultural characteristics reflect socioeconomic factors influencing psychiatric disability and treatment. Prior to World War II, large numbers of mentally retarded, demented, and schizophrenic patients were confined to publicly funded custodial institutions, where they were maintained by teams of health professionals headed by psychiatrists. At present, many more people with chronic or recurrent psychotic disorders are treated in community mental health centers, receiving short-term acute hospital care in their own locality and maintenance care via patient services in their catchment districts. Middle-class patients from a variety of ethnic backgrounds tend to be seen in private clinics, hospitals, and offices for a wide range of psychiatric conditions. Although sometimes offered on a "sliding scale" according to ability to pay, such treatments are on a fee-for-service basis, and the patients may be partially or completely reimbursed by third-party health insurers.

For severe psychiatric disabilities, patients from the upper middle and upper classes might use these same facilities, although some might seek care in a few expensive private hospitals. This trend is not unique to the USA; in all societies, the privileged classes have access to the most sophisticated medical services. What is distinctive to American psychiatric practice is the large number of clients and patients who also use counseling and psychiatric services for the resolution of characterologic, situational, and existential problems of varying degrees of severity. By social and functional criteria, many of these persons are not seriously disabled in their social roles (as students, workers, homemakers, professionals) but seek help for the resolution of long-standing or current conflicts that reduce their capacity for happiness and achievement or fulfillment.

This exensive use of psychotherapeutic services (ranging from counseling to psychoanalysis) both exemplifies and reinforces the acceptability of psychiatry as a discipline in North America. In a society that stresses emotional independence from family, the need for technical solutions to personal problems is increased. Again reflecting cultural values, such needs call for secular and professional rather than spiritual or mystical solutions. As Daly (1973) has pointed out, preferences for rational and technical systems of treatment tend to become belief systems in themselves. Because blatantly magical beliefs are culturally unacceptable, they become covertly expressed as a kind of "scientism" or an inflated regard for medicine and technology.

Magical thinking in the USA thus becomes less conspicuous but nevertheless is irrepressible. Like all human beings, Americans who are sick may unrealistically feel guilty and look for "reasons" why they have been "made sick" at this time. Despite their conscious belief in scientific medicine, they may yearn for or pursue magical relief or cure (eg, through DMSO, laetrile/amygdalin, megavitamins, colonic flushes, etc). Although they "know better," they may secretly wish that other people might fall ill (or even die) and relish the fact that some people become sick (on the basis that "they probably deserve it").

Since the postwar period, the endorsement of specialty medicine has become ascendant in the teaching and practice of medicine. Some opposing trends have appeared during the past 20 years. Specialization is now seen as increasing medical costs, since patients with more than one problem may have to consult more than one doctor. This also decreases the bond of intimacy and understanding between doctor and patient, since no one professional is looking at the "whole patient" or family. Federally supported programs in community medicine, family practice, and the promotion of "primary care" have somewhat modified this trend. Reflecting broader social changes, there has also been a growth of folk and "holistic" medicine. Physical and psychiatric methods of treatment are available involving combinations of exercise, diet, and vitamins along with preventive and inspirational methods, either alone or in conjunction with conventional medical treatment. Within medicine itself, programs to train physician assistants, nurse practitioners, midwives, and other paraprofessionals have gained some acceptance. The growth of consumerism has made patients more critical and selective in their attitudes toward health professionals. Policy affecting the availability and quality of medical service now involves a complex of decision makers, including government agencies, insurance carriers, health planners, and consumer boards. Reflecting these developments, psychiatrists and other physicians have surrendered the exaggerated trust and even revered status they were accorded in former times.

In patterns of communication, American physicians and their patients tend to work together on a pseudoegalitarian basis, where the doctor's authority is implicitly assumed but not exploited. Cooperation is expected, and a friendly but parental intimacy is inherent in clinical encounters.

In summary, American medicine and psychiatry are becoming increasingly self-conscious about the institutional and cultural features of their own modes of practice.

SUMMARY

The study of human nature and of the behavior of human beings is currently going forward from a broad scientific base in a number of physical, medical, and social sciences. In the health sciences, those disciplines that explain normal and pathophysiologic processes of the body (eg, anatomy, pathology, biochemistry, pharmacology) are of primary importance for comprehending these complexities and pursuing methods for prevention and treatment of disease. The insights of the social sciences have provided greater understanding at all levels of health care—from research illuminating the characteristics of individual and group experience of disease to studies of the factors relating to efficiency, cost-effectiveness, and actual delivery of services. The present chapter has reviewed some of the real and potential contributions of anthropology both to psychiatry and general medicine. These are briefly summarized below.

The most general contribution from anthropologic theory derives from the principle of **cultural relativism.** This principle accentuates the diversity of human adaptation secondary to differences in physical and ecologic habitat, customary practices, language, socialization practices, and worldview. Methodologically, cultural relativism lends itself to the cross-national study of health and disease with the objective of attaining a deeper grasp of the potentials for treatment and prevention of illness among diverse populations. Humanistically, the principle of relativism is a reminder that diversity of adaptation and custom may lead to superficial conclusions (such as ethnic stereotypes) and act to conceal universal features characteristic of all humans and all societies. Such an insight is helpful in blunting the force of another universal human vulnerability—the tendency to distrust, hold in contempt, and feel prejudice toward individuals and groups who are "different."

Another important general contribution is present in the rich **qualitative** complexity revealed in anthropologic studies. This consists of detailed examinations of how people behave, how they explain their behavior, and what they believe in as well as what they "know" to be true. Given this qualitative emphasis, the techniques of anthropologic research complement the **quantitative** techniques of political science, economics, and sociology in the study of patients, caretakers, and health institutions. Anthropologic contributions also complement the scientific work of psychologists, psychoanalysts, and clinical psychiatrists in seeking explanations of behavior based upon **group** beliefs and socialization practices, which are related to **individual** conscious and unconscious motivations underlying human behavior.

Perhaps the most practical contributions to medicine and psychiatry, in particular, are the anthropologic insights concerning communication between healers and their patients. Beyond the obvious necessity of clearly transmitting and receiving information about the historical and symptomatic aspects of illness, the effectiveness of treatment (for both the practitioner and the patient) is a function of the success of mutual understanding, leading to the choice of appropriate physical and pharmacologic therapies. In psychotherapeutic transactions, exceptional communication is essential to successful outcomes.

Finally, as a science for the qualitative study of human beings and human organizations, anthropology provides a mirror for health institutions in which otherwise inapparent features of their own beliefs, practices, policies, and idiosyncrasies can be viewed and improved. Attempts to facilitate health care ordinarily focus on the external, objective improvement of procedures, practitioners, and facilities. Just as important, however, are the internalized search and critical examination of practice styles, professional mystique, and "traditions" that may obstruct the continuing refinement of medical care.

REFERENCES

Bureau of the Census: *Statistical Abstract of the United States.* US Department of Commerce, 1981.

Carr JE: Ethnobehaviorism and the culture-bound syndromes: The case of amok. *Cult Med Psychiatry* 1978;**2**:269.

Caudill N, Doi T: Interrelations of psychiatry, culture and emotion in Japan. Pages 374–422 in: *Man's Image in Medicine and Anthropology.* Gallston I (editor). Internat Univ Press, 1963.

Daly R: The spectres of technicism. Pages 341–359 in: *Alienation: Concept, Term and Meanings.* Johnson FA (editor). Seminar Press, 1973.

Diagnostic and Statistical Manual of Mental Disorders (DMS-III), 3rd ed. American Psychiatric Association, 1980.

Engel GE: The clinical application of the biopsychosocial model. *Am J Psychiatry* 1978;**137**:535.

Favazza AR: Anthropology and psychiatry. Chap 5.1 in: *Comprehensive Textbook of Psychiatry/IV,* 4th ed. Kaplan HI, Freedman AM, Sadock BJ (editors). Williams & Wilkins, 1985.

Foulkes E: *The Artic Hysterias of the North Alaskan Eskimos.* American Anthropological Association, 1972.

Harwood AE: *Ethnicity and Medical Care.* Harvard Univ Press, 1981.

Hollender M, Hirsch S: Hysterical psychosis. *Am J Psychiatry* 1964;**120**:1066.

Jackson JJ: Urban black Americans. Pages 37–130 in: *Ethnicity and Medical Care.* Harwood AE (editor). Harvard Univ Press, 1981.

Kay MA: Classification of illness among Mexican-Americans. In: *Ethnicity and Medical Care.* Harwood AE (editor). Harvard Univ Press, 1981.

Kleinman A: *Patients and Healers in the Context of Culture.* Univ of California Press, 1980.

Kroeber AL, Kluckhohn C: *Culture.* Vintage Books, 1952.

Manual of the International Statistical Classification of Diseases, Injuries and Causes of Death (ICD-9), 9th ed. World Health Organization, 1977.

Murphy JM: Psychiatric labeling in cross-cultural perspective. *Science* 1976;**191**:1019.

Novak M: *The Rise of the Unmeltable Ethnics.* Macmillan, 1971.

Offer D, Sabshin M: *Normality.* Basic Books, 1966.

Parsons T: *The Social System.* Free Press, 1951.

Starr P: *The Social Transformation of American Medicine.* Basic Books, 1983.

Tanaka-Matsumi J: Taijin kyofusho: Diagnostic and cultural issues in Japanese psychiatry. *Cult Med Psychiatry* 1979; **3**:231.

Townsend JM: *Cultural Conceptions and Mental Illness: A Comparison of Germany and America.* Univ of Chicago Press, 1978.

Willie CV: The black family and social class. *Am J Orthopsychiatry* 1974;**44**:50.

Zborowski M: *People in Pain.* Jossey-Bass, 1969.

Section II. Psychiatric Assessment

16 — Introduction to Clinical Assessment: The Mayor of Wino Park

Howard H. Goldman, MD, PhD

Wino Park is an unoccupied rectangle of land "south of Market" in San Francisco, open on 2 sides, which has been somewhat crudely developed as a temporary haven for a shifting population of about 50 men and a few older women who lounge there out of the wind during the day and are allowed to sleep in metal shelters at night if they have no better bed to go to. The police leave them alone if they stay quiet. There have been a few assaults and small-change robberies in Wino Park but no murders, no rapes, no drug dealing that anyone knows of.

John Francis ("Red") Kimball, self-appointed Mayor of Wino Park, whose full story is told in more detail in Chapter 22, has lived in the park for 4 or 5 months. After a night in jail, he is now in restraints in a police ambulance on his way to Memorial Hospital Emergency. As the ambulance backs to the unloading dock he shouts and struggles, complains loudly of brutal treatment, threatens legal action, invokes retribution by powerful "friends downtown." With professional skill and no hard feelings, the attendants transfer the Mayor from the ambulance litter to a hospital gurney, strap him down, exchange paperwork and a few words of explanation with hospital intake personnel, and depart along a beam of revolving blue light in a crackle of radio code words.

In the reception area the Mayor alternately scowls and cajoles. He wants a cigarette. He wants to be liked and knows he won't be, a trashy Irish drunk in a bored, intolerant time and place, a burden on the taxpayers, uncared for, welcome nowhere, all but homeless. He was married once but drank too much, was impotent, hit his wife, and lost her to California's smoothly functioning no-fault marital dissolution system. He lived for a while in a hotel in the Tenderloin district where the night manager agreed to receive and hold monthly SSDI checks by arrangement with adult protective services workers. The Mayor now lives in Wino Park as his life slowly worsens. He drinks only wine, and not a lot of that by skid row standards—"up to 2 quarts a day" in Chapter 22. When not somnolent with drink he postures and harangues his fellows in the Park, turning

away scorn with knowing glances. In occasional bursts of resolve he holds "news conferences" at downtown crosswalks, speaking right into nonexistent microphones, raising an arm to take questions from the less favored correspondents in the back rows, fielding tough questions with quotable quips, expounding plans to extend ever grander services to his threadbare constituency if only the supervisors had the guts, the vision. Now there is talk of closing Wino Park. Nothing is so fierce as the functionary's loyalty to his function. The Mayor gets wild sometimes thinking about it.

• • •

The Mayor has been to Memorial before, but he's worse this time. His assaults are more than bluster, and he gets 3 injections of diazepam that night. When he wakes he is nervy, somehow jaunty, sexually aggressive with the nurses. He is assigned to a senior medical student not yet at ease with psychiatric patients whose job it is to deal with the Mayor until a decision can be made about what to do with him. Dealing with him means first of all recording vital signs and starting some tests for the Mayor's bulging file. With help from a technician, blood is drawn and sent for analysis. A urine sample is taken, a stool sample. There is much vulgar comment and protest. The student has an ophthalmoscope and would like to use it. It's his favorite instrument but not an easy one to use. You have to get close, and this patient smells. You have to focus, and this patient jerks around. He stands uncertainly with it in his hand, wondering what to do, for all the world like a television reporter with a field mike. Tomorrow is Father's Day and he hasn't sent a card. Why is this rumball "mayor" standing there as if he wants something? Without thinking he asks the most interesting question the Mayor has ever heard: "Mr Kimball, what brings you to the hospital at this time?"

182

● ● ●

THE MAYOR GRANTS
AN INTERVIEW*

"I am the Mayor of Wino Park. They talk about closing me down. That's how I started drinking more and got real bad, turning yellow, blacking out. Next thing I know, I'm staring you in the face, like old times, we're buddies from way back, I remember last night, everything. You were scared, I could tell. I was a mess, right? But I walked in under my own steam, right? The Mayor don't need help. I see double, did you know that? I have pains in my belly, too.

"I wasn't always like this. They didn't elect me Mayor for nothing. I have the gift. Sometimes I talk too much, give away my secrets. Like that cop, moving me along. I wasn't causing nobody any trouble. I was doing God's own work. It's my secret fate to help people, I whispered that to the cop, I shouldn't have touched him, you can't touch cops these days, they

---

*The Mayor's account here varies somewhat from the facts developed in Chapter 22.

overact, like my old man, *he just couldn't stop hitting me sure I talked back to him the way he yelled at Ma then he was sorry, she couldn't have kids after me, something was wrong, she didn't come home with me from the hospital they said.* [Long pause.] He died in one of these places. God damn him. [Starting to cry.] God damn him."

● ● ●

INTRODUCTION TO CLINICAL
ASSESSMENT

This was the first of many interviews with the Mayor. He stayed at the hospital for 3 weeks, undergoing extensive diagnostic evaluation, beginning treatment, and continuing in monitored rehabilitation after discharge. His evaluation included daily interviews, examinations and tests, and a personality assessment. These subjects are discussed in Chapters 17–21. Chapter 22 consists of the details of the assessment procedure and its results presented in one commonly used case study format.

17

The Psychiatric Interview

David E. Reiser, MD

Patient interviewing is a core skill in medicine. Despite technical advances, the bedrock of diagnosis and treatment continues to be communication. The doctor and patient must talk. Both, but especially the doctor, must also know how to listen. No diagnostic test or apparatus can ever replace the human bond that forms the basis of medical practice, the doctor-patient relationship. The primary tool the physician utilizes to cement that relationship is a skillful and sensitive interview.

SIMILARITIES BETWEEN THE PSYCHIATRIC INTERVIEW & THE GENERAL MEDICAL INTERVIEW

The goal of all communication between doctor and patient is to facilitate **diagnosis and treatment** and further the aims of the **working alliance** between doctor and patient. Because of this, the psychiatric interview is similar in many ways to the general medical interview. It is useful to review the similarities before underscoring important differences.

Diagnosis

Diagnosis and individualized assessment (formulation) are major goals of medical interviewing. An accurate diagnosis is at the heart of every evaluation, and the diagnosis becomes the benchmark against which treatment success or failure is subsequently measured. This may seem obvious. What is not always appreciated, however, is the relationship between effective interviewing and accurate diagnosis.

Many patients withhold important medical information, fearing that it is too trivial or perhaps embarrassing to bring up. This is most apt to occur if the physician appears busy or impatient. For example, a modest girl in her teens presents to her family practitioner with complaints of fatigue. She has only recently entered puberty and is bashful about her sexuality. A brusque and hurried interview that focuses too quickly on a checklist of her symptoms may fail to elicit a symptom that embarrasses her—she has frequent urges to urinate. To the physician, this information is vital to a possible diagnosis of diabetes. To the patient, however, it is embarrassing, and it will be disclosed only in an atmosphere of openness and trust.

The interview also determines *what* is diagnosed. In a hurried, narrowly focused interview, for example, a physician might be able to elicit symptoms of congestive heart failure in a 60-year-old man. This information will do little good, however, if the physician notices nothing about the temperament and coping style of the patient. A skilled interviewer might go on to learn that for the past year this patient has been despondent over the death of his wife. Since her death, in fact, he has been noncompliant in the matter of taking medications, including digitalis. He says, "They gave my wife drugs toward the end, and that's what killed her." Bringing out these fears and attitudes is just as critical as eliciting a 10-day history of severe orthopnea.

Thus, good interviewing is essential both in establishing an accurate diagnosis and in gaining insight into the personality and coping style of the patient.

Treatment

Effective interviewing is also essential for effective treatment. For example, a physician makes a diagnosis of pneumococcal pneumonia in a 78-year-old widow living in a hotel for pensioners. He prescribes oral ampicillin; his receptionist schedules a return visit; and he considers his job done. Five days later, he learns that the patient has been admitted to the hospital in severe respiratory distress. What the physician failed to appreciate was the presence of Alzheimer's disease (discussed in Chapters 10 and 24). Not only had the patient failed to take her medication—she had never had the prescription filled, forgetting all about it as soon as she left the physician's office.

Studies of patient compliance show that only 50–70% of patients comply with the therapeutic regimens prescribed by their physicians (Davis, 1966). Distrust, unexpressed anxiety, and confusion about physicians' instructions are the common reasons for noncompliance. *Most instances of noncompliance, in fact, seem to stem from breakdowns in the doctor-patient relationship.* Doctors think they communicate clearly to their patients, and patients think they understand what their physicians tell them—yet serious breakdowns in communication still occur.

The interview can be therapeutic in its own right. The prospect of help, the experience of being understood, and the impact of new insight offered by a trusted and respected physician all can have a therapeutic effect.

Effective interviewing must include, at a minimum, creation of an atmosphere conducive to a patient's expression of questions and concerns, opportunities for appropriate patient education, and meaningful follow-up. The doctor who walks out the door saying, "Call me if you have any questions," has not done enough. Patient education pamphlets, videotapes, and reprints can all be helpful. Yet there seems to be no substitute for an effective doctor-patient relationship, with the interview being the agent that cements it.

The Working Alliance

No treatment protocol is maximally effective if a good doctor-patient relationship has not been established. Regardless of our biotechnical skills, success depends to a great extent on the patient's compliance and trust. The working alliance can be defined as an agreement between physician and patient, based on mutual rapport and trust, to undertake treatment *together*. Steps in that process may entail discomfort and risk; they are deemed worth the risk when both believe that such steps may improve the patient's condition. In some treatments, this working alliance may simply be assumed. In others, it must not be taken for granted. A physician prescribing penicillin for streptococcal sore throat is not apt to read the patient every paragraph of a pharmacology textbook concerning adverse drug reactions. At the other extreme, in the realm of "heroic medicine," there are dramatic instances of high technology being applied to medical conditions once thought to be unmanageable by any means. In such cases, patients may have to be given detailed information about all potential risks of treatment, and the working alliance obviously entails much communication between physician and patient regarding numerous critical details. Between such extremes lie most of medicine's daily challenges. In almost all cases, however, a physician's success with patients depends on the ability to establish an alliance based on trust and to communicate the necessary facts effectively.

As the foregoing is intended to suggest, there are many similarities between the psychiatric interview and the medical interview. This deserves emphasis, for the psychiatric interview is too often set apart in the clinician's mind as something abstract and specialized, based on knowledge and principles that need to be grasped only by psychiatrists. But as Harry Stack Sullivan (1962) has said, "Man is more simply human than otherwise." Psychiatric patients are not so different from other patients: Something has gone wrong, and they are seeking help. But like most patients, they are ambivalent about help, wanting it yet fearful of what might lie in the future—knowing that they need an expert to intervene yet unhappy with the realization that they cannot handle the problem themselves.

DIFFERENCES BETWEEN THE PSYCHIATRIC INTERVIEW & THE GENERAL MEDICAL INTERVIEW

The psychiatric interview differs from the medical interview in that the psychiatric patient must communicate personal concerns about disturbed mental functioning through language that can only be formed as a process of mentation. Depending on the psychiatric condition, this problem can be great or small; but in all cases, special tact and sensitivity are required of the psychiatric interviewer.

Diagnosis

The impediments to diagnosis posed by a psychiatric condition can vary considerably. A patient with a nonpsychotic disorder characterized by anxiety or depression may be able to communicate with no greater difficulty than any other patient. Many psychiatric conditions, however, affect the patient's ability to communicate and comprehend what is going on, as shown in the following examples:

(1) A patient suffering from a psychotic disorder such as paranoid schizophrenia may be experiencing a flood of derogatory and frightening auditory hallucinations at the time of the interview. He may be convinced that someone is plotting to poison him and steal all of his possessions. The physician who walks into the room, extends a hand, and begins with a friendly introduction may be in for a rude surprise. Instead of smiling back obligingly, the patient may back into a corner, raise his fists in front of him, and say, "You're not coming near me with that poison!"

(2) A manic patient may rush about the examination area uttering profanities, hardly able or willing to heed the doctor's reassurances. She may be busy testing all of the water faucets in the emergency area, convinced she has a magic formula for converting tap water into liquid uranium.

(3) A demented patient may be outwardly cooperative. He will sit compliantly, nod when asked if he understands, and smile affably. Unfortunately, he thinks it is 1924 and is firmly convinced that the doctor interviewing him is his high school football coach.

(4) A sociopathic patient may give a heart-wrenching story about the anguish of narcolepsy, leading the physician to miss the twinkle in her eyes as she asks for a prescription for 100 dextroamphetamine capsules, "just like my doctor gives me back home."

The psychiatric interview may require multiple evaluations over time. A patient suffering from a psychiatric disorder, especially in its acute stage, may not be able to tolerate a detailed, lengthy interview at the first meeting. A depressed patient may be too despondent and withdrawn to be helpful at this stage of the illness as a detailed informant. A manic patient may be more interested in reeling off profit projections from her latest scheme to establish a nationwide chain of boutiques than in reporting that she stopped taking her lithium. A paranoid patient may eye the clinician suspiciously, convinced that there are microphones strapped to his body. In all such cases, the clinician must be prepared to terminate the interview and resume it later when the patient's condition improves. Nothing is gained by attempting to force patients to endure the interviewing process beyond a comfortable limit.

The more acutely impaired a psychiatric patient is, the more the science of observation becomes critical. The science of observation will be elucidated further in the next section. It will suffice here to note that words are not the only source of information during an interview. Communication in a variety of other modes—including facial expressions and body language—conveys the underlying mood. If a clinician walks into the examining room and finds a disheveled, tense young man with clenched fists darting fearful glances around the room, the clinician has observed a great deal though the patient has not yet said anything.

The psychiatric interviewer must be prepared to seek out ancillary sources of data. People are usually part of a social network. Important members of this network will often be present in the emergency or acute care setting with the patient—friends, employers, spouses, ex-spouses, etc. When such people come with the patient to the acute care setting, it is usually worthwhile to spend some time talking with them, always with the patient's knowledge. Even when no one comes in with the patient, it is often good practice to seek such people out later for the help they can give as informants. Stresses in a relationship often underlie psychiatric decompensation. The collateral information from people who know the patient is often invaluable.

Similarly, the physician should search old medical records, call prior treating physicians, and seek out other potential sources of data (school, military, employment records, etc) that may help in understanding the patient now. The patient's confidentiality, dignity, and trust must always be respected, but data obtained from collateral sources may be critical for effective diagnosis.

Treatment

There was a time when little other than communication was available to a psychiatrist for treating patients. Antipsychotic drugs, effective antidepressants, and benzodiazepines are quite recent developments. The future holds prospects for effective somatic and pharmacologic treatments, but communication will not doubt continue to play a central role.

The Working Alliance

Psychiatric patients, like many medical patients, are ambivalent about needing professional help. Even though they want help with problems they are unable to solve, they may feel humiliated and defeated by the mere fact of needing assistance. Wanting to change patterns of behavior, they nevertheless fear giving up familiar ways of coping. Patients who have great hopes for the results of treatment may also have great fear of failure. Cultural proscriptions and taboos about psychiatry and the "stigma" of psychiatric treatment reinforce such attitudes. A patient with a diseased heart or kidney usually does not feel shame to the same degree a patient with alcoholism or psychosis does. For these reasons, the interviewer must be sensitive to the importance of empathy, respect, and trust in order to develop a good working alliance with the patient. Regardless of what patients say or how they behave, the interviewer should assume that seeking psychiatric help is a distressing and conflict-laden event for all patients.

THE SCIENCE OF OBSERVATION

Illustrative case

A group of medical students and their preceptor went to interview a 79-year-old woman in the orthopedics unit. She was in a semiprivate room and had a visitor, a woman in her mid 40s. Flowers, cards, and a framed photograph on the bedside table—of a handsome man in his late 50s wearing clothes styled in the late 1950s—showed that the patient was not alone in the world. She was in good spirits, with a hip that was only sprained and not more seriously injured. She asked her visitor to return another time—happy, she said, "to have some young people to talk to."

The preceptor was then unexpectedly called away to an emergency and urged the students to proceed with the interview for at most 20 minutes.

Later, the preceptor offered to anticipate the students' impressions of the old woman though he had been with her less than a minute before he was called away. The students were astonished at how much he had been able to observe in that time: that she was a widow, because she wore a wedding band and the picture would have been more recent—or there would have been none—if her husband were still alive; that she had grown children and maintained close ties with them, because a greeting to "the kids" (her grandchildren?) had gone with the visitor, who said, "Goodbye, Mom," and because the patient related so well to the young medical students; and that she belonged to several clubs and social groups, because there were so many flowers and cards—some with a great many signatures—in the room.

Most students think of the interview chiefly as something that they *do, perform,* and *conduct.* This is true, of course, but the interview is also a time to *observe, perceive,* and *take in.* The first concept of the interview is active and intrusive; the second is passive and receptive. In fact, the interview involves both, but most physicians err in the direction of being too active. One of the essential skills of observation is staying quiet so the patient can talk and so things can happen that need to be noted.

There are 2 phases to the observation component of the interview: active vigilance, and what Freud (1912) called even-hovering attention.

Active vigilance is most appropriate during the first few minutes of the interaction. The "first few" minutes begin right away, as soon as the therapist and patient see each other, and not when they have settled down, with names exchanged and notes taken, so that the interview can formally "start." In the illustrative case above, the phase of active vigilance began the instant the group walked to the patient's bedside. During this phase of the interview, the student should take in as much as possible, actively and aggressively processing data that come in through all of the senses. How does the patient first greet the interviewer? Does he or she offer a hand or sit passively? Does the patient make eye contact? Is the handclasp firm and warm, or is it cold and clammy? Are there any books on the bed or table? What is the patient wearing? What are the first jokes and casual banter uttered by the patient? Are there any unusual sounds or smells in the room?

When the interview formally begins, the phase of active vigilance continues for the first few minutes of the dialogue. The student should make an effort to remember *everything* the patient says. What was the *very first* thing the patient said? What was the accompanying emotional tone? The following illustrate the importance of the patient's initial remarks:

(1) "Whatever it is they're accusing me of, I didn't do it!" one patient "joked" at the start of an interview. It turned out that this man had been riddled with guilt since the suicide of his son 2 years previously. That is when his health began to fail.

(2) "I wouldn't have nothin' to offer anyhow! Go away and leave me alone!" This patient turned out to be deeply tormented and embittered by her children's recent decision to place her in a nursing home.

After the phase of active vigilance, the student should shift to **even-hovering attention.** Students will discover, especially if they have been vigilant in the first few minutes of the interaction, that they can remember the rest of the interview without resorting to detailed notes. Note taking is in fact discouraged except in order to jot down a few key facts, since a student with head lowered over a notepad is not looking at the patient and paying attention.

After the first few minutes, simply adopt a relaxed and receptive stance. *Listen!* Allow whatever the patient is saying to come into your mind freely. Allow yourself also to attend the thoughts, ideas, and random associations that you yourself are having while the patient is talking. There will be time for more focused and directive interviewing later.

Many students have conceptual difficulties that interfere with observation. One involves finding a balance between skeptical inquiry and jumping to conclusions. Another is an almost universal tendency to attribute what transpires in an interview to how well the interview was conducted. In the illustrative case, although most of the students were impressed by the preceptor's acumen, a few of them were angered by it and even felt the preceptor had jumped to conclusions. This does happen, and students are right to be cautious. Any conclusions drawn from limited data should be regarded as hypotheses, not certainties, and physicians should not hesitate to modify or expand their ideas about patients' problems as more data become available. At the same time, they should give the science of observation the benefit of the doubt before dismissing all hunches that can be extracted from small pieces of observable data. To be nonjudgmental and resist premature appraisal is laudable, but physicians cannot afford to ignore the clinical data the initial interaction so often provides.

The converse of this is that physicians should never assume that the data a patient provides are always perceived by them and the patient in the same way. Just as some interviewers ignore small yet important facts, others erroneously assume that they understand what the patient means even when the patient speaks in ambiguous terms. Patients talk about "not being myself lately" or being "out of sorts," "without get-up-and-go." The clinician should never assume that these and similar phrases are automatically clear. "Not being myself" could mean "I've been sexually impotent," or it could mean "I cry all night, and I've just bought a gun to kill myself with." It never hurts to ask, "What do you mean when you say you are not yourself?" "Out of sorts in what way, specifically?" "What do you mean by get-up-and-go?" The clarifying responses the patient then provides may startle the physician, who thought the patient meant something else entirely.

Regarding the student's second concern—that he or she is always responsible for how an interview goes—only experience will teach that the interview is less influenced by what the examiner does than by the temperament and mood of the patient. It is primarily patients who shape the interview—and they do so with the same coping styles, wishes, fears, and conflicts with which they shape (or fail to shape) their lives. This is precisely why the interview provides such valuable data: It *replicates* the coping pattern and difficulties of the patient.

Students are always eager to learn how to correct what they did wrong and to understand what they could have done to make an interview go better. Interviewing technique is important, and students are right to ask for constructive criticism. But they must also sooner or later understand that how an interview goes usually says more about the patient than about the student. To assert this principle is not to deny responsibility for contemplating one's own limitations but to recognize an important diagnostic principle of psychiatry.

CONTENT & PROCESS

Illustrative case

A 51-year-old construction foreman was being evaluated on a neuropsychiatry unit for symptoms of forgetfulness. He had had only a sixth-grade education but was highly regarded on the job and boasted of being a "self-made man." A medical student was conducting the initial evaluation interview. In responding to a question about the family, the patient began to speak derisively about his son, whom he had sent to college but who was now staying at home, collecting unemployment insurance, and playing a guitar and dreaming of riches on the rock scene. "He may have a college degree, but there's things I know that only life can teach!"

The medical student listened attentively and respectfully. Then he said, "It sounds like your son doesn't always respect what you know, what experience has taught you."

"That's right!"

The medical student then made an important intuitive connection. "I'm probably about the same age as your son," he said. "I hope I don't come across as a know-it-all with you. I'm a student—I told you that. Be sure to let me know if I'm not understanding something."

"No, doc, you're doing all right. You're all right."

All interpersonal communication has both a content and a process (Reiser and Schroder, 1980). Everyone is accustomed to focusing on the **content** of communication, but it is often the **process** that communicates what is most important. Music offers a good analogy: The content forms the basic notes of communication, while process comprises the rhythm, timing, chord structure, and harmony. Content is the literal *what* that is being said; process is the timing and flow, the all-important *way* in which something is said.

While there is process communication in all interactions, its importance obviously varies. If one is asking a store clerk how much something costs, the process is hardly important unless local custom encourages bargaining. In the doctor-patient interaction, however, process is always important. Regardless of what the problem is, the patient will always have concerns about the doctor. "Can this person help me?" "Does he care about me?" "Does she find my problem disgusting?" "Trivial?" "Has he ever seen anyone with my problem before?" The foreman in the illustrative case had an important concern: Would the young "doctor" treat him with understanding and respect? While the specifics may vary, the concerns are universal, and addressing them sympathetically will help establish a good working alliance. Because patients can rarely express these concerns directly, they almost always do so through process, though they are not always aware of it.

Mastering and understanding the process level of communication is an exacting skill that takes time and experience to acquire. The interviewer can usually detect the process level of a patient's communications by asking 3 questions: (1) What is the patient telling me about his or her concerns *right now?* (2) What is the patient telling me about his or her feelings *right now?* (3) What is the patient telling me about his or her feelings concerning what is going on between us *right now?*

This is how the student understood his patient's concerns in the illustrative case. *Right now,* the patient was saying he was concerned about whether the young student would patronize him. *Right now,* he was saying that he wanted to be treated with respect even though he was not an educated man.

Attention to process often answers another key question in the psychiatric interview: *Why now?* A 46-year-old man with a 20-year history of manic-depressive illness comes to the emergency room markedly depressed. *Why now?* A young college senior develops a delusion that he is part of an international scheme. *Why now?*

What has been going on in the patient's life? The answer is always critical. More often than not, it will be found in the process of a patient's communication more than in the content. In the case of one very depressed man, for example, the process level of his communication dwelt extensively on themes of rejection and loss. He even told a sad joke about a man who was a cuckold. This process unfolded while the patient ostensibly disclosed only content. "I've been married 15 years to a good woman." This prompted the interviewer to inquire further about the patient's marriage and enabled him to learn that the patient suspected his wife had started an affair. This was the *why now?* for this patient's illness.

Finally, the concept of process is closely related to the phenomenon of **transference,** discussed in Chapter 3. In the psychiatric relationship, the intense feelings a patient has toward his or her therapist may be critical. Success in psychotherapy often depends on the skillful handling of these feelings. In certain forms of therapy, such as psychoanalysis and psychoanalytically oriented psychotherapy (see Chapter 43), an understanding of the patient's transference actually becomes an integral part of the process of treatment itself. With few exceptions, the nature and extent of the transference will also be communicated in process.

THE "A.R.T." OF INTERVIEWING

Every psychiatric interview may be conceptualized as having 3 phases: *A*ssessment, *R*anking, and *T*ransition (Reiser and Schroder, 1980).

Assessment

The assessment phase of the interview is the maximally open-ended, nondirective phase of the interaction. The setting should be a quiet and private place where doctor and patient can talk in an unhurried manner. Both should be seated and able to interact in normal tones at about the same eye level. If such a setting is not available, an empathic interview can go a long way toward overcoming the disadvantages of noise and lack of privacy. In all cases, the interviewer should try to ensure the best setting possible under the circumstances.

The interviewer should introduce and identify himself or herself, clearly explain the purpose of the meeting with the patient, and then invite the patient to begin in as open-ended a manner as possible. Some interviewers use a standard phrase, eg, "What sort of troubles have you been having?" Or, "Tell me about the problem that brings you here." Some simply begin with a look of interest and an inviting gesture of the hand.

There are several reasons why it is important to start in an open-ended manner. First, an invitation to talk tells the patient, "You're important to me. I am interested in everything about you. Everything that concerns you is potentially of concern to me." Communicating this attitude is always important in medi-cine but is even more so when working with patients who have problems that damage their sense of self-worth and their ability to trust others. Second, the clinician can often discern subtle but important clues to disturbances in thought processes. In response to the open-ended beginning of the interview, does the patient proceed to tell his or her story in a logical, goal-directed manner? Or does the patient ramble in a loose and incoherent way about seemingly unrelated concerns? Or does the patient start to cry and seem unable to articulate any story at all? Is there inappropriate laughter? Is there a rush of language amounting to pressure of speech? These and similar incongruities of affect and cognitive disturbances (see Chapters 12 and 18) can be readily diagnosed if the interviewer is appropriately nondirective. If the examiner too quickly launches into a content-intensive, checklist style of interviewing, such data may be missed. A third reason for beginning in an open-ended manner is perhaps the most important of all. The physician may be wrong in assuming he or she knows what is most important in the patient's presentation. If a patient entering an emergency room appeared belligerent and paranoid and expressed fears of gangland revenge, the physician may have initially assumed that the person was suffering from a psychosis of the paranoid type, probably schizophrenia. Yet this conclusion would have to be reassessed if, in the course of an open-ended interview, the patient began to talk about his activities as a drug dealer and his recent heavy use of cocaine.

During the assessment phase, the patient will raise concerns, describe symptoms, and offer other clues the clinician will wish to investigate further. These will range from the patient's medical and past psychiatric history to family relations and vocational and financial difficulties. After a time—usually 3–10 minutes—the clinician will be ready to begin the second phase of the interview process.

Ranking

During the ranking phase of the interview, the physician makes decisions about the order in which different areas of inquiry should be examined. During the 3- to 10-minute assessment phase, the patient may introduce a half-dozen areas of interest worth pursuing. What comes first? It is common practice to proceed first with the medical history, especially the present illness, but this is seldom necessary (except of course in true emergencies) and may be ill-advised. It is best to postpone the medical history if it is suspected that the patient has apprehensions about the doctor-patient relationship itself. These concerns are usually expressed in process (as in the illustrative case described above). When these concerns are significant, they need to be dealt with before other data are obtained.

Thus, the physician might rank a given patient's problems as follows: (1) concerns about whether I will understand that he is afraid to come to the hospital, (2) a 3-week history of depression and suicidal ideation, (3) breakup of marriage, and (4) loss of job after 20 years. The physician might then proceed by saying, "Before we talk further about your depression, Mr Smith, do I get the feeling you're afraid I'll insist you be hospitalized tonight?"

Within each ranked area, the examiner should proceed from an open-ended, nondirective style to progressively more focused and defined inquiry. Thus, the physician might say, "Tell me more about this feeling of hopelessness." After the patient has attempted to do so, the clinician's inquiry would become progressively more directive: "Have you lost any weight over the past few weeks?" . . . "How many pounds would you say you've lost?" etc. Finally, questions that require the most specific type of responses may be asked: "Would you say you've lost a couple of pounds or 10 pounds in the last 2 weeks?"

A good rule in ranking is to let the *patient's* priorities control whenever possible. The physician may be eager to elicit data concerning sleeplessness and euphoria or a 20-year drinking history. The patient may be much more troubled by concerns about being hospitalized or perhaps by something else altogether—something concerning the family or changes in employment or health.

Transition

Assessment and ranking are complex clinical skills that develop gradually as experience and knowledge increase; transitions are fairly easy from the first day. A transition consists of telling the patient when and why the subject of the interview is being changed. After the assessment phase, for example, the clinician may say, "It sounds like you're very concerned about the effect your drinking is having on your wife. But right now I'd like to hear more about why you think you want to end it all." In this instance, the clinician has properly given assessment of suicidal ideation a very high priority. The clinician ranked this consideration first after listening to many of the patient's concerns and then made a transition by telling the patient exactly what the focus of attention was and why.

Transitions may also be used to return to a more open-ended interview, after a specific line of inquiry has run its course. After a careful review of systems, the clinician might say, "Now that I've gotten the basics I need concerning your medical history, perhaps we could return to something you mentioned earlier—that your grandmother was hospitalized once for a psychiatric problem and things didn't go well. Could you tell me more about that?"

The line of questioning is usually clear in the clinician's mind, but the patient cannot be expected to understand what the clinician is up to. Great care must be taken to avoid confusion in changing the topic of inquiry.

"A.R.T." Sequence

Although assessment, ranking, and transition have been presented here in that sequence, all 3 actually go on simultaneously. For example, during a review of systems, the clinician may come upon a new fact that should be assessed more thoroughly then and there, indicating a need to return to the assessment phase of the interview. As the doctor-patient relationship proceeds, new facts are always emerging that require reassessment and ranking.

SPECIFIC INTERVIEWING TECHNIQUES

The foundation of good psychiatric interviewing—indeed all medical interviewing—is a working alliance between doctor and patient in a spirit of growing mutual trust. No amount of skill in technique can compensate for basic defects in this alliance. Conversely, a patient will usually forgive the doctor any number of mistakes if basic trust is there. The most potent single interviewing technique, therefore, is **empathy,** an appreciation of what the patient is going through. It is far more important than any special technique, more meaningful to the patient than anything learned from this or any other book. With that understood, the remainder of this chapter can be given over to comments about "tricks of the trade" of interviewing adapted from Reiser and Rosen (1984).*

(1) Pay attention to the patient's comfort. Too often, students see patients in crowded institutional settings where their dignity, privacy, and comfort are neglected. Doctors converge around the bedside in large groups and literally "talk down" to the supine patient. Introductions are mumbled or omitted altogether. Perhaps some of this is inevitable, but the psychiatric interviewer should be more meticulous in such matters. A quiet and private setting should be found if possible. Doctor and patient should both be comfortable and able to interact at eye level. Perhaps this sort of courtesy should not be called a technique at all. But its benefits for the patient and the interviewing process are so frequently overlooked that it must be underscored.

(2) Remember the basics. As emphasized in previous sections, *understanding* the patient is more important than rigid adherence to classic technique. Nevertheless, a few of the standard interviewing rules and nostrums are helpful. (a) Don't ask 2 questions at the same time. ("Have you ever been bothered by voices or odd beliefs?") (b) An open-ended question is usually preferable to a closed-ended one. (c) Don't ask questions calling for negative answers. ("You haven't had any experience with 'voices,' have you?") (d) Avoid being judgmental. ("Have you had any disgust-

ing or obscene thoughts?") (e) Make liberal use of facilitating remarks. ("I see. . . . Tell me more. . . . How was that for you? . . . Go on. . . . ") (f) Ask for clarification. ("Can you explain what you meant by that? I'm not sure I exactly followed that.")

(3) Don't be afraid to be yourself. The student should not try to imitate a portrait of Freud in a double-breasted suit. If a patient tells a joke and the joke is funny, go ahead and laugh. If the patient wants to know something about you—where you come from, whether you are married and have children—go ahead and answer. It is an unfortunate myth that the doctor-patient relationship should be totally unilateral, with the patient telling all and the doctor nothing. In an unselfconscious way, always respecting the patient's dignity, you should feel free to tell who you are, both in the facts you disclose and the attitude you convey. There are times when it is appropriate—indeed indicated—to touch a patient on his or her hand or shoulder. That may be perceived as "phony" if you are naturally reserved, and so you may not be able to bring it off. If that is the case, don't force it. But you should never be afraid to reach out and be human. Physical contact is a potent "drug" which—like any drug—may have major side effects. It takes experience to know when to touch as well as when not to. Still, too much has been written about the psychiatrist as iceberg—silent, cold, unbending. Remember also that a patient can be "touched" in many ways. An empathic expression of understanding or a sincere look of concern on your face can often touch a patient more deeply than your hand on his or her shoulder. Be yourself. When you communicate, whether through words or by laying on of your hands, be guided by your answer to the question, "Am I doing this for my patient?"

(4) Encourage the expression of feelings. Some patients are under strong cultural proscriptions against public displays of affect, especially grief and rage. Physicians may have the same attitude, and if so may believe that if a patient starts to cry, for example, something must have gone wrong with the interview. Most psychiatric patients are in emotional states they feel they cannot express—usually rage and sorrow. Almost without exception, they should be encouraged to let these feelings come out. ("There are tears in your eyes. His death has left you *very* sad, hasn't it?") The only case in which encouraging expression of affect is contraindicated is when a patient is in danger of total loss of control, signaled by escalating behavior—a louder and louder voice, tenser body habitus, etc. In such circumstances, the interviewer should demand that affect be controlled.

(5) Consider the patient in developmental terms. As this textbook makes clear, growth and development do not cease at age 21. It is often useful to consider the patient's stage of development. Might this depressed 50-year-old woman be suffering from "empty nest syndrome" (depression because the children have all left home)? Might this agitated psychotic young man be struggling with emotional conflicts related to sexual intimacy and separation from his

---

*Adapted and reproduced with permission of the copyright holder, University Park Press.

family? A developmental perspective can assist the interviewer in understanding the patient's concerns, especially if the patient and interviewer are of widely disparate ages.

(6) Remember that the patient is more scared than you are. A young man is nervous about meeting you and about the implications of having a psychiatric disturbance. Will you read his mind? Will you find him unlikable? Is he on a course leading to incurable insanity? Or do you find his problems laughably trivial, not worthy of serious attention or compassion? Inexperienced clinicians are often apprehensive in approaching a psychiatric patient but not nearly so apprehensive as the patient usually is, and knowing this may enable you to be of help sooner than otherwise.

(7) Tell the patient what you think he or she is feeling. Imagine that you yourself are suffering from a psychiatric disorder—eg, that you have developed severe phobic symptoms. You have become afraid to travel by air, then by car, and now are afraid even to leave your home on foot. Which of the following would seem more empathic to you? "Can you describe your reaction to these events?" or "You must feel like a prisoner! How painful for you!" Some clinicians argue against what may seem like putting words in a patient's mouth. That is a pitfall to be avoided, but the risk is exaggerated. If you are occasionally wrong about what a patient is feeling, the patient will tell you so. If you are consistently wrong, something has prevented you from forming an empathic bond with that patient. If you are not sure you know what the patient is feeling, it is easy enough to ask, "What is this like for you?" or "How was that for you?" in order to elicit a report of the patient's affective experience. Clinicians miss a good opportunity to interact therapeutically when they do know how the patient is feeling but fail to communicate their insight to the patient.

(8) When an interview bogs down, try repeating the patient's last words. This technique was first popularized by the psychologist Carl Rogers (1951), who felt it was maximally nondirective and encouraged patients to proceed in the direction they preferred. Overreliance on this technique, however, is counterproductive. All psychiatric interviews have a purpose, which is not restricted to letting a patient go wherever he or she wants. The interview should follow the patient's lead, but sometimes the physician must be directive. Repeating the patient's last words is a technique that can be effective and should be used when needed. Encouraging nods of the head or supportive murmurs can accomplish the same thing. Periods of silence should be permitted also.

(9) Go ahead and ask the "unaskable." If you are in touch with your own feelings as well as those of your patient, you may realize that a patient is very scared, angry, or depressed. It may even occur to you that the patient is thinking of committing suicide. Fortunately, most do not, but even if a patient does not act on suicidal thoughts, he or she may feel terribly isolated and alone. Many patients think about death but

feel they cannot tell anyone. A similar burden is imposed by other intense affects patients dread sharing. If you think that a patient might be suicidal, ask the question, tactfully and respectfully. It is impossible to put such an idea into a patient's head, which is what interviewers sometimes fear; but it is quite possible and very dangerous to ignore a patient's nonverbal signals. Most people who attempt suicide have seen a physician recently, often without indicating their intent, and many go on to use medications prescribed by the physician in the attempt. Thus, in the case of suicide, clinicians must always ask the "unaskable."

The same principle applies to many other areas—if you suspect alcoholism, drug abuse, child battering, or some other socially "delicate" problem, you must not be afraid to inquire. Occasionally you may give offense, but less often than one might think. Special note should be made of the subject of sexuality. Despite our "liberated" times, it is surprising how often interviewers overlook inquiring about sexual concerns. Sex is part of being human and is frequently affected by illness, especially psychiatric illness. Usually, however, the physician must inquire firmly and directly if he or she hopes to be of any help in this aspect of the patient's welfare. Ultimately, it is not just suicide and sex but all taboos to which the admonition *ask!* applies: fear of death, mutilation, sexual dysfunction, madness, suicide. A patient will let you know if you should back off. More often, the patient will open up with an outpouring of gratitude and relief.

(10) Learn to be quiet. When patients come to a point in their story where they are about to disclose something uncomfortable, they will often fall silent. Silence can be socially awkward, but as a psychiatric interviewer you must learn to take advantage of it. When a patient falls silent, be silent too. The pressure does build, and it may seem awkward for a time, but the patient usually goes on to tell the interviewer what is really bothering him or her. Most interviewers would do well to listen more and talk less. If silence becomes unduly protracted, it may be useful to say something neutral—"Go ahead. . . . Yes, go on. . . . I'm listening"—to relieve awkwardness and encourage the patient to continue.

(11) Pay attention to body language. Body language is one of many ways in which patients try to communicate. This subject has received considerable attention in both medical and lay publications, perhaps more than it deserves. Yet body language is an important way in which both patients and doctors express themselves. And unlike the tongue, the body seldom lies.

Body language can be particularly revealing at the beginning of the interview. Observe how patients position themselves and move. Watch how they sit or stand, seek or avoid eye contact, etc. Body language is a reliable form of communication that everyone uses. The trick, as with other observational skills, lies in being *conscious* of what is observed.

(12) Start broadly and then focus in. As the above discussion of the *"A.R.T."* of interviewing makes clear, it is rarely necessary to focus narrowly on any agenda at the outset of an interview. Allow the patient at least 3–10 minutes for assessment, the most open-ended phase of the interview. Books about interviewing list many techniques for staying broadly focused or narrowing in. They speak of open-ended versus closed-ended questions, of compound versus simple sentences, of facilitating responses, etc. While such labeling may be useful for some students, most do not find this kind of analysis helpful. Instead, as in cinematography, the interviewer should think of technique as involving a gradual focusing in, from wide-angle distance shots to narrow-angle close-ups. The interviewer's responses during the assessment phase are broadly focused wide-angle responses consisting of empathic silences, repeating the patient's last words, identifying the patient's affect ("That must have made you very sad!"), requesting clarification, etc. As the interviewer begins to focus in, questions become more directed: "Tell me more about this depression, Mr Jones." Or, "You mentioned that you and your wife have been fighting. Tell me more about what's going on there." As the camera angle narrows progressively, the questions naturally become more constricting: "How long have you been feeling that life

was hopeless?" "How many pounds have you lost?" Now the emphasis is on specific data, chronology of symptoms and their nature and severity, their relations to other symptoms, etc. At this stage, the interviewer inquires about symptoms and signs directly related to the diagnostic criteria for specific mental disorders. Finally, the interviewer may focus in on the most narrowly directed question of all—those that can only be answered yes or no: "Have you ever had blackouts?" "Have you found yourself thinking that everyone is against you?"

SUMMARY

The 12 interviewing techniques discussed above, coupled with an understanding of the content/process distinction and the *"A.R.T."* of interviewing, should enable the psychiatric interviewer to obtain a meaningful story from the patient. The interviewer should always remember, however, that technique is invariable secondary to the human dimension of interviewing—above all, establishing empathy, respect, and trust.

REFERENCES

Balint M: *The Doctor, His Patient, and the Illness.* Internat Univ Press, 1972.

Davis M: Variations in patients' compliance with doctors' orders: Analysis of congruence between survey responses and results of empirical investigations. *J Med Educ* 1966;**41:** 1037.

Freud S: Recommendations to physicians practicing psychoanalysis (1912). In: *Standard Edition of the Complete Psychological Works of Sigmund Freud.* Vol 12. Hogarth Press, 1958.

MacKinnon RA, Michels R: *The Psychiatric Interview in Clinical Practice.* Saunders, 1971.

Reiser DE, Rosen DH: *Medicine as a Human Experience.* University Park Press, 1984.

Reiser DE, Schroder AK: *Patient Interviewing: The Human Dimension.* Williams & Wilkins, 1980.

Rogers CL: *Client-Centered Therapy.* Houghton Mifflin, 1951.

Sullivan HS: *Schizophrenia as a Human Process.* Norton, 1962.

The Mental Status Examination

18

Jonathan Mueller, MD, Ralph J. Kiernan, PhD, & J.W. Langston, MD

The mental status examination (MSE) is an instrument the clinician uses to assess a patient's orientation, attention, feeling states, speech, thought patterns, and specific cognitive skills. Like a lens or filter, it allows the clinician to perceive details and patterns whose nature might otherwise be only vaguely delineated. This examination, along with a careful history, physical examination, and laboratory examination, provides the foundation for psychiatric diagnosis and clinical assessment. Table 18–1 lists the major elements of the mental status examination organized in hierarchical format.

As Hughlings Jackson pointed out, functions most recently evolved (phylogenetically and ontogenetically) are the most vulnerable to disruption. Psychiatrists study disruption of thoughts, feelings, and behaviors that emerge from the organic functioning of the brain. The hierarchical structure of the mental status examination reflects the fact that higher cortical functions, such as abstract thought, may be distorted or disrupted by pathologic processes at many levels. It is obvious that one cannot test a stuporous patient's appreciation of abstract similarities, but it is often forgotten that other factors also constrain assessment of thought processes. For example, a patient who is unable to attend because of fever or metabolic disturbance cannot make new memories, although the neuronal substrate for "memory making" may be structurally intact. Among the factors that affect the interpretation and conduct of the mental status examination are disturbances of attention, vigilance, or concentration; emotional turmoil; perceptual disturbances (impaired vision or hearing); and receptive or expressive language disorders. A patient unwilling to cooperate with the examination will neither reveal intact functions nor disclose deficits. Failure to recognize limitations at any of these levels will lead to errors both in diagnostic formulation and in determination of appropriate treatment.

Although the mental status examination will be presented here as a separate part of the clinical examination (chief complaint, history of present illness, past medical, psychiatric, and social history, etc), it must be emphasized that the mental status examination is not simply an encapsulated or isolated part of the evaluation. Information noted throughout the interview will later be reported in the mental status examination, and information gained during formal mental status testing may prompt the physician to reevaluate the medical history or to seek confirmation of details by returning to specific items later in the examination. When a patient has a memory disorder, for example, the clinician should suspect omissions and inconsistencies in the history and investigate other sources if needed.

Physicians do not always have multiple opportunities to evaluate patients and may be called on for urgent decisions about a patient's capacity for self-care, potential for violence, suicidal risk, or hold on reality. Especially in emergency room and consultation/liaison settings, there is a premium on prompt assessment. To maximize the yield of the mental status examination, the clinician must be ever mindful of the privileged nature of the relationship with the patient and of the impact specific questions may have on the patient. Initially, the examiner should explain the purpose of the mental status examination, indicating that it is part of every complete patient evaluation. It may help reduce the patient's anxiety and avoid offending the patient to add, "You may find some of the questions very easy and some quite difficult to answer." The clinician must be able to note subtle behavioral clues (a change in voice tone, averted gaze, a tear, a swallow, a sigh, or hesitancy to discuss a particular matter) without losing track of material that must be covered in order to complete the examination. Although the examiner should have a structured scheme for covering all aspects of the mental status examination, a "shopping list" approach is not appropriate. Nevertheless, certain complaints, signs, or symptoms do require that a mental checklist be consulted. For example, if a patient experiences hallucinations, it is essential to obtain a detailed description of the phenomenon. (1) Are hallucinations auditory, visual, tactile, olfactory, or gustatory? (2) Are they elementary (simple points or lines) or complex (formed figures)? (3) Do visual hallucinations occur only in one part of the visual field? (4) Are they disturbing or comforting? (5) Is the hallucinating patient com-

Table 18–1. Organizing the mental status examination (hierarchical format).

1. Presentation.
2. Motor behavior and affect.
3. Cognitive status.
4. Thought.
5. Mood.

manded to perform certain acts (eg, do things harmful to self or others), and if so can the commands be resisted? (6) Do the hallucinations seem to emanate from a particular source?

GENERAL FORMAT OF THE MENTAL STATUS EXAMINATION

The goal of the mental status examination is to assess—both qualitatively and quantitatively—a range of mental functions at a specific time. A clear record of the data provides a baseline for future examinations. Quantification of elements of the mental status examination enables the clinician to assess deterioration or improvement in specific functions over time.

Assessment of cognitive strengths and weaknesses traditionally has been done by psychologists. Physicians who wish to benefit from precise measurement of cognitive function must either master the psychologic literature on the subject or learn to make their own assessments. Quantitative assessment of higher cortical functions (cognitive status examination) is a process that is essential for proper diagnosis and management of organic mental disorders. Specifically, attention, language, constructional ability, recent memory, calculation, and reasoning abilities such as appreciation of similarities and practical judgment can all be assessed in a graded fashion.

One practical way to characterize cognitive dysfunction is to systematically probe areas of intellectual functioning with **screening** questions difficult enough that a right answer implies an adequate level of function in that area and renders further testing of that area unnecessary. If the patient fails the screening item, the examiner presents a very easy question followed by a series of increasingly difficult ones (the **metric**). This "screen/metric" approach provides a graded quantitative measure of the degree of functional impairment in specific areas. Such an approach is rapid and efficient, since time is not wasted examining areas in which the patient has obvious strengths.

Several standardized brief mental status examinations serve as cognitive screening devices but are insensitive to important aspects of mental status. Textbooks often provide very detailed "laundry list" approaches to mental status examinations that may exhaust both patient and examiner when used rigidly and in their entirety. Such mental status examination formats are rarely presented hierarchically and do not provide quantifiable results. The following approach to the standardized and quantified mental status examination is recommended for routine use in single or serial assessments. Although its organization differs from that of standard examinations in current use, it contains the same elements. A detailed outline of this mental status examination and a standardized work sheet and report form are provided in Table 18–3 and Figures 18–4 and 18–5 at the end of this chapter. Many of the terms are defined in the Glossary of Psychiatric Signs & Symptoms or elsewhere in the text.

PRESENTATION

Level of Consciousness

Fluctuations in degree of alertness should be documented as precisely as possible. (For example, "Patient yawning and drowsy but responds to verbal encouragement with cooperation that never lasts more than 20 seconds.") Level of consciousness can be described along a continuum from coma to full alertness. **Coma** is a state in which neither verbal nor motor responses can be elicited by noxious stimuli. (In moderate to light coma, motor reflexes may be elicited but not psychologic responses.) **Stupor** is a state in which vigorous and repeated stimulation is required to rouse the patient. **Somnolence** and **lethargy** are less obtunded states in which drowsy, inactive, and indifferent patients respond to stimulation in delayed or incomplete fashion. **Drowsiness** is a sleeplike state from which the patient cannot be roused fully by minor stimuli. **Alert wakefulness** is a state in which responses to auditory, tactile, or visual stimuli are prompt and appropriate.

The Glasgow Coma Scale (Table 18–2) developed by Teasdale and Jennett (1974) is a graded approach to assessment of impaired consciousness on the basis of eye opening and verbal and motor responses to various stimuli. The scale ranges from 3 for deep coma to 14 for alert wakefulness. It has demonstrated great value for assessing and predicting degree of recovery.

General Appearance

The examiner notes clothing, personal hygiene, and any use of cosmetics, documenting details of fastidiousness or inattention (eg, "a 3-day growth of beard with food spilled on his nightshirt"). Is the pa-

Table 18–2. Glasgow Coma Scale.

	Coma Scale
Eyes open (E)	
Spontaneously	4
To speech	3
To pain	2
None	1
Best motor response (M)	
Obeys commands	5
Localizes pain	4
Flexion to pain	3
Extension to pain	2
None	1
Best verbal response (V)	
Oriented	5
Confused	4
Inappropriate words	3
Incomprehensible sounds	2
None	1

Summed Glasglow Coma Scale = E + M + V.

Range: From 3 for deep coma to 14 for alert wakefulness.

tient robust in appearance? Does he or she appear physically ill, with signs of alcoholism (eg, palmar erythema, facial flushing, spider angiomas) or endocrine disease (eg, cushingoid)? Special attention is paid to idiosyncrasies of appearance. These details should be recorded carefully enough so that a third party would be able to recognize the patient from the description without having seen the patient.

Attitude

Is the patient cooperative, evasive, arrogant, bemused, or apathetic? The patient's attitude toward the examiner and the examination situation determines to a large extent how much and what kind of information will be derived.

MOTOR BEHAVIOR & AFFECT

Motor Behavior

Are the patient's movements rapid, abrupt, clumsy, graceful, or totally absent? Is the level of motor activity fairly constant, or do abrupt periods of fitful hyperactivity alternate with apathetic withdrawal? If the patient displays unusual responses, how are they provoked? Are movements coherent and goal-directed, or do they have no discernible purpose? Are there bizarre repetitive stereotyped movements? Does behavior include nail biting (anxiety), tapping the feet (anxiety or akathisia), or sticking out the tongue and licking the lips repetitively (buccolingual-masticatory syndrome of tardive dyskinesia)?

If the patient is mute, does he or she consistently avoid the examiner's gaze, closing eyes tightly and resisting efforts to lift the lids (catatonic negativism or malingering)? Do the patient's movements repeat those of the examiner (echopraxia)? Will the patient's limbs remain in unnatural positions if placed there (called catalepsy, or "waxy flexibility")? Is a mute patient able to write if handed a pencil or to nod yes or no in response to certain questions (indicating either aphemia or hysterical mutism)? Is there any change in behavior depending upon whether the examiner discusses nonpersonal events rather than more personal issues such as the health of either the patient or the patient's immediate family?

Affect

"Affect" may be considered the observable correlate of emotion, ie, the outer manifestation of inner states. It may be characterized as bright, sluggish, voluble, expansive, anguished, tearful, etc. The examiner pays particular attention to the range, intensity, lability, and appropriateness of affective behavior.

Affect has 3 components: facial expression, gestures, and speech. Although speech and language are often described together, there is a rationale for considering the flow, volume, pressure, rhythm, and intonation of speech as kinetic phenomena apart from language. The emotional coloring (prosody) of speech may be impaired in major depression, in dysfunction of the basal ganglia, in Broca's aphasia ("motor" aphasia), or secondary to damage of the right cerebral hemisphere (see Chapter 10).

The term "witzelsucht" refers to a facetious jocularity sometimes observed in association with frontal lobe lesions.

"Blunted" affect is grossly diminished in range of emotional expression.

Explosions of tears or anger ("catastrophic reactions") can occur in organically impaired individuals confronted with tasks once simple but now difficult or impossible to perform.

COGNITIVE STATUS

Arguments can be made for assessing the patient's cognition at either the outset or the conclusion of the mental status examination. The authors believe that a structured assessment of the patient's cognitive status is best performed immediately after the clinician has noted the patient's initial presentation, motor behavior, and affect, before an attempt is made to assess thought and mood. Impairments in cognitive ability may masquerade as either thought disorder (aphasia may appear as "concreteness of thought") or mood disturbance (an amnestic patient given the diagnosis of cancer 2 days previously may make no spontaneous mention of this and may therefore appear to deny or be indifferent to the diagnosis).

Attention

Is the patient so preoccupied or easily distracted that cooperation with the examiner is impossible? Is there a visual field cut, inattention to a visual hemifield in the absence of a field cut, or neglect of one side of the body?

A. Immediate Recall: Immediate recall refers to the retention of small amounts of information for up to 30 seconds. Material "in" immediate recall requires further processing before it can enter more permanent memory stores.

Proper assessment of attention is of great importance, since it may have implications for further evaluation and treatment. In the presence of an attentional deficit, the examiner must be wary of drawing inferences from further testing of higher cortical functions. Since inattention is a hallmark of acute confusional state, its presence should prompt a search for remediable (toxic, metabolic, or infectious) medical problems. However, inattention may also be seen in nonorganic mental disorders such as brief psychotic reaction and posttraumatic stress disorders. As a general rule, digit span (see below) is preserved in the early stages of dementia, and it is not until cortical degeneration is well advanced that one finds impaired attention.

Attention span may be assessed by having the patient repeat a list of words or a digit sequence presented at the rate of one digit per second. It is important that the digits not be grouped (by rhythmic clusters or intonation) and that they be somewhat random (eg, not all odd or all even). This should be practiced, since it is difficult to present a string of digits in this fashion without clustering. Intact repetition of 6 digits forward rules out major attentional disturbance. Inability to repeat at least 5 digits is considered abnormal.

Patients who fail the initial screening task of 6-digit repetition are presented with a metric: digit sequences of increasing length, beginning with 3-digit numbers. The examiner discontinues this task only after the patient has missed twice at a given level (eg, 2 mistakes at the 5-digit level).

B. Concentration & Vigilance: The ability to sustain attention over a longer period may be referred to as "concentration" or "vigilance." Serial 7s (see p 199) or repetition backward of a digit sequence or the months of the year (or days of the week) may be used to assess concentration. Psychiatric disorders such as anxiety, depression, and schizophrenia may impair vigilance without disrupting digit repetition.

Orientation

Orientation is assessed with reference to person, place, and time. Orientation to **person** (ability to give one's own name when asked to do so) reflects "overlearned" information and is seldom if ever lost in organic brain disease. Failure to give one's own name occurs in hysterical dissociation and most often reflects negativism, confusion, distraction, hearing impairment, or receptive language disorder.

Orientation to **place** can be tested with reference to country, state, county, city, type of building, name of building, location of building, and location in the building. A patient may know he or she is in a hospital but not know the city or state.

Orientation to **time** may be tested with reference to year, season, month, day of week, and date. Because time changes more frequently than location, it is more vulnerable to disruption and thus is the most sensitive index of disorientation. (One cannot, however, use time of day as a screen for orientation to time, since patients may know or guess the time of day from numerous cues but have no idea of the month or year.)

Language

Failure to assess language in a systematic fashion is a shortcoming of many mental status examinations and can lead to diagnostic confusion. Word-finding difficulty (anomia), for example, may be mistakenly thought to reflect a disorder of memory or judgment. Aphasia (see Chapter 10) is a language disorder often mistakenly attributed to confusion, dementia, hysteria, or psychosis.

Language proficiency is assessed by testing 4 parameters: fluency, comprehension, repetition, and naming. (Reading and writing will not be discussed here.)

A. Fluency: Fluency refers to the ability to produce sentences of normal length, rhythm, and melody. It is commonly assessed by listening to the patient's spontaneous speech. Is speech hesitant, stammering, or inarticulate? Are words mumbled or spoken too softly to be heard? Is the volume constant, or does it decrease toward the end of the sentence? Does the patient use bizarre syntax resulting in nonsense? What is the range of vocabulary? Is speech "empty," consisting of few substantive words and frequent circumlocutions? (The function or some particular attribute of an item may be offered as a substitute for its name—eg, "the thing that holds it on your shirt," rather than "the clip of the pen.") Patients may become adept at masking word-finding difficulty by skirting certain issues or using unobtrusive circumlocutions.

A helpful method for assessing fluency is to have the patient describe what he or she observes in a picture such as the "fishing picture" (Fig 18–1). Although this is not truly spontaneous speech, there are distinct advantages to presenting each patient with a uniform speech stimulus. The examiner quickly learns to note neglect of details and to recognize subtle word-finding difficulties. Upon completion of the patient's description, the examiner can return to specific details of the picture that have been omitted or incorrectly described. Verbatim recording of a patient's description of the picture is essential. Special attention is paid to paraphasic errors, which consist of distortions involving either individual letters ("brain clumor") or whole words (eg, "stick" for pencil). Speech is described for clinical purposes in an all-or-nothing fashion as either "fluent" or "nonfluent."

B. Comprehension: Just as intact auditory perception is essential for optimal interactions between geriatric patients and friends or hospital staff, language comprehension is also crucial. Since repetition and comprehension may be "dissociated" in language disorders that spare the perisylvian speech areas (see Chapter 10), it is dangerous to infer intact comprehension from a patient's ability to repeat what is said. Thus, any tendency by the patient to consistently echo or repeat should actually raise a question of comprehension deficit. It is as if these patients are trying to "run the tape by" one more time in order to extract from it as much information as possible.

There are many ways to assess comprehension at the bedside. The patient can be asked to point to objects the examiner names or whose function is described. This method is limited by objects that are at hand and by the examiner's skill in abstract description of common objects. Another approach is to present questions that can be answered yes or no. If this is done, the examiner must ask at least 6 questions, since the patient has a 50–50 chance of answering any one question correctly. (It should also be noted that some aphasic patients are unable to say yes or no even when they know the answer.)

A graded screening and metric approach to testing comprehension that has proved useful is as follows:

The screening item consists of obeying a 3-step command. At least 5 objects are placed in front of the patient, who is told to "turn over the paper, hand me the pen, and point to your nose." A patient who fails this task is asked to perform the metric, which consists

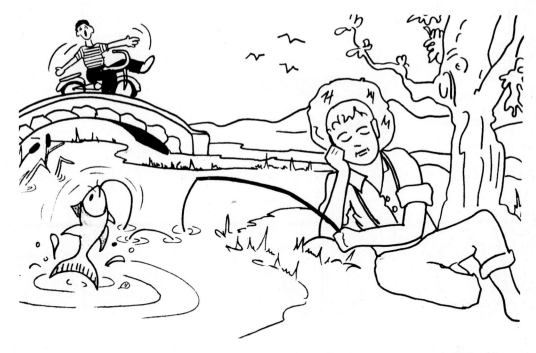

Figure 18–1. "Fishing Picture." (Reproduced with permission of the Northern California Neurobehavioral Group, Inc.: *Neurobehavioral Mental Status Examination Test Booklet and Stimulus Booklet.* Copyright © 1983.)

of three 1-step commands, two 2-step commands, and one 3-step command. Success in performing each of the one-step commands rules out major apraxic problems. (See Chapter 10 for discussion of ideomotor apraxia.)

The metric is performed (for example) as follows:

One-step commands: (1) Pick up the pen. (2) Point to the floor. (3) Hand me the keys.

Two-step commands: (1) Point to the pen and pick up the keys. (2) Hand me the paper and point to the coin.

Three-step command: Point to the keys, hand me the pen, and pick up the coin.

A surprising number of patients are unable to perform a 3-step command despite intact cooperation, attention, and auditory acuity. Careful documentation of inability to comprehend and comply with complex requests (ie, subclinical language disorder) is of great value to the nursing staff and others who manage the patient on the ward. Documentation of such deficits minimizes the risk that these patients will be wrongfully considered negativistic or uncooperative.

C. Repetition: Sentences that are short and contain high-frequency ("everyday") words are the easiest to repeat. Longer sentences that contain low-frequency words or short grammatical function words with no objective referents ("from," "and") are more difficult to repeat. An appropriate screening sentence for repetition might be "The beginning movement revealed the composer's intention." The patient who fails this is given a series of phrases or sentences of graded difficulty as the metric: "Out the window." "He

swam across the lake." "The winding road led to the village." "He left the latch open." "The honeycomb drew a swarm of bees." "No *ifs, ands,* or *buts.*"

Because the bizarre speech of patients with Wernicke's aphasia is fluent, the physician may incorrectly conclude that these patients are psychotic or in a confusional state. Demonstration of paraphasic errors on repetition tasks provides elegant proof of primary language dysfunction. Repetition is impaired in all of the major perisylvian aphasic syndromes.

D. Naming: Naming parts of an object (eg, "tentacle") is even more difficult than naming the object itself ("octopus"). Thus, an appropriate screening question turns out to be naming a pen and its parts on visual confrontation: cap or cover, point or nib, and clip. (The patient who can name a pen and its parts has intact naming ability and does not have aphasia.) A patient unable to pass the screening question is confronted with a metric consisting of 8 pictured items that are increasingly difficult to name (Fig 18–2). Thus, one obtains a graded estimate of the degree of word-finding difficulty.

Although an individual who names items correctly does not have aphasia, not every patient who manifests naming difficulties has aphasia. Otherwise healthy individuals who are physically exhausted or sleep-deprived often manifest dysnomia. Dysnomia may be an early nonspecific sign of generalized cerebral dysfunction secondary to metabolic disturbance. Aphasic dysnomia may occur as an isolated and dramatic deficit with localized left hemispheric lesions, or it may exist as part of a larger aphasic syndrome.

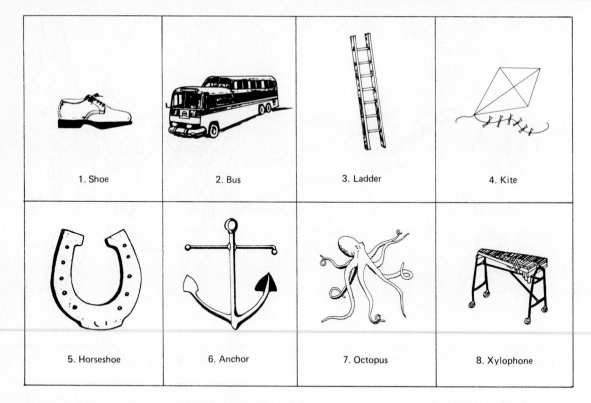

Figure 18–2. Eight pictures from the metric test of naming ability. (Reproduced with permission of the Northern California Neurobehavioral Group, Inc.: *Neurobehavioral Mental Status Examination Test Booklet and Stimulus Booklet.* Copyright © 1983.)

Unless naming is carefully assessed, the clinician runs the risk of mistaking word-finding difficulty for "thought blocking," amnesia, or impaired judgment. Accordingly, language is assessed prior to memory.

Memory

A. Verbal Memory: A general impression of the patient's memory can be gained from the way in which he or she presents the history. Is there internal consistency, or are there gaps and contradictions? Does the patient remember the physician's name from a past encounter, or does the patient confabulate, claiming to have met an individual whom he or she has never seen before? Is there a period for which the patient has poor recall? If so, is the patient unable to recall either personal or general information from that period (organic amnesia), or is there selective inability to recall personally relevant information (psychogenic amnesia)?

1. Recent memory–Ability to recall events of the past minutes or days reflects recent memory. (Orientation to place and time also actually reflects memory.) Recent memory is assessed clinically by asking the patient to learn new information. This is commonly done by presenting 4 unrelated words. The patient is told that he or she will be asked for these words later in the examination. The examiner must be certain the patient can repeat all 4 words before going on with other parts of the examination, which constitute

"interference material." (The number of trials required to learn 4 words is another measure of attention.) Failure to make sure that the patient can repeat all 4 words invalidates any conclusions about recent memory as a specific ability area—the patient may simply not have been attending to the task, and apparent failure to recall may really reflect initial failure to register material.

For each word a patient is unable to recall after 5 or 10 minutes, a category prompt (eg, "a color" or "an animal") is given. If the patient is still unable to recall the word, a list of 3 or 4 words—one of which is the test word—is presented. Points are assigned on the basis of whether a word is recalled on command (3 points), following a prompt (2 points), or recognized from a list (1 point).

Five to 10 minutes after a depressed patient or a severely amnestic alcoholic has been given 4 words to learn, neither may be able to recall any of the words when asked to do so. The depressed patient, however, will usually respond to category prompts or recognize the words from lists, whereas an alcoholic patient with Korsakoff's syndrome may not even recall having been given a list of words to learn. The examiner who simply records "none of 4 words recalled at 5 minutes" for both of these patients fails to distinguish 2 very different situations. Moreover, a maximum 12-point scoring system (4 items, each rated 0–3) allows the clinician to monitor improvement or deterioration of memory following administration of agents such as thiamine, digitalis and diuretics, or tricyclic antidepressants. Clinicians who ask patients what they had for breakfast should verify the answer by asking the nursing staff also. It is worth repeating that the distinction between attentional and amnestic deficits is crucial. *The diagnosis of amnestic syndrome cannot be made in the presence of an attentional deficit.*

2. Remote memory–Ability to recall the events of weeks or years ago is difficult to assess clinically, since the examiner seldom knows enough about the patient to ask pertinent or verifiable questions. Unless the examiner is prepared to seek corroboration (such as what schools the patient actually attended or the dates of military service), there is no point in asking such questions. Questions about past presidents, dates of wars, and events that affect everyone (such as President Kennedy's assassination) are helpful, but evaluation of responses remains problematic, since failure to recall may reflect increasing forgetfulness (as in senile dementia) or a period of time during which the patient was unable to lay down memories. With resolution of memory problems (eg, following traumatic amnesia secondary to head injury, or in response to thiamine treatment of Wernicke-Korsakoff syndrome), older memories tend to return before more recent ones (Ribot's law).

B. Visual Memory: Patients may be asked to reproduce designs or report details of pictures after delays of seconds or minutes. Alternatively, the examiner may ask the patient to remember a series of items (eg, clock, window, chair) or where the examiner places or hides an item such as a dollar bill (eg, behind a picture).

Constructional Ability

While testing of constructional ability is frequently omitted from the routine mental status examination, it may be helpful in the detection of organic brain disease. Patients may be asked to copy drawings, manipulate blocks, or reconstruct a figure using tokens. Before the examiner draws conclusions about a patient's constructional ability, it is essential to assess visual acuity, motor functions (strength, praxis, and coordination), and tactile sensation.

As a screening test for constructional ability, the patient is instructed to study 2 figures for 10 seconds and is then asked to reproduce them from memory. Successful completion of the screen requires intact immediate visual recall as well as significant visual-spatial ability. The screening test and examples of acceptable and unacceptable responses are shown in Fig 18–3.

Individuals who fail the screen are asked either to copy a series of increasingly difficult figures or to reconstruct geometric figures using tokens (Fig 18–3).

Calculations

The patient's education and professional background should be considered before calculating ability

is tested. The traditional "serial 7s" task, in which the patient is asked to "subtract 7 from 100 and then continue, subtracting 7 from each answer," is a difficult task for many high school graduates (ie, over two-thirds are unable to get into the 50s without an error in less than 30 seconds). In addition to calculating ability, the task requires sustained concentration and is easily disrupted by anxiety; for this reason, difficulty with serial 7s should not be taken as evidence of dyscalculia. Simple addition, subtraction, and multiplication often assess rote learning (a type of remote recall) rather than calculating. Thus, an appropriate assessment of calculations involves tasks that fall somewhere between the 2 examples. As a screening device, the question "How much is 5×13?" is appropriate. Examples of metric items are shown below.

How much is $5 + 3$?
How much is $15 + 7$?
How much is 39 divided by 3?
How much is $31 - 8$?

Reasoning

Cognition can be subdivided into 2 areas: practical judgment and abstraction (similarities and proverb interpretation).

A. Practical Judgment: Assessing practical judgment is especially important in the evaluation of thought disorders, character disorders, or dementia. This area is difficult to appraise because many judgment questions can be answered "correctly" by the aid of simple memory (remembering what one's parents or teachers said should be done in a given situation). Practical judgment also reflects the patient's social and financial background. (A prosperous physician who loses his wallet in the airport in Denver, Colorado, might call home to have money wired to him, whereas an adolescent runaway might turn to Traveler's Aid, go to a local church, or try to hitchhike.)

1. Screening question–The patient is asked, "What would you do if you were stranded in the airport in Denver, Colorado, with only a dollar in your pocket?" Acceptable answers are calling a friend or family member to wire money and going to Traveler's Aid. If the patient claims to know people in the Denver area, the examiner should say, "For the purposes of this question, imagine you are in an airport far away from anyone you know." If the patient suggests using credit cards, the examiner should say, "For the purposes of this question, imagine you do not have credit cards." Patients should be asked to explain their answers further when vague or partially correct answers are given.

2. Metric–The patient is asked the following series of questions. A score of 2 points is given for a fully correct answer, 1 point for a partially correct or vague answer, and no points for an incorrect answer. Examples of 2-point, 1-point, and 0-point answers for each item are given below.

a. What would you do if you woke up at 1 minute before 8:00 AM and remembered an appointment

Screening test: Copy these figures:

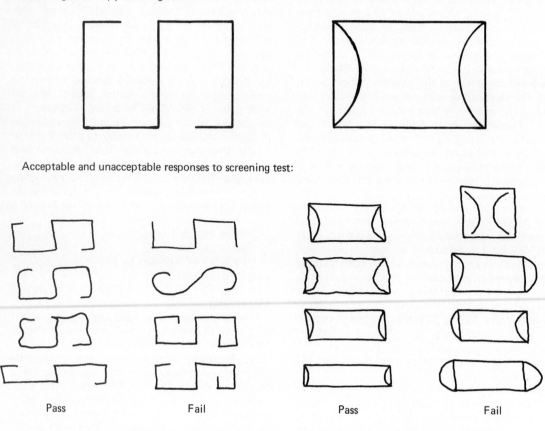

Acceptable and unacceptable responses to screening test:

Pass   Fail   Pass   Fail

Metric test for constructions:

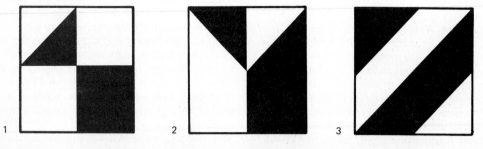

1   2   3

Figure 18–3. Testing constructional ability. (Reproduced with permission of the Northern California Neurobehavioral Group, Inc.: *Neurobehavioral Mental Status Examination Test Booklet and Stimulus Booklet.* Copyright © 1983.)

downtown at 8:00 AM? *Answers:* 2 points–call the person; 1 point–dress as quickly as I can and rush downtown; 1 point (vague)–cancel the appointment; 0 points–go back to bed.

b. What would you do if while walking beside a lake you saw a 2-year-old child playing alone at the end of a pier? *Answers:* 2 points–remove the child from the pier and look for the parents; 1 point–tell the child to get away from the water; 1 point (vague)– make sure the child is not harmed; 0 points–yell for help; look for a lifeguard; go for help.

c. What would you do if you came home and found

a broken pipe was flooding the kitchen? *Answers:* 2 points–shut off the main water valve; 1 point–call the plumber; 1 point (vague)–stop the water; 0 points– mop up the mess.

B. Abstraction: (Similarities and proverb interpretation.)

1. Similarities–Ability to appreciate the commonality between 2 objects is tested as part of the Wechsler Adult Intelligence Scale. Low native intelligence, psychosis, distraction, or dementia may produce impairment in abstracting ability.

a. Screening question–The patient is told, "I

am going to ask you how some things are alike." A specific example is then given: "For example, a hat and a coat are alike because they are both clothing." As a screening item, the patient is asked, "In what way are painting and music alike?" Only the abstract responses "art" or "forms of art" are passing. Less specific abstract responses, such as both are "artistic" or "created," are not passing answers.

b. Metric–The patient is told, "I have some other pairs of items. Again, I want you to tell me how they are alike. In what way are a rose and a tulip alike?" Each item is similarly introduced. The first time a patient responds with a difference between the items, that response is recorded and the patient is told, "That is how they are different. I want you to tell me how they are alike." Regardless of whether the patient goes on to give a good answer, no credit is given. Subsequent "difference" responses are not corrected or credited with points.

(1) Rose–tulip: 2 points–flowers; 1 point–grow, have petals, need water, smell nice; 0 points–pretty, same color, fresh, outdoors.

(2) Bicycle–train: 2 points–vehicles, means of transportation; 1 point–ride them, wheels, toys; 0 points–go fast, have tracks.

(3) Watch–ruler: 2 points–measuring instruments; 1 point–have numbers, tell how much; 0 points–are useful, have many parts.

(4) Corkscrew–hammer: 2 points–tools; 1 point– used by humans, made of metal, do work; 0 points–cut into things, are strong.

2. Proverb interpretation–Another means of assessing a patient's capacity to abstract is to ask for the patient's interpretation of a proverb. Proverbs such as "There's no use crying over spilled milk" and "The grass is always greener on the other side of the street" are easier than "People who live in glass houses shouldn't throw stones" or "Every cloud has a silver lining." Proverb interpretation is strongly influenced by culture, educational level, and socioeconomic class.

THOUGHT

Assessment of thought may be divided into several areas: process, content, cognitive functions (abstraction and judgment), fund of knowledge, and insight. Each will be discussed briefly.

Thought Process
Process of thought is assessed by noting coherence of speech and reflects the way in which mental associations are made. Thought process may be described as concrete, tangential (getting off the track of the subject and failing to return), circumstantial (digressive but able to return to the subject), perseverative (sticking to a single thought, phrase, or word), loose (absence of logical thought progression), or incoherent. Thought "blocking" refers to sudden cessation of thought or speech. It may occur in schizophrenia, and lesser de-

grees are seen in anxiety states such as obsessive compulsive disorders. In rare instances, thought process may be so disrupted that the examiner has little or no idea of the content of a patient's thought.

Thought Content
In assessing the content of a patient's thought, the examiner notes preoccupations, ambitions, phobias, and perceptual disturbances (such as illusions and hallucinations). Patients may be asked, "Do you have the feeling that you control your own thoughts?" On careful questioning, patients may admit that they believe thoughts are inserted into or withdrawn from their minds or broadcast to others, or that their thoughts are controlled by outside forces.

Specific fears or beliefs should not be taken at face value, but their origins should be explored. A statement such as "I don't want to go out of my house," for example, may have widely different meanings. A patient with a right parietal lobe tumor may no longer be able to find the way home after walking to a nearby store. One suffering from a major depressive disorder may feel too tired to go for a walk or may have lost all interest in former sources of pleasure. A schizophrenic patient may fear being overtaken by enemies and tortured. Yet another individual may fear open streets or becoming trapped in a crowd.

Patients who deny specific delusions may still claim to have a special relationship with God. It is often helpful to ask patients, "How do you think others feel about you?" (admired, shunned, unappreciated, etc).

Although visual and olfactory hallucinations may occur in "functional" psychoses such as schizophrenia or affective disorder, they tend to occur more frequently in association with organic disease. Patients should be asked to describe how vivid and frequent their hallucinations are, in what circumstances they occur (on falling asleep or waking), and whether they are pleasant, comforting, or terrifying. They should be asked to identify the source of the hallucination (whether it originates within the patient or is projected from some outer source). If hallucinations consist of commands, patients should be asked whether they are able to resist the commands. Patients who are asked if they have special bodily feelings may respond that they feel dead or unreal inside.

Insight
The patient's degree of understanding of his or her medical or psychologic problems is a measure of insight. The patient may be asked, "How do you understand your problems?" or "What has been most helpful to you in dealing with this problem in the past?" Although insight and understanding are often essential to working with patients, some patients are able to acquire insight only after their behavior has changed. It is always important to look for cognitive, perceptual, or informational explanations of "poor insight" before imputing to patients psychodynamic defenses against insight.

MOOD

The term "mood" denotes a persisting subjective state of feeling tone as reported by the patient. If the patient does not volunteer a description of his or her mood, the examiner may ask, "How are you feeling inside?" or "What are your spirits like?" Mood may be characterized (for example) as blue, despondent, anxious, fearful, bored, exuberant, irritable, or restless.

Are there dissociations between affect and reported mood? Does the patient with immobile facies say that he or she feels nothing inside or report that he or she feels sad but cannot cry? Does the facial expression of a schizophrenic patient who describes inner feelings of fear or emptiness reflect this, or does he or she wear a "silly" smile while describing inner turmoil? Patients with pseudobulbar palsy (due to disruption of fibers connecting frontal motor cortex with brain stem nuclei subserving emotional expression) may report episodes of laughing or crying uncontrollably, breaking into laughter when they feel blackly depressed, or crying when amused.

MENTAL STATUS & INTELLIGENCE

Mental status examination and intelligence testing are often combined. Elements of the mental status examination are tested in formal tests of intelligence. Abnormalities in mental status (eg, attention or memory) clearly affect ability to complete tests of intelligence (see Chapter 20 for a detailed discussion of tests of intelligence). Conversely, some rough measures of intelligence, especially fund of knowledge, often are included in mental status examinations. Our formal examination format does not include measurement of fund of knowledge, but it is briefly described here for the sake of completeness.

The patient's **fund of knowledge** may be assessed by asking questions about a wide range of subjects (politics, literature, art, history, geography, etc). In addition to reflecting educational level, the questioning may also help evaluate recent and remote memory. Although intelligence often manifests itself in a wide range of interests, some individuals with superior intelligence actually have very restricted interests. Vocabulary (noted under speech) represents a particular example of fund of knowledge and correlates highly with intelligence.

Table 18–3. Detailed elements of the mental status examination (hierarchical format).

1. **Presentation:**
   Level of consciousness: coma to alert wakefulness (Glasgow Coma Scale; see Table 18–2).
   General appearance: body habitus; hygiene; cosmesis; dress.
   Attitude: degree of cooperation and effort.
2. **Motor behavior and affect:**
   Motor behavior: akinesia; involuntary movements; mannerisms.
   Affect: facial expression; gestures; speech characteristics; pressure, volume, prosody.
3. **Cognitive status:**
   Attention:
      Attention span: digit span; number of trials required to learn 4 words.
      Concentration and vigilance: serial subtraction; letter cancellation tasks; months of year backwards.
   Orientation: for personal identity; place; time.
   Language:
      Fluency: spontaneous speech; description of picture.
      Comprehension: of spoken or written language; performing commands of graded complexity; response to "yes/no" questions; pointing to named or described items.
      Repetition: sentences of graded difficulty; isolated words; letters; numbers.
      Naming: objects and parts of objects to visual confrontation (or on tactile presentation).
      Reading: aloud vs for comprehension; paragraph; sentence; words; letters; numbers.
      Writing: written description of picture; write name and address; write from dictation; copy a written phrase, word, or letter.
      Spelling: words of graded difficulty.
   Memory:
      Verbal memory: 4 unrelated words recalled after 5 minutes; recall of short story or paired words.
      Visual memory: reproduction of figures; recall of where examiner hides object.
   Constructional ability: reproducing figures from memory; copying figures; constructing blocks or token designs.
   Calculations: addition, subtraction, multiplication, and division.
   Reasoning:
      Practical judgment.
      Abstraction: similarities and proverb interpretation.
4. **Thought:**
   Process: coherence; goal directedness; logicality.
   Content: hallucinations; delusions; preoccupations; suicidal or homicidal ideation.
   Insight: nature of illness and awareness of factors that affect the course of the illness.
5. **Mood:**
   Relation to affect and congruence with thought content.

TEST BOOKLET
for
THE NEUROBEHAVIORAL COGNITIVE STATUS EXAMINATION
(NCSE)

Addressograph

NAME:_____

AGE AND DATE OF BIRTH: _____

NATIVE LANGUAGE: _____

HANDEDNESS (circle):   L   R

LEVEL OF EDUCATION: _____

OCCUPATIONAL STATUS: _____

DATE: _____

TIME: _____

EXAMINER: _____

EXAMINATION LOCATION: _____

COGNITIVE STATUS PROFILE*

	LOC	ORI	ATT	LANGUAGE			CONST	MEM	CALC	REASONING	
				COMP	REP	NAM				SIM	JUD
							--6--			--8--	--6--
† AVG. RANGE	-ALERT-	--12--	-(S)8-	-(S)6-	--(S)--	--(S)--	-(S)5-	--12--	-(S)4-	-(S)6-	(S)5-
					--12--	--8--					
		--10--	--6--	--5--	--11--	--7--	--4--	--10--	--3--	--5--	--4--
MILD	--IMP--	--8--	--4--	--4--	--9--	--5--	--3--	--8--	--2--	--4--	--3--
MODERATE		--6--	--2--	--3--	--7--	--3--	--2--	--6--	--1--	--3--	--2--
SEVERE		--4--	--0--	--2--	--5--	--2--	--0--	--4--	--0--	--2--	--1--
Write in lower scores		⊠					⊠		⊠		

ABBREVIATIONS

ATT	-	Attention	JUD	-	Judgment	ORI	-	Orientation
CALC	-	Calculations	LOC	-	Level of Consciousness	REP	-	Repetition
COMP	-	Comprehension				S	-	Screen
CONST	-	Constructions	MEM	-	Memory	SIM	-	Similarities
IMP	-	Impaired	NAM	-	Naming			

*The validity of this examination depends on administration in strict accordance with the NCSE Manual.

†For patients over age 65 the average range extends to the "mild impairment level" for Constructions, Memory and Similarities.

Note: Not all brain lesions produce cognitive deficits that will be detected by the NCSE. Normal scores, therefore, cannot be taken as evidence that brain pathology does *not* exist. Similarly, scores falling in the mild, moderate, or severe range of impairment do not *necessarily* reflect brain dysfunction (see the section of the NCSE Manual entitled "Cautions in Interpretation").

The Northern California
Neurobehavioral Group, Inc.
P.O. Box 460
Fairfax, CA 94930
Telephone: (415) 457-6400

Figure 18-4. Neurobehavioral Cognitive Status Examination Test Booklet. (Reproduced with permission of the copyright holder. Material provided courtesy of J Mueller, MD, RJ Kiernan, PhD, and JW Langston, MD.)

THE NEUROBEHAVIORAL COGNITIVE STATUS EXAMINATION (NCSE)
Record patient's responses verbatim.

I. LEVEL OF CONSCIOUSNESS: Alert_____ Lethargic_____ Fluctuating_____
    Describe patient's condition: _____

II. ORIENTATION (Score 2, 1, or 0.)

		Response	Score
A. Person	1. Name (0 pts.)		____
	2. Age (2 pts.)		____
B. Place	1. Current location (2 pts.)		____
	2. City (2 pts.)1		____
C. Time	1. Date: mo. (1 pt.)____ day (1 pt.)____ yr. (2 pts.)____		
	2. Day of week (1 pt.)		____
	3. Time of day within one hour (1 pt.)		____

Total Score _____

III. ATTENTION
    A. Digit Repetition
        1. Screen: 8-3-5-2-9-1   Pass____   Fail____
        2. Metric: Graded digit repetition (Score 1 or 0; discontinue after 2 misses at one level.)

Score	Score	Score	Score
3-7-2____	5-1-4-9____	8-3-5-2-9____	2-8-5-1-6-4____
4-9-5____	9-2-7-4____	6-1-7-3-8____	9-1-7-5-8-2____

Total Score _____

    B. Four Word Memory Task
        Give the four unrelated words from Section VI: robin, carrot, piano, green.
        (Alternate list: table, lion, orange, glove.) Have patient repeat the four words twice correctly (see Manual) and record the number of trials required to do this:_____ .

IV. LANGUAGE
    A. Speech Sample
        1. Fishing Picture (Record patient's response verbatim.)

        _____
        _____
        _____
        _____

    B. Comprehension (Be sure to have at least 3 other objects in front of the patient for this test.) If a, b, and c are successfully completed, praxis for these tasks is assumed normal.
        1. Screen: 3-step command: "Turn over the paper, hand me the pen, and point to your nose."
                                                          Pass____   Fail ____
        2. Metric: (Score 1 or 0.) If incorrect, describe behavior.

	Response	Score
a. Pick up the pen.		____
b. Point to the floor.		____
c. Hand me the keys.		____
d. Point to the pen and pick up the keys.		____
e. Hand me the paper and point to the coin.		____
f. Point to the keys, hand me the pen, and pick up the coin.		____

Total Score ____

    C. Repetition
        1. Screen: The beginning movement revealed the composer's intention.

        _____
                                                          Pass____   Fail____
        2. Metric: (Score 2 if first try correct; 1 if second try correct; 0 if incorrect.)

	Response	Score
a. Out the window.		____
b. He swam across the lake.		____
c. The winding road led to the village.		____
d. He left the latch open.		____
e. The honeycomb drew a swarm of bees.		____
f. No ifs, ands, or buts.		____

Total Score ____

Figure 18–4 (cont'd). Neurobehavioral Cognitive Status Examination Test Booklet.

D. Naming
   1. Screen: a) Pen_____   b) Cap or Top_____   c) Clip_____   d) Point, Tip, or Nib_____

   Pass_____   Fail_____

   2. Metric: (Score 1 or 0.)

	Response	Score			Response	Score
a. Shoe	_____	_____	e.	Horseshoe	_____	_____
b. Bus	_____	_____	f.	Anchor	_____	_____
c. Ladder	_____	_____	g.	Octopus	_____	_____
d. Kite	_____	_____	h.	Xylophone	_____	_____

Total Score _____

V. CONSTRUCTIONAL ABILITY
   A. Screen: Visual Memory Task (Present stimulus sheet for 10 seconds, then have patient draw the two figures from memory. Must be perfect to pass. The examiner may wish to have patients who fail the screen copy the two figures.)

   Pass_____   Fail _____

   B. Metric: Design Constructions (Score 2 if correct in 0-30 seconds; 1 if correct in 31-60 seconds; 0 if correct in greater than 60 seconds or incorrect.)

Total Score _____

VI. MEMORY (Score 3 if recalled without prompting; 2 if recalled with category prompt; 1 if recognized from list; 0 if not recognized.) Check if correct.

Words	Check	Category Prompt	Check of Response	List (circle)	Score
Robin	_____	Bird	_____	Sparrow, robin, bluejay	_____
Carrot	_____	Vegetable	_____	Carrot, potato, onion	_____
Piano	_____	Musical instrument	_____	Violin, guitar, piano	_____
Green	_____	Color	_____	Red, green, yellow	_____

Incorrect initial response: _____   Total Score _____

VII. CALCULATIONS
   A. Screen: 5 × 13   Response:_____   Time:_____   (Must be correct within 20 seconds.)

   Pass_____   Fail _____

   B. Metric: (Score 1 point if correct within 20 seconds.) Problems may be repeated, but time runs continuously from first presentation.

	Response	Time	Score
1. How much is 5 + 3?	_____	_____	_____
2. How much is 15 + 7?	_____	_____	_____
3. How much is 39 ÷ 3?	_____	_____	_____
4. How much is 31 − 8?	_____	_____	_____

Total Score _____

VIII. REASONING
   A. Similarities (Explain: "A hat and a coat are alike because they are both articles of clothing." If patient does not respond, encourage; if patient gives differences, score 0.)

   1. Screen: Painting-Music (Must be abstract—only "art," "artistic," or "forms of art" are acceptable.)

   _____   Pass_____   Fail _____

   2. Metric: (Score 2 if abstract; 1 if imprecisely abstract or concrete; 0 if incorrect.) See manual for examples. Check if abstract.

	Check	Abstract Concept	Other Responses	Score
a. Rose-Tulip	_____	Flowers	_____	_____
b. Bicycle-Train	_____	Transportation	_____	_____
c. Watch-Ruler	_____	Measurement	_____	_____
d. Corkscrew-Hammer	_____	Tools	_____	_____

Total Score _____

Figure 18–4 (cont'd). Neurobehavioral Cognitive Status Examination Test Booklet.

B. Judgment
    1. Screen: What would you do if you were stranded in the Denver Airport with only $1.00 in your pocket?

          _____

          _____

                                                    Pass_____   Fail_____

    2. Metric: (Score 2 if correct; 1 if partially correct; 0 if incorrect.)
        a. What would you do if you woke up one minute before 8:00 a.m. and remembered an important appointment downtown at 8:00?

          _____

          _____

                                                        Score_____

        b. What would you do if you were walking beside a lake and you saw a two-year-old child playing alone at the end of a pier?

          _____

          _____

                                                        Score_____

        c. What would you do if you came home and found that a broken pipe was flooding the kitchen?

          _____

          _____

                                                        Score_____

IX. MEDICATIONS   Total Score _____

List *all* current medications and dosages:

1. _____ 2. _____ 3. _____ 4. _____

5. _____ 6. _____ 7. _____ 8. _____

X. GENERAL COMMENTS

Note any known or observed motor, sensory or perceptual deficits that may affect test performance (e.g., impaired visual or auditory acuity, tremor, apraxia, dysarthria):

_____

_____

_____

Note "process features" such as distractability, frustration, exhaustion, and nature of cooperation. The patient's impression of his or her performance should also be noted here.

_____

_____

_____

Space for Visual Memory Task

Figure 18–4 (cont'd). Neurobehavioral Cognitive Status Examination Test Booklet.

Range of Typical Cognitive Status Profiles in
Mild to Moderate Presenile Dementia

COGNITIVE STATUS PROFILE

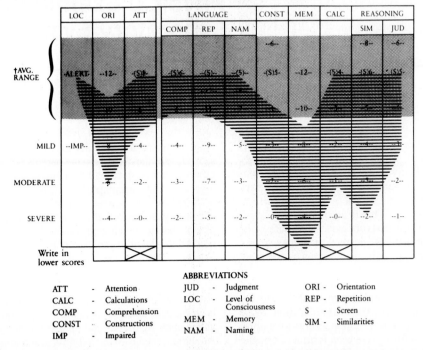

ABBREVIATIONS

ATT	-	Attention	JUD	-	Judgment	ORI - Orientation
CALC	-	Calculations	LOC	-	Level of	REP - Repetition
COMP	-	Comprehension			Consciousness	S - Screen
CONST	-	Constructions	MEM	-	Memory	SIM - Similarities
IMP	-	Impaired	NAM	-	Naming	

Figure 18–5. Range of typical scores for mild to moderate dementia (from Cognitive Status Profile of the Neurobehavioral Cognitive Status Examination Booklet [see Fig 18–4]). Reproduced with permission of the copyright holder.

REFERENCES

Benson DF: *Aphasia, Alexia and Agraphia.* Churchill Livingstone, 1979.

Cummings JL: *Clinical Neuropsychiatry.* Grune & Stratton, 1985.

Diagnosis and psychiatry. Chap 12 in: *Comprehensive Textbook of Psychiatry/IV,* 4th ed. Kaplan HI, Freedman AE, Sadock BJ (editors). Williams & Wilkins, 1985.

Hinsie LE, Campbell RJ: *Psychiatric Dictionary,* 4th ed. Oxford Univ Press, 1970.

Kiernan RJ, Langston WJ, Mueller J: The neurobehavioral mental status examination. Presented at the American Psychological Association meetings, Oct, 1983.

Taylor J (editor): *Selected Writings of John Hughlings Jackson.* Basic Books, 1958.

Teasdale G, Jennett B: Assessment of coma and impaired consciousness: A practical scale. *Lancet* 1974;**2**:81.

Van Dyke C, Mueller J, Kiernan RJ: The case for psychiatrists as authorities on cognition. *Psychosomatics* 1987;**28**:87.

Walsh KW: *Neuropsychology.* Churchill Livingstone, 1977.

19

Physical Examination & Laboratory Evaluation

Jonathan Mueller, MD

The ability to perform a physical examination is, like any other skill, acquired and maintained by frequent practice. Many psychiatrists who have completed their training—and particularly those who have exclusively outpatient practices—do not perform physical examinations. This is unfortunate, since internists and other specialists often perform abbreviated neurologic examinations despite neuropsychiatric symptoms. As the role of the neurosciences and other branches of medicine becomes increasingly important in the practice of modern psychiatry, the psychiatrist's ability to perform relevant examinations should become a central concern of psychiatric education. Since the purpose of the physical examination is to confirm or refute hypotheses that have been formulated on the basis of the patient's history and a review of systems, these areas will be considered first.

MEDICAL HISTORY & REVIEW OF SYSTEMS

Medical History

Detailed attention to the medical history reassures patients that they are being seen by a physician who recognizes the interplay between physical and mental distress. As an expression of concern for the patient's reactions to and feelings about illness, history taking serves to initiate a working alliance between patient and therapist. The medical history obtained from a psychiatric patient may provide clues to the actual cause of changes in mental status and inevitably sheds light on the patient's biologic limitations—limitations of what existential psychotherapists term the patient's "being in the world."

The earliest events that influence central nervous system development are experienced in utero. These may include physical assaults and deprivation endured by the mother during pregnancy and maternal addiction to substances such as alcohol, heroin, nicotine, or other psychoactive drugs. Patients are often unaware of major prenatal events. Thus, documentation from previous medical records and history obtained from siblings, parents, or other relatives may be crucial.

Early childhood illnesses may be significant either because of enduring effects on major organ systems or because of suspicions they raise about immunologic compromise. **Major medical illnesses** in a child or other members of the family may result in prolonged separation of the child from the parents or a significant decrease in time spent with and interest shown in a developing child's accomplishments or difficulties.

Surgical procedures, regardless of the age at which they are performed, have special importance as events during which control of the body is relinquished to a team of professionals. Hip fracture in an elderly patient may precipitate a series of physical and psychologic events culminating in loss of autonomy. Any major surgical procedure exposes the patient to risks of hypotension and anesthesia. "She has never been the same since her operation" is a frequent observation made by friends and family of elderly patients. All current medications and dosage schedules should be listed, along with past and present use of alcohol and other substances.

Special attention should be devoted to documenting the occurrence of **neurologic disturbances.** Seizures, head trauma, blackouts, loss of consciousness, and language or memory problems all have great bearing on psychiatric assessment. Likewise, **endocrine disturbances** in patients with diabetes, thyroid or parathyroid disease, or hyper- or hypofunction of the adrenal glands can present as psychiatric illness.

Review of Systems

The following list is not exhaustive but provides examples of physical dysfunction with major implications for psychiatric assessment and management.

A. Nervous System and Sensory Organs: Complaints of headache may arise from a wide range of causes, including stress, migraine, hypoxia, brain tumor, subarachnoid hemorrhage, and meningitis. Since diplopia very rarely represents a conversion phenomenon, complaints of double vision should always trigger a search for disorders of neurologic origin, such as Wernicke's encephalopathy, multiple sclerosis, or diabetic cranial nerve palsy. Visual hallucinations or illusions may arise from structural damage to any part of the visual system, eg, from lesions of the retina, the optic nerve, tract, visual radiations, or the occipital cortex. Hallucinations confined to one visual hemifield or one visual quadrant always suggest structural damage from disease or injury. Older patients should be asked about changes in hearing or vision, since correction of these deficits (hearing aid or glasses) can improve patient's ability to care for themselves and lead independent social lives. Loss of hearing may lead to paranoid ideation.

B. Cardiovascular System: Recurrent anxiety may reflect cardiac arrhythmia (especially paroxysmal atrial tachycardia), angina, or mitral valve prolapse. Worsening of congestive heart failure with attendant drowsiness or hypoxemia may be easily mistaken for depression. Any history of angina, arrhythmia, or myocardial infarction should be noted. Heart disease may impose significant limitations on the patient's life-style, and cardiac medications may have psychoactive effects.

C. Respiratory System: Episodic shortness of breath or hyperventilation may occur secondary to panic attacks or may be seen in the context of general anxiety disorders. Conditions such as chronic obstructive pulmonary disease, congestive heart failure, pulmonary embolism, and pneumonia must always be excluded when anxiety is assessed.

D. Gastrointestinal System: Vague recurrent abdominal symptoms may be seen in patients with somatoform disorders (eg, conversion disorder and somatization disorder), but abdominal distress due to organic causes (eg, regional enteritis, ulcerative colitis, and porphyria) may be accompanied by prominent psychologic distress. Anorexia is a vegetative sign of depression, but loss of appetite may also arise from numerous organic causes, particularly cancer. Hyperphagia with weight gain may be a sign of diabetes mellitus (eating habits reflect rapidly changing blood glucose levels) or may occur in atypical cases of depression or rare cases of ventromedial hypothalamic disorders. Diarrhea may be due to irritable bowel syndrome or a malabsorption syndrome. Diarrhea accompanied by nausea, polyuria, and polydipsia may be a sign of lithium toxicity. Hypomotility or atony of the bowel, on the other hand, may be caused by use of psychiatric medications with anticholinergic properties (eg, tricyclic antidepressants, low-potency neuroleptics, and antiparkinsonism medications).

E. Genitourinary System: Frequency of urination is a cardinal symptom of diabetes mellitus but may also reflect anxiety states, use of diuretics, or lithium toxicity. Inability to initiate urination should suggest anticholinergic toxicity in patients taking psychiatric medications and is a major concern in elderly men with prostatic hypertrophy. Episodes of incontinence, if accompanied by loss of consciousness, suggest either vasovagal phenomena or seizures. Spinal cord lesions (eg, secondary to trauma or multiple sclerosis) above the S1–2 level can produce a spastic bladder. The triad of dementia, ataxia, and incontinence in an elderly individual should raise the question of normal-pressure hydrocephalus—a potentially reversible condition.

PHYSICAL EXAMINATION

The patient's general appearance tells the clinician a great deal about the severity and acuteness or chronicity of the illness. Failure to note subtle or obvious signs of physical illness may lead to prolonged, costly, and unnecessary or inappropriate treatment. Detection of a physical sign, on the other hand, may afford the physician unexpected leverage in treating an illness that was initially thought to be psychiatric. It is the rule rather than the exception that medical illnesses have behavioral manifestations and emotional consequences. In addition, some somatic illnesses present with psychiatric symptoms.

Vital Signs

It is essential to record vital signs early in therapy with psychiatric patients—if possible before medications are started or before they are changed. Orthostatic measurements (with the patient lying supine and then standing) of pulse and blood pressure are particularly valuable.

A. Pulse: Tachycardia may reflect anxiety, pain, or ingestion of adrenergic agonists or anticholinergic substances. Furthermore, some arrhythmias (especially paroxysmal atrial tachycardia) produce marked anxiety. Bradycardia is common in patients with anorexia nervosa. Return of the pulse rate to the normal range in these patients is one means of monitoring protein ingestion.

B. Blood Pressure: Hypertension has multiple medical causes and places the patient at significant risk of cerebrovascular and cardiovascular accidents as well as renal complications. Situational stress may elevate blood pressure on a transient or chronic basis. Concurrent ingestion of monoamine oxidase inhibitors and wines or cheeses containing tyramine may lead to dangerous episodes of hypertension. Some antihypertensive drugs can produce episodes of major depression and may also cause impotence. In addition, psychotropic medications may produce postural hypotension via peripheral blockade of alpha-adrenergic receptors.

C. Temperature: Hypothermia is a potentially dangerous complication of antipsychotic medications in the elderly. Hyperpyrexia may reflect infection anywhere in the body (including the central nervous system), atropine poisoning, toxicity due to dopamine-blocking agents ("neuroleptic malignant syndrome"), or the hypermetabolic state of delirium tremens.

D. Respiratory Rate: While hyperventilation may arise in the context of stress disorders, anxiety states, or panic attacks, it may also reflect metabolic acidosis with a compensatory respiratory drive. Central respiratory drive may be diminished by barbiturates, benzodiazepines, alcohol, or brain stem compression or lesions.

Head

Evidence of head trauma such as skull deformities or scars should be noted. Patients may be amnestic for the actual event if the trauma was associated with loss of consciousness. An increase in cranial circumference or an unusual cranial shape suggests congenital abnormalities or developing hydrocephalus.

A. Face and Mouth: Hyper- or hypotelorism

(wide- or narrow-set eyes) may suggest congenital central nervous system abnormalities. Adenoma sebaceum (multiple papules over the bridge of the nose and cheeks) occurs in tuberous sclerosis. A "port wine" stain over the second division of the fifth cranial nerve suggests Sturge-Weber syndrome. A "butterfly" rash over the nose and cheeks suggests the possibility of systemic lupus erythematosus. A round or moon-shaped face may reflect idiopathic Cushing's disease or ingestion of corticosteroids. Hair loss from the lateral eyebrows occurs in syphilis, leprosy, and hypothyroidism. A sore, raw tongue reflects vitamin deficiency; a large tongue, hypothyroidism; and greenish discoloration of the tongue, brominism. Repetitive tongue movements are common in edentulous patients but may also be seen in patients with involuntary buccal, lingual, and masticatory movements (tardive dyskinesia), which may occur as a late complication of neuroleptic drug use. Regular tremor of the lips (an early parkinsonian complication of dopamine-blocking drugs) has been termed the "rabbit syndrome." Lack of facial expression may be a symptom of schizophrenia, major affective disorder, dementia, or idiopathic Parkinson's disease or may reflect drug-induced akinesia.

B. Eyes: Dilated pupils may reflect stress, anticholinergic toxicity, or hyperadrenergic states secondary to amphetamine abuse. Constricted pupils suggest ingestion of a narcotic, but brain stem lesions at the pontine level may also cause pinpoint pupils. Herniation of the uncus (a structure on the medial aspect of the temporal lobe) secondary to increased intracranial pressure compresses the pupilloconstrictor fibers of the third cranial nerve, causing the ipsilateral pupil to become fixed and dilated. Extraocular muscles may be affected in Wernicke's encephalopathy, in progressive supranuclear palsy, or following ingestion of phencyclidine, phenytoin, or barbiturates. Copper-colored rings at the limbus of the iris (Kayser-Fleischer rings) are a hallmark of Wilson's disease.

Neck

Thyroid enlargement or tenderness is significant, since symptoms of both hyper- and hypothyroidism can be mistaken for primary psychiatric disease. Carotid bruits suggest advanced atheromatous disease and have special significance if the individual has a history of transient ischemic attacks, reversible neurologic deficits due to ischemia, or stroke. Neck stiffness with pain on flexion (meningismus) suggests meningeal irritation. Involuntary torsion of the head and neck to one side (toricollis) may occur as drug-induced dystonia or in association with dystonia musculorum deformans, a rare neurologic disorder.

Heart

Congestive heart failure (characterized by a third or fourth heart sound on auscultation) may be associated with hypoxia, anergy, and agitation. Unless the cardiac condition is recognized, "psychiatric signs" may be mistakenly treated with antianxiety, antipsychotic, or antidepressant medications. The midsystolic click of a prolapsed or "floppy" mitral valve is increasingly recognized in association with anxiety attacks, a syndrome for which propranolol may provide effective treatment. Tachycardia can arise secondary to anxiety or to use of psychoactive medications.

Lungs

Hypoxia from any cause (including asthma, congestive heart failure, pneumonia, pneumothorax, or pulmonary embolism) may produce either quiet or agitated confusional states. Pneumonia is a reversible cause of dementia syndromes in the elderly.

Abdomen

The presence of multiple surgical scars may suggest any of a number of psychiatric illnesses (eg, conversion disorder, somatization disorder, chronic factitious illness, repeated ingestion of foreign bodies by schizophrenic individuals or by patients with borderline personality disorder) or may suggest the numerous abdominal crises seen in acute intermittent porphyria. Hepatomegaly and vascular spiders suggest chronic alcohol abuse.

Skeleton

Bony abnormalities may reflect congenital defects or may have arisen slowly in the context of collagen vascular disease. The cranioskeletal abnormalities of gigantism most frequently arise secondary to pituitary dysfunction.

Extremities

Palmar erythema suggests collagen vascular disease or hepatic disease. Multiple laceration scars over the inner aspects of the forearms or wrists are stigmas of multiple suicidal gestures occasionally seen in severely ill patients with borderline personalities. Clubbing of the digits may reflect cardiac or pulmonary disease. Yellowish staining of the fingertips suggests a smoking habit. The tremor of Parkinson's disease is initially a resting tremor of the hands and may be unilateral. Other forms of tremor may be seen with lithium use, in hyperadrenergic states (eg, anxiety, amphetamine abuse, alcohol withdrawal), or in benign familial (essential) tremor. The central obesity of Cushing's disease is accompanied by peripheral loss of fatty tissue, with the skin of the hands taking on the quality of parchment.

NEUROLOGIC EXAMINATION

Cranial Nerves

A. Cranial Nerve I (Olfactory): Is there unilateral or bilateral anosmia secondary to trauma and disruption of the olfactory bulb fibers as they travel through the cribriform plate, or is there unilateral anosmia secondary to a meningioma of the olfactory groove? Does the patient report olfactory hallucinations (schizophrenia versus irritation of the medial temporal lobe)?

B. Cranial Nerve II (Optic): If visual acuity is poor, does it improve if the patient puts on glasses or looks through a pinhole (the pinhole corrects for refractive errors)? Is the patient taking anticholinergic drugs that impair the pupillary constriction required for near vision? Is there a homonymous visual field cut, suggesting a lesion of the optic chiasm or tract, visual radiations, or visual cortex; or is there monocular blindness, suggesting lesions anterior to the chiasm (ie, damage to the optic nerve or retina)? Examination of the fundi may demonstrate blurring of the disk margins (associated with increased intracranial pressure) or arteriolar narrowing that suggests hypertension.

C. Cranial Nerves III (Oculomotor), IV (Trochlear), and VI (Abducens): If nystagmus is present, does it reflect therapeutic or toxic levels of drugs (eg, barbiturates or phenytoin) or alcohol intoxication or withdrawal? Is the nystagmus secondary to phencyclidine ingestion? If gaze paralysis is present, is it caused by thiamine deficiency associated with Wernicke's encephalopathy or by abducens palsy (often a nonspecific sign of increased intracranial pressure), or does it reflect the internuclear ophthalmoplegia seen in multiple sclerosis? Is there limitation of vertical gaze, as seen in progressive supranuclear palsy or with pineal tumors (Parinaud's syndrome)?

D. Cranial Nerve V (Trigeminal): Is facial sensation intact over all 3 branches of the trigeminal nerve? In cases of conversion (hysterical) anesthesia, sensory loss usually extends to the mandibular angle (innervated by the second cervical nerve).

E. Cranial Nerve VII (Facial): Is there facial asymmetry either at rest or on spontaneous motion? Is the entire hemiface involved (peripheral lesion), or is the forehead spared (central lesion)? Is a cortical lesion suggested by aphasia with right facial paralysis or by aprosody (loss of speech melody) with left facial palsy?

F. Cranial Nerve VIII (Acoustic and Vestibular Components): Is there sensorineural or conductive hearing loss? High-frequency hearing loss (presbycusis) is common in the elderly. Before diagnosing "hysterical" gait disorder, be certain the patient does not have position-induced vertigo secondary to labyrinthine dysfunction.

G. Cranial Nerves IX (Glossopharyngeal) and X (Vagus): Is the gag reflex intact, absent (patient at risk for aspiration), or overly brisk (associated with the "emotional incontinence" of pseudobulbar paralysis)? Swallowing is a complex act and may be grossly impaired despite an intact gag reflex.

H. Cranial Nerve XI (Accessory): Is there asymmetry of sternocleidomastoid muscle strength or diminished bulk of the trapezius muscle on palpation? In cases of conversion (hysterical) weakness, patients often complain of inability to turn the head toward the side of weakness. Patients with hemispheric lesions producing true weakness of limb movement and head turning will demonstrate weakness on turning the head away from the side of weakness.

I. Cranial Nerve XII (Hypoglossal): Does the tongue deviate from the midline? If so, is this a sign of a brain stem lesion, or does it reflect a supranuclear lesion of cranial nerve VII?

Motor System

A. Muscle Mass: Is there asymmetry of face, body, or limb muscle mass (congenital versus disuse atrophy following stroke versus neuropathic or myopathic)?

B. Muscle Tone: Is there parkinsonian cogwheel rigidity, lead pipe rigidity of an upper motor neuron disease, or the flaccidity of a lower motor neuron disease? Are muscles rigid secondary to dystonia? Is there the "waxy flexibility" of cataleptic catatonia or the rigid resistance of negativistic catatonia? Does the examiner encounter the ratchetlike gegenhalten (paratonia) of frontal lobe disease, characterized by increasing resistance in response to the examiner's attempts to passively move the patient's limbs at increasing speeds?

C. Strength: Strength may be graded on a 6-point scale in which 5 = normal strength, 4 = movement against gravity and applied force, 3 = movement against gravity only, 2 = movement with gravity eliminated, 1 = trace movement, and 0 = no movement. Attention is paid to comparisons of left versus right, proximal versus distal, and upper versus lower motor strength.

D. Coordination: Is performance impaired on testing of finger-to-nose, heel-to-shin, and rapidly alternating (rhythmic) movements (all suggesting cerebellar hemispheric disorders), or does ataxia affect chiefly the lower limbs and trunk (suggesting midline cerebellar disorders)? Beware of inferring coordination deficits in the presence of weakness.

E. Reflexes:

1. Deep tendon reflexes–Are tendon reflexes symmetric or asymmetric? Is there hyperreflexia consistent with upper motor neuron disease, or does areflexia accompany flaccid paralysis? A brisk jaw jerk suggests bifrontal disease. Diffusely brisk reflexes may be seen in withdrawal from alcohol, benzodiazepine, or barbiturates; catatonic excitement; hyperthyroidism; or magnesium or calcium deficiency. Diffusely sluggish reflexes may be seen in hypothyroidism and barbiturate or benzodiazepine intoxication.

2. Pathologic reflexes–

a. Babinski's sign–Does stimulation of the plantar surface of the foot produce plantar flexion ("down-going" toe) or dorsiflexion (extension) of the great toe? An "upgoing toe" suggests pyramidal tract (upper motor neuron) lesions that may be at the level of the spinal cord, brain stem, or brain.

b. Primitive reflexes–Can reflexive sucking, grasping, rooting, or snouting be elicited? Reappearance of these reflexes suggests diffuse frontal lobe disorders. A unilateral grasping reflex may indicate involvement of one frontal hemisphere.

F. Gait and Station: Does the patient walk in a stooped fashion, with slow shuffling steps and diminished arm swing? If so, is this parkinsonian picture drug-induced or idiopathic? Is gait wide-based and ataxic? Gait ataxia may be due to alcoholic intoxication, permanent ataxia secondary to alcoholic cerebellar degeneration, or intoxication with antipsychotic agents such as phenobarbital. Is one leg moved forward in circumduction and the arm on that side held in flexion over the chest? This occurs most commonly following stroke of the contralateral hemisphere.

G. Movements: Is there asymmetry of movement (paralysis, neglect), poverty of movement, or excess of movement? Are there spontaneous dyskinetic movements (Huntington's chorea, tardive dyskinesia, levodopa-induced dyskinesia, Wilson's disease), tremors (resting parkinsonian tremor, benign familial tremor, cerebellar "intention" tremor), myoclonic jerks, or fasciculations?

Sensation

Sensory loss is characterized with reference to location and to the modalities involved. Does the patient fail to respond only to pinprick and changes of temperature, or is there also diminshed proprioceptive sensation? Is the deficit limited to one extremity, or are upper and lower extremities involved symmetrically (evidence of polyneuropathy)? Is the loss of sensation a "crude" inability to perceive the stimulus, or is it instead a specific inability to localize or recognize the stimulus? Tests of sensory extinction (failure to perceive sensation on one side of the body when bilateral areas are simultaneously stimulated), stereognosis (ability to recognize and name an object after feeling its shape), or graphesthesia (ability to recognize a number or letter "written" on the skin) allow the clinician to recognize syndromes of cortical sensory loss associated with parietal lesions.

LABORATORY EXAMINATIONS & OTHER DIAGNOSTIC TESTS

Just as the physical examination provides an opportunity to confirm or refute hypotheses formulated on the basis of the history and review of systems, the request for laboratory and other diagnostic tests should also derive from and be dictated by findings in the history, review of systems, and physical examination. If utilized in this way, the laboratory provides relevant diagnostic and prognostic data that benefit the patient and allow clinicians to sharpen their observational skills. Indiscriminate ordering of laboratory tests, on the other hand, is costly, short-circuits the traditional medical practice of careful examination leading to formulation of hypotheses, and can be detrimental to the patient-physician relationship.

Laboratory tests are essential elements of the modern psychiatrist's diagnostic and therapeutic resources. Even as recently as a decade ago, this was not the case.

Biologic tests in psychiatry may be anatomic (CT scan of the head), functional (electroencephalogram, dexamethasone suppression test, thyroid function tests, creatinine clearance, positron emission tomography), or diagnostic (Venereal Disease Research Laboratories [VDRL] test for syphilis). Advances in psychopharmacology in the last 2 decades have demanded refined quantitative measures of medication levels. Over the next decade, research advances in psychiatry and neuroimmunology may require psychiatrists to become conversant with biologic probes of the immune system.

This section discusses the role of laboratory and other diagnostic studies in general psychiatric practice. It cannot be emphasized too strongly that negative test results do not constitute proof that organic disease is not present. Normal findings on neurologic examination, for example, do not rule out a demyelinating process that is in remission any more than negative findings on electroencephalography rule out a seizure disorder. Thus, test results must always be viewed as part of the larger clinical picture.

Diagnostic Workup

A. Delirium: The workup of a delirious patient is similar to that of a demented patient (see below). Special concern, however, is directed toward the toxicology screen. Among the substances for which psychiatrists most often screen are the following: heavy metals (mercury, lead, arsenic); hallucinogens (LSD, phencyclidine, tetrahydrocannabinol); atropinic substances (phenothiazines, antidepressants, sedatives, antiparkinsonism drugs); stimulants (amphetamines, cocaine, methylphenidate); central nervous system depressants (alcohol, phenobarbital, phenytoin); anxiolytics (benzodiazepines, meprobamate); and pain medications (morphine, heroin, hydromorphone, meperidine).

B. Dementia: The following is a list of tests that should be considered before the diagnosis of senile dementia of the Alzheimer type is made.

1. Blood, plasma, or serum values–Hemoglobin, hematocrit, white blood cell count, vitamin B_{12}, folic acid (red blood cell), sodium, calcium, magnesium, creatinine, urea nitrogen, glucose (fasting), bilirubin (direct and indirect), total protein, partial thromboplastin time, glutamic-oxaloacetic transaminase, thyroxine, erythrocyte sedimentation rate, arterial blood gases, and ceruloplasmin (in patients under 50 years of age).

2. Antigen and antibody tests–Fluorescent antinuclear antibody (FANA test, VDRL test for syphilis, *Treponema pallidum* hemagglutination (TPHA) test, and fluorescent treponemal antibody (FTA-ABS) test.

3. Other studies–

a. Chest x-ray.

b. Electrocardiography.

c. Electroencephalography–The electroencephalogram may be helpful in documenting dysrhythmia or epileptic discharge. Provocative maneuvers such as sleep, sleep deprivation, and photic stimulation may be used to lower the seizure threshold. Nasopharyngeal leads may facilitate detection of medial temporal lobe spike activity. The electroencephalogram is particularly helpful in assessing toxic, metabolic, and infectious causes of confusion. It can also aid in differentiating catatonia from stuporous states of uncertain cause.

Epilepsy is ultimately a clinical diagnosis, and findings on the electroencephalogram may or may not corroborate the diagnosis. Abnormal electroencephalographic tracings may be seen in patients who never have clinical seizures. Likewise, patients with frank clinical seizure disorders may have unremarkable electroencephalographic tracings. Many patients with hysterical seizures (pseudoseizures) also have a history of true seizures. Observation of a clinical seizure with concomitant electroencephalographic tracings that show no epileptic discharge makes possible a diagnosis of pseudoseizure. It does not exclude a coexisting true seizure disorder, however.

d. Computerized tomography (CT)–CT scan of the head allows the clinician to examine serial sections of brain. Computerized calculation of tissue density not only identifies abnormal structures but also indicates their nature (eg, cerebrospinal fluid, air, bone, blood). The psychiatric evaluation of any patient over the age of 40 years with no prior psychiatric illness should include a CT scan of the head.

CT scan of the head is an essential tool in the investigation of dementia syndromes. Although generalized atrophy of the brain correlates poorly with the degree of cognitive dysfunction, focal atrophy of the frontal and temporal lobes may suggest a history of Pick's disease or significant closed head injury. Isolated infarction of strategic brain regions (eg, dominant inferior parietal lobe, hippocampus, or dorsomedial thalamus) may produce dementia or amnestic syndromes, whereas numerous infarctions can combine to produce the picture of multi-infarct dementia. Other structural abnormalities to be excluded in the workup of dementia include brain tumors (primary or metastatic), subdural hematomas, and normal-pressure hydrocephalus.

Chronic abusers of alcohol, some schizophrenics, and a subpopulation of elderly patients with depression (but without dementia) have abnormal findings on CT scan of the head. Findings such as these, along with possible applications in the treatment of patients with neurobehavioral disorders, indicate that brain imaging will become increasingly important in psychiatric assessment.

e. Magnetic resonance imaging (MRI)–The advent of MRI presents an attractive alternative to CT scanning. Because this new imaging method does not rely on ionizing radiation, it may be safely performed on the same individual repeatedly. Other advantages of MRI over CT scanning include (1) enhanced resolution of gray-white boundaries; (2) greater sensitivity to

edema; and (3) absence of bone-induced artifact in studies of the spinal cord, posterior fossa (brain stem and cerebellum), and orbital frontal regions (which are frequently contused in closed head injury).

f. Lumbar puncture–This procedure is usually performed to detect evidence of hemorrhage, infection, or cancer involving the central nervous system. In the presence of an unrecognized space-occupying lesion of the brain, a sudden drop in cerebrospinal fluid pressure following lumbar puncture may result in herniation of the uncus through the tentorial notch. This in turn compresses the brain stem, leading to stupor, coma, or death. Therefore, lumbar puncture is performed only after a CT scan of the head has been done. A needle is inserted in the L4-5 interspace, and 5–10 mL of fluid is withdrawn. Opening and closing pressures, as well as gross appearance (color and turbidity) of the fluid, are noted. Samples are assayed for cell count, cell type, and protein and glucose levels; submitted for VDRL and FTA-ABS tests for syphilis; and stained and cultured for bacterial and fungal organisms. Special studies such as protein electrophoresis and viral antigen tests may also be performed.

g. Positron emission tomography (PET)–In contrast to the CT scan of the head, which provides static or structural information, the PET scan (currently a research tool) offers a means of monitoring local central nervous system metabolism, ie, examining brain function in vivo. PET scanning offers tremendous promise for finding physiologic correlates of psychiatric disorders in which no gross structural deficits exist.

h. Pneumoencephalography–This procedure essentially has been replaced by CT scan of the head.

C. Depression:

1. Levels of 3-methoxy-4-hydroxyphenylglycol (MHPG)–In the mid 1970s, it was suggested that urinary or cerebrospinal fluid levels of MHPG (a metabolic breakdown product of norepinephrine in the central nervous system) could be useful to the clinician in selecting an appropriate tricyclic antidepressant. Original hypotheses suggested that patients with low urinary MHPG levels would be more likely to respond to imipramine than to amitriptyline. Recent work has shown that amitriptyline and imipramine both increase serotonin levels at the synaptic cleft, while their demethylated analogs (nortriptyline and desipramine) primarily potentiate increases in norepinephrine. Thus, it seems reasonable that depressed individuals with low MHPG levels may respond best to tricyclic antidepressants such as nortriptyline and desipramine, which have relative specificity for noradrenergic systems.

2. Dexamethasone suppression test–The development of the dexamethasone suppression test as a biologic probe of the hypothalamic-pituitary-adrenal axis (eg, for diagnosis of Cushing's disease) was initially hailed as a landmark for biologic psychiatry. Proceeding from the observation that some depressed patients have high serum cortisol levels, researchers soon discovered that these levels failed to be suppressed in response to exogenous corticosteroid administration, a response also found in patients with Cushing's disease.

The dexamethasone suppression test (as modified for psychiatric use) is performed by giving 1 mg of dexamethasone orally at 11:30 PM, obtaining serum samples at 4 and 11 PM the following day, and measuring serum cortisol levels. If either of these 2 cortisol levels is 5 μg/dL or greater, the patient is described as "failing to suppress" and thus is said to have a positive, or abnormal, response.

Although at first the test was thought to have high specificity (few false-positive results), it is now known that many patients with dementia (without depression) have abnormal dexamethasone suppression test results. Moreover, the test is only 50% sensitive, yielding a significant number of false-negative results.

Because of the increasing number of false-positive results (eg, in patients with dementia and schizophrenia), no clear indications exist at present for clinical diagnostic use of the dexamethasone suppression test. Nevertheless, since suppression of cortisol levels correlates with a good response to antidepressant agents, serial tests may be helpful in monitoring drug responses.

a. Causes of false-positive results–These include pregnancy (high doses of estrogens), Cushing's disease or syndrome, major physical illness (as well as trauma, fever, dehydration, nausea), severe weight loss (malnutrition, anorexia nervosa), hepatic enzyme induction (eg, with use of phenytoin, barbiturates, meprobamate), and uncontrolled diabetes mellitus.

b. Causes of false-negative results–These include Addison's disease, corticosteroid therapy, hypopituitarism, and therapy with high doses of benzodiazepines.

3. Thyrotropin-releasing hormone (TRH) stimulation test–TRH, a tripeptide released from the hypothalamus, stimulates secretion of thyroid-stimulating hormone (TSH) from the pituitary. In normal patients, injection of synthetic TRH (protirelin) produces an increase in TSH level of about 5 μU/mL. About 25% of depressed patients have an increase of less than 5 μU/mL, and 60–70% have an increase of less than 7 μU/mL. Recent work suggests that the TRH stimulation test and the dexamethasone suppression test detect different *subpopulations* of depressed patients, since there is only a 30% overlap in results.

The protocol is as follows: The patient should be instructed to take nothing by mouth for 8 hours prior to the test. A baseline TSH level is obtained before administration of protirelin, 0.5 mg intravenously, infused over 1 minute. The TSH level is determined at 30 minutes. An increase of less than 5 μU/mL (blunted response) is abnormal.

A major question about the test is whether it detects trait or state abnormalities, since blunted TSH responses persist following treatment.

Psychiatric conditions that may cause false-positive results (blunted response) include mania, alcohol withdrawal, and anorexia nervosa. Other conditions causing false-positive results include old age, starvation, chronic renal failure, Klinefelter's syndrome, and testing repeated too frequently (pituitary TSH levels may be depleted if the test is done more often than once a week).

Monitoring Therapeutic Drug Levels

A. Lithium: Careful monitoring of serum lithium levels is essential in the management of any patient receiving this medication. Different individuals tolerate or require different levels of lithium. While acutely manic patients may require and tolerate blood levels of 1–1.8 meq/L, a therapeutic blood level for one individual may be a toxic blood level for another. Elderly individuals, for example, are occasionally maintained effectively at a blood level of 0.4 meq/L and show signs of toxicity when levels rise to 0.6 or 0.7 meq/L. Because lithium is cleared from the central nervous system more slowly than from the peripheral circulation, it may be prudent to discontinue (rather than simply lower the dosage of) lithium if toxicity occurs. There are well-documented reports of toxicity continuing for as long as 1 week after serum lithium levels have fallen well below the therapeutic range.

B. Tricyclic Antidepressants: Methods to evaluate blood levels of tricyclic antidepressants have been available in research settings since the early 1970s. With the exception of nortriptyline, however, they have generally not been used. Nortriptyline is unique in that it appears to possess a "therapeutic window." Specifically, it has been observed that depressed patients do best when they have nortriptyline blood levels of 50–150 ng/mL.

Studies of tricyclic antidepressants have indicated that there may be as much as a 20-fold difference in blood levels among age-matched individuals receiving the same dosage. Thus, failure to respond to an antidepressant medication may reflect not only lack of patient compliance but also individual differences in absorption, metabolism, or excretion of the drug.

C. Anticonvulsants: Methods are available to evaluate blood levels for all of the well-known anticonvulsant medications. Regular monitoring of serum levels is essential in managing individuals with seizure disorders. Levels may fluctuate, depending on other drugs taken by the patient. The physician should determine patient compliance before evaluating whether seizures are refractory to certain medications. Carbamazepine (Tegretol) is a tricyclic anticonvulsant medication that also has psychotropic effects and is emerging as a mainstay in the treatment of complex partial (temporal lobe) seizures. Early reports suggest that a subset of individuals with bipolar affective disorder (manic-depressive illness) also respond to treatment with carbamazepine.

REFERENCES

Bailey H: *Demonstration of Physical Signs in Clinical Surgery,* 15th ed. J. Wright & Sons (Bristol), 1973.

DeJong RN: *The Neurologic Examination,* 4th ed. Harper & Row, 1979.

Fisher CM: Quantitation of deficits in clinical neurology. *Trans Am Neurol Assoc* 1969;**94:**263.

Lee SH, Rao KCVG: *Cranial Computed Tomography.* McGraw-Hill, 1983.

Patten J: *Neurological Differential Diagnosis.* Harold Starke, 1978.

Plum F, Posner JB: *The Diagnosis of Stupor and Coma,* 3rd ed. Davis, 1982.

Rowland LP (editor): *Merritt's Textbook of Neurology,* 7th ed. Lea & Febiger, 1984.

Weiner HL, Levitt LP: *Neurology for the House Officer,* 2nd ed. Williams & Wilkins, 1978.

20 Intelligence Testing & Neuropsychologic Assessment

Edward L. Burke, PhD

A diagnostic test, in the broadest sense, may be defined as an attempt to ascertain the presence or absence—or the excess or deficiency—of some function or condition. Medical research has led to the development of a great number of tests for a wide variety of conditions, and a parallel development can be traced in psychology during the last century.

The attempt to apply scientific methods to human behavior, which gave rise to the modern discipline of psychology, began in the latter part of the 19th century. Wilhelm Wundt is generally credited with having established the first psychology laboratory—in 1876 at the University of Leipzig—and his work had a decisive influence on the development of psychology in the USA, since a number of Americans who studied under him returned home to found some of the first departments of psychology here.

INTELLIGENCE TESTING

The early "psychologists" received their first professional training in a variety of other disciplines. Many were educators with special interests in the applications of psychology to the problems of the mentally retarded or of the gifted. Wundt devoted considerable attention to the measurement of individual differences, and the classification of students according to differences in intelligence, which was done by later psychologists, was a logical outgrowth of his interests. They set out to define the criteria for intelligence and to normalize them on large samples of subjects, but controversies arose—still not entirely resolved—concerning the nature of intelligence and how it might be measured. The most basic argument was whether intelligence consisted of a single general factor, designated **g**, which might manifest itself in a variety of ways, or whether what we call intelligence in fact consists of a number of correlated but distinct skills.

However one resolves the controversy theoretically, in practice the most widely used individually administered intelligence tests measure performance in several different areas. The Wechsler intelligence scales serve as an example.

The original Wechsler-Bellevue Intelligence Scale (1939) has gone through several stages of change. The currently used tests are the **Wechsler Adult Intelligence Scale–Revised** (WAIS-R) and the **Wechsler Intelligence Scale for Children–Revised** (WISC-R). The scales for adults and children have the same structural design, but the material used is adapted to different age levels. The WAIS-R and the WISC-R are each divided into 2 sections, verbal and performance, each with its separately computed intelligence quotient (IQ). These sections are further divided into subtests, the verbal section into information, comprehension, similarities, arithmetic, digit span, and vocabulary; the performance section into digit symbol, block design, picture completion, object assembly, and picture arrangement. Each of these subtests has also been normalized, with a mean score of 10 and a standard deviation of 3.

Administration of the test to children has the advantage of providing indications for remedial or educational interventions. While such interventions may also be available for adults, they inevitably become less useful with the passage of time.

The Wechsler scales yield a standardized IQ that is normalized separately for each age group. The Stanford-Binet test based the IQ on "mental age" as a percentage of "chronologic age." For example, IQ = 100 when mental age and chronologic age are the same; IQ = 150 when mental age is 1.5 times chronologic age; and IQ = 50 when mental age is 0.5 times chronologic age. As a result, IQ declines steadily as chronologic age increases once adult mental age has been achieved. On the Wechsler scales, subjects' IQ scores are compared with those of other individuals in the same age group. This makes the WAIS-R useful in measuring the intelligence of older people.

Controversies regarding intelligence tests have not been limited to the question of whether or not what we call intelligence is a single factor or a function of many. Important social issues have been raised regarding the cultural bias of tests (in favor of certain ethnic or socioeconomic groups) and the way in which test scores might be used in decisions about access to educational opportunities.

The stratification of the sample used to normalize the 1981 edition of the WAIS-R represents an attempt to eliminate such bias. For the most part, data from the 1970 United States census were used. The standardization sample was divided into 9 age groups corresponding to categories used by the Census Bureau.

Equal numbers of men and women were included for each age group. Whites and nonwhites were included in approximately the same proportion as they occur in the population, as reflected in census data collected in 1975 and 1977. The population samples were drawn pro rata according to population density from 4 major geographic areas specified in the United States census reports. The sample was additionally stratified according to 6 occupational groups drawn from the census, as well as for 5 educational levels. Obviously, even after all these efforts, the sample would not be a perfect one in every respect, but the complexity involved shows the problems that confront test designers and the ways in which they try to overcome them. Examples of updating and cultural broadening of material in the information subtest are questions related to Amelia Earhart, Marie Curie, Martin Luther King, Albert Einstein, and Louis Armstrong, replacing questions regarding Longfellow, Homer, and others.

The distribution of IQ scores in the actual sample of the WAIS-R very closely parallels that of a theoretical normal curve. With a score of 100 as the mean and a standard deviation of 15, scores from 90 to 109 are described as "average." Scores from 80 to 89 and 110 to 119 are called "low average" and "high average," respectively. Scores from 70 to 79 are referred to as "borderline"; from 120 to 129, the corresponding scores on the upper side, are referred to as "superior." Finally, scores of 69 or below are categorized as "mentally retarded," whereas at the upper end, scores of 130 and above are called "very superior." About 2.5% of the total sample falls in each of the last-mentioned categories.

The most obvious misuse of an intelligence test such as the Wechsler would be to reduce its findings to a single numerical result: the IQ. From what has been said about the standardization of each subtest, it is clear that a person might conceivably have a mean score of 100 but subtest scores almost entirely in the "very superior" and "borderline" ranges.

It should be clear also that factors other than intelligence may influence performance on an IQ test. Consider the apathetic or rebellious adolescent who is required to take the test. Fatigue, illness, or medication may also adversely affect performance, as well as personality traits that cause one subject to "freeze" at the sight of a stopwatch while another becomes energized by the prospect of a timed test.

In practice, the WAIS-R or WISC-R is most frequently administered as one part of a battery of psychologic tests. Just how the test results are used will depend upon what the diagnostic question is. As with all other tests, the results are most meaningful in the context of a carefully elicited history.

The information and vocabulary subtests strongly reflect educational experience and family milieu. A bright person might score low on these subtests if illness, isolation, or other factors have impoverished these aspects of life. Arithmetic and digit span can be interfered with by anxiety. Similarities test the capacity for abstraction, while comprehension tests the subject's understanding of what is appropriate or effective in a variety of problem situations. All of these subtests are called **verbal tasks** because the medium of the response is words. In contrast, the **performance tasks**—such as reproducing designs with blocks, arranging pictures in a meaningful sequence, and assembling parts of a puzzle—are responded to in nonverbal ways.

While almost everyone will do better on one section of the test than the other, scores for the verbal and the performance sections are usually in the same general range. Any notable disparity (eg, 15 points) requires investigation. Given the mainly left-brain and right-brain tasks of the respective parts of the test, one might suspect organic brain damage in such cases, but the possible interpretations are by no means limited to that one explanation. Thought disorders may be detected in bizarre or idiosyncratic answers on the information, comprehension, similarities, or picture arrangement subtests.

Although the Weschler scales are not expressly designed to detect organic deficits as such, they can be useful as screening devices. As discussed in the next section, Weschler performance subtests such as digit symbol, block design, and object assembly may confirm or refine findings on simple neuropsychologic tests.

NEUROPSYCHOLOGIC TESTING

Impairment of psychologic functions such as perception, concentration, memory, reasoning, or speech may occur at any age, suddenly or gradually, and may be transient or permanent. Impairment may be related to some event such as an injury or accident or may not be attributable to any apparent cause.

In such cases it is important to establish, to the extent possible, the relative contributions of psychologic and organic factors. Since these factors may interact in complex ways, most test batteries include tests aimed at identifying both elements. A test battery may be designed to explore the area suspected of being more important, with additional tests aimed at picking up indications of other deficits. If such indications are positive, the lead can then be pursued further by additional tests.

Screening Tests for Gross Organic Deficits

A number of relatively simple tests frequently included in psychologic test batteries are helpful in identifying gross indications of organic mental disorder. One of the most frequently used tests of this type is the **Bender Gestalt Test,** which consists of a series of 9 geometric patterns to be copied from models by the subject. Most people can draw the figures without great difficulty. The size and arrangement of the figures may occasionally suggest specific personality characteristics, but one may also encounter rotations of figures or gross distortions suggestive of perceptual or motor difficulties.

A simple test that presents little difficulty for most subjects but may prove extremely difficult or impossible for organically impaired patients to perform is the **Trail-Making Test,** which has 2 parts. The first part (Trails A) consists of a series of numbers, each enclosed in a circle, spread out on a page. The task is to connect the numbers in proper sequence by drawing a line from one circle to the next until all the circles have been joined. The second part (Trails B) presents a more complicated variant of the same task: The subject is asked to connect the circles in sequence alternating back and forth between numbers and the letters of the alphabet—1, A, 2, B, 3, C, etc.

Several subtests of the WAIS-R (described above) are useful in picking up gross organic deficit. Examples are **block design** (reproducing designs with blocks), **object assembly** (arranging parts of a puzzle), and **digit symbol** (pairing arbitrarily assigned symbols with numbers), the latter being the most sensitive. If scores on these subtests are notably low either absolutely or relative to verbal subtests or to previous scores on these same subtests, organic impairment is strongly suggested.

Halstead-Reitan Battery

The tests and subtests described above are used mainly as screening devices. Other tests explicitly intended to assess neuropsychologic impairment in greater detail are available but are costly and time-consuming; they are not ordinarily requested unless there is clear evidence of an organic deficit that requires more detailed examination. The best known set of tests of this type is the Halstead-Reitan battery, an elaborate and complicated series of tests that requires extensive training in its administration and interpretation. It is usually done on referral to a specialist in neuropsychology.

The Halstead-Reitan battery grew out of Ward C. Halstead's research, begun at the University of Chicago in the 1930s. Halstead employed a battery of 27 behavioral tests in his studies of the effects of brain lesions. About 10 have come to be known as the **Halstead Impairment Index.** The impairment index for an individual subject is determined simply by counting the number of tests on which the results fall in the range characteristic of the performance of brain-damaged rather than of normal subjects.

Ralph Reitan set up a program at Indiana University Medical Center aimed at an experimental study of the effects of brain lesions, using several of Halstead's tests. Reitan and his associates administered this elaborate battery individually to almost 2000 patients (usually requiring 1–1½ days for testing each subject). In addition to assessing the presence or absence of brain damage on the basis of test findings, Reitan has gone on to investigate patterns of psychologic test results that seem to identify locations and types of brain lesions.

The battery includes the Minnesota Multiphasic Personality Inventory (see Chapter 21); the Wechsler-Bellevue Intelligence Scale (Form I); both parts of the Trail-Making Test (see above); and the following tests:

A. Category Test: This test utilizes a projection apparatus for presenting stimulus material. It is a complex concept-formation test that requires the subject to note similarities and differences in stimulus material; to put forward hypotheses to explain recurring similarities and differences in the stimulus material; to test these hypotheses following positive and negative reinforcement; and to adapt hypotheses as a function of the reinforcement received. The main purpose of the test is to determine the subject's ability to use both negative and positive experiences as a basis for altering performance. Each successful interpretation of the set pattern receives a positive score.

B. Test of Critical Flicker Frequency: The subject is asked to indicate the point at which a variably intermittent light is perceived as a steady light. An additional score is based on the subject's deviation from the first score on 5 successive trials. This test by itself, unlike the others in the battery, shows no significant differences between groups with and without brain damage. It remains, however, as an element in the Halstead-Reitan battery.

C. Tactual Performance Test: This test utilizes blocks of various shapes, each of which has a correspondingly shaped space cut into a board. The subject is blindfolded and not permitted to see the board or blocks at any time. The subject first fits the blocks into the proper spaces with the dominant hand, then repeats the procedure with the other hand, and then performs the task a third time using both hands. After the board and blocks have been put out of sight and the blindfold removed, the subject is required to draw a diagram of the board representing the blocks in their proper spaces. The subject is given 3 scores: one for the total time needed to place the blocks on the board, one for the number of blocks reproduced in the drawing of the board (memory component), and one for the number of blocks correctly localized (localization component). The ability to place the variously shaped blocks in their proper spaces depends upon tactile form discrimination, kinesthesia, manual dexterity, and visualization of the spatial configuration of the shapes in terms of their spatial interrelationships on the board.

D. Rhythm Test: This is a subtest of the Seashore Test of Musical Talent. The subject is required to differentiate between pairs of rhythmic beats that are sometimes the same and sometimes different. The subject receives a positive score for each correct discrimination. The test requires alertness, sustained attention to the task, and the ability to perceive and compare rhythmic sequences.

E. Speech-Sounds Perception Test: This test consists of 60 spoken nonsense words that have a syllable containing the sound of "ee." The words are played from a tape recorder. Several variant spellings of each word are listed on a printed sheet (theeks, zeeks, theets, zeets). The subject listens to each word and then selects the corresponding spelling from the multiple-choice form. The test requires the subject to maintain attention through 60 items, to perceive the spoken sound stimulus through hearing, and to relate the perception through vision to the correct configuration of letters on the test form. The score consists of the number of correct pairings.

F. Finger Oscillation Test: This test is a measure of tapping speed, using the index finger, first of the dominant hand and then of the other hand. The subject is allowed 5 consecutive trials of 10 seconds each for both hands. Performance on this test is dependent almost purely on motor speed. This subject's score is the average of the 5 trials.

G. Time Sense Test: In this test of visual perception and memory, the subject is required to depress a key that permits a sweep hand to rotate on the face of a clock. The task is to allow the hand to rotate 10 times and then to stop it as close to the starting position as possible. The visual component is scored as the number of errors in 40 trials. The face of the clock is then turned away, and the subject is asked to duplicate the visually controlled performace as closely as possible. The visual component of this test requires the subject to maintain alertness and coordinate counting from 1 to 10 with the rotation of the clock's sweep hand. The memory component requires estimation of how long it took for the hand to make 10 revolutions; the subject uses initial perception of this interval as a reference point. The memory component score consists of the number of deviations from the initial perception.

H. Aphasia Examination: This is an adaptation of the Halstead-Wepman Aphasia Screening Test. Some items of the latter, which rarely yield positive results, have been omitted, while other procedures related to aphasia—such as finger agnosia, fingertip number-writing recognition, and tactile, auditory, and visual suppression phenomena—have been added. This test provides a survey of possible aphasia and related deficits. It samples the subject's ability to name common objects, spell, identify individual numbers and letters, read, write, calculate, enumerate, understand spoken language, identify body parts, and differentiate between right and left. Each of these various abilities is examined in terms of the particular sensory modalities through which the stimuli are perceived. The test also provides an opportunity for judging whether the deficit is receptive or expressive in character. (See Chapters 10 and 18 for more information on aphasia and aphasia testing.)

The interpretation of test battery results is a complex procedure that cannot be described briefly. In a study of 50 patients with brain damage and 50 control subjects with no evidence of brain damage (matched in pairs for race, age, sex, and education), Reitan found that none of the brain-damaged persons had lower impairment indices than their matched controls. Using the best cut-off point in the 2 raw score distributions, he determined that only 4% of the brain-damaged group had been misclassified. He concluded that the Halstead Impairment Index serves as a valid and reliable basis for inferring the presence or absence of brain damage in individual subjects.

One cannot predict in individual instances which test or tests may be of crucial help. While the impairment index, category test, and localization component of the tactual performance test are generally the most helpful measures, one of the other tests sometimes proves to be particularly important for individual patients. For the fine points of the clinical application of the individual tests, one may consult Reitan's extensive writings (see references).

Reitan's work has not been limited to an effort to determine the type and location of brain lesions. Additional investigations in his laboratory have been invaluable not only in providing hypotheses for formal investigation but also in furnishing insights into the complexity of brain-behavior relationships in human beings and the limitations and qualifications that must accompany most generalizations.

Batteries Based on Luria's Approach

An alternative approach to the evaluation of local injuries to the brain has been developed by A. R. Luria of the Soviet Union. In Luria's opinion, current psychologic tests are too complex and provide no more than gross evaluations of cognitive processes. He has assumed that complex behavioral processes are in fact not localized but distributed in broad areas of the brain and that the contribution of each cortical zone to the organization of the whole functional system is quite specific. He has accordingly undertaken a careful analysis of specific disturbances in the neuropsychologic examination for diagnosis of focal brain injury. Luria's approach has been gaining adherents, but his methods are not yet widely used in the USA.

On the basis of Luria's approach and techniques, Christensen (1979) developed a battery to test 10 neuropsychologic functions: (1) motor skills, (2) acoustic-motor organization, (3) higher cutaneous and kinesthetic functions, (4) visual perception, (5) receptive speech, (6) expressive speech, (7) reading and writing, (8) arithmetic, (9) memory, and (10) function of intellectual processes. Many common tests are incorporated into this battery, including elements of the mental status examination such as digit span, certain memory tests, and serial sevens (see Chapter 18). Detailing the variety of tests in Christensen's adaptation of Luria's neuropsychologic investigation is beyond the scope of this text. The reader is referred to the writings of Christensen (1979) and Lezak (1983).

Christensen's battery adapts its tests to the needs of each patient (as does Luria's "experimental" approach); thus, the results are difficult to interpret. The battery is not comprehensive, and most patients will require further testing—eg, of intelligence and some memory functions not already covered in the battery.

Golden and his colleagues at the University of Nebraska (1981) developed a standardized battery from the many tests used by Luria and Christensen. The battery, called the **Luria-Nebraska Neuropsychological Battery,** tests the 10 functions listed above. The scales for scoring correspond to the 10 functions but with reading and writing placed on separate scales and with motor and tactile functions scored on right-hemisphere, left-hemisphere, and pathognomonic scales. Although standardized, this battery suffers from some of the same limitations as Christensen's battery. The Luria-Nebraska battery distinguishes between normal controls and neurologically impaired patients, but its reliability and usefulness have been questioned (Lezak, 1983).

Luria's contributions to neuropsychologic assessment are the flexibility and individualized approach to test subjects. Christensen's battery captures the process; the Luria-Nebraska battery standardizes the tests used.

Other Batteries

In *Neuropsychological Assessment,* Lezak (1983) describes several other batteries and composite tests for brain damage, including one of her own design. In addition, she describes many other neuropsychologic tests. Of interest and relevance are the aphasia tests developed by Kaplan and associates (Goodglass and Kaplan, 1972; Kaplan and coworkers, 1978). The reader is referred to these references and to the discussions on aphasia testing in Chapters 10 and 18.

REFERENCES

Bender L: *A Visual Motor Gestalt Test and Its Clinical Use.* Research Monograph No. 3. American Orthopsychiatric Association, 1938.

Christensen AL: *Luria's Neuropsychological Investigation,* 2nd ed. Wiley, 1979.

Golden CJ et al: A standardized version of Luria's neuropsychological tests. Pages 608–642 in: *Handbook of Clinical Neuropsychology.* Filskov S, Boll TJ (editors). Wiley, 1981.

Goodglass H, Kaplan E: *Assessment of Aphasia and Related Disorders.* Lea & Febiger, 1972.

Halstead W: *Brain and Intelligence: A Quantitative Study of the Frontal Lobes.* Univ of Chicago Press, 1947.

Kaplan E, Goodglass H, Weintraub S: *The Boston Naming Test.* Lea & Febiger, 1978.

Lezak MD: *Neuropsychological Assessment,* 2nd ed. Oxford Univ Press, 1983.

Matarazzo JD: *Wechsler's Measurement and Appraisal of Adult Intelligence,* 5th ed. Oxford Univ Press, 1972.

Reitan R: The comparative effects of brain damage on the Halstead Impairment Index and the Wechsler-Bellevue Scale. *Clin Psychol* 1959;**15**:281.

Reitan R: An investigation of the validity of Halstead's measures of biological intelligence. *Arch Neurol Psychiatry* 1955;**73**:28.

Reitan R: The relation of the Trail Making Test to organic brain damage. *J Consult Psychol* 1955;**19**:393.

Reitan R: The validity of the Trail Making Test as an indicator of organic brain damage. *Percept Mot Skills* 1958;**8**:271.

Reitan R, Davison L (editors): *Clinical Neuropsychology: Current Status and Applications.* Winston, 1974.

Wechsler D: *The Measure and Appraisal of Adult Intelligence.* Williams & Wilkins, 1961.

Wechsler D: *Wechsler Adult Intelligence Scale–Revised.* Harcourt Brace Jovanovich, 1981.

Wechsler D: *Wechsler Intelligence Scale for Children–Revised.* Harcourt Brace Jovanovich, 1981.

Zimmerman I, Woo-Sam J: *Clinical Interpretation of the Wechsler Adult Intelligence Scale.* Grune & Stratton, 1973.

Personality Assessment

21

Daniel S. Weiss, PhD

When Osler suggested that the patient was more important than the disease, he was emphasizing the importance of understanding the life circumstances and personality of the individual patient. When physicians make diagnoses, whether of somatic or psychiatric disorders, they must also consider the nature of the person who has the disorder. Concern with the psychologic context in which the symptoms appear helps the clinician understand the meaning and implications of the presenting complaint and the particular symptom pattern. What the current episode of illness means to the patient and what coping resources and personal strengths and weaknesses the patient possesses will influence the clinician's approach to evaluation, setting of treatment objectives, and choice of treatment plans.

Personality is the composite of enduring attributes of an individual's psychologic makeup. The importance assigned to personality today is not new. There is a long history of observations testifying to the central place individual differences in personality have been accorded for understanding both health and illness. The early Greeks employed a classification based on the 4 humors of the body: phlegm, black bile, blood, and yellow bile. The particular balance of the bodily substances determined personality characteristics, psychologic identity, and even health and disease. The phrenology of Franz Josef Gall (1835), which represented an attempt to relate similarities in skull structure to similarities in personality, is noteworthy because it was empirical as well as theoretic. Today, despite agreement on the importance of a patient's personality in understanding the presentation of symptoms and the choice of treatment for virtually any mental disorder, there are still fundamental questions about what personality is and how it should be defined.

Is personality best understood as a process occurring in hypothesized psychologic structures, ie, the id, ego, and superego? Or are the constituents of personality synonymous with these psychologic structures? Or is personality both the structures and the processes? Although this is now a purely theoretic issue, many psychologic tests for assessment of personality rest on just such theoretic notions of personality. As a result, these theoretic positions have influenced how personality assessment has developed and changed.

DEFINITIONS OF PERSONALITY

There are probably as many definitions of personality as there are authors who have written about the subject. Allport's (1937) definition is as apt as any: "Personality is the dynamic organization within the individual of those psychophysical systems that determine his unique adjustments to his environment." Two German terms, representing 2 views of personality, further explain the concept. *Persönlichkeit* denotes the distinctive impression that someone makes on another. This word derives from the Latin *persona* and connotes the sense we get about how individuals choose and perform their social roles. Behind the mask, however, is a complex player donning various roles. The term *Personalität* denotes this more fundamental or basic concept of personality used in psychiatric clinical situations. This definition of personality, which goes beyond exhibited behaviors to reach the core of identity, is considered by some to be synonymous with the term *self* and is the key concern in the field of depth psychology.

DSM-III CLINICAL EVALUATION OF PERSONALITY TRAITS & DISORDERS

In *DSM-III*, axis II used to record observations about personality, including personality traits and, when appropriate, personality disorders. **Personality traits** are defined as "enduring patterns of perceiving, relating to, and thinking about the environment and oneself, and are exhibited in a wide range of important social and personal contexts." The diagnosis of **personality disorder** is made "only when personality traits are inflexible and maladaptive and cause either significant impairment in social or occupational functioning or subjective distress." In addition, a person may meet diagnostic criteria for a personality disorder (eg, borderline personality disorder) and also demonstrate histrionic or avoidant personality traits. All of this information is recorded on axis II in a complete clinical evaluation according to *DSM-III*.

The major clinical and diagnostic dilemma is determining when (at what point or under what circumstances) a set of personality traits (or the patient's "personality") becomes "maladaptive" or is "overly rigid." This is a valid clinical question and not just a theoretic point for argument by students in the field of personality assessment. When does the clinician diagnose a personality disorder? At what point is intervention necessary? These difficult clinical judgments contribute to the so-called unreliability of psychiatric diagnosis on axis II. Personality assessment is one tool the clinician employs in making decisions about the nature and range of a patient's personality.

PERSONALITY ASSESSMENT PROCEDURES

This chapter will focus on the standardized procedures used by properly trained and experienced clinicians to describe an individual's personality. This description may be in terms of either the more overt impression made by the patient (*Persönlichkeit*) or the more basic temperament of character (*Personalität*). Most frequently, assessments incorporate aspects of both views of personality. The goals of assessment usually consist of one or more of the following: (1) to assess psychologic processes, (2) to assess personality traits, (3) to assess psychologic structures, (4) to aid in diagnosis, and (5) to formulate treatment plans. This chapter concentrates on the use of psychologic tests for achieving these objectives. The use of other techniques (such as structured diagnostic interviews) to diagnose personality disorders is discussed briefly in Chapter 13.

FEATURES OF PSYCHOLOGIC TESTS FOR PERSONALITY ASSESSMENT

Standardization

The greatest advantage of using psychologic tests for personality assessment is that both the stimuli used to elicit information and the conditions under which the stimuli are administered are standardized. This means that differences in response may be attributed to differences in the respondents. Compare this situation to that of the usual clinical interview. If one clinician compared the answers of 2 patients interviewed by another clinician, the conclusions about the personalities of the 2 patients could be influenced very much by how the interviews were conducted. Using standardized procedures eliminates this undesirable source of variability in personality assessment.

Another important feature of standardization is the use of "fixed-choice" responses. This limitation on how responses may be made—for example, answering only "true" or "false" to the questions on the Minnesota Multiphasic Personality Inventory (MMPI)—facilitates comparison of personality assessments by one individual with that of others. Because another source of information that might vary is held constant, other types of information about personality are made clearer.

In personality assessment tools with fixed-response formats, the scoring or keying of responses is also fixed. For example, the patient may respond only "true" or "false" to item 181 on the MMPI: "When I get bored, I like to stir up some excitement." The manner in which the choice affects the score is also standardized: If the patient responds "true," this scores a point on the basic clinical scale measuring hypomania. If the patient answers "false," the score on this and all other scales is not affected. The meaning of this single response in terms of personality assessment is not subject to interpretation by the examiner or by the clinician. With the MMPI, the clinician's contribution lies in interpreting the pattern of scale scores (see below).

A final advantage of standardizing procedures, response formats, and scoring is that it is easier to collect data that can provide norms for comparing individual results to other data. In the same way that normal ranges are established for blood pressure, weight, and serum cholesterol levels, the measures of personality in particular reference populations may be standardized and norms developed. These norms have been used to identify patterns or profiles or scores (within a given test and among different tests) to categorize patients. Norms permit a clinician to identify personality traits that deviate significantly from the average, to assess the severity of these traits, and occasionally to make a diagnosis of a personality disorder, given other supporting data.

Although stimuli (eg, the 10 inkblot cards of the Rorschach test) are standardized, each card is not just one more of the same thing; ie, the stimuli are not interchangeable. In the Rorschach inkblots, there is a range of variation in certain dimensions (color, clarity, form). Used as a set, they are standardized, but certain stimuli tap certain personality processes. Similarly, in the MMPI, some items are scored on more than one scale (eg, on scales of depression and schizophrenia), while others are scored only on one scale or only on the other. In personality assessment, this explains the usual clinical practice of using a battery of psychologic tests that vary in types of procedures, stimuli, response formats, and scoring methods. The end result is a test battery that evokes a wide range of responses indicating different aspects of personality.

Reliability

Physicians are accustomed to using diagnostic indices derived from "hard" sources of data (eg, temperature, blood counts) without questioning the reliability of measurements, since the instruments (thermometers, Coulter counters) are standardized for reliability. Instruments for assessing personality must also be calibrated for reliability, and that is difficult. Without proper attention to reliability, measurements may be worthless because the results are not consistent. The reliability of a psychologic measure is a function of its **reproducibility of results** from one administration to the next. Other terms used for reliability are **consistency of measurement** and **stability of measurement.** For example, if a patient takes the Rorschach test twice, his or her responses in the second test should be very similar to those of the first (assuming that nothing about the patient's personality has changed). The results of personality assessment should change only if the patient has changed.

In psychologic measurement, there are several forms of reliability coefficients. Most are based on some form of correlation. A **correlation** is a statistic that numerically conveys the strength of a relationship between 2 variables. The correlation ranges from +1.00 through zero to −1.00. A correlation of +1.00 is a perfect positive relationship; scores on one variable are perfectly predictable from the other. A correlation of zero indicates that no relationship exists; and a correlation of −1.00 indicates a perfect negative relationship. (The following is an example of correlation: In a general unselected population, measured intelligence and annual income yield a correlation of about 0.40, whereas measured intelligence and years of education show a correlation of 0.65−0.75.)

For purposes of personality assessment, the most relevant method of indexing reliability is known as **test-retest reliability.** Simply stated, the test-retest reliability coefficient is the correlation between 2 sets of scores on the same test taken after an interval of time has elapsed between administrations. A moment's reflection shows that although this is the desired ideal, in actual practice the method has some problems. The shorter the time between administrations, the more likely individuals are to remember their previous responses. Hence, results may be affected by memory as well as by the fidelity of the test. On the other hand, the longer the time between administrations, the greater the possibility that there may indeed be some kind of personality change that will lower the correlation between the 2 sets of results. Despite these concerns, reliability is indexed in this manner, and cautious use of psychologic measures requires that estimates of reliability be available or known to the clinician before confidence is placed on the results. Typically, reliability coefficients of 0.70 and above are deemed acceptable. It is very rare to obtain test-retest reliability coefficients greater than 0.90.

Validity

If 2 different instruments are used to measure the same thing, the results should be consistent with each other. A ruler and a tape measure should give the same measurement of a given distance or dimension. Moreover, rulers and tape measures should be used to measure distance but not temperature. If both instruments actually measure distance, they are valid measures of the construct "distance." For psychologic tests, *a measure has validity if it is measuring what it purports to measure.* Evidence of validity for psychologic tests is not obvious, however, and certainly not self-evident. How can it be determined, for example, that fantasy stories made up in response to a Thematic Apperception Test (TAT) picture are actually measures of "a need for achievement"? The mere fact that the test author offers the measure as an index of some personality trait or characteristic does not make it so. Hence, psychologists have endeavored to develop procedures that would validate psychologic tests. Although the fine details of such procedures are beyond the scope of this discussion, some broad terms are helpful.

Evidence of validity can be grouped into 3 broad categories: (1) content (face) validity; (2) predictive, concurrent, or postdictive validity; and (3) construct validity.

Content validity is the desired correspondence between the test material and the concept or domain the test intends to measure. Questions about assertiveness, deference, argumentativeness, stubbornness, and submissiveness are relevant as measures of the trait of dominance but not as measures of activity level or intelligence. When the questions or items of a test look like they measure what they are supposed to measure, the test is said to have **face validity.** This is essentially equivalent to content validity.

Predictive validity is a second kind of evidence. If the scores on the depression scale of the MMPI predict the patient's response to treatment with tricyclic antidepressant medication or predict the results of the dexamethasone suppression test, then the scale possesses predictive validity. If 2 tests are given at the same time, then predictive validity is known as **concurrent validity.** If responses to a test administered today show a relationship with responses to a childhood event (eg, loss of a parent), then the test has **postdictive validity.** It is essential to assemble empirical evidence and document the relationship between the psychologic test and some outcome, regardless of when the outcome is assessed. The outcomes to be predicted by a psychologic test are not always obvious but may be derived from theory. In such cases, assessing validity is more complicated and sophisticated.

Construct validity is the term assigned to the complex network of interrelationships between psychologic tests, outcomes, demographic variables, and other factors that theoretically relate to one another in specified ways. Many of the concepts utilized in psychology and psychiatry are not directly measurable ("operationalizable") in the way that operational concepts such as blood pressure and body temperature are. Concepts such as "ego strength," "free-floating anxiety," and "resistance" are frequently postulated in theories of psychopathology but cannot be physically measured. When, however, theories specify what tests should be positively (or negatively) related to each other and an instrument provides evidence that substantiates these presumed relationships, the tests are said to have construct validity. Such validation supports the use of the measures and strengthens the theory as well.

Barron's (1953) ego strength scale developed from

the MMPI is an example of a measure with construct validity. Barron demonstrated that scores on this scale were predictive of the outcome of outpatient psychotherapy, a result confirming the hypothesis of writers such as Otto Fenichel. Patients with higher scores on the ego strength scale before beginning treatment showed more improvement (on the average) than those with lower scores. Barron showed that the scale was moderately related to intelligence ($r = 0.40$), as was predicted by several psychoanalytic theoreticians. The general theory of ego psychology was that a negative relationship exists between ego strength and general psychiatric distress. Barron's data showed a median correlation (about -0.50) to the other MMPI scales. This pattern of evidence (supplemented by considerably more data not mentioned here) was consistent with the construct of ego strength. Barron concluded that the MMPI test had construct validity and that the theoretic observations about ego functioning and its relationship to symptoms were also confirmed in his study.

Evaluation of validity evidence is difficult in psychiatry, since the criterion against which a test is assessed for validity is often no better—or no more firmly scientifically established—than the measure itself.

Under these circumstances, about the best the clinician can do is to take the stance of a juror in a civil legal proceeding: What does the preponderance of evidence indicate? What is the consensus from all of the relevant sources of information that are available? In spite of their limitations, psychologic tests for personality assessment will continue to provide an important source of information that is not wholly dependent upon the clinician's judgment about a patient's clinical condition.

CLASSIFICATION OF PSYCHOLOGIC TESTS FOR PERSONALITY ASSESSMENT

Psychologic tests are most easily classified as either objective or projective. A clever explanation of the distinction is offered by the psychologist George Kelly (1958): "When the subject is asked to guess what the examiner is thinking, we call it an objective test; when the examiner tries to guess what the subject is thinking, we call it a projective device." There are, of course, psychologic tests and assessment devices that do not neatly fit into these categories, but most are predominantly one or the other.

Objective Tests

Objective tests are tests whose scoring (numerical results) can be produced mechanically. This generally implies that the response format is standardized. Examples of such tests in personality assessment are the MMPI, the California Psychological Inventory (CPI), and the Sixteen Personality Factor Questionnaire (16 PF). Another objective test familiar to medical

students is the Medical College Admission Test. What is not objective in such tests is the meaning of the results or scores. As shown in the clinical example in Chapter 22, the training, experience, and skill of the psychologist come into play in the interpretation and synthesis of the results of the various tests.

Projective Tests

Projective tests are less structured than objective tests in response format and in scoring. The term projective was coined by Frank (1939), based on the following assumption: Because of the unstructured and ambiguous nature of the stimuli and response options available to the respondent, the responses must be *projections* of the patient's "way of seeing life, his meanings, significances, patterns, and especially his feelings." In projective methods, the kinds of responses are not fixed, scoring is usually time-consuming, several scoring systems often exist for each technique, scoring may differ from clinician to clinician, and the interpretation of the results of projective methods frequently requires integrative thinking on the part of the clinician. The best-known examples of projective techniques are the set of inkblots developed by Rorschach, the Thematic Apperception Test (TAT) developed by Morgan and Murray (1935) at the Harvard Psychological Clinic, Draw-a-Person techniques, and Sentence Completion tasks. Less favored today are Word Association tasks.

The Sentence Completion tasks, Draw-a-Person techniques, and Word Association tasks are somewhat more idiosyncratic and are less standardized than the other projective techniques. A common use of these tasks is to provide information for psychodynamic formulations about personality and intrapsychic conflicts. Another technique sometimes used in this manner is the Bender Gestalt Test (see Chapter 20). Although it was originally designed to tap visual-motor coordination and assess development and maturational growth, some clinicians use the test symbols as a projective technique. This use is probably not warranted and is not supported by data.

MINNESOTA MULTIPHASIC PERSONALITY INVENTORY (MMPI)

The MMPI is the most thoroughly researched objective personality assessment instrument. Item development and testing began in the late 1930s. The test authors, Hathaway and McKinley (a psychologist and a psychiatrist), undertook the mammoth task of test construction, recognizing the acute need for an objective measure of various dimensions of psychopathologic disorders to aid clinicians in diagnosis and treatment planning. The MMPI was designed to provide for multiphasic assessment of psychopathologic changes in much the same way that medical checkups are multiphasic.

Administration

The original MMPI consisted of a set of 550 items, each printed on a separate card. The directions to the patient were to read the statement and decide whether "it is true as applied to you or false as applied to you." The patient sorted these cards into one of 3 piles: true, false, or cannot say. In later versions of the MMPI, items were arranged in a booklet so that the test could be administered in a group format rather than an individual format. In the most popular version, the first 399 items comprise all of the items used in the 10 basic clinical and 3 validity scales. The remaining items are used for scoring special scales.

Scales & Scoring

The MMPI basic clinical scales were constructed empirically—ie, several diagnosed criterion groups were formed (hypochondriasis, depression, etc; see below), and items that differentiated the patients with characteristics of these groups from the normal controls were retained. In this manner of test construction, the clinician does not decide a priori how, for example, paranoid patients will respond to items and does not have to make any assumptions about scoring. The direction of scoring comes from data that indicate how paranoid patients differ from controls in answering items.

A. Scoring: Computing scores on any MMPI scale follows this procedure: Items are grouped into different clinical scales (see below) measuring different dimensions of psychopathologic conditions and personality. Raw scores are obtained by summing the number of items answered in the "scored direction" (responses deviating from the norm). These raw scores are then converted to a standardized T score with a scale from 0 to 100, the average score being 50. The MMPI profile is plotted in terms of these T scores. Separate standardizations are used for male and female test subjects. Higher scores mean higher levels of psychopathologic characteristics. A T score of 70 or above is generally considered abnormal.

Two confusing aspects of the MMPI item pool relate to scoring items that appear on more than one scale. If a patient responds "true" to a given item, this may add points to one scale but not to another scale—ie, the "scored direction" of one scale differs from that of another scale. Also, since items were selected empirically, it is not always clear what scale an item is scored on. Some MMPI items lack face validity.

B. Clinical Scales: The following are the basic clinical scales, the profile abbreviation, the number of items, and a short description of content and function of each scale, as adapted from unpublished materials prepared by Gough in 1971:

1. Hypochondriasis (Hs) [33] taps complaints about bodily functioning, physical health, and disease. Patients with actual physical disease show minor elevations in score. Diffuse, scattered, nonspecific complaints are associated with T scores of 60–70. Higher scores indicate fixation and organization of symptoms. The scale is negatively related to intellect, and high scorers are usually pessimistic and touchy.

2. Depression (D) [60] reflects the patient's current morale. It is the best single indicator of adjustment but is responsive to minor fluctuations as well as major trends. Depression can be interpreted directly (ie, without referring to any other scale). High scores indicate hopelessness, helplessness, discouragement, and loss of morale.

3. Hysteria (Hy) [60] provides an estimate of the underlying psychologic aspects of hysteria more than the likelihood of symptomatic expression. High scorers tend to be self-centered, demanding, immature, and somatically preoccupied, alternately suggestible and deeply skeptical. Low scores are also significant, usually reflecting a tart and prickly social style and hardheadedness.

4. Psychopathic deviate (Pd) [50] refers to a patient who is asocial and antisocial rather than retarded or psychotic. High scores are associated with impulsiveness, acting-out behavior, and insensitivity (but not hostility toward others), and where intellect is high, high scores are associated with easy, effortless social technique. Low scores are dependably indicative of constraint, unwarranted self-satisfaction, and conformity.

5. Masculinity-femininity (Mf) [60] is the only scale that is scored differently for men and women. Feminine scores (high scores for men, low scores for women) indicate breadth of interest, intellectuality, personal scope, and self-awareness. Masculine scores (high scores for women, low scores for men) connote aggressiveness, inflexibility, coarseness, and a general tendency to think and behave in a crude vulgar manner.

6. Paranoia (Pa) [40] is, like hysteria, a gauge of predispositions rather than a direct measure of the symptoms. It is a complicated scale, including emphasis on rationality and objectivity as well as heightened interpersonal sensitivity. Contrary to expectation, persons with T scores in the range of 52–62 are typically described very favorably by others. Persons with low scores ($<$ 45) and those with high scores ($\geq$ 70) are described as stubborn, touchy, and difficult to get along with.

7. Psychasthenia (Pt) [48] shows its strongest relationships with other measures of neurotic tendency. It provides an index of agitation, perplexity, self-doubt, apprehension, and anxiety. Just as many patients with medical illnesses have elevated temperatures, nearly everyone with a psychiatric problem shows elevated psychasthenia scores.

8. Schizophrenia (Sc) [78] includes items assessing ego deterioration and breakdowns of self-direction, along with feelings of isolation, worry, and inferiority. It is therefore important to determine the degree to which psychotic items are endorsed in individuals with T scores in the range of 65–75. Many persons with mild social incapacity score in this range. Higher scores reflect considerable affect and tension and are associated with acute clinical syndromes rather than with a schizoid personality style.

9. Hypomania (Ma) [46] measures spontaneity, expansiveness, enthusiasm, and frankness, which are characteristic of those with elevated scores. Irritability, lack of control, and defects of judgment may also be suggested, depending on scores in other scales. Low scores can frequently be interpreted as signs of inertia and apathy.

10. Social introversion (Si) [70] is a scale that was developed somewhat later by Drake (1946) in Wisconsin. Clinical evidence indicates that this scale is a general index of neuroticism, with higher scores signaling moodiness, anxiety, lack of confidence, and worry.

C. Validity Scales: The MMPI is scored for 3 validity scales, which serve the following functions: (1) to identify results that are likely to be invalid because of accidental errors (skipping an item on the answer sheet) or deliberate manipulation of responses and (2) to aid in clinical interpretation of the scale scores.

1. Lie scale (L) [15] consists of improbable and naive claims to virtue. Lack of insight, overevaluation of moral worth, and inflexibility are suggested by scores in the higher range. Extremely high scores flag the record for a possible "fake good." A "fake good" record is one in which the patient has not been candid and truthful and has deliberately tried to look extremely well adjusted and "good." An example of a lie scale item is a "false" response to "I gossip a little at times."

2. Frequency scale (F) [64] consists of items answered in the same direction by more than 90% of subjects. The scored direction is opposite to the popular response. Content is varied, ranging from unconventional beliefs and attitudes to outright eccentricity and bizarreness. Moderately elevated scores (6–9 in raw scores) suggest counteractiveness and independence of thought. Higher scores indicate either disinterest, misunderstanding of directions, or "fake bad" responses; in a psychotic profile, they suggest ego dysfunction. An example of a frequency scale item is a "true" response to "No one cares much what happens to me."

3. Correction scale (K) [30] is an ego functioning scale. High scores are related to prudence, reserve, and circumspection. Low scores indicate self-criticality, lack of confidence in self and others, and bluntness in social style. An example of a correction scale item is a "false" response to "I certainly feel useless at times."

Interpretation

Although it was hoped that the MMPI scales could each be used individually to demarcate the areas of a particular psychopathologic condition, it became clear quite early in their use that the MMPI scales were not each pure measures of the pathologic dimension that the scale names indicated. Instead, both clinical and research use turned to the analysis of profiles and profile patterns.

Early clinical use of the MMPI revealed that there were consistent patterns of scores associated either with diagnostic categories or with common clinical syndromes. A system of coding the profiles was developed as a shorthand to indicate patterns associated with the highest T scores (> 70) and other scores. These codings were eventually organized into a series of interpretive rules for generating clinical descriptions of patients. The interpretive rules were assembled into manuals known as MMPI "cookbooks," which offer "recipes" for clinical descriptions.

An example of one of the classic code-type patterns of scores is the so-called conversion pattern (Fig 21–1). This profile is one in which scores on both the Hs and Hy scales are elevated, while those on the D scale are distinctly lower. Persons exhibiting this pattern admit having somatic complaints and problems in living yet deny that these problems affect their mood. Generally, they are using an external (bodily) solution to psychologic difficulties. Another very common pattern is one of elevated scores on the F, D, Pd, and Sc scales. These profiles mark the distrust, anger, lack of affiliation, disaffection, and oddity of patients with schizoid or schizophrenic disturbances.

Appropriate use of the MMPI requires training and experience, as well as an understanding of psychometrics and methods used for profile analysis. Although the "cookbooks" are available, their blind use will not be particularly helpful. The skilled interpreter of MMPI profiles will sometimes decide that the cookbook formula is wrong and some other clinical picture is more accurate. The "clinical lore"of the MMPI, and other instruments as well, consists of sensing from the *comparison of the profile pattern with other characteristics known about the patient* that the cookbook description does not fit.

However, there are some general observations that will help the novice understand MMPI results. In general, patients presenting with neurotic disorders will show higher scores on the Hs, D, Hy, Pd, and Mf scales than on the Pa, Pt, Sc, Ma, and Si scales. The profile curves will slope downward from left to right. Conversely, patients with more serious psychotic disorders will show a slope downward from right to left. Patients with character problems will show curves higher in the middle of the profile with a dropping off on either end. These are very gross trends, however, and should not be considered inflexible rules.

Many users of the MMPI currently employ commercial scoring and interpretive services to process patients' responses. The scoring services provide all the standard clinical and validity scales, as well as cer-

---

Figure 21–1. Minnesota Multiphasic Personality Inventory profile of idealized female patient with conversion neurosis. (Reproduced, with permission, from Minnesota Multiphasic Personality Inventory, copyright © 1943 by the University of Minnesota, renewed 1970. This profile Form 1948, 1976, 1982.)

[see legend on facing page]

tain special scales of interest such as Barron's ego strength scale (1953), Taylor's manifest anxiety scale (1953), and Navran's dependency scale (1954). Additionally, the scoring service provides a narrative summary of interpretation of the meaning of the profile, along with responses to certain key items such as alcohol abuse and hearing voices. The computer-generated narrative summaries are an outgrowth of the code-type profile pattern analyses and cookbooks discussed above.

Reliability & Validity

The reliability coefficients for the MMPI are quite satisfactory. Some scales, such as the depression scale, are not as stable (ie, consistent or reliable) as others, such as the paranoia scale; however, no one questions the reliability of the basic clinical scales. Test-retest correlations range from 0.61 to 0.87 in a sample of female psychiatric patients.

The considerations for validity of the MMPI are more complex. As discussed above, the scales are not pathognomonic of the psychopathologic conditions whose names they bear. A T score above 70 on the schizophrenia scale is *not necessarily* diagnostic of schizophrenia. Nonetheless, the MMPI has proved useful in clinical formulation, treatment planning, and prediction of outcome. On the whole, there is evidence for concurrent, predictive, and construct validity, with the strength of the evidence following that order.

Issues in the Use of the MMPI

Three issues are currently the focus of concern for clinical use of the MMPI.

The first issue is the use of commercial services for interpretation of the profile (see above). Prudent clinicians will wish to occasionally compare interpretations from these services with their own interpretations.

The second issue regards norms. There is still controversy regarding the applicability of the published "Minnesota" norms for patients from different ethnic and cultural backgrounds as well as for older and younger patients. The most detailed work has concerned separate norms for black Americans. An informed position suggests the use of both national and local or special norms for profile interpretation. Failing that, a general rule is to interpret cautiously any mildly elevated curves in profiles from minority patients.

The third issue is the proliferation of short forms of the MMPI. Versions such as Mini-Mult, Midi-Mult, and Faschingbauer's (1974) Abbreviated MMPI (FAM) all promise results comparable to those of the full MMPI for less time and trouble. Although a generally acceptable correlation has been shown between scale scores on the full MMPI and those on the short forms, the short forms do a poor job in reproducing the profile codes that are the heart of MMPI use and interpretation. Hence, most authorities and reviewers discourage the use of the short forms for assessment of patients with potentially serious clinical disorders.

In his review of the MMPI in the *Eighth Mental Measurements Yearbook,* a compendium of reviews of almost all published psychologic tests, King (1978) concluded as follows:

> The MMPI remains matchless as the objective instrument for the assessment of psychopathology. The clinician who uses the MMPI clinically is finding his endeavor being made both more difficult and easier. It is being made easier by the continued and high quality elaboration of actuarial interpretive systems to aid in the clinical decision-making process. It is becoming more complicated because the clinician must pay attention to increasing numbers of moderating variables, such as age and possibly race, in his interpretations. In addition, the possible applications of the instrument are increasing to include alcoholics, drug abusers, parents of emotionally disturbed children, and medical patients.

RORSCHACH PSYCHODIAGNOSTICS

The set of 10 published Rorschach inkblots is part of a series developed and used by the Swiss psychiatrist Hermann Rorschach in his clinical research. Rorschach was interested in fantasy, and he noticed that specfic kinds of blots evoked fairly consistent responses from certain groups of patients. These findings were published in his monograph (1942), but his work was cut short by his death at the age of 38.

The Rorschach technique is probably the best-known personality assessment measure. This is due not only to the extremely widespread use of the technique but also to early claims and hopes that it could and would provide an "x-ray" of the mind. Despite this mystique about the Rorschach technique, it is actually among the most thoroughly researched measures used in all of psychologic testing, and today there is good documentation of its range and limitations for use.

Administration

The 10 inkblots are ambiguous stimuli that provoke associations. The standard series is reproduced on cards that are 18 × 24 cm (7 × 9 ½ inches) and numbered from I to X. Card I is shown in Fig 21-2. Five of the blots (I, IV, V, VI, and VII) are in black and white; the others include colors. The examiner gives the patient a statement of directions such as the following and stresses that there are no right or wrong answers: "I have a series of cards with inkblots on them. They look like different things to different people. I'll show them to you, one at a time, and I'd like for you to tell me everything that each one looks like, everything that each one reminds you of. After you've finished with the first card, hand it back and we'll go on to the next one."

During the first phase of the test, the **free association phase,** the examiner records each response as nearly verbatim as possible, notes the orientation of the blot for each response (eg, upside down), and

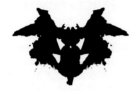

Figure 21–2. Card I of the Rorschach Psychodiagnostics, reduced to one-sixth of actual size. (Reproduced with permission of the copyright holder, Hans Huber AG Buchhandlung Verlag.)

notes the elapsed time from the presentation of the blot to the first response.

After all 10 blots have been presented, there is usually an **inquiry phase.** Each blot is given back to the patient, and the examiner reads back the patient's response and asks what about the blot prompted that response. During this phase of the procedure, patients may give additional responses. These are noted, and the same inquiry procedure is followed for these additional responses. Even though new responses may be made during the inquiry phase, *only free association responses are scored.*

Scoring

The great bulk of the work is devoted to scoring the responses. There is no one "official" scoring procedure. Major scoring systems were developed in the late 1930s and early 1940s and published by Beck (1944), Klopfer and coworkers (1942, 1954), and Rapaport and colleagues (1946). More recently, Exner (1974) has proposed an integrative scoring system with more detailed normative data, and it is likely that this system will become the standard for scoring the Rorschach technique.

All of the major scoring systems follow Rorschach's original scheme in noting these 4 categories: (1) location, (2) determinants, (3) contents, and (4) popularity. Exner uses 2 other categories: organizational activity and form quality. Exner's scoring system is presented below.

A. Location: Scoring of location is based on the part of the inkblot used as the basis for the response. The common categories of location are (1) the whole blot, (2) a common detail, (3) an unusual detail, and (4) the white space around or in the middle of the blot. (All of the scoring categories use abbreviated symbols, such as W for whole, but the full set is only of interest to advance examiners.)

B. Determinant: Scoring of determinants is based on the qualities of the blot that were used in forming the percept, ie, what made it look like the object described by the patient. The major categories of determinants are (1) form, (2) movement, (3) color (chromatic), (4) color (achromatic), (5) texture (shading-derived), (6) dimensionality (shading-derived), (7) shading (general or diffuse), (8) dimensionality (form-derived), and (9) pairs and reflections.

C. Content: There are 27 content categories. Examples with Exner's numbers are (1) whole human, (7) animal detail, (14) blood, (19) fire, (25) sex, and (26) x-ray.

D. Popularity: There are specific responses given frequently to specific cards. Exner has tabulated 13 popular responses; several are listed here, with popularity number shown in parentheses and Rorchach card number shown in brackets: (1) [1] bat or butterfly; (6) [IV] animal skin or human figure dressed in fur; (10) [VII] human heads or faces, usually those of women or children; and (13) [X] crab, lobster, or spider.

E. Organizational Activity: The scoring of organizational activity is indexed by the symbol Z. It is a complex feature to score, and it deals with the patient's process of integrating the various features of the inkblot to form an organized and coherent percept.

F. Form Quality: Most scoring systems evaluate how well the percept "fits" the actual blot. Exner uses a 4-level system for scoring quality of fit: superior (+), ordinary (o), weak (w), and minus (−). The minus response is defined as "the distorted, arbitrary, unrealistic use of form as related to the content offered, where an answer is imposed on the blot area with total, or near total, disregard for the structure of the area."

Interpretation

Despite the heavy and involved emphasis on scoring, conclusions about personality structure and functioning have come less from formal scoring and more from a movement back and forth between what theory suggests about psychopathologic disorders and what the responses to the Rorschach inkblots suggest about the patient's style of processing information. Although Exner's scoring system is quite detailed and empirically based, his instructions for interpretation are much less mechanical. They emphasize a 2-stage process of (1) initially generating many hypotheses about defenses, contact with reality, intelligence, fantasy life, and sexuality, based on the formal scoring of the whole record, the specific scoring of each response, the sequence of responses, and the content of the verbalization; and (2) integrating the hypotheses and modifying or ruling out the contradictory ones. After this process, a coherent personality description is written.

Although some writers have argued that interpretation of the Rorschach record should be blind, without reference to any other information about the patient, this method is *not* recommended. The Rorschach technique is not a parlor game; it is an aid to understanding personality functioning. As such, all available information about the person's functioning is useful. If several psychologic tests have been used, Exner recommends that the Rorschach record be examined first, so that some hypotheses are not prematurely ruled out by non-Rorschach information.

Reliability & Validity

The reliability of Rorschach scoring systems has been examined and found to be adequate. In this instance, reliability is taken to mean that 2 clinicians generate the same formal scoring from a Rorschach protocol. The reliability of the *clinical summary write-ups,* however, has not been routinely examined and must therefore remain questionable. The validity of the Rorschach technique is also difficult to evaluate, owing to variations in administering the test and interpreting results. Most reviews suggest that the Rorschach technique adds interesting and perhaps important information to the clinical assessment, but a rigorous evaluation of *how much more* it adds has not been conducted. Most research using the Rorschach technique compares groups on the basis of mean scores rather than by generating specific clinical predictions to be tested. Hence, the Rorschach technique is best viewed as an extremely well researched technique that suggests important themes of personality and psychodynamics—themes that should be considered during treatment planning and confirmed or disproved during the treatment.

Issues in the Use of the Rorschach Technique

Despite the great strides made by Exner in standardizing scoring, the value of the Rorschach technique in personality assessment continues to depend almost exclusively on the clinician's write-up of the record, which involves some degree of subjectivity. This makes it difficult to evaluate the technique, but some conclusions are possible.

First, by itself, the Rorschach record *cannot* provide a diagnosis. Hypotheses about personality styles or defenses can be entertained, but it is inappropriate to use the Rorschach record to validate these hypotheses. Second, Exner's work amply demonstrates that there are *no universal meanings* for any card. There is no "father card," "mother card," or "sex card," as many writers have argued. Third, the administration process is as ambiguous as the blots are. The record of responses may be influenced by characteristics of the examiner or by the context in which the examination takes place. Fourth, like psychodynamic formulations of conflict and defense, the yield from a Rorschach record must be viewed as a working formulation to be modified on the basis of other information as it becomes available.

Other Uses of the Rorschach Technique

One other productive use of the Rorschach technique has been the scoring of communication deviances (noted in the patient's responses during both phases of administration) to evaluate signs of thought disorder. Singer and Larson (1981) have been primarily responsible for this work, which has focused on patients with schizophrenia or borderline personality disorder. This approach has promise and illustrates a way in which the Rorschach technique can be modified to illuminate different areas of personality.

THEMATIC APPERCEPTION TEST (TAT)

The TAT was designed to elicit important personality themes from fantasy-based stories told by the patient in response to somewhat ambiguous pictures. Like the Rorschach technique, the TAT is a projective test designed to assess underlying personality processes—in this case, underlying needs. The procedure was developed by Morgan and Murray (1935) as part of a study of normal personality done at the Harvard Psychological Clinic.

Administration

The test materials consist of 31 cards (30 drawings and fuzzy photographs plus one blank card). Murray suggested that each subject be shown only 20 cards, and he designated some to be used only for boys (B), others for girls (G), and others for male or female adults (M or F). The following are a few examples of pictures (descriptions and numbers are taken from the TAT manual): *Card 2:* Country scene: In the foreground is a young woman with books in her hand; in the background, a man is working in the fields and an older woman is looking on. *Card 3BM:* On the floor against a couch is the huddled form of a boy with his

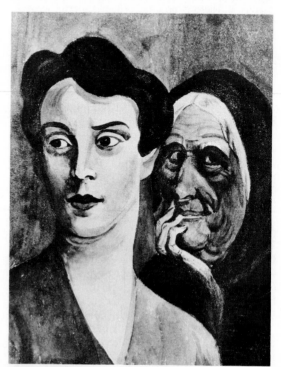

Figure 21–3. Card 12F of the Thematic Apperception Test. (Reprinted, by permission of the publishers, from Henry A. Murray, *Thematic Apperception Test.* Cambridge, Mass.: Harvard University Press, copyright © 1943 by the President and Fellows of Harvard College; copyright © 1971 by Henry A. Murray.)

head bowed on his right arm. Beside him on the floor is a revolver. *Card 6GF:* A young woman sitting on the edge of a sofa looks back over her shoulder at an older man with a pipe in his mouth who seems to be addressing her. *Card 12F:* The portrait of a young woman. A weird old woman with a shawl over her head is grimacing in the background (Fig 21–3). *Card 13MF:* A young man is standing with downcast head buried in his arm. Behind him is the figure of a woman lying in bed.

Murray proposed 2 series of administrations (10 cards each), with the following directions: "This is a test of imagination, one form of intelligence. I am going to show you some pictures, one at a time, and your task will be to make up as dramatic a story as you can for each. Tell what has led up to the event shown in the picture, describe what is happening at the moment, what the characters are feeling and thinking, and then give the outcome. Speak your thoughts as they come to your mind. Do you understand? Since you have 50 minutes for 10 pictures, you can devote about 5 minutes to each story. Here is the first picture." The subject would respond to the other 10 cards at a later sitting.

In clinical practice today, most examiners use fewer than 20 pictures and limit the testing to a single administration. The pictures selected depend upon the examiner's personal preference and intuitive notions about what important dynamic areas of the patient's personality may be illuminated by particular cards. The examiner records verbatim the story given by the patient and should attempt to be as unobtrusive as possible throughout the session. Some writers recommend that patients be prompted to give outcomes for their stories if these are not produced spontaneously; opinions on this procedure vary.

Scoring & Interpretation

Unlike the Rorschach technique, the TAT does not separate scoring from interpretation. Murray's original suggestions involved conceptualizing the story material in terms of (1) the **hero** of each story (presumably the individual with whom the subject identifies); (2) the **needs** (inner states) of the subject for various activities or gratifications (need for aggression, need for achievement); (3) the **press,** ie, the environmental context in which the subject assumes the hero is operating and which influences the hero's needs; and (4) the **thema,** a term indicating the motivational trends of the hero in responding to the combination of needs and stress.

Other methods of interpreting the TAT are linked to conceptual or theoretic systems, such as psychoanalysis or jungian typologies, or to specific content areas of academic research in psychology, such as motivation to achieve and need for power.

Reliability & Validity

Fewer studies have been conducted on the reliability of the scoring systems of the TAT, partially because there has been less systematization of scoring. Some studies show that raters agree; others show marked divergence. The reliability of the TAT is therefore questionable. The validity of the TAT is also questionable in the sense that in many cases the stories given are not, as Murray hoped, "an x-ray picture" of the "inner self." Many stories pertain to overt themes in a patient's life, rather than to unconscious fantasied ideas. Some research shows that the sex of the examiner influences the type of responses, depending upon the sex of the patient. The TAT may give clues to the personality needs and wishes of patients, but it does not do so invariably. It is best used as an adjunctive technique to generate hypotheses or confirm hypotheses from other sources. Basing a diagnosis or a treatment plan solely on the TAT is not recommended.

BROAD ISSUES IN PERSONALITY ASSESSMENT BY PSYCHOLOGIC TESTING

Three themes have run through the discussion of psychologic tests in this chapter.

(1) Despite the search for standardization and uniformity in the use of psychologic tests for personality assessment, different clinicians have different systems. Thus, the interpretation of a battery of psychologic tests depends upon who does the interpreting. In an analogous fashion, the test results depend upon who the patient is; results may be accurate indicators of personality, or they may reflect *individual differences in responses that are not primarily indicative of personality.* This is why tests do not have perfect predictability and why it is difficult to determine with high accuracy a complete picture of a patient's personality.

(2) The research evidence about the utility of testing has been disappointingly mixed. It is not clear how much more information is gained by using the MMPI, the Rorschach technique, and the TAT, for example, rather than just one or 2 of the tests. In this area, clinicians have been somewhat resistant to take seriously the research evidence, viewing it as simplistic, naive, and not in touch with clinical realities. There are clinical examples in which results of the battery of tests have suggested a personality assessment that is not what any one test would have suggested. The issue here is one of cost- and time-effectiveness. Like laboratory tests in clinical medicine, psychologic tests must be evaluated for redundancy, cost, and possibility of yielding incremental information.

(3) The major area requiring more careful scrutiny is the area of agreement among clinicians—not in scoring of psychologic tests but in interpreting the results. If trained clinicians cannot reach an acceptable level of agreement about interpretation, then more structured formats for interpretation must be developed to aid in standardizing the kinds of categories used and inferences made from the testing results.

REFERENCES

Allport GW: *Personality: A Psychological Interpretation*. Holt, 1937.

Barron FX: An ego strength scale which predicts response to psychotherapy. *J Consult Psychol* 1953;**17:**327.

Beck SJ: *Rorschach's Test*. Vol 1: *Basic Processes,* 1944; Vol 2: *A Variety of Personality Pictures,* 1949. Grune & Stratton.

Bender L: *A Visual Motor Gestalt Test and Its Clinical Use*. American Orthopsychiatric Association, 1938.

Drake LE: A social introversion scale for the MMPI. *J Appl Psychol* 1946;**30:**51.

Exner JE: *The Rorschach: A Comprehensive System*. Vol 1. Wiley, 1974.

Faschingbauer TR: A 166-item written short form of the group MMPI: The FAM. *J Consult Clin Psychol* 1974;**42:**645.

Fenichel O: *The Collected Papers of Otto Fenichel*. Vol 2. Norton, 1954.

Frank LK: Projective methods for the study of personality. *J Psychol* 1939;**8:**839.

Gall FG: *On the Functions of the Brain and Each of Its Parts*. Marsh, Capen, & Lyon, 1835.

Gough HG: *Brief Descriptive and Interpretational Summary of the Scales on the Minnesota Multiphasic Personality Inventory*. [Unpublished manuscript.]

Hathaway SR, McKinley JC: *Minnesota Multiphasic Personality Inventory Manual*. Psychological Corporation, 1951.

Kelly GA: Man's construction of his alternatives. In: *The Assessment of Human Motives*. Lindzey G (editor). Rinehart, 1958.

Kelly GA: *The Psychology of Personal Constructs*. Norton, 1955.

King GD: Review of the Minnesota Multiphasic Personality Inventory. In: *The Eighth Mental Measurements Yearbook*. Buros OK (editor). Gryphon Press, 1978.

Klopfer B, Kelley D: *The Rorschach Technique*. World Book, 1942.

Klopfer B et al: *Developments in the Rorschach Technique*. Vol 1. World Book, 1954.

Morgan CD, Murray HA: A method for investigating fantasies: The Thematic Apperception Test. *Arch Neurol Psychiatry* 1935;**34:**289.

Murray HA: *Thematic Apperception Test Manual*. Harvard Univ Press, 1943.

Navran L: A rationally derived MMPI scale for dependence. *J Consult Psychol* 1954;**18:**192.

Rapaport D, Gill M, Schafer R: *Psychological Diagnostic Testing*. Vol 2. Year Book, 1946.

Rorschach H: *Psychodiagnostics*. Huber, 1942; Grune & Stratton, 1951.

Singer MT, Larson DG: Borderline personality and the Rorschach test. *Arch Gen Psychiatry* 1981;**38:**693.

Taylor JA: A personality scale of manifest anxiety. *J Abnor Soc Psychol* 1953;**48:**285.

The Clinical Case Summary: The Mayor of Wino Park

22

Howard H. Goldman, MD,PhD

The following is a case study of the Mayor of Wino Park, briefly introduced as a character sketch in Chapter 16. The standard sequence for presenting clinical psychiatric cases is set forth in Table 22–1. The hypothetical data needed to complete this clinical case summary would have been collected during the Mayor's 3-week hospitalization, when he underwent an extensive evaluation, including all of the elements presented in Chapters 17–21. Although the case is presented here primarily to demonstrate the form and content of a case summary, the details of the case also illustrate the complex interaction of biologic, psychologic, and social factors in medicine and psychiatry.

CASE SUMMARY

Identifying data: John F. ("Red") Kimball is 54 years old, divorced, unemployed, currently subsisting on Social Security Disability Insurance (SSDI) benefits, and living on the streets or in Wino Park, a protected urban camping ground in San Francisco. The night manager of the Billings Hotel on Pine Street receives and holds the patient's monthly check. The patient prefers to be addressed as Mayor and referred to as the Mayor.

Table 22–1. Suggested format for a clinical case summary.

Identifying data
Informant (sources of information) and assessment of reliability
Chief complaint
History of the present illness
Past medical and psychiatric history
Review of systems
Habits
Family history
Social history
Developmental history
Physical examination
Neurologic examination
Mental status examination
Diagnostic tests
Differential diagnosis
Provisional psychosocial formulation
Hospital course
Multiaxial diagnosis
Psychosocial formulation
Continuing treatment plan and disposition

Informant: The patient is a poor historian. Throughout his hospital stay, his responses to inquiries have been marked by inconsistencies, gaps, and confabulation. His ability to give a useful past history has improved as his attention span increases with treatment, but his history of the present illness continues to be marred by deficits in short-term memory.

To supplement the history, we obtained medical records from previous hospitalizations, outpatient clinic records, and school and military records. No work history documentation could be obtained, nor could any family member be located to verify the history. During an earlier admission, a lifelong acquaintance corroborated much of the patient's early life history as presented in this case study.

Chief complaint: "They closed Wino Park—and I'm yellow, have the shakes, and somebody's trying to poison me . . ."

History of the present illness: While living in Wino Park off and on for the past 5 years, the Mayor had been in good health except for a few episodes of depression treated with tricyclic antidepressants and supportive psychotherapy. During the past year, he appointed himself mayor of all of the homeless alcoholics and other unemployed and mentally ill people who slept in the park. He felt he was their spokesman, and during the past 3 months, after it was announced that the park was to be closed, he felt under constant pressure to "save" their haven. He began giving impromptu "news conferences" to anyone who would listen at downtown intersections during rush hour—or before groups of tourists waiting for cable cars. He also began to drink more heavily than ever at that time, consuming several quarts of wine daily.

About 10 weeks prior to the present admission, the Mayor was arrested for threatening an officer who attempted to take him into custody when he was found drunk, wandering the streets. He was released the next morning, but the desk sergeant thought he seemed depressed and perhaps in need of medical evaluation, so he was sent to the hospital in a police ambulance. He admitted he had been in a "black mood" for the past couple of weeks, with no appetite, and had been losing weight, waking up at night, and then unable to get back to sleep. He was obviously agitated and said he could not concentrate and thought a lot about death when he wasn't casting about for some magical solution to the Wino Park "crisis," as he saw it. His preoccupation with death and veiled threats of suicide ("Maybe I'll 'end it'") led to his admission to a psychiatric inpatient unit for observation and protective detention. He signed himself out after 72 hours, proclaiming, "There's nothing wrong with me!" His discharge diagnosis was recurrent unipolar depression. He refused to stay in the hospital for a trial of treatment with antidepressant medication. He could not be committed, because he denied suicidal intentions and had not developed delirium tremens. He also refused referral to an outpatient clinic.

The Mayor continued to be depressed and drank "to kill the pain of going insane" and to stop the "shakes." There was no apparent change in his condition until 2 weeks before the present admission, when he became jaundiced, more agitated, confused, and paranoid. He was afraid that someone had contaminated the wine with some kind of poison or "Yellow Dye Number Nine," and he was organizing people to march to the liquor stores to pull the wine off the shelves. At that point he was sleeping only a few hours a night. He became extremely irritable (euphoric one moment, angry the next), and his scheming, grandiosity, and paranoid ideation increased. His speech was pressured, tangential, and at times almost incomprehensible. The "people's press conferences" at downtown intersections became disruptive, and the police were called on several occasions, but there were no arrests or contacts with the health care system until the day of admission.

On the day of admission, Wino Park was closed, and all of the homeless men and women were being turned out or relocated. The Mayor refused to go. When the police said they would have to arrest him if he did not leave, he became agitated, running around furiously and talking loudly. All of the pathologic thought, affect, and behavior of the previous 2 weeks intensified. He threatened loudly that he would kill anyone who touched him and then kill himself. When he seemed close to collapse from exhaustion, the police grabbed him, handcuffed him, called for an ambulance, and drove him to the hospital again.

Past medical and psychiatric history: Medical records indicate that the patient was the 35-week product of a difficult pregnancy and labor complicated by abnormal maternal bleeding secondary to multiple small uterine fibroid tumors. The patient's mother had a hysterectomy following delivery; she was separated from her baby for 4 weeks, unable to nurse him, and then was hospitalized for depression for 4 months postpartum.

During childhood, the patient had measles, mumps, and chickenpox but no other infectious diseases except for an occasional cold. A fractured clavicle at age 8 years was inflicted by his alcoholic father. He had an appendectomy at age 13, shortly after his mother died. (The appendix was normal, according to the pathology report.)

At age 20, the patient received a medical discharge from the navy for a "character disorder" and was noted to be an alcoholic and occasional binge drinker. Between the ages of 20 and 35, he was working, married, and in excellent health. He was divorced at age 35, and his drinking increased. (For details, see Social History.) For the next 5–10 years, his work history was interrupted by several admissions to alcohol treatment centers, outpatient alcohol counseling, and periods of ambulatory psychiatric treatment for depression. Once, while depressed, he was treated with thyroid hormone; he became acutely psychotic and agitated and was thought to have bipolar affective disorder (manic-depressive illness).

At age 45, the patient became severely depressed and suicidal. He was committed to a state mental hospital because he had refused treatment in a voluntary general hospital psychiatric unit. On admission, he was heavily sedated with antipsychotic medication because of agitation and auditory hallucinations consisting of voices commanding him to kill himself. Because of the imminent danger of suicide, he underwent a course of 12 electroconvulsive treatments, which dramatically improved his mental status, especially his agitation and suicidal ideation. He remained somewhat depressed and stayed in the hospital for 3 months. A trial of tricyclic antidepressants and supportive psychotherapy was successful in further reducing his symptoms, and he was discharged with a prescription for amitriptyline, 200 mg daily at bedtime. He went to live in a single-room occupancy hotel in the "Tenderloin district" of San Francisco. He was seen as an outpatient for several years in a clinic operated by the county, but his drinking was not controlled, and he stopped his medication. He was readmitted to various hospitals several times. As noted earlier, his sole source of support was SSDI funds. The night manager at the hotel serves as his conservator.

The patient became so mentally disorganized, paranoid, and unmanageable that he could no longer stay at the hotel. He was accepted at a board and care home for alcoholic men but would not agree to the restrictions. He could not be committed to a hospital, because he was not dangerous to himself or others, and so he began his life on the streets and in Wino Park 5 years prior to the current admission.

The Mayor has no documented history of endocrine disorders, including thyroid disease and Cushing's syndrome. He has no history of acute liver disease, gastritis, or other gastrointestinal disorders, although his liver enzyme levels have been elevated in the past. There is no record of jaundice prior to this illness. He has never had delirium tremens or any seizure disorder, and he has no known allergies.

Review of systems: In addition to having the symptoms and signs mentioned in the history of the present illness, the patient admits to seeing double from time to time and losing his footing occasionally. Pertinent negative findings include the absence of focal neurologic and endocrinologic signs and symptoms (other than those mentioned above, eg, diplopia, tremor) and no abnormalities in stool color.

Habits: The Mayor drinks up to 2 quarts of wine daily. He has been drinking since he was 12 years old; he admits to having been a binge drinker as a teenager and an alcoholic since his 20s. There is no other history of drug abuse. He has smoked one package of cigarettes daily since age 15, plus occasional cigars.

Family history: The patient is the only child of Francis Kimball and Jean-Marie Thibodeau Kimball. Francis Kimball died at age 55, when the patient was 35, of injuries sustained in an accident at the state mental hospital where he had been a patient for nearly 5 years. Mr Kimball had been away without leave from the hospital, had gotten drunk, started a fight with another patient, was pushed over a wall, and fell 10 feet and struck his head. He had been hospitalized for bipolar affective disorder (manic-depressive illness) and alcoholism. He had no other known disorders. Jean-Marie Kimball died at age 32 of breast cancer. She had no other known illnesses other than postpartum depression and uterine fibromyomas. All of the grandparents died before they reached age 50: one by suicide, one from "heart disease," one from influenza in 1918, and one from tuberculosis.

Social history: As a child, John F. Kimball lived with both parents, although their occasional extended absences from home (due to parents' illnesses and father's alcoholism) necessitated informal foster care with neighbors and with "aunts and uncles" for up to 3 months at a stretch. John attended parochial school for 6 years and then completed junior high and attended high school in the public schools in San Francisco. His performance was uneven; he did well with some subjects and teachers and poorly with others. He was good in dramatics, athletics, and public speaking, had many friends, and was elected class treasurer as a sophomore. He became depressed as a senior, did poorly, and dropped out before graduation. He entered the navy and served for 3 years. He spent time in the "brig" for insubordination, drunkenness, and being AWOL. He was never promoted above the rank of Seaman First-Class and was discharged for medical reasons with a diagnosis of "character disorder and alcoholism."

Building on some skills he learned in the navy and on his persuasive manner, the patient got a union card and a job as a machinist. He worked in a dry dock, repairing ships. He was liked by his workmates; they drank and caroused together, and Kimball became union shop steward. For a time he was involved in union politics and attended local election rallies.

"Red" Kimball married a girl from his old neighborhood shortly after discharge from the navy. They lived in a flat and "got along fine," but he insisted they have no children. She acquiesced reluctantly until she turned 30. At that time, she began to complain about "feeling empty" and wanting a family. He began to spend less time at home, more time with the "boys," and his drinking increased. He became impotent, and they stopped having sexual relations altogether. Their marriage slowly deteriorated as he became more depressed and his alcoholism worsened. They began to fight, and he abused her physically on 2 occasions. She filed for dissolution of the marriage, and the patient had not seen his wife since the decree became final.

The remainder of the social history is conveyed along with the past history, discussed earlier. As noted, the patient is homeless, unemployed, and supported by SSDI.

Developmental history: The Mayor's life began with a 5-month separation from his mother, who was hospitalized with postpartum complications, including a hysterectomy and postpartum depression. As a newborn, he was raised by a neighbor and supported by his father, whose alcoholism made him an undependable caretaker. Mrs Kimball returned home and took up the child-rearing responsibility with renewed energy, but she never seemed able to get emotionally close to her son. The same was true of Mr Kimball, although when he was sober, he was a great "pal" to his son, teaching him to box and play games.

Little is known of the Mayor's childhood from age 2 to 6 years. In spite of never feeling emotionally close to her son, his mother tended to "spoil him" with small favors and took him with her everywhere. As his father's absences became more frequent and longer in duration, "Red" Kimball became protective of his mother. The Mayor's earliest traumatic memories are of his father's physical assaults on his mother. He was terrified and felt guilty that he couldn't help her. Once he did step in the way of his father's blows and sustained a fractured clavicle. He began to "hate" his "old man" and felt confused when his father confessed to him in tears—drunk and begging forgiveness. The image of the "pal" was incongruent with the hated "old man." As a child, "Red" thought almost everything was his fault because he had been "bad."

Ages 7–12 were marked by minor school difficulties and further troubles at home. "Red" took his first drink at age 12 and became drunk easily at first but soon developed tolerance to large quantities of alcohol. His mother died when he was 13 years old, and he was extremely quiet, withdrawn, and guilty. He had no one to talk to, and his sadness turned to anger and resentment toward his parents, who had neglected him. And the anger turned quickly to guilt for having hateful feelings toward his parents. A few months later, he complained of intense stomach cramps and was operated on for suspected appendicitis, but the surgical specimen was normal.

The patient reached puberty at about age 14, engaged in homosexual horseplay (group masturbation) with some friends at age 15, and had his first heterosexual experience at age 16. He related no history of sexual dysfunction other than episodes of impotence during his marriage (described above) and while drunk.

Other details of social and sexual relationships are discussed in the social history.

Physical examination: On admission the patient was a plethoric man who seemed older than his stated age, with a barrel chest, thin limbs, and protruding abdomen. He was in apparent distress, shouting and waving his arms. His scleras were yellow and his skin jaundiced where it was not tanned from prolonged exposure.

Vital signs: Pulse 120 and regular, respiration 24, labored; blood pressure 160/90 left arm, sitting; temperature 100 °F. At the time of admission, only a limited examination could be performed because of the patient's lack of cooperation. A cursory examination of the lungs, heart, and abdomen revealed no acute disease. The examination was completed the following morning, when pulse was 88 and regular, respiration 12 and regular, blood pressure 140/90 in both arms with orthostatic drop of 25 mm Hg, and temperature 99 °F.

Head, eyes, ears, nose, and throat: Several scars on the face and scalp healed by secondary intention, marked scleral icterus, spider angiomas and injected veins on the nose, nasopharyngeal congestion.

Neck: Supple, no thyromegaly, no lymphadenopathy.

Thorax and lungs: Increased anteroposterior diameter, lungs clear to percussion and auscultation, although breath sounds were distant and the chest was slightly hyperresonant. No gynecomastia.

Heart and great vessels: The point of maximum impulse was felt in the fifth intercostal space 2 fingerbreadths to the left of the midclavicular line; the impulse was hyperdynamic. Heart sounds were all within normal limits, with no murmurs, rubs, or clicks. All peripheral pulses were felt; no bruits.

Abdomen: Icteric skin, appendectomy scar. Abdomen distended with ascites fluid wave (1/4). Tenderness in the right upper quadrant, with an enlarged liver felt 4 cm below the costal margin. No splenomegaly, no masses, no costovertebral angle tenderness. Bowel sounds were normal.

Rectum: Prostatic hypertrophy (2/4) with no discrete mass. Stool test for occult blood was negative.

Genitourinary tract: Normal adult male with slight testicular atrophy. Normal pattern of pubic hair.

Extremities: No bony abnormalities, full range of motion.

Neurologic examination:

Mental status: (See below.)

Cranial nerves: I, II, V, VII–XII tested and all within normal limits; III, IV, VI, pupils equal, round, and reacting to light and accommodation, but abduction and conjugate gaze were paralyzed; diplopia was evident.

Motor system:

   Muscle mass and tone–Normal.

   Strength–Full strength (5/5).

   Coordination–Slight asterixis and dysdiadochokinesia, demonstrated in difficulties with finger-to-nose and heel-to-shin tests.

   Reflexes–All 3/4 without clonus, except that ankle jerks were absent; Babinski, Hoffmann absent.

   Gait and station–Wide-based gait.

   Movements–Normal fluidity without tics, chorea, or dyskinesia; mild resting tremor in both hands (1/4).

Sensation: Diminished pain and vibration sense in the extremities, feet worse than hands; no extinction on simultaneous stimulation.

Mental status examination:

Overview: Exaggerated alertness and easy distractibility; disheveled, with poor personal hygiene but a certain flair to his carriage and disarray; uncooperative at times but with perseverance able to complete the exam; hyperactive, unable to sit for more than 3–4 minutes at a time.

Emotion: Labile, expansive, irritable, with rapid shifts from tearful sadness to red-faced anger. Affect was appropriate. (Thoughts were consistent with affect.)

Attention: Failed the 7-digit screening test, only able to recall 3 digits on second try. Unable to perform serial 7s or 3s.

Orientation: To person, place (that it was a hospital only), and time (only to year, not month or day).

Memory: Attention deficit made memory assessment difficult. With effort and repetition, the patient was able to immediately recall 3 items, but he could not remember any of them at 5 minutes even with prompting and reinforcement. Visual memory was similarly impaired.

The patient confabulated to fill in the gaps in recent memory. Long-term memory was adequate for a period prior to 4 or 5 years ago. He knew the United States presidents and current events of the period.

Speech and language: Pressured and incessant, but fluent, with normal comprehension; repetition and naming both intact. Two-and 3-step commands could not be assessed because of memory deficits.

Constructional ability: Unable to perform tests requiring memory. The patient was able to copy test figures when they were in front of him.

Calculations: Able to pass the screening test (5 × 13).

Thought:

> *Thought process*–Thought process markedly disturbed, occasionally incoherent. When coherent, the patient had flight of ideas, was tangential, but did not demonstrate looseness of association.

> *Thought content*–Content marked by mood-congruent auditory hallucinations saying "you are to blame" or laughing derisively. The patient was preoccupied by guilt and images of death alternating with "grandeur." He had paranoid delusions that someone was trying to poison the wine in the liquor stores: "Yellow Dye Number Nine is making me yellow all over!" He denied ideas of reference, thought broadcasting, or other delusions of control. He also denied complex hallucinations of several voices conversing and had no visual, tactile, or gustatory hallucinations, illusions, or other preoccupations.

> *Congnitive functions*–Refused to interpret proverbs or answer screening questions: "Don't bother me with that nonsense. . . . My time is too valuable." Judgment grossly impaired. Did demonstrate some ability to abstract when he tried to take over a nurse's responsibility of explaining to a patient why he should take his medication. He implored the patient, "Take that stuff and your mood might get to be like mine. Besides, it'll help you get out of here quicker if you do like they say!"

> *Fund of knowledge*–Knew the presidents and current events up to 4–5 years ago.

> *Insight*–Aware of the reasons for hospitalization but expended considerable energy denying problems and displacing them onto the politics of the demise of Wino Park.

Diagnostic tests:

Laboratory tests: Serum electrolytes and blood urea nitrogen were normal. Blood ammonia was trivially elevated to 120 μg/dL on admission but fell into the normal range within 3 days. Thyroid studies were normal. Serum aspartate aminotransferase, alkaline phosphatase, and bilirubin were all elevated on admission and returned toward normal by discharge. Bilirubin fell from 4.1 mg/dL to 1.8 mg/dL (mostly direct). Serum albumin was depressed; gamma globulin was elevated. Prothrombin time was in the high normal range. Hematologic evaluation showed a mild macrocytic anemia and moderate leukocytosis with a shift to the left. Erythrocyte sedimentation rate was mildly elevated. Serum iron was normal; serum folate was low. Urinalysis and electrocardiography were normal.

X-rays: Chest films showed slight cardiomegaly and evidence of mild emphysema; there was no evidence of congestive heart failure. A CT scan of the head was normal, with no evidence of tumor, infarct, or subdural hematoma.

Neuropsychologic tests: Full-scale WAIS had been 110 on a previous evaluation. On this admission, the patient's concentration and memory were so impaired that a complete reexamination was impossible. All tests requiring short-term memory were failed. Results of the screening Bender Gestalt Test, however, were normal. The examiner noted that when the patient was tested near the end of his manic episode, he copied the test figures flamboyantly and large in size.

Personality assessment: No testing was done on this admission. Previous tests included an MMPI; results showed high scores on psychasthenia, masculinity, paranoia, and hysteria. On one administration, he also showed an elevation on the depression scale; at another time, the hypomania scale was elevated.

Differential diagnosis: The differential diagnosis on admission was not complicated, because of the well-established prior diagnoses of affective disorder and alcohol dependence, the recurrence of classic symptoms and signs during this episode of illness, and a strong family history of affective illness. For the sake of completeness, other diagnoses were considered: organic affective syndrome, delirium tremens, and especially the nonaffective psychotic disorders (eg, schizophrenia, acute paranoid disorder). No organic cause could be identified, although it is possible that encephalopathy and transiently elevated blood ammonia levels associated with the patient's alcoholic hepatitis may have exacerbated or precipitated his psychosis. The same may be said of his alcohol intoxication. Upon alcohol withdrawal, there was no worsening of his mental status, no increase in tremor, and no seizures—effectively eliminating delirium tremens from the diagnosis. The pattern of the Mayor's illness without persistent psychosis and with prolonged intervals free of illness precluded a diagnosis of schizophrenia; acute paranoid disorder and the other psychotic illnesses were ruled out only by the presence of the full-blown manic episodes and depressive episodes in the Mayor's history and by current findings on mental status examination. On admission, he demonstrated most of the symptoms and signs of manic episode (Table 30–1); shortly after admission, he developed a major depressive episode (Table 30–1). This pattern replicated at least one earlier cycle of bipolar affective disorder.

A diagnosis of alcohol dependence could also be made unequivocally (Table 25–3). The diagnosis of alcohol amnestic syndrome was straightforward (see Chapter 24 and Table 25–3), having been made in the presence of a gaze palsy characteristic of Wernicke's encephalopathy often associated with Korsakoff's psychosis (amnestic syndrome). The diagnosis of alcoholic hepatitis was based on the acute onset of jaundice in an alcoholic and marked abnormalities in hepatic function. Alcoholic cirrhosis was suggested by the presence of ascites; however, *definitive* diagnosis can only be based on liver biopsy, which was not performed, since it was considered too dangerous and because the Mayor was uncooperative. Hematologic evaluation revealed a macrocytic anemia, also probably due to chronic alcoholism.

Provisional psychosocial formulation: Too little information was available on admission to develop a formulation, although the initial psychologic themes centered on losses and self-esteem.

Hospital course:

Week 1: The first week was devoted to a thorough evaluation, reported in this case summary, and to initial treatment of the patient's many problems. Treatment of agitation and insomnia began with oxazepam, 30 mg 4 times daily, reduced to 15 mg 3 times daily by the end of the week. When baseline renal and endocrine studies were completed, the patient was started on lithium carbonate, 600 mg orally 3 times daily for 5 days until a therapeutic level of 1.1 meq/L was achieved, and a maintenance dose of 300 mg 3 times daily was established. In evaluative and supportive psychotherapy, the patient revealed many important losses and separations in his life. The psychologic themes are discussed in the psychosocial formulation below. The Mayor appeared to become depressed by the end of the first week, as his manic signs and symptoms abated with aggressive treatment. During this period, he was confined to the ward. Attempts to contact family and friends were unsuccessful. Social service personnel set about finding the patient a place to live after discharge.

Oxazepam had been selected initially for the control of agitation for 2 reasons: It is less toxic to the liver than the antipsychotic medications,

and it would help to control alcohol withdrawal symptoms and seizure activity associated with delirium tremens if any of these should occur. The patient was observed closely for delirium tremens, but this did not develop. He was also given thiamine, 50 mg intravenously on admission, followed by 50 mg intramuscularly daily thereafter to reverse the Wernicke-Korsakoff syndrome (gaze paralysis and memory disturbance). The gaze paralysis cleared rapidly, but the patient was left with an impairment in memory. Folic acid was given orally, 1 mg daily, for the anemia.

It was decided not to treat the apparent alcoholic hepatitis and hope that abstinence and improved nutrition would permit the patient's liver to heal and that laboratory values would return toward normal and the jaundice would subside. A definitive diagnosis could not be made; a biopsy was not advisable owing to poor cooperation and the risk of excessive bleeding (prothrombin time in high normal range).

Week 2: The Mayor's affect deteriorated into a depressive episode. He complained of a return of agitation, loss of appetite, thoughts (but no plans) of death and suicide, and difficulty concentrating. Feelings of guilt and failure dominated his individual therapy sessions and his comments in ward group therapy meetings. At the beginning of the week, he was involved in ward activities; by the end of the week, he had lost interest in everything and seldom left his room. He was watched closely to prevent a suicide attempt. In spite of only 1 week of symptoms and signs of depression, he was started on amitriptyline, 150 mg orally at bedtime, since this drug had been effective in treating his depressive episodes in the past. Although a higher dose had been necessary before, a lower dose was advised because of the impaired hepatic function. Oxazepam was discontinued.

Week 3: The third week was characterized by slow improvement in mental status. Concentration and attention improved. There was no psychosis. Affect lightened slightly. The patient's sleep improved, and he was taking 2 meals daily by the end of the week. He still felt guilty and was negative, but he stopped ruminating about death and suicide. Arrangements were made for him to go to a board and care home for alcoholics, but he could not obtain a bed for 2 weeks. Plans to keep him until his depression had completely resolved had to be dropped because he insisted on discharge, as did the utilization review committee at the hospital. He was not suicidal and could not be committed involuntarily to a state mental hospital for further care. His conservator at the single-room occupancy hotel agreed to look after him and let him stay there again. The

Mayor also agreed to take his medication and continue in treatment in the hospital's outpatient department. He was making progress in treatment and was beginning to see that he needed to forgive himself for his imagined wrongdoings and to develop a less intense and extreme style in dealing with other people.

By the time of discharge, the patient still had signs of impaired memory and depressed affect, but he was free of psychosis, and his attention span was normal. His jaundice was clearing, and his liver function was returning toward normal.

Multiaxial discharge diagnosis:

Axis I: Bipolar affective disorder (Table 30–1). Manic episode on admission. Depressive episode by discharge. Alcohol dependence (Table 25–3). Alcohol amnestic syndrome (Korsakoff's psychosis) (Chapter 24 and Table 25–3).

Axis II: Histrionic and passive-aggressive traits are probably secondary to affective disorder.

Axis III: Alcoholic hepatitis with jaundice. Wernicke's syndrome (gaze palsy and encephalopathy). Alcoholic cirrhosis (suspected clinically). Peripheral neuropathy. Macrocytic anemia.

Axis IV: Psychosocial stressors rated severe—5/7. Loss of "home" and status as "Mayor." Acute physical illness perceived as threat.

Axis V: Global assessment of function. Current: 2/9 (in danger of harm). Past year: 3/9 (inability to function).

Psychosocial formulation: The Mayor is an angry, guilt-ridden man with bipolar affective disorder complicated by alcoholism and its psychologic and physiologic concomitants. His life story represents a cyclic struggle to achieve a sense of self-worth and self-forgiveness in the face of hardships, losses, separations, and failures. One can only speculate on the interplay of heredity and environment in the evolution of this man's psychopathology; he has a strong family history of affective disorder and alcoholism. In many ways he has repeated the history of his father—in his illness and in his personal life.

The Mayor's depression may be viewed as a response to his losses and separations, beginning at birth: His mother's hospitalizations and depression, his father's repeated absences and ultimate institutionalization and death, and his mother's death all provoked sadness, anger, and a feeling that perhaps he was unloved, unlovable, or perhaps even so "bad" that he made these terrible events and problems happen. The anger fed his guilt, and when it became too intense, it triggered a morbid retreat into depression and alcohol abuse or an angry flight into

mania. Manic euphoria, grandiosity, and the projection of his anger onto others in paranoid fantasies briefly protected him from pain and guilt. (For example, *others* were trying to poison him with Yellow Dye Number Nine, not *he* who was intoxicating himself and his liver with wine.)

The Mayor's sense of guilt and inadequacy appears to stem from the confusion, terror, and helplessness he felt while witnessing his mother's abuse at the hands of his father. He also fell victim to his father's wrath, which hurt him and confused him further. His alliance with his mother may be viewed as overdetermined (ie, having many causes.) His failure to develop a bond with his mother during infancy and her resentment at the loss of her ability to have more children following his birth set up a cycle of reaction formations leading to a studied closeness between them. In other words, they tried unconsciously to overcome their own unconscious resentments toward each other and to compensate for the bond that did not develop in infancy.

The father, too, worked at being a "pal" when he wasn't drunk, depressed, or "away." During childhood, the patient felt doubly guilty about his mother (causing her unhappiness and not protecting her from attack)—a pain he says he felt in his "gut." In retrospect, his symptoms of appendicitis shortly following his mother's death may be seen as a manifestation of this pain. In spite of anger toward his father, he emulated him—all the way to the hospital.

The patient's marriage was also in many respects patterned after that of his parents. It was a hostile-dependent relationship lasting 15 years. In contrast, the Mayor's marriage ended not with the death of his wife but in divorce following injury and abuse. In this case, the abusiveness stemmed from his wife's wish to have children and the Mayor's adamant opposition. One can speculate that his violent opposition derived from a fear that were he to be a father, he might abuse his "son" (he could only imagine a boy child) and disappoint him ("as my father disappointed me").

The Mayor wants everyone to love him but is unable to get close to anyone. He lacks the capacity for intimacy. His charm, dramatic style, and engaging personality have brought him no closeness and no increase in self-esteem. These he has manufactured in flights into mania—an escape from his severe depression. His disappointments, failures, and anger he projects onto others out to get him, especially authority figures, teachers, superiors in the navy, his bosses at work, the police, alcohol manufacturers, his wife, and his doctors.

Bipolar affective disorder and alcoholism have isolated the Mayor from the things he wanted most but were denied him by fate, circumstance, and heredity. A biologic predisposition to affective disorder coupled with environmental circumstances and emotional deprivation and trauma combine to explain the man and his illness.

The patient's sensitivity to loss and stress precipitated this episode of illness with the loss of his "home" in the park and his status as Mayor. He says, "I *was* the Mayor of Wino Park!" The park had been an asylum for a homeless man who needed his expansive fantasies to feel a sense of worth.

The Mayor will soon be 55, the age at which his father died in a mental hospital. Whether the Mayor survives will depend in part on the ability of health care professionals to control his disorder biomedically, understand his illness and his defenses psychologically, help him find a new home and social support, and capitalize on his strengths in his wit, charm, and capacity for leadership.

Continuing Treatment Plan & Disposition:

Biomedical treatment plan:

Lithium carbonate, 300 mg orally 3 times daily.

Amitriptyline, 150 mg orally at bedtime.

Thiamine, 100 mg orally 3 times daily.

Folic acid, 1 mg orally daily.

General internal medicine follow-up in 2 weeks.

Psychotropic medications to be monitored by psychiatrist.

Lithium levels to be determined weekly or until stabilized.

Psychologic treatment plan:

Continue in weekly individual supportive treatment focusing on interpersonal skills; sessions limited to 30 minutes, as tolerated.

Referral to Alcoholics Anonymous.

Visit from nurse if patient fails to comply with his appointments.

Social treatment plan:

Transfer to alcoholism board and care home from his discharge residence at the hotel in San Francisco.

Alcoholics Anonymous will help him to build a new social network as well as reinforce his abstinence.

SSDI checks to be transferred from the hotel to the board and care home after a 1-month trial. Conservatorship might also be transferred to the board and care home operator.

Section III. Mental Disorders

Classifying Mental Disorders: *Diagnostic and Statistical Manual of Mental Disorders: (DSM-III-R)*, Third Edition (Revised)

23

Howard H. Goldman, MD, PhD, & Jack A. Grebb, MD

Note to Reader on Use of *DSM-III-R* in This Text

By arrangement with the American Psychiatric Association, the authors of *Review of General Psychiatry* have borrowed freely from *DSM-III-R*. Most of what we have taken from *DSM-III-R* is identified as such in the tabular matter, eg, "Table 13–4. *DSM-III-R* diagnostic criteria for cyclothymia." Language from the diagnostic criteria of *DSM-III-R* reproduced in this text otherwise than in the tables is in quotes. The quoted passages are reproduced exactly as they appear in *DSM-III-R*. The tables have been normalized to the style of the book in small matters of punctuation and spelling.–HHG.

The *Diagnostic and Statistical Manual of Mental Disorders* (*DSM-III*), 3rd edition (American Psychiatric Association, 1980), together with its 1987 revision (*DSM-III-R*), contains a standard classification of mental disorders widely used in North America and gaining international acceptance. It is the product of a thorough review of the current state of psychiatric nosologic data and thus serves as a valuable guide to the diagnosis of mental disorders. It contains no information about treatment, individual or family psychodynamics, social issues, or—except in a few specific cases described below—the causes of the syndromes. The word "statistical" in the title refers only to the numbering system used for coding purposes and not to statistical data. The *DSM-III-R* diagnoses and their appropriate code designations are presented on pp 247–251.

As discussed in Chapter 12, diagnosis is the process of evaluating patterns of signs and symptoms and thus identifying specific disorders. The diagnostic model implies the existence of some problem severe enough to require professional intervention. Therefore, a compendium of psychiatric diagnoses should not include normal variations in personality styles, mood, or anxiety. For example, normal grief following the death of a close friend or family member is not an entity in *DSM-III*, and an antisocial act (eg, stealing

a car) by a person with no psychopathologic symptoms does not justify a diagnosis of mental disorder.

Until *DSM-III* was published, the lack of an explicit inventory of mental disorders with specified diagnostic criteria was an impediment to research in the field. The most dramatic demonstration of this was documented in the United States-United Kingdom Diagnostic Project in the early 1960s (Cooper and coworkers, 1972). This study was undertaken to explain the higher rate of diagnosis of schizophrenia in the USA compared with that in the United Kingdom. The report showed that psychiatrists in the USA were painting with a much broader "schizophrenia brush" than their colleagues in the United Kingdom—ie, the difference in reported prevalence was a difference in diagnostic practices and not a difference in occurrence of the disorder in the 2 populations. It is safe to assume that major differences in diagnostic concepts also existed among clinicians and researchers in the USA. Without a common classification system, clinicians and researchers purporting to talk to each other about "schizophrenia" (for example) might not be talking about the same condition at all.

The Diagnostic Project highlights the primary purpose of a standard classification system: clear communication between professionals. Other aims are to facilitate clinical decision making and research. Accurate diagnosis is the essential first step toward predicting the course and outcome of mental illness, planning treatment, and devising strategies for prevention. A precise classification system focuses attention on more homogeneous populations of sick people, permitting more refined tests of theories of etiology and pathogenesis of the mental disorders. These characteristics make *DSM-III* a valuable resource for research, clinical care, and psychiatric education. Although *DSM-III* facilitates diagnosis, it does not help with the process of psychosocial formulation. There is a danger that a preoccupation with precise diagnosis, embodied in *DSM-III*, will distract the student and clinician from individual psychosocial assessment. Both processes are essential; only diagnosis has been standardized in *DSM-III*. (See Chapter 12.)

RECENT HISTORY OF OFFICIAL CLASSIFICATIONS

DSM-III is the third classification system to be published by the American Psychiatric Association (APA). *DSM-I* (1952) emphasized the concepts of "reaction" and "defense mechanisms." The former term sprang from Adolf Meyer's (1957) psychobiologic theory of mental disorders as reactions of the individual's personality to psychologic, social, and biologic factors. The use of "defense mechanisms" reflected the strong influence of psychoanalysis in the development of *DSM-I. DSM-II* (1968) dispensed with the term "reaction" and tried (with some success) to avoid implying a specific theoretic framework. Whereas *DSM-I* discouraged multiple diagnoses, *DSM-II* clearly encouraged them.

DSM-III was published in 1980 and represents the most exhaustive attempt to date to reach a consensus about psychiatric diagnosis. The Task Force on Nomenclature and Statistics, headed by Robert L. Spitzer, coordinated the efforts of advisory committees, consultants, general APA members, and representatives of other mental health professions in the development of the *Manual*. Extensive field trials involving 550 clinicians also were conducted. A revision, *DSM-III-R,* was initiated in 1983 to "clarify ambiguities, resolve inconsistencies, and incorporate factual changes" and was published in 1987.

The history of the *International Statistical Classification of Diseases, Injuries, and Causes of Death (ICD)* has somewhat paralleled that of the *DSM*. The *ICD* is published by the World Health Organization and contains the official system for recording all diseases, injuries, impairments, symptoms, and causes of death. Nine editions, *ICD-I* through *ICD-9*, have been published. The latest version of *ICD-9*—clinical modification (*ICD-9-CM*)—includes some of the new categories from *DSM-III;* however, it retains many of the old categories from *DSM-II* that were not included in *DSM-III*.

BASIC CONCEPTS

Table 23–1 lists the 3 basic concepts underlying the philosophy of *DSM-III*. Each of these concepts is further discussed below.

Table 23–1. Basic concepts and major characteristics of *DSM-III*.

Basic concepts
  Definition of mental disorder
  Descriptive and nontheoretic approach
  Reliable and valid categories and criteria
Major characteristics
  Diagnostic criteria (inclusion and exclusion)
  Levels of diagnostic certainty
  Hierarchical organization of diagnostic classes
  Multiaxial diagnosis (and multiple diagnoses)
  Complete and systematic descriptions of diagnostic classes
  Glossary of technical terms

Definition of Mental Disorder

According to *DSM-III*, ". . . each of the mental disorders is conceptualized as a clinically significant behavioral or psychological syndrome or pattern that occurs in an individual and that is typically associated with either a painful symptom (distress) or impairment in one or more important areas of functioning (disability). In addition, there is an inference that there is a behavioral, psychological, or biological dysfunction, and that the disturbance is not only in the relationship between the individual and society. (When the disturbance is *limited* to a conflict between an individual and society, this may represent social deviance, which may or may not be commendable, but is not by itself a mental disorder.)" The concept of "disorder" represents a level of diagnostic and theoretical conceptualization (see Chapter 12). Table 23–2 lists other levels of conceptualization, along with their definitions and examples from *DSM-III-R*. Although most *DSM-III-R* conditions are in fact syndromes, they are called disorders somewhat in the hope that they represent relatively homogeneous conditions.

Table 23–2. Levels of diagnostic conceptualization.-

Level	Definition	*DSM-III-R* Examples
Sign	An objective manifestation of a pathologic condition. Signs are objectively observed by an examiner and not reported subjectively by the patient.	Catatonia, as in schizophrenia, catatonic type.
Symptom	A subjective manifestation of a pathologic condition. Correctly refers to subjective complaints by the patient; however, often used to include the concept of "sign" as well.	Phobia, as in phobic disorder.
Dysfunction	General term for difficult or abnormal function. Can be synonymous with sign or symptom.	Functional vaginismus (could also be sign or symptom).
State	General term for the current status of a patient's signs and symptoms.	Psychosis, as in atypical psychosis.
Trait	General term for an enduring characteristic of an individual, presumably one that distinguishes him or her from other individuals.	Paranoid personality traits.
Syndrome	A group of signs and symptoms that occur together in a recognizable pattern.	Dementia or any of the organic brain syndromes.
Disorder	Similar to a syndrome but implying more certainty regarding the discreteness of the condition as well as the possibility that it *may* represent a single disease.	Bipolar affective disorder.
Disease	A syndrome with a known cause or pathophysiologic process.	Alcohol hallucinosis.

Descriptive & Nontheoretic Approach

Only the patient's behavior and subjective reports about his or her internal state provide data for the formulation of *DSM-III* diagnoses. There are no biologically based diagnostic criteria in *DSM-III*. *DSM-III* describes the phenomenology of the disorders; therefore, its approach is often called "descriptive" or "phenomenologic."

DSM-III does not explain how or why a certain disorder exists. The cause of most mental disorders is simply not known, and their descriptions do not properly include theories of origin. In this way, *DSM-III* avoids stating more than is known about mental disorders and makes itself acceptable to mental health professionals with different theoretical backgrounds. Table 23–3 lists the 4 *DSM-III-R* conditions that do in fact include etiologic considerations in their descriptions and diagnostic criteria.

Reliable & Valid Categories & Criteria

DSM-III was written with a commitment toward increased reliance on actual data rather than completely subjective impressions. Existing research data were used to ensure the soundness of specific diagnostic categories and criteria. This led to the exclusion of several previously recognized diagnostic categories and the inclusion of several new ones.

The concept of reliability refers to the extent to which different users of a classification system can agree on diagnoses in a series of cases (see Chapter

Table 23–3. *DSM-III-R* conditions with specific etiologic considerations.

Condition	Etiologic Factor
Organic Organic mental disorders associated with a specific substance (eg, barbiturate withdrawal)	Specific substance (eg, barbiturate).
Psychologic Conversion disorder	"Psychologic factors are judged to be etiologically related to the symptoms." This criterion clearly describes an intrapsychic dynamic problem as the cause of the condition.
Stressor (rare and extreme) Posttraumatic stress disorder	"The person has experienced an event. . . distressing to almost anyone." This criterion clearly describes an environmental event leading to a mental disorder.
Stressor (common) Adjustment disorders	"A reaction to an identifiable psychosocial stressor." An environmental or social event is considered to be part of the cause of the syndrome.

13). The concept of diagnostic validity has different levels of meaning (see Chapter 13). The lowest level is a consensus among professionals that certain characteristics describe a specific subgroup of patients and that these characteristics are somewhat specific to this subgroup. This is the level of validity of most of *DSM-III* and is the result of the many meetings and discussions of the Task Force on Nomenclature and Statistics. The next step in the process of validating the *DSM-III* categories is the focus of much current research addressing the following questions: (1) Does a specified disorder have a single course or outcome? (2) Does it respond consistently to a specific treatment? (3) Does it have a genetic or other biologic basis? (4) Does it have a common psychosocial basis? Affirmative answers to these questions indicate higher levels of validity. The advance *DSM-III* makes is that it reliably defines the subgroups of patients about whom these questions can be asked.

MAJOR CHARACTERISTICS OF *DSM-III*

The major characteristics of *DSM-III* are listed in Table 23–1 and described below.

Diagnostic Criteria

For each disorder in *DSM-III-R,* there are specific diagnostic criteria. Most of these are inclusion criteria describing signs or symptoms that must be present before the diagnosis can be made. For example, criterion A of organic hallucinosis is "prominent persistent or recurrent hallucinations." Other criteria are exclusion criteria which, if present, exclude the individual from that particular diagnostic category. For example, criterion C for organic hallucinosis is "not occurring exclusively during the course of delirium."

The criteria are presented as guidelines. Although strict adherence to the criteria is suggested, clinical judgment will of course enter into the diagnostic process. The more research-oriented the situation, the less variation should be permitted in interpretation of the criteria. The criteria themselves are presented at the lowest level of inference, which means that very little should have to be "read into" them; however, for some diagnostic categories, particularly the personality disorders, more interpretation and subjective judgment are required. For example, criterion 7 of obsessive compulsive personality disorder is "restricted expression of affection." Here the clinician must evaluate what is a normal versus an abnormal expression of affection.

Levels of Diagnostic Certainty

DSM-III-R allows the user to state the diagnosis at the level of certainty appropriate to the amount of information available about a particular patient. Table 23–4 summarizes these levels. The physician should never decide on a diagnosis beyond a level of certainty that is justified by the information (subjective and ob-

Table 23–4. *DSM-III-R* diagnoses representing levels of diagnostic certainty.

When even the presence or absence of a mental disorder is uncertain:
  Diagnosis deferred on axis I or axis II.
When general class of disorder is known but more specific diagnosis cannot be made:
  Atypical psychosis.
  (Personality) disorder not otherwise specified.
When specific diagnosis is strongly suspected but not confirmed:
  Specific diagnosis (provisional, rule out . . .). *Example:* Schizophrenia, paranoid, unspecified (provisional, rule out amphetamine delusional disorder).
When a specific diagnosis is known:
  Specific diagnosis.
When a mental disorder is definitely not present:
  Codes for conditions not attributable to a mental disorder that are a focus of attention or treatment, eg, malingering.
  No diagnosis on axis I or axis II.

Table 23–5. Summary of 5 *DSM-III-R* axes.

Axis	Content
I	All mental disorders (except 2 classes contained on axis II). Conditions not attributable to mental disorders that are a focus of attention or treatment (V codes). Additonal codes: unspecified mental disorder (non-psychotic): no diagnosis; diagnosis deferred.
II	Developmental disorders. Personality disorders. Personality traits (no numerical diagnostic codes).
III	Any current physical disorder or condition that is potentially relevant to the understanding of the individual.
IV	Severity of psychosocial stressors.
V	Global assessment of functioning (GAF).

jective) available. The reader should note that Conditions Not Attributable to a Mental Disorder That Are a Focus of Attention or Treatment (also called the "V" codes) are coded on axis I (see Chapter 35).

Hierarchical Organization of Diagnostic Classes

Reading from the beginning toward the end of *DSM-III*, the diagnostic classes are arranged in descending order of inclusiveness of symptoms. In other words, diagnostic groups near the beginning may include the symptoms described in subsequent groups. The presence of a disorder listed or discussed early in *DSM-III* often serves as an exclusion factor for a disorder listed later. For example, a patient with an organic mental disorder associated with the signs and symptoms of major depression is usually considered to have an organic disorder with secondary depression (organic affective disorder) and not major depressive episodes. The presence of an organic mental disorder is an exclusion criterion for many disorders listed in the sections of *DSM-III-R* following the discussion of organic mental disorder. Similarly, a diagnosis of schizophrenia precludes a diagnosis of delusional (paranoid) disorder discussed in a section following the schizophrenic disorders in *DSM-III-R*.

Multiaxial Diagnosis

There are 5 diagnostic axes in *DSM-III-R*, and the inclusion of all appropriate diagnoses (ie, multiple diagnoses) is encouraged on the first 3 of these. Table 23–5 summarizes the 5 axes.

Axes I and II contain all of the mental disorders listed in *DSM-III-R*, with axis II containing only the developmental disorders and personality disorders. In addition, personality *traits,* which are not officially coded, are recorded on axis II when a patient does not meet the criteria for a personality *disorder*. All diagnostic classifications for which a patient meets the criteria should be included on these 2 axes.

Axis III is operationally defined as potentially including all of the diagnoses in *ICD-9-CM* not listed in its section on mental disorders. Given the current state of knowledge, it is better to be overinclusive on axis III, since most physical conditions are likely to have some effect on mental functioning (via the brain, in particular). Some conditions on axis III might have a direct relationship to axis I, eg, hepatic failure on axis III resulting in delirium on axis I. Other axis III diagnoses (eg, diabetes mellitus or Cushing's disease) might have a less obvious or accepted relationship with the axis I diagnoses (eg, generalized anxiety disorder or major depressive episodes).

Axes IV and V are for use in special clinical or research settings. The code numbers for axis IV are listed in Table 23–6. Axis V is presented in Table 23–7. Specific clinical examples for each code level on these 2 axes are given in *DSM-III-R*. In the formal *DSM-III* diagnosis, the major psychosocial stressors should actually be listed. Clinicians should distinguish between acute events and enduring circumstances. Axis V, Global Assessment of Functioning, should assess the period of best function lasting at least a few months during the past year as well as the current status. Social relations, occupational functioning, and the use of leisure time should be taken into account in this assessment. This optimum period may in fact be due to optimum treatment at that time, eg, when a patient with neuroleptic-responsive schizophrenia is taking his or her medication. Axes IV and V may have

Table 23–6. *DSM-III* codes for axis IV.

Axis IV*	
Code	Term
1	None
2	Minimal
3	Mild
4	Moderate
5	Severe
6	Extreme
7	Catastrophic
0	Inadequate information or no change in condition

*Severity of psychosocial stressors.

Table 23–7. Axis V: Global assessment of functioning (GAF).

Consider psychologic, social, and occupational functioning on a hypothetic continuum of mental health–illness. Do not include impairment in functioning due to physical (or environmental) limitations. Use intermediate codes when appropriate, eg, 45, 68, 72.

Code	Level of Functioning
90–81	Absent or minimal symptoms (eg, mild anxiety before an examination, an occasional argument with family member), good functioning in all areas, interested and involved in a wide range of activities, socially effective, generally satisfied with life, no more than everyday problems or concerns.
80–71	If symptoms are present, they are transient and expectable reactions to psychosocial stressors (eg, difficulty concentrating after family argument); no more than slight impairment in social, occupational, or school functioning (eg, temporarily falling behind in schoolwork).
70–61	Some mild symptoms (eg, depressed mood and mild insomnia, occasional truancy, or theft within the household) OR some difficulty in social, occupational, or school functioning, but generally functioning pretty well, has some meaningful interpersonal relationships.
60–51	Moderate symptoms (eg, few friends and conflicts with peers, flat affect and circumstantial speech, occasional panic attacks) OR moderate difficulty in social, occupational, or school functioning.
50–41	Serious symptoms (eg, no friends, unable to keep a job, suicidal ideation, severe obsessional rituals, frequent shoplifting) OR any serious impairment in social, occupational, or school functioning.
40–31	Some impairment in reality testing or communication (eg, speech is at times illogical, obscure, or irrelevant) OR major impairment in several areas, such as work or school, family relations, judgment, thinking, or mood (eg, depressed man avoids friends, neglects family, and is unable to work; child frequently beats up younger children, is defiant at home, and is failing at school).
30–21	Behavior is considerably influenced by delusions or hallucinations OR serious impairment in communication or judgment (eg, sometimes incoherent, acts grossly inappropriately, suicidal preoccupation) OR inability to function in almost all areas (eg, stays in bed all day; no job, home, or friends).
20–11	Some danger of hurting self or others (eg, suicide attempts without clear expectation of death, frequently violent, manic excitement) OR occasionally fails to maintain minimal personal hygiene (eg, smears feces) OR gross impairment in communication (eg, largely incoherent or mute).
10–1	Persistent danger of severely hurting self or others (eg, recurrent violence) OR persistent inability to maintain minimal personal hygiene OR serious suicidal act with clear expectation of death.

important prognostic implications. In general, the more specific the stressor and the higher the recent level of functioning, the better the prognosis. (See Chapters 12 and 41 for cases illustrating the use of multiaxial diagnosis.)

APPLICATION

DSM-III-R sets forth the following procedural guidelines for arriving at a diagnosis for a particular patient: (1) Record all diagnoses from *DSM-III-R* for which the patient meets the criteria on axes I and II; (2) record all pertinent physical disorders (listed in *ICD-9-CM*) on axis III; (3) if appropriate, assess psychosocial stressors and global assessment of functioning on axes IV and V; and (4) state diagnoses at the appropriate level of certainty. By convention, diagnoses should be listed in descending order of importance within each category or axis. The first axis I diagnosis is considered the major focus of treatment unless the words "principal diagnosis" in parentheses follow an axis II diagnosis. Two examples of complete *DSM-III-R* diagnoses, complete with *DSM-III-R* code numbers, are presented below.

Example 1:
Axis I:	295.14	Schizophrenia, disorganized, chronic, with acute exacerbation.
	305.02	Alcohol abuse, episodic.
	305.33	Hallucinogen abuse, in remission.

Axis II:	V71.09	No diagnosis on axis II.
Axis III:		Right lower lobe pneumonia, unspecified organism.
Axis IV:		Psychosocial stressors: (1) Lost disability check; (2) evicted from apartment. Severity: 5–Severe. Acute.
Axis V:		Current GAF: 25. Highest GAF past year: 30.

Example 2:
Axis I:	300.90	Unspecified mental disorder (nonpsychotic).
	305.62	Cocaine abuse, episodic.
Axis II:	301.81	Narcissistic personality disorder.
Axis III:	None.	
Axis IV:		Psychosocial stressors: No information. Severity: 0–Inadequate information.
Axis V:		Current GAF: 75. Highest GAF past year: 85.

Decision Trees for Differential Diagnosis

DSM-III Appendix A contains 7 examples of decision trees for *DSM-III* diagnoses covering the following presentations: psychotic features; irrational anxiety and avoidance behavior; mood disturbances; antisocial, aggressive, defiant, or oppositional behavior; physical complaints and irrational anxiety about physical illness; academic or learning difficulties; and organic brain syndromes. Reviewing these decision trees will give the user of *DSM-III* practice in the logic of the *Manual*.

Caution Regarding Use

The clinician must remember 3 major caveats when using *DSM-III*. First, treatment for any specific patient must be individualized regardless of the *DSM-III* diagnosis. For example, not every patient with a diagnosis of major depression is a suitable candidate for treatment with antidepressant drugs. Second, clinicians, researchers, and students must avoid grouping people together as "schizophrenics" or "autistics," since this implies homogeneity in all aspects of their lives. A *DSM-III* diagnosis refers to only part of a patient's functioning. It is much more accurate to refer to an individual as "the patient with schizophrenia," for example. Third, researchers and theorists must not assume that each *DSM-III* disorder has a single cause. As already noted, these actually are syndromes that may have multiple causes.

Interface With Problem-Oriented Medical Record

The problem-oriented medical record is a list of all problems (both active and resolved) stated at the most accurate level of diagnostic formulation. A problem is operationally defined as any biopsychosocial issue that requires separate assessment. Therefore, all *DSM-III* diagnoses on axes I, II, and III are suitable for inclusion on a patient's problem list. A lower level of diagnostic certainty, eg, atypical psychosis, can be "updated" by a note in the progress notes to a higher level of diagnostic certainty, eg, schizophrenia, undifferentiated. Axis I diagnoses that are no longer active can be listed as resolved/inactive on problem lists.

SUMMARY & FUTURE DIRECTIONS

The *Manual* is an evolving document. It has already been revised. Nothing in *DSM-III* is written in stone. In fact, the major purpose of being clear and specific in *DSM-III* is to facilitate further examination of the disorders and continued testing of the validity and reliability of the diagnostic criteria.

INTRODUCTION TO FOLLOWING CHAPTERS

This text largely conforms to *DSM-III-R* in its classification of disorders, use of diagnostic criteria, and format. Chapters 24–40 generally follow the sequence and content of *DSM-III-R,* including discussions of most of the disorders. There are, however, a few exceptions: Because of their importance in general medicine as well as psychiatry, substance use disorders are discussed separately from the other organic mental disorders in Chapter 25, and alcoholism is discussed in both Chapter 25 (organic aspects of alcohol abuse) and Chapter 26. Psychologic factors affecting physical conditions are discussed in Chapter 4 as well as in Chapters 5 and 56. The sexual disorders are divided into separate chapters on sexual dysfunction (Chapter 37) and gender identity disorders and the paraphilias (Chapter 38).

The disorders of infancy, childhood, and adolescence are discussed in Chapter 41. Although *DSM-III-R* nomenclature is also used, the chapter takes its organization from the Group for the Advancement of Psychiatry classification system. The *DSM-III-R* diagnostic criteria of several important or common childhood disorders are presented, but the chapter provides an overview of child psychopathology through a series of illustrative cases. The eating disorders, listed with these disorders in *DSM-III-R,* are discussed separately in Chapter 39—again because of their significance in general medical practice.

This text goes beyond *DSM-III* in its discussion of each of the mental disorders. In addition to a presentation of the clinical features of each disorder (ie, symptoms and signs, including diagnostic criteria and natural history or course), differential diagnosis, and prognosis, there is usually an illustrative case, followed by a discussion of epidemiology, etiology and pathogenesis, and treatment. Occasionally, some of these sections (eg, natural history or prognosis) are deleted or condensed because of lack of information, but this format is the general pattern of Chapters 24–40.

REFERENCES

American Psychiatric Association: *Diagnostic and Statistical Manual of Mental Disorders (DSM-III),* 3rd ed. American Psychiatric Association, 1980.

American Psychiatric Association: *Diagnostic and Statistical Manual of Mental Disorders (DSM-III-R),* 3rd ed. (revised). American Psychiatric Association, 1987.

American Psychiatric Association: *Reference to the Diagnostic Criteria from DSM-III-R.* American Psychiatric Association, 1987.

Cooper JE et al: *Psychiatric Diagnosis in New York and London.* Oxford Univ Press, 1972.

Kendell RE: The choice of diagnostic criteria for biological research. *Arch Gen Psychiatry* 1982;**39:**1334.

Meyer A: *Psychobiology: A Science of Man.* Thomas, 1957.

Spitzer RL, Endicott J, Robins E: Research diagnostic criteria: Rationale and reliability. *Arch Gen Psychiatry* 1978;**35:**773.

Spitzer RL, Williams JBW: Classification of mental disorders. Chap 14.1 in: *Comprehensive Textbook of Psychiatry/IV,* 4th ed. Kaplan HI, Freedman AM, Sadock BJ (editors). Williams & Wilkins, 1985.

Spitzer RL, Williams JBW, Skodol AE: *International Perspectives on DSM-III.* American Psychiatric Press, 1983.

Williams JBW, Spitzer RL: Research diagnostic criteria and *DSM-III. Arch Gen Psychiatry* 1982;**39:**1283.

DSM-III-R CLASSIFICATION: AXES I & II CATEGORIES & CODES

All official DSM-III-R codes are included in ICD-9-CM. Codes followed by an asterisk are used for more than one DSM-III-R diagnosis or subtype in order to maintain compatibility with ICD-9-CM.

A long dash following a diagnostic term indicates the need for a fifth digit subtype or other qualifying term.

The term specify following a diagnostic category indicates qualifying terms that clinicians may wish to add in parentheses after the name of the disorder.

NOS = Not Otherwise Specified

The current severity of a disorder may be specified after the diagnosis as:

mild ———
moderate ⎤ currently meets diagnostic criteria
severe ———

in partial remission
(or residual state)
in complete remission

DISORDERS USUALLY FIRST EVIDENT IN INFANCY, CHILDHOOD, OR ADOLESCENCE

DEVELOPMENTAL DISORDERS
Note: These are coded on Axis II.

Mental Retardation
317.00	Mild mental retardation
318.00	Moderate mental retardation
318.10	Severe mental retardation
318.20	Profound mental retardation
319.00	Unspecified mental retardation

Pervasive Developmental Disorders
299.00	Autistic disorder
	Specify if childhood onset
299.80	Pervasive developmental disorder NOS

Specific Developmental Disorders
Academic skills disorders
315.10	Developmental arithmetic disorder
315.80	Developmental expressive writing disorder
315.00	Developmental reading disorder

Language and speech disorders
315.39	Developmental articulation disorder
315.31*	Developmental expressive language disorder
315.31*	Developmental receptive language disorder

Motor skills disorder
315.40	Developmental coordination disorder
315.90*	Specific developmental disorder NOS

Other Developmental Disorders
315.90*	Developmental disorder NOS

Disruptive Behavior Disorders
314.01	Attention-deficit hyperactivity disorder

	Conduct disorder,
312.20	group type
312.00	solitary aggressive type
312.90	undifferentiated type
313.81	Oppositional defiant disorder

Anxiety Disorders of Childhood or Adolescence
309.21	Separation anxiety disorder
313.21	Avoidant disorder of childhood or adolescence
313.00	Overanxious disorder

Eating Disorders
307.10	Anorexia nervosa
307.51	Bulimia nervosa
307.52	Pica
307.53	Rumination disorder of infancy
307.50	Eating disorder NOS

Gender Identity Disorders
302.60	Gender identity disorder of childhood
302.50	Transsexualism
	Specify sexual history: asexual, homosexual, heterosexual, unspecified
302.85*	Gender identity disorder of adolescence or adulthood, nontranssexual type
	Specify sexual history: asexual, homosexual, heterosexual, unspecified
302.85*	Gender identity disorder NOS

Tic Disorders
307.23	Tourette's disorder
307.22	Chronic motor or vocal tic disorder
307.21	Transient tic disorder
	Specify: single episode or recurrent
307.20	Tic disorder NOS

Elimination Disorders
307.70	Functional encopresis

Specify: primary or secondary
type

307.60   Functional enuresis
Specify: primary or secondary
type
Specify: nocturnal only, diurnal
only, nocturnal and diurnal

Speech Disorders Not Elsewhere Classified

307.00*   Cluttering
307.00*   Stuttering

Other Disorders of Infancy, Childhood, or Adolescence

313.23   Elective mutism
313.82   Identity disorder
313.89   Reactive attachment disorder of infancy or early childhood
307.30   Stereotype/habit disorder
314.00   Undifferentiated attention-deficit disorder

ORGANIC MENTAL DISORDERS

Dementias Arising in the Senium & Presenium

Primary degenerative dementia of the Alzheimer type, senile onset,
290.30   with delirium
290.20   with delusions
290.21   with depression
290.00*   uncomplicated
(Note: Code 331.00 Alzheimer's disease on axis III)

Code in fifth digit:
1 = with delirium, 2 = with delusions, 3 = with depression, 0* = uncomplicated
290.1x   Primary degenerative dementia of the Alzheimer type, presenile onset,
_____
(Note: Code 331.00 Alzheimer's disease on axis III)
290.4x   Multi-infarctdementia, _____

290.00*   Senile dementia NOS
Specify etiology on axis III if known
290.10*   Presenile dementia NOS
Specify etiology on axis III if known (eg, Pick's disease, Jacob-Creutzfeldt disease)

Psychoactive Substance-Induced Organic Mental Disorders

Alcohol
303.00   intoxication
291.40   idiosyncratic intoxication (128)
291.80   Uncomplicated alcohol withdrawal
291.00   withdrawal delirium
291.30   hallucinosis
291.10   amnestic disorder
291.20   Dementia associated with alcoholism

Amphetamine or similarly acting sympathomimetic
305.70*   intoxication
292.00*   withdrawal
292.81*   delirium
292.11*   delusional disorder

Caffeine
305.90*   intoxication

Cannabis
305.20*   intoxication
292.11*   delusional disorder

Cocaine
305.60*   intoxication
292.00*   withdrawal
292.81*   delirium
292.11*   delusional disorder

Hallucinogen
305.30*   hallucinosis
292.11*   delusional disorder
292.84*   mood disorder

Posthallucinogen
292.89*   perception disorder

Inhalant
305.90*   intoxication

Nicotine
292.00*   withdrawal

Opioid
305.50*   intoxication
292.00*   withdrawal

Phencyclidine (PCP) or similarly acting arylcyclohexylamine
305.90*   intoxication
292.81*   delirium
292.11*   delusional disorder
292.84*   mood disorder
292.90*   organic mental disorder NOS

Sedative, hypnotic, or anxiolytic
305.40*   intoxication
292.00*   Uncomplicated sedative, hypnotic, or anxiolytic withdrawal
292.00*   withdrawal delirium
292.83*   amnestic disorder

Other or unspecified psychoactive substance
305.90*   intoxication
292.00*   withdrawal
292.81*   delirium
292.82*   dementia
292.83*   amnestic disorder
292.11*   delusional disorder
292.12   hallucinosis
292.84*   mood disorder
292.89*   anxiety disorder
292.89*   personality disorder
292.90*   organic mental disorder NOS

Organic Mental Disorders Associated With Axis III

Physical Disorders or Conditions, or Whose Etiology Is Unknown

293.00	Delirium
294.10	Dementia
294.00	Amnestic disorder
293.81	Organic delusional disorder
293.82	Organic hallucinosis
293.83	Organic mood disorder
	Specify: manic, depressed, mixed
294.80*	Organic anxiety disorder
310.10	Organic personality disorder
	Specify if explosive type
294.80*	Organic mental disorder NOS

PSYCHOACTIVE SUBSTANCE USE DISORDERS

	Alcohol
303.90	dependence
305.00	abuse
	Amphetamine or similarly acting sympathomimetic
304.40	dependence
305.70*	abuse
	Cannabis
304.30	dependence
305.20*	abuse
	Cocaine
304.20	dependence
305.60*	abuse
	Hallucinogen
304.50*	dependence
305.30*	abuse
	Inhalant
304.60	dependence
305.90*	abuse
	Nicotine
305.10	dependence
	Opioid
304.00	dependence
305.50*	abuse
	Phencyclidine (PCP) or similarly acting arylcyclohexylamine
304.50*	dependence
305.90*	abuse
	Sedative, hypnotic, or anxiolytic
304.10	dependence
305.40*	abuse
304.90*	Polysubstance dependence
304.90*	Psychoactive substance dependence NOS
305.90*	Psychoactive substance abuse NOS

SCHIZOPHRENIA

Code in fifth digit: 1 = subchronic, 2 = chronic, 3 = subchronic with acute exacerbation, 4 = chronic with acute exacerbation, 5 = in re-mission, 0 = unspecified.

	Schizophrenia,
295.2x	catatonic, _____
295.1x	disorganized, _____
295.3x	paranoid, _____
	Specify if stable type
295.9x	undifferentiated, _____
295.6x	residual, _____
	Specify if late onset

DELUSIONAL (PARANOID) DISORDER

297.10	Delusional (paranoid) disorder
	Specify type: erotomanic
	grandiose
	jealous
	persecutory
	somatic
	unspecified

PSYCHOTIC DISORDERS NOT ELSEWHERE CLASSIFIED

298.80	Brief reactive psychosis
295.40	Schizophreniform disorder
	Specify: without good prognostic features or with good prognostic features
295.70	Schizoaffective disorder
	Specify: bipolar type or depressive type
297.30	Induced psychotic disorder
298.90	Psychotic disorder NOS (atypical psychosis)

MOOD DISORDERS

Code current state of major depression and bipolar disorder in fifth digit:
   1 = mild
   2 = moderate
   3 = severe, without psychotic features
   4 = with psychotic features (*specify* mood-congruent or mood-incongruent)
   5 = in partial remission
   6 = in full remission
   0 = unspecified

For major depressive episodes, *specify* if chronic and *specify* if melancholic type.

For bipolar disorder, bipolar disorder NOS, recurrent major depression, and depressive disorder NOS, *specify* if seasonal pattern.

Bipolar Disorders

	Bipolar disorder,
296.6x	mixed, _____
296.4x	manic, _____
296.5x	depressed, _____
301.13	Cyclothymia
296.70	Bipolar disorder NOS

Depressive Disorders

	Major Depression,
296.2x	single episode, _____

296.3x	recurrent, _____
300.40	Dysthymia (or depressive neurosis)
	Specify: primary or secondary type
	Specify: early or late onset
311.00	Depressive disorder NOS

ANXIETY DISORDERS (or Anxiety & Phobic Neuroses)

	Panic disorder
300.21	with agoraphobia
	Specify current severity of agoraphobic avoidance
	Specify current severity of panic attacks
300.01	without agoraphobia
	Specify current severity of panic attacks
300.22	Agoraphobia without history of panic disorder
	Specify with or without limited symptom attacks
300.23	Social phobia
	Specify if generalized type
300.29	Simple phobia
300.30	Obsessive compulsive disorder (or obsessive compulsive neurosis)
309.89	Posttraumatic stress disorder
	Specify if delayed onset
300.02	Generalized anxiety disorder
300.00	Anxiety disorder NOS

SOMATOFORM DISORDERS

300.70*	Body dysmorphic disorder
300.11	Conversion disorder (or Hysterical neurosis, conversion type)
	Specify: single episode or recurrent
300.70*	Hypochondriasis (or Hypochondriacal neurosis)
300.81	Somatization disorder
307.80	Somatoform pain disorder
300.70*	Undifferentiated somatoform disorder
300.70*	Somatoform disorder NOS

DISSOCIATIVE DISORDERS (or Hysterical Neuroses, Dissociative Type)

300.14	Multiple personality disorder
300.13	Psychogenic fugue
300.12	Psychogenic amnesia
300.60	Depersonalization disorder (or depersonalization neurosis)
300.15	Dissociative disorder NOS

SEXUAL DISORDERS

Paraphilias

302.40	Exhibitionism
302.81	Fetishism
302.89	Frotteurism
302.20	Pedophilia
	Specify: same sex, opposite sex, same and opposite sex
	Specify if limited to incest
	Specify: exclusive type or nonexclusive type
302.83	Sexual masochism
302.84	Sexual sadism
302.30	Transvestic fetishism
302.82	Voyeurism
302.90*	Paraphilia NOS

Sexual Dysfunctions

Specify: psychogenic only, or psychogenic and biogenic (Note: If biogenic only, code on axis III
Specify: lifelong or acquired
Specify: generalized or situational

	Sexual desire disorders
302.71	Hypoactive sexual desire disorde
302.79	Sexual aversion disorder
	Sexual arousal disorders
302.72*	Female sexual arousal disorder
302.72*	Male erectile disorder
	Orgasm disorders
302.73	Inhibited female orgasm
302.74	Inhibited male orgasm
302.75	Premature ejaculation
	Sexual pain disorders
302.76	Dyspareunia
306.51	Vaginismus
302.70	Sexual dysfunction NOS

Other Sexual Disorders

302.90*	Sexual disorder NOS

SLEEP DISORDERS

Dyssomnias

	Insomnia disorder
307.42*	related to another mental disorder (nonorganic)
780.50*	related to known organic factor
307.42*	Primary insomnia
	Hypersomnia disorder
307.44*	related to another mental disorder (nonorganic)
780.50*	related to a known organic factor
780.54*	Primary hypersomnia
307.45	Sleep-wake schedule disorder
	Specify: advanced or delayed phase type, disorganized type, frequently changing type
307.40*	Other dyssomnias

Parasomnias

307.47	Dream anxiety disorder (nightmare disorder)

307.46*	Sleep terror disorder
307.46*	Sleepwalking disorder
307.40*	Parasomnia NOS

FACTITIOUS DISORDERS

	Factitious disorder
301.51	with physical symptoms
300.16	with psychological symptoms
300.19	Factitious disorder NOS

IMPULSE CONTROL DISORDERS NOT ELSEWHERE CLASSIFIED

312.34	Intermittent explosive disorder
312.32	Kleptomania
312.31	Pathological gambling
312.33	Pyromania
312.39*	Trichotillomania
312.39*	Impulse control disorder NOS

ADJUSTMENT DISORDER

	Adjustment disorder
309.24	with anxious mood
309.00	with depressed mood
309.30	with disturbance of conduct
309.40	with mixed disturbance of emotions and conduct
309.28	with mixed emotional features
309.82	with physical complaints
309.83	with withdrawal
309.23	with work (or academic) inhibition
309.90	Adjustment disorder NOS

PSYCHOLOGICAL FACTORS AFFECTING PHYSICAL CONDITION

| 316.00 | Psychological factors affecting physical condition *Specify*: physical condition on axis III |

PERSONALITY DISORDERS
Note: These are coded on axis II.
Cluster A

301.00	Paranoid
301.20	Schizoid
301.22	Schizotypal

Cluster B

301.70	Antisocial
301.83	Borderline
301.50	Histrionic
301.81	Narcissistic

Cluster C

301.82	Avoidant
301.60	Dependent
301.40	Obsessive compulsive

| 301.84 | Passive aggressive |
| 301.90 | Personality disorder NOS |

V CODES FOR CONDITIONS NOT ATTRIBUTABLE TO A MENTAL DISORDER THAT ARE A FOCUS OF ATTENTION OR TREATMENT

| V62.30 | Academic problem |
| V71.01 | Adult antisocial behavior |

| V40.00 | Borderline intellectual functioning (Note: This is coded on axis II.) |

V71.02	Childhood or adolescent antisocial behavior
V65.20	Malingering
V61.10	Marital problem
V15.81	Noncompliance with medical treatment
V62.20	Occupational problem
V61.20	Parent-child problem
V62.81	Other interpersonal problem
V61.80	Other specified family circumstances
V62.89	Phase of life problem or other life circumstance problem
V62.82	Uncomplicated bereavement

ADDITIONAL CODES

300.90	Unspecified mental disorder (nonpsychotic)
V71.09*	No diagnosis or condition on axis I
799.90*	Diagnosis or condition deferred on axis I.

| V71.09* | No diagnosis or condition on axis II |
| 799.90* | Diagnosis or condition deferred on axis II |

MULTIAXIAL SYSTEM

Axis I	Clinical Syndromes V Codes
Axis II	Developmental Disorders Personality Disorders
Axis III	Physical Disorders and Conditions
Axis IV	Severity of Psychosocial Stressors
Axis V	Global Assessment of Functioning

24 Organic Mental Disorders

Renee L. Binder, MD

The term "organic mental disorder" denotes psychologic and behavioral abnormalities resulting from transient or permanent cerebral dysfunction. Organic mental disorders are distinguished from functional disorders such as schizophrenia and affective illness in that they have known biologic causes and pathophysiologic mechanisms, whereas the functional disorders do not.

The term "organic brain syndrome" denotes a specific array of signs and symptoms. There are a variety of different organic brain syndromes. Eight of them—delirium, dementia, amnestic syndrome, organic delusional syndrome, organic hallucinosis, organic mood syndrome, organic anxiety syndrome, and organic personality syndrome—will be considered in this chapter.

Terminology of Organic Mental Disorders

In previous classification systems (*DSM-I* and *DSM-II*), certain terms that are no longer considered useful were used in describing organic brain syndromes; their definitions are important because they are still in the older medical literature. The terms "psychotic" and "nonpsychotic" were used to characterize severe and nonsevere brain syndromes, respectively. In current usage, the term "psychotic" denotes inability to distinguish what is real from what is unreal; ie, a psychotic patient is one who lacks "reality testing." The terms "acute" and "chronic" were used to characterize reversible and irreversible brain syndromes, respectively. The prototype of acute brain syndrome was delirium, and the prototype of chronic brain syndrome was dementia. This was confusing, because delirium may progress to irreversible brain damage and dementia may in some cases be reversible. It was also confusing because the terms "acute" and "chronic" were being used differently than in medicine generally, where the words refer to mode of onset and duration rather than reversibility.

Symptoms & Signs of Organic Mental Disorders

A. Common Symptoms and Signs: In the evaluation of a patient with a psychologic or behavioral disturbance, certain symptoms and signs suggest an organic rather than a functional origin.

1. Fluctuating performance on serial mental status examinations.

2. Memory impairment.

3. Disorientation.

4. Cognitive impairment—eg, dyscalculia, or reduced fund of information.

5. Visual hallucinations or illusions.

6. Formication (sensation of bugs crawling under the skin).

7. Floccillation/carphologia (picking at nightclothes or covers).

8. Prior physical illness or current physical symptoms.

9. Autonomic symptoms (tachycardia, fever, sweating, hypertension).

10. History of recent drug or medication intake.

11. Sudden onset without any previous personal or family psychiatric history—at any age, but especially in a patient over 40.

12. Lack of expected response to traditional treatment.

Although any of these symptoms and signs may be present in a functional disorder, when they are elicited, it is important to at least consider an organic cause of behavioral and psychologic disturbances.

B. Syndromes of Same Origin: The same cause can result in different organic brain syndromes in different patients. For example, neurosyphilis can cause delirium, dementia, organic delusional syndrome, organic hallucinosis, organic affective syndrome, or organic personality syndrome. Even in the same patient, a given cause may lead first to one organic brain syndrome and then to another. For example, neurosyphilis may first present as an organic affective syndrome or an organic personality syndrome and then progress to dementia.

C. Factors Affecting Symptoms and Signs: Even if a specific organic cause is present, the severity and type of signs and symptoms of organic brain syndromes depend on physical, psychologic, and social factors.

1. Physical factors affecting symptoms and signs include the following:

a. The degree of organic insult. For example, brain tumor is manifested differently depending on the size and location of the tumor and whether intracranial pressure is increased. Pernicious anemia is manifested differently depending on the serum level of vitamin B_{12}.

b. The rate at which brain involvement occurs. For example, brain tumor is manifested differently depending on whether it grows slowly or rapidly. In the case of heavy metal poisoning, effects depend on whether intoxication is gradual or acute.

c. The physical condition of the patient.

2. Psychologic factores affecting symptoms and signs include the following:

a. The patient's personality and psychologic defense mechanisms. For example, in response to the same organic insult, a patient with a paranoid personality may become more paranoid and one with an obsessive personality more obsessive. An obsessive medical student developed a steroid psychosis after she was treated for systemic lupus erythematosus. Her symptoms included pinning notes all around her bed and ruminating obsessively, wondering whether she should put a drinking glass 2 inches or 5 inches from the edge of her nightstand.

b. The patient's intelligence and education.

c. The patient's level of premorbid psychologic adjustment. For example, a patient who was relatively well adjusted before developing organic brain syndrome may be able to tolerate a mild deficit better than can a patient with preexisting difficulties.

d. Current psychologic stress and conflict. For example, a patient who has recently lost a spouse or been forced to retire may already be depressed and have difficulty tolerating even mild organic deficits.

3. Social factors affecting symptoms and signs include the following:

a. Degree of social isolation versus support. For example, a patient with senile dementia functioned adequately while living with his wife, who took care of him; but when she entered the hospital for treatment of medical problems, his condition deteriorated.

b. Degree of familiarity with the environment. For example, patients with organic brain syndrome often function poorly and become easily confused in an unfamiliar hospital environment, although they may be able to take care of themselves fairly well at home.

c. Either insufficient or excessive sensory input may cause confusion in a patient with organic brain syndrome.

DELIRIUM

Symptoms & Signs

The *DSM-III-R* criteria for the diagnosis of delirium are shown in Table 24–1.

One aspect of delirium is a deficit in the capacity to maintain and shift attention. Thus, the patient has difficulty answering a question because of difficulty remembering the content or because of perseveration about a previous question. Another method of testing for attention deficit is to ask the patient to recite the months or spell a word backward or count backward from 100 by 3s (100, 97, 94, etc). (See Chapter 18 for formal tests of attention.)

Visual hallucinations are especially common. For example, a patient will report seeing his or her dead mother in the room. Patients sometimes report feeling as if they are dreaming when they know they are awake. A patient may attempt to get out of bed, pick at the bedclothes, or strike out at nonexistent objects. On the other hand, the patient may be sluggish or stuporous. The same patient may alternate from one of these extremes to the other.

In delirium, disorientation to time is worse than disorientation to name or place. For example, a patient may know that his name is John Smith and that he is in a hospital but will have no idea what time it is. As he becomes more delirious, he may still know that his name is John Smith, but he may think that he is in school and still have no idea what time it is. Memory impairment is usually tested by asking the patient to repeat the names of 3 or 4 objects and then recall them after 5 minutes. Memory testing may be impossible if the patient is uncooperative or mute or cannot attend to questions.

Natural History

According to *DSM-III-R*, the clinical features "develop over a short period of time (usually hours to days) and tend to fluctuate over the course of a day." In fact, the fluctuating course is one of the most significant clinical aspects of delirium. A patient may be totally disoriented during one mental status examination and have a fairly coherent lucid period later in the day.

The duration of an episode of delirium is usually brief—about a week, rarely more than a month. The duration and course depend upon identification and correction of the underlying cause. If the underlying

Table 24–1. *DSM-III-R* diagnostic criteria for delirium.

A. Reduced ability to maintain attention to external stimuli (eg, questions must be repeated because attention wanders) and to appropriately shift attention to new external stimuli (eg, perseverates answer to a previous question).

B. Disorganized thinking, as indicated by rambling, irrelevant, or incoherent speech.

C. At least 2 of the following:
   (1) Reduced level of consciousness, eg, difficulty keeping awake during examination.
   (2) Perceptual disturbances: misinterpretations, illusions, or hallucinations.
   (3) Disturbance of sleep-wake cycle with insomnia or daytime sleepiness.
   (4) Increased or decreased psychomotor activity.
   (5) Disorientation to time, place, or person.
   (6) Memory impairment, eg, inability to learn new material, such as the names of several unrelated objects, after 5 minutes, or to remember past events, such as history of current episode of illness.

D. Clinical features develop over a short period of time (usually hours to days) and tend to fluctuate over the course of a day.

E. Either (1) or (2):
   (1) Evidence from the history, physical examination, or laboratory tests of a specific organic factor (or factors) judged to be etiologically related to the disturbance.
   (2) In the absence of such evidence, an etiologic organic factor can be presumed if the disturbance cannot be accounted for by any nonorganic mental disorder, eg, manic episode accounting for agitation and sleep disturbance.

disorder persists, delirium may lead to dementia or some other form of organic brain syndrome or may end in death.

Differential Diagnosis

The differential diagnosis of delirium includes functional disorders such as schizophrenia and affective disorder. Both delirium and these functional disorders may include perceptual disturbances, disorganized thinking, disturbances of the sleep-wakefulness cycle, and abnormal psychomotor activity. However, in delirium, delusions and hallucinations tend to be more random and not organized into a delusional system. Also in delirium, there is a fluctuating course with cognitive impairment, and there may be a reduced level of consciousness.

Both delirium and dementia are characterized by cognitive impairment. However, in delirium, there is a fluctuating course, whereas in dementia there is a relatively stable cognitive impairment. It is important to realize that both delirium and dementia may be present in the same patient.

A factitious disorder with psychologic symptoms in which the patient tries to simulate delirium must also be ruled out. The patient's ability to simulate delirium will depend on knowing what true delirium looks like. In factitious disorder, the symptoms are worse when the patient is aware of being observed; this is not true of delirium.

In true delirium, there is usually generalized slowing of electroencephalographic background activity; this slowing is absent in delirium tremens.

Prognosis

The prognosis of delirium depends on identification and treatment of the underlying cause. If the underlying disorder is treated successfully, complete recovery is the rule. If it persists without treatment or in spite of treatment, the delirium may lead to dementia or other organic brain syndrome or even death.

Illustrative Case

A 43-year-old woman was brought to the hospital by members of her family, who reported that for the last few days she had become increasingly frightened and suspicious. She felt that the people who lived upstairs were threatening her and that it was unsafe to be at home. She said she had seen babies being lowered from the window of the upstairs apartment. Her family stated that these ideas had no basis in reality.

On initial mental status examination, the patient was observed to be agitated and frightened, with pressure of speech, and preoccupied with ideas of persecution. She was fully oriented to time and place, and memory was intact. The admitting third-year medical student and resident thought the patient was having a paranoid reaction. She was admitted to hospital for evaluation and observation. At that time, an organic cause was not suspected.

On the first day of hospitalization, there was a marked change in the patient's mental status, which seemed to improve and then worsen. She became more agitated and tremulous and developed tachycardia, diaphoresis, and hypertension. This progressed to disorientation (she did not know where she was or what time it was), visual hallucinations (she saw her mother in her room), illusions (shadows on the wall were misinterpreted as a person), and problems in memory (she could not recall 3 objects).

Urine and serum chemical tests showed high barbiturate levels, though the patient had denied chronic drug use. A diagnosis of delirium secondary to barbiturate withdrawal was then made, and the patient was successfully treated with gradually decreasing doses of barbiturates to prevent seizures.

Epidemiology

Delirium is a common condition. It may occur in any patient entering or recovering from comma or recovering from anesthesia. It may also occur in any patient who is overmedicated with psychoactive drugs. Delirium is especially common in children and in persons over age 60, since the immature or aging brain is more susceptibe to delirium. Preexisting brain damage, drug or alcohol addiction, and a history of delirium also appear to increase the chances of developing delirium.

Etiology

A. Common Causes:

1. Metabolic imbalance–Examples are hypoxia, hypercapnia, hypoglycemia, hepatic or renal disease, hyper- or hypothyroidism, porphyria, and electrolyte abnormalities such as excess or deficiency of sodium, potassium, calcium, and magnesium.

2. Substance abuse, drug toxicity, withdrawal syndrome–The classic presentation is delirium tremens from alcohol withdrawal or the delirium of barbiturate withdrawal, as in the illustrative case. A cause of delirium not uncommonly seen in emergency rooms is anticholinergic intoxication. Such patients have been traditionally described as "red as a beet, dry as a bone, mad as a hatter, and blind as a stone"—because of peripheral vasodilatation, dry mucous membranes and lack of sweating, delirium, and impaired visual accommodation. Common agents involved in anticholinergic intoxication are scopolamine, antiparkinsonism drugs (trihexyphenidyl, benztropine), tricyclic antidepressants (amitriptyline, imipramine), and antipsychotic medications (thioridazine, chlorpromazine). There are opportunities for diagnostic confusion when a hallucinating patient is known to be taking antipsychotic medication, so that the clinician does not know if the psychosis is a schizophrenic symptom or a toxic drug reaction. However, in the case of psychosis due to anticholinergic drug toxicity, hallucinations are usually visual (sometimes auditory or tactile), and the patient has the additional somatic symptoms mentioned above.

3. Trauma–Head trauma.

B. Less Common Causes:

1. Infections–Either systemic (pneumonia, typhoid fever, malaria) or intracranial (encephalitis, meningitis, encephalomyelitis).

2. Space-occupying lesions in the brain– Neoplasms, abscesses, tumors, hematomas, aneurysms, parasitic cysts.

3. Thiamine deficiency– Wernicke's encephalopathy.

4. Hypertension– Hypertensive encephalopathy.

5. Seizures– Postictal state.

6. Environmental causes– Either sensory deprivation or overstimulation may cause delirium. Two examples of delirium caused by sensory deprivation are "black patch delirium" and "iron lung delirium." When patients underwent bilateral cataract surgery (both eyes done at the same time to decrease the anesthetic risk), they often became delirious when both eyes were patched postoperatively; ophthalmologists now operate on one eye at a time. Patients with poliomyelitis in body respirators had limited visual fields and sometimes became delirious; this was prevented by using mirrors to increase the field of vision. Some patients become delirious in intensive care units, perhaps from a combination of sensory overstimulation (frequent attention by nursing and medical staff, noises of life support equipment, and resuscitation efforts in nearby beds), sleep deprivation, and fear of death.

7. Fever– High fever.

Pathogenesis

The pathogenesis of delirium is not clearly understood, but it appears to involve dysfunction of both the cerebral cortex and the subcortical structures that serve arousal, alertness, attention, information processing, and maintenance of the normal sleep-wakefulness cycle. In delirium, the integrated activity of these anatomic structures is disturbed. Studies of the pathogenesis of delirium sometimes give conflicting results, revealing the heterogeneity of the disorder. For example, delirium is often associated with a reduced cerebral metabolic rate, but in delirium associated with hyperthermia, the rate is increased. Again, delirium is usually associated with slowing of background electroencephalographic activity, but this does not occur in delirium tremens.

Treatment

A. Specific Measures: The most important aspect of management is to identify and treat causative factors. This involves a complete medical history and physical examination and appropriate laboratory tests, including complete blood count and urinalysis, metabolic screening battery (for renal, adrenal, and hepatic disease and for abnormalities in blood glucose and electrolytes, including calcium and magnesium), thyroid function tests, a serologic test for syphilis, toxicology screens, and chest x-ray. An electroencephalogram, CT head scan, lumbar puncture, and other tests such as bromide levels, heavy metal screen, serum vitamin B_{12} levels, and an antinuclear antibody

(ANA) test should be considered depending on the clinical situation.

Once the cause is identified, prompt treatment should be given. In the illustrative case (see above), barbiturates in diminishing doses were administered for delirium associated with barbiturate withdrawal.

B. General Measures: Ensure sleep, maintain fluid and nutritional intake, and provide supportive nursing care. This involves monitoring vital signs and watching for hyperthermia or circulatory collapse. The patient should be at rest in a quiet, well-lighted room, with a clock and calendar to help maintain orientation. The nursing staff should periodically reorient the patient to time, location, and reason for hospitalization. The restless, agitated, fearful patient should be mildly sedated with haloperidol, 5–10 mg every hour, or a similar sedative drug.

DEMENTIA

The *DSM-III-R* criteria for dementia (Table 24–2) include loss of intellectual abilities and impairment of memory. These symptoms will be noted on testing of comprehension, calculation, knowledge, and memory during the mental status examination (see Chapter 18). The patient with dementia is forgetful, has difficulty learning new material, and will often try to minimize or deny deficits. Recent memory is worse than remote memory. The patient may not be able to recall the names of 3 objects after 5 minutes but may have excellent recall of events that occurred in childhood.

Impairment of abstract thinking can be tested by asking the patient to interpret proverbs or state how a chair and a desk or a dog and a cat are similar or different. Other disturbances of higher cortical function (Table 24–2) can also be identified by means of the mental status and neurologic examinations. Two good tests for constructional difficulty are to ask the patient to draw a clock face and set the hands at a certain time or to copy a figure such as those shown below:

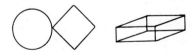

Often, the patient will have an accentuation of premorbid character traits, so that a normally suspicious patient will become more paranoid as dementia develops. With frontal lobe disease, there is loss of inhibition, and the patient may tell obscene jokes or make sexual advances to strangers.

Lability or shallowness of affect may also be noted.

Natural History

Dementia may have a progressive, static, or remitting course. The mode of onset and subsequent course depend on the cause. For example, primary degenerative dementia of the Alzheimer type has a slow onset

Table 24–2. *DSM-III-R* diagnostic criteria for dementia.

A. Demonstrates evidence of impairment in short- and long-term memory. Impairment in short-term memory (inability to learn new information) may be indicated by inability to remember 3 objects after 5 minutes. Long-term memory impairment (inability to remember information that was known in the past) may be indicated by inability to remember past personal information (eg, what happened yesterday, birthplace, occupation) or facts of common knowledge (eg, past presidents, well-known dates).

B. At least one of the following:
   (1) Impairment in abstract thinking, as indicated by inability to find similarities and differences between related words, difficulty in defining words and concepts, and other similar tasks.
   (2) Impaired judgment, as indicated by inability to make reasonable plans to deal with interpersonal, family, and job-related problems and issues,
   (3) Other disturbances of higher cortical function, such as aphasia (disorder of language), apraxia (inability to carry out motor activities despite intact comprehension and motor function), agnosia (failure to recognize or identify objects despite intact sensory function), and "constructional difficulty" (eg, inability to copy 3-dimensional figures, assemble blocks, or arrange sticks in specific designs).
   (4) Personality change, ie, alteration or accentuation of premorbid traits.

C. The disturbance in criterion A or criterion B significantly interferes with work or usual social activities or relationships with others.

D. Not occurring exclusively during the course of delirium.

E. Either (1) or (2):
   (1) There is evidence from the history, physical examination, or laboratory tests of a specific organic factor (or factors) judged to be etiologically related to the disturbance.
   (2) In the absence of such evidence, an etiologic organic factor can be presumed if the disturbance cannot be accounted for by any nonorganic mental disorder, eg, major depression accounting for cognitive impairment.

and progresses to death over a period of several years. Dementia due to head trauma may begin quite suddenly and then remain static for a long time. Dementia due to neurosyphilis or normal pressure hydrocephalus may be completely reversible.

Differential Diagnosis

Normal aging and age-related forgetfulness are part of the differential diagnosis of dementia. In normal aging, memory losses are slight and do not interfere with daily activities. Dementia is not synonymous with aging. In dementia, loss of intellectual abilities is of sufficient severity to interfere with social or occupational functioning.

Delirium is distinguished from dementia by the presence, in delirium, of a widely fluctuating clinical course. In dementia, the cognitive impairment tends to be relatively stable.

Schizophrenia may be confused with dementia, since both conditions are associated with deterioration from previous levels of functioning, impairment of abstract thinking and judgment, and inappropriate affect. In schizophrenia, however, the onset is usually during adolescence and young adulthood, whereas dementia occurs predominantly in the elderly (although dementia may occur at any age, depending on the cause). In schizophrenia, there is no identifiable brain lesion that accounts for the symptoms, and schizophrenia typically presents with no disturbance in sensorium, whereas in dementia there is global cognitive impairment.

Factitious disorders with psychologic symptoms may rarely be confused with dementia. In factitious disorders, the symptoms are worse when the patient is aware of being observed, and the symptoms are not consistent with what is observed in dementia. For example, the patient simulating memory impairment will often show equal difficulty with recent and remote memory, whereas in true dementia recent memory is usually worse.

The major differential diagnostic problem in a patient who complains of memory impairment, difficulty in concentrating, and decline in intellectual functioning is between depression and dementia. Much has been written about the syndrome of "pseudodementia," a disorder in which dementia is mimicked or caricatured by functional psychiatric illness, often depression (Table 24–3). Patients who are depressed may perform poorly on mental status examinations and on neuropsychologic testing, and patients who are demented may also appear depressed. In depression, there is usually a more sudden onset of cognitive deficit, and its onset can be dated with some precision; in dementia, the onset of cognitive loss is usually more gradual. In depression, there may be a history of previous mental illness; in dementia, this is usually lacking. In depression, there is often a history of vegetative signs, such as appetite and sleep disturbances; in dementia, these are usually lacking. In depression, patients expose and exaggerate their defective cognitive performance; in dementia, patients conceal, rationalize, minimize, and compensate for their deficits.

On mental status examination, patients with depression make little effort to perform even simple tasks and will often answer, "I don't know." There will also be marked variability in performance of tasks of similar difficulty. In dementia, patients will struggle to perform tasks and often give near-miss answers,

Table 24–3. Differentiation of pseudodementia and dementia.

Pseudodementia	Dementia
Sudden onset.	Gradual onset.
Prior psychiatric illness.	No prior psychiatric illness.
Vegetative signs.	No vegetative signs.
Patients expose cognitive deficits.	Patients conceal cognitive deficits.
Patients respond "I don't know."	Patients give near-miss answers.
Marked variability in cognitive performance.	Consistently poor in cognitive performance.
Recent and remote memory equally poor.	Recent memory worse than remote memory.
Sundowning rare.	Sundowning common.

and there will be consistently poor performance on tasks of similar difficulty. In depression, memory loss for recent and remote memory is usually equally severe; in dementia, memory loss for recent events is usually more severe than for remote events. "Sundowning" is rare in depression and common in dementia—ie, the patient becomes more confused and has more cognitive difficultly when the sun goes down at night.

Even with all of these clues to differentiation between pseudodementia of depression and true dementia, it may be difficult to make the distinction. The only definitive way of distinguishing between depression and dementia may be to actively treat the depression and see if the patient continues to show signs of dementia well after the depressive episode ends.

Prognosis

The prognosis of dementia depends on the underlying cause. About 5–15% of all dementias are reversible, and if their cause is identified and is treatable, the prognosis is good. However, Alzheimer's disease (the most common cause of dementia in the elderly) is progressive and usually leads to death in several years. Death is usually preceded by poor nutrition, dehydration, and respiratory infection.

Illustrative Case

The patient was a 65-year-old married and recently retired dentist whose chief complaint was depression. He had experienced a series of professional difficulties over the years, including a prosecution for fraud after billing 2 insurance companies for the same service. He had never done anything like this in the past, and at a pretrial hearing he claimed he had been confused, and the charges were dropped. The patient later decided to retire and sold his practice impulsively and, as his family thought, improvidently. In retirement, the patient became depressed and suicidal and decided to seek psychiatric help.

The mental status examination showed depressed affect. However, the patient had no vegetative signs and no history of mental illness. He had problems in recent memory and calculation and could not remember where his daughter lived. He had difficulty finding the psychiatrist's office and went to the wrong part of the building several times. A complete medical history revealed that the patient had minor problems with urinary incontinence as well as ataxia. CT scan revealed ventricular dilatation consistent with normal-pressure hydrocephalus. A neurosurgical shunt to divert cerebrospinal fluid from the cerebral ventricular space to the atrium of the heart reversed his dementia as well as his secondary depression.

In the above case, the incident of billing 2 insurance companies was probably an early sign of deterioration of previously good judgment.

Epidemiology

Dementia is found predominantly in elderly persons, although certain specific etiologic factors may cause dementia at any age. The diagnosis may be made at any time after the IQ is fairly stable (usually by age 3 or 4).

In the USA, 5% of people over the age of 65 have severe dementia (unable to care for themselves), and 10% have mild dementia. Therefore, in 1980, with 25 million people over 65, there were 1.2 million individuals with severe dementia and 2.5 million with milder dementia. By 1990, 32 million will be over 65.

Dementia affects 58% of the more than 1 million individuals in nursing homes in the USA. More than half of patients over age 65 in state and county mental hospitals also have a diagnosis of dementia.

Etiology & Pathogenesis

The most common cause of dementia is Alzheimer's disease, which accounts for 65% of dementias in persons over age 65. In Alzheimer's disease, progressive dementia occurs with no identifiable cause (other than aging) and no abnormal laboratory findings. The electroencephalogram is often diffusely slow, and CT scan often shows cerebral cortical atrophy and slight to moderate ventricular dilatation. No correlation has been found between the extent of cerebral cortical atrophy and severity of dementia, and some patients with Alzheimer's disease show no evidence of atrophy. However, most studies have revealed some correlation between the extent of ventricular dilatation and the severity of dementia. Clinically, the diagnosis of Alzeimer's disease is made by excluding other causes of dementia.

The histopathologic changes in Alzheimer's disease consist of microscopic senile plaques, neurofibrillary tangles, and granulovacuolar degeneration of neurons. In some texts, a distinction is made between the presenile form of Alzheimer's disease (below age 65) and the senile form (over age 65). However, there is no convincing evidence of morphologic or biochemical differences between these 2 forms of Alzheimer's disease.

About 10% of cases of dementia in persons over age 65 are so-called multi-infarct dementias, in which cerebral softening occurs following multiple infarctions of brain tissue. There is typically an abrupt onset and a stepwise deteriorating course and patchy distribution of deficits, depending upon which regions of the brain have been destroyed. There are focal neurologic signs and symptoms and a history of hypertension and strokes.

Other common causes of dementia are alcoholism and head trauma. *It is important to look for reversible causes of dementia, since 5–15% of all dementias are reversible.*

Examples of causes of reversible dementia include intracranial conditions (meningiomas, subdural hematomas, normal-pressure hydrocephalus), systemic illnesses (pulmonary insufficiency, severe anemia, uremia, hyponatremia, Wilson's disease, porphyria), deficiency states (vitamin B_{12} deficiency, thiamine deficiency, pellagra), endocrinopathies (Addison's disease, myxedema, hyperthyroidism, hypo- or hyperparathyroidism), heavy metal poisoning (mercury, lead, arsenic, thallium), infections (neurosyphilis, chronic tuberculous or cryptococcal meningitis, cerebral abscess), collagen vascular disorders (systemic lupus erythematosus), and drug toxicity (disulfiram, bromides).

In normal-pressure (occult) hydrocephalus, there is usually a triad of dementia, ataxia, and urinary incontinence. The disorder may be idiopathic or due to subarachnoid hemorrhage, meningitis, or head trauma. There is obstruction to the flow of cerebrospinal fluid over the convexities of the cerebral hemispheres, and cerebrospinal fluid absorption through the usual pathways at the superior sagittal sinus is impaired. The ventricles are enlarged, but there is no increase in cerebrospinal fluid pressure. As in the illustrative case (see above), this type of dementia can sometimes be completely reversed with a neurosurgical shunt procedure that relieves the obstruction.

The deficits in dementia result from widespread damage to any part of the brain, but especially the cerebral cortex. There may not be structural changes, but cerebral dysfunction is always present. Neurochemical investigations of patients with Alzheimer's disease have shown that central cholinergic neurotransmission is reduced. In consequence, there has been an attempt to treat Alzheimer's disease with acetylcholine precursors such as choline and lecithin, with cholinergic agonists such as arecoline, or with anticholinesterase agents such as physostigmine. All of these methods of treatment have given mixed results and are still experimental.

Treatment

A. Specific Measures: Reversible causes should be sought aggressively in any patient who presents with dementia. This involves a complete history and physical examination, including a history of drug, alcohol, and medication intake. In addition, the following minimal workup should be ordered: complete blood count (look for anemia and evidence of collagen vascular disease); urinalysis; chest x-ray (look for pulmonary disease and congestive heart failure); metabolic screening battery (look for renal, adrenal, and hepatic disease and electrolyte or glucose imbalance); thyroid function tests; serologic tests for syphilis, including the Venereal Disease Research Laboratories (VDRL) test and the fluorescent treponemal antibody (FTA-ABS) test (one-third of patients with neurosyphilis have nonreactive serum VDRLs, but FTA-ABS will be positive); serum vitamin B_{12} (in pernicious anemia, central nervous system findings may exist without anemia); and CT scan (look for space-occupying lesions, evidence of infarct, and normal-pressure hydrocephalus). Depending on the clinical situation, other tests such as lumbar puncture, toxicology screen, heavy metal screens, serum bromides, and ANA tests should also be considered.

B. General Measures: Simple advice or psychotherapy will help the patient deal with anxiety and depression. The patient should be given information about the illness as tolerated, help with the process of grieving over losses, and help with the effort to maintain faltering self-esteem. In appropriate circumstances, the patient should be offered advice about a change of situation (job, domicile) and about full utilization of available skills.

Social stimulation and structure must be sustained. The patient should be in a stimulating environment to maximize intellectual capacities. Patients in nursing homes should have free access to television and newspapers and recreational activities, and pets if possible. A structured schedule during the day is important to give a comfortable sense of predictability in life.

Family intervention (such as giving support and advice to the family) is an important part of the treatment of dementia, since family members usually have questions and concerns and may express shame or guilt if given the opportunity.

Prescribe *low-dose* medication for symptomatic relief. Symptoms that may respond to pharmacologic therapy include anxiety, agitation, hyperactivity, depression, irritability, disturbed sleep, and psychotic behavior. (See Chapters 52–54 for details.)

AMNESTIC SYNDROME

Symptoms & Signs

Table 24–4 sets forth the *DSM-III-R* diagnostic criteria for amnestic syndrome.

Memory loss is both anterograde and retrograde. With anterograde amnesia, the patient cannot recall recent events since the insult to the brain; with retrograde amnesia, the patient cannot recall events before the insult occurred. It is useful to distinguish 4 kinds of memory: immediate, recent, intermediate, and remote. Memory deficit in amnestic syndrome involves recent and intermediate memory and spares immediate and remote memory. Immediate memory involves the ability to retain new material as long as attention is not distracted—eg, the patient should be able to recite 6 digits forward. Recent memory involves the ability to retain new material after attention is distracted—eg, by asking the patient to recall the names of 3 objects after 5 minutes of further interviewing. Impairment of recent memory leads to anterograde amnesia—inability to recall events that have occurred since the insult to the brain, since the patient has not been able to retain new material. Anterograde amnesia covers a vari-

Table 24–4. *DSM-III-R* diagnostic criteria for amnestic syndrome.

A. Both short-term memory impairment (inability to learn new information) and long-term memory impairment (inability to remember information that was known in the past) are the predominant clinical features.

B. No clouding of consciousness, as in delirium; no general loss of major intellectual abilities, as in dementia.

C. Evidence, from the history, physical examination, or laboratory tests, of a specific organic factor that is judged to be etiologically related to the disturbance.

able period of time in different patients, and testing of recent memory is impaired during the period of anterograde amnesia. The somewhat arbitrary term intermediate memory is for events that occurred in the past 3–20 years. This can be tested by asking the patient about events in his or her life or newsworthy events that occurred in the last decade.

Retrograde amnesia is inability to recall events that occurred before the insult to the brain, because of difficulties in intermediate memory. Retrograde amnesia covers variable periods of time in different patients. Remote memory is for events in the more distant past, sometimes arbitrarily defined as what was learned before age 12. This can be tested by asking the patient about events in early life.

In amnestic syndrome, there is no general loss of major intellectual abilities. However, there may be confabulation, where the patient recites imaginary events to fill in gaps in memory. Confabulation is not a constant feature of amnestic syndrome. It tends to occur early in Korsakoff's psychosis but disappears later on. (Korsakoff's psychosis is an amnestic syndrome secondary to thiamine deficiency. Etiology is discussed later.)

Disorientation may be present but is not an invariable feature of amnestic syndrome. Disorientation is usually present in Korsakoff's psychosis but not in amnestic syndrome due to other causes.

Natural History

The mode of onset and the course of amnestic syndrome depend on the underlying cause. Amnestic syndrome secondary to head trauma has a sudden onset with gradual but incomplete recovery. Amnestic syndrome secondary to thiamine deficiency in alcoholics has an acute or subacute onset and may be irreversible, especially if well established.

Differential Diagnosis

The distinction between Wernicke's encephalopathy (a delirium) and Korsakoff's psychosis (an amnestic syndrome) should be clarified, since Korsakoff's psychosis typically appears concomitantly with or following Wernicke's encephalopathy. Wernicke's encephalopathy comes on subacutely in a patient with a history of many years of alcohol abuse. The signs and symptoms include delirium, ataxia, ophthalmoplegia, and nystagmus. The delirium clears in about a month, and in about 85% of survivors the amnestic syndrome becomes manifest if it has not been evident all along. A few patients with thiamine deficiency develop amnestic syndrome without a preceding episode of Wernicke's encephalopathy.

In delirium, there is a fluctuating course; this is absent in amnestic syndrome. In dementia, there are other major intellectual deficits, whereas in amnestic syndrome, only memory deficit is involved. In factitious disorder with psychologic symptoms or functional amnesia, there is often a stressful precipitating event, but this may be hard to elicit and, in any case, may also be present in amnestic syndrome. In func-

tional amnesia, the patient may show selective memory impairment (eg, deny being married), although other recent and remote memories are preserved. In another kind of functional amnesia, the patient has global amnesia, ie, professes total amnesia for all events in past life. Failure of a patient without aphasia to state his or her own name is usually functional, and this may help distinguish functional amnesia from amnestic syndrome. Anterograde amnesia is rarely psychogenic and strongly suggests amnestic syndrome.

Prognosis

The prognosis for a patient with amnestic syndrome depends on the underlying cause. Gradual but incomplete recovery may follow amnestic syndrome secondary to head trauma, subarachnoid hemorrhage, bilateral hippocampal infarction, carbon monoxide poisoning, or other hypoxic states. Permanent memory loss may follow amnestic syndrome secondary to herpes simplex encephalitis and Korsakoff's psychosis. In one study of Korsakoff's psychosis, 21% of patients recovered completely, 53% had incomplete recovery, and 25% showed no appreciable memory improvement. Complete recovery usually occurred within a year. Incomplete recovery may take 5 years to reach its limit.

Illustrative Case

The patient was a 28-year-old married construction worker who was transferred to the psychiatric hospital from a medical ward. Ten days before admission, after learning that his wife was having an affair, he went to the basement and hanged himself with a rope looped over a water pipe. His wife saw him hanging and became confused about what to do. She tried unsuccessfully to burn the rope with a match and then ran to a neighbor for help. By the time the patient was cut down, he had suffered a pulmonary and cardiac arrest and had dilated pupils. He had been hanging by the neck for about 10 minutes. He was resuscitated and was having spontaneous respirations within 24 hours of the anoxic episode. Ten days later, he was transferred to the psychiatric unit. Initial mental status examination revealed a patient who was conscious, alert, and feeding himself. He was oriented as to self but disoriented as to place and time. Reading, writing, and spelling were not affected.

The patient was able to repeat 6 digits forward. However, his recent memory was impaired, and he was unable to recall any of 3 objects after 5 minutes. Intermediate memory was also impaired, and he did not know he was married and remembered nothing about the suicide attempt. He did not remember past presidents or details of his work history. His remote memory was better, in that he remembered his birthplace and some details of his early life, eg, physical punishment by his stepfather. He was also able to abstract proverbs.

Physical and neurologic examinations were within normal limits except for an elevated right hemidiaphragm and right upper extremity weakness from the traction injury of the patient's upper brachial plexus, primarily the C5 root. This weakness improved during the course of his 2-week hospitalization, although the memory impairment remained. The patient was transferred to a long-term rehabilitation hospital. When evaluated 3 months later, he was able to learn new material but had no memory for the period during which he was not storing new information. Intermediate memory had also improved, and he was able to remember more details of his past life.

Since some of this patient's intermediate memory has returned, it appears that his retrograde amnesia was a disorder of retrieval rather than storage.

Epidemiology

Amnestic syndrome is uncommon, and no epidemiologic data are available.

Etiology & Pathogenesis

Amnestic syndrome may result from any pathologic process that causes bilateral damage to certain diencephalic and medial temporal structures, eg, mamillary bodies, fornix, or hippocampal complex. The most common cause is thiamine deficiency associated with chronic alcoholism. However, thiamine deficiency causing Wernicke's encephalopathy or Korsakoff's psychosis may also result from protracted vomiting, carcinoma of the stomach, and voluntary starvation. The lesions in Korsakoff's psychosis involve the mamillary bodies, the inner portions of the dorsomedial, anteroventral, and pulvinar nuclei of the thalamus, and often the terminal portions of each fornix.

Other causes of amnestic syndrome include head trauma, subarachnoid hemorrhage, surgical trauma, carbon monoxide poisoning, other causes of hypoxia, infarction in the region of the posterior cerebral arteries, bilateral hippocampal infarction, and herpes simplex encephalitis. A syndrome called transient global amnesia has been described (see Chapter 10). Temporal lobe seizures and postconcussive states can also cause an amnestic syndrome of sudden onset and brief duration followed by complete spontaneous recovery.

Treatment

The treatment of amnestic syndrome is supportive, consisting mainly of giving advice and information to the patient and family to help them deal with the deficits. Depending on the severity of the symptoms and the supports available, the patient may or may not be able to lead a supervised existence in the community. Memory therapy, where patients have been taught to use mnemonics, has been successful in some patients.

In a patient with Wernicke's encephalopathy, it is important to prevent or minimize the development of Korsakoff's psychosis. Give thiamine, 100 mg intramuscularly daily for the first 3 days and then 100 mg orally daily until a normal diet is established. Other B complex vitamins should be given for general nutrition.

ORGANIC DELUSIONAL SYNDROME

Symptoms & Signs

Delusions, which are the predominant feature of organic delusional syndrome, may or may not be systematized and may be of different types, eg, delusions of jealousy, grandeur, or persecution. Persecutory delusions are the most common type.

Additional clinical features are outlined in Table 24–5.

Natural History

The mode of onset and the course depend on the underlying cause.

Differential Diagnosis

The differential diagnosis includes delirium, dementia, organic hallucinosis, organic affective syndrome, and the functional psychoses such as schizophrenia or the paranoid disorders. However, in delirium, there is a fluctuating course; in dementia, a significant loss of intellectual abilities; in organic hallucinosis, a predominance of hallucinations; and in organic affective syndrome, a predominance of affective symptoms. The difference between organic delusional syndrome and the functional disorders is that organic delusional syndrome is caused by a specific organic factor. Organic delusional syndrome should be suspected in any patient who presents with a paranoid psychosis with no previous personal or family psychiatric history, especially if the patient is over 40. It should also be suspected if the patient has any physical symptoms, autonomic symptoms, or a history of recent drug or medication intake or an atypical clinical course in terms of mode of onset and responsiveness to treatment.

Prognosis

The prognosis of organic delusional syndrome depends on identification and treatment of the underlying cause. The syndrome often lifts after withdrawal of the toxic agent or recovery from the physical illness; however, delusional psychoses may persist after phenocyclidine or amphetamine ingestion and in some other cases, either as a direct effect of the drug or because the drug has unmasked an existing predisposition to a paranoid psychosis such as schizophrenia.

Illustrative Case

An 83-year-old widow whose behavior had become increasingly paranoid during the past year was

Table 24–5. *DSM-III-R* diagnostic criteria for organic delusional syndrome.

A. Delusions are the predominant clinical feature.
B. Evidence, from the history, physical examination, or laboratory tests, of a specific organic factor that is judged to be etiologically related to the disturbance.
C. Does not occur exclusively during the course of delirium.

brought to the hospital by her daughter. Neighbors had been complaining about the patient's abusive behavior, including throwing excrement at neighbors and their homes, chopping down trees at a local parochial school, and wandering aimlessly around the neighborhood, screaming about how the Catholics and Communists were trying to kill her. She refused to eat anything unless she bought and cooked it herself, because she thought her daughter was trying to poison her.

On initial mental status examination, the disheveled woman was spitting, biting, and kicking. She threatened to kill the staff with an axe and called them Catholics and Communists. She was oriented to person, place, and time. It was difficult to assess her memory and fund of knowledge because of her lack of cooperation; however, her daughter reported that they were not severely impaired. Her insight and judgment were poor.

The medical history revealed that 10 years before, the patient had undergone total gastrectomy for leiomyoma of the stomach. She took vitamin B_{12} injections for 5 years but discontinued them because she felt she did not need them anymore. Laboratory studies on admission were normal except that her serum vitamin B_{12} level was 91 pg/mL (normal: > 148 pg/mL). She did not have anemia.

The patient was initially given haloperidol, which caused a decrease in her agitation; however, her paranoid thinking persisted. She was then given vitamin B_{12}, 100 μg intramuscularly daily, and 3 days later her paranoid thinking markedly decreased. The haloperidol dosage was gradually decreased to see if psychotic symptoms would recur. After 3 months of maintenance on monthly vitamin B_{12} without haloperidol, she remained free of psychotic symptoms. Her family and friends all felt that she was back to her normal self.

As this case demonstrates, psychiatric symptoms can occur without hematologic manifestations in vitamin B_{12} deficiency.

Epidemiology

The prevalence of organic delusional syndrome depends on the underlying cause.

Etiology & Pathogenesis

The causes of organic delusional syndrome include drugs such as amphetamines, phencyclidine, sympathomimetic amines, LSD, corticosteroids, and bromides; alcohol (causing alcoholic paranoia); epilepsy (especially temporal lobe epilepsy); brain tumor; encephalitis; neurosyphilis; head trauma; pernicious anemia; systemic lupus erythematosus; endocrine diseases such as hypo- or hyperthyroidism, Cushing's syndrome, Addison's disease, hyperinsulinism, and hypopituitarism; porphyria; and Huntington's chorea.

The pathogenesis of delusional symptoms in these disorders is not well understood.

Treatment

A. Specific Measures: Causative factors must be identified and treated. A patient suspected of having organic delusional syndrome—eg, an older patient with no personal or family psychiatric history who complains of physical or autonomic symptoms and gives a history of recreational drug or medication intake or an atypical clinical course—should have an organic workup including a complete medical history and physical examination, complete blood count, urinalysis, metabolic screening battery, thyroid function tests, serologic test for syphilis, serum vitamin B_{12} determination, toxicology screen, and chest x-ray. Lumbar puncture, electroencephalography, ANA test, test for urinary porphyrins, and CT scan should also be considered.

B. General Measures: Give symptomatic relief with medications until the underlying cause can be identified and treated. Chlorpromazine or haloperidol is often used to reduce paranoid symptoms.

ORGANIC HALLUCINOSIS

Symptoms & Signs

Table 24–6 lists the *DSM-III-R* criteria for organic hallucinosis.

Hallucinations vary from simple and unformed to highly complex and organized. Patients may or may not believe the hallucinations are real. Hallucinations may occur in any modality, but certain causes tend to produce hallucinations in certain spheres; eg, alcohol and otosclerosis tend to induce auditory hallucinations, and hallucinogens and cataracts tend to induce visual hallucinations.

Natural History

The mode of onset and the course of organic hallucinosis depend on the underlying cause. For example, organic hallucinosis secondary to alcohol (alcohol hallucinosis) usually comes on acutely while the patient is drinking or after a period of abstinence lasting from a few hours to weeks but usually within 2 days following the last drink. Alcohol hallucinosis improves spontaneously within days to weeks, although hallucinations may last for months or may even be permanent. Patients who are blind as a result of bilateral cataracts may develop chronic visual hallucinations, and patients who are deaf as a result of otosclerosis may develop chronic auditory hallucinations.

Table 24–6. *DSM-III-R* diagnosis criteria for organic hallucinosis.

A. Persistent or recurrent hallucinations are the predominant clinical feature.

B. Evidence, from the history, physical examination, or laboratory tests, of a specific organic factor that is judged to be etiologically related to the disturbance.

C. Does not occur exclusively during the course of delirium.

Differential Diagnosis

The differential diagnosis includes delirium, dementia, organic delusional syndrome, hypnagogic (upon going to sleep) and hypnopompic (upon waking up) hallucinations, and the functional psychoses such as schizophrenia and affective disorders.

In delirium, there is a fluctuating course; in dementia, a significant loss of intellectual abilities; and in organic delusional syndrome, delusions are the predominant feature, though hallucinations may be present also. Delusions in organic hallucinosis syndrome are restricted to the content of the hallucinations or to the belief that the hallucinations are real. The difference between organic hallucinosis and the functional disorders is that organic hallucinosis is caused by a specific organic factor.

It is sometimes not clear whether a patient with hallucinations and a history of alcohol abuse is experiencing alcoholic hallucinosis or paranoid schizophrenia. Patients with alcoholic hallucinosis tend to be older (40s and 50s); have an acute onset of symptoms; have no personal or family history of schizophrenia; have derogatory, persecutory auditory hallucinations or formless hallucinations such as cackling, knocking, whispering, or roaring sounds; have an anxious, depressed affect rather than a flat affect; display logical, coherent thought processes; and improve spontaneously. The distinction from delirium tremens is based on the visual rather than auditory hallucinations and the clouded sensorium in the latter syndrome.

Prognosis

The prognosis of organic hallucinosis depends on the underlying cause. Alcoholic hallucinosis or hallucinogen-induced hallucinosis usually resolves spontaneously but will recur with additional bouts of drinking or exposure to hallucinogens. Hallucinosis associated with otosclerosis and cataracts usually is chronic. Patients may harm themselves attempting to flee from terrifying hallucinations.

Illustrative Case

A 45-year-old unemployed man was brought to the hospital by the police after he broke into a stranger's house and asked for help in defending himself against some people who were trying to kill him. The patient was separated from his wife and had been drinking heavily for several years, averaging over a pint of whiskey plus wine and beer every day. He quit drinking 2 days before admission and began having auditory hallucinations consisting of voices criticizing him and threatening to kill him. The patient denied any personal or family history of mental illness.

On initial mental status examination, the patient was cooperative but quite anxious. His thought processes were logical and coherent. He was fully oriented, with intact immediate, recent, and remote memory. He was able to do serial 7s and abstract proverbs. He spoke of hearing voices that told him men were pursuing him and were going to kill him,

and he had an unshakable belief that these men were running after him.

The patient was admitted to the hospital and given chlordiazepoxide for sedation and multivitamins and thiamine, since he had a history of alcoholism and poor nutrition. On the second hospital day, he reported that he was no longer having auditory hallucinations, and his paranoid ideation had disappeared. He was discharged and referred to Alcoholics Anonymous for help with his drinking.

Epidemiology

The prevalence of organic hallucinosis depends on the underlying cause. Alcoholic hallucinosis is rare and occurs in people who have been drinking for many years.

Etiology & Pathogenesis

The most common causes of this syndrome are prolonged use of alcohol and the use of hallucinogens such as LSD, psilocybin, and mescaline. Other causes include bilateral blindness or bilateral deafness, drug toxicity (levodopa, bromocriptine, amantadine, ephedrine, propranolol, methylphenidate, pentazocine), brain tumors and other space-occupying lesions (temporal lobe tumors, meningioma of the olfactory groove, chromophobe adenoma, craniopharyngioma, aneurysm, abscess), temporal arteritis, migraine, hypothyroidism, neurosyphilis, Huntington's chorea, cerebrovascular disease, and seizure foci—especially in the temporal and occipital lobes.

The pathogenesis is unclear, but hallucinations are thought to be related to stimulation of specific cerebral sites or to disinhibition of brain areas that store sensory perceptions which are then released and experienced as hallucinations.

Treatment

A. Specific Measures: Identify any underlying causes. If a patient presents with isolated visual, olfactory, tactile, or auditory hallucinations, an organic cause should be suspected and ruled out. The workup should incude a complete medical history and physical examination, toxicology screen, thyroid function tests, serologic tests for syphilis, and perhaps an electroencephalogram and CT scan.

B. General Measures: When indicated, reassure the patient that the hallucinations are temporary and not a sign of impending mental breakdown. For example, explain that the hallucinations are caused by migraine or hallucinogens.

Antipsychotic medications such as haloperidol or sedative-hypnotics such as chlordiazepoxide are often used in patients with alcoholic hallucinosis.

ORGANIC MOOD SYNDROME

Symptoms & Signs

Organic mood syndrome is characterized by a depressive or manic mood disorder. Symptoms consistent with major depressive disorder include dysphoric mood, appetite disturbance, sleep disturbance, anhedonia, lack of energy, psychomotor retardation, feelings of worthlessness, and suicidal ideation. Those consistent with mania include elated or irritable mood, hyperactivity, pressure of speech, racing thoughts, grandiosity, decreased sleep, distractibility, buying sprees, and reckless decisions.

Table 24–7 lists additional criteria for organic mood syndrome.

Natural History

The mode of onset and the course depend on the underlying cause.

Differential Diagnosis

The differential diagnosis includes delirium, dementia, organic hallucinosis, organic delusional syndrome, and the functional affective psychoses.

In delirium, there is clouding of consciousness; in dementia, a significant loss of intellectual abilities (mild cognitive impairment can occur in the organic affective syndrome); in organic hallucinosis, a predominance of hallucinations; and in organic delusional syndrome, a predominance of delusions.

The difference between organic mood syndrome and the functional affective disorders is that the former should be suspected in any patient who presents with an affective psychosis with no personal or family psychiatric history, especially if the patient is over 40. It should also be suspected if the patient has any physical symptoms or a history of recent medication intake or an atypical clinical course in terms of mode of onset and responsiveness to treatment.

Prognosis

The prognosis of organic mood syndrome depends on identification and treatment of the underlying cause.

Illustrative Case

A 59-year-old married woman, a retired nurse's aide, was brought to the hospital by her family because of a "personality change" during the preceding 3 months. She had not been sleeping well and stopped cooking family meals, repeatedly called the police and fire departments, and made several unnecessary purchases of expensive items. She had no psychiatric history, and her baseline personality was described as quiet and motherly. There was no family history of mental illness. During initial questioning, she denied any history of syphilis, but after positive laboratory re-

sults were obtained, she admitted with embarrassment that she had been treated for syphilis in 1941.

Initial mental status examination revealed pressure of speech, flight of ideas, and tangentiality. The patient's mood was labile, ranging from irritable to tearful. She was oriented as to person, place, and time. Her immediate, recent, intermediate, and remote memory as well as calculations and fund of knowledge were good, although her insight and judgment were poor.

Initial laboratory results were normal except for the positive VDRL and FTA-ABS. Lumbar puncture revealed neurosyphilis with an elevated protein and white blood cell count and a reactive VDRL. The patient was given penicillin and chlorpromazine and discharged. Follow-up lumbar punctures 2 and 7 months after discharge revealed a significant decrease in the number of white blood cells and protein. The patient and her husband reported that she had returned to her baseline functioning 2 months after discharge. Chlorpromazine was discontinued at 5 months, and by 14 months her psychiatric symptoms had not returned.

Epidemiology

The prevalence of organic mood syndrome depends on the underlying cause.

Etiology

A. Drugs: Reserpine, methyldopa, guanethidine, clonidine, propranolol, and oral contraceptives can all cause depression. Amphetamines, cimetidine, isoniazid, levodopa, and bromides can cause mania. Corticosteroids can cause either depression or mania.

B. Endocrine Diseases: Hypothyroidism, hyperparathyroidism, and Addison's disease can cause depression. Cushing's syndrome can cause mania or depression.

C. Infectious Diseases: Infectious mononucleosis and other viral infections can cause depression; influenza and neurosyphilis can cause depression or mania.

D. Neoplastic Diseases: Carcinoma of the pancreas is associated with depression. Brain tumors can cause depression or mania.

E. Miscellaneous Diseases: Pernicious anemia and parkinsonism are associated with depression.

Pathogenesis

Although the pathogenesis of affective symptoms and signs in these disorders is not well understood, many hypotheses exist. Some of these are discussed elsewhere in this text. (See Chapters 10, 11, and 30 for examples.)

Treatment

A. Specific Measures: Identify and treat causative factors. A patient who presents with late age at onset, physical symptoms, no personal or family psychiatric history, a history of medication intake, or an atypical clinical course should have an organic workup, including a complete medical history and

Table 24–7. *DSM-III-R* diagnostic criteria for organic mood syndrome.

A. The predominant disturbance is a persistent depressed, elevated, or expansive mood.

B. Evidence, from the history, physical examination, or laboratory tests, of a specific organic factor that is judged to be etiologically related to the disturbance.

C. Does not occur exclusively during the course of delirium.

physical examination, complete blood count, urinalysis, metabolic screening battery, thyroid function tests, serologic tests for syphilis, serum vitamin B_{12} determination, toxicology screens, and chest x-ray. CT scan should also be considered.

B. General Measures: Symptomatic relief with medications and psychotherapy should be provided until the underlying cause can be identified and treated. Antipsychotic medication such as chlorpromazine, haloperidol, or lithium carbonate can be used to control manic symptoms. Antidepressant medication can sometimes alleviate depressive symptoms.

ORGANIC ANXIETY SYNDROME

The diagnostic criteria for organic anxiety syndrome are listed in Table 24–8. Little is known about this syndrome, which resembles the anxiety disorders but has a variety of specific organic causes, including hyperthyroidism, pheochromocytoma, fasting hypoglycemia, hypercortisolism, intoxication with stimulants (eg, caffeine, amphetamine), withdrawal from central nervous system depressants (eg, alcohol, sedatives), brain tumors of the third ventricle, and epilepsy involving the diencephalon.

Specific treatment requires identification and treatment of the causative factors. Symptomatic treatment with anxiolytic drugs before specific treatment is started may prove helpful.

ORGANIC PERSONALITY SYNDROME

Symptoms & Signs

The *DSM-III-R* criteria for organic personality syndrome are listed in Table 24–9. Patients with emotional lability, impairment of impulse control, and marked indifference often have frontal lobe lesions and may be referred for investigation of "frontal lobe signs." Patients with frontal lobe disease are difficult to manage when they are apathetic, euphoric, and irritable. (See Chapter 10.)

Natural History

The mode of onset and the course of organic personality syndrome depend on its underlying cause.

Differential Diagnosis

The differential diagnosis includes delirium, dementia, organic mood syndrome, organic delusional

Table 24–8. *DSM-III-R* diagnostic criteria for organic anxiety syndrome.

A. Prominent, recurrent, panic attacks or generalized anxiety.

B. Evidence from the history, physical examination, or laboratory tests of a specific organic factor that is judged to be etiologically related to the disturbance.

C. Does not occurr exclusively during the course of delirium.

Table 24–9. *DSM-III-R* diagnostic criteria for organic personality syndrome.

A. A persistent personality disturbance, either lifelong or representing a change or accentuation of a previously characteristic trait, involving at least one of the following:
 (1) Affective instability, eg, marked shifts from normal mood to depression, irritability, or anxiety.
 (2) Recurrent outbursts of aggression or rage that are grossly out of proportion to any precipitating psychosocial stressors.
 (3) Markedly impaired social judgment, eg, sexual indiscretions.
 (4) Marked apathy and indifference.
 (5) Suspiciousness or paranoid ideation.

B. Evidence from the history, physical examination, or laboratory tests of a specific organic factor that is judged to be etiologically related to the disturbance.

C. This diagnosis is not given to a child or adolescent if the clinical picture is limited to the features that characterize attention deficit hyperactivity disorder (see Table 41–9).

D. Does not occur exclusively during the course of delirium and does not meet the criteria for dementia.

syndrome, organic hallucinosis, and the functional psychoses such as schizophrenia and the affective disorders.

In delirium, there is a fluctuating course; in dementia, significant intellectual deterioration; in organic affective syndrome, signs and symptoms of an affective disorder that dominate the clinical picture; in organic delusional syndrome, predominant delusions; and in organic hallucinosis, predominant hallucinations. The difference between organic personality syndrome and the functional disorders is that in the former there is an organic factor that antedates the personality change and is etiologically related to it. Schizophrenia and affective disorders also cause other symptoms—eg, in schizophrenia, there are delusions, hallucinations, and looseness of associations; in mania or depression, changes in sleep patterns, reduced levels of motor activity and energy, and loss of self-esteem.

Prognosis

The prognosis depends on the underlying cause. The syndrome may be reversible in the case of chronic intoxication, neurosyphilis, benign brain tumors, or temporal lobe epilepsy; may be static with traumatic injury to the frontal lobes; or may progress to dementia with multiple sclerosis or Huntington's chorea.

Illustrative Case

A 32-year-old unemployed divorced man had had repeated psychiatric hospitalizations since age 15, each one following a "rage attack" during which he became hyperactive and violent, with inappropriate affect and emotional lability. He was maintained on phenothiazines with moderately successful control of behavior. A month prior to the current admission, he began to complain of severe generalized headaches. He denied nausea and vomiting, weakness, numbness, incontinence, and seizures.

The mental status examination revealed normal memory, calculations, and fund of information. The patient's thought processes were logical and coherent. Neurologic examination was completely normal except for chronic papilledema of the optic disks. CT scan and angiography revealed a large bilateral occipital meningioma of the falx cerebri. This was surgically removed except for a residual 1% of tumor. Pathologic examination showed a 75-g fibroblastic meningioma.

Six years later, the patient and his family were contacted for follow-up. The patient had had no further psychiatric hospitalizations or "rage attacks." The family said he had some difficulty concentrating, but they verified that he had had no more violent episodes. He was planning to remarry and was taking college courses.

Epidemiology

The incidence and prevalence depend on the underlying cause.

Etiology & Pathogenesis

The most common causes of this syndrome are brain neoplasms; head trauma, including postconcussive syndrome; and subarachnoid hemorrhage, especially with anterior communicating artery aneurysm. Other causes include temporal lobe epilepsy, in which the organic personality syndrome is an interictal phenomenon; postencephalitic parkinsonism; Huntington's chorea; multiple sclerosis; endocrine disorders, especially thyroid or adrenocortical disease; chronic poisoning (manganese, mercury); neurosyphilis; arteritis such as in systemic lupus erythematosus; chronic use of drugs such as marihuana, which may cause an amotivational syndrome; and space-occupying lesions of the brain such as abscess or granuloma.

The pathogenesis of personality change in organic disorders is unknown. Some theories about a neuroanatomic basis of these changes are discussed in Chapter 10.

Treatment

In addition to identifying and treating the underlying cause, the clinician should counsel the patient and family with respect to prognosis and other aspects of management. Psychotropic medications such as lithium or phenothiazines may be required to help control violent behavior.

SUMMARY

Important points relevant to the diagnosis and treatment of organic mental disorders can be summarized as follows:

(1) It is often hard to distinguish by clinical presentation whether psychiatric symptoms have an organic or functional basis. Symptoms and signs that suggest organic causes are reviewed on pp 252 and 253.

(2) In all cases that may have an organic basis, it is important to search vigorously for the cause. With appropriate specific treatment, some or all of the psychiatric symptoms can be reversed.

(3) Two other aspects of treatment are supportive treatment and psychoactive medication to control symptoms.

(4) Organic mental disorders are common. It is important not to miss them in diagnosis, because they are treatable and sometimes curable.

REFERENCES

Beck JC et al: Dementia in the elderly: The silent epidemic. *Ann Intern Med* 1982;**97**:231.

Caine ED: Pseudodementia. *Arch Gen Psychiatry* 1981; **38**:1359.

Coyle JT: Alzheimer's disease: A disorder of cortical cholinergic innervation. *Science* 1983;**219**:1184.

Cummings J, Benson DF, LoVerme S: Reversible dementia: Illustrative cases, definition and review. *JAMA* 1980;**243**:2434.

Dietch JT, Zetin M: Diagnosis of organic depressive disorders. *Psychosomatics* 1983;**24**:971.

Dubin WR, Weiss KJ, Zeccardi JA: Organic brain syndrome: The psychiatric imposter. *JAMA* 1983;**249**:60.

Katzman R: Alzheimer's disease. *N Engl J Med* 1986;**314**:964.

Kokmen E: Dementia: Alzheimer type. *Mayo Clin Proc* 1984; **59**:35.

Kosik KH, Growdon JH: Aging, memory loss and dementia. *Psychosomatics* 1982;**23**:745.

Krauthammer C, Klerman GL: Secondary mania: Manic syndromes associated with antecedent physical illness or drugs. *Arch Gen Psychiatry* 1978;**35**:1333.

Lipowski ZJ: Delirium updated. *Compr Psychiatry* 1980; **21**:190.

Lipowski ZJ: A new look at organic brain syndromes. *Am J Psychiatry* 1980;**137**:674.

Lipowski ZJ: Transient cognitive disorders (delirium, acute confusional states) in the elderly. *Am J Psychiatry* 1983; **140**:1426.

Mackenzie TB, Popkin MK: Organic anxiety syndrome. *Am J Psychiatry* 1983;**140**:342.

Peters BH, Levin HS: Effects of physostigmine and lecithin on memory in Alzheimer disease. *Ann Neurol* 1979;**6**:219.

Rabins PV: Reversible dementia and the misdiagnoses of dementia: A review. *Hosp Community Psychiatry* 1983; **34**:830.

Reisberg B, Ferris SH, Gershon S: An overview of pharmacologic treatment of cognitive decline in the aged. *Am J Psychiatry* 1981;**138**:593.

Schneck MK, Reisberg B, Ferris SH: An overview of current concepts of Alzheimer's disease. *Am J Psychiatry* 1982; **139**:165.

Seltzer B, Sherwin I: Organic brain syndromes: An empirical study and critical review. *Am J Psychiatry* 1978;**135**:13.

Surawicz FG: Alcoholic hallucinosis: A missed diagnosis. *Can J Psychiatry* 1980;**25**:57.

Wells CE: Pseudodementia. *Am J Psychiatry* 1979;**136**:895.

25 Psychoactive Substance Use Disorders: Drugs & Alcohol*

David E. Smith, MD, & Mim J. Landry

Overview

Substance abuse is one of the major public health problems in the USA. Deaths associated with alcohol abuse and alcoholism now rank third, behind heart disease and cancer. Alcoholism, the most common substance use disorder, affects millions of people each year. Use and cultural acceptance of other psychoactive substances including illegal drugs are increasing significantly. Certain basic principles of diagnosis and treatment apply to all psychoactive substance use disorders. The physician should be familiar with these principles and with the psychopharmacology and toxicology of specific substances. This chapter provides information on the diagnosis and treatment of disorders associated with the use of the following psychoactive substances: alcohol, stimulants, sedative-hypnotics, exotic drugs (eg, "crack"), hallucinogens, phencyclidine (PCP), opiates, psychotomimetic amphetamines, (eg, "Ecstasy"), and marihuana.

Patterns of Psychoactive Drug Use

Use of nonprescription psychoactive drugs can be categorized into 5 patterns based on the designations utilized by the National Commission on Marijuana and Drug Abuse:

(1) Experimental use is defined as short-term, nonpatterned trials of a drug. The users are motivated chiefly by curiosity and a desire to experience the anticipated effect. Experimental use generally begins socially among friends.

(2) Social-recreational use occurs in social settings among friends or acquaintances who wish to share an experience perceived as acceptable and pleasurable. The primary motivation is social, and use is voluntary.

(3) Circumstantial-situational use is defined as self-limited use of variable pattern, frequency, intensity, and duration. Use is motivated by a perceived need to achieve a known drug effect in order to cope with a specific condition or situation.

(4) Intensified use is characterized by long-term patterned use at least once a day. Such use is motivated by a perceived need or desire to obtain relief from a persistent problem or stressful situation.

(5) Compulsive use is characterized by frequent and intense use of relatively long duration, producing some degree of psychologic dependence; ie, the user cannot discontinue use at will without experiencing physiologic discomfort or psychologic disruption.

Persons at all levels of society (including physicians and other health professionals, who have a disproportionately high rate of alcoholism and prescription narcotic addiction) may fall victim to substance abuse. Addiction to psychoactive substances is not restricted to any particular subgroup or subculture of the population, and proper treatment of addictive disorders requires objective criteria based on clinically sound procedures.

Part of the difficulty in dealing with substance abuse is that recreational drug use is so widespread. Any pattern of drug use involves a complex interaction of physical, psychologic, pharmacologic, and sociocultural variables. Use of certain psychoactive drugs such as alcohol and tobacco, although culturally accepted, may pose substantial health hazards, while use of other recreational drugs may be illegal and culturally unacceptable but may pose less of a health hazard. The difficulty of defining what constitutes substance abuse causes confusion in diagnosis and treatment.

Definitions

In this chapter, **drug abuse** is defined as use of a psychoactive drug to such an extent that it *seriously interferes* with health or occupational and social functioning. The definition emphasizes "dysfunction" in a way that some definitions of the term "drug abuse" do not. For example, some writers would define as abuse even casual infrequent recreational use of small doses of psychoactive drugs for the pleasurable effects anticipated or for the purpose of enhancing performance. Other definitions are based on cultural norms; eg, Jaffe (1980) defines drug abuse as "the use usually by self-administration of any drug in a manner disapproved by medical or social norms of a given culture." The problem with these definitions is that they offer no objective, nonjudgmental criteria that can be used in deciding when intervention and treatment are required.

Although the emphasis in this chapter is on "recreational" drugs, prescribed psychoactive medications can be abused also. Physicians who prescribe such drugs have the responsibility to monitor their ef-

---

*For alcohol abuse, see also Chapter 26.

fects on the patient to make certain that toxicity and dependence are not developing.

Symptoms of drug abuse (eg, psychologic dependence) may evolve into chronic use and physical dependence. Physical dependence, however, is not the chief criterion for defining addictive disease. The key characteristics of addictive disease are compulsion, loss of control, and continued use of the drug despite the adverse physical and social consequences. Compulsive drug abuse is similar in many ways to chronic relapsing physical disease, and emphasis in management should be on the addictive disease as such.

Different individuals may respond in different ways to the same dosage of a particular drug. For example, although diazepam is usually safe in therapeutic doses, individuals with a psychobiologic predisposition to addictive disease, as evidenced (for example) by a past or family history of alcoholism, may develop dependence even at ordinary therapeutic dosages. Other predisposed groups may rapidly escalate dosage and develop tolerance, with associated adverse physical, psychologic, and behavioral consequences. The psychobiologic predisposition of dependency-prone individuals is currently being investigated.

Addiction, as defined by the World Health Organization, is "a behavioral pattern of drug use characterized by overwhelming involvement with the use of a drug, compulsive drug-seeking behavior, and a high tendency to relapse after withdrawal." The World Health Organization stresses that "addiction should be viewed on a continuum relative to the degree where drug use affects the total life quality of the drug user and to the range of circumstances in which it controls his behavior."

Compulsive abuse of certain drugs such as the sedative-hypnotics and narcotic analgesics may produce **physical dependence.** Although stimulants such as amphetamines and cocaine are quite toxic, compulsive abuse does not produce a well-defined pattern of physical dependence; however, it does represent the addictive disease process, since the user becomes compulsive and continues such compulsive use despite adverse effects on health and on occupational and social functioning. Therefore, focusing only on physical dependence is inappropriate because (1) some drugs do not produce the familiar alcohol/heroin dependence and withdrawal phenomena; (2) there may be an absence of physical dependence in spite of compulsive and dysfunctional use of a drug that does cause physical dependence; (3) physical dependence often represents a late stage of addictive disease; and (4) addictive disease is often manifested by binge patterns of use.

Common symptoms of the progression of dependence on a psychoactive substance (eg, cocaine) are charted in Table 25–1. The progression and symptoms described for cocaine are almost identical for alcohol and the other drugs. Toxicologic and pharmacologic differences are pronounced during acute crises and acute medical management.

Addiction and physical dependence have different mechanisms of action, which are only beginning to be understood. Developments in brain chemistry research hold much promise for explaining the addictive process and suggesting treatment strategies. For example, Blum and Trachtenberg (1986) found that the depletion and alternation of neurotransmitter receptor sites in the central nervous system following chronic cocaine and alcohol use may help to explain cocaine and alcohol hunger (treatment involving the use of amino acids was proposed). Some drugs have a higher potential for abuse than others—the potential for abuse of a single drug can vary according to its purity, route of administration, dose, effective duration, and psychopharmacology (including, but not limited to, the user's tolerance and dependence). The mental stability and expectations of the user, other medical and psychologic factors, and even social factors affect a drug's potential for abuse.

Principles of Diagnosis

Drug categories associated with substance abuse and dependence are discussed in separate sections below: alcohol; sedative-hypnotics, including barbiturates and benzodiazepines; opiates and opioids; central nervous system stimulants, including amphetamine and cocaine; and hallucinogens, including substances as diverse as LSD, phencyclidine (PCP), and cannabis. Table 25–2 outlines the *DSM-III-R* criteria for abuse of and dependence on these substances, including multiple drug abuse (polysubstance abuse). This section also discusses multiple psychopathologic disorders associated with substance abuse.

It is important to note that in polysubstance abuse and addiction, one substance may be the "primary" drug which has more desirable effects (eg, cocaine euphoria). The person often uses a "secondary" drug (eg, alcohol) in order to ease the negative side effects of the primary drug. Thus, the self-described cocaine addict may actually be addicted to both cocaine *and* alcohol. Many people use several drugs simultaneously in order to experience the *combined effect.* Such persons may not describe their intake of cocaine, alcohol, and marihuana as significant, since the intake of each drug may not be very high. The physician should thus focus on **dysfunction** rather than tolerance, physical dependence, or amount when making a diagnosis.

In 1954, the American Medical Association defined alcoholism as a primary disease. Similarly, the American Medical Society on Alcoholism and Other Drug Dependencies (AMSAODD), the largest organization of physicians in the field of addiction treatment, stated in 1987 that all drug dependencies are diseases and should be considered and treated as primary illnesses. In this **disease concept of addiction,** addiction is a pathologic process in its own right, with characteristic signs and symptoms, a reliable diagnosis, prognosis, and treatment and recovery strategies. Traditional psychiatric approaches, however, regard addiction as a symptom of an underlying psychopathologic process. In this **psychiatric orientation of addiction,** treatment plans would involve an explo-

Table 25–1. Cocaine abuse: progression and recovery.*

	Experimental	Compulsive	Dysfunctional	Rehabilitation	Recovery
Social	Most friends are nonusers. Uses cocaine only when offered. Normal relationships.	More friends are users. Begins to buy cocaine. Does not keep promises. Makes attempts to change. Increased social disruption and distance.	All friends use cocaine. Begins to deal cocaine. Increased lying, borrowing. Stealing. Possibility of violence and divorce. Possible high-dose use in isolation.	Stops all psychoactive drug use. Receives treatment for medical complications. Regains proper nutrition and sleep. Learns about addictive disease. Becomes involved in 12-step program (Alcoholics Anonymous, Narcotics Anonymous, Cocaine Anonymous). Learns addiction can be treated. Meets recovering addicts. Learns recovery process.	Normal thinking begins. Begins healthy, meaningful relationships. Continues 12-step program for spiritual needs. Increased psychologic sophistication. Family and friends participate in recovery process. Return to work expectations explored. Spiritual and emotional growth.
Hygiene	Average, normal health. Rare sleep and nutritional losses.	Regular nutritional and sleep problems. Tendency to use more cocaine. Increased chance of toxic problems and polysubstance abuse.	Serious medical symptoms, risk of seizure. Chronic sleep and nutritional problems. Haggard appearance. Toxic psychosis, paranoia, delusions, hallucinations. Serious polysubstance abuse, including overdose.		
Work	Rare impairment of duties.	Regularly late and "sick." Poor performance, disciplinary problems. Regular pay advances. Tendency to work alone.	Loses job, status, or professional license. Engages in embezzlement, theft of drugs.		
Money	Little or no impact.	Frequent overspending. Unpaid debts accumulate.	Chronic overspending, financial ruin.		
Feelings	Uses cocaine to enhance feelings or out of curiosity	Uses cocaine to repress feelings or to ward off depression and guilt; experiences mood swings.	Uses cocaine to feel normal and cover guilt. Total preoccupation with using cocaine. Compulsion, loss of control, inability to stop despite adverse consequences.		

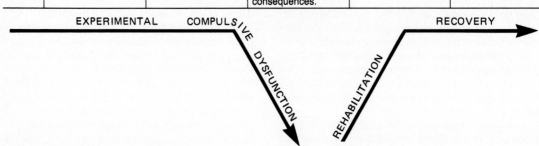

*Modified and reproduced, with permission, from Smith DE; Cocaine-alcohol abuse: Epidemiological, diagnostic and therapeutic considerations. *J Psychoactive Drugs* 1986;**18(2)**:119.

Table 25–2. *DSM-III-R* diagnostic criteria for psychoactive substance dependence and abuse.

Psychoactive substance dependence:
A. At least 3 of the following:
  (1) Substance often taken in larger amounts or over a longer period than the person intended.
  (2) Persistent desire or one or more unsuccessful efforts to cut down or control substance use.
  (3) A great deal of time spent in activities necessary to get the substance (eg, theft), taking the substance (eg, chain-smoking), or recovering from its effects.
  (4) Frequent intoxication or withdrawal symptoms when expected to fulfill major role obligations at work, school, or home (eg, does not go to work because hung over, goes to school or work "high," intoxicated while taking care of his or her children), or when substance use is physically hazardous (eg, drives when intoxicated).
  (5) Important social, occupational, or recreational activities given up or reduced because of substance use.
  (6) Continued substance use despite knowledge of having a persistent or recurrent social, psychologic, or physical problem that is caused or exacerbated by the use of the substance (eg, keeps using heroin despite family arguments about it, cocaine-induced depression, or having an ulcer made worse by drinking).
  (7) Marked tolerance: need for markedly increased amounts of the substance (ie, at least a 50% increase) in order to achieve intoxication or desired effect, or markedly diminished effect with continued use of the same amount.
  Note: The following items may not apply to cannabis, hallucinogens, or phencyclidine (PCP):
  (8) Characteristic withdrawal symptoms (see specific withdrawal syndromes under psychoactive substance-induced organic mental disorders).
  (9) Substance often taken to relieve or avoid withdrawal symptoms.
B. Some symptoms of the disturbance have persisted for at least 1 month or have occurred repeatedly over a longer period of time.

Psychoactive substance abuse:
A. A maladaptive pattern of psychoactive substance use indicated by at least one of the following:
  (1) Continued use despite knowledge of having a persistent or recurrent social, occupational, psychologic, or physical problem that is caused or exacerbated by use of the psychoactive substance.
  (2) Recurrent use in situations in which use is physically hazardous (eg, driving while intoxicated).
B. Some symptoms of the disturbance have persisted for at least 1 month or have occurred repeatedly over a longer period of time.
C. Never met the criteria for psychoactive substance dependence for this substance.

Polysubstance dependence:
A. A period of at least 6 months during which the person was repeatedly using at least 3 categories of psychoactive substances (not including nicotine and caffeine), but no single psychoactive substance predominated.
B. During this period, the dependence criteria were met for psychoactive substances (as a group) but not for any specific substance.

cation and cooperation between health care professionals.

One of the key differences between the 2 concepts described above centers on their approach to treatment and the importance of complete abstinence from psychoactive drugs. The disease concept of addiction emphasizes sobriety as a tool and as a goal, whereas the psychiatric orientation concept of addiction leaves the door open for learning to use psychoactive drugs responsibly after exhibiting addiction. A problem arises when an individual must be described as having both an addiction and one or more psychiatric disorders (**dual diagnosis**). Some addicts and alcoholics began using psychoactive drugs in an attempt to alleviate psychiatric or social problems, eg, using alcohol to relieve anxiety or cocaine to offset depression. However, once the basic criteria of addiction have been met (compulsion, loss of control, and continued use despite adverse consequences), the addiction should be the primary focus of treatment. Clinical experience has shown that addicts respond best to a treatment approach that emphasizes abstinence.

Guide to Management of Substance Abuse Crises
  A. Assessment: This should include the following:
  1. Substance used–
  a. Type of substance (or availability of sample for identification or testing if the patient does not know the type).
  b. Route of administration (inhaled, ingested, injected, etc).
  2. Pattern and circumstances of substance use–
  a. Self-medication because of physical, mental, or emotional problem.
  b. Concomitant use of prescription or over-the-counter medications.
  c. Concomitant use of alcohol (type, quantity, duration) and drugs.
  d. Alternating or concomitant use of other drugs in the same drug group.
  e. Identifiable events, such as loss or celebration, precipitating the substance abuse crisis.
  f. If drug is used habitually, pattern of development and method of maintenance of habit.
  3. Extent of potential support system–
  a. Family or friends available to help the patient follow through on treatment.
  b. Community groups or agencies specifically addressing the patient's abuse pattern.
  4. History of previous treatment–
  a. Type and duration of treatment.
  b. Results.
  5. Other–
  a. Effect of drug use on the patient's life (eg, financial problems, changes in physical appearance).
  b. Physical infirmity that could exacerbate the problem.
  c. Willingness to change abuse habits.

ration of underlying illness in the hope that addiction could be overcome indirectly. This controversy regarding the diagnosis and treatment of addiction has a profound effect on treatment as well as on communi-

B. Initial Management of the Crisis: Before treatment is begun, it is important to assure the patient of confidentiality and explain the rationale for treatment and what to expect. The patient's behavior is observed carefully, vital signs are monitored, and the patient is given only symptomatic treatment before the substance is identified. No medication should be given if there is any question about identification of the drug.

The goal of the 3 approaches listed below is to achieve an alteration in the patient's status or a favorable resolution of the crisis. Judgment must be used in selecting the most appropriate approach in the circumstances.

1. Assistance– The involvement of another individual or authority in the substance abuse crisis often helps patients endure the crisis and work out a personal solution. This gives them an opportunity for growth through mastery of the crisis. Psychiatric emergency clinicians often directly involve others or ask patients to recommend someone with whom they are comfortable to reassure and guide them during the crisis.

2. Complete management– Some cases require complete management of the crisis by the clinician, as in the active treatment of drug overdose. This approach (called "taking over") is direct and often necessary, but the patient does not participate in resolution of the crisis.

3. Patient education– In some instances, clinicians provide additional information or resources so that patients can resolve their own substance abuse crisis.

C. Follow-Up Strategies: After crisis intervention for the drug overdose, medical management of the complications, and appropriate detoxification procedures (see later sections on specific drugs), the physician should evaluate the patient to determine if there are any associated physical problems, persistent organic mental disorders, or major underlying psychopathologic conditions. In most cases, the substance use disorder must be viewed as the primary disease process. Fewer than 10% of patients who have addictive disease have a major underlying psychopathologic condition. However, if an underlying problem exists, it is difficult to follow a drug-free abstinence-oriented approach to treatment, since the patient will often require psychotropic medication for management of the psychopathologic disorder. Antidepressants may be prescribed for a major depressive episode, or an antipsychotic drug may be given for an underlying thought disorder. For some patients with primary addictive disease, a drug maintenance program (eg, with methadone) may be implemented, but abstinence-based recovery-oriented strategies should be tried first.

Maintenance programs with drugs such as methadone are not considered recovery-oriented strategies, since recovery is defined as living a responsible and comfortable life without the use of psychoactive drugs. However, other drug maintenance strategies that represent exceptions to this definition can facilitate recovery. Clinicians should consider using disulfiram (Antabuse), which blocks the effects of alcohol and produces an adverse reaction when alcohol is used; or naltrexone, which blocks the effects of self-administered opiates. Disulfiram and naltrexone should be used as adjuncts to a full recovery program and should *not* be considered the full extent of treatment.

Most follow-up strategies are psychosocial in nature and include family therapy and individual psychotherapy. Successful strategies include participation in nonmedical self-help groups, such as Alcoholics Anonymous and Narcotics Anonymous; other types of recovery support groups, such as the Cocaine Recovery Support Group and the Impaired Health Professional Support Group, are also available. These programs focus on abstinence and emphasize the principles of recovery, with the group process supporting and maintaining recovery. On occasion, the addict will require residential therapy, typically in a highly structured behavior modification self-help community.

Follow-up care must be tailored to the individual's addictive disease process and must be flexible enough to change as the patient's needs change. The physician should recognize that addiction is a chronic, relapsing disease with potentially fatal consequences but that recovery is possible.

Physicians should be able to diagnose addictive disease both in their patients and in their colleagues, since drug addiction in health professionals is 2–3 times the national average. Once the diagnosis is established, a treatment plan should be formulated to deal with all aspects of the addictive disease disorder, including crisis intervention, drug detoxification, and follow-up. Consultation with a multidisciplinary health care team is often required to implement such a diverse treatment plan.

ALCOHOL ABUSE
(See also Chapter 26.)

Alcoholism has all of the qualities of substance abuse and dependence. The impairment may involve physiologic, psychologic, or social dysfunction. As tolerance for alcohol increases, it is common for alcoholics to engage in multiple drug use, typically with barbiturate and other sedative-hypnotic drugs. Alcoholism is progressive, so that alcoholics may organize and orient their lives around drinking. Medical authorities and organizations such as the AMA have concluded that alcoholism should be treated as a disease.

Because of its prevalence, alcoholism is discussed in detail in Chapter 26. In this chapter, basic information and diagnostic criteria will be introduced.

Clinical Features
DSM-III-R diagnostic criteria for the various disorders associated with alcohol use are outlined in Table 25–3. Additional diagnostic considerations are discussed below.

A. Alcohol Abuse and Dependence: A wide range of symptoms and signs of alcoholism may be

Table 25–3. *DSM-III-R* diagnostic criteria for disorders associated with abuse of alcohol.

Alcohol intoxication:
A. Recent ingestion of alcohol (with no evidence suggesting that the amount was insufficient to cause intoxication in most people).
B. Maladaptive behavioral changes, eg, disinhibition of sexual or aggressive impulses, mood lability, impaired judgment, impaired social or occupational functioning.
C. At least one of the following signs: (1) slurred speech; (2) incoordination; (3) unsteady gait; (4) nystagmus; (5) flushed face.
D. Not due to any physical or other mental disorder.
Alcohol idiosyncratic intoxication:
A. Maladaptive behavioral changes, eg, aggressive or assaultive behavior, occurring within minutes of ingesting an amount of alcohol insufficient to induce intoxication in most people.
B. The behavior is atypical of the person when not drinking.
C. Not due to any physical or other mental disorder.
Uncomplicated alcohol withdrawal:
A. Cessation of prolonged (several days or longer) heavy ingestion of alcohol or reduction in the amount of alcohol ingested, followed within several hours by coarse tremor of hands, tongue, or eyelids, and at least one of the following: (1) nausea or vomiting; (2) malaise or weakness; (3) autonomic hyperactivity, eg, tachycardia, sweating, elevated blood pressure; (4) anxiety; (5) depressed mood or irritability; (6) transient hallucinations or illusions; (7) headache; (8) insomnia.
B. Not due to any physical or other mental disorder, such as alcohol withdrawal delirium.
Alchohol withdrawal delirium:
A. Delirium developing after cessation of heavy alcohol ingestion or a reduction in the amount of alcohol ingested (usually within one week).
B. Marked autonomic hyperactivity, eg, tachycardia, sweating.
C. Not due to any physical or other mental disorder.
Alcohol hallucinosis:
A. Organic hallucinosis with vivid and persistent hallucinations (auditory or visual) developing shortly (usually within 48 hours) after cessation of or reduction in heavy ingestion of alcohol in a person who apparently has alcohol dependence.
B. No delirium as in alcohol withdrawal delirium.
C. Not due to any physical or other mental disorder.
Alcohol amnestic disorder:
A. Amnestic syndrome following prolonged heavy ingestion of alcohol.
B. Not due to any physical or other mental disorder.
Dementia associated with alcoholism:
A. Dementia following prolonged heavy ingestion of alcohol and persisting at least 3 weeks after cessation of alcohol ingestion.
B. Exclusion of all causes of dementia other than prolonged heavy use of alcohol by history, physical examination, and laboratory tests.

observed in all parts of the body and may include anxiety, depression, insomnia, impotence, frequent infections, pancreatitis, hypertension, multiple gastrointestinal problems, ulcers that do not heal, behavior disorders and social symptoms indicative of a disrupted life-style, aggressive behavior, and suicide attempts or threats. Laboratory tests may reveal abnormal liver function; decreased levels of serum protein, albumin, magnesium, and potassium; increased levels of blood ammonia; elevated serum uric acid; elevated hemoglobin and red blood cell counts, with or without

folic acid or vitamin B_{12} deficiency; drug screen positive for other chemicals; and increased blood alcohol levels.

B. Alcohol Intoxication: The signs of intoxication correlated with progressive blood alcohol levels are summarized in Table 25–4. The relationships between the ingestion of alcohol, the blood ethanol concentration, and the signs of intoxication vary and depend on the history of use, rate of ingestion, and alterations in absorption, metabolism, and excretion. Alcohol is fully absorbed within 30 minutes to 2 hours, depending on the beverage ingested and on food intake.

C. Alcohol Withdrawal: The most common neurologic sign of withdrawal is **tremor.** The tremor of alcohol withdrawal must be differentiated from that of anxiety or thyrotoxicosis and from familial tremor. Tremor from alcohol withdrawal is an exaggeration of a mild tremor that many people have after being frightened, after drinking too much coffee, or after "a night on the town." This tremor is usually benign but slowly worsens as the individual continues to drink over time. Because alcohol "cures" the tremor of alcohol withdrawal, it is important that the clinician ask the patient if drinking alcohol eliminates tremor. Some alcoholics claim that the immediate effect of alcohol in stopping their "shakes" is the reason they continue to drink. Their tremors can be so severe that they cannot walk or bring a glass to their lips. After several days of withdrawal, the tremor ceases.

The "rum fit," or **seizure,** is generalized and nonfo-

Table 25–4. Signs of intoxication correlated with blood alcohol levels.*

Blood Alcohol Level (mg/dL)†	Signs of Intoxication
20–99	Muscular incoordination Impaired sensory function Changes in mood, personality, and behavior
100–199	Marked mental impairment Incoordination Prolonged reaction time Ataxia
200–299	Nausea and vomiting Diplopia Marked ataxia
300–399	Hypothermia Severe dysarthria Amnesia Stage I anesthesia
400–700	Coma Respiratory failure Death

*Reproduced, with permission, from Becker CE, Roe RL, Scott RA: *Alcohol as a Drug.* Medcom Press, 1974. Copyright © 1974 by Williams & Wilkins.
†Lethal dose varies. For adults, it is 5 – 8 g/kg; for children, 3 g/kg. If there is no food intake, lethal dose occurs before above doses are absorbed. Signs of intoxication are more apparent when blood alcohol level is rising than when it is falling.

cal. It may be a single seizure but usually is followed by one or more further seizures with interim recovery of consciousness. The postictal period is short, and although multiple seizures and even **status epilepticus** occur in 3% of cases, most of the seizures are over within 6 hours. It is prudent to include a lumbar puncture, electroencephalogram, and skull x-rays in the initial evaluation. Further tests (pneumoencephalography, cerebral angiography, brain scan, etc) are unnecessary if the seizures are clearly the result of withdrawal and the neurologic examination is negative for other significant pathologic findings.

D. Alcohol Hallucinosis: Clinicians may categorize the hallucinations resulting from withdrawal according to their content (eg, hallucinatory threats) and associated mental state (eg, anxiety in response to these threats). Becker and coworkers (1974) claim that alcoholics have visual or auditory hallucinations or a mixture of both types during withdrawal. Although auditory hallucinations are also typical of functional psychosis, a definitive diagnosis cannot be based on hallucinatory content alone. Final diagnosis can be made only after all signs of alcohol withdrawal have resolved. It is important to rule out a diagnosis of paranoid schizophrenia; this can be done on the basis of the history. The usual age (about 40 years) at the onset of alcohol hallucinosis is later than in schizophrenia, and neither family backgrounds nor premorbid personalities are similar to those of schizophrenic patients.

Hallucinations in an alcohol-dependent patient with a clear sensorium (except for disorientation to time) are indicative of **alcohol hallucinosis.** Hallucinatory behavior is likely to be transient and intermittent, and it usually increases in the evening. The mental status examination shows disorientation only to time, and patients are able to converse rationally and are often aware that they are hallucinating (unlike patients with psychotic disorders).

Patients with **atypical delusional-hallucinatory states** may have relatively secure orientation but may demonstrate marked paranoid ideation and often deny obvious hallucinatory behavior. The type of behavior demonstrated by these patients varies, depending on their premorbid personality, the abruptness of withdrawal, and the meaning of the hallucinations for the patient. Many patients who have hallucinated during prior periods of withdrawal become familiar with the experience and seem able to ignore the hallucinations. Others never seem comfortable with their hallucinations and fear for their sanity.

Transient hallucinosis, like withdrawal seizure activity, is self-limited and tends to occur during the first 24 hours after the patient stops drinking. Many withdrawing alcoholics know that taking a few drinks, diazepam, or other sedative-hypnotic drugs will stop or diminish these hallucinations. However, because most experienced alcoholics also know that alcohol or other sedative drugs will only temporarily alleviate their hallucinations, they will seek medical help once the hallucinations start. Although most patients are usually not a danger to themselves or others during alcoholic hallucinations, some may try to hurt themselves in response to frightening internal voices.

There is a clear difference between the signs of **delirium tremens (DTs)** and the signs of alcohol hallucinosis. Patients with the former have hallucinations and are greatly disoriented and agitated; those with the latter have hallucinations but a clear sensorium. Patients with delirium tremens are disoriented in 2 or 3 spheres—time, place, and person. The characteristic hallucinations of delirium tremens are constant, and patients have no awareness that they are hallucinating. There is no means of determining which patients will experience serious delirium tremens and which will have no more than several days of tremulousness with or without transient hallucinations.

E. Alcohol Amnestic Disorder: Psychiatric emergency room staff members occasionally encounter patients who claim that they do not remember how they arrived in this "strange location." These patients may have developed enough tolerance to the effects of alcohol so that they can complete complex tasks and travel many miles but yet have no recollection of having done so. The amnesia results from a thiamine deficiency, and the first stage is called **Wernicke's disease.** Wernicke's disease is a neurologic disorder manifested by confusion, ataxia, and abnormalities in eye movement (gaze palsies, nystagmus, and other neurologic signs). If Wernicke's disease is not treated with massive doses of thiamine, memory impairment may be permanent (**Korsakoff's psychosis**). Patients who suffer from a confirmed diagnosis of alcohol amnestic disorder usually do not recover but may improve slightly with time. After obtaining a detailed history from these patients (or from their relatives or close friends), particularly regarding drinking habits, the clinician should help the patients reorient themselves. Since amnestic periods caused by drinking are indicators of severe alcohol abuse and since continued drinking jeopardizes brain functioning, it is important that patients with alcohol amnestic disorder seek further treatment for their drinking problem. (See also Chapters 10, 24, and 26.)

F. Drug-Alcohol Interaction: Since approximately 60–70% of the adult population consumes various amounts of alcohol, it is predictable that other drugs, whether prescribed or not, will be taken with alcohol or while alcohol is still present in the body. Clinicians considering the possibility of drug-alcohol reaction should remember that many over-the-counter drugs, including cough remedies, mouthwashes, tonics, and liquid vitamin formulations, contain high concentrations of alcohol. These over-the-counter drugs—as well as sedative-hypnotics, tranquilizers (particularly the phenothiazines), antihistamines, tricyclic antidepressants, and narcotics—have additive depressant effects when taken with alcohol.

Psychiatric emergency room staff may frequently need to assess individuals who have ingested ethanol with methanol (wood alcohol). Methanol is often consumed as a cheap substitute for other alcoholic beverages and is an ingredient in some household and industrial chemical preparations, so that it may be ingested accidentally. Methanol itself is toxic, but its metabolites (formaldehyde and formic acid) are even more toxic, causing metabolic acidosis and damage to the central nervous system and retina. Hyperventilation (precipitated by the acidosis) and visual loss within 12–24 hours of ingesting methanol are the chief signs of methanol poisoning. The patient with methanol poisoning is given ethanol. Alcohol dehydrogenase, the enzyme that metabolizes both ethyl alcohol and methyl alcohol, has a greater affinity for ethanol than for methanol. If an adequate blood concentration of ethanol is maintained, alcohol dehydrogenase will combine preferentially with ethanol. As a result, methanol is not metabolized but safely excreted in the urine.

Table 25–5 summarizes some alcohol-drug combinations and the resulting reactions that can be used to assess individuals who appear to have combined drugs with alcohol.

Treatment

Treatment for the various forms of alcohol abuse is discussed in detail in Chapter 26.

Supportive care, fluid and electrolyte replacement, and monitoring and maintenance of vital signs are basic elements in the management of acute alcohol intoxication. Becker and coworkers (1974) have noted that

Table 25–5. Summary of selected alcohol-drug combinations and resulting reactions.*

Concomitant Drugs	Resultant Reactions
Alcohol-sensitizing agents Calcium carbimide (Temposil)† Disulfiram (Antabuse)	Blockade of the metabolism of alcohol, resulting in flushed face, tachycardia, and nausea and vomiting. Reactions thought to be caused by accumulation of acetaldehyde.
Antidepressants	Potentiation of central nervous system effects of alcohol. Deaths have been reported with amitriptyline.
Barbiturates	Additive effects, with enhanced sedation and respiratory depression. Occasionally, death results.
Central nervous system stimulants	Probable potentiation of central nervous system depressant effects of alcohol.
Chlorpromazine (Thorazine, many others)	Potentiation of central nervous system depressant effects of alcohol. Significant impairment of psychomotor function. All phenothiazines have same potential.
Opiates Propoxyphene (Darvon, others)	Potentiation of central nervous system depressant effects of alcohol.

*Modified and reproduced, with permission, from Becker CE, Roe RL, Scott RA: *Alcohol as a Drug.* Medcom Press, 1974. Copyright © 1974 by Williams & Wilkins.
†Not available in the USA.

fructose can be effective in reducing the blood alcohol level in intoxicated individuals who can tolerate this simple sugar, including those with idiosyncratic intoxication. Fructose is converted to D-glyceraldehyde, which is metabolized to nicotinamide adenine dinucleotide, a substance needed to oxidize more ethanol. It is believed that fructose increases the elimination rate of alcohol from the blood by as much as 80%.

Patients with alcohol hallucinations should *not* be given phenothiazines or other antipsychotic drugs. Phenothiazines lower the seizure threshold, and antipsychotic drugs generally exacerbate the problem.

AMPHETAMINE & STIMULANT ABUSE

General nervous system stimulants are widely used in the USA; the 2 most prevalent are **nicotine** in tobacco products and **caffeine** in coffee or tea. (Although given diagnostic codes and diagnostic criteria in *DSM-III-R,* tobacco and caffeine abuse are not discussed separately in this text.) Stimulant abuse has become a serious problem, with the major stimulants of abuse being **cocaine** (a derivative of the coca plant) and synthetic stimulants such as **amphetamine** and **amphetaminelike drugs** (eg, methylphenidate) (Table 25–6). Most of the substances have legitimate medicinal value. Cocaine is approved in medicine for topical anesthesia. Amphetamines and amphetaminelike drugs are approved for narcolepsy, hyperkinesia, and short-term diet control.

The management of stimulant abuse is complicated by the availability of cocaine "look-alikes" (eg, ephedrine, lidocaine) that resemble cocaine in appearance, contain no controlled substance, and may themselves be toxic. The potent central nervous system stimulants have a high potential for abuse. In the drug culture, the primary routes of cocaine administration are nasal insufflation, smoking "free base" ("crack") cocaine, and injection. Administration of amphetamines is by the oral route or injection. Dependence on the stimulant can develop but is primarily of a psychologic nature, with no well-defined abstinence symptoms other than depression or lethargy. However, the stimulants can lend themselves to compulsive use and high-dose abuse. Since high-dose abuse of short-acting stimulants such as cocaine lends itself to compulsion, loss of control, and continued use despite adverse consequences, it represents a form of addictive disease.

Because **crack** cocaine is prepared by a simplified basification technique that yields free base cocaine in small, proportionately less expensive dosage units, there are fewer obstacles to involvement with this rapid delivery form of cocaine. Free base cocaine vaporizes at approximately 100°C and can be easily smoked. The pulmonary route enhances rapid and thorough plasma cocaine concentration. Euphoria is swift and marked, followed by severe depression, which is typically self-medicated with additional cocaine, which in turn leads to a progression and worsening of symptoms (Table 25–1).

Table 25–6. Characteristics of depressants, hallucinogens, opiates and opioids, and stimulants.

Drug	Usual Route of Administration	Duration of Effects	Potential for Physical Dependence	Potential for Psychologic Dependence	Potential for Tolerance
Depressants					
Barbiturates					
Pentobarbital (Nembutal; "yellow jackets")	Oral (pill or capsule)	4 h	High to moderate	High to moderate	Yes
Secobarbital (Seconal; "reds")					
Barbituratelike substances Glutethimide (Doriden)	Oral (pill or capsule)	4 h	High	High	Yes
Methaqualone (Quaalude and others; "ludes," "quaads")*					
Benzodiazepines					
Diazepam (Valium)	Oral (tablet)	8–12 h	Low	Low	Yes
Lorazepam (Ativan)	Oral (tablet)	4–6 h	Low	Low	Yes
Carbamates					
Meprobamate (Equanil, Miltown, others)	Oral (pill or capsule)	4 h	Moderate	Moderate	Yes
Other depressants					
Chloral hydrate (Noctec, Oradrate)	Oral (pill or capsule)	4 h	Moderate	Moderate	Possible
Hallucinogens†					
Indolealkylamines					
DET, DMT ("businessman's special")	Oral (inhalation or smoking)	Up to days	Unknown	Degree unknown	Yes
LSD ("acid," "blotter," "sunshine," "windowpane")	Oral (liquid, pill, capsule, or sugar cube)	12 h	None	Degree unknown	Yes
Psilocin ("magic Mexican mushroom")	Oral (pill, capsule, or sugar cube)	6 h	None	Degree unknown	Possible
Phenylethylamines					
Mescaline ("mescal," "cactus")	Oral	4 h	None	Degree unknown	Yes
Phenylisopropylamines DOB, DOM, MDA, MMDA, MDMA, MDE, PCP	Oral (pill or capsule)	4 h–up to days	Unknown	Degree unknown	Yes
Opiates and opioids					
Codeine	Oral (liquid or tablet); injection	3–6 h	Moderate	Moderate	Yes
Heroin	Injection in muscle or vein; inhalation	3–6 h	Very high	Very high	Yes
Methadone	Oral (liquid); injection	12–24 h	High	High	Yes
Morphine	Injection; oral (liquid or tablet)	4 h	High	High	Yes
Opium	Oral (smoking)	4 h	High	High	Yes
Other opioids					
Diphenoxylate with atropine (Lomotil)	Oral (liquid)	4 h	Low	Low	Yes
Hydromorphone (Dilaudid)	Injection	4 h	High	High	Yes
Meperidine (Demerol)	Injection	4 h	High	High	Yes
Propoxyphene hydrochloride (Darvon)	Oral (tablet)	4 h	Moderate	Moderate	Yes
Miscellaneous cough syrups	Oral (liquid)	4 h	Moderate	Moderate	Yes
Stimulants					
Amphetamines	Oral (pill or capsule); injection	4 h	Possible	High	Yes
Cocaine	Inhalation; oral (capsule or smoking)	2 h	Possible	High	Possible
Methylphenidate	Oral (tablet)	4–6 h	Possible	High	Yes
Phenmetrazine	Oral (tablet)	4–6 h	Possible	High	Yes

*Withdrawn in 1983. Not legally available after 1984.
†DET = diethyltryptamine; DMT = dimethyltryptamine; LSD = lysergic acid diethylamide; DOB = 4-bromo-2,5-dimethoxyamphetamine; DOM = 4-methyl-2,5-dimethoxyamphetamine; MDA = methylenedioxyamphetamine; MDMA = N-methyl-3,4-methylenedioxymethamphetamine; MDE = N-ethyl-3,4-methylenedioxyamphetamine; and MMDA = 3-methoxy-4,5-methylenedioxyamphetamine.

Amphetamine may be taken orally in low doses to enhance physical or emotional performance; or it may be taken in high doses, either orally or intravenously, to produce euphoria and a "rush" (ie, a burst of energy accompanied by a physical sensation in the head and neck). High-dose oral use can also produce psychotic reactions. Even moderate doses of amphetamine in conjunction with physical exertion at high environmental temperatures may contribute to heat stroke through interference with regulation of body temperature. Several deaths of bicyclists have been attributed to this phenomenon.

Many people are occasional amphetamine users who take low oral doses while studying for an examination or for "treatment" of their obesity. Although obese patients are often under medical care, they are not always carefully supervised, and some actually abuse the drug. Amphetamine is at times used orally or intravenously to counteract effects of other drugs. Once a pattern of amphetamine use is established, the drug is frequently used to counteract the effects of amphetamine abstinence.

In addition to the effects of euphoria, stimulation, relief of fatigue, and suppression of appetite, other possible effects of stimulant use include excitation, increased pulse rate and blood pressure, and insomnia. Massive overdoses of amphetamine occasionally occur in suicide attempts, in intravenous users who obtain unusually potent preparations, and in children who inadvertently ingest the drug. Patients may be unconscious following seizures, with hypertensive crises or even cerebrovascular accidents.

Clinical Features

DSM-III-R diagnostic criteria for abuse, dependence, intoxication, delirium, delusional disorder, and withdrawal are set forth in Table 25–7.

Differential Diagnosis

There are numerous difficulties in diagnosing acute amphetamine toxicity. Amphetamine use is concealed in some cases, and the clinician encounters an acutely agitated, anxious, paranoid, perhaps belligerent patient whose abnormal behavior is not due to any obvious cause. Differential diagnosis includes the following: (1) paranoid schizophrenia; (2) bipolar affective disorder during the manic phase; (3) anxiety disorders, especially with panic attacks; (4) amphetamine-precipitated psychotic reaction; (5) drug intoxication with psychedelics, phencyclidine (PCP), or other sympathomimetics (eg, ephedrine, cocaine); (6) hyperthyroid crisis, including ingestion of thyroid preparations; and (7) pheochromocytoma.

A history from friends or relatives may provide important clues. A history of recurrent episodes of hyperactivity and paranoia treated for long periods with antipsychotic medication suggests paranoid schizophrenia; however, chronic amphetamine use may account for the recurrent episodes and should be considered. Urine tests may be negative for amphetamine if the urine is alkaline due to markedly reduced urinary excretion. Blood testing for amphetamine is most helpful in confirming the diagnosis; however, results may not become available for several days.

On physical examination, pupils are usually dilated and heart rate and blood pressure increased. However, psychiatric disorders associated with increased epinephrine or norepinephrine secretion may also dilate pupils or increase heart rate and blood pressure. If the patient's behavior is within tolerable limits for a psychiatric ward and if blood pressure is not dangerously high, a period of observation is frequently helpful in establishing a correct diagnosis. Antipsychotic medications are effective in reducing agitated, hostile behavior but may further obscure the diagnosis, especially if toxicologic analysis is not ordered. For this reason, benzodiazepine sedatives are preferred initially for control of behavior. If the individual is suffering from amphetamine toxicity, abnormal behavior will subside over 1–3 days as the blood level of amphetamine falls. An individual who remains actively psychotic after blood and urine amphetamine levels are normal has some other psychiatric disorder rather

Table 25–7. *DSM-III-R* diagnostic criteria for disorders associated with abuse of cocaine and amphetamines or similarly acting sympathomimetics.*

Intoxication due to amphetamine or similarly acting sympathomimetic:
 A. Recent use of amphetamine or a similarly acting sympathomimetic.
 B. Maladaptive behavioral changes, eg, fighting, grandiosity, hypervigilance, psychomotor agitation, impaired judgment, impaired social or occupational functioning.
 C. At least 2 of the following signs within 1 hour of use: (1) tachycardia; (2) pupillary dilation; (3) elevated blood pressure; (4) perspiration or chills; (5) nausea or vomiting; (6) visual or tactile hallucinations (cocaine).
 D. Not due to any physical or other mental disorder.

Withdrawal from amphetamine or similarly acting sympathomimetic:
 A. Cessation of prolonged (several days or longer) heavy use of amphetamine or a similarly acting sympathomimetic, or reduction in the amount of substance used, followed by dysphoric mood (eg, depression, irritability, anxiety) and at least one of the following, persisting more than 24 hours after cessation of substance: fatigue; insomnia or hypersomnia; psychomotor agitation.
 B. Not due to any physical or other mental disorder, such as amphetamine or similarly acting sympathomimetic delusional disorder.

Delirium due to amphetamine or similarly acting sympathomimetic:
 A. Delirium developing within 24 hours of use of amphetamine or a similarly acting sympathomimetic.
 B. Not due to any physical or other mental disorder.

Delusional disorder due to amphetamine or similarly acting sympathomimetic:
 A. Organic delusional syndrome developing shortly after use of amphetamine or a similarly acting sympathomimetic.
 B. Rapidly developing persecutory delusions are the predominant clinical feature.
 C. Not due to any physical or other mental disorder.

*Diagnostic criteria for cocaine abuse and intoxication are the same as those for amphetamine abuse and intoxication.

than—or in addition to—an acute toxic reaction to amphetamine.

Experimental studies confirm the clinical observation that sufficiently large doses of amphetamine will induce paranoid psychosis in all individuals. Methylphenidate (Ritalin) produces a similar reaction. Amphetamine psychosis results from prolonged high-dose amphetamine abuse, often in association with sleep deprivation. The clinical manifestations of full-blown amphetamine psychosis resemble those of a functional paranoid psychosis but are dose-related and have a much shorter course. Unless the individual suffers from a persistent psychotic disorder such as schizophrenia, the psychotic reaction will resolve as the amphetamine or methylphenidate is excreted from the body. When amphetamine is withdrawn, these patients become depressed and anxious and their sleep difficulties intensify. Clinical experience has demonstrated that they do not respond well to phenothiazines, lithium, or antidepressants. Patients arriving at the psychiatric emergency clinic with amphetamine dependence should be referred for outpatient treatment.

Amphetamines can also precipitate latent psychotic reactions that do not necessarily subside on cessation of drug use. It is important to distinguish carefully between acute toxic reactions that are dose-related and amphetamine-precipitated psychotic reactions that continue after blood and urine tests are negative for amphetamine (see above). The prognosis, as well as the long-term treatment, is quite different. A period of observation (24–48 hours) will usually be necessary to differentiate between the 2 conditions. With a drug-precipitated psychotic reaction, long-term maintenance with antipsychotic medication in conjunction with therapy is the treatment of choice. Therefore, these patients are usually hospitalized.

Treatment

Treatment strategies are largely determined by the initial signs and symptoms (see Guide to Management of Substance Abuse Crises, p 269). Strategies to reduce the amount of drug in the patient's system in cases of acute intoxication (overdose) include emesis in conscious patients, gastric lavage with an acidic solution (ion trapping) in unconscious individuals, and acidification of the urine with ascorbic acid or ammonium chloride to enhance excretion. Hypertensive crises are treated with an alpha-adrenergic blocking agent such as phentolamine. There is an evolving trend toward the use of beta-adrenergic blocking agents such as propranolol in managing acute stimulant reactions. The current antipsychotic drug of choice in treating amphetamine toxicity is haloperidol.

PHENCYCLIDINE (PCP) ABUSE

The phencyclidines are "dissociative anesthetics" and have a mechanism of action quite different from that of other hallucinogens. In the drug culture, they are used for "mind-altering" experiences. These substances have a high potential for chronic toxicity.

PCP and its analogs, including ketamine, are the "bogeyman" drugs of the present day. They can be produced cheaply and easily with readily accessible ingredients. Their use has increased among minority groups and less affluent young people but is rare among "substance-sophisticated" populations. About 95% of users experience no crisis, but the 5% who become seriously intoxicated present a difficult management problem. Without warning, the user may alternate between coma and violence.

Clinical Features

DSM-III-R criteria for PCP intoxication, delirium, delusional disorder, mood disorder, and organic mental disorder are presented in Table 25–8.

The term "PCP syndrome" has been used to describe the pattern of PCP toxicity. The PCP syndrome

Table 25–8. *DSM-III-R* diagnostic criteria for disorders associated with abuse of phencyclidine (PCP) or similarly acting arylcyclohexylamines.

Intoxication due to PCP or similarly acting arylcyclohexylamine:
A. Recent use of phencyclidine or a similarly acting arylcyclohexylamine.
B. Maladaptive behavioral changes, eg, belligerence, assaultiveness, impulsiveness, unpredictability, psychomotor agitation, impaired judgment, impaired social or occupational functioning.
C. Within 1 hour (less when smoked, insufflated ["snorted"], or used intravenously), at least 2 of the following signs: (1) vertical or horizontal nystagmus; (2) increased blood pressure or heart rate; (3) numbness or diminished responsiveness to pain; (4) ataxia; (5) dysarthria; (6) muscle rigidity; (7) seizures; (8) hyperacusis.
D. Not due to any physical or other mental disorder.

Delirium due to PCP or similarly acting arylcyclohexylamine:
A. Delirium developing shortly after use of phencyclidine or a similarly acting arylcyclohexylamine.
B. Not due to any physical or other mental disorder.

Delusional disorder due to PCP or similarly acting arylcyclohexylamine:
A. Organic delusional syndrome developing shortly after use of phencyclidine or a similarly acting arylcyclohexylamine, or emerging up to 1 week after an overdose.
B. Not due to any physical or other mental disorder, such as schizophrenia.

Mood disorder due to PCP or similarly acting arylcyclohexylamine:
A. Organic mood syndrome developing shortly after use of phencyclidine or a similarly acting arylcyclohexylamine (usually within 1 or 2 weeks) and persisting more than 24 hours after cessation of substance use.
B. Not due to any physical or other mental disorder.

Organic mental disorder not otherwise specified due to PCP or similarly acting arylcyclohexylamine:
A. Recent use of phencyclidine or a similarly acting arylcyclohexylamine.
B. The resulting illness involves features of several organic mental syndromes or a progression from one organic mental syndrome to another, eg, initially there is delirium, followed by an organic delusional syndrome.
C. Not due to any physical or other mental disorder.

is manifested in the following 4 stages, which may or may not be successive:

A. Stage 1 (Acute PCP Toxicity): Reactions of acute PCP toxicity are a direct result of PCP intoxication and may include coma, hypertension, seizures, respiratory depression, and psychosis and agitation. Patients with acute toxicity may report to psychiatric emergency units with symptoms of paranoia, thought disorder, negativism, hostility, and grossly altered body image or may be referred for treatment as a result of their assaultive and antisocial behavior.

B. Stage 2 (PCP Toxic Psychosis): Stage 2, development of prolonged toxic psychosis, is apparently not related to toxic blood levels of PCP and does not inevitably follow stage 1.

C. Stage 3 (PCP-Precipitated Psychotic Episodes): In some individuals, PCP may precipitate a psychotic reaction that lasts a month or more and appears to be clinically similar to functional psychosis. Characteristics of PCP-precipitated psychotic episodes are of the schizoaffective type (see Chapter 29), with paranoid features and a waxing and waning thought disorder. Most individuals in stage 3 have psychotic or prepsychotic personalities, and this is the major prognostic indicator.

D. Stage 4 (PCP-Induced Depression): PCP frequently produces a depressive reaction with severe cognitive impairment. Depression may follow any of the previous stages, but the diagnosis is missed by many clinicians, particularly when depression follows stage 3. The condition lasts from a day to several months but is usually completely reversible with abstinence from PCP.

Treatment

PCP can be stored in various tissues, including fat cells, for long periods and is subject to reabsorption from the intestine. Abusers of PCP and its analogs should have long-term treatment and be monitored for recurring symptoms (see also Guide to Management of Substance Abuse Crises, p 269). The following protocol is recommended for the various stages of PCP toxicity:

A. Stage 1 (Acute PCP Toxicity):

1. Coma– As in management of any comatose patient, the first step is to stabilize the cardiovascular and respiratory systems and protect the individual from bodily harm, such as may occur during convulsions.

2. Hypertension– Treatment with diazoxide (Hyperstat IV) has been recommended.

3. Seizures– Convulsions may occur and are not necessarily limited to one or 2 episodes. Therefore, recommended treatment is administration of intravenous diazepam over a period of 2 minutes following the seizure.

4. Respiratory depression– Occurrence of respiratory depression is unusual with pure PCP except in very high dosages. However, respiratory depression may be marked when PCP is taken in combination with alcohol, other sedative-hypnotics, or opiates. If respiration is sufficiently depressed, assisted breathing with a mechanical respirator may be necessary.

5. Psychosis and agitation– Luisada and Brown (1976) have delineated the following 5 immediate goals of treatment: preventing injury to the patient or others, ensuring continuing treatment, providing a supportive environment with reduced external stimuli, ameliorating the psychosis, and reducing agitation. The reduction of external stimulation through the use of seclusion or a quiet room is of prime importance.

6. Elimination of PCP from the body– Although many clinicians prefer conservative supportive management, Aronow and coworkers (1978) describe the successful use of continuous gastric suction, acidification of the urine with vitamin C and cranberry juice, and a potent diuretic such as furosemide to enhance elimination.

PCP is recycled through the enterohepatic circulation, and introducing a slurry of activated charcoal into the intestine may decrease reabsorption of PCP from the small intestine. This should not be used instead of gastric suction in a comatose patient. However, 100 mg of activated charcoal slurry should be introduced into the stomach just before the nasogastric tube is removed from a comatose patient. The slurry may be given orally to a noncomatose patient.

B. Stage 2 (PCP Toxic Psychosis): After the acute PCP toxicity stage has passed, some individuals develop a prolonged toxic psychosis. Most clinicians recommend the use of haloperidol or other tranquilizer that is not a phenothiazine. Others recommend sedative-hypnotic medication. There is no sound research basis for the use of either of these medications, nor is there any indication that these drugs shorten the course of acute PCP psychosis. It does appear, however, that they make patients more manageable in the ward, which is probably the major reason these medications are used.

C. Stage 3 (PCP-Precipitated Psychotic Episodes): Immediate goals for treatment of psychosis and agitation are the same as those described for acute PCP toxicity, including prevention of injury and reduction of external stimuli.

D. Stage 4 (PCP-Induced Depression): In this form of depression, the individual is at high risk of suicide or may use other types of drugs to alleviate the depression. If antidepressants are prescribed on an outpatient basis, dosage for only 2 or 3 days should be dispensed at one time. The patient should be cautioned about possible interaction of tricyclic antidepressants with PCP, alcohol, and other drugs and should be advised to discontinue the tricyclic antidepressants if PCP use is resumed. The underlying basis of PCP-induced depression is unknown, and there is disagreement among experienced clinicians about what constitutes the best treatment.

PSYCHOTOMIMETIC AMPHETAMINE ABUSE

Some of the amphetamines include among their properties some that are similar to those of "psychedelic" drugs. MDA (3,4-methylenedioxyamphetamine), MDMA (M-methyl-3,4-methylenedioxymethamphetamine), and MDE (N-ethyl-3,4-methylenedioxymethamphetamine) are some of the more popular psychotomimetic drugs. MDA is known in some areas as the "love drug." MDMA is referred to as "Ecstasy," and MDE is called "Eve." These "designer" drugs have 2 basic qualities: they enhance insight/empathy and stimulate the central nervous system.

At low doses, MDMA and MDE can produce a state of well-being and self-insight, heightened empathy, and lowered psychologic defenses, leading to open communication. These effects have led to their use in therapy by some psychotherapists and psychiatrists. However, at higher doses, the stimulant properties of these drugs emerge.

Research has revealed acute MDMA toxicity syndromes (at low, medium, and high doses), prolonged toxicity syndromes (at high and low doses), and MDMA-induced anxiety syndromes. The acute and prolonged toxicity syndromes are dose-related and can be treated as for stimulant toxicity. However, the MDMA-induced anxiety syndromes, which emerge some time after MDMA ingestion or persist in the absence of MDMA in the bodily fluids, should be treated as anxiety disorders. Landry (1987) hypothesized that MDMA-induced anxiety syndromes are the result of the drug's ability to bring to the surface important unresolved psychodynamic conflicts. Unless dysfunctional, patients with these anxiety syndromes should respond to psychotherapy and protocols for nonpsychoactive anxiety. At the upper dosage limits, or in people with underlying cardiac problems, MDMA, MDE, and MDA can result in death caused by hypothermia, cardiac fibrillation, or other complications.

BARBITURATE & OTHER SEDATIVE-HYPNOTIC ABUSE

The category of depressant drugs includes a wide variety of substances which differ markedly in their physical and chemical properties but which share the common characteristic of causing generalized depression of the central nervous system. This drug group includes sedative-hypnotics (eg, barbiturates) and antianxiety agents (eg, benzodiazepines), which are widely prescribed in the USA. Some drugs, such as the barbiturates, are diffuse depressants of the central nervous system, with no specific receptors. Others, such as the benzodiazepines, have a specific receptor in the brain and have more specific action (see Chapter 54).

Depressant drugs listed in Table 25–6 include the barbiturates, barbituratelike substances, benzodiazepines, carbamates, and chloral hydrate. In addition to the effects of euphoria and reduction of aggressive or sexual drives, other possible effects of these drugs include drowsiness, respiratory depression, and nausea. Although drugs classified as central nervous system depressants differ in their pharmacologic actions and the onset and duration of their effects (Table 25–6), all exhibit some degree of cross-tolerance and cross-dependence. These depressant drugs are also cross-tolerant to alcohol, and their concomitant use with alcohol increases the risk of abuse and overdose.

Barbiturates

The barbiturates are the oldest of the sedative-hypnotics and can be classified as ultrashort-, short-, intermediate-, and long-acting (see Chapter 53). Ultrashort-acting barbiturates such as thiopental are used for anesthesia because of their rapid onset and brief duration of action. As a consequence, the ultrashort-acting barbiturates are rarely abused. The short- and intermediate-acting barbiturates include secobarbital and pentobarbital and are used primarily for insomnia. Their short duration of action and short to intermediate duration of disinhibition make them the most commonly abused drugs in the barbiturate class. The long-acting barbiturates have an onset of effects of up to 1 hour, and their duration of action is up to 16 hours; thus, they are very useful as anticonvulsant agents. They have a very low abuse potential.

Patients who have taken an overdose of barbiturates or other sedative-hypnotics arrive at emergency units with a variety of signs and symptoms that must be interpreted quickly and accurately. A sedative-hypnotic overdose is a life-threatening emergency that cannot be treated definitively by nonmedical personnel. Signs and symptoms of sedative-hypnotic overdose include slurred speech, staggering gait, sustained vertical or horizontal nystagmus, slowed reactions, lethargy, and progressive respiratory depression characterized by shallow and irregular breathing and leading to coma and possibly death.

Most patients treated for an overdose of sedative-hypnotics are acutely intoxicated or in coma following ingestion of a single large dose, but they are not usually physically dependent on the drug. Unless the sedative-hypnotic has been used daily for more than a month in an amount equivalent to 400–600 mg of a short-acting barbiturate, a severe withdrawal syndrome will not develop.

Benzodiazepines

Benzodiazepines have become the most widely used drug group in the USA. The indications for their use are anxiety, muscle spasm, seizures, and treatment of acute alcohol withdrawal symptoms. Benzodiazepines are representative of the broad sedative-hypnotic class (see Chapter 54). Often inappropriately called "minor tranquilizers" (in contrast to the neuroleptics, or "major tranquilizers"), the benzodiazepines have varying durations of action, including short-acting benzodiazepines such as lorazepam and long-acting ones such as diazepam. All, however, have approximately equal abuse potential.

One of the major reasons for the popularity of benzodiazepines is that they have a much wider therapeutic index than the barbiturates. It is almost impossible to kill oneself with an overdose of benzodiazepines, although the therapeutic index and danger from overdose are greatly altered when benzodiazepines are taken in combination with alcohol. Most cases of benzodiazepine-related overdose seen in emergency rooms are associated with alcohol ingestion.

Dependence

There are substantial variations in individual reactions to the use of benzodiazepines in dosages within the therapeutic range. Most individuals who take benzodiazepines within therapeutic range over long periods experience no significant withdrawal. However, individuals with a psychobiologic predisposition to addiction (often with a past history or family history of alcoholism) who take benzodiazepines in dosages within the therapeutic range for over 3 months may manifest severe withdrawal psychosis and seizure upon abrupt cessation of their use.

Some physicians switch from a medium- or longer-acting benzodiazepine such as diazepam to a shorter-acting benzodiazepine such as alprazolam in the mistaken belief that the shorter-acting drug has less potential for abuse. They may lower the equivalent dose as well, prompting the emergence of a sedative-hypnotic abstinence syndrome (anxiety and insomnia) throughout the day and at night. All benzodiazepines have the same potential for abuse; the use of shorter-acting benzodiazepines should be limited to their intended therapeutic purpose (eg, relief of panic). Patients with benzodiazepine dependence should enroll in a formal program of gradual detoxification. Alternatives to psychoactive medications should be sought for patients with both a dependence on benzodiazepines and a diagnosis of anxiety disorder. Thera-

peutically effective medications that have a lower potential for dependence (eg, imipramine rather than alprazolam in a drug-dependent patient with a history of panic disorder) should also be sought. If these alternatives, as well as stress reduction education, relaxation training and exercise, and biofeedback fail, and if major dysfunction is present, then a benzodiazepine is the drug of choice.

If a benzodiazepine is taken at several times the therapeutic dosage for approximately 1 month, physical dependence can develop, and abrupt cessation can produce sedative-hypnotic withdrawal symptoms such as withdrawal psychosis and seizures. Table 25–9 describes the different signs and symptoms associated with benzodiazepine withdrawal, including symptom generation and symptom reemergence. The characteristics of symptom generation and symptom reemergence upon withdrawal from a long-acting benzodiazepine such as diazepam are illustrated in Fig 25–1.

Clinical Features

DSM-III-R diagnostic criteria for intoxication, withdrawal, withdrawal delirium, and amnestic disorder are shown in Table 25–10.

Treatment

A. Overdose: Fig 25–2 outlines the ways in which an acute sedative-hypnotic overdose can be managed in an emergency situation. For additional information see Guide to Management of Substance Abuse Crises, p 269.

B. Withdrawal: It should be stressed that both the barbiturate and nonbarbiturate sedative-hypnotics can produce physical dependence on the drug for the duration of withdrawal sequelae, determined in part by the differing metabolic properties and duration of action of the primary drug dose. For example, physical dependence on large doses of a short-acting barbiturate may be produced when the drug is abruptly stopped. The peak risk of seizure occurs at about the

Table 25–9. Comparison of syndromes related to benzodiazepine withdrawal.*

Syndrome	Symptoms	Time Course	Response to Reinstitution of Benzodiazepine
Sedative-hypnotic-type withdrawal	Anxiety, insomnia, nightmares, seizures, psychosis, hyper-pyrexia, death.	Symptoms begin 1–2 days after stopping short-acting benzodiazepine or 2–4 days after stopping long-acting benzodiazepine.	Reversal of symptoms 2–6 hours after reinstituting hypnotic level doses.
Receptor site-mediated withdrawal	Anxiety (including somatic manifestations), insomnia, nightmares, muscle spasm, psychosis.	Symptoms begin 1 day after stopping benzodiazepine. They may continue for weeks to months but will improve with time.	Reversal of symptoms within 45–90 minutes of taking small doses of benzodiazepine.
Symptom reemergence	Variable but should be same as symptoms present prior to taking benzodiazepine.	Symptoms emerge when benzodiazepine is stopped and will continue unabated with time.	Responsiveness of symptoms within 45–90 minutes of taking usual therapeutic doses of benzodiazepine.

*Reproduced, with permission, from Smith DE, Wesson DR: Low dose benzodiazepine withdrawal: Receptor site mediated. *California Society for the Treatment of Alcoholism and Other Drug Dependencies News* (San Francisco) 1982;9:1.

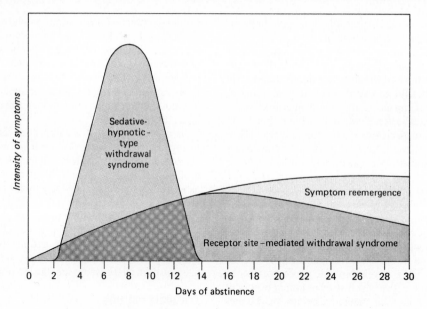

Figure 25–1. Comparison of relative intensity and time course of benzodiazepine withdrawal syndromes. (Reproduced, with permission, from Smith DE, Wesson DR: Low dose benzodiazepine withdrawal: Receptor site mediated. *California Society for the Treatment of Alcoholism and Other Drug Dependencies News* [San Francisco] 1982;**9:**1.)

Table 25–10. *DSM-III-R* diagnostic criteria for disorders associated with abuse of sedative, hypnotic, or anxiolytic drugs.

Intoxication due to sedative, hypnotic, or anxiolytic:
  A. Recent use of a sedative, hypnotic, or anxiolytic.
  B. Maladaptive behavioral changes, eg, disinhibition of sexual or aggressive impulses, mood lability, impaired judgment, impaired social or occupational functioning.
  C. At least one of the following signs: (1) slurred speech; (2) incoordination; (3) unsteady gait; (4) impairment in attention or memory.
  D. Not due to any physical or other mental disorder.
Uncomplicated withdrawal from sedative, hypnotic, or anxiolytic:
  A. Cessation of prolonged (several weeks or more) moderate or heavy use of a sedative, hypnotic, or anxiolytic, or reduction in the amount of substance used, followed by at least 3 of the following: (1) nausea or vomiting; (2) malaise or weakness; (3) autonomic hyperactivity, eg, tachycardia, sweating; (4) anxiety or irritability; (5) orthostatic hypotension; (6) coarse tremor of hands, tongue, and eyelids; (7) marked insomnia; (8) grand mal seizures.
  B. Not due to any physical or other mental disorder, such as sedative, hypnotic, or anxiolytic withdrawal delirium.
Withdrawal delirium due to sedative, hypnotic, or anxiolytic:
  A. Delirium developing after the cessation of heavy use of a sedative, hynotic, or anxiolytic, or a reduction in the amount of substance used (usually within 1 week).
  B. Autonomic hyperactivity, eg, tachycardia, sweating.
  C. Not due to any physical or other mental disorder.
Amnestic disorder due to sedative, hypnotic, or anxiolytic:
  A. Amnestic syndrome following prolonged heavy use of a sedative, hypnotic, or anxiolytic.
  B. Not due to any physical or other mental disorder.

second day. Conversely, with a longer-acting nonbarbiturate sedative-hypnotic such as diazepam, a large or even standard therapeutic dose over a long period of time produces physical dependence. Abrupt cessation can cause withdrawal seizures as well as withdrawal psychosis, with the peak danger time being the fifth or sixth day. All of these withdrawal syndromes from sedative-hypnotics can be managed by detoxification with phenobarbital, a long-acting barbiturate. In this program of treatment, 30 mg of phenobarbital is initially substituted for each hypnotic dose of a sedative-hypnotic to which the individual is addicted. For example, a 30-mg sedative dose of phenobarbital is substituted for each 100-mg hypnotic dose of the drug to which the individual is addicted. This "phenobarbital stabilization period" should continue for 2 days, followed by graded reduction of phenobarbital dosage over 7–20 days.

If the history of barbiturate abuse is variable or if the patient is using multiple sedative-hypnotics, then a challenge of short-acting pentobarbital (100–200 mg) or of long-acting phenobarbital (100–200 mg) can be used to test the individual's tolerance before starting the detoxification schedule. A person who does not have sedative-hypnotic tolerance will respond to the challenge with signs of sedation, ataxia, and mild intoxication; one who has developed tolerance will show minimal effect.

Addiction to a wide variety of other nonbarbiturate sedative-hypnotic substances—prescribed primarily for insomnia—that have a high abuse potential can oc-

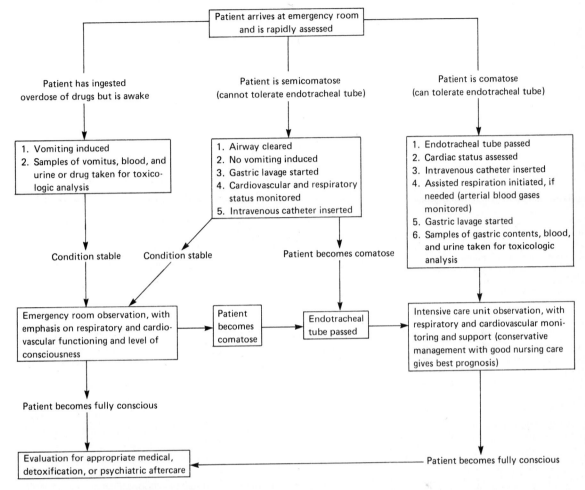

Figure 25–2. Acute treatment for barbiturate or other sedative-hypnotic overdose. (Reproduced, with permission, from Smith DE, Wesson DR, Seymour RB: The abuse of barbiturates and other sedative-hypnotics. In: *Handbook on Drug Abuse.* DuPont RL, Goldstein A, O'Donnel J [editors].)

cur if the individual takes 5–10 times the therapeutic dose for approximately 1 month. This group includes glutethimide, ethchlorvynol, and methaqualone.* Physical dependence on barbiturates and barbiturate-like substances can cause an extremely severe withdrawal syndrome with features of psychosis, seizure, and amnestic disorder. If the individual has been taking these medications for longer than 1 month or has been self-administering them in high doses, they should not be abruptly stopped, and the medication should be either gradually reduced or the phenobarbital substitution and withdrawal technique (detoxification) initiated.

HALLUCINOGEN DRUG ABUSE

Hallucinogen abuse escalated in the 1960s and continues to be a problem. The pharmacologic and clinical properties of hallucinogens are presented in Table 25–6. In addition to effects for which hallucinogens are used (euphoria and altered perception of visual and auditory stimuli), other possible effects include illusions and hallucinations, poor judgment, and impaired perception of time and space.

Clinical Features
A. Acute Toxicity: *DSM-III-R* criteria for abuse and hallucinogen hallucinosis are shown in Table 25–11. In acute hallucinogenic drug toxicity, individuals are aware of having taken a drug (eg, LSD) but are in a state of severe anxiety and panic. They feel they cannot control the drug's effects and want to be rescued immediately. The diagnosis depends on a thor-

---

* Withdrawn in 1983. Not legally available after 1984.

Table 25–11. *DSM-III-R* diagnostic criteria for disorders associated with abuse of hallucinogens.

Hallucinogen hallucinosis:
A. Recent use of a hallucinogen.
B. Maladaptive behavioral changes, eg, marked anxiety or depression, ideas of reference, fear of losing one's mind, paranoid ideation, impaired judgment, impaired social or occupational functioning.
C. Perceptual changes occurring in a state of full wakefulness and alertness, eg, subjective intensification of perceptions, depersonalization, derealization, illusions, hallucinations, synesthesias.
D. At least 2 of the following signs: (1) pupillary dilation; (2) tachycardia; (3) sweating; (4) palpitations; (5) blurring of vision; (6) tremors; (7) incoordination.
E. Not due to any physical or other mental disorder.

Hallucinogen delusional disorder:
A. Organic delusional syndrome developing shortly after hallucinogen use.
B. Not due to any physical or other mental disorder, such as schizophrenia.

Hallucinogen mood disorder:
A. Organic mood syndrome developing shortly after hallucinogen use (usually within 1 or 2 weeks), and persisting more than 24 hours after cessation of hallucinogen use.
B. Not due to any physical or other mental disorder.

Posthallucinogen perception disorder:
A. The reexperiencing, following cessation of use of a hallucinogen, of one or more of the perceptual symptoms that were experienced while intoxicated with the hallucinogen, eg, geometric hallucinations, false perceptions of movement in the peripheral visual fields, flashes of color, intensified colors, trails of images from moving objects, positive afterimages, halos around objects, macropsia, and micropsia.
B. The disturbance in criterion A causes marked distress.
C. Other causes of the symptoms have been ruled out, such as anatomic lesions and infections of the brain, delirium, dementia, sensory (visual) epilepsies, schizophrenia, entoptic imagery, and hypnopompic hallucinations.

ough understanding of the phases of the hallucinogenic experience. The course of the hallucinogenic "trip" (based on ingestion of 100–250 μg of LSD) can be described in 3 overlapping phases. The precise duration of each phase is dependent on dosage, individual idiosyncrasies, and the setting in which the drug is taken.

1. Phase 1 (sensory phase)–This phase, lasting from ingestion to the fifth hour, is characterized by sensory changes—visual, auditory, tactile, olfactory, gustatory, and kinesthetic effects—and awareness of internal bodily functions.

2. Phase 2 (symbolic, recollective, and analytic phase)–From the second to eighth hours, manifestations include visual imagery characterized by vivid colors, "hallucinations" (illusions), and altered visual perceptions; mood and affect changes; and altered communication.

3. Phase 3 (heightened sensibility phase)–From the second to tenth hours, insight, integration, and transformation of perceptions are heightened. Manifestations include concern with philosophy, religion, and cosmology; exaggeration of character traits and psychodynamic conflicts; exaggerated emotion;

and feelings of heightened psychologic perception and insight.

B. Chronic Toxicity: There are 4 recognized chronic reactions to hallucinogens or psychedelics: prolonged psychotic reactions, flashbacks, depression severe enough to be life-threatening, and exacerbation of preexisting psychiatric illness.

DSM-III-R describes hallucinogen delusional disorder, hallucinogen mood disorder, and posthallucinogen perception disorder (Table 25–10).

Treatment

See Guide to Management of Substance Abuse Crises, p 269. External stimuli such as bright lights, loud music, and strangers coming or going may be interpreted as hostile by the patient having a "bad trip." A quiet room in a supportive environment (with "trusted" individuals) is a good place to "talk down" a frightened patient. Sitting on pillows on the floor is recommended for both patient and clinician. A nonthreatening physical setting also allows the clinician to avoid adopting an overly authoritative or threatening style.

Empathy and self-confidence are essential attributes of physicians or others called upon to deal with people undergoing hallucinogenic crises. Anxiety or fear is almost certain to be communicated to the patient, who may perceive the fear in an amplified manner. Physical contact often is reassuring but may be misinterpreted. When approaching patients who have been "tripping," the clinician must be guided by judgment and previous experience.

Psychotic reactions usually occur in patients with preexisting psychologic problems. These reactions are similar to functional psychotic states and can be severe and prolonged. Appropriate treatment often requires residential care and then outpatient counseling.

"Flashbacks" are transient, spontaneous recurrences of drug effects long after the hallucinogenic intoxication has dissipated. These episodes cease with time, but in extreme cases the patient should be referred for antipsychotic medication and outpatient therapy.

MARIHUANA ABUSE

Marihuana, hashish, and other cannabis preparations have hallucinogenic and sedative properties. The active constituent is tetrahydrocannabinol (THC). At low to moderate doses, marihuana usually produces a sense of well-being, relaxation, and emotional disinhibition. A range of sensory and perceptual distortions, milder than those associated with LSD, may occur. Increased heart and pulse rates and a small drop in blood pressure are common.

At high doses, marihuana produces LSD-like effects such as hallucinations, disorganized thought, panic, paranoia, agitation, and rare psychotic reactions sometimes accompanied by rage and violence. *DMS-III-R* describes cannabis intoxication and cannabis-induced delusional disorder. Tolerance to cannabis can develop, and a mild withdrawal syndrome of insomnia, anxiety, restlessness, perspiration, loss of appetite, and upset stomach is also seen. Chronic heavy use compromises pulmonary functioning; it also suppresses testosterone (a particular problem for adolescents). Marihuana also suppresses the immune system. The effects of marihuana and alcohol are additive. Because marihuana is a sedative-hypnotic as well as a hallucinogen, use of marihuana by a person who has developed a tolerance to alcohol will ward off symptoms of alcohol withdrawal. Moreover, a person who has developed tolerance to marihuana or to alcohol may use one drug during abstinence from the other in an attempt at self-medication for symptoms of withdrawal. This practice by persons unsophisticated in the combined use of alcohol and marihuana often leads to alcohol-marihuana overdose.

A small subgroup of chronic marihuana users fulfills the *DSM-III-R* diagnostic criteria for marihuana dependence. These users typically smoke marihuana daily and have family and personal histories of psychoactive substance dependence. Sometimes an individual with a dependence on another drug (eg, alcohol or cocaine) may perceive marihuana as benign and attempt to use it in a controlled fashion while abstaining from the other drug. Invariably, this person will return to the use of the primary drug after using marihuana. It is important to help persons with a dependence upon psychoactive substances to understand that abstinence from all mood-altering drugs is the most critical aspect of recovery.

OPIATE & OPIOID ABUSE

Drugs in the opiate and opioid class include the natural substances derived from the opium poppy, such as opium, morphine, and codeine; semisynthetics, such as diacetylmorphine (heroin); and synthetic narcotic analgesics (opioids), such as meperidine, methadone, and propoxyphene (Table 25–6). Opiates have been used as analgesics since ancient times, and some of them are still the analgesics of choice for severe pain. These drugs are also prescribed for reduction of aggressive or sexual drives. The effects for which these drugs are used illicitly include euphoria and "escape." Adverse effects are drowsiness, respiratory depression, constricted pupils, and nausea.

Clinical Features

DSM-III-R diagnostic criteria for abuse, dependence, intoxication, and withdrawal are presented in Table 25–12.

The combination of pinpoint pupils and a declining level of consciousness is presumptive evidence of overdose of an opiate (eg, heroin or morphine) or an opioid. While pinpoint pupils are an important diagnostic sign, the pupils may be dilated as a consequence of hypoxia in cases of advanced coma.

Medical complications associated with the direct pharmacologic effects of opiates and opioids are relatively rare and include constipation, decrease in sexual desire, and impairment of sexual functioning. However, in the drug culture, opiates such as heroin are usually administered intravenously, producing a broad range of "needle diseases" including abscesses, hepatitis, and endocarditis. Addicts (such as physicians and nurses) who inject meperidine (Demerol) or other pharmaceutical opioids rather than heroin and who use sterile needles have a much lower incidence of "needle disease."

Treatment

A. Overdose: See Guide to Management of Substance Abuse Crises, p 269. Fortunately, overdose with either an opiate or an opioid can be reversed by administration of the narcotic antagonist naloxone (Narcan). This is usually done in the emergency unit. The intravenous route is preferred, with 2–3 mg given initially. If the patient is in shock and has low blood pressure, 1 mg can be injected sublingually initially and the injection repeated sublingually or intravenously to gain a response. The sublingual injection site must be carefully watched for oozing blood, which may be aspirated and cause serious consequences.

In opiate or opioid overdose, pupillary dilation and an elevation in the level of consciousness will occur within 20 seconds to 1 minute following intravenous administration of naloxone. If this response is obtained, a second injection of naloxone, 2 mg intravenously, should follow for prolonged effect. However, for overdose by methadone or propoxyphene napsylate, both long-acting preparations, repeated doses of naloxone will be required every 1–2 hours. (Naloxone is a short-acting narcotic antagonist, and the opiate effect will outlast the antagonist effect of a single dose.)

Table 25–12. *DSM-III-R* diagnostic criteria for disorders associated with abuse of opioids.

Opioid intoxication:
  A. Recent use of an opioid.
  B. Maladaptive behavioral changes, eg, initial euphoria followed by apathy, dysphoria, psychomotor retardation, impaired judgment, impaired social or occupational functioning.
  C. Pupillary constriction (or pupillary dilation due to anoxia from severe overdose) and at least one of the following signs: (1) drowsiness; (2) slurred speech; (3) impairment in attention or memory.
  D. Not due to any physical or other mental disorder.
Opioid withdrawal:
  A. Cessation of prolonged (several weeks or more) moderate or heavy use of an opioid, or reduction in the amount of opioid used (or administration of an opioid antagonist following a brief period of use), followed by at least 3 of the following: (1) craving for an opioid; (2) nausea or vomiting; (3) muscle aches; (4) lacrimation or rhinorrhea; (5) pupillary dilation, piloerection, or sweating; (6) diarrhea; (7) yawning; (8) fever; (9) insomnia.
  B. Not due to any physical or other mental disorder.

The availability of a specific reversal agent does not mean that general supportive measures such as clearing the airway, maintaining respiration, keeping the patient warm, and elevating the feet can be neglected.

B. Dependence: Detoxification from opiate dependence usually requires inpatient hospital facilities. In this program of treatment, a long-acting narcotic such as methadone is substituted for the opiate to which the patient is addicted. The methadone dosage during the first 2 days is usually 10–40 mg; this is followed by a gradual dosage reduction over a 3- to 21-day period, until the patient is drug-free. Methadone itself can produce dependence; it is a long-acting narcotic and a drug of abuse in the same drug group.

Nonnarcotic medication may be used on an outpatient basis to relieve symptoms of narcotic withdrawal. This includes the use of a sedative, a hypnotic, and an antispasmodic for relief of anxiety, insomnia, and gastrointestinal upset, respectively. There is a growing trend in outpatient detoxification centers toward the use of effective but less potent narcotic medication, such as propoxyphene. Acupuncture and other nondrug approaches have also been utilized on an outpatient basis for detoxification.

SUBSTANCE ABUSE & AIDS

The substance abuser risks various health complications ranging from drug-related violence and automobile accidents to liver disease. The sharing of needles by addicts carries the risk of direct transmission of hepatitis and acquired immunodeficiency syndrome (AIDS). Unfortunately, psychoactive drug use increases a person's risk-taking behavior, including unsafe sexual practices. For example, the use of intravenous amphetamines is often associated with sexual activity, especially in some homosexual men who use stimulants to sustain erections for many hours. As of the first quarter of 1987, 16.7% of AIDS patients in the USA were intravenous drug abusers, and an additional 7.7% were homosexual intravenous drug abusers. It is critical that such high-risk individuals receive access to both AIDS education and substance abuse education and treatment.

The emergence of AIDS and AIDS-related complex (ARC) adds another dimension to differential diagnosis of chemical dependence and psychiatric disorders. The astute clinician must assess whether psychiatric symptoms (especially anxiety or depression) are (1) symptoms of drug use (or withdrawal); (2) symptoms of an endogenous disorder; (3) a psychologic reaction to, or fear of, AIDS; or (4) an indication of the effects (eg, depression and delirium) of the human immunodeficiency virus on the central nervous system. The psychiatrist who has no experience with psychoactive substance use disorders or with AIDS-related psychologic disorders should engage in multidisciplinary cooperation with other health care professionals, including paraprofessional substance abuse and AIDS counselors, when treating psychoactive substance abusers in this high-risk category.

REFERENCES

Aronow R, Miceli JN, Done AK: Clinical observations during phencyclidine intoxication and treatment based on ion-trapping. In: *National Institute on Drug Abuse Research Monograph 21*, 1978.

Becker CE, Roe RL, Scott RA: *Alcohol as a Drug*. Medcom Press, 1974.

Blum K, Trachtenberg MC: Neurochemistry and alcohol craving. *California Society for the Treatment of Alcohol and Other Drug Dependencies* 1986,**13:**1.

Done AK, Aronow R, Miceli JN: The pharmacokinetics of phencyclidine in overdosage and its treatment. In: *National Institute on Drug Abuse Research Monograph 21*, 1978.

Dowling GP, McDonough ET, Bost RO: "Eve" and "Ecstasy": A report of five deaths associated with the use of MDEA and MDMA. *JAMA* 1987;**257:**1615.

Griffith JS, Cavanaugh J, Oates J: Schizophreniform psychosis induced by large dose administration of amphetamine. *J Psychedelic Drugs* 1969;**2:**42.

Hayner GN, McKinney HE: MDMA: The dark side of Ecstasy. *J Psychoactive Drugs* 1986;**18:**341.

Inaba D et al: *Pharmacological and Toxicological Perspectives on Commonly Abused Drugs*. Medical Monograph Series. Vol 5. National Institute on Drug Abuse, 1982.

Jacobs PE: Emergency room drug abuse treatment. *J Psychedelic Drugs* 1975;**7:**43.

Jaffe JH: Drug addiction and drug abuse. Chapter 23 in: *Goodman and Gilman's The Pharmacological Basis of Therapeutics*, 6th ed. Gilman AG, Goodman LS, Gilman A (editors). Macmillan, 1980.

Katzung BG (editor): *Basic & Clinical Pharmacology,* 2nd ed. Lange, 1984.

Landry ML: MDMA use: A typology for abuse and treatment. *J of Subst Abuse Treat*. [In press.]

Luisada PV, Brown BI: Clinical management of the phencyclidine psychosis. *Clin Toxicol* 1976;**9:**539.

Manual on Alcoholism. American Medical Association, 1977.

Marks J: The benzodiazepines: An international perspective. *J Psychoactive Drugs* 1983;**15:**145.

National Commission on Marijuana and Drug Abuse: *Drug Use in America. Problem and Perspective*. US Government Printing Office, 1973.

Pittel SM, Oppedahl MC: The enigma of PCP. In: *Handbook on Drug Abuse*. DuPont RL, Goldstein A, O'Donnel J (editors). Basic Books, 1979.

Sapira JD, Cherubin CE: *Drug Abuse: A Guide for the Clinician*. Excerpta Medica, 1976.

Schick JFE, Freedman DX: Research in non-narcotic drug abuse. In: *American Handbook of Psychiatry: New Psychiatric Frontiers*, 2nd ed. Vol 6. Arieta S (editor). Basic Books, 1975.

Schick JFE, Smith DE, Meyers FH: Patterns of drug use in the Haight-Ashbury neighborhood. *Clin Toxicol* 1970;**3:**19.

Schick JFE, Smith DE, Wesson DR: Analysis of amphetamine toxicity and patterns of use. *J Psychedelic Drugs* 1972;**5:**32.

Schuckit MA: *Drug and Alcohol Abuse: A Clinical Guide to Diagnosis and Treatment*. Plenum Press, 1979.

Seymour RB, Gorton JG, Smith DE: The client with a substance abuse problem. In: *Practice and Management of Psychiatric Emergency Care*. Gorton JG, Partridge R (editors). Mosby, 1982.

Showalter CV, Thornton WE: Clinical pharmacology of phencyclidine toxicity. *Am J Psychiatry* 1977;**134:**1234.

Siegel RK: Cocaine and sexual dysfunction: The curse of mama coca. *J Psychoactive Drugs* 1982;**14:**71.

Smith DE: Benzodiazepine dependence potential: Current studies and trends. *J Subst Abuse Treat* 1984;**1:**163.

Smith DE: Cocaine-alcohol abuse: Epidemiological, diagnostic and treatment considerations. *J Psychoactive Drugs* 1986;**18:**117.

Smith DE, Gay GR (editors): *It's So Good, Don't Even Try It Once*. Prentice-Hall, 1972.

Smith DE, Milkman HB, Sunderwirth SG: Addictive disease: Concept and controversy. In: *The Addictions: Multidisciplinary Perspectives and Treatments*. Lexington Books, 1985.

Smith DE, Wesson DR: Benzodiazepine dependency syndromes. *J Psychoactive Drugs* 1983;**15:**85.

Smith DE, Wesson DR: Low dose benzodiazepine withdrawal: Receptor site mediated. *California Society for the Treatment of Alcoholism and Other Drug Dependencies News* (San Francisco) 1982;**9:**1.

Smith DE et al: The diagnosis of the PCP abuse syndrome. In: *National Institute on Drug Abuse Research Monograph 21*, 1978.

Smith DE et al (editors): *A Multicultural View of Drug Abuse*. G. K. Hall & Co. and Schenkman Publishing Co., 1978.

Smith DE et al (editors): *PCP: Problems and Prevention*. Kendall/Hunt Publishing Co., 1980.

Snyder SH: Amphetamine psychosis: A "model" schizophrenia mediated by catecholamines. *Am J Psychiatry* 1973;**130:**61.

Wesson DR, Ling W: Naltrexone and its use in treatment of opiate dependent physicians. *California Society for the Treatment of Alcoholism and Other Drug Dependencies News* (San Francisco) 1980;**7:**1.

Wesson DR, Smith DE: A clinical approach to the diagnosis and treatment of amphetamine abuse. In: *Amphetamine Use, Misuse, and Abuse: Proceedings of the National Amphetamine Conference*. Smith DE et al (editors). G. K. Hall & Co., 1978.

Wesson DR, Smith DE, Linda KL: Drug crisis intervention: Conceptual and pragmatic considerations. *J Psychedelic Drugs* 1974;**6:**135.

Whitfield DC, Smith DE, Seymour RB: Psychedelics. In: *The Patient With Alcoholism and Other Drug Problems: A Clinical Approach for Physicians and Helping Professionals*. Whitfield DC (editor). Year Book, 1980.

Wilford BB (editor): *Drug Abuse: A Guide for the Primary Care Physician*. American Medical Association, 1981.

Williams MH: *Drugs and Athletic Performance*. Thomas, 1973.

26

Psychoactive Substance Use Disorders: Alcohol*

Nick Kanas, MD

Alcoholism is a major problem worldwide. In the USA, over 13 million people—7% of the adult population—are alcoholics. Alcoholism costs the nation an estimated $43 billion annually in lost production, health care, accidents, and crime, and it is a major contributor to half of the motor vehicle fatalities and nearly 30% of motor vehicle injuries. Alcohol is by far the most commonly abused drug among adolescents—even more so than marihuana. The health care system is greatly affected by alcoholism, since 10% of adults entering a private physician's office are alcoholic and 15–40% of adult admissions to general hospitals are for alcohol-related problems. Over 12 million children of alcoholics are at high risk for hyperactivity, low IQ, emotional problems, alcoholism, and child abuse.

There is no single cause of alcoholism. Biomedical, psychologic, and social factors (Fig 26–1) all play a role in its development, and stressful events sometimes serve as catalysts of drinking behavior. Increased alcohol use can lead to both psychologic and physical dependence, which result in a number of important biomedical, psychologic, and social sequelae such as cirrhosis, depression, marital problems, and occupational problems. These sequelae themselves are stressful and lead to more drinking, further dependence, and additional sequelae—and the cycle continues. Treatment should be directed first at the stage of dependence on drinking, then to the important sequelae of drinking, and finally should attempt to explore and modify predisposing causes.

Definitions

The *DSM-III-R* diagnostic criteria for disorders associated with alcohol use are presented in full in Chapter 25, Table 25–3. The following is a brief review of criteria for alcohol dependence and abuse:

Alcohol dependence is characterized by at least 3 of 9 specific signs or symptoms (eg, inability to control the amount consumed; interference with work, school, or social activities; tolerance; withdrawal) and duration of problems for at least 1 month. **Tolerance** is defined as a need for greatly increased amounts of a substance in order to become intoxicated, or decreased

effect with use of the same amount of the substance. **Withdrawal** denotes the development of characteristic signs and symptoms (eg, tremor, tachycardia, restlessness) after cessation or reduction in amount of a substance consumed.

Alcohol abuse is characterized by a maladaptive pattern of alcohol use, duration of problems for at least 1 month, and failure to meet the criteria for alcohol dependence. This is a residual category most applicable to people who have only recently begun to abuse alcohol.

Both "alcohol dependence" and "alcohol abuse" denote addiction and its sequelae. The direct effects of alcohol on the central nervous system are categorized in *DSM-III-R* under "alcohol-induced organic mental disorders" and include such entities as alcohol intoxication, alcohol withdrawal delirium (DTs), alcohol hallucinosis, and dementia associated with alcoholism. (See Chapter 25 for *DSM-III-R* criteria.)

Diagnostic Workup

Some effects of alcoholism are encompassed in the *DSM-III-R* criteria for alcohol dependence and abuse. Table 26–1 lists several biomedical, psychologic, and social sequelae.

A. History and Mental Status Examination: Essential to the workup are a complete history and mental status examination in the course of which the possibility of alcoholism is explored in a nonthreatening manner. One should not raise the issue of alcoholism directly at first but instead should look for clues and responses that might indicate a problem with alcohol. For example, the following should alert the physician to the possibility of alcoholism: a history of gulping drinks, blackouts, morning tremor, defensiveness, or dependence on other drugs; a positive family history; or marital or job problems. Indirect questions such as "Do you drink alcohol?" or "When and in what settings do you like to drink?" are much less threatening initially than direct questions such as "Is alcohol a problem for you?" or "Are you an alcoholic?" It is important to start asking questions in general terms and gradually become more specific. If alcoholism is suspected to be a problem, an interview with the spouse or other family members is indicated.

1. Level of alcohol consumption– In the USA, beer accounts for 49% of alcohol consumed, hard

---

* See also Chapter 25.

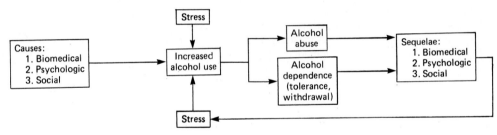

Figure 26–1. A conceptual model of alcoholism.

liquor for 39%, and wine for 12%.* Daily alcohol consumption can be estimated using the following conversion: one 12-oz can of beer (4% ethanol) = one 1-oz shot of hard liquor (43% ethanol) = one 4-oz glass of wine (12% ethanol)—each contains 12–15 mL of ethanol. Alcoholics with tolerance to alcohol may consume the equivalent of a liter or more of hard liquor per day. A high daily consumption rate is but one indication that an alcohol problem exists and should be used in conjunction with other symptoms and signs in making the diagnosis.

2. Denial of drinking problems—Alcoholics usually deny the presence and extent of their problem. In some cases, denial is a characteristic defense mechanism the individual uses in other contexts also. Extreme forms of denial may represent reactions to stress from past traumatic events, sequelae of alcoholism, or even stress associated with the treatment process itself. Denial may vary in intensity, and a patient may deny problems he or she acknowledged previously. If denial is confronted too vigorously, increased anxiety and anger may result, producing more denial or a flight from treatment. Confrontation should be modified in accordance with the therapist's assessment of the patient's ability to face the problem.

3. Blackouts—Blackouts occur in 64–94% of alcoholics. They are a form of anterograde amnesia in which the patient is unable to recall events that occurred during a bout of drinking even though he or she was conscious and active at that time. Blackouts last for minutes to days, and their frequency is an index of the severity and duration of alcoholism. Predisposing factors include gulping drinks on an empty stomach and going without sleep. Blackouts are generally unrelated to organic disturbances as measured by neuropsychologic testing. The differential diagnosis of alcoholic blackouts includes head trauma, carbon monoxide poisoning, hysteria, and malingering.

B. Physical Examination: A complete physical examination should be performed after the history and mental status examination.

1. Signs—In early stages of alcoholism, pertinent physical findings may be limited to evidence of hep-

atomegaly, tremor, or mild peripheral neuropathy. In more advanced stages, there may be a number of physical signs consistent with the sequelae listed in Table 26–1.

2. Laboratory and x-ray findings—Useful laboratory measurements include the blood alcohol level (see Chapter 25 and Table 25–4); serum levels of aspartate aminotransferase (AST, SGOT), alkaline phosphatase, gamma-glutamyl transpeptidase, and bilirubin (increased levels indicate liver damage); and erythrocyte mean corpuscular volume (macrocytosis indicates liver disease, folate deficiency, or the toxic effect of alcohol on the developing erythroblast). Urinalysis and chest x-ray should be performed in all cases. Fractures, subdural hematomas, pneumonia, tuberculosis, and lung cancer from smoking are often found.

C. Adjuncts to Diagnosis: Useful aids in making a diagnosis of alcoholism include the CAGE Ques-

Table 26–1. Sequelae of alcoholism.

Biomedical	Biomedical (cont'd)
Birth defects	Sexual dysfunction
Blackouts	(impotence,
Bone fractures	amenorrhea)
Cardiomyopathy	Subdural hematoma
Cerebellar degeneration	Tuberculosis
Cirrhosis	Wernicke's syndrome
Delirium tremens	**Psychologic**
Dementia	Angry outbursts
Esophageal varices	Anxiety
Esophagitis	Craving for alcohol
Fatty liver	Denial
Gastritis	Dependency
Hepatitis	Depression
Hypertension	Guilt
Hypothyroidism	Hallucinosis
Increased risk of cancer	Loneliness
(mouth, pharynx, larynx,	Paranoia
esophagus, liver, pancreas)	Suicidal ideation
Intoxication	Use of other drugs
Korsakoff's syndrome	**Social**
Myopathy	Automobile accidents
Nutritional deficiency, espe-	Family problems (marital,
cially vitamin (thiamine,	child abuse)
folate) deficiency	Financial problems
Pancreatitis	Inadequate shelter
Peripheral neuropathy	Legal problems
Pneumonia	Social isolation
Portal hypertension	Vocational problems
Seizures	

* Data from the *Special Report to the US Congress* cited on p 297.

tionnaire (Mayfield and coworkers, 1974), the Michigan Alcoholism Screening Test, and the MacAndrews Alcoholism Scale. Neuropsychologic tests are helpful in assessing the degree and location of brain damage. These procedures should be viewed as adjuncts to a careful history, mental status examination, and physical examination.

Illustrative Case

A divorced man in his late 40s presented to the emergency room and requested treatment for alcoholism. He had been drinking a fifth of liquor or a gallon of wine a day since being fired from his job 3 months before. He had exhausted his resources and had been sleeping in his car. Over the past month, he had experienced dark-colored urine, increasing abdominal girth, and a 10-lb weight gain despite eating poorly. Two years previously, he had been hospitalized for leg edema and weight gain secondary to ascites from alcoholic liver disease. He was admitted to the hospital for medical detoxification and evaluation for possible recurrence of ascites and liver disease.

The patient had had an unremarkable childhood and had completed 2 years of college. He began drinking heavily during his military service tour of duty. His drinking continued after discharge from the army and averaged a fifth of hard liquor every 3 days for the next 20 years. He experienced marital problems related to his drinking and had been divorced twice. After his second divorce, his drinking increased, and this led to performance problems at work. He was fired from his job as a computer programmer a year prior to admission to the hospital, and since that time he had lived alone and held temporary jobs. The last temporary job was managing a fast-food outlet. He denied having had blackouts, seizures, or delirium tremens. He had stopped drinking 3 times on his own, and withdrawal resulted in tremor; he also had had 2 abstinent periods in the past 6 years, the longest lasting 6 months. He had attended Alcoholics Anonymous meetings in the year prior to admission, but he left the group after a month because he did not like it. The patient denied having a personal or family history of psychiatric or other drug abuse problems, although he said his father was a heavy drinker.

Findings at the time of admission to the hospital included tremor; palmar erythema; a reddish complexion with spider angiomas; occasional expiratory wheezes; a distended abdomen with a fluid wave and shifting dullness; a liver 18 cm in width, with a hard, nontender edge; and decreased sensations of pain, vibration, and touch in the lower third of his legs. AST (SGOT), alkaline phosphatase, bilirubin, and glucose levels were all elevated. Results of pulmonary function tests were consistent with those of a mild form of chronic obstructive pulmonary disease. Liver and spleen scan revealed hepatosplenomegaly consistent with hepatocellular disease. Liver biopsy showed fatty metamorphosis, cirrhosis, and resolving hepatitis. The patient was given oral diazepam for the first few

days of withdrawal and, except for some tremulousness, had an uneventful course. He seemed motivated for further treatment of his alcoholism and was transferred to the alcohol rehabilitation unit after 16 days on the medical ward. At the time of his transfer, the patient was noted to be anxious, depressed, worried about his future, and obsessive in his thinking.

During the 28 days the patient was in the rehabilitation unit, his medical status stabilized, and results of his liver function tests returned to normal, although his plasma glucose level remained slightly high. He became less anxious and depressed and more extroverted as a result of participating in ward activities and group therapy 4 times a week. He also received individual counseling twice a week, which assisted him in setting up his treatment plan. He obtained disability insurance and saw a vocational counselor, who gave him a list of agencies where he could seek work as a computer programmer. He participated in Alcoholics Anonymous and seemed to enjoy the experience this time. In the week before discharge from the hospital, he began treatment with disulfiram and was accepted into a halfway house for alcoholics.

After discharge from the hospital, the patient was followed in the alcohol rehabilitation clinic. His initial treatment included individual counseling and group therapy once a week and attendance at group sessions of Alcoholics Anonymous 3 times a week. Although he initially demonstrated a depressed mood and some denial of personal problems, he seemed motivated for treatment. Over the next few months, he became less depressed, began making friends, and became active in his church, in a teenage outreach organization, and in the rehabilitation unit alumni group. This resulted in improved self-esteem and more assertive behavior. He found a job as a computer programmer and began paying off his debts. As his life stabilized, disulfiram was discontinued, and he was able to remain abstinent without it.

Ten months after beginning outpatient treatment in the alcohol clinic, the patient moved into an apartment and continued to see some of the abstinent friends he had met in the halfway house. Because he was able to remain abstinent and demonstrated continued improved self-confidence, his individual counseling sessions were cut back to once a month; he continued in group therapy on a weekly basis. One year after entering the clinic, he was found to have adult-onset diabetes mellitus, which was treated with an oral hypoglycemic agent. During his second year in the outpatient clinic, his mood and social skills continued to improve, and he remained abstinent and fully employed. Near the end of his second year, he accepted a job as a senior computer programmer in another city. He terminated treatment from the clinic without difficulty after 2 years.

Epidemiology

It is difficult to give exact prevalence rates of alcoholism, since estimates are determined from associated factors, such as cirrhosis rates or the percentage of patients in treatment who are alcoholic, and since the accuracy and comparability of such figures vary in different geographic areas.

A. Cultural and Social Factors: One commonly reported figure is the adult per capita consumption rate of alcohol: In a recent survey of 26 countries, Portugal, France, and Italy were the top 3 countries; the USA was 15th; and Israel was 26th. More alcohol is consumed per capita in the Pacific Coast and New England regions of the USA than in other regions. However, per capita consumption figures give only approximate correlations with alcoholism rates. For example, the incidence of alcoholism in Portugal is lower than its high consumption rate would indicate. Social and cultural factors play a role in determining not only how much people drink but also whether or not they abuse alcohol. As a general rule, alcoholism rates are considered to be high in the USA, northern France, Poland, northern Russia, Sweden, and Switzerland; they tend to be low in China, southern France, Greece, Italy, Israel, Portugal, and Spain.

Per capita consumption rates may also be deceiving in regard to their association with alcoholism and socioeconomic status. Consumption levels tend to increase with increasing socioeconomic status; for example, the highest levels of *abstinence* are reported in the lower socioeconomic classes. However, alcoholism is more frequent in the middle socioeconomic ranges. Kissin (1977) estimated that 20–25% of alcoholics are in the upper and middle social classes; 40–50% are in the lower-middle and upper-lower social classes; and 25–30% are in the inner-city and skid row populations. Despite the high incidence of problem drinking in the middle socioeconomic ranges— particularly among semiprofessional technical workers and semiskilled laborers—the important point is that alcoholism occurs among all socioeconomic groups.

Other factors that correlate positively with problem drinking include living in urban or suburban areas, having a history of childhood disruptions or alcoholic parents, being separated or divorced, and lacking affiliation with religious organizations. Among churchgoers, the proportion of heavy drinkers is higher among Catholics than Protestants. There is no overall difference in drinking rates of whites and blacks; however, more black women than white women are either abstainers or heavy drinkers. The alcoholism rate among American Indians is at least twice the national average, and incidences of 25–50% have been reported on some reservations. The per capita consumption rate among Latinos is relatively low, but in one survey the proportion of those who drank heavily was high (28%). Alcoholism is uncommon among Asians.

B. Sex and Age Factors: The male/female ratio of alcoholics has been equalizing in recent years. Whereas earlier surveys estimated a ratio of 7:1, more recent surveys reveal a ratio of 2–3:1. This trend probably reflects better case reporting of female alcoholics. It is also likely that the changing social role of women

allows them to admit having a drinking problem rather than seek help for anxiety or depression.

In men, heavy drinking is highest at ages 18–20, drops somewhat in the early 20s, and then begins to increase to a second peak at ages 35–39. In women, heavy drinking is highest at ages 21–29, dips slightly in the early 30s, and then increases and levels off in the late 30s and early 40s.

About 30–60% of high school students use alcohol at least once a month, and 1–3% report daily use. Adler and Kandel (1981) found evidence of a developmental sequence of drug abuse in adolescents: Use of beer and wine led to use of hard liquor, and use of legal drugs led to use of illegal drugs. Eisterhold and coworkers (1979) found that over half of high school students who used alcohol also used another drug and that use of beer or wine by parents was significantly related to such use by their children.

There is a general drop in the rate of heavy drinking in both sexes in the 50s and early 60s. This is in part attributable to financial limitations and the early death of alcoholics. However, about half of the people over 60 who once were heavy drinkers become abstinent after age 44, chiefly out of fear of damaging their health. This number, added to the number of people who never took up drinking, gives an abstinence rate of over 50% in the population 65 years and older. Elderly alcoholics typically drink in isolation on a daily basis and consume small amounts of alcohol per episode. About two-thirds of elderly alcoholics have a history of long-standing problems with alcohol and neurotic and personality difficulties; the remaining third develop drinking problems later in life in association with problems of aging, such as bereavement, retirement, loneliness, and illness.

C. Associated Psychiatric Problems: It is difficult to estimate the prevalence of other psychiatric problems in alcoholics, since most surveys are done in psychiatric settings. A review of several surveys of patients in whom both alcoholism and an additional psychiatric disorder were diagnosed reveals that the additional psychiatric disorder in 70–80% of cases was a personality disorder (antisocial, dependent, schizoid, or borderline personality); in 10–15%, it was a psychotic condition (schizophrenia, major depression, or bipolar disorder); and in 10–15%, it was a neurotic condition (generalized anxiety or obsessive compulsive disorder).

An interesting survey of 510 adults in the community was reported by Weissman and colleagues (1980). Of the 6.7% who were alcoholics, 71% had a history of at least one other psychiatric disorder. Over 75% of these people had a depressive disorder. The risk for suicide was much higher in alcoholics than in patients with other psychiatric disorcers but not alcoholism.

D. Associated Abuse of Other Drugs: There is a strong association between alcoholism and other forms of drug abuse. Over half of high school students using alcohol use another drug also, and 60% of adolescent polydrug abusers drink alcohol at least once a week. Among adults, about 20% of polydrug abusers have diagnosable alcoholism, and Weissman and coworkers (1980) found the prevalence of drug misuse to be 12% among adult alcoholics. From these figures, one may conclude that polydrug abuse is more common among adolescents than adults and that more drug abusers misuse alcohol than vice versa. Nevertheless, in evaluating an alcoholic patient, one must always consider the possibility of addiction to other drugs.

Using the Minnesota Multiphasic Personality Inventory (MMPI), Sutker and associates (1979) studied personality characteristics in 175 male alcoholics (mean age 44 years) and 125 male heroin addicts (mean age 25 years). They concluded that both populations demonstrated behavioral and cognitive nonconformity but that alcoholics appeared to be more neurotic (anxious, depressed, etc). Although total group statistics showed heroin addicts to be more antisocial than alcoholics, this distinction disappeared when age-matched groups of heroin addicts and alcoholics were compared.

There is a question whether alcoholics and patients with other drug addictions should be treated in separate or combined treatment programs. Baker and coworkers (1977, 1982) found that alcoholic patients preferred treatment in separate programs. Although small but significant advantages for both alcoholics and drug addicts in separate rather than combined programs were noted at 6-month follow-up, the differences became less significant after 2 years. Nevertheless, many therapists prefer separate programs, particularly for alcoholics.

E. Alcoholism in Physicians: Alcoholism is a major problem in physicians. Murray (1976) found that 29–39% of British physicians discharged from hospitals in England and Scotland had a problem with alcohol; in addition, first admission rates for alcoholism in his Scottish sample were 2.7 times higher in physicians than in other patients from the same socioeconomic class. In his English sample, 46% of the 41 alcoholic physicians had a family history of psychiatric disorders or alcohol abuse (or both); 29% had attempted suicide; 37% had an additional diagnosed psychiatric disorder; and 56% abused other drugs in addition to alcohol. Thirty-six of these physicians were followed for a mean total of 63 months; 80% continued to have difficulty with alcohol, 67% required further treatment, and 51% were not practicing medicine.

The prognosis for alcoholic physicians is improved if the problem is identified early and they receive intensive treatment for their alcoholism. Bissell and Jones (1976) interviewed 98 United States and Canadian physicians who were members of Alcoholics Anonymous and had been abstinent for at least a year. Many of their characteristics were similar to the physicians studied by Murray, but 75% were able to continue practicing medicine, although one-third of these reported some decline in work status. Kliner and coworkers (1980) studied 67 alcoholic physicians 1 year after they had completed an intensive Alcoholics

Anonymous-oriented inpatient program. They found that 76% had been abstinent since treament; 79% had reported improvement in their professional performance as a result of treatment; and more than 75% reported improvement in all areas surveyed. Experiences such as these have led many states in the USA to establish programs for alcoholic physicians, with emphasis on early identification, adequate treatment, and long-term follow-up.

Etiology, Pathogenesis, & Natural History

Numerous factors have been identified as potential causes of alcoholism. In some patients, one factor may predominate; in others, several factors interact; and in many, no clear-cut cause can be found. In addition, a stressful event may be the final precipitant that initiates the addictive cycle (Fig 26–1).

A. Biomedical Factors: Evidence supporting a role of biomedical factors in alcoholism comes from genetic, physiologic, biochemical, and prenatal data.

1. Genetic factors–There have been a number of twin, genetic marker, and adoption studies that support the conclusion that susceptibility to adverse effects of alcohol and predilection for uncontrollable drinking are hereditary. Particularly intriguing are the studies showing that alcoholism is more likely to occur in adopted children whose biologic parents were alcoholics than in those whose biologic parents were nonalcoholics. Such studies control for environmental factors, although the role of in utero and neonatal influences cannot be completely excluded. The exact nature of this genetic susceptibility has not been defined, although it seems stronger for males than for females.

2. Physiologic factors–Physiologic studies have correlated alcoholism with hypofunction of an endocrine gland, eg, the adrenal cortex or the thyroid. In these studies, it is unclear wheather endocrine hypofunction leads to alcoholism or vice versa; thus, a clear causal relationship is still unproved. It has been suggested that deficits in the hypothalamus lead to an uncontrollable thirst for alcohol, but there is little evidence to support this hypothesis.

3. Biochemical factors–Because of the association of alcoholism and depression, numerous studies have attempted to relate alcoholism to levels of monoamine oxidase. These studies have generally measured monoamine oxidase levels in platelets and have found that levels are lower in alcoholics than in controls. Since platelet levels of monoamine oxidase are strongly affected by genetic factors, some have speculated that this may be an important biochemical link between hereditary influences and the affective state of alcoholics. Data are still accumulating in this promising line of research. Cerebrospinal fluid levels of 5-hydroxyindoleacetic acid in alcoholics have been found to be significantly lower than those in controls, again suggesting an association between adrenergic neurotransmitters and alcoholism.

4. Prenatal factors–Infants whose mothers

drink heavily during pregnancy often show biologic defects such as decreased size and weight. Fetal alcohol syndrome, a neonatal condition characterized by neurophysiologic dysfunction and various anatomic malformations, has been described. Some workers have hypothesized that offspring of alcoholic mothers develop physical dependence on alcohol in utero and that this dependence becomes reactivated on exposure to alcohol during adolescence or adulthood; however, this notion remains speculative.

B. Psychologic Factors: Data supporting psychologic causes of alcoholism are from 3 sources: (1) psychoanalytic case studies, (2) personality assessments using psychologic testing, and (3) theories of learning.

1. Emotional conflicts–Psychoanalytic theory holds that early developmental deprivation and trauma may result in painful conflicts that are repressed. Symptoms such as anxiety and depression may occur when these conflicts begin to enter conscious awareness. Reactivation of conflicts may be triggered later in life by stress or by events that are reminiscent of the original conflicts (see Role of Stress, below). Alcohol is seen as releasing inhibitions and allowing for the expression of these repressed conflicts. During treatment, many analysts have noted the presence of recurring themes involving oral-dependent, aggressive, and depressive impulses. Most of the published data are from retrospective psychoanalytic case studies; data from prospective studies are lacking.

2. Personality traits–Psychologic testing has been used to explore common personality characteristics found in alcoholics. Several studies using the MMPI have shown that alcoholics demonstrate an abnormal elevation on the D (depression) and Pd (psychopathic deviance) scales. Some of these data on personality traits support the notion that alcoholics exhibit oral-dependent and depressive character traits, which is consistent with the psychoanalytic position mentioned above. Despite the fact that groups of alcoholics typically show these patterns, there is much individual variation, with some alcoholics not showing significant abnormalities. In addition, since psychologic tests are often administered to adults already identified as being alcoholics, one must be wary of concluding that the results describe personality traits predating the onset of alcoholism, since it is possible that years of drinking may encourage the emergence of clinically abnormal character traits later in life. For example, Vaillant (1980) has presented prospective data supporting the notion that oral-dependent traits may result from rather than cause alcoholism.

3. Learned behavior–Learning theory has also been used to develop a causal model of alcoholism. Many alcoholics report that being intoxicated reduces anxiety and replaces it with a feeling of well-being. Since people are drawn toward pleasurable states, drinking behavior is reinforced and gradually becomes a learned behavior (a habit). This theory does not explain why some drinkers become alcoholics and others remain social drinkers. Nevertheless, it has received some empirical support in studies involving rats.

C. Social Factors: The importance of social factors as a cause of alcoholism is supported by data from surveys and field studies that show relationships between the particular social variable under study and the rates of alcohol consumption or alcoholism. Some of the most important variables, such as sex, age, and ethnicity, are discussed in the section on epidemiology (above). The relevance of social factors is unclear, since it is sometimes difficult to isolate social factors from other variables. For example, immigrants to the USA who grow up in ethnically isolated neighborhoods tend to demonstrate alcoholism rates typical of those of their native lands rather than of the USA at large. It is difficult to determine how much of this is sociocultural and how much might reflect the influence of a genetic pool or important psychologic characteristics.

Alcoholism rates in societies where the attitudes toward drinking are varied (such as in the USA) tend to be higher than in societies such as Israel, where drinking is part of traditional cultural or religious practices. National or local social influences also affect alcohol preference: Germans prefer beer, and the southern French prefer wine.

Family structure also plays an important role in alcoholism. Using general systems theory, one may conceptualize the alcoholic's family as a maladaptive system whose stability depends on one member fulfilling a sick role. Although the family is dysfunctional, it is in a homeostatic state. Any attempt on the part of the physician, therapist, or others to change the behavior of one family member will disturb the other family members and result in an increase in their anxiety and an attempt by them to resist the disturbing influence. This "systems" view has important implications for treatment, and the entire family should therefore be considered in the treatment plan.

D. Role of Stress: An interaction of biomedical, psychologic, and social factors may lead to the gradual development of alcoholism. In many alcoholics, the addictive process is insidious and takes place over months or years. In some alcoholics, however, an acute traumatic life event (eg, the death of a spouse, physical illness, or even delayed posttraumatic stress syndrome) leads to increased drinking as a coping mechanism in dealing with resultant anxiety and depression. In predisposed individuals, the drinking behavior can escalate into addiction, even when the cause of stress is removed. In the diagnostic workup of alcoholic patients, it is useful to look for a history of drinking escalations after stressful events, since the presence of a stress response syndrome such as this may affect treatment planning. For example, alcoholics particularly vulnerable to stress can be taught how to avoid stressful situations in life or to prevent escalation of drinking by seeking help immediately following a traumatic event.

Treatment & Prognosis

A. Effect of the Physician's Attitude on Treatment: The physician's attitude affects the treatment of alcoholics. Attitudinal barriers include moralistic views that alcoholics are "bad" people; frustration over the fact that alcoholics are difficult, time-consuming patients who often leave treatment prematurely or offer little financial or ego reward; and pessimism over the "revolving-door syndrome" whereby, despite great expenditure of time and energy on the part of the physician, the patient may later return for treatment in an inebriated state. It is also true that physicians tend to treat those problems that interest them. For example, internists focus on biomedical issues and psychiatrists on psychosocial issues. To properly treat alcoholics, one must give equal attention to biomedical, psychologic, and social issues; this is a difficult conceptual stance for many physicians.

Attitudinal barriers begin in the medical school and house staff years. Fisher and coworkers (1975) found a general tendency for pessimism and negative moral views to be expressed as students and physicians ascended the ladder of medical training: House staff members were more negative than second-year medical students, and they, in turn, were more negative than first-year medical students. Chappel and colleagues (1977) found that a course in substance abuse taught to second-year medical students significantly improved their attitudes, so that they took a less moralistic and more therapeutic view of the problem. Since the prognosis for cure of alcoholism is better than for cure of many other conditions, it is important to educate physicians about alcoholism and its treatment so they will know how to deal with this problem.

B. Abstinence Versus Controlled Drinking: One of the most controversial issues in the treatment of alcoholics is whether the goal should be permanent abstinence or moderate, controlled drinking. Alcoholism has been conceptualized by some as a loss of ability to control consumption, perhaps due to a neurophysiologic feedback dysfunction that affects the ability to regulate alcohol intake based on interoceptive cues. If this view is accepted, it follows that alcoholics must be regarded as inherently unable to control their drinking behavior, so that attempts at controlled drinking are doomed to failure. Furthermore, strict abstinence in the treatment of alcoholics has a long tradition and is a basic philosophic stance of Alcoholics Anonymous, one of the oldest and most successful treatment programs. Traditions die hard, particularly when time and experience have proved their merit. Finally, the fantasy of the majority of alcoholics is that they will someday be able to become "normal" drinkers. Because clinical experience has shown that most alcoholics who attempt controlled drinking ultimately fail, most workers in the field are skeptical about controlled drinking as a basic treatment goal.

Several studies give support to the view that 10–15% of alcoholics can achieve a moderate, controlled drinking pattern for long periods. Some of these studies may be criticized on methodologic grounds. These results must be viewed cautiously in any case, since controlled drinkers have higher relapse rates than abstainers. Finally, successful controlled drinkers have less severe drinking problems and more stable family and work situations prior to entering treatment than most alcoholics and so perhaps had a better prognosis to begin with. There are some patients for whom controlled drinking might be beneficial— eg, geriatric patients who developed alcoholism later in life. In a controlled environment such as a nursing home, moderate drinking in a social context has been shown to be beneficial for some elderly patients. However, for the vast majority of alcoholics, total abstinence is the key to successful treatment.

C. Disulfiram (Antabuse): In the late 1930s, it was noted that workers in the rubber industry developed unpleasant reactions shortly after drinking alcohol. Inadvertent absorption of the antioxidant disulfiram was identified as the cause. In the late 1940s, disulfiram was introduced as a therapeutic agent in the treatment of alcoholism. Since it produces an unpleasant reaction in the presence of alcohol, it is now used as a deterrent to drinking; at one time, its use was advocated in aversive conditioning.

1. Mechanisms of action–As shown in Fig 26–2, disulfiram acts by blocking 2 important enzymes. Its primary action is in blocking aldehyde dehydrogenase in the liver. When a patient taking disulfiram drinks ethyl alcohol, acetaldehyde cannot be converted to acetate, and the level of acetaldehyde in the blood may increase 5- to 10-fold. It is thought that the alcohol-disulfiram reaction is due to this increased level of acetaldehyde. A second important clinical action of disulfiram is actually due to one of its metabolites, diethyldithiocarbamate, which blocks the enzyme dopamine β-hydroxylase and thereby results in increased dopamine levels in the brain.

Some of the characteristics of the alcohol-disulfiram reaction are shown in Table 26–2. Nausea and flushing usually occur within 30 minutes, and the full-blown reaction—which may include many of the symptoms and signs in the first column of Table 26–2—usually lasts 30–90 minutes. More serious reactions may occur in individuals who are unusually sensitive or have consumed large amounts of alcohol. For this reason, patients undergoing an alcohol-disulfiram reaction should be carefully monitored in an emergency room, and appropriate treatment for possible convulsions, myocardial infarction, or cardiovascular collapse should be available. Hypertension may be observed early in the reaction and hypotension later. Hypertension is thought to result from the direct effect of acetaldehyde on the release of norepinephrine peripherally, causing vasoconstriction. However, since norepinephrine levels are believed to be already low owing to the action of diethyldithiocarbamate on dopamine β-hydroxylase, vasoconstriction is followed by vasodilatation and hypotension as norepinephrine levels are depleted.

2. Side effects–As shown in Table 26–3, disulfiram has a number of potential side effects. Most

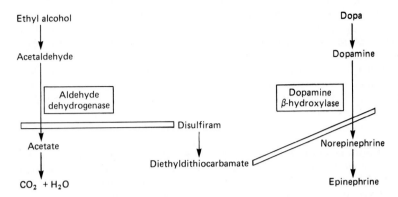

Figure 26–2. Enzymatic blocking effects of disulfiram. Disulfiram blocks aldehyde dehydrogenase in the liver, thereby preventing conversion of acetaldehyde to acetate and resulting in increased blood levels of acetaldehyde. Diethyldithio-carbamate (a metabolite of disulfiram) blocks dopamine β-hydroxylase, thereby preventing conversion of dopamine to norepinephrine and resulting in increased dopamine levels in the brain. Dopa = dihydroxyphenylalanine.

of these are rare, with the most common being drowsiness, metallic or garlic taste in the mouth, fatigue, and headaches. Some of the neurologic side effects are probably due to a metabolite of disulfiram (carbon disulfide), and they appear to be dose-related. Other side effects such as hypersensitivity hepatitis are idiosyncratic. Disulfiram has a number of important interactions with commonly prescribed medications, and its use in pregnant women has been associated with fetal abnormalities.

Disulfiram has been shown to produce psychotic reactions in vulnerable alcoholics. Those at risk include patients with low cerebrospinal fluid levels of dopamine β-hydroxylase; patients receiving 500 mg or more of disulfiram daily; and patients with a history of major depression, mania, borderline personality, or schizophrenia. It is thought that psychosis occurs through the blockage of dopamine β-hydroxylase, which leads to increased levels of dopamine in the brain. Since increased dopamine has been implicated in psychotic conditions such as schizophrenia, this hypothesis makes clinical sense.

3. Dosage and indications–The usual dose of disulfiram is 250 mg/d, usually taken in the evening because of the drowsiness it causes. Sensitivity to alcohol develops within 12 hours of taking the first dose,

although antacids and iron decrease its absorption and may prolong this time frame. Disulfiram is eliminated slowly from the body, and patients should be warned that they cannot drink for 1–2 weeks after stopping medication.

Disulfiram works best in older, motivated, compulsive alcoholics who do not suffer from a potentially psychotic condition and who tend to follow a binge pattern in their drinking. It is especially useful as a means of helping the patient get through stressful periods without taking a drink or as an inducement to remaining abstinent during entry into a treatment program. Disulfiram should seldom be prescribed continuously for more than 3–6 months, because side effects are time-related. Since many of the side effects

Table 26–3. Side effects of disulfiram.

Disulfiram taken alone
Arteriosclerotic cardiovascular disease
Birth defects (limb reduction abnormalities)
Cramps
Drowsiness
Fatigue
Headache
Hypercholesterolemia
Hypersensitivity hepatitis
Hypertension
Metallic or garlic taste
Nausea and vomiting
Optic neuritis
Peripheral neuropathy
Psychosis, particularly in predisposed individuals (history of major depression, mania, borderline personality, schizophrenia)
Rash
Disulfiram taken with other drugs
Additive or synergistic effects with barbiturates, cholordiazepoxide, diazepam, isoniazid, monoamine oxidase inhibitors, paraldehyde, phenytoin, sympathomimetics, tricyclic antidepressants, warfarin
Confusion and alcohol-disulfiram type of reaction with paraldehyde
Psychosis with metronidazole
Disulfiram taken with alcohol
See Table 26–2

Table 26–2. Alcohol-disulfiram reaction.

Common effects	Less common effects
Anxiety and feelings of impending doom	Coma
Blurred vision	Confusion
Dyspnea	Convulsions
Face and neck flushing	Death due to myocardial infarction or cardiovascular collapse
Headaches	
Hypertension or hypotension	Electrocardiographic changes (T wave flattening, S–T segment depression, Q–T prolongation)
Nausea and vomiting	
Orthostatic syncope	
Palpitations	
Sweating	
Tachycardia	Esophageal rupture
Thirst	Shock
Vertigo	

are also dose-related, the dose should rarely exceed 250 mg/d. Alcoholics taking disulfiram should be carefully cautioned about side effects, the risks of the alcohol-disulfiram reaction, and perhaps unrecognized sources of alcohol such as wine and vinegar sauces and medications that contain alcohol (eg, cough syrup). Occasionally, patients are sensitive to the alcohol in after-shave lotion or aerosol deodorants; therefore, use of talcum powder and alcohol-free deodorants may be advisable.

D. Treatment Settings and Effectiveness: Based on his extensive review, Baekeland (1977) concluded that only 2–15% of untreated alcoholics improve. This is in sharp contrast to the better prognosis for the estimated 15% of alcoholics and problem drinkers who are involved in formal treatment. There are 3 types of treatment settings for alcoholics: (1) specialized alcoholism treatment programs, (2) Alcoholics Anonymous, and (3) treatment by the individual physician. Each of these settings accounts for treatment of about one-third of the total population in treatment.

1. Specialized alcoholism treatment programs–The number of specialized treatment programs serving the alcoholic population has increased in recent years. Patients are self-referred to these programs or are referred by community agencies, physicians, and other professionals. Many of these programs include detoxification facilities, an inpatient rehabilitation unit, and an outpatient clinic.

a. Detoxification facilities–Detoxification may be done in one of 3 settings. To prevent late withdrawal reactions, patients should be carefully observed for at least 5 days.

Severely ill patients should be hospitalized and treated in a **general medical ward** or **specialized unit** capable of dealing with potential complications. Indications for admission include impending or frank delirium tremens; medical problems that might be aggravated by the stress of withdrawal; and severe functional problems, such as suicidal or homicidal ideation or a psychotic condition. Patients with a history of medical complications or delirium tremens during previous withdrawals should also be considered for hospitalization.

Since only 5% of alcoholics require hospitalization for detoxification, most can be managed in a **social model detoxification setting.** These centers provide a nonthreatening environment where the patient is kept active and provided with support and attention. Since the centers are usually staffed by nonprofessionals and are not licensed or staffed to handle severe illness or to dispense medications, patients referred to such settings should be ambulatory and physically well.

Finally, some alcoholics may be managed in an **outpatient clinic,** with withdrawal aided by use of benzodiazepines. This type of withdrawal program should be reserved for physically and psychologically stable patients who are well motivated and have friends or relatives who can give them support and monitor their use of minor tranquilizers.

b. Inpatient rehabilitation units–Inpatient rehabilitation units have become important settings for dealing with the sequelae of alcoholism. The length of stay may vary from 2 to 4 weeks or even longer. Rehabilitation units offer a variety of services, including general medical workups; disulfiram treatment; individual, group, and family therapy; recreational therapy; educational films and discussions; vocational testing and counseling; Alcoholics Anonymous groups; and careful attention to discharge planning, eg, help with finding a place to live and a temporary source of financial aid. Individuals referred to these units include patients who cannot remain abstinent outside a controlled setting, patients who need a period of hospitalization to stabilize their social situation, and patients who might benefit from an intensive therapeutic experience that may involve up to 10 hours a day. Alcoholics with severe psychiatric or medical disorders do not do well in these intense, demanding programs.

c. Outpatient alcohol clinics–Many of the treatment services offered by outpatient alcohol clinics parallel those described above. However, since patients often spend years enrolled in outpatient programs, the focus is on long-term management and the uncovering of predisposing causes. Alcoholics in outpatient programs must be able to function outside a controlled environment.

d. Effectiveness of programs–In several reviews of specialized treatment programs, 30–40% of alcoholics were found to be significantly improved after 1–2 years. These results were adjusted statistically to account for program dropouts and patients whose improvement was "spontaneous" (ie, could not be attributed to the treatment program). Success was measured as continuous abstinence or improved biomedical or psychosocial status. Outpatient programs are slightly more successful than inpatient programs, although combined programs give the best results. Treatment programs vary greatly, depending on patient motivation and treatment setting. Poorly motivated alcoholics who are ordered by a judge to participate as a way of retaining a license or staying out of jail improve at a rate of about 10%, whereas improvement rates approaching 70% have been reported in highly motivated patients enrolled in multifaceted programs and receiving support from family and employers. (Programs sponsored by employers to help alcoholic workers are discussed in Chapter 60.)

2. Alcoholics Anonymous–This organization was founded in 1935 by 2 recovering alcoholics. There are now almost 500,000 members in the USA and Canada alone. Alcoholics Anonymous is a self-help organization of nonprofessionals that emphasizes group support and surrender to a "higher power" to achieve permanent total abstinence. Sponsors and program members are available to help alcoholics 24 hours a day, and sober interactions are encouraged through frequent meetings and club activities.

Although Alcoholics Anonymous surveys usually report a 1-year continuous abstinence rate of nearly

60%, dropout rates are high, approaching 50% in the first 3 months. When these data are considered in the analysis, the 1-year improvement rate approximates that of specialized alcoholism treatment programs. Nevertheless, for those who accept the Alcoholics Anonymous model and remain in treatment, the program offers an important and often lifesaving source of support and abstinence. About half of those who participate for 3 months will be abstinent and continue to participate throughout the next year, and a member who has been abstinent for 1–5 years has a good chance (86%) of completing the following year without drinking. Spin-offs of Alcoholics Anonymous—such as Al-Anon and Alateen for adults and teenagers living with alcoholics—have been helpful in providing support.

3. Treatment by an individual physician–Individual physicians in private, clinic, or hospital based settings are an important treatment source for alcoholics. Although most physicians concern themselves with aspects of alcoholism treatment that represent their area of expertise, a growing number are taking an eclectic view that integrates biomedical, psychologic, and social factors in the treatment plan. It is critical that physicians familiarize themselves with community resources and establish channels for referrals to other professionals who may have more expertise in some aspects of treatment. Treatment approaches should be flexible, supportive, and nonjudgmental. Physicians should remember that alcoholism is a disorder characterized by loss of control over drinking behavior, frequent relapses, a chronic course, and a variety of causes and effects. The physician who takes

responsibility for constructing and coordinating all aspects of the patient's care (emotional, physical, etc) will be more likely to have a successful treatment plan.

E. Phases of Treatment for Alcoholism: In planning treatment for the alcoholic, the physician should base priorities on each patient's biomedical, psychologic, and social needs. The discussion below approaches treatment in terms of 4 sequential phases, each with typical problems and possible solutions (Table 26–4). However, not all patients enter treatment in phase 1 or 2, and some patients may skip a phase depending on individual needs.

1. Phase 1 (acute crisis)–In evaluation of an alcoholic, the first consideration is whether or not the patient is experiencing a life-threatening crisis (Table 26–4). The possibility of an acute medical or psychiatric emergency should be considered in *every* alcoholic. Although the specific details of treatment are beyond the scope of this chapter, measures usually include immediate hospitalization and vigorous medical or psychiatric intervention (eg, administration of intravenous fluids, precautions against suicide attempts, one-on-one nursing care). If family violence has occurred, family therapy and even a home visit by the staff may be useful. Alcoholic patients hospitalized for some other problem must be observed for the appearance of withdrawal symptoms.

2. Phase 2 (withdrawal from alcohol)–After acute crisis is ruled out, safe withdrawal from the effects of alcohol can be started (Table 26–4). Patients admitted to the hospital with delirium tremens should be placed in a well-lighted room and will require frequent observation (and possibly restraints). The prin-

Table 26–4. Phases of treatment for alcoholism.

Phase of Treatment	Typical Problems	Possible Solutions
Phase 1 (acute crisis)	Biomedical: Gastrointestinal bleeding; pneumonia; delirium tremens.	Hospitalization; appropriate medical intervention.
	Psychologic: Hallucinosis; paranoia; suicidal ideation.	Hospitalization; appropriate psychiatric intervention.
	Social: Family violence.	Hospitalization; appropriate psychiatric intervention; family therapy; home visit.
Phase 2 (withdrawal from alcohol)	Biomedical: Impending delirium tremens; withdrawal effects; acute medical problems.	Medical or social model detoxification; outpatient detoxification; appropriate medical intervention.
	Psychologic: Denial; worry about health; stressful life events.	Counseling; brief individual or group therapy.
	Social: Inadequate shelter; financial problems.	Counseling; social services referral.
Phase 3 (sequelae of alcoholism)	Biomedical: Chronic medical problems; malnutrition.	Appropriate medical intervention; vitamin supplements, proper diet, and exercise; disulfiram.
	Psychologic: Denial; depression; guilt; stressfull life events; psychologic craving for alcohol.	Counseling; brief individual or group therapy; antidepressants; lithium carbonate; behavior modification techniques.
	Social: Family, housing, vocational, and legal problems; loneliness; unfilled leisure time.	Counseling; social services referral; family therapy; recreational therapy; Alcoholics Anonymous, Al-Anon, or Alateen; alcoholic halfway house.
Phase 4 (focus on predisposing causes)	Biomedical: Genetic factors.	Counseling.
	Psychologic: Neurotic and personality disorders; major affective disorders; schizophrenia.	Long-term individual or group therapy; antidepressants; lithium carbonate; major tranquilizers.
	Social: Sociocultural and familial influences.	Counseling.

ciples of care include reassurance, careful monitoring of vital signs, and intravenous fluids with electrolytes and vitamins. Most alcoholics have low thiamine stores, and glucose solutions may cause further depletion of thiamine; therefore, thiamine should be added to intravenous fluids to prevent Wernicke's syndrome. Intravenous benzodiazepines are generally used, often in high doses, for delirium tremens. The physician must be alert to complications associated with delirium tremens (eg, seizures and marked autonomic hyperactivity) as well as the possibility of associated medical problems (eg, pneumonia or subdural hematoma). With treatment, most alcoholics recover from delirium tremens, although the mortality rate may reach 15%.

In addition to biomedical problems during the withdrawal period, psychosocial issues should also be addressed. Many alcoholics deny or minimize the extent of psychologic or social problems. Others are legitimately worried about their health or are recovering from a stressful life event, such as a death in the family or a divorce, that served as the occasion for the latest drinking spree. Supportive counseling or brief individual or group therapy may be instituted as soon as the patient's sensorium clears and the medical status improves. Since compliance with treatment may be affected by problems such as having no money and nowhere else to go, the physician may wish to offer advice about such matters or make referral to appropriate social service agencies.

3. Phase 3 (sequelae of alcoholism)– After acute problems and withdrawal have been dealt with, concern should focus on the sequelae of alcoholism. Some patients in this phase of treatment may be admitted directly to an outpatient clinic. Others with more tenuous biomedical and psychosocial status should first be admitted to an inpatient rehabilitation unit. As shown in Table 26–4, chronic medical problems such as peripheral neuropathy, cirrhosis, or organic brain syndrome should be managed appropriately. Vitamins and suitable instructions on the importance of diet and exercise will improve physical status. Disulfiram (Antabuse) should be prescribed for patients who need this added incentive to avoid alcohol.

Psychologically, many alcoholics experience depression, guilt, or the impact of stressful life events during this phase, particularly as the defense of denial begins to crumble. Counseling or brief individual or group therapy may help. Antidepressants or lithium carbonate may be useful for alcoholics with major affective disorders.

Newly abstinent alcoholics are particularly prone to experience a psychologic craving for alcohol. The intensity of the craving is correlated with anxiety or environmental factors such as seeing an advertisement for alcohol or experiencing a stressful life event. Behavior modification techniques that utilize aversive conditioning have been used to reduce craving. Mild electric shock or emetics such as apomorphine or emetine are given while the patient drinks in a controlled setting, usually an inpatient or rehabilitation

unit. The goal of such treatment is to create an aversion to alcohol that will persist after treatment. Aversive and other behavioral techniques are not effective as the sole form of treatment, but they have been used with success in multifaceted programs that address both drinking behavior and associated psychosocial problems. Covert sensitization (see Chapter 46) and other newer behavioral techniques that use fantasy and imagination to develop conditioned aversion to alcohol have also shown promise, although not all patients can be successfully trained to use these techniques.

Years of alcoholism may lead to family difficulties, inadequate shelter, a poor job history, legal and financial problems, loneliness, and trouble filling leisure time in a nonalcohol context. The physician may wish to counsel the patient on these matters or make referral to appropriate social agencies for food stamps, vocational counseling, etc. Family therapy may be helpful, since patterns of family interaction become more rigid when an alcoholic member is drinking than when he or she is sober. Recreational activities and hobbies may help the alcoholic fill leisure time. Alcoholics Anonymous is useful in giving support as well as encouraging and reinforcing abstinence. Al-Anon and Alateen may be useful for the spouse and children of alcoholics.

In some communities, another referral source is the alcoholic halfway house, which Rubington (1977) defines as "a transitional place of indefinite residence of a community of persons who live together under the rule and discipline of abstinence from alcohol and other drugs." This setting provides the abstinent alcoholic with a sober environment in the company of other recovering alcoholics able to offer support and advice. Food and shelter are provided, and many halfway houses have their own therapeutic programs that may include vocational counseling and informal "rap" groups. Although the stay is usually limited to a few months, many alcoholics are functioning at a higher level by this time and are ready to live independently.

4. Phase 4 (focus on predisposing causes)– After the sequelae of alcoholism have been managed, it is appropriate to focus on predisposing causes of the problem (Table 26–4). The physician should be sensitive to the patient's concerns involving genetic and sociocultural factors. Some alcoholics feel that genetic factors doom them to a life of alcoholism and approach treatment pessimistically for that reason. Others blame their religious or cultural background or are reluctant to seek treatment from physicians of different ethnic backgrounds. Counseling that emphasizes support and reassurance may be effective in alleviating concern, exploring stereotypes, and breaking cultural barriers.

For many alcoholics, psychologic issues are important predisposing causes of drinking. Diagnostically, these may include neurotic problems such as dysthymic and generalized anxiety or posttraumatic stress disorder; personality problems such as antisocial, dependent, or borderline disorder; major affective problems such as bipolar or major depressive disorder; and schizophrenia. For alcoholics with neurotic and borderline personality disorders, long-term individual therapy may be useful. Alcoholics with other personality disorders do best in group therapy. Therapy that emphasizes insight and interpersonal learning tends to be stressful for alcoholics, so they need additional group experiences providing support and emphasizing abstinence, such as that offered by Alcoholics Anonymous or a "rap" group. Kanas and Barr (1982) have recently described a therapeutic group for alcoholics that fosters insight and interpersonal learning as well as emphasizing support and sobriety. Assertiveness training groups have also been useful for many alcoholics. Finally, for alcoholics with major affective disorders or schizophrenia, treatment with antidepressants, lithium carbonate, or major tranquilizers may be helpful. Minor tranquilizers such as the benzodiazepines have addictive potential and should not be used for long periods.

SUMMARY

Alcoholism is a serious disorder characterized by loss of control over drinking; a chronic, relapsing course; and a number of biomedical, psychologic, and social causes and effects. *DSM-III* describes 2 forms of alcoholism: alcohol abuse and alcohol dependence. In the diagnostic workup, a complete history, mental status examination, and physical examination are essential, along with appropriate laboratory tests. Since alcoholism affects both sexes and people of all ages, races, and socioeconomic classes, the physician should be alert to its possibility when evaluating any patient. Case finding is made difficult by denial of alcoholism by patients, negative physician attitudes, and the presence of alcoholism among physicians.

Permanent abstinence is a major treatment goal for alcoholics. Therapeutic approaches should be flexible, supportive, and nonjudgmental. Important treatment settings include inpatient and social model detoxification units, inpatient rehabilitation wards, outpatient alcohol clinics, and alcoholic halfway houses. Disulfiram (Antabuse) and Alcoholics Anonymous are important adjuncts to treatment. By addressing issues involving acute crises, withdrawal, and sequelae and causes of alcoholism, the physician may play a key role in coordinating the treatment of alcoholic patients.

REFERENCES

General
US Department of Health, Education, and Welfare: *Special Report to the US Congress on Alcohol and Health*. [First, Second, Third, and Fourth Special Reports.] US Government Printing Office, 1971, 1974, 1978, and 1981.

Diagnostic Workup
Eckhardt MJ et al: Health hazards associated with alcohol consumption. *JAMA* 1981;**246:**648.

Kanas N: Stress and alcoholic denial. *J Drug Education* 1984;**14:**105.

Mayfield D, McLeod G, Hall P: The CAGE Questionnaire: Validation of a new alcoholism screening instrument. *Am J Psychiatry* 1974;**131:**1121.

Tarter RE, Schneider DU: Blackouts. *Arch Gen Psychiatry* 1976;**33:**1492.

Epidemiology
Adler I, Kandel DB: Cross-cultural perspectives on developmental stages in adolescent drug use. *J Stud Alcohol* 1981;**42:**701.

Baker SL Jr: The Veterans Administration Alcoholism Program. *Psychiatr Ann* 1982;**12:**443.

Baker SL Jr et al: The Veterans Administration Comparison Study: Alcoholism and drug abuse—Combined and conventional treatment settings. *Alcoholism: Clin Exp Res* 1977;**1:**285.

Bissell L, Jones RW: The alcoholic physician: A survey. *Am J Psychiatry* 1976;**133:**1142.

Eisterhold MJ et al: Multiple-drug use among high school students. *Psychol Rep* 1979;**44:**1099.

Kissin B: Theory and practice in the treatment of alcoholism. In: *The Biology of Alcoholism*. Vol 5: *Treatment and Rehabilitation of the Chronic Alcoholic*. Kissin B, Begleiter H (editors). Plenum Press, 1977.

Kliner DJ, Spicer J, Barnett P: Treatment outcome of alcoholic physicians. *J Stud Alcohol* 1980;**41:**1217.

Mirin SM, Weiss RD, Michael J: Alcohol abuse in patients dependent on other drugs. *Psychiatr Ann* 1982;**12:**430.

Murray RM: Alcoholism amongst male doctors in Scotland. *Lancet* 1976;**2:**729.

Murray RM: Characteristics and prognosis of alcoholic doctors. *Br Med J* 1976;**2:**1537.

Sutker PB et al: Alcoholics and opiate addicts: Comparison of personality characteristics. *J Stud Alcohol* 1979;**40:**635.

Weissman MM, Myers JK, Harding PS: Prevalence and psychiatric heterogeneity of alcoholism in a United States urban community. *J Stud Alcohol* 1980;**41:**672.

Etiology, Pathogenesis, & Natural History
Alexopoulos GS et al: Platelet MAO during the alcohol withdrawal syndrome. *Am J Psychiatry* 1981;**138:**1254.

Ballenger JC et al: Alcohol and central serotonin metabolism in man. *Arch Gen Psychiatry* 1979;**36:**224.

Goodwin DW: Alcoholism and heredity: A review and hypothesis. *Arch Gen Psychiatry* 1979;**36:**57.

Kanas N: Alcoholic liver disease: An eclectic approach to the treatment of the chronic alcoholic. In: *Hepatology*. Zakim D, Boyer T (editors). Saunders, 1982.

Kolakowska T, Swigar ME: Thyroid function in depression and alcohol abuse: A retrospective study. *Arch Gen Psychiatry* 1977;**34:**984.

Vaillant GE: Natural history of male psychological health. 8. Antecedents of alcoholism and orality. *Am J Psychiatry* 1980;**137:**181.

Treatment & Prognosis

Baekeland F: Evaluation of treatment methods in chronic alcoholism. In: *The Biology of Alcoholism*. Vol 5: *Treatment and Rehabilitation of the Chronic Alcoholic*. Kissin B, Begleiter H (editors). Plenum Press, 1977.

Chappel JN et al: Substance abuse attitude changes in medical students. *Am J Psychiatry* 1977;**134**:379.

Costello RM: Alcoholism treatment and evaluation: In search of methods II. *Int J Addict* 1975;**10**:857.

Finney JW, Moss RH: Characteristics and prognoses of alcoholics who become moderate drinkers and abstainers after treatment. *J Stud Alcohol* 1981;**42**:94.

Fisher JC et al: Physicians and alcoholics: The effect of medical training on attitudes toward alcoholics. *J Stud Alcohol* 1975;**36**:949.

Goldstein M, Nakajima K: The effect of disulfiram on catecholamine levels in the brain. *J Pharmacol Exp Ther* 1967;**157**:96.

Kanas N: Alcoholism and group psychotherapy. In: *Encyclopedic Handbook of Alcoholism*. Pattison EM, Kaufman E (editors). Gardner Press, 1982.

Kanas N: Multi-factor group therapy for alcoholics. *Curr Psychiatr Ther* 1982;**21**:149.

Kanas N, Barr MA: Outpatient alcoholics view group therapy. *Group* (Spring) 1982;**6**:17.

Kitson TM: The disulfiram-ethanol reaction: A review. *J Stud Alcohol* 1977;**38**:96.

Kwentus J, Major LF: Disulfiram in the treatment of alcoholism: A review. *J Stud Alcohol* 1979;**40**:428.

Ludwig AM et al: Loss of control in alcoholics. *Arch Gen Psychiatry* 1978;**35**:370.

Major LF et al: Dopamine-beta-hydroxylase in the cerebrospinal fluid: Relationship to disulfiram-induced psychosis. *Biol Psychiatry* 1979;**14**:337.

Matthew RJ, Claghorn JL, Largen J: Craving for alcohol in sober alcoholics. *Am J Psychiatry* 1979;**136**:603.

Nathan PE, Briddell DW: Behavioral assessment and treatment of alcoholism. In: *The Biology of Alcoholism*. Vol 5: *Treatment and Rehabilitation of the Chronic Alcoholic*. Kissin B, Begleiter H (editors). Plenum Press, 1977.

Pendery ML, Maltzman IM, West LJ: Controlled drinking by alcoholics? New findings and a reevaluation of a major affirmative study. *Science* 1982;**217**:169.

Rubington E: The role of the halfway house in the rehabilitation of alcoholics. In: *The Biology of Alcoholism*. Vol 5: *Treatment and Rehabilitation of the Chronic Alcoholic*. Kissin B, Begleiter H (editors). Plenum Press, 1977.

Shapiro RJ: A family therapy approach to alcoholism. *J Marriage Fam Counsel* 1971;**3**:71.

Thompson WL: Management of alcohol withdrawal syndromes. *Arch Intern Med* 1978;**138**:278.

Schizophrenic Disorders

27

Stuart R. Schwartz, MD, & Bruce Africa, MD, PhD

Schizophrenia is a major psychiatric disturbance that includes a wide range of severely disordered behavior. The clinical picture invariably shows thought disturbances, often with characteristic symptoms such as hallucinations and delusions, bizarre behavior, and deterioration in the general level of functioning. Schizophrenia is often discussed as though it were a single entity, but it is more appropriately considered a group of disorders of unknown cause that result in severe and prolonged mental distubance. For this reason, the *DSM-III-R* heading is schizophrenic disorders rather than schizophrenia. Both terms are used in this chapter.

In the USA, the number of persons who will be hospitalized at some point for treatment of schizophrenia is one in 100. An estimated 2 million new cases occur throughout the world each year at enormous human and financial cost.

History of Schizophrenia

Although the diagnostic definition of schizophrenia continues to be the subject of study and debate, descriptions of an apparently schizophrenic disorder have been found that date back to 1400 BC. In 1852, the Belgian psychiatrist Benedict Augustine Morel described a condition in which a young person experienced severe emotional and intellectual disturbance, which he labeled *"démence précoce."* Other European psychiatrists in the late 19th century described similar severe, disabling mental disturbances and classified them as distinct diseases, eg, catatonia, paranoia, and hebephrenia.

In 1896, Emil Kraepelin, a German psychiatrist, classified several previously described major psychiatric disorders into 2 groups based on outcome and course. He used the term "manic-depressive psychosis" for the group of disorders characterized chiefly by exacerbations and remissions in disturbances of affect rather than thinking. "Dementia praecox" was the term used for the other major group of disorders, which featured severe disturbances in functioning (eg, catatonia, hebephrenia) that began in adolescence and progressively worsened. Kraepelin did note that there were variations in course and that some 13% of those people with apparent dementia praecox recovered without residual deficit.

Eugen Bleuler, a Swiss psychiatrist, introduced the term schizophrenia, which means "splitting of the mind," to describe a syndrome marked by autism (a turning inward away from the world), ambivalence, and primary disturbances in affect and associations. Bleuler provided an excellent picture of the psychologic characteristics of the disorder, although, like Kraepelin, he assumed that eventually an underlying biologic determinant would be discovered.

In the early 20th century, Adolf Meyer, working in the USA, emphasized the importance of stress in the genesis of all mental illness and applied his unified psychobiologic approach to understanding the major psychotic disorders as well as the neurotic disorders. In the 1930s and 1940s, Harry Stack Sullivan contributed to an understanding of how interpersonal relationships are influenced by and causally related to schizophrenia. Kurt Schneider, in post-World War II Germany, highlighted certain characteristic disturbances of thinking which, though not pathognomonic, have proved useful in assisting in the diagnosis of schizophrenia.

A great deal of controversy and confusion has risen over the years about the definition and meaning of the term "schizophrenia." The marked variability in the clinical picture seen over an individual's lifetime leads to contradictory impressions on the part of different observers, who may see the patient at different times and thereby gain dissimilar perspectives. The more recent diagnostic consensus of *DSM-III-R* may serve to clarify the picture for both clinicians and researchers, since it provides a synthesis between a focus on symptoms (Bleuler, Schneider) and on clinical course (Kraepelin) (Table 27–1).

The currently accepted concept of the schizophrenic disorders recognizes disorganization of a previous level of functioning, characteristic symptoms involving multiple psychologic processes, clear-cut psychotic features during the active phase of the illness, and a tendency toward chronicity.

Symptoms & Signs

Schizophrenia always involves disorganization of a previous level of functioning. Family and friends observe that the person has changed and is no longer the same ("She's not herself anymore"). The individual functions poorly in significant areas of routine daily living, such as work and social relations. There is often a notable lack of concern for self-care in an individual who has previously been capable of it. As they lose their grip on reality, patients experience the following feelings:

Table 27–1. *DSM-III-R* diagnostic criteria for schizophrenic disorders.

A. Presence of characteristic psychotic symptoms in the active phase: either (1), (2), or (3) for at least 1 week (unless the symptoms are successfully treated):
  (1) Two of the following: delusions; prominent hallucinations (throughout the day for several days or several times a week for several weeks, each hallucinatory experience not being limited to a few brief moments); incoherence or marked loosening of associations; catatonic behavior; flat or grossly inappropriate affect.
  (2) Bizarre delusions (ie, involving a phenomenon that the person's culture would regard as totally implausible, eg, thought broadcasting, being controlled by a dead person).
  (3) Prominent hallucinations (as defined above) of a voice with content having no apparent relation to depression or elation, or a voice keeping up a running commentary on the person's behavior or thoughts, or 2 or more voices conversing with each other.
B. During the course of the disturbance, functioning in such areas as work, social relations, and self-care is markedly below the highest level achieved before onset of the disturbance (or when the onset is in childhood or adolescence, failure to achieve expected level of social development).
C. Schizoaffective disorder and mood disorder with psychotic features have been ruled out, ie, if a major depressive or manic syndrome has ever been present during an active phase of the disturbance, the total duration of all episodes of a mood syndrome has been brief relative to the total duration of the active and residual phases of the disturbance.
D. Continuous signs of the disturbance for at least 6 months. The 6-month period must include an active phase (of at least 1 week, or less if symptoms successfully treated) during which there were psychotic symptoms characteristic of schizophrenia (symptoms in criterion A), with or without a prodromal or residual phase, as defined below.
  Prodromal phase: A clear deterioration in functioning before the active phase of the disturbance that is not due to a disturbance in mood or to a psychoactive substance use disorder and that involves at least 2 of the symptoms listed below.
  Residual phase: Following the active phase of the disturbance, persistence of at least 2 of the symptoms noted below, these not being due to a disturbance in mood or to a psychoactive substance use disorder.
  Prodromal or Residual Symptoms:
  (1) Marked social isolation or withdrawal.
  (2) Marked impairment in role functioning as wage-earner, student, or homemaker.
  (3) Markedly peculiar behavior (eg, collecting garbage, talking to self in public, hoarding food).
  (4) Marked impairment in personal hygiene and grooming.
  (5) Blunted or inappropriate affect.
  (6) Digressive, vague, overelaborate, or circumstantial speech, or poverty of speech, or poverty of content of speech.
  (7) Odd beliefs or magical thinking, influencing behavior and inconsistent with cultural norms, eg, superstitiousness, belief in clairvoyance, telepathy, "sixth sense," "others can feel my feelings," overvalued ideas, ideas of reference.
  (8) Unusual perceptual experiences, eg, recurrent illusions, sensing the presence of a force or person not actually present.
  (9) Marked lack of initiative, interests, or energy.
  Examples: Six months of prodromal symptoms with 1 week of symptoms from criterion A; no prodromal symptoms with 6 months of symptoms from criterion A; no prodromal symptoms with 1 week of symptoms from criterion A and 6 months of residual symptoms.
E. It cannot be established that an organic factor initiated and maintained the disturbance.
F. If there is a history of autistic disorder, the additional diagnosis of schizophrenia is made only if prominent delusions or hallucinations are also present.

(1) Perplexity– At the onset of illness, patients report a sense of strangeness about the experience as well as confusion about where the voices are coming from and why their everyday experience is so markedly changed.

(2) Isolation– The schizophrenic person experiences an overwhelming sense of being different and separate from other people. The work of Frieda Fromm-Reichmann (1950) highlights the intense loneliness experienced by these patients.

(3) Anxiety and terror– A general sense of discomfort and anxiety often pervades the experience. It is sharpened by periods of intense terror caused by a world within that is experienced as dangerous or uncontrollable.

In schizophrenia, severe disturbances occur in several of the following areas: language and communication, content of thought, perception, affect, sense of self, volition, relationship to the external world, and motor behavior. Any of these symptoms may be seen in other psychologic disturbances, and none by itself is pathognomonic of schizophrenia. Furthermore, individuals who are well adapted and who have no evidence of any underlying psychopathologic disorder may when under stress exhibit a symptom that is similar to that seen in schizophrenic persons. It is the number of psychologic processes involved and the degree of impairment over time that characterize schizophrenia. Disabling symptoms characteristic of schizophrenia do not preclude development of other psychiatric disorders, nor are schizophrenic patients devoid of ordinary human characteristics—feelings, thoughts, and actions.

A. Disturbances in Language and Communication: The schizophrenic individual thinks and reasons according to private and often idiosyncratic rules of logic. The form of thinking is disordered (formal thought disorder). The individual cannot maintain a consistent train of thought. Ideas slip from one track to another, and communication is severely impaired (so-called **derailment** or **looseness of associations**). **Circumstantiality** (irrelevant detours in speech) or **tangentiality** (continuing digression in speech, so that the conversion fails to reach the anticipated goal) may also occur. There may be **poverty of content of speech,** in which little information is communicated, because many words are vague, overabstract, overconcrete, repetitive, or stereotyped. A more severe symptom is the formation of **neologisms;** the schizophrenic individual's speech is filled with "new words" formed by condensing and combining several known words in a manner unique to the individual, who may often be able to provide a precise definition that may have personal magical or wish-fulfilling properties. Complete incoherence of speech (**word salad**) may occur, with a mixture of words lacking meaning and logical coherence.

The disorder in thought permeates many areas of the patient's life and may be shown not only in language but also in work and personal creative efforts (eg, arts, crafts). Maher (1972) has offered a few excellent examples of the thought disorder of the schizophrenic patient:

> The subterfuge and the mistaken planned substitutions for that demanded American action can produce nothing but the general results of negative contention and the impractical results of careless application, the natural results of misplacement of mistaken purpose and unrighteous position, the impractical serviceabilities of unnecessary contradictions.

Another patient wrote:

> If things turn by rotation of agriculture or levels in regards and timed to everything: I am referring to a previous document when I made some remarks that were facts also tested and there is another that concerns my daughter she has a lobed bottom right ear, her name being Mary Lou. . . . Much of abstraction has been left unsaid and undone in this product/milk syrup, and others due to economics, differentials, subsidies, bankruptcy, tools, buildings, bonds, national stocks, foundation craps, weather, trades, government in levels of breakages, and fuses in electronics to all formerly "stated" not necessarily factuated.

In a case reported by McGhie and Chapman (1961), the patient describes the experience of tangentiality and looseness of association as follows:

> My thoughts get all jumbled up. I start thinking or talking about something but I never get there. Instead, I wander off in the wrong direction and get caught up with all sorts of different things that may be connected with the things I want to say but in a way I can't explain. People listening to me get more lost than I do.

It is important to emphasize that the disturbance in language and communication described above cannot be attributed to lack of education, low intelligence, or a certain cultural background.

B. Disturbances in Content of Thought: Things go on in the mind of a schizophrenic patient that do not go on in the minds of other people. Distortions of reality lead to incorrect conclusions.

A **delusion** is a false belief that may be fixed (ie, maintained over an extended period) or temporary. Certain delusions are particularly characteristic of schizophrenia, such as the notion that one's thoughts are being broadcast into the external world so that others can hear them; or that thoughts are inserted into one's mind by another individual or superior force; or that an individual or machine is dominating and controlling one's life (**delusion of influence**).

Ideas of reference are also common in schizophrenia; ie, events that are in reality unrelated to the patient are invested with a personal significance (eg, a newspaper article or television program may be seen to have a special personal message that relates directly to the patient). Delusional themes are often persecutory (belief that one is being watched, followed, or plotted against); grandiose (belief that one has special powers, influence, or wealth); or somatic (belief that something is rotting inside one's body). In normal adolescence, people often experience a feeling of heightened self-consciousness and the feeling that others can read their private feelings. The schizophrenic patient experiences similar feelings with far greater intensity, distress, and conviction.

In the autobiography *Memoirs of My Nervous Illness,* Schreber (1955) states:

> I can put this point briefly: everything that happens is in reference to me. Writing this sentence, I am aware that other people may be tempted to think that I am pathologically conceited: I know very well that this tendency to relate everything to oneself, to bring everything that happens into connection with one's own person is a common phenomenon among mental patients. But in my case, the very reverse obtains. Since God entered into nerve-contact with me exclusively, I become in a way for God the only human being or simply the human being around whom everything turns, to whom everything that happens must be related and who, therefore, from his own point of view, must also relate all things to himself.

McDonald (1960) described the thought disturbances as follows:

> Not knowing that I was ill, I made no attempt to understand what was happening, but felt that there was some overwhelming significance in all of this, produced either by God or Satan. . . . The walk of a stranger on the street could be a "sign" to me which I must interpret. Every face in the windows of a passing streetcar would be engraved on my mind, all of them concentrating on me and trying to pass me some sort of message.

C. Disturbances in Perception: Hallucinations are false perceptions in the absence of an external stimulus. In schizophrenia, these are usually auditory. Visual, tactile, and olfactory hallucinations are more common in organic mental states. In auditory hallucinations, voices seem to speak directly to the patient or make comments (frequently negative) on the patient's behavior. Hallucinations must be distinguished from **illusions,** which are false interpretations of a real stimulus.

D. Disturbances in Affect: Affect, or "feeling tone," refers to the outward expression of emotion, as opposed to mood, which is inferred from affect or the patient's own statements. In schizophrenia, affect may be inappropriate, ie, inconsistent with the topic or context of communication. It may be extremely labile, showing rapid shifts from tears to joy for no obvious reason. It may be flattened, with virtually no signs of emotional expression; the voice may be monotonous and the face immobile. Patients may state that they no longer respond to life with normal intensity or that they are "losing their feelings."

Physicians must be cautious in evaluating the affect of a schizophrenic patient, because prior use of antipsychotic drugs to treat severe agitation may often produce a state that is nearly identical to the flattening of the affect described above.

E. Disturbances in Sense of Self: Schizophrenic patients have lost touch with who they are. They may have doubts, concerns, and worries about the very nature of their identity. They may feel that the very core of their identity is vulnerable or changing in some mysterious way. The overwhelming sense of perplexity about this feeling is then translated into concerns about the meaning of existence. Two patients' statements, as reported by Mendel (1976), were as follows:

> I have experienced this process chiefly as a condition in which the integrating mental picture in my personality was taken away and smashed to bits, leaving me like agitated hamburger, distributed evenly throughout the universe.

> I am like a zombie living behind a glass wall. I can see all that goes on in the world, but I can't touch it. I can't reach it. I can't be in contact with it. I am outside. They are inside, and when I get inside, they aren't there. There is nothing there, absolutely nothing.

F. Disturbances in Volition: In schizophrenia, disturbance in self-initiated, goal-directed activity is invariable and may grossly impair work performance or functioning in other roles. The disruption takes the form either of inadequate interest or drive or of inability to complete a course of action successfully. Overwhelming ambivalence, which directs the individual toward 2 diametrically opposed courses of action, may lead to a stalemate with no goal-directed activity. In contrast, in the early stages of schizophrenia, there may sometimes be a sense of mission, with a resulting outpouring of energy to complete a particular task, which is often bizarre.

G. Disturbances in Relationship to the External World: The individual with schizophrenia tends to withdraw from involvement with other people and to direct attention inward toward egocentric and illogical ideas and fantasies. The word autistic (derived from the Greek word *autos,* meaning *self*) has been used to describe the overwhelming, self-centered concerns of the patient with a schizophrenic disorder.

H. Disturbances in Motor Behavior: Motor disturbances range from a markedly decreased reaction to the environment to almost total reduction of spontaneous movements and activity (catatonic stu-

por), in which the individual acts like a zombie. The schizophrenic individual may assume strange postures with bizarre mannerisms. At other times, individuals may become wildly aggressive and difficult to control; they may move about constantly, stopping only when exhaustion sets in.

Types of Schizophrenia

Schizophrenic disorders are divided into 5 subtypes on the basis of distinctive clustering of symptoms.

A. Disorganized Type: (Formerly called hebephrenia.) Features include incoherence; lack of systematized delusions; and blunted, inappropriate, or silly affect. The clinical picture is usually associated with a history of poor functioning and poor adaptation even before illness, an early and insidious onset, and a chronic course without significant remissions. Social impairment is usually extreme.

B. Catatonic Type: Features include either excitement or stupor and mutism, negativism, rigidity, and posturing.

C. Paranoid Type: Features include persecutory and grandiose delusions, delusional jealousy, and persecutory or grandiose hallucinations. Associated features include anger, argumentativeness, violence, fearfulness, delusions of reference, and concerns about autonomy, gender identity, and sexual preference. Onset occurs later in life than in other types of schizophrenia, and symptoms persist more than in other types, with no waxing and waning. Functioning also remains at a more or less constant level and is not marked by deterioration and recovery. Patients in this subgroup may be quite intelligent and well informed.

D. Undifferentiated Type: Features include grossly disorganized behavior, hallucinations, incoherence, or prominent delusions.

E. Residual Type: Features include current lack of schizophrenic symptoms but definite experience of at least one schizophrenic episode in the past. There may be some delusions and hallucinations, but the person is "burned-out" and is not immersed in the fresh turmoil of the florid, active phase. These patients often function as long-term outpatients but are incapable of maintaining gainful employment.

In the 1980s, more emphasis has been placed on a simplified but useful distinction between type I and type II schizophrenia (Crow, 1985). **Type I schizophrenia** is characterized by the "positive symptoms" of hallucinations or delusions, bizarre, agitated behavior, and disorganized speech. These symptoms are more frequently seen in the earlier years of psychosis and are usually suppressed by conventional neuroleptics. **Type II schizophrenia** is characterized by emotional blunting, social withdrawal, poverty of speech and motor activity, and cognitive deficits; these symptoms indicate a poor prognosis, even in an acute episode, and they become more common in chronic illness. Type II schizophrenia usually is associated with a family history of schizophrenia, deficits in premorbid development, and less favorable response to conventional neuroleptics (Kay and coworkers, 1986).

Natural History

The onset of schizophrenia usually occurs in adolescence, although paranoid schizophrenia may appear for the first time in childhood or when patients are in their early 30s. In some patients, the onset of illness is sudden; in others, prodromal symptoms are present for days, weeks, or months before clear-cut schizophrenic symptoms appear. Depression, anxiety, suspiciousness, hypochondriasis, marked difficulty in concentrating, and restlessness are the usual prodromal symptoms. The patient often presents initially to a family physician and emphasizes hypochondriac concerns or bizarre somatic delusions. There is commonly some event in the person's life that triggers the development or worsening of schizophrenia. Such psychosocial sources of stress are often understated as the individual deals with retreat from a painful reality. In other patients, it is impossible to define a clear-cut precipitating event or stressful happening.

The characteristic presentation of schizophrenia is a gradual withdrawal from people, activities, and social contacts, with increasing concern for abstract and sometimes idiosyncratic ideas. The acute stage of psychosis may be florid, with prominent hallucinations, delusions, and severe disorders in thinking. After the active psychotic period, there is often a stage of postpsychotic depression that may last many months, even when treated. Gradually, symptoms may disappear, and the person may recover with no residual deficits; a long remission may follow. Some patients experience only a single recurrence and remain symptom-free for most of their lives. Although the course of illness can fluctuate over several decades following its onset in early adulthood, a characteristic and relatively stable expression of illness is usually established in each individual within the first 5 years.

Each recurrence of illness leads to increasing impairment. Patients who are severely affected are able to function only marginally in the community and usually have periodic relapses requiring rehospitalization. Those patients whose illnesses are chronic, progressive, and deteriorating require lifetime hospitalization or continuous supervision.

Zubin and Spring (1977) have emphasized that the one feature all schizophrenic patients have in common is not persistent illness but rather persistent vulnerability. Some patients are highly vulnerable and have repeated or almost continual episodes of illness, whereas others are less vulnerable and have few episodes. When episodes develop in this latter group, they are not lifelong. Eventually, they remit, with or without treatment. Most schizophrenic patients today spend most of their lives in the community and are superficially indistinguishable from the rest of the population.

After the active phase of illness, impairment may vary widely. During the acute stage, psychotic symptoms are always associated with significant impairment. The individual may require hospitalization to ensure that basic needs are met and that poor judgment does not lead to complications, such as marked failure in social relations, work, and education; gross personal neglect; suicide; and violent behavior. Although there are many sensationalized accounts of violent acts committed by psychotic individuals, most people with schizophrenia are not dangerous to others. It is not known whether the incidence of violent acts is higher in patients with schizophrenia than in the nonschizophrenic population. The suicide rate is higher than that in the general population, and life expectancy is lower even when only nonsuicidal deaths are considered.

Two prospective studies have followed the development of schizophrenia over more than 20 years. Though one took place before the widespread use of antipsychotic medications (Bleuler, 1978), both found that only 40% of patients with diagnosed schizophrenia are overtly ill throughout their lifetime; 40% have a phasic course; and 20% recover without deficit, usually after a single episode (Huber & coworkers, 1975).

Differential Diagnosis

The differential diagnosis must consider organic mental disorders, which often have a bizarre presentation with delusions and hallucinations similar to those of schizophrenia. Disorientation and memory impairment strongly suggest an organic mental disorder. Toxic psychosis associated with use of amphetamines, LSD, or phencyclidine may have symptoms identical to those of schizophrenia. Any history of drug use provided by such a patient is notoriously unreliable, but the diagnosis becomes apparent when a toxic condition clears up dramatically after only a few days of closely supervised observation. Organic disorders associated with alcohol use may mimic schizophrenia, particularly a chronic paranoid type. Metabolic and circulatory diseases such as hyperthyroidism or cerebral arteriosclerosis must be ruled out.

It is important to distinguish schizophrenia from major affective disorders, since the course and appropriate treatment of these disorders differ markedly. Until 10 years ago, it was not appreciated that patients with affective disorders, particularly when they were acutely psychotic, could present the signs and symptoms of schizophrenia (Pope and Lipinski, 1978). The course of disease in a typical patient with an affective disorder is generally intermittent, with symptom-free intervals between episodes of illness. The course in schizophrenia, on the other hand, is usually downhill, and the schizophrenic patient is always markedly vulnerable to stress. A family history of affective disorder helps to establish the diagnosis of affective psychosis rather than schizophrenia. Other conditions such as schizophreniform or atypical psychoses may resemble schizoprenia at one point in the clinical picture but have a different course. Occasionally, severe neuroses such as obsessive compulsive disorder or phobic disorder may seem to have a delusional component similar to that of schizophrenia. Severe personality disorders may have transient psychotic symptoms similar to those of schizophrenia, but in contrast to schizophrenia, there are periods of much better levels of functioning. In mental retardation, the low level of functioning and odd behavior with impoverished affect may suggest long-standing chronic schizophrenia.

Individuals who are members of subcultural or religious groups may have beliefs or experiences that are difficult to distinguish from pathologic delusions or hallucinations. When such experiences can be explained because of their known association with such subcultural groups or values, they should not be considered evidence of schizophrenia. The developmental struggles of adolescence may also resemble the onset of a pattern of abnormal thinking. Even an experienced observer may have difficulty making the correct clinical diagnosis of schizophrenia.

Psychologic tests such as the Rorschach (inkblots), TAT (Thematic Apperception Test), or MMPI (Minnesota Multiphasic Personality Inventory) may assist in diagnosis (see Chapter 21).

Prognosis

There are 2 schools of thought regarding the prognosis of schizophrenia. The first, derived from Kraepelin's original concept, views schizophrenia as an irreversible, deteriorating disorder with a negative prognosis. If the individual recovers, therefore, it is assumed that the wrong diagnosis was made. A second, more favorable view emphasizes that schizophrenic individuals may have extended remissions with improvements in functioning, although social function does not return to the level shown before the patient became ill. Both schools of thought regard schizophrenia as a chronic disorder, characterized by deterioration and impaired function.

The clinician attempting to provide a prognosis for a schizophrenic patient must consider not only the symptoms but also the total picture of that individual: abilities, as well as disabilities, and assets as well as liabilities, as Mendel (1976) pointed out. The clinician must evaluate the stresses and demands made on the patient, the world in which the patient lives, and the one the patient creates for himself or herself.

The prognosis is good if the onset of illness is sudden and a precipitating stress is clearly identifiable. The outcome is also more favorable if the patient's social functioning was at least adequate before illness developed and if the patient performs successfully in a work situation outside the family environment.

The prognosis is poor if the onset of illness is insidious, with slowly emerging symptoms and no clearly identifiable precipitating stress. Likewise, if the individual was not functioning adequately (socially, economically, or intellectually) before the onset of illness, the outlook is unfavorable. The major conclusion of many studies is that poor prior functioning predicts poor outcome and that current chronicity predicts future chronicity. Recent data from a 20-year prospective study indicate that as this chronic illness progresses, the significance of certain prognostic factors (predictors) changes. For example, in the first decade, the social level of functioning reached by the patient before the onset of illness is a positive predictor. In the second decade, the presence of affective symptoms (especially depression) is a positive predictor, whereas symptoms of paranoia or assaultiveness and family overinvolvement are negative predictors. Beyond the second decade, a family history of schizophrenia is the most important negative prognostic factor.

Illustrative Case

A 25-year-old divorced woman with no personal or family history of psychiatric treatment entered a psychiatric hospital only after coercion by her employer, who had discovered that she was the author of several vaguely threatening but clearly psychotic anonymous notes to her coworkers; when faced with the choice of losing her job or accepting treatment, the patient reluctantly entered the hospital. She was articulate, and she appeared to be "normal" except for her allusions to "months of torment," which she blamed on a neighbor. In the first days of hospitalization, she stated that her treating physician looked like the neighbor; she then decided that he was indeed her persecutor, and another psychiatrist was asked to assume care of the patient. Insisting that there was nothing wrong with her, the patient refused to take any medication that might lessen her alertness or sense of control as she attempted to defend herself from her ongoing torment.

The patient was the third of 4 children of a "pseudomutual" family, wherein family members seemed to be mutually helping each other and getting along well but in actuality were intruding on and intensely involved with each other's business, often making decisions "for your own good" and denying the existence of any conflict. The patient described her increasing loneliness over the 4 years since her divorce and her frustration over becoming more and more dependent on her family for any social contact ouside of work. Nine months before admission to the hospital, the patient was appropriately approached by a male neighbor, who invited her out for a social drink. Within 24 hours, the patient was immersed in a world in which planes were dive-bombing her house, other people could read her mind, she was being physically subjected to pains from unseen radiation sources, and the actions of other people all seemed to fit into a pattern which she could not understand but which clearly was directed at her. For over 8 months, the patient continued to exist in this world and to work as a secretary. Her paranoid fears, however, led her to write threatening notes. The notes were discovered by her employer, and she was hospitalized.

Although the patient acknowledged that she was able to talk and relate openly to the therapist, she felt that she remained safe only because she was in the hospital. The patient had also revealed during the course of therapy that she had a handgun at home. She said that her torment was so severe that she had no choice but to attempt to end either her own life or that of the other physician, whom she now identified as her persecutor. This last statement provided the rationale for an involuntary transfer to a locked psychiatric unit, where the patient was told that she could either take pills or receive injections of haloperidol. The transfer between wards within the same hospital was personally supervised by the psychiatrist, who continued to be the psychotherapist throughout treatment. The patient was able to tolerate 15 mg of haloperidol during the first day; this was rapidly increased to 30 mg a night during the rest of her hospital stay. Within 3 days, it appeared that the patient still had a good working relationship with the therapist, and within 1 week after medication was started, the patient returned to an open unit. A month after haloperidol had been started, the patient exhibited acceptable behavior on a weekend pass away from the hospital, and she was discharged from the hospital the following week.

The life course of this patient, who is profoundly disturbed but possesses great potential in terms of intelligence, willingness to work, and goals admired and sanctioned by society, largely depends on 2 factors. One is the extent to which the patient can maintain a therapeutic relationship with the one person who she agrees seems to understand her situation and whom she trusts at this point. The other factor is whether the patient will gradually accept the idea that a maintenance dose of haloperidol is required to reduce the severity of symptoms and prevent the psychotic episodes that have interrupted her life. She may never achieve all of her goals and may require future hospitalization but need not be institutionalized indefinitely.

Epidemiology

Studies of the epidemiology of schizophrenia have made possible useful estimates of the extent of schizophrenia within a given society, identification of subgroups of the population that appear to be more at risk, and characteristics of these populations that may predispose them to this illness. These results have been achieved despite the fact that the schizophrenic disorders have a wide range of clinical presentations and outcomes. The major difficulties in epidemiologic studies have been the differences in diagnostic criteria, absence of a definitive conceptual framework, and lack of a clearly established cause.

The importance of diagnostic criteria in epidemiologic studies was made clear by the 1968 United States-United Kingdom study, which showed that schizophrenia was diagnosed twice as often in New York as in London (Cooper and coworkers, 1972). It was subsequently established that these supposed major differences in the rates of prevalence of schizophrenia and manic-depressive disease reflected differences in diagnostic criteria, not differences in the clinical presentations within the 2 cultures. Further confidence in epidemiologic data was established by the 1973 World Health Organization study, which demonstrated that investigators in 9 widely different world cultures could achieve high reliability among themselves (80–90%) when they used agreed-upon diagnostic criteria both within their own cultures and in each of the other cultures studied.

The best current source of treated prevalence data in the USA comes from the Monroe County (NY) Psychiatric Case Register (Babigian, 1980). (Treated prevalence data involve the number of people who receive treatment for a particular problem, in contrast to the true prevalence of a disease, ie, the number of people who have the disease, whether or not they receive treatment.) Begun in 1960, the case register continues to report on patient care in a county of about 800,000 people, which includes the city of Rochester, New York. The data base is unusually complete, including all patients treated in both private and public facilities.

Data from Monroe County are consistent with those from many other sources and are summarized below. Data from different sources usually differ by no more than a factor of 1.5–2, and there have never been discrepancies that approach an order of magnitude.

The incidence of schizophrenia within the total population would appear to be from 0.3 to 0.6 per 1000, and the treated prevalence rate for any given year is about 4 per 1000. The lifetime treated prevalence rate in the Monroe County study was 13 per 1000, from which it was calculated that there is about a 1% lifetime risk of developing schizophrenia in the general population. The incidence of first treatment is highest for men aged 15–24 years; for women, the peak appears between 25 and 34 years of age (Loranger, 1984). It is not known if these figures reflect a difference in the time of onset of psychosis, a difference in society's tolerance of disturbed behavior in men compared with women, or difference in treatment between the sexes. For both sexes, however, the number of those in treatment peaks between the ages of 35 and 44 years, reflecting the chronicity of the disease. Of those schizophrenics who are in treatment, 90% are between the ages of 15 and 54 years.

The incidence of schizophrenia apparently remained stable in the USA over the 100-year period ending in 1950, but this is expected to change (Erlenmeyer-Kimling and coworkers, 1966). The reproductive rate of schizophrenic individuals has always been much lower than that of the population as a whole until recently, and this was thought to reflect both the high mortality rate associated with schizophrenia and the limitations on family formation caused both by the disease and by hospitalization for treatment. A comparison of reproductive rates in the schizophrenic population shows that the rate had almost doubled between 1934–1936 and 1954–1956 and was approaching that of the nonschizophrenic population. Most of this increase may be attributed to increased rates of marriage and childbirth among schizophrenic patients living in the community after hospital discharge. Since it is known that the incidence of schizophrenia is higher among the biologic families of schizophrenics, an increase in the incidence of schizophrenia can be anticipated. The overall number of patients with schizophrenia will also increase because of the post-World

War II baby boom, which generated a large cohort of patients now in their 20s and 30s who are at great risk for the development of schizophrenia.

Although patients with schizophrenia represent fewer than 40% of those requiring psychiatric hospitalization, the chronicity of the disease and the massive, all-encompassing difficulties in function experienced by schizophrenic patients have made it the most serious and disabling mental illness. At any given time, about half of the beds assigned to psychiatric patients in hospitals are occupied by patients whose diagnosis is schizophrenic disorder, and this figure increases to two-thirds if geriatric patients with organic brain syndromes are excluded. The appearance of schizophrenia during the early adult years and its persistence throughout life heighten the loss to society of productive human beings and underscore the personal tragedy for affected patients and their families.

Etiology & Pathogenesis

The schizophrenic disorders are characterized by various attributes, which are actually descriptions of behaviors that are themselves complex end products of central nervous system activity. Despite intensive research, a single causative factor has not been discovered for these schizophrenic syndromes.

Studies from the following areas have improved our understanding of schizophrenia and have led to major innovations in treatment: (1) genetics; (2) development of the individual before the illness became apparent, in terms of both personal psychology and psychosocial environment, with the primary focus on the family; and (3) the biopsychosocial state of the person at the time of illness. Although information from each of these areas is important, none can exclusively explain the development of schizophrenia.

A. Biologic Factors:

1. Genetics–Genetic studies of schizophrenia have focused on the elements of consanguinity, twins, and adoption. Consanguinity studies have been the most frequently employed; these compare the incidence of schizophrenia in the relatives of an index case with the incidence in control families (Wiener, 1980). Results indicate that closer consanguinity correlates with a higher incidence of schizophrenia (Table 27–2).

Since it was recognized that biologic families (ie, those with the same gene pool) also usually provided

Table 27–2. Genetic relationship correlated with incidence of schizophrenia.*

Relationship	Incidence
General population	0.8%
Sibling schizophrenic	8%
One parent schizophrenic	12%
Dizygotic twin schizophrenic	14%
Both parents schizophrenic	39%
Monozygotic twin schizophrenic	47%

*Data from Gottesman and Shields (1976), Kety and coworkers (1976), and Kringlen (1976).

the parenting during development, the 2 variables of genetics and nurturing were isolated by studying children who had been adopted shortly after birth and who had subsequently developed schizophrenia. In this way, it was hoped that the enviornmental effects of nurturance could be separated from the genetic effects of nature. These studies confirmed the existence of a genetic component in the predisposition to schizophrenia. Nine percent of the biologic family members of schizophrenic children were themselves schizophrenic, whereas only 2% of the biologic family members of nonschizophrenic adopted children were schizophrenic; the incidence of schizophrenia in the adopting families of these 2 groups of children was the same (Kety and coworkers, 1971). In some of the families studied, one of the adopting parents developed schizophrenia after the adoption, but this trait did not seem to be passed on to the adopted child with a frequency greater than that seen in the general population. Whether the schizophrenic parent was the father or the mother made no difference. Schizophrenic disorders are weakly associated between generations. The strongest association between parents with schizophrenic-type disorders and their offspring is that between parents with *chronic* schizophrenia and their offspring, in whom there is a high chance of schizophrenic disorder.

More recent analyses of these data using *DSM-III* criteria have confirmed the original findings while suggesting that genetic expression can manifest itself in the "schizophrenia spectrum" of schizoid, schizotypal, and paranoid personality disorders. Patients with acute psychoses, including schizophreniform disorder, have no higher incidence of a family history of schizophrenia than do controls.

A summary of these studies makes clear that although a genetic factor is involved in the predisposition to schizophrenia, it is not sufficient to ensure development of the disorder, as is shown by the considerable discordance in incidence in monozygotic twins.

The stress-diathesis model of schizophrenia assumes that there is an inherited gene for schizophrenia that is expressed about 20 years later. According to this model, an innate vulnerability (the diathesis) is shaped throughout childhood and adolescent development by a host of psychosocial and environmental factors. The stresses of young adulthood may precipitate schizophrenia in an individual with this innate vulnerability. The phenotype of the disorder is expressed only after years of interaction between the environment and the individual with the schizophrenic genotype.

Mathematical analyses of data accumulated from genetic studies have also established that there is no simple mendelian pattern of inheritance and that the incidence of schizophrenia cannot be explained by a single-gene theory. Unfortunately, the data do not distinguish between various theories of multiple gene interaction.

2. Specific abnormalities–Many specific biochemical aspects—metabolic pathways and hormonal responses in particular—seem to be different in schizophrenic patients as opposed to normal patients, especially during acute illness. It has been impossible to distinguish between physiologic cause and effect in most studies of schizophrenia. Individual biochemical abnormalities have been prematurely announced to be causal factors in schizophrenia, as illustrated by a widely published report that enkephalins caused schizophrenia and that hemodialysis was the cure. Within 6 months, however, controlled experiments eliminated the enkephalins as causative agents (Lewis and coworkers, 1979).

Some investigators have suggested that because of the heterogeneity of the schizophrenic disorders, this pattern of proposing causative agents—and then withdrawing the claim after research fails to validate the proposal—is bound to be repeated. This is another way of saying that if schizophrenia does represent a syndrome of multiple causes and discrete subtypes, research attempting to arrive at a "unitary hypothesis" of the disorder will continue to be unproductive. Comparing schizophrenic patients with controls in pursuit of a single causative agent may be as fruitless as comparing "the retarded" with controls or comparing febrile with afebrile patients. Although interest in the heterogeneity of schizophrenia is high, the search for a single cause or neuropathologic correlate continues.

a. Anatomic and physiologic factors— Schizophrenia has been viewed as an illness in which thoughts and behavior are disordered without the gross dysfunction in cognition or sensorium that is associated with organic brain syndromes. Although there have been attempts to establish neuroanatomic or structural differences in the brains of schizophrenic patients as opposed to those of normal controls, such differences either have not been demonstrated or have later been found to be the result of exogenous factors. CT scans have indicated that persons with chronic schizophrenia may have enlarged lateral ventricles and atrophy of the frontal cortex. In a subgroup of schizophrenic patients, enlarged third ventricles (which imply changes in the periventricular limbic-striatal area) have been demonstrated on CT scanning independently of duration of illness or treatment (Schulsinger and coworkers, 1984). Patients with schizophrenia also showed decreased utilization of prefrontal cortical areas that was independent of current medication. Magnetic resonance imaging (MRI) studies showed that the frontal lobes of schizophrenic patients are smaller than those of controls.

Within the last decade, a physiologic difference between schizophrenic patients and normal controls has been established (Holzman and coworkers, 1984). Abnormalities in saccadic eye movements (seen when the eye tracks a moving object such as a pendulum) are highly associated with schizophrenia. The movements are abnormally jerky in 80% of schizophrenic patients who are not taking medication, in 45% of nonschizophrenic relatives of schizophrenic patients, and in only 7% of controls. The concordance is 71% for

monozygotic twins and 54% for dizygotic twins; both rates are higher than the concordance for actual development of schizophrenia. At present, the significance of these findings is unclear. However, abnormal saccadic eye movements represent a potential phenotypic marker for schizophrenia.

b. Biochemical factors—Many elements have been proposed and investigated in the search for a biochemical abnormality in schizophrenia. These biochemical elements are grouped below on the basis of a proved relationship to schizophrenia and on the significance of that relationship.

(1) Established relationship of demonstrated significance—Alterations in the amount of dopamine in the brains of patients with schizophrenia and in normal people have frequently been implicated in the etiology of schizophrenia (Snyder, 1981). Attention was originally focused on dopamine because it was found that the phenothiazines improved schizophrenia but worsened Parkinson's disease, already recognized as a dopamine deficiency disease. It was subsequently found that levodopa, a direct precursor of dopamine that enters the brain, exacerbates schizophrenia, as do chemicals such as disulfiram that block the conversion of dopamine to norepinephrine. Furthermore, it has been suggested that the psychosis produced in normal people by amphetamine is related to the blocking of dopamine reuptake (Janowsky and Davis, 1976).

Dopamine receptors are blocked in vitro by antipsychotic drugs, and there is a linear correlation of this blocking of the dopamine receptor and the established clinical potencies of the individual drugs. Recent studies using positron emission tomography (PET) have proved that the number of dopamine receptors in the basal ganglia of patients with chronic schizophrenia is markedly elevated relative to the number in controls. Similar elevations were found in patients who had been treated with neuroleptics as well as in those who had not.

It should be emphasized, however, that altered levels of dopamine are not considered a "cause" of schizophrenia, but they do seem to be implicated in the manifestation of symptoms. In fact, drugs that affect dopamine levels are equally effective in reducing psychotic symptoms regardless of whether these are manifested as schizophrenia, mania, or certain psychoses (eg, psychoses developing in patients treated with corticosteroids or patients with complex metabolic or environmental derangements who are being treated in intensive care units).

(2) Established relationship of uncertain significance—The first biochemical abnormality established with certainty in schizophrenia was worsening of symptoms after administration of "methyl donors" such as methionine. This finding is reproducible, but its clinical significance remains uncertain despite vigorous investigative efforts.

Elevated levels of serum creatinine phosphokinase have also been consistently associated with schizophrenia. The greatest elevations occur in the prodromal period. The isoenzyme involved in this phenomenon originates in muscle; because of this fact, the abnormality is unlikely to be a causal factor in schizophrenia, and its association with schizophrenia is only slightly greater than its association with other functional psychoses (Meltzer and coworkers, 1980).

Recent studies of phenylethylamine have shown that levels of this metabolite of phenylalanine are elevated in the cerebrospinal fluid of patients with paranoid schizophrenia and that other metabolites of phenylethylamine are found in higher concentrations in the urine of these patients than in the urine of normal controls. The recent discovery in brain tissue of an "amphetamine receptor" with high specificity for phenylethylamines highlights the potential importance of these chemicals (Paul and coworkers, 1982).

The search for an "internal hallucinogen" as a cause of schizophrenia—which evolved after the realization that some long-term psychoses occurred in patients with a history of LSD use—has established that normal humans may produce at least trace amounts of one such compound. Dimethyltryptamine, a very short-acting, powerful, and once widely used psychedelic, is synthesized by enzymes that can be found in human platelets and in the pineal gland (Gillin and coworkers, 1976).

(3) Disproved relationships of historical significance only—The recognition that the psychedelic drug mescaline was an analogue of the catecholamine neurotransmitters dopamine and norepinephrine led to a search for an "internal hallucinogen." The major candidate was adrenochrome, which could be chemically synthesized from the catecholamines. Adrenochrome was also thought to be related to various "pink spots" that appeared when components of the urine or serum of schizophrenic patients were subjected to chromatography. Studies subsequently showed that these abnormal chemicals either resulted from incidental factors in the environment of schizophrenic patients, eg, inadequate amounts of vitamin C in the diet of institutionalized patients, or occurred as laboratory artifacts. The catecholamines are chemically unstable, and it has been established that there are no human metabolic pathways that could produce adrenochrome or the other putative abnormal neurotransmitters, except dimethyltryptamine, as previously described.

It has been suggested that various serum proteins, particularly immunoglobulins, exist in abnormal levels in patients with schizophrenia. The original and best known of such factors was thought to be taraxein, but neither its precise identity nor its initially reported ability to produce schizophrenic symptoms has ever been established.

The class of chemical agents known as psychedelics or hallucinogens has been investigated for its relationship to schizophrenia (Rosengarten and Friedhoff, 1976). LSD is the most potent drug in this class, which also includes mescaline and psilocybin, among others. All of these substances are chemical analogues of either the catecholamines or indoleamines. However, careful clinical observations and examination of subjective experience during drug use (by normal controls and subjects with functional psychoses) have led to the conclusion that the altered states of consciousness produced acutely by these drugs are distinctly different from those occurring in either schizophrenia or mania. Visual distortions and fully developed visual hallucinations are much more common with the drug-induced states. These states also often include an ecstatic sense of awe. Acute effects pass within 12–24 hours. Unlike patients with functional psychoses, almost all normal subjects who used these drugs failed to show any residual psychologic disturbance or discomfort.

(4) Unproved relationship of unknown significance—The discovery of a new class of peptide neuroregulators (of which the endorphins and enkephalins are the best known) has made understanding of the integration of the central nervous system even more complex. As mentioned above, however, there is presently no evidence that these peptides are significantly related to schizophrenia.

B. Psychosocial Factors:

1. Development of the individual—Attempts have been made to explain the occurrence of schizophrenia in terms of the intrapsychic development of the child, usually using models of psychoanalytic psychology (see Chapters 2, 3, 6, and 7). According to this theory, schizophrenia results from the young child's failure to develop a mature ego capable of interpreting reality and coping with inner drives. Contemporary theories of the pathogenesis of schizophrenia focus on the failure of the infant to psychologically "separate" from the mother during the first and second years of life (Mahler and coworkers, 1975). The normal child goes through a stage of individuation at this time and begins to function independently. This process is thought to be essential for the formation of a stable sense of self as separate from others. In theory, the deficits in identify seen in schizophrenia result from a failure in psychologic separation from the parents.

It is clear that the onset of schizophrenia in young adults coincides with developmental stages of leaving home. This period is for finding a place in society, forming peer relationships, and developing a work role. The onset of schizophrenia is often associated with failure to adapt successfully to the necessary changes required by these new social roles. Once illness begins, a decrease in integration of ego functions and the development of regressive behavioral patterns are almost inevitable.

Traditionally, theories of schizophrenia based on the development of "the self" focus on the individual patient with symptoms. However, the patient is part of a family system that may also influence the pathogenesis of schizophrenic disorders.

2. Development within the family—Some theories of the pathogenesis of schizophrenia have focused on the immediate environment of the family. The patient is seen as a reflection of disturbed interactions among family members, some of whom may themselves be disturbed. Lidz and coworkers (1965) have identified 2 patterns in families that were dysfunctional and yet remained superficially intact.

In one pattern, Lidz identifies a marked schism between the parents, with one parent often forming an inappropriately close relationship with a child of the opposite sex, who later becomes schizophrenic. The other pattern is characterized by a skewed power relationship, in which one parent is clearly dominant, although this is not always acknowledged by the rest of the family.

A related set of patterns is identified by Wynne (1978), who describes families as either "pseudomutual" or "pseudohostile"; ie, the family insists that all members relate to one another in the emotional tone characteristic of the family, and members actively suppress any expression of alternative feelings.

A more specific type of presumably psychotogenic communication is the "double bind." As described by Bateson and colleagues (1956), this is the discordance between the overt communication of verbal speech and the covert message of the emotional tone or nonverbal actions that directly contradict the verbal message. In such a situation, the patient cannot win, regardless of the reply or course of action chosen. Rosenbaum (1970) includes the following classic example of the double bind:

> A young man who had fairly well recovered from an acute schizophrenic episode was visited in the hospital by his mother. He was glad to see her and impulsively put his arm around her shoulders, whereupon she stiffened. He withdrew his arm and she asked, "Don't you love me anymore?" He then blushed, and she said, "Dear, you must not be so easily embarrassed and afraid of your feelings."

In all of these patterns of disturbed family relationships, the family also has a covert injunction against commenting on this double-bind behavior, so that the patient is effectively trapped in a situation that is both unbearable and unchangeable. These logically inconsistent patterns, which are often inconclusive and incomprehensible, have been termed communication deviance. Another variable, expressed emotion, is defined as "high" when the family consistently directs intrusive, hostile, and overtly critical comments toward the patient. A 15-year prospective study indicates that high levels of communication deviance and expressed emotion are predictors of schizophrenia in persons at high risk, eg, the children of schizophrenic patients.

Although these environmental studies have focused on the family as the immediate and most important influence in the development of schizophrenia, other factors ranging from the uterine environment to the larger social environment must also be considered. For example, retrospective studies of the perinatal histories of schizophrenic patients have found a higher-than-expected frequency of difficult births when compared to nonschizophrenic normal controls. Many explanations, including poor maternal nutrition, have

been suggested, but no definitive study has been completed. A hint of the importance of the uterine environment comes from studies of those monozygotic twins who were discordant for schizophrenia; in 10 of 12 cases, the child with the smaller birthweight became schizophrenic. Many other environmental influences have been explored; none has provided an adequate explanation for the pathogenesis of the schizophrenic disorders.

3. Development within society and the larger environment—The epidemiologic studies discussed above not only provide information about the prevalence of schizophrenia within the general population but also identify several factors in addition to those concerned with the patient or the patient's family that clearly have a strong association with schizophrenia. These factors appear to have a major impact on the emergence of schizophrenia in those who are genetically susceptible to its development.

a. Population density—Population density has been correlated with prevalence, though in a manner that seems applicable only to urban settings. Specifically, there is a strong correlation between the prevalence of schizophrenia and the local population density within districts of cities that have a total population greater than 1 million. In smaller cities of 100,000–500,000 people, the correlation is weaker, and it disappears altogether in smaller towns. Data from an unrelated study of the incidence of schizophrenia among the children of schizophrenic mothers consistently show that the prevalence of schizophrenia in mothers in rural settings is only half that found in cities (Reisby, 1967). These data may reflect urban-rural differences in environmental stress, differences in diagnostic and treatment facilities, or differences in the tolerance of deviant behavior. The relative importance of these factors remains unclear, however.

b. Socioeconomic class—As discussed in Chapter 14, a second factor consistently confirmed by many studies is the association of schizophrenia and lower socioeconomic class. One major explanatory theory states that the conditions of life in lower socioeconomic classes (with the inherently greater stress and reduced flexibility in choice of personal response to stress) are causal factors in the development of schizophrenia.

Another explanation suggests that those who develop schizophrenia tend to drift into the lower social classes or fail to rise above the class of their parents because of their inability to perform adequately in many life functions. They have difficulty engaging in economically productive work and in forming social networks. This "drift hypothesis" is supported by the finding that schizophrenic individuals are more likely to be of a lower social class than their parents. The argument remains unsettled.

c. Date of birth—A third factor affecting the incidence of schizophrenia is a birthdate in the winter months (January, February, March). In both Europe and the USA, incidence of schizophrenia is significantly increased in those born between January and

April; and a complementary peak in incidence is found in South Africa during the months corresponding to winter in the southern hemisphere (July, August, September). This finding has led to many intriguing hypotheses, of which the occurrence of prenatal infections in the mother seems best supported by current data.

d. Other factors−Several other factors have been proposed as possible influences on the development of schizophrenia. The data are not as consistent and well established as those for the factors mentioned above. The first of these elements is **stress,** as subjectively perceived by the patient and reported after the development of illness. Although it is hard to defend the argument that stress causes schizophrenia, it has been shown that the number of identifiable stressful events (particularly loss of a meaningful person or relationship) clearly increases during the time just before the onset of schizophrenia.

Emigration and the resulting obvious **cultural dislocation** have also been proposed as causes likely to increase the incidence of schizophrenia. This suggestion has not been uniformly confirmed by various studies, so the impact of emigration on the incidence of schizophrenia remains uncertain.

Industrialization is another factor that seems to affect the incidence of schizophrenia. It has been noted that the incidence of schizophrenia has risen in developing countries as they have increased their contact with industrialized nations. As industrial development proceeds, an even more definite difference in the presenting symptoms of schizophrenia occurs. In developing countries, catatonic schizophrenia is far more common; with greater industrialization, paranoid schizophrenia becomes more common. This pattern is consistent with the shift that has occurred in the USA over the last 50 years, in which the number of people presenting with catatonic symptoms has dramatically decreased, while the number of those showing paranoid symptoms has increased.

Treatment

The consequences of schizophrenia are painful and unacceptable both to the patient and to the surrounding community. The magnitude of these consequences has led to a wide range of treatments and protective strategies. Even before the development of a conceptual framework to explain schizophrenia, physical methods were used to protect society and to help families and caretakers minimize the disruption caused by schizophrenia. The earliest treatments involved sedation, restraint, confinement, and the removal of the patient from society to a distant institution. Patients could be observed and treated, and society could avoid contact with these frightening and disturbing people. Hospital treatment was a long process often ending in continuous institutionalization. Occasionally, a combination of psychologic, social, and somatic treatments was followed by remission.

The probability of eventual discharge from hospitals for patients who have developed schizophrenia for the first time has increased over each decade of this century. Social attitudes and nondrug therapies have played a major role in this process. However, the dramatic increase in these release rates since the late 1950s could not have occurred without the introduction of phenothiazines in the mid to late 1950s. Drug treatment controlled acute symptoms and reduced the length of hospitalization from years and months to weeks and days.

A. Historical Treatment: The history of the treatment of schizophrenia has included many physical treatments which were thought to help the patient and which undoubtedly did affect the patient, who was forced to pay attention to the somatic treatment and those administering it. Of all of these treatments, only 3 are worth discussing now.

1. Coma−The earliest chemical treatment of schizophrenia induced prolonged coma, either by injection of insulin and subsequent production of hypoglycemia or by continuous infusion of barbiturates. The first method has obvious dangers related to the lowering of blood glucose levels below those associated with coma to those that produce permanent brain damage. Both insulin and barbiturate coma therapies apparently do improve schizophrenic symptoms, but neither is now used to any extent.

2. Electroconvulsive therapy (ECT)−It was originally noted that some institutionalized schizophrenic patients had fewer symptoms after a grand mal seizure. This postictal effect was mistakenly thought to show that epilepsy was incompatible with schizophrenia (and therefore that epileptic convulsions might prevent schizophrenia), and researchers looked for ways to produce seizures in schizophrenics. Initially, seizures were induced by pentylenetetrazol (Metrazol), but much better control over the induction of seizures was obtained by the use of electric current. Before the use of phenothiazines, electroconvulsive therapy was the treatment of choice for schizophrenia, and many patients improved sufficiently to return to the community. In controlled comparison with antipsychotic drugs, however, electroconvulsive therapy has been proved to be significantly less effective, and it is rarely indicated now for schizophrenia. Although electroconvulsive therapy remains an accepted treatment for major depressive illnesses, particularly in the elderly, its use in schizophrenia is now limited to those occasional patients who fail to improve after all major antipsychotic medications have been tried and who nonetheless require continued care. Electroconvulsive therapy is also occasionally used in schizophrenic patients who exhibit either catatonic excitement or suicidal impulses, since either of these conditions can be suppressed in a few days by this therapy.

3. Psychosurgery−Psychosurgery—the severing of tracts between the frontal lobe and the midbrain—was developed in the mid 1930s and widely used for about 20 years after that. The chances of creating a patient who was apathetic and lacked distinctive personality lessened as improved surgical techniques made possible more precise ablations.

Nonetheless, the procedure has fallen from favor now that the efficacy of antipsychotic medications has been established. Recent US government reports have acknowledged that some conditions may benefit from psychosurgery; however, fewer than 400 such surgeries were performed in the USA in 1977, and psychosurgery is now rarely used in the USA (see Chapter 10).

B. Contemporary Treatment: Appropriate treatment of schizophrenia now always uses a combination of biologic, psychologic, and social methods. The psychiatrist usually works as part of a treatment team, and in many cases the family is actively incorporated into the treatment plan.

1. Supportive psychotherapy–The first consideration should always be the safety of the patient and the patient's associates. Often, 24-hour supervision is necessary during the more fulminant stages of illness. With the increasing use of antipsychotic drugs during the past 20 years and the emphasis on treating patients in the least restrictive environment, most schizophrenic patients have been managed within their own communities after comparatively brief hospitalization.

The establishment of a trusting "working alliance" with the patient is of major importance. If the clinician's goal is to stablize the patient's symptoms and reduce dysfunction, the doctor-patient relationship must guide all treatment methods. This relationship also holds the key to success. Schizophrenic individuals are vulnerable and are exquisitely sensitive to their environment even when they are apparently out of touch with reality. Special care must therefore be taken in all interpersonal transactions.

Working with schizophrenic patients requires a great deal of patience on the part of the psychiatrist and the treatment team. The psychiatrist must make every effort to take the time to understand these patients even though much of their behavior and verbal interaction may be initially repellent. The psychiatrist must accept these patients as they are and take the position that although patients will not be asked to conform in a way that is impossible for them, they must nevertheless abandon the maladaptive behaviors associated with their schizophrenia and learn to function in the reality accepted by normal people. Thus, once the acute phase of illness has passed, patients should begin to attend to their own basic needs and to participate in therapeutic group activities.

Work with schizophrenic patients is termed **supportive treatment** in that it not only emphasizes positive reinforcement (appreciation, approval, or justifiable praise) but also supports the basic personality structure. Therapy does not try to break down or restructure an already weak and vulnerable ego. The therapist avoids overloading the individual with information about inner motives and fearful impulses, since this type of insight cannot be usefully assimilated by the schizophrenic patient. Discussion should focus instead on solving immediate problems and helping to develop social skills. Relief of painful

symptoms is essential to successful adaptation; therefore, the psychiatrist does not make interpretations that bring up earlier anxiety-laden, threatening memories. Rather, the psychiatrist listens carefully but interactively and attempts to understand each patient in a way that fosters development of a more adaptive, mature personality. In effect, the psychiatrist takes the role of a concerned but nonintrusive parent who uses understanding and skill to promote the maximum possible development in a vulnerable individual. Although the diagnosis of schizophrenia carries a guarded prognosis, the situation is never hopeless, and much can be improved. The psychiatrist must communicate this feeling to both the patient and the family.

The methods and goals of family therapy in the treatment of schizophrenia have been reconsidered in the last 5 years, following the discovery that high expressed emotion levels in patients' families contributed significantly to relapse. A team approach is usually used to educate the family and patient about the nature of schizophrenia, the avoidance of stressors, and the recognition of early signs of relapse. The exploration of past emotional conflicts is intentionally avoided; instead, the family learns to develop problem-solving techniques. The team approach thus attempts to lower high expressed emotion levels within the family while directly coaching the patient in social skills. This approach, in conjunction with the use of neuroleptics, appears to have as significant an impact on delaying relapse as did the introduction of neuroleptics in producing remission 30 years ago. The benefits derived from 9 months of this psychoeducational method were found to extend through a subsequent year when appropriate medications were continued.

2. Drug treatment–(See also Chapter 52.) Initially, phenothiazines emerged as the major drug used in acute hospital treatment of psychosis, and they were also widely used in the long-term stabilization of schizophrenic patients after their subsequent return to the community. Controlled prospective studies of 1965–1975 confirmed what had become clinically apparent a decade earlier: that use of phenothiazines achieved remission of symptoms in weeks rather than years in 90% of those experiencing an acute schizophrenic episode; that recovery was sufficient to enable patients to return to the community; and that the likelihood of rehospitalization could be reduced by half in those patients who had been treated with phenothiazines in the hospital—regardless of the type of treatment received following discharge (May and coworkers, 1981).

The antipsychotic drugs now used include several other classes of drugs besides the phenothiazines originally used. All of the presently available antipsychotics appear to block the dopamine receptor of the nerve membrane. Table 27–3 shows the relative potencies of several commonly used drugs standardized against that of chlorpromazine, the original antipsychotic still widely used.

When the antipsychotics listed in Table 27–3 are

used, many factors must be considered in selection of the best drug regimen for a given patient.

a. Choice of drugs—Although the effective therapeutic dose required to treat a patient varies in relation to the drug's ability to block the dopamine receptor (as reflected in the relative potencies in Table 27–3), it is essential to recognize that all of these drugs have been found to be equally effective among large groups of patients. Just as the relative potencies reflect the drug's ability to block the dopamine receptor, the relative side effects reflect binding at other known neurotransmitter receptors. Individual patients may respond to one drug better than another, and a history of a favorable response to treatment with a given drug in either the patient or a family member should lead to use of that particular drug as the drug of first choice. If the initial choice is not effective in 2–4 weeks, it is reasonable to try another antipsychotic drug with a different chemical structure. Aside from milligram potencies, the chief differences among the antipsychotic agents are those of side effects, which may affect compliance or may be used to advantage by the patient (eg, to produce nighttime sedation).

Useful generalizations may be made about the differences between the low- and high-potency antipsychotics. The low-potency drugs have much greater sedative and hypotensive properties, to which the patient usually becomes more tolerant within a few weeks, but the greater risk of malignant hyperthermia and obesity associated with this group of drugs continues throughout the period of active drug use (ie, not more than 2 weeks after the discontinuation of oral medications). Low-potency drugs also are inherently anticholinergic, so that the use of additional anticholinergic drugs to prevent extrapyramidal symptoms is often unnecessary.

The high-potency drugs, which have been widely used since the 1970s, have little inherent anticholinergic activity and frequently produce extrapyramidal symptoms or dystonia, so that anticholinergic drugs are usually required, at least in the initial weeks of treatment. They may be more likely to produce **neuroleptic malignant syndrome,** a devastating acute illness characterized by fever, delirium, autonomic dysfunction, and muscle rigidity. The incidence of this iatrogenic disease may be as high as 1%, but as with schizophrenia, the "disease" may be a grouping of various medical conditions.

The only long-acting depot antipsychotics available in the USA are the esters of fluphenazine and haloperidol, which may be given as infrequently as every 2 weeks to establish adequate drug levels. This type of drug treatment decreases relapse rates for previously stable outpatients but is not as effective immediately following treatment of an acute psychotic episode.

b. Dosage—The proved efficacy of antipsychotics in reducing relapse rates led at first to some untoward consequences, in that patients who had been treated with high doses of antipsychotic drugs to control acute psychotic symptoms continued to receive high doses as maintenance levels in the absence of known contraindications to long-term use and in the belief that this would prevent relapse. Many patients suffered from unacceptable side effects such as tardive dyskinesia (see below), and the psychiatric community recognized that it was essential to determine the minimum effective dose of antipsychotic medications. Fortunately, it was found that except during acute exacerbations of psychosis, lower doses of antipsychotic medications are consistent with excellent long-term control of symptoms in schizophrenia.

In the early 1970s, tardive dyskinesia, an often irreversible disfiguring movement disorder, was shown to be a frequent side effect of chronic administration of antipsychotics (see Chapter 52). Tardive dyskinesia is characterized by repetitive, involuntary movements, usually of the mouth and tongue, but often of the thumb and fingers and occasionally of a limb or the whole trunk (Granacher, 1981). Although tardive dyskinesia occasionally occurs spontaneously, it usually occurs later, because major risk factors are older age and total cumulative exposure to dopamine antagonists, of which antipsychotic drugs are the most widely used.

Tardive dyskinesia is thought to result from dopamine receptor supersensitivity following chronic receptor blockade by the antipsychotic agent. The question whether tardive dyskinesia is a later manifestation of changes initially expressed as extrapyramidal symptoms has not yet been answered. Anticholinergic drugs do not improve tardive dyskinesia and may make it worse. The recommended treatment of tardive dyskinesia is to lower the dosage of antipsychotic drugs and hope for gradual remission of the choreoathetoid movements. Increasing the dosage of an antipsychotic briefly masks the symptoms of tardive dyskinesia, but symptoms will reappear later as a reflection of the progression of receptor supersensitivity.

Studies with both a low-potency drug (chlorpromazine) and a high-potency drug (trifluoperazine) clearly established that acute psychotic symptoms respond more quickly to high doses (600–1000 mg of

Table 27–3. Relative binding to human brain receptors of neuroleptics at equivalent therapeutic dosages.[*]

Drug	Dosage (mg)[†]	Receptor[†]			
		α_1	α_2	H_1	Muscarinic
Chlorpromazine	100	100	100	100	100
Thioridazine	100	53	92	55	400
Mesoridazine	51	66	24	250	50
Molindone	7	0.007	8.6	0.0005	0.00006
Thiothixene	5	1.2	19	7.8	0.12
Trifluoperazine	3	0.33	0.87	0.45	0.33
Haloperidol	1.6	0.67	0.32	0.006	0.005
Fluphenazine	1.2	0.35	0.59	0.53	0.046

[*]Adapted from Richelson (1984).
[†]Adapted from Davis (1976).

chlorpromazine or equivalent drug) than to low doses (< 400 mg of chlorpromazine or equivalent). Although megadoses of fluphenazine equivalent to over 50,000 mg of chlorpromazine were safely given to a group of acutely psychotic individuals, their improvement was neither better nor worse than that of a comparable group given standard high doses (Quitkin and coworkers, 1975). This clinical experiment demonstrated the high therapeutic index of this class of drugs, but the increased risk of eventual tardive dyskinesia and the absence of substantial benefit indicate that such dosages should never be used.

New dosage strategies have been developed in order to balance the need for high levels of neuroleptics for the treatment of acute episodes with the risk associated with higher total lifetime dosage. Three strategies ("low dose," "targeted symptom," and "drug holiday") may be used to lower the maintenance doses in the years of illness following acute hospitalization. The "low-dose" approach attempts to find the minimum effective dose in preventing relapse. Studies have shown that the minimum parenteral dose of fluphenazine decanoate is 5 mg intramuscularly every 2 weeks, but this guideline cannot be easily translated into oral dosages. The "targeted symptom" strategy calls for close monitoring of the patient by a treatment team and the use of medications only for specific symptoms. The use of "drug holidays" (when a long-acting drug is not taken for 1–2 days) has fallen into disfavor, both because it seems to decrease patient compliance and because it may exacerbate tardive dyskinesia.

c. Duration of drug treatment–The agitated patient with a functional psychosis can almost invariably be calmed in 1–2 days. Hourly doses of antipsychotics may be administered until symptoms abate. The psychosis gradually resolves only after 2–6 weeks of a high-dose drug regimen as outlined above. The dosage used in the hospital should be continued through the time of discharge and the accompanying stress of changing to a new and less structured environment. Major reductions in the dosage at discharge should be avoided for at least 4 weeks and are best attempted about 2–4 months after discharge. These decreases should be achieved in stages, and it should be recognized that any new equilibrium in body concentration of the drug will not be reached for at least 2 weeks after the change has been made (since these drugs have half-lives of 1–2 days). The patient should be alerted to note any signs of returning symptoms, so that modest increases in dosage may be made, if necessary, to abolish recurrent symptoms (Hansell and coworkers, 1977). Gradual reduction in dosage should approach a minimum that enables the patient to function as well as possible at a level that is in accord with the patient's wishes and is also socially acceptable. The ideal minimum is obviously no medication at all, and for many schizophrenic patients, this may gradually become true. There are also many patients who must accept the fact that reduction below a certain minimum dose (usually equivalent to 100–400 mg of

chlorpromazine) causes return of psychotic symptoms within weeks. For many patients, lifelong maintenance treatment with antipsychotic medications is a necessary part of existence.

d. Context of drug therapy–Although antipsychotic medication may effectively normalize a patient's overt behavior, thought processes, and ability to communicate coherently, it does little to help a patient achieve those factors considered to be essential for enhancing the quality of life: the ability to relate to friends or loved ones and the ability to obtain adequate food, clothing, and shelter by performing work for recompense. The true task of the long-term treatment of schizophrenia is 2-fold: (1) to establish a psychologically stable baseline free from recurrent psychotic episodes, and (2) to help the patient build upon this baseline to lead a life that is qualitatively enriched by reasonable personal, social, and vocational achievements.

3. Combined drug and supportive therapy–Most schizophrenic patients benefit from prudent use of antipsychotic medication in combination with supportive psychotherapy and work with the patient's family. Physicians may restrict their involvement to adjusting the dosage of medication, but a therapist may find that increased psychotherapeutic support may make additional medications unnecessary. Unfortunately, although medication is relatively inexpensive, a therapist's time is not. Institutions are rarely able to provide the needed consistency provided by continuing interaction with the same therapist. For many chronically ill schizophrenic patients, one way of obtaining this desired constancy is to maintain a relationship with a family physician who understands their vulnerability and needs. The psychiatrist can be available to consult with the family doctor when required. During initial hospitalization, there is an involuntarily imposed social structure, constant companionship of trained personnel, and supervised medication. Upon return to the community, patients become responsible for complying with medication requirements, although that task involves at least some loose association with a prescribing physician. Patients usually remain in contact with a treating physician or a treatment institution over months to years. During this time, patients should assume increasing responsibility for their own well-being and understanding of their illness and life situation.

A major goal in the treatment of patients after discharge from the hospital is to help them recognize what kinds of stressful situations or internal stimuli indicate that a relapse is beginning. When patients become aware of these early signs of psychosis, they can often regain control of their lives merely by increasing the dosage of antipsychotic medication for a few weeks and by increasing their contact with the professionals treating them. This self-help is of major therapeutic benefit to patients, who find that they can exercise some measure of control over their illness and hope for a life that is not interrupted by recurrent hospitalization.

Changes observed in improved schizophrenic patients are as follows:

(1) Ability to be alone and yet feel secure.

(2) Development of a more distinct sense of self independent of other people.

(3) Greatly improved modulation of affect.

(4) Ability to feel genuine pleasure both in aesthetic pursuits and in interpersonal situations.

(5) Improvement in thought disorder, ranging from marked diminution to outright absence of symptoms.

(6) Lessened susceptibility to transient psychotic symptoms.

(7) Realistic scaling down of personal ambitions.

(8) Ability to take credit for personal accomplishments.

(9) Improvements in social judgment.

SUMMARY

Schizophrenic disorders comprise a complex syndrome characterized by a disturbance in reality testing, marked impairment of social functioning, and severe personality disorganization involving disturbances in thought, affect, and behavior. There is no known cause, although genetic factors clearly play a significant role. Psychosocial factors play an important part in development of schizophrenic disorders, and there may also be biochemical bases for these illnesses. Treatment should consist of various methods and should include the formation of a therapeutic alliance with the schizophrenic person as well as with friends and family. Although schizophrenia is one of the most serious psychiatric disturbances, a comprehensive approach to the care and treatment of schizophrenic disorders can improve the quality of life of patients and their families.

REFERENCES

General

Arieti S: *Interpretation of Schizophrenia*, 2nd ed. Basic Books, 1974.

Green H: *I Never Promised You a Rose Garden*. Signet, 1964.

Kaplan B: *The Inner World of Mental Illness*. Harper & Row, 1964.

Laing RD: *The Divided Self*. Pelican, 1965.

Sechehaye MA: *Autobiography of a Schizophrenic Girl*. Signet, 1970.

History of Schizophrenia

Bleuler E: *Dementia Praecox, or The Group of Schizophrenias*. Internat Univ Press, 1950.

Fromm-Reichmann F: *Principles of Intensive Psychotherapy*. Univ of Chicago Press, 1950.

Kraepelin E: *Dementia Praecox*. Livingstone, 1919.

Schneider K: *Clinical Psychopathology*. Grune & Stratton, 1959.

Schreber DP: *Memoirs of My Nervous Illness*. Dawson & Sons, 1955.

Sullivan HS: *Schizophrenia as Human Process*. Norton, 1962.

Symptoms & Signs, Natural History, & Prognosis

Bleuler M: *The Schizophrenic Disorders*. Yale Univ Press, 1978.

Crow TJ: The two-syndrome concept: Origins and current status. *Schizophr Bull* 1985;**11**:471.

Harrow M, Marengo, JT: Schizophrenic thought disorder at follow-up: Its persistence and prognostic significance. *Schizophr Bull* 1986;**12**:373.

Huber G, Gross G, Schuttler R: A long-term follow-up study of schizophrenia: Psychiatric course of illness and prognosis. *Acta Psychiat Scand* 1975;**52**:49.

Kay SR, Opler LA, Fiszbein A: Significance of positive and negative syndromes in chronic schizophrenia. *Br J Psychiatry* 1986;**149**:439.

Maher BA: The language of schizophrenia: A review and interpretation. *Br J Psychiatry* 1972;**120**:3.

McDonald N: Living with schizophrenia. *Can Med Assoc J* 1960;**82**:218.

McGhie A, Chapman J: Disorders of attention and perception in early schizophrenia. *Br J Med Psychol* 1961;**34**:218.

McGlashan TH: Predictors of shorter-, medium-, and longer-term outcome in schizophrenia. *Am J Psychiatry* 1986;**143**:50.

Mendel W: *Schizophrenia: The Experience and Its Treatment*. Jossey-Bass, 1976.

Pope HG Jr, Lipinski JR Jr: Diagnosis in schizophrenia and manic-depressive illness. *Arch Gen Psychiatry* 1978;**35**:811.

Strauss JS et al: *The Psychotherapy of Schizophrenia*. Plenum Press, 1980.

Zubin J, Spring B: Vulnerability: A new view of schizophrenia. *J Abnorm Psychol* 1977;**86**:103.

Epidemiology

Babigian HM: Schizophrenia: Epidemiology. Chapter 15.2 in: *Comprehensive Textbook of Psychiatry/IV*, 4th ed. Kaplan HI, Freedman AM, Sadock BJ (editors). Williams & Wilkins, 1985.

Cooper JE et al: *Psychiatric Diagnosis in New York and London*. Oxford Univ Press, 1972.

Erlenmeyer-Kimling L, Rainer JD, Kallman FJ: Current reproductive trends in schizophrenia. In: *Psychopathology of Schizophrenia*. Hoch PH, Zubin J (editors). Grune & Stratton, 1966.

Etiology & Pathogenesis

Bateson G et al: Towards a theory of schizophrenia. *Behav Sci* 1956;**1**:251.

Gillin JC et al: The psychedelic model of schizophrenia: The case of N,N-dimethyltryptamine. *Am J Psychiatry* 1976;**133**:203.

Gottesman I, Shields J: A critical review of recent adoption, twin, and family studies of schizophrenia: Behavioral genetics perspectives. *Schizophr Bull* 1976;**2**:360.

Grinspoon L, Bakalar JB: Psychedelics and acylcyclohexylamines. Chapter 12 in: *APA Annual Review, Vol 5*.

Frances AJ, Hales RE (editors). American Psychiatric Press, 1986.

Holzman PS et al: Pursuit eye movement and dysfunctions in schizophrenia. *Arch Gen Psychiatry* 1984;**41**:136.

Janowsky DS, Davis JM: Methylphenidate, dextroamphetamine and levamfetamine: Effects on schizophrenic symptoms. *Arch Gen Psychiatry* 1976;**33**:304.

Kety SS et al: Mental illness in the biological and adoptive families of adopted schizophrenics. *Am J Psychiatry* 1971;**128**:302.

Kety SS et al: Studies based on a total sample of adopted individuals and their relatives: Why they were necessary, what they demonstrated and failed to demonstrate. *Schizophr Bull* 1976;**2**:413.

Kringlen E: Twins: Still our best method. *Schizophr Bull* 1976;**2**:429.

Lewis RV et al: On β_H Leu^5-endorphin and schizophrenia. _H Leu^5-endorphin and schizophrenia. *Arch Gen Psychiatry* 1979;**36**:237.

Lidz T, Fleck S, Cornelison A: *Schizophrenia and the Family*. Internat Univ Press, 1965.

Mahler MS, Pine F, Bergman A: *The Psychological Birth of the Infant: Symbiosis and Individuation*. Basic Books, 1975.

Meltzer HT, Ross-Stanton J, Schlessinger S: Mean serum creatine kinase activity in patients with functional psychoses. *Arch Gen Psychiatry* 1980;**37**:650.

Paul SM, Hulihan-Giblin B, Skolnick P: (+) − Amphetamine binding to rat hypothalamus: Relation to anorexic potency for phenylethylamines. *Science* 1982;**218**:487.

Reisby N: Psychosis in children of hospitalized schizophrenic mothers. *Acta Psychiatr Scand* 1967;**43**:8.

Rosenbaum PC: *The Meaning of Madness*. Science House, 1970.

Rosengarten H, Friedhoff AJ: A review of recent studies of the biosynthesis and excretion of hallucinogens formed by methylation of neurotransmitters or related substances. *Schizophr Bull* 1976;**2**:90.

Schulsinger F et al: Cerebral ventricular size in the offspring of schizophrenic mothers. *Arch Gen Psychiatry* 1984;**41**:602.

Snyder SH: Dopamine receptors, neuroleptics, and schizophrenics. *Am J Psychiatry* 1981;**138**:460.

Watson CG et al: Schizophrenia birth seasonality in relation to the incidence of infectious disease and temperature extremes. *Arch Gen Psychiatry* 1984;**41**:85.

Wiener H: Schizophrenia: Etiology. Chapter 15.3 in: *Comprehensive Textbook of Psychiatry/IV*, 4th ed. Kaplan HI,

Freedman AM, Sadock BJ (editors). Williams & Wilkins, 1985.

Wong DF et al: Positron emission tomography reveals elevated D-2 dopamine receptors in drug-naive schizophrenics. *Science* 1986;**234**:1558.

Wynne LL (editor): *The Nature of Schizophrenia*. Wiley, 1978.

Treatment

Anderson CM et al: Family treatment of adult schizophrenic patients: A psychoeducational approach. *Schizophr Bull* 1980;**6**:490.

Carpenter WT Jr: Thoughts on the treatment of schizophrenia. *Schizophr Bull* 1986;**12**:527.

Davis JM: Comparative doses and costs of antipsychotic medication. *Arch Gen Psychiatry* 1976;**33**:858.

Falloon IRH et al: Family management in the prevention of morbidity in schizophrenia. *Arch Gen Psychiatry* 1985;**42**:887.

Granacher RP Jr: Differential diagnosis of tardive dyskinesia: An overview. *Am J Psychiatry* 1981;**138**:1288.

Gunderson J, Mosher L: *Psychotherapy of Schizophrenia*. Jason Aronson, 1975.

Hogarty GE et al: Family psychoeducation, social skills training and maintenance chemotherapy in the aftercare of schizophrenia. *Arch Gen Psychiatry* 1986;**43**:633.

Kane JM et al: Low-dose neuroleptic treatment of outpatient schizophrenia. *Arch Gen Psychiatry* 1983;**40**:893.

Leff J et al: Life events, relatives' expressed emotion and maintenance neuroleptics in schizophrenic relapse. *Psychol Med* 1983;**13**:799.

May PRA et al: Schizophrenia: A follow-up study of the results of five forms of treatment. *Arch Gen Psychiatry* 1981;**38**:776.

Peroutka SJ, Snyder SH: Relationship of neuroleptic drug effects at brain dopamine, serotonin, alpha-adrenergic, and histamine receptors to clinical potency. *Am J Psychiatry* 1980;**137**:1518.

Quitkin F, Rifkin A, Klein DE: Very high dosage versus standard dosage fluphenazine in schizophrenia. *Arch Gen Psychiatry* 1975;**32**:1276.

Richelson E: Neuroleptic affinitives for human brain receptors and their use in predicting adverse effects. *J Clin Psychiatry* 1984;**45**:331.

Vaughn CG, Leff JP: The influences of family and social factors in the course of psychiatric illness. *Br J Psychiatry* 1976;**129**:125.

28 Delusional (Paranoid) Disorders

Edward L. Merrin, MD

DSM-III-R dramatically changed the organization and conceptualization of the paranoid disorders, renaming them delusional disorders. This change emphasizes that paranoid ideation was not always prominent in delusional disorders previously categorized as "paranoid disorders." Such disorders were characterized by delusions but by none of the other criteria for schizophrenia or the other psychotic disorders. Table 28–1 lists the new criteria for delusional disorders, subsuming the more detailed and specific *DSM-III* criteria for the paranoid disorders.

Delusions are unrealistic fixed ideas that resist modification when confronted with objective contradictory evidence or logic. Delusions are commonly found in patients with virtually all forms of organic or functional psychotic disorders. They can be characterized by their thematic content (eg, delusions of persecution, of having sinned, of having special powers or abilities), by their degree of realism or implausibility, and by their internal consistency (the patient's beliefs can be explained in a way that others can understand).

Special attention has long been directed toward the relatively small proportion of psychotic patients whose delusions are the most prominent or the only manifestation of their illness. The origin of this interest probably lies in the otherwise largely intact personality of the patient who firmly, passionately, and stubbornly clings to an idea that seems clearly unlikely to the physician, family, and friends. Throughout most of the history of psychiatry, the terms "paranoia" and "paranoid disorder" have been used to describe this malady. The term paranoia was originally applied by Kahlbaum in 1863 to delusional patients without deterioration of affect or intellectual function. Kraepelin incorporated paranoia as a category of illness in his 1912 textbook, emphasizing an insidious onset and chronic course. These early writers are still influential in our understanding of these disorders.

Since it is the delusional beliefs of a persecutory nature that are most commonly described, in some countries the term paranoia is used to describe cases where suspiciousness or persecutory themes predominate. More recently, it has become clear that this was not the intent of the early writers, nor does this use of the term appear to be clinically valid. In developing the criteria for *DSM-III-R*, a decision was made to substitute the term "delusional disorder." This is in keeping with the practice in many European countries of including patients with any systematized delusion (erotic, religious, grandiose, somatic) in this group. It also avoids confusing the adjective "paranoid," often used to denote excessive suspiciousness, with the nosologic entity "paranoid disorder."

Delusional disorders, as defined in *DSM-III-R*, have no known organic cause and are characterized by persistent delusional beliefs. The emotions and behavior exhibited by patients with delusional disorders are understandable in the context of these beliefs. For example, patients who believe that they have a physical malady will continue to seek medical care and will not be reassured by unproductive diagnostic workups. When patients with delusions of persecution become

---

Table 28–1. *DSM-III-R* diagnostic criteria for delusional (paranoid) disorder.

A. Nonbizarre delusion(s) (ie, involving situations that occur in real life, such as being followed, poisoned, infected, loved at a distance, having a disease, being deceived by one's spouse) of at least 1 month's duration.

B. Auditory or visual hallucinations, if present, are not prominent (as defined in schizophrenia, criterion A[1][b]).

C. Apart from the delusion(s) or its ramifications, behavior is not obviously odd or bizarre.

D. If a major depressive or manic syndrome has been present during the delusional disturbance, the total duration of all episodes of the mood syndrome has been brief relative to the total duration of the delusional disturbance.

E. Has never met criterion A for schizophrenia, and it cannot be established that an organic factor initiated and maintained the disturbance.

Specify type: The following types are based on the predominant delusional theme. If no single delusional theme predominates, specify as other type.

Erotomanic type: the predominant theme of the delusion(s) is that a person, usually of higher status, is in love with the subject.

Grandiose type: the predominant theme of the delusion(s) is one of inflated worth, power, knowledge, special identity, or special relationship to a deity or famous person.

Jealous type: the predominant theme of the delusion(s) is that one's sexual partner is unfaithful.

Persecutory type: the predominant theme of the delusion(s) is that one (or someone to whom one is close) is being malevolently treated in some way. People with this type of delusional disorder may repeatedly take their complaints of being mistreated to legal authorities.

Somatic type: the predominant theme of the delusion(s) is that the person has some physical defect, disorder, or disease.

Other type: does not fit any of the previous categories, eg, persecutory and grandiose themes without a predominance of either; delusions of reference without malevolent content.

convinced that they are in danger, they may become frightened and engage in avoidant or confrontational behavior. Hallucinations may be present, but they are not persistent and are not a prominent part of the clinical picture.

Delusional disorders differ from schizophrenic or schizophreniform disorders in several ways. There are no bizarre or absurd delusional beliefs, no Schneiderian first-rank symptoms (eg, delusions of being controlled by an external force, hearing 2 voices discussing oneself in the third person, or believing that one's thoughts are "broadcast" in some way so that others can hear them [see Chapter 27]), and no incoherence or loosening of associations. Despite their delusional thinking, these patients do not manifest the extensive disturbances of thinking, perception, and behavior characteristic of schizophrenic disorders. Their affect is neither blunted nor inappropriate. Unlike schizophrenic patients, they seem to function normally outside their circumscribed area of abnormal thinking. Delusional disorders differ from affective disorders in that the full clinical syndrome of mania or depression is not present or is brief in comparison with the delusional symptoms.

A duration of at least 1 month is required for a diagnosis of delusional disorder. Six types are included in *DSM-III-R,* classified by the predominant delusional theme: erotomanic, grandiose, jealous, persecutory, and somatic (Table 28–1). Some patients exhibit features of more than one type and are subsumed under an "other" type. Since most literature has focused on patients with predominantly persecutory delusions, much of the detailed descriptions below will focus on that type.

Symptoms & Signs

The disorder is marked by an insidious onset of persecutory delusional ideas that gradually become the focus of the patient's life. The delusional beliefs themselves are internally consistent; in fact, the clinician may have difficulty deciding where legitimate grievances or misfortunes end and psychotic fantasies begin. What may begin as a frustrating experience with a government agency or employer may become a complex delusion, including everyone in the patient's surroundings in a terrifying drama of persecution and harassment. These patients may resort to litigation or appeal to public authorities for assistance. As these efforts are frustrated, the patient perceives those agencies and individuals as having joined the ranks of the enemy. A sense of self-importance and of messianic mission may develop over time as patients see themselves standing alone against evil forces.

Patients with erotomanic delusional disorder have developed a fixed belief that a particular person is deeply in love with them. This person is usually of higher social status than the patient (eg, a film or rock star, prominent politician, or college professor). The patient may attempt to communicate with this person by letter, by telephone, or even by forced intrusion into the person's home. The patient will often provide idiosyncratic interpretations of the public statements or gestures of the target person as evidence that the person is in love with and trying to communicate with the patient.

Patients with delusional disorder of the grandiose type believe that they are unusually special or have very important talents or abilities. Such patients may spend much of their time working on ideas for great inventions. These may be presented as having important potential benefits for humanity but will seem lacking in substance to the listener.

Patients with delusional disorder of the jealous type will often believe that their spouse is "carrying on " with various lovers, and significant clues seem to appear everywhere. They may read special significance into random events, pieces of conversation, or misplaced household items.

In delusional disorder of the persecutory type, patients believe they are victims of an organized plot. They may feel that they are being pursued, that their telephone is being tapped, or that their reputation is being purposely maligned. Often the reason why someone might treat them this way is unclear to these patients.

Patients with predominant somatic delusions may believe they have some dreaded disease or are dying. In one particular manifestation of this type of delusional disorder, patients complain of infestation with insects or parasites; such patients are likely to present for treatment at a dermatologist's office rather than in a psychiatric setting.

The "other" type of delusional disorder is reserved for patients with more than one type of delusion, without any one clearly predominating. In some cases grandiose, jealous, and persecutory delusions may share the spotlight. For example, the patient may feel persecuted because the patient's tormentors see the patient's superior talents as obstacles to their evil plans. There are also other forms of delusions that do not clearly fit the other categories (eg, the delusion of doubles [Capgras's syndrome], in which patients believe that a loved one is a double or imposter and is not to be trusted).

Remarkably, normal social functioning in spite of complex delusional beliefs persists. These patients behave and communicate in a normal fashion outside of their delusional concerns. Their emotional responses conform to our expectations of a normal person facing the same threat or danger. During an interview, the patient may feel strongly motivated to discuss delusional beliefs and engage the clinician as an ally. The patient may be excited, demonstrating mild pressure of speech and perhaps mild circumstantiality or tangentiality. These features are not prominent, however, and are limited to the attempt to woo an audience. The patients rarely have insight into the fact that they are ill, and their attendance in a psychiatric setting is often the result of pressure from family or the courts. In some cases, a desperate patient requests hospitalization for protection. Depression, perhaps with suicidal ideation, may be present in a patient who has exhausted all personal resources coping with a life that has become a nightmare.

The age at onset is later than in most cases of schizophreniform or schizophrenic disorders but is similar to that of affective disorders. Most patients are first diagnosed after age 40, although the illness may have been developing undetected for some time. Frank delusions are often precipitated by life events that are perceived as threatening or isolating (eg, loss of an established position at work, divorce, recent immigration). Older patients with impaired hearing or other physical disabilities that limit social contacts are particularly at risk.

Differential Diagnosis

A diagnosis of delusional disorder is appropriate if the following criteria are met: (1) nonbizarre, superficially plausible delusions have been present for at least 1 month; (2) hallucinations, if present, are neither prominent nor persistent; (3) there is an absence of strange or bizarre behavior; and (4) schizophrenia, affective disorder, and organic disorders are ruled out.

Schizophrenia differs in that it tends to have an earlier onset (although there is considerable overlap); it has a duration of at least 6 months; and it is associated with additional symptoms of psychosis at some time during the illness. These include prominent auditory hallucinations, marked loosening of associations or poverty of speech, markedly illogical thinking, or other delusional content of a bizarre or absurd nature. Schizophreniform disorder is distinguished from delusional disorder in a similar fashion with the exception that the duration of an episode of illness is limited to 6 months. Organic mental disorders (eg, cerebral neoplasm and organic delusional disorders associated with psychostimulant drug abuse) can also present with prominent delusions.

Differentiation from affective disorders can be difficult. Patients with delusional disorder can become clinically depressed; careful history taking will reveal that depressive symptoms developed long after the onset of delusional ideation or were transient. Some clinicians have stressed that persecutory ideation in depressed patients is usually based on an exaggerated feeling of guilt; they are being punished for their crimes or otherwise deserve the treatment they believe they are receiving. This is not, however, an ironclad rule in clinical practice, since depressed patients may display virtually any type of delusion.

Differentiation from mania can also be difficult. In both disorders, patients may present with exaggerated feelings of self-importance and belligerence. When delusional patients feel they have a sympathetic audience, they may display loud, pressured speech as they try to convince the listener of their beliefs and the dangers they face. More careful clinical evaluation will indicate the circumscribed nature of these signs as well as the absence of increased motor activity, excessive plans, hypersexuality, decreased need for sleep (as opposed to inability to sleep because of fear and anxiety), or other symptoms required to meet the criteria for

manic disorder. Despite the application of these guidelines, it may be difficult to rule out a diagnosis of affective disorder. As a final test, some clinicians advise a trial of treatment with antidepressants or lithium, particularly when there is a family history of affective disorder.

Chronic delusional symptoms are often present in patients with histories of alcohol abuse. In the past, such patients were thought to suffer from a specific disorder called alcoholic paranoia, or alcoholic paranoid state. Some psychiatrists believe that alcohol plays an important role in the pathogenesis of paranoia in alcoholic patients. However, the illness is phenomenologically identical to that seen in nonalcoholic patients, and there is no evidence of a different pathogenetic process. The clinician should not confuse delusional disorder with alcoholic hallucinosis, a syndrome of acute onset clearly related to alcohol withdrawal but occurring in the absence of severe symptoms of excessive autonomic discharge (tachycardia, postural hypotension, diaphoresis) or disorientation. Unlike delusional disorder, there are florid and persistent auditory hallucinations; most cases resolve in a few days to several weeks.

A more subtle distinction is between delusional disorder, persecutory type, and paranoid personality. In the case of the latter, the patient may be generally suspicious of the motives of others but does not have an organized delusional system. In practice, however, it may be difficult to extract delusional ideas from paranoid patients, since they are able to conceal the extent of their suspiciousness when they do not trust the examiner.

In induced psychotic disorder (shared paranoid disorder), the patient has acquired a belief system from another person with whom he or she shares a close personal relationship. The person with the dominant role has a more pernicious psychiatric disorder, whereas the other often becomes nonpsychotic if separated from the partner (see Chapter 29).

Prognosis

The prognosis of delusional disorder is poor. Patients rarely give up their delusional beliefs entirely, and engaging them in treatment is difficult. A satisfactory outcome is achieved if they can function in the community without feeling the need to act upon or discuss their abnormal beliefs.

Illustrative Case No. 1

A 59-year-old divorced man requested hospital admission because he feared for his life. While working as a power company engineer, he had become convinced that the design for a new nuclear power plant was faulty and unsafe. Despite 11 years with the company, he was fired for repeatedly annoying his superiors with these concerns. He filed suits against the company, some protesting his firing, some to stop construction of the power plant, and even some to stop utility rate increases. He became well known to company and public officials, who saw him as a comic but somehow tragic figure.

Meanwhile, the patient developed the belief that he was now an attorney because of a "grandfather" clause in the state law, since he had filed so many suits on his own behalf. He also began to believe that his attempts to publicize engineering defects in the power plant blueprints had made him unpopular with certain powerful groups, including the Mafia, the Bank of America, the FBI, and even the Vatican. He had squandered his savings on a trip to Europe, where he attempted to pursue his investigations, finally selling his antique jewelry collection, piece by piece, until he was deported from England. Whenever local authorities would intervene, he would assume that they were involved, helping to keep track of his whereabouts. A month prior to admission, he had been committed briefly after trying to convince police that a contract was out on his life. He was treated with neuroleptics, without apparent effect, and was released.

At the time of hospital admission, the patient was well groomed and articulate. He rambled on about his delusions and fears unless interrupted firmly. There was no evidence of hyperactivity, hallucinations, or other delusional thinking. On the ward, he was neither talkative nor socially intrusive. He slept peacefully, believing that he was safe in the hospital. After treatment with moderate doses of a neuroleptic drug, he felt safe leaving the hospital for a halfway house. Careful questioning revealed his continued belief in the conspiracy against him. He became depressed after realizing that some of his actions may have been excessive. A trial of antidepressant treatment was not effective, but these feelings diminished over time.

From the patient's perspective, a theme of injustice ran through his life. He was the younger of 2 boys reared in a small northeastern community. His older brother often bullied him, and he vividly recalled being punished by his mother for acts committed by his brother. At school, he was often the butt of jokes because of his small stature. His wife of 21 years had left him, taking their 3 children and getting the better part of the property settlement. Thus, it seemed that even before his illness, he had a propensity for seeing himself as a victim of unfair treatment.

Illustrative Case No. 2

A 31-year-old merchant seaman with no history of psychiatric disturbances came to the hospital with the conviction that a "contract" had been made on his life. He claimed to have been well until the 14th day of a 25-day voyage, 2 weeks before admission. On that day, he drank some liquid antacid for indigestion and thought he heard fellow crew members whispering, "He took it." Fearing foul play, he locked himself in his cabin for the remainder of the voyage, knife at hand, waiting for an attack to occur. When the ship reached port, he took the antacid to a commercial laboratory for analysis. He called an aunt long-distance, and she suggested he seek hospitalization.

At the time of admission, the patient asserted that he had been watched closely on board ship. He believed the first mate was responsible for the harassment. He related an incident in which he and a friend had engaged in "nonverbal" communication in front of the mate as if to indicate that they were having a homosexual affair. The purpose was to embarrass the mate, whom they suspected of being gay because he had discontinued showings to the crew of sexually explicit films. On close questioning, the patient admitted that he had never discussed this with the friend but that it was somehow understood between them. As a result of their action, the first mate set out to destroy him, first by poison and later by enlisting the aid of the FBI and other government agencies.

Psychiatric examination revealed no other delusions or hallucinations. Speech was well organized and understandable, the range of affect was normal, and there was no evidence of mania or depression. History, physical examination, and laboratory studies ruled out organic mental disorder, alcoholism, and drug abuse. Treatment with small doses of haloperidol was welcomed by the patient, who found it allowed him to relax and sleep at night. All psychotic symptoms resolved within 2 weeks.

This man was a self-described loner. He was resentful of his family and would say little about them. He had worked in a variety of occupations and had never had an intimate relationship. His illness may have been precipitated by awareness of homosexual attraction to the shipmate. Being trapped on board ship, he was unable to distance himself from the source of these feelings. As a result, he projected both sexual and aggressive ideas onto the first mate.

Illustrative Case No. 3

A 65-year-old man, a former prizefighter, had been making the rounds of local hospitals for 2 years with the complaint that his nose was shrinking. He feared that if this process progressed too far, he would not be able to breathe and would subsequently die. Although he was at times depressed about this, the depression was transient, whereas his frantic concerns about his nose continued unabated. Multiple attempts by ENT specialists to reassure him that there was nothing wrong had failed. He had been treated on psychiatric units with unsuccessful trials of neuroleptics and antidepressants several times. An attempt at electroconvulsive therapy had failed when the patient left against medical advice. He had since refused any psychiatric referral. At no time had there been evidence of hallucinations, other delusions, or disorganized thought. His behavior and level of self-care were totally appropriate. Multiple mental status examinations, neurologic studies, and laboratory screenings failed to disclose evidence of organic mental disorder.

Epidemiology

Kendler (1982) has reviewed the epidemiology of delusional disorder. This corresponds closely to the *DSM-III-R* concept but includes some patients with prominent hallucinations. Delusional disorder is relatively uncommon, representing 1–4% of all psychiatric hospital admissions. The incidence of the disorder is between 1 and 3 per 100,000 population annually, while the prevalence is between 0.02 and 0.03%. Onset is typically in middle life or later, with few first hospitalizations before age 35. Women are affected more often than men but not as predominantly as in affective disorders. Low socioeconomic status and recent immigrant status are common associated factors. Most patients have been married. Full recovery is unusual. Genetic studies indicate a lack of familial relationship to either schizophrenia or affective disorder.

Etiology & Pathogenesis

The cause of delusional disorder is unknown, but a number of theories have been proposed, most of which emphasize psychologic mechanisms and are particularly relevant to the persecutory type. Kraepelin and Kretschmer postulated that the disorder resulted from overwhelming stress in premorbid personality characterized by distrustfulness and hypersensitivity to slights. Later writers have postulated a developmental deficit in the ability to trust in others. Cameron (1974) stressed that individuals with delusional disorder have an inability to compare the perspectives of others with their own. They thus seem to be isolated, asocial people who must be vigilant lest something potentially threatening happen.

Freud made a major contribution to the understanding of paranoid thinking when he described the psychologic mechanism of **projection,** a process whereby ideas or feelings unacceptable to conscious awareness are disowned and attributed to (projected upon) others. In his analysis of the Schreber case in 1911, Freud argued that persecutory delusions were specifically the result of projected homosexuality, which had been latent in the patient. Modern writers actually consider Schreber to have been a paranoid schizophrenic. They also point out that although homosexual themes are common in male patients with persecutory symptoms, they are not universally present. Therefore, although Freud's thesis can aid in the understanding of an individual patient's psychodynamics, it is no longer considered a sufficient explanation for the pathogenesis of delusional disorder, persecutory type.

Salzman (1960) offered an alternative explanation based on the clinical observation that many paranoid patients exhibit pronounced grandiosity. It is often assumed that patients conclude they are important because of the attention they are receiving. Salzman believes that the reverse is actually true—ie, patients adopt an unrealistic view of their importance and abilities in order to compensate for feelings of vulnerability and worthlessness. The resulting arrogance antagonizes others, leading to rejection and humiliation. These events foster suspiciousness and distrust, finally setting the stage for overt paranoia.

Cameron (1974) has described the sequence of events leading to the development of a persecutory delusional system. Initially, the patient experiences feelings of being personally threatened and vulnerable. The source of these feelings may be a real or imagined problem such as deafness or unwanted homosexual fantasies. These patients try to explain their responses by looking for and identifying hostility in those around them. They try to discuss their suspicions with others, who only argue and try to convince them of their foolishness. Such people then become suspect also. By this process, patients become increasingly isolated, and the size of the hostile group enlarges. Increasingly puzzled about what is going on around them, they search for clues. As they begin to construct an explanation, they may see evidence of being followed, monitored, or subjected to tests. Everyone seems to indicate by comments or gestures that they know something about what is going on. Everywhere they go, people may be making remarks, casting glances, and so on. Newspapers or television programs may contain concealed messages or references to them. Cameron coined the term "pseudocommunity" to describe the organized group the patient believes is coordinating this effort. The delusional system becomes crystallized when patients develop a hypothesis to account for being singled out and when they decide who is behind the persecution. They may then act on their beliefs by filing lawsuits, trying to evade their enemies, or even counterattacking. It is usually at this point that such patients come to the attention of psychiatrists.

These psychologic formulations have significant shortcomings. They lack diagnostic specificity; similar psychologic issues are identifiable in patients with a variety of psychiatric disorders who happen to have persecutory delusions. Many patients with hypersensitive, asocial personalities develop other disorders (such as schizophrenia). In addition, similar phenomena may occur in otherwise normal individuals, sometimes under conditions of subjectively perceived vulnerability such as drug intoxication or fatigue or in social or religious groups whose values isolate them from the larger community. In some circumstances, overvigilant scanning of the environment for danger or treachery may be adaptive. Nonetheless, social isolation, whether due to maladaptive personality functioning, physical limitations, or cultural dislocation, seems to be an important etiologic factor in the pathogenesis of persecutory symptoms and delusional disorders in general. Additional contributory causes obviously are present but are beyond our current understanding.

Treatment

Although a trial of antipsychotic medication is nearly always indicated, the patient will be unlikely to participate willingly in any treatment program unless there is some basis for trust in the physician. Therefore, establishing rapport and a trusting relationship with the patient is more crucial to treatment of delusional disorder than any other specific treatment measure. Patients with this disorder are wary of any situation they do not control. To take medication as prescribed, they must fully trust the physician's competence, judgment, and motives. Suspicious patients often believe that medication may be designed to harm them or lower their resistance to outside influence. Any side effect, real or imagined, may frighten the patient into refusing further treatment. In the case of a committed patient, medications may be administered against the patient's protests, but the wisdom of doing so must be weighed against the possibility that the patient's mistrust and resistance to future treatment efforts may increase. In more acute psychotic disorders, a brief period of chemotherapy may return the patient to a state in which insight and cooperation are enhanced, and the patient may even be grateful that the physician took firm measures. However, in a chronic disorder, the response to chemotherapy is typically limited. Real improvement will depend on the long-term combination of continued neuroleptic therapy and a developing relationship with the clinician.

Paranoid patients feel that they have been disappointed by people who at first seem to be on their side but later betray them. Because of their hypersensitivity and vulnerability to perceived rejection or loss of face, they approach new relationships in a guarded fashion. At the same time, they are desperate for human contact and friendship and may wish to find someone to trust who can help them. To take advantage of this, the physician must assume a professional and respectful attitude toward these patients. A paternalistic approach will be perceived as insulting; an informal manner may imply that the physician does not take their concerns seriously. Complete frankness is called for—pretending to believe their delusional ideas leads to the appearance of betrayal when the physician's true feelings become apparent. Therapists should make it clear that they disagree with these patients but respect their opinions. There should be no attempt to argue with them or talk them out of their delusions by logical reasoning. As trust in the therapist deepens, the patients will feel better "understood," and the evidence for and against the validity of their delusional beliefs can be mutually explored in the

hope that the patients will begin to question the validity of the delusional beliefs. In essence, the therapist helps the patient overcome a deficiency in reality testing.

SUMMARY & CONCLUSIONS

Delusional disorders, whether acute or chronic, are characterized by prominent delusions and by the relative absence of hallucinations, disorganized thought and behavior, or deterioration of affect. Although not as common as other functional psychoses, they are consistently encountered in psychiatric settings. A premorbid personality beset by hypersensitivity, low self-esteem, distrustfulness, and feelings of resentment is common, as well as other conditions conducive to social isolation. Particular psychologic processes such as projection and hypervigilance are found in many cases. Patients may be difficult to treat because of their suspiciousness and lack of insight. Epidemiologic and genetic studies suggest that delusional disorders are distinct from both schizophrenia and affective disorder.

Because of the frequency of delusional symptoms in many forms of organic and functional mental disorders, careful diagnostic assessment is always important. In particular, proper diagnosis of organic mental disorder or affective disorder may result in a different choice of more specific treatment.

Delusional thinking has persisted as a subject of curiosity and mystery. It seems to reflect the operation of mental mechanisms that are ubiquitous in health as well as in disease. It is often difficult to distinguish between what constitutes an appropriate attitude of caution and distrust and pathologic paranoid ideation. Instances of excessive suspiciousness and overinterpretation of coincidental events are common in everyday life, yet they can also signal the presence of serious mental disorder. They physician must use a combination of clinical judgment, common sense, and familiarity with clinical psychopathologic concepts to arrive at an appropriate diagnosis and treatment plan.

REFERENCES

Cameron NA: Paranoid conditions and paranoia. Pages 676–693 in: *American Handbook of Psychiatry*. Vol 3. Arieti S, Brody EB (editors). Basic Books, 1974.

Kendler KS: Demography of paranoid psychosis (delusional disorder): A review and comparison with schizophrenia and affective illness. *Arch Gen Psychiatry* 1982;**39:**890.

Kendler KS: The nosological validity of paranoia (simple delusional disorder): A review. *Arch Gen Psychiatry* 1980;**37:**699.

Kendler KS, Gruenberg AM, Strauss JS: An independent analysis of the Copenhagen sample of the Danish Adoption Study of schizophrenia. The relationship between paranoid psychosis (delusional disorder) and the schizophrenia spectrum disorders. *Arch Gen Psychiatry* 1981;**38:**985.

Kendler KS, Hays P: Paranoid psychosis (delusional disorder) and schizophrenia: A family history study. *Arch Gen Psychiatry* 1981;**38:**547.

Lewis A: Paranoia and paranoid: A historical perspective. *Psychol Med* 1970;**1:**2.

Meissner WW: *The Paranoid Process*. Jason Aronson, 1978.

Munro A: Monosymptomatic hypochondriacal psychosis manifesting as delusions of parasitosis. *Arch Dermatol* 1978; **114:**940.

Munro A: Paranoia revisited. *Br J Psychiatry* 1982;**141:**344.

Salzman L: Paranoid state: Theory and therapy. *Arch Gen Psychiatry* 1960;**2:**679.

Swanson DW, Bohnert PJ, Smith JA: *The Paranoid*. Little, Brown, 1970.

29

Other Psychotic Disorders

Edward L. Merrin, MD

The presence of psychotic symptoms does not always warrant a diagnosis of schizophrenia. Many patients with psychotic symptoms are now considered to be suffering from major affective disorders with psychotic features or from certain types of personality disorders. However, some patients who present with obvious psychotic symptoms (delusions, hallucinations, disorganized speech or thought) for which there is no known organic cause fail to meet the criteria for any of the personality disorders, for schizophrenia, or for major affective disorders with psychotic features. These patients present the clinician with an important challenge, since accurate assessment and diagnosis may have critical consequences in choosing treatment and estimating prognosis.

The *DSM-III-R* categories of psychotic disorders discussed here represent an attempt to provide the practitioner with diagnoses that reflect the status of current knowledge. Each diagnosis has its own implications for treatment and prognosis, so that differential diagnosis both within and outside this group of disorders is crucial.

SCHIZOPHRENIFORM DISORDER

Symptoms & Signs

The term "schizophreniform disorder" was coined by Gabriel Langfeldt in 1939 to describe psychotic disorders in which typical symptoms of schizophrenia were present but without a chronic course. In *DSM-III-R*, the concept has been narrowed to exclude patients whose affective symptoms are severe enough to suggest a diagnosis of affective disorder. To satisfy the diagnostic criteria for schizophreniform disorder, patients must display psychotic symptoms sufficient to meet *DSM-III-R* criteria for the active phase of schizophrenia, but they must return to their previous level of functioning within 6 months. In older texts, some of these patients were termed "acute," "good-prognosis," or "remitting" schizophrenics.

Natural History

The long-term course of schizophreniform disorder is variable. In some patients, there is only a single psychotic episode, whereas in others, there are repeated episodes separated by varying lengths of time. First episodes usually occur in late adolescence or early adulthood, often in association with a specific precipi-

tating crisis. A better prognosis is often associated with adequate social and occupational functioning before the onset of illness, an abrupt rather than insidious onset, and confusion or disorientation during the most acute phase of the episode. Blunted or flat affect is a poor prognostic sign.

The diagnosis may have to be changed as the patient is followed over a period of months or years. Apparently, the majority of patients eventually develop schizophrenia, with recovery from subsequent episodes being less complete. In others, later episodes may take the form of depression or mania, with or without psychotic features. Particularly in adolescent patients, what appears to be schizophreniform illness often develops into an affective disorder as the patient matures into young adulthood.

Differential Diagnosis

Schizophreniform disorder is distinguished from schizophrenia by its short course (longer than 1 week but no longer than 6 months) and by the absence of any residual schizophrenic symptoms. Brief reactive psychosis is always related temporally to a significant psychosocial stressor and does not persist beyond 1 month. Unlike the mood disturbances in major depression or bipolar disorder, those in schizophreniform disorder, if present, are not accompanied by enough of the symptoms necessary for a diagnosis of affective disorder. Schizoaffective disorder differs from schizophreniform disorder in that a full affective syndrome is present. Affective symptoms may be difficult to evaluate in an acutely psychotic patient, however. As in schizophrenia, all organic or toxic factors (eg, psychostimulant or hallucinogenic drug intoxication, encephalitis) should be ruled out by appropriate history, physicial and mental status examination, and laboratory tests.

Prognosis

On long-term follow-up, about half of all patients with schizophreniform disorder will either improve or recover, whereas only one-third of schizophrenic patients will substantially improve. The length of illness is a factor in estimating short-term prognosis; patients whose illness lasts only 1 month do better than those with longer-lasting illnesses. Patients whose illness lasts closer to 6 months are eventually more likely to have an illness similar to schizophrenia, with a similar outcome. On longer-term follow-up, schizophreniform illnesses have outcomes intermediate between those of schizophrenia and affective disorder, but closer to the former. Patients with schizophreniform disorder are particularly more likely than schizophrenic patients to have good functioning in marital and social relationships.

Illustrative Case

A 31-year-old man recently fired from his job was admitted to the hospital with a recurrence of symptoms he had had on 2 previous occasions. He complained of difficulty in focusing his thoughts, speeded-up and intrusive thoughts of a bizarre nature ("there's a telepath in my old lady's body"), and auditory hallucinations of the voices of "telepaths" who controlled his body movements. During the interview, he manifested pressured speech, loose associations, and occasional idiosyncratic usage of words. Various tics and twitches occurred that were attributed to the influence of the "telepaths." His symptoms cleared entirely after several weeks of treatment with antipsychotic drugs, and he was able to return to living with his girlfriend. He also sought a new job as a licensed vocational nurse.

During his earlier life, the patient had always formed friendships and seemed well adjusted despite frequent family moves. His first episode of psychosis, which occurred at age 25 years, followed a romantic disappointment. A second episode occurred 3 years later during a period of unemployment and economic distress. His father was a salesman who was interested in the occult. A younger brother and sister had both suffered from psychotic illnesses of an unknown type.

Epidemiology

The prevalence of schizophreniform disorder is not known, although epidemiologic studies are currently under way in various population groups. It does appear to be less common than schizophrenia, at least among patients admitted to psychiatric hospitals. In one recent survey, schizophreniform disorder was diagnosed about half as often as schizophrenia. Although adequate data are lacking, it is a fair guess that schizophreniform disorder that shares the same causative factors as schizophrenia occurs with equal frequency in men and women. Such a disorder often represents the earliest stage of true schizophrenia. In a subgroup of patients with schizophreniform disorder that is related to affective disorder, women are probably more likely to be affected.

Etiology & Pathogenesis

As in the other major functional psychotic disorders, the cause of schizophreniform disorder is unknown. Some authorities have suggested that many patients with schizophreniform disorder actually suffer from an atypical affective disorder. The episodic course of the disorder and the effectiveness of lithium treatment in some patients support this hypothesis. However, other evidence indicates a link between schizophreniform disorder and schizophrenia. A recent study that used *DSM-III* criteria for schizophreni-

form disorder showed that the risk of developing schizophrenia in first-degree relatives of patients with schizophreniform disorder was similar to that of relatives of patients with schizophrenia (2% and 3%, respectively). In contrast, relatives of patients with affective disorder had almost no risk of developing schizophrenia. The same type of analysis indicated that in first-order relatives of patients with schizophreniform disorder, the risk of developing affective disorder was about 6%, a figure similar to that for relatives of schizophrenic patients but far less than the risk reported for relatives of patients with affective disorders (13%). As many as 20% of patients with schizophreniform disorders also appear to have unusually large cerebral ventricles, a finding frequently reported in studies of schizophrenic patients as well.

Treatment

A. Specific Measures: The main emphasis of treatment of schizophreniform disorder is somatic rather than psychologic. During the acute phase, the most frequently used medications are the neuroleptics—phenothiazines, butyrophenones, and similar drugs. A few patients improve without medication, possibly because the episode is self-limited. Occasionally, the supportive environment of a hospital alone is sufficient to terminate the psychotic episode. For this reason, some physicians prefer (if economically feasible) to observe the patient for several days before beginning treatment. This strategy permits the physician to verify the diagnosis and to better evaluate the need for treatment. It also exposes the patient to less risk of developing side effects such as tardive dyskinesia from long-term treatment with antipsychotic medications. Treatment itself proceeds in a fashion identical to that used for schizophrenia, with doses of antipsychotic drugs being gradually increased over a period of days or weeks until maximum benefit is achieved. Symptoms such as insomnia, agitation, suspiciousness, and disorganized thoughts may recede dramatically during the first few days of treatment, but auditory hallucinations and delusions may clear more gradually.

Alternative drugs have been used. Lithium may be effective in up to 30% of patients with schizophreniform disorder, who may constitute a subgroup with atypical presentation of an affective disorder. A trial of lithium may be worth considering in patients with recurrent psychotic episodes. Some clinicians have found benzodiazepine agents such as lorazepam or clonazepam useful in providing rapid control of acute agitation without the excessive sedation and parkinsonism associated with high-dose neuroleptic therapy. Electroconvulsive therapy has been used effectively in patients with dramatic, florid symptoms of abrupt onset. In patients who are extremely agitated, assaultive, or dangerously suicidal, electroconvulsive therapy has the advantage of achieving quick results. Patients in catatonic stupor also respond well; when dehydration and poor nutrition become serious problems in such patients, electroconvulsive therapy may be lifesaving.

In the first episode of schizophreniform disorder, neuroleptic medication rather than lithium is probably the wisest choice for initial drug treatment. A good rule of thumb is to gradually withdraw neuroleptic drugs after 6 months and—as long as symptoms do not recur—to continue to follow the patient who is not taking medication. Maintenance drugs may be required if subsequent episodes occur with any frequency but are free from residual symptoms suggesting a schizophrenic process. If residual symptoms do occur, treatment is as for schizophrenia. For patients who respond to both lithium and neuroleptics, lithium may be a better treatment choice, since it does not carry the risk of tardive dyskinesia or cause extrapyramidal symptoms, which may be socially detrimental even in mild forms. However, lithium therapy also carries certain risks and complications (see Chapter 52).

Not all patients with schizophreniform disorder need be hospitalized; if family members are willing to help administer medications and if the patient shows no signs of suicidal ideation or violent, destructive behavior, outpatient treatment may be possible. Frequent repeat office visits or telephone contacts enable the clinician to monitor progress and adjust medication. However, in the first episode of schizophreniform illness, it is preferable to hospitalize the patient in order to rule out illness that has a clear organic cause.

Suicide is of critical concern in the treatment of patients with schizophreniform disorder, particularly after psychotic symptoms have subsided. Many patients enter into a prolonged depression after psychotic symptoms have cleared. There are several possible explanations for this phenomenon: (1) It is part of the natural history of the disorder; (2) it is caused by neuroleptic drugs; (3) it indicates an underlying affective disorder; or (4) it represents a psychologic reaction to the realization that one has been mentally ill. These so-called postpsychotic depressions respond poorly to antidepressant treatment, and the risk of suicide is high. Patients should therefore be followed closely after discharge from the hospital and rehospitalized if suicidal ideation becomes apparent.

B. General Measures: Psychologic management varies from patient to patient but follows a general pattern. During the acute phase, providing a simplified, nonambiguous, structured environment is important. Every opportunity should be taken to remind the patient that the illness will be of limited duration. As the patient improves, it becomes possible to explore the psychologic, family, and other environmental issues that may have precipitated or contributed to the episode. The patient should also be helped to understand the nature of schizophreniform disorder and to recognize early signs of future episodes in order to obtain help quickly.

SCHIZOAFFECTIVE DISORDER

Ever since Emil Kraepelin first described the 2 major syndromes of dementia praecox (schizophrenia) and manic-depressive illness (bipolar affective disorder), clinicians have recognized that many patients cannot be assigned exclusively to either one group or the other. Eugen Bleuler suggested that any schizophrenialike features indicated a schizophrenic illness, regardless of what affective symptoms might also be present. Other writers noted that patients with affective symptoms had better-adjusted personalities before onset of illness and were more likely to achieve total remission from a given episode of illness than patients who had psychotic symptoms alone. Some authors felt that patients with both psychotic and affective symptoms suffered from another illness altogether. Cycloid psychosis, atypical schizophrenia, good-prognosis schizophrenia, and remitting schizophrenia have been some of the diagnoses assigned to these patients.

Symptoms & Signs

Jacob S. Kasanin coined the term "schizoaffective disorder" in 1933, and it has achieved widespread use as a description of psychotic illness with an admixture of schizophrenialike and affective symptoms. The diagnosis of schizoaffective disorder is appropriate when the clinician is unable to determine which symptoms represent the patient's primary underlying disease process. At some time during the illness, a full affective syndrome (manic episode or major depressive episode) is accompanied by psychotic symptoms that meet criterion A for schizophrenia. If the psychotic symptoms persist 2 weeks beyond the resolution of the affective symptoms, the diagnosis of affective disorder is ruled out. Similarly, if the duration of the affective symptoms is not brief in relation to the total duration of the patient's illness, schizophrenia is ruled out. In practice, this diagnosis is often used on a provisional basis and may reflect some uncertainty about the most appropriate diagnosis.

Natural History & Prognosis

On long-term follow-up, it appears that the age at onset and the degree of recovery for patients with schizoaffective disorder are intermediate between those for patients with affective disorders and those for patients with schizophrenia. When patients with schizoaffective disorder are divided into those with and those without psychotic symptoms for significant periods (weeks or months) between affective episodes, a clearer picture emerges. Patients with chronic psychotic symptoms do about as well as schizophrenic patients, and those without persistent psychotic symptoms have courses similar to those of patients with affective disorders.

Differential Diagnosis

The term "schizoaffective disorder" has been used to describe a wide variety of disorders, many of which meet the *DSM-III-R* criteria for other maladies. When a patient is evaluated, clarification of the temporal relationship between the 2 types of symptoms is important.

Patients with a predominantly schizophrenic clinical picture but with occasional periods of depression or elation that meet the *DSM-III-R* criteria for affective disorder should be diagnosed as having schizophrenia with atypical affective disorder. Patients who suffer from an illness with a remitting course with or without recurrences are considered to have affective disorders with psychotic features. The psychotic features should clear as the mood disturbance resolves and should not dominate the clinical picture. If the thematic content of any delusions or hallucinations is related to the patient's mood of depression or elation, the most appropriate diagnosis is major depression or bipolar affective disorder with mood-congruent psychotic features. (Examples would include the belief by a depressed woman that she has sinned or a manic individual's belief that he or she is the Messiah.) If the psychotic symptoms are not related to the theme of the patient's predominant mood, a diagnosis of major depression or bipolar affective disorder with mood-incongruent psychotic features is appropriate. Other diagnoses that must be considered are schizophreniform disorder—when the illness is not chronic and affective symptoms are not as prominent as in schizoaffective disorder—and brief reactive psychosis, which is always preceded by severe psychosocial stressors and resolves within 1 month.

Illustrative Case No. 1

A 65-year-old man of German descent requested outpatient psychiatric follow-up at the urging of his sister. His history included frequent hospitalizations since his 30s for an illness characterized in part by auditory hallucinations and paranoid delusions. After each hospitalization, he recovered enough to return to his full-time job. Upon retiring, he moved to the West Coast, where his sister lived, and took up residence in a downtown hotel.

In the clinic, the patient continued to receive the injections of depot phenothiazines that he had been receiving elsewhere. Within a few months, he became markedly depressed. A trial of tricyclic antidepressant drugs resulted in a euphoric mood accompanied by pressured speech, insomnia, and poor judgment. The antidepressant medication was discontinued, but the depression returned within a few months, and the patient was subsequently hospitalized.

Upon admission to the hospital, the patient was severely slowed in his movements and speech and walked with a stooped gait. He slept poorly and had little appetite. When interviewed, he insisted that therapeutic efforts were best spent on other patients, because he was a worthless person for whom there was no hope. He wanted to be dead but lacked the initiative or courage to commit suicide. There were no delusions or hallucinations, and his speech was well organized and logical. Results of a dexamethasone suppression test showed failure to suppress cortisol secretion. The patient responded dramatically within 10 days of resumption of the antidepressant drug in a lower dosage. Results of a second dexamethasone suppression test were normal. The history suggested a manic component to his previous illness, and prophylactic lithium treatment was begun. The depot phenothiazine was discontinued.

Several months after he was discharged from the hospital, the patient stopped taking the lithium because of a tremor. He also began to pace around his hotel, slept poorly, and ate only one small meal daily. He also stopped bathing and shaving. After 1 month, he was coaxed with tremendous effort by his hotel manager and clinic staff to return to the hospital. There he presented in a filthy, disheveled state; he was lice-ridden and had lost 20 lb. He was not visibly depressed or elated, however. He was extremely negativistic and turned his head and glared frequently as if responding to a voice. After several days of treatment with moderate doses of haloperidol, he began to respond to questioning by his physician. He denied having been depressed and insisted that nothing was wrong with him. He admitted hearing women singing happy German children's songs and often sang along with them. He also discussed his belief that Jews were attempting to harm him and his children and grandchildren as retaliation for what the Germans had done to them during World War II. He claimed that he had felt this way for years but often avoided discussing it with his doctors. He described a series of seemingly ordinary incidents that had happened through the years that he felt proved his point.

Illustrative Case No. 2

A 44-year-old divorced man presented with a 20-year history of various psychiatric hospitalizations. During this period, he abused alcohol frequently, traveled about the country, and received inpatient care at least once annually. The usual diagnosis had been paranoid schizophrenia. Two months before his latest request for inpatient care, he had started lithium treatment at a hospital in southern California. He claimed that unlike the neuroleptic drugs he had been given in the past, lithium had cleared up his thinking considerably. However, after discharge, he became concerned about increased urination and dysuria; he was frightened that the lithium might be causing renal damage, and he discontinued the drug. He also stopped taking the chlorpromazine that had been prescribed. He complained of sleeplessness and weight loss and became loud and belligerent when his need for hospitalization was questioned.

Mental status examination revealed a guarded, somewhat sarcastic, thin man who spoke in increasingly loud tones with a considerable degree of pressure and circumstantiality. His behavior on the ward was intrusive and loud, and he slept little. His mood was irritable, and he was frequently pacing, talking, or otherwise active. When questioned about auditory hallucinations, he became extremely defensive and insisted that he did not hear voices. He did say, however, that sometimes he picked up information from the "wrong channel" but ignored it. He had gotten "into trouble" in the past when he paid attention to what he had heard.

Initial treatment consisted of lithium. Small doses of haloperidol had to be added temporarily because his pressured, irritable manner caused conflicts with other patients. After 1 week, his behavior was considerably subdued, but it became apparent that he was hallucinating constantly. He spent most of his day off the ward in animated conversation with nonexistent persons. Serum lithium levels at that point were within the therapeutic range. Addition of haloperidol in standard doses eliminated the hallucinations, but withdrawal of lithium resulted in a return of manic behavior. He clearly required both medications.

In contrast to the patient described in the first illustrative case, who presented with mainly affective symptoms on most occasions, this patient occasionally developed an agitated, overly talkative state superimposed upon a chronic hallucinosis. Neither lithium nor neuroleptics alone were able to alleviate both aspects of his illness.

Epidemiology

Because it has been difficult to establish standardized diagnostic criteria, the incidence and prevalence of schizoaffective disorder are unknown. Limited knowledge suggests that schizoaffective disorder is probably less prevalent than either schizophrenia or affective disorder. Women are probably more commonly affected than men.

Etiology & Pathogenesis

It seems unlikely that all schizoaffective disorders arise from a unique cause. Causative factors in schizoaffective disorder are probably related to those of schizophrenia when chronic mood-incongruent psychotic symptoms are prominent, and probably also to affective disorders when a remitting course or chronic mood-congruent symptoms are present. Early-onset affective disorders often show many schizophrenialike features. There is no evidence that any of these patients suffer from a combination of both disorders. However, genetic studies of patients with schizoaffective disorder usually indicate family histories of alcohol abuse or affective disorder.

Treatment

The treatment of schizoaffective disorder is empirical. During a manic phase, lithium, neuroleptics, or both are often used. Some evidence indicates that schizoaffective manic patients may take longer than manic patients to respond to lithium. In highly active patients, the onset of action of lithium is too long, and unless they are treated with neuroleptics they either leave treatment or become unmanageable. However, less active patients do well on lithium, together with small doses of neuroleptics initially to promote sleep and curb restlessness. Other drugs in current use are lorazepam, a short-acting sedative, and the anticonvulsant clonazepam for short-term control of manic excitement. They offer the advantage of minimizing the occurrence of excessive extrapyramidal effects associated with neuroleptic use.

Complete remission may occur in some of these patients treated with lithium alone; some clinicians then change the diagnosis to mania. Other patients continue to experience delusions or hallucinations unless a neuroleptic is added to the treatment regimen. Whether or not both drugs should be used together is a matter of clinical judgment. On the one hand, there is some evidence that a combination of an antipsychotic (eg, haloperidol) and lithium is somewhat more efficacious than an antipsychotic alone—regardless of whether the course of the patient's illness is more like that of an affective disorder or more similar to that of schizophrenia. Lower dosages of neuroleptics may also be possible when given adjunctively with lithium. On the other hand, lithium treatment carries an additional set of risks (see Chapter 52), and lithium-neuroleptic combinations may produce severe extrapyramidal reactions or confusion in some patients.

In earlier reports, lithium was found to produce a toxic confusional state in some patients with schizophrenia, but these reports have not been uniformly confirmed, and many schizoaffective and schizophrenic patients with atypical affective disorder have been treated with lithium without suffering this problem. When lithium is not effective or is not well tolerated, the anticonvulsant carbamazepine may be indicated. It is clearly an effective antimanic agent, particularly in patients who have not reponded to lithium. Certain precautions in its use are necessary, since granulocytopenia can occur during the first few weeks of treatment. Calcium channel blockers are currently under evaluation for use in control of manic symptoms and may be a third major clinical option. However, neither carbamazepine nor calcium channel blockers have been systematically evaluated in schizoaffective patients.

The treatment of the schizoaffective depressed patient has not been as well studied as that of the schizoaffective patient with mania. As in major depression with psychotic features, treatment with antidepressant drugs alone—even at relatively high doses—is not often effective. Administration of a neuroleptic drug is usually required, at least initially. The neuroleptic may often be tapered after psychotic symptoms have abated and the patient's mood has lifted. The combined drug treatment may often have to be continued indefinitely. Some schizoaffective depressed patients may fail to demonstrate suppression of cortisol secretion after the administration of dexamethasone. It is not known whether the dexamethasone suppression test can be used to monitor clinical progress in schizoaffective disorder as it is apparently possible to do in major depression.

It has been noted that some patients with schizophrenia have become more psychotic when treated with antidepressants; this untoward response may have made clinicians reluctant to use the same treatment in patients with schizoaffective depression. The cause of these adverse effects is unclear. Some of them may have represented toxic psychoses resulting from the simultaneous administration of multiple psychotropic drugs, all with anticholinergic activity. Others may have represented manic responses to the antidepressant. Both of these adverse effects are relatively common. Patients who are receiving combined treatment of this type should be monitored closely for emergence of untoward symptoms. If problems develop, a review of the patient's medications and reduction in dose or discontinuation of the antidepressant or other agents should be considered.

The use of lithium in schizoaffective depression is not clearly indicated. Because only a few unipolar depressive illnesses respond to lithium, the use of lithium as a first-line antidepressant is probably not justified. It may be indicated when there is a history of previous positive response or when other drugs have failed. Lithium may also be indicated when the history strongly suggests previous manic periods. Lithium prophylaxis has not been proved effective in treatment of recurrent schizoaffective depression. If the patient has depressive episodes only, maintenance treatment with drugs such as tricyclic antidepressants or monoamine oxidase inhibitors is probably a more prudent choice.

BRIEF REACTIVE PSYCHOSIS

Psychiatrists have long recognized that otherwise well-functioning people may develop psychotic symptoms when they are confronted with overwhelming stress. In certain cultures, symptoms conform to certain patterns that are recognized by the individual's group as a valid signal of the person's distress. In Western society, several forms of presentation of brief reactive psychosis have been described, and terms such as reactive psychosis, psychogenic psychosis, and hysterical psychosis have all been applied to basically similar reactions.

Unfortunately, a tendency to lump all "psychotic" disorders together has interfered with the recognition and understanding of brief reactive psychosis and has often stood in the way of appropriate treatment. For example, the term "3-day schizophrenia" has been used to describe brief psychotic illnesses such as those seen in young soldiers involved in combat operations in the South Pacific during World War II. On occasion, massive doses of psychotropic drugs were used, and the remarkable clearing of symptoms was subsequently attributed incorrectly to the drug therapy.

Symptoms & Signs

Brief reactive psychoses may take many forms, but they always have certain features in common. First, there is a precipitating stress. This may be quite obvious, eg, an automobile accident, natural catastrophe, combat, or the sudden death of a loved one. The patient's personality structure is an important consideration in determining how much stress is necessary to precipitate a psychotic reaction. Patients with certain personality disorders (eg, histrionic or borderline personality) may be prone to develop psychotic symptoms more easily. It should be noted that the psychosocial stressor must be sufficiently severe to provoke signs of distress in almost anyone in order for the diagnosis of brief reactive psychosis to be warranted.

The second feature common to reactive psychoses is abrupt onset of symptoms, often within a few hours of the precipitating event. There is no history of a gradually developing prodrome, as is often seen in schizophreniform disorder or schizophrenia.

The psychotic symptoms themselves may be of various types. Delusions, hallucinations (auditory hallucinations are common but visual hallucinations occur occasionally), loose or disconnected verbalization, and bizarre and disorganized behavior are all possible. A clinical picture resembling bipolar affective disorder has also been described. Symptoms are often dramatic and florid and are usually thematically related to the precipitating event.

Natural History & Prognosis

The duration of the disorder is brief (no longer than 1 month), and there is no residual deficit. However, many patients will have repeat episodes in response to future stresses, especially if a basic personality disorder leads to a maladaptive life-style that subjects the individual to intolerable situations.

Differential Diagnosis

Brief reactive psychosis may be distinguished from various other mental disorders. The presence of toxic factors, such as withdrawal from alcohol or drugs, should be ruled out by appropriate history taking, physical examination, and laboratory tests. Schizophreniform disorder generally lasts longer than 1 month, and this diagnosis may be considered if symptoms persist. If prominent affective symptoms are present after 1 month, a diagnosis of affective or schizoaffective disorder may be warranted. In schizophrenia, the patient should show signs of a chronic disorder without a return to the level of functioning seen before the onset of illness. Some schizophrenic patients with chronic, low-level symptoms may experience a brief worsening of psychotic symptoms in response to stress; this should *not* be diagnosed as brief reactive psychosis. If no precipitating event can be identified but symptoms clear within 1 month, a diagnosis of atypical psychosis may be appropriate. Transient psychotic symptoms may be present in patients with borderline or schizotypal personality disorders, but these are fleeting and not associated with a clear psychosocial stressor (see Atypical Psychosis, below). A few patients may present with factitious symptoms or may be outright malingerers.

Illustrative Case

A 60-year-old widower was admitted to the urology service for evaluation of acute onset of inability to void. While a physician was explaining the nature of a planned diagnostic procedure, bright red blood appeared in the catheter bag in full view of the patient. He became extremely frightened and, despite the physician's attempts to reassure him, developed the conviction that he would not survive the upcoming procedure. When a psychiatric consultant visited him several hours later, he was sobbing uncontrollably and was unable to lie still. He overheard messengers from God telling him he would be dead soon, and he saw visions of his deceased wife, who promised him a reunion. While in this state, he refused to accept information contrary to what he was experiencing in his hallucinations. He also professed guilt about exaggerating his emotional problems over the years in order to obtain disability compensation.

The patient's psychiatric history dated back to World War II, when he had experienced 2 episodes of psychogenic amnesia and had traveled long distances before finding himself in a strange city. Since then, he had had periods of anxiety, particularly in crowded public situations, and he had finally stopped working at age 50 years. He had never been psychotic.

After 2 days of treatment and frequent reassurance from the medical staff, his symptoms disappeared almost as dramatically as they had begun. A week later he claimed amnesia for the entire event, including his "confession" of guilt.

Epidemiology

The incidence and sex distribution of brief reactive psychosis are unknown.

Etiology & Pathogenesis

Brief reactive psychosis is thought to be mainly psychologic in origin (rather than social or biologic), although the latter factors probably contribute. When confronted with a stressful situation, the natural response is to use familiar problem-solving behavior patterns either to achieve a resolution or to maintain psychologic equilibrium until external events change. If an individual's usual coping strategies are not effective, anxiety increases. Psychotic symptoms may emerge when the patient's psychologic defenses are completely overwhelmed. How much stress is necessary to reach this point is partly determined by the patient's structure of defenses. For some patients, only chaotic events such as natural disasters or combat experiences are severe enough to upset the equilibrium; other people may be overwhelmed by divorce, physical illness, or financial disaster. Some patients with character defects (ie, personality disorder) may be unable to cope with transitions or disappointments that most other people would be able to handle, even though they might find them unsettling.

Besides signaling psychologic collapse, brief reactive psychosis may provide secondary gain for the patient and may become a regular method of evading responsibility or unpleasant circumstances in the future. The dramatic psychotic symptoms make it clear to oth-

ers that the patient is helpless. Since the symptoms are accepted as part of legitimate illness and not as evidence of shirking, others can rush in to the rescue without having any negative feelings toward the patient. In patients confronted with a chronically intolerable situation, occasional emotional collapses when the situation gets worse provide a brief escape.

Treatment

A. Drug Treatment: The treatment of psychotic symptoms should be approached conservatively and should be individualized for each patient. Psychotropic medications have a place in controlling agitation and insomnia. If brief reactive psychosis is suspected initially, neuroleptic medications should be limited to short-term use only and then only when absolutely necessary. If the diagnosis is suspected after neuroleptic treatment has already started, medications should be discontinued as soon as possible. Symptomatic treatment with benzodiazepines (which are not associated with the risk of tardive dyskinesia) will often make the patient more comfortable, although these agents may not relieve all symptoms in some patients.

B. Psychologic Treatment: Psychologic treatment may take several forms. Simply being removed from the crisis and having the care and attention of the hospital staff may allay the patient's anxiety enough to permit constructive discussion and problem solving. Once the resources of the staff become available, the stress may no longer seem overwhelming. Enlisting the aid of family members may also be important for the same reason. In individual psychotherapy, encouraging the patient to recount the events that led to the breakdown and to discuss their impact and meaning will facilitate recovery. Such discussion has 2 effects: It allows the patient to control anxiety by breaking down the experience into understandable units, and it offers the patient a model for dealing with crises in the future. Longer-term psychotherapy directed at more fundamental psychologic conflicts may be indicated for some patients.

INDUCED PSYCHOTIC DISORDER (Shared Paranoid Disorder)

Symptoms & Signs

Induced psychotic disorder is an uncommon disorder characterized by uncritical acceptance by one person of the delusional beliefs of another, usually more psychotic, individual. Although 2 people are most commonly involved (*folie à deux*), cases have been reported involving 3 or more and in some instances an entire family. The patients are always relatives or persons who have lived in intimate contact for a long time.

A characteristic feature of induced psychotic disorder is a complex dependent relationship between the parties; a pattern of dominance and submission is usually apparent. The dominant partner is more seriously ill, suffering from a delusional psychosis—usually paranoid schizophrenia or delusional disorder—but sometimes an affective disorder. This individual is the originator of the delusions, passing them on to the passive partner. The submissive partner may have a history of less severe emotional disturbance but is often not otherwise psychotic, although there are exceptions. Being extremely suggestible and overly dependent on the more forceful personality of the dominant partner, the submissive partner is ready to suspend critical thinking in order to share the imagined comforts of the delusional world. Thus, the psychosis is virtually imposed upon or transmitted to the submissive partner. The content of the delusions is usually persecutory or hypochondriacal. The delusions underscore the perceived hostility of the outside world, reinforcing the social isolation and interdependence of the parties. This marked isolation becomes a strong motivation to maintain the close relationship at all costs.

Cases involving large families have unique features. One dominant member suffers from a psychotic disorder and is the source of the delusions. However, family members may differ greatly in the degree to which they share the psychotic beliefs, depending upon the presence and severity of psychopathologic changes in each member. Once again, the delusions become a unifying bond, serving to buttress the family against the hostility of an outside world from which they are isolated and estranged.

Differential Diagnosis

Organic delusional disorder should be ruled out in both patients. If the submissive partner suffers from schizophrenia, schizophreniform disorder, or schizoaffective disorder, this diagnosis will eventually become more important. Significant personality disorder should also be noted, if present. None of these diagnoses are incompatible with induced psychotic disorder, however.

Prognosis

The prognosis for the submissive "recipient" is quite good when the underlying psychopathologic condition is not of psychotic proportions. Simple separation from the dominant partner results in clearing of delusional thinking. When both parties suffer from psychotic disorders, additional treatment specific for the underlying illness is necessary, with the final outcome depending on the diagnosis. In approximately 40% of reported cases, the recipient patient has responded to separation from the dominant partner alone.

Illustrative Case

A hotel manager in a small town called the police because a guest family had stopped paying its bills and had been acting strangely. A 48-year-old man, his 25-year-old wife, and their infant son had registered 2 weeks previously and had not left the room except for the wife's trips to the grocery store. These forays also had ceased a week before. The rent for the second week had not been paid despite frequent demands.

Other guests complained of chanting and yelling during the night.

The husband was an unemployed laborer with a history of psychiatric hospitalizations and arrests for drunkenness and assault. He professed to be receiving messages from God directing him and his family to await the destruction of the world and the beginning of "the new order." His family would be among the few survivors and would play a leading role in the future of mankind. He heard the voice of God and of various angels who gave him explicit instructions to follow.

His wife was an extremely introverted, socially awkward woman whose mother abandoned her to an orphanage at the age of 5. She had never dated before her husband took an interest in her after meeting her in a shop where she worked as a clerk. They were married after a short courtship, and soon after she broke off contact with all former associates. She was dependent on her husband for income and all decision making, accompanying him as he moved from town to town in search of work. Jobs were usually lost because of arguments with his employers or drinking. She rarely had contacts with other adults without her husband being present; on those occasions, he would invariably speak for her.

The husband had to be forcibly removed from the hotel room by the police and was eventually committed to a state hospital. His wife initially resisted offers of help, fearing that if she left the hotel she would not be saved from the impending holocaust. She gradually gave up these beliefs in response to simple reassurance. The child was placed in a foster home. The wife and husband were reunited after his release from the hospital and were lost to follow-up.

Epidemiology

There are no data on the incidence or prevalence of induced psychotic disorder. It is thought to be quite rare. Over 90% of cases involve members of a single family. The most common cases involve 2 sisters. Mother and child are next in frequency of occurrence, followed by father/child and husband/wife combinations. Pairings between friends and fellow mental patients are infrequent but have occurred.

Approximately 25% of the submissive (recipient) partners are suffering from a physical disability such as hearing loss or stroke, which may increase their susceptibility to domination by their partners.

Etiology & Pathogenesis

Induced psychotic disorder is believed to arise as a result of interdependency between the partners and serves to preserve their relationship. In order for the mechanism to work, several conditions must be met. The inducing partner, already mentally ill, must be dominant in the relationship and be able to influence the submissive partner. There must be a distinct advantage to both partners in sharing the delusions. For the inducing partner, maintaining at least one human contact represents a chance to avoid complete isolation. The delusions are the only currency of communication that allows a tie with the partner so that alienation from outside reality can be endured. For the submissive partner, the delusions become a compromise, allowing continuation of a dependent relationship.

Some authors have emphasized the role of identification in induced psychotic disorder. The recipient patients admire the strength and will of their partners. By identifying with them, they can acquire these characteristics for themselves. In order to do so, they pay the price of withdrawal from reality, since in the process of identification they also acquire the psychotic thinking of the partner. The submissive party comes to hate the dominant one and unfortunately becomes full of self-blame for being weak and dependent. This further reduces self-esteem, thus increasing dependency and strengthening the pathologic process.

Treatment

The first step in treatment is separation from the dominant partner. In many cases, the patient then becomes accessible to rational discussion and soon gives up the delusional system. However, since many patients will return to the same relationship, other steps may be indicated. These might include family or conjoint therapy as well as assistance with developing activities and interests outside the relationship.

When the recipient patient also suffers from a psychotic disorder, more specific treatment will be necessary in addition to separation. Depending on the underlying diagnosis, this may include antipsychotics, antidepressants, or electroconvulsive therapy.

ATYPICAL PSYCHOSIS

Symptoms & Signs

Atypical psychosis is basically a diagnosis for those disorders which are characterized by psychotic symptoms (delusions, hallucinations, disorganized speech or behavior) but which do not otherwise meet the criteria for more specific disorders. The diagnosis of atypical psychosis is appropriate when results on history and clinical examination are incomplete or puzzling or when there are unusual features. When evaluating an acutely psychotic patient, the physician may only be able to manage the patient's agitated or unruly behavior and must forgo more careful diagnostic analysis until later. A diagnosis of "atypical psychosis" is preferred to "diagnosis deferred," because it communicates more information by noting the presence of psychotic symptoms.

One appropriate use of the diagnosis of atypical psychosis is for patients who present with brief periods of psychotic symptoms that do not bear any relationship to a recognizable psychosocial stressor. Some of these patients have serious personality disorders that predispose them to psychotic reactions to events that would be insignificant to most individuals. Their overreactions are sometimes based on misinterpretation of events around them.

The diagnosis of atypical psychosis is also called for when symptoms consistent with the diagnosis of schizophrenia first occur after age 45. Some psychiatrists have termed this disorder **paraphrenia.**

Illustrative Case

A 28-year-old man presented with feelings of depression and fearfulness. He usually dealt with such feelings by giving in to the strong urge to flee his environment and start over. This time a friend advised him to seek help. He was a chronically unhappy person who felt he should be a woman and who lived a homosexual life-style. He had previously been married in what he felt had been a brief attempt to produce a child "for my mother." His homosexual relationships were short-lived and caused him great pain as he desperately sought the chance "to be a woman" to someone. He had gone through frequent periods of depression, several suicide attempts by drug overdose, and numerous psychiatric hospitalizations of short duration.

On this occasion, the patient complained of depression, difficulty in sleeping, and a feeling of fear, which came over him daily. There were no apparent signs of psychosis until about 2 weeks after his hospital admission. At that time, he began to believe that all of the other patients and staff knew about his sexual life and were discussing it. He was convinced that the contents of his private discussions with his therapist were being disclosed to the entire ward, and he interpreted the actions and comments of both staff and patients accordingly. He began to feel uncomfortable in the hospital, and he requested discharge. The request was refused, and after several days of these symptoms, he was given small doses of haloperidol, with improvement occurring almost overnight. A week later, the medication was discontinued, and the symptoms did not recur.

SUMMARY

The appropriate diagnosis of functional psychosis depends upon both careful clinical observation and description and a detailed history. The following characteristics are particularly important in the differential diagnosis of the psychotic disorders discussed in this chapter: (1) the presence or absence of both psychotic and affective symptoms and their temporal relationships; (2) the duration and degree of recovery from each episode of illness; and (3) the presence or absence of significant precipitating events.

REFERENCES

Biederman J et al: Combination of lithium carbonate and halo-peridol in schizo-affective disorder: A controlled study. *Arch Gen Psychiatry* 1979;**36**:327.

Brotman AW, Farhadi AM, Gelenberg AJ: Verapamil treatment of acute mania. *J Clin Psychiatry* 1986;**47**:136.

Carman JS, Bigelow LB, Wyatt RJ: Lithium combined with neuroleptics in chronic schizophrenic and schizoaffective patients. *J Clin Psychiatry* 1981;**42**:124.

Cavenor JO et al: A clinical note on hysterical psychosis. *Am J Psychiatry* 1979;**136**:830.

Coryell W, Tsuang MT: *DSM-III* schizophreniform disorder: Comparisons with schizophrenia and affective disorder. *Arch Gen Psychiatry* 1982;**39**:66.

Coryell W, Tsuang MT: Outcome after 40 years in *DSM-III* schizophreniform disorder. *Arch Gen Psychiatry* 1986;**43**:324.

Dempsey GM et al: Treatment of schizo-affective disorder. *Compr Psychiatry* 1975;**16**:55.

Enoch MD, Trethowan WH: Folie à deux (et folie à plusieurs). Pages 134–157 in: *Uncommon Psychiatric Syndromes,* 2nd ed. John Wright & Sons, 1979.

Fogelson DL et al: A study of *DSM-III* schizophreniform disorder. *Am J Psychiatry* 1982;**139**:1281.

Goodnick PJ, Meltzer HY: Treatment of schizoaffective disorders. *Schizophr Bull* 1984;**10**:30.

Grossman LS, Harrow M, Fudala JL, Meltzer HY: The longitudinal course of schizoaffective disorders: A prospective followup study. *J Nerv Ment Dis* 1984;**172**:140.

Himmelhoch JM et al: When a schizoaffective diagnosis has meaning. *J Nerv Ment Dis* 1981;**169**:277.

Hirsch SJ, Hollender MH: Hysterical psychosis: Clarification of the concept. *Am J Psychiatry* 1969;**125**:909.

Hirschowitz J et al: Lithium response in good prognosis schizophrenia. *Am J Psychiatry* 1980;**137**:916.

Hollender MH, Hirsch SJ: Hysterical psychosis. *Am J Psychiatry* 1964;**120**:1066.

Kasanin JS: The acute schizoaffective psychoses. *Am J Psychiatry* 1933;**90**:97.

Leonhard K: Cycloid psychoses: Endogenous psychoses which are neither schizophrenic nor manic-depressive. *J Ment Sci* 1961;**107**:633.

Levinson DF, Levitt MEM: Schizoaffective mania reconsidered. *Am J Psychiatry* 1987;**144**:415.

Maj M: Evolution of the American concept of schizoaffective psychosis. *Neuropsychobiology* 1984;**11**:7.

McGlashan TH, Carpenter WT: An investigation of the postpsychotic depressive syndrome. *Am J Psychiatry* 1976;**133**:14.

Modell JG, Lenox RH, Weiner S: Inpatient clinical trial of lorazepam for the management of manic agitation. *J Clin Psychopharmacol* 1985;**5**:109.

Prien RF et al: A comparison of lithium carbonate and chlorpromazine in the treatment of excited schizo-affectives: Report of the Veterans Administration and National Institute of Mental Health Collaborative Study Group. *Arch Gen Psychiatry* 1972;**27**:182.

Procci WR: Schizo-affective psychosis: Fact or fiction? *Arch Gen Psychiatry* 1976;**33**:1167.

Rosenthal NE et al: Toward the validation of RDC schizoaffective disorder. *Arch Gen Psychiatry* 1980;**37**:804.

Victor BS et al: Use of clonazepam in mania and schizoaffective disorders. *Am J Psychiatry* 1984;**141**:1111.

Weinberger DR et al: Computed tomography in schizophreniform disorder and other acute psychiatric disorders. *Arch Gen Psychiatry* 1982;**39**:778.

30

Affective Disorders

Victor I. Reus, MD

About 55 years ago, the British physician Aubrey Lewis noted that the history of the diagnosis and treatment of melancholia could serve as a history of psychiatry itself. That observation seems particularly relevant today, since advances in the diagnosis and treatment of affective disorders have led to a dramatic increase in their perceived prevalence and to more rigorous criteria for placement in competing nosologic categories.

The hallmark of the affective disorders is a primary pervasive disturbance in mood (affective disorders are now called mood disorders in *DSM-III-R*). In this context, the term "mood" denotes an emotional state that may affect all aspects of the individual's life. The syndromes are characterized by pathologically elevated or depressed mood and should be regarded as existing on a continuum with normal mood. A diagnosis of affective disorder is appropriate when the mood disturbance is "primary" and central to the illness and not secondary to some other physical or psychologic state. In the latter instance, the diagnosis would be incomplete without a reference to the precipitating cause. Although historically a precipitating stressful event was thought to be a critical element in the differential diagnosis of affective disorders, current opinion is that data of this sort lack diagnostic specificity and prognostic validity. Even so, when a mood disturbance following a stressful life event is a mild one that does not meet the criteria for any of the disorders discussed in this chapter, a diagnosis of **adjustment disorder with depressed mood** is warranted (see Chapter 35).

In this chapter, the class of affective disorders is divided into disorders in which there is a full major affective syndrome; disorders in which there is only a partial but persistent syndrome; and disorders that cannot be classified in either of these 2 ways (Table 30–1). Major affective disorders are further classified according to whether the patient has a history of a manic episode. A past or present history of a manic episode justifies a diagnosis of **bipolar disorder,** which may be further subdivided on the basis of the presenting affective state **(manic, depressed,** or **mixed).** Some investigators have suggested that within the spectrum of bipolar illness are distinct subtypes characterized by prominence of either mania or depression. If there is no history of manic episode and if the criteria of severity are met, a diagnosis of **major depressive disorder** is warranted. Major depression is further subclassified according to whether it is a first

episode or a recurrence. Additional clinical features such as the presence of psychotic ideation or vegetative signs should also be specifically recorded. Although not authorized by *DSM-III*, the term "unipolar" is sometimes used in describing this group of disorders.

Other specific affective disorders include cyclothymic disorder and dysthymic disorder. In **cyclothymic disorder,** the symptoms resemble those of bipolar disorder but are neither severe enough nor of sufficient duration to meet the criteria for diagnosis of bipolar or major depressive disorder. The term **dysthymic disorder** partially encompasses the group of individuals historically classified as suffering from depressive neurosis. Individuals with this diagnosis have chronic depression that is not of sufficient severity or duration to meet the criteria for major depressive episode.

The terms **atypical bipolar disorder** and **atypical depression** are reserved for individuals who do not precisely meet any of the criteria just described. One example would be patients with a history of major depressive episodes and episodes with some manic features not of sufficient severity or duration to meet the criteria for bipolar affective disorder, mixed type.

BIPOLAR DISORDER

Symptoms & Signs

One essential criterion for a diagnosis of bipolar disorder is a past or present history of a manic episode. Primary manic episodes are characterized by a predominantly elevated, expansive, or irritable mood that presents as a prominent or persistent part of the illness. "Secondary" mania is identical behaviorally to "primary" mania but is limited to situations in which the precipitating cause is known, as in amphetamine-stimulated manic and hyperthyroid manic states. Manic patients classically have abundant resources of energy and engage in multiple activities and ventures. At baseline and between episodes, the bipolar manic patient may indeed function at a high level of productivity, particularly in areas requiring creative talent. In the intial stages of an episode—and sometimes in attenuated episodes—the ventures may appear genuinely creative and perhaps only mildly eccentric. In time, however, as the investment in these activities becomes excessive, the individual loses the capacity to

Table 30–1. *DSM-III-R* diagnostic criteria for affective disorders.*†

Manic episode:
Note: A "manic syndrome" is defined as including criteria A, B, and C, below. A "hypomanic syndrome" is defined as including criteria A and B, but not criterion C, ie, no marked impairment.
   A. A distinct period of abnormally and persistently elevated, expansive, or irritable mood.
   B. During the period of mood disturbance, at least 3 of the following symptoms have persisted (4 if the mood is only irritable) and have been present to a significant degree: (1) inflated self-esteem or grandiosity; (2) decreased need for sleep, eg, feels rested after only 3 hours of sleep; (3) more talkative than usual or pressure to keep talking; (4) flight of ideas or subjective experience that thoughts are racing; (5) distractibility, eg, attention too easily drawn to unimportant or irrelevant external stimuli; (6) increase in goal-directed activity (either socially, at work or school, or sexually) or psychomotor agitation; (7) excessive involvement in pleasurable activities which have a high potential for painful consequences that the person does not recognize, eg, buying sprees, sexual indiscretions, foolish business investments.
   C. Mood disturbance sufficiently severe to cause marked impairment in occupational functioning or in usual social activities or relationships with others, or to necessitate hospitalization to prevent harm to self or others.
   D. At no time during the disturbance have there been delusions or hallucinations for as long as 2 weeks in the absence of prominent mood symptoms (ie, before the mood symptoms developed or after they have remitted).
   E. Not superimposed on schizophrenia, schizophreniform disorder, delusional disorder, or psychotic disorder NOS.
   F. It cannot be established that an organic factor initiated and maintained the disturbance.
Note: Manic episodes that are apparently precipitated by somatic antidepressant treatment (eg, drugs, ECT) should be diagnosed as mood disorders.

Major depressive episode:
Note: A "major depressive syndrome" is defined as criterion A below.
   A. At least 5 of the following symptoms have been present during the same 2-week period and represent a change from previous functioning; at least 1 of the symptoms is either (1) depressed mood or (2) loss of interest or pleasure. (Do not include symptoms that are clearly due to a physical condition, mood-incongruent delusions or hallucinations, incoherence, or marked loosening of associations.): (1) depressed mood (or can be irritable mood in children and adolescents) most of the day, nearly every day, as indicated either by subjective account or observation by others; (2) markedly diminished interest or pleasure in all, or almost all, activities most of the day, nearly every day (as indicated either by subjective account or observation by others of apathy most of the time); (3) significant weight loss or weight loss or weight gain when not dieting (eg, more than 5% of body weight in a month), or decrease or increase in appetite nearly every day (in children, consider failure to make expected weight gains); (4) insomnia or hypersomnia nearly every day; (5) psychomotor agitation or retardation nearly every day (observable by others, not merely subjective feelings of restlessness or being slowed down); (6) fatigue or loss of energy nearly every day; (7) feelings of worthlessness or excessive or inappropriate guilt (which may be delusional) nearly every day (not merely self-reproach or guilt about being sick); (8) diminished ability to think or concentrate, or indecisiveness, nearly every day (either by subjective account or as observed by others); (9) recurrent thoughts of death (not just fear of dying), recurrent

suicidal ideation without a specific plan, or a suicide attempt or a specific plan for committing suicide.
   B. (1) It cannot be established that an organic factor initiated and maintained the disturbance; (2) the disturbance is not a normal reaction to the loss of a loved one (uncomplicated bereavement).
   C. At no time during the disturbance have there been delusions or hallucinations for as long as 2 weeks in the absence of prominent mood symptoms (ie, before the mood symptoms developed or after they have remitted).
   D. Not superimposed on schizophrenia, schizophreniform disorder, delusional disorder, or psychotic disorder NOS.

Diagnostic criteria for melancholic type:
The presence of at least 5 of the following: (1) loss of interest or pleasure in all, or almost all, activities; (2) lack of reactivity to usually pleasurable stimuli (does not feel much better, even temporarily, when something good happens); (3) depression regularly worse in the morning; (4) early morning awakening (at least 2 hours before usual time of awakening); (5) psychomotor retardation or agitation (not merely subjective complaints); (6) significant anorexia or weight loss (eg, more than 5% of body weight in a month); (7) no significant personality disturbance before first major depressive episode; (8) one or more previous major depressive episodes followed by complete, or nearly complete, recovery; (9) previous good response to specific and adequate somatic antidepressant therapy, eg, tricyclics, ECT, MAOI, lithium.

Bipolar disorder, mixed:
   A. Current (or most recent) episode involves the full symptomatic picture of both manic and major depressive episodes (except for the duration requirement of 2 weeks for depressive symptoms) intermixed or rapidly alternating every few days.
   B. Prominent depressive symptoms lasting at least 1 full day.

Bipolar disorder, manic:
Currently (or most recently) in a manic episode. (If there has been a previous manic episode, the current episode need not meet the full criteria for a manic episode.)

Bipolar disorder, depressed:
   A. Has had one or more manic episodes.
   B. Currently (or most recently) in a major depressive episode. (If there has been a previous major depressive episode, the current episode need not meet the full criteria for a major depressive episode.)

Cyclothymia:
   A. For at least 2 years (1 year for children and adolescents) presence of numerous hypomanic episodes (criteria A and B but not criterion C of manic episode) and numerous periods with depressed mood or loss of interest or pleasure that did not meet criterion A of major depressive episode.
   B. During a 2-year period (1 year in children and adolescents) of the disturbance, never without hypomanic or depressive symptoms for more than 2 months at a time.
   C. No clear evidence of a major depressive episode or manic episode during the first 2 years of the disturbance (or 1 year in children and adolescents).
Note: After this minimum period of cyclothymia, there may be superimposed manic or major depressive syndromes, in which case the additional diagnosis of bipolar disorder or bipolar disorder NOS should be given.
   D. Not superimposed on a chronic psychotic disorder, such as schizophrenia or delusional disorder.
   E. It cannot be established that an organic factor initiated and maintained the disturbance, eg, repeated intoxication from drugs or alcohol.

*In order to avoid redundancy, *DSM-III-R* lists criteria for manic and major depressive episodes and their subclassifications and then offers criteria for major affective disorders and other specific affective disorders. This table follows the *DSM-III-R* outline but omits criteria for some subclassifications of episodes.
†Affective disorders are now called mood disorders in *DSM-III-R*.

Table 30–1 (cont'd). *DSM-III-R* diagnostic criteria for affective disorders.*†

Bipolar disorder not otherwise specified:
Disorders with manic or hypomanic features that do not meet the criteria for any specific bipolar disorder. *Examples:* (1) at least one hypomanic episode and at least one major depressive episode, but never either a manic episode or cyclothymia (such cases have been referred to as "bipolar II"); (2) one more hypomanic episodes, but without cyclothymia or a history of either a manic or a major depressive episode; (3) a manic episode superimposed on delusional disorder, residual schizophrenia, or psychotic disorder NOS.
Specify if seasonal pattern.

Major depression, single episode:
  A. A single major depressive episode.
  B. Has never had a manic episode or an unequivocally hypomanic episode.

Major depression, recurrent:
  A. Two or more major depressive episodes, each separated by at least 2 months of return to more or less usual functioning. (If there has been a previous major depressive episode, the current episode of depression need not meet the full criteria for a major depressive episode.)
  B. Has never had a manic episode or an unequivocally hypomanic episode.

Dysthymia (or depressive neurosis):
  A. Depressed mood (or can be irritable mood in children and adolescents) for most of the day, more days than not, as indicated either by subjective account or observation by others, for at least 2 years (1 year for children and adolescents).
  B. Presence, while depressed, of at least 2 of the following: (1) poor appetite or overeating; (2) insomnia or hypersomnia; (3) low energy or fatigue; (4) low self-esteem; (5) poor concentration or difficulty making decisions; (6) feelings of hopelessness.
  C. During a 2-year period (1 year for children and adolescents) of the disturbance, never without the symptoms in criterion A for more than 2 months at a time.
  D. No clear evidence of a major depressive episode during the first 2 years (1 year for children and adolescents) of the disturbance.

Note: There may have been a previous major depressive episode, provided there was a full remission (no significant signs or symptoms for 6 months) before development of the dysthymia. In addition, after these 2 years (1 year in children or adolescents) of dysthymia, there may be superimposed episodes of major depressive syndrome, in which case both diagnoses are given.
  E. Has never had a manic episode or an unequivocally hypomanic episode.
  F. Not superimposed on a chronic psychotic disorder, such as schizophrenia or delusional disorder.
  G. It cannot be established that an organic factor initiated and maintained the disturbance, eg, prolonged administration of an antihypertensive medication.

Depressive disorder not otherwise specified:
Disorders with depressive features that do not meet the criteria for any specific mood disorder or adjustment disorder with depressed mood. *Examples:* (1) major depressive episode superimposed on residual schizophrenia; (2) recurrent mild depressive disturbance that does not meet the criteria for dysthymia; (3) depressive episodes unrelated to stress that do not meet the criteria for a major depressive episode.

Diagnostic criteria for seasonal pattern:
  A. There has been a regular temporal relationship between the onset of an episode of biopolar disorder (including biopolar disorder NOS) or recurrent major depression (including depressive disorder NOS) and a particular 60-day period of the year (eg, regular appearance of depression between the beginning of October and the end of November). Do not include cases in which there is an obvious effect of seasonally related psychosocial stressors, eg, regularly being unemployed every winter.
  B. Full remissions (or a change from depression to mania or hypomania) also occurred within a particular 60-day period of the year (eg, depression disappears from mid February to mid April).
  C. There have been at least 3 episodes of mood disturbance in 3 separate years that demonstrated the temporal seasonal relationship defined in criteria A and B; at least 2 of the years were consecutive.
  D. Seasonal episodes of mood disturbance, as described above, outnumbered any nonseasonal episodes of such disturbance that may have occurred by more than 3 to 1.

behave with reasonable caution and judgment and to conform with social expectations and norms. In many manic episodes and particularly in initial stages, the predominant mood is euphoria. The mood is often accompanied by a sense of absolute conviction or certitude, usually involving a self-perceived talent or perception but occasionally centering around more metaphysical and cosmic matters. A newly discovered or dramatically enhanced interest in religious or sexual experiences is a common feature. The euphoria experienced by the manic patient has an infectious quality and may mislead some people—even close associates—into accepting types of behavior that otherwise might not be tolerated. Manic patients can be quite engaging, and their well-known proclivity for buying sprees and improvident business ventures is often accompanied, at least for a time, by a remarkable ability to obtain loans or gifts of money and encouragement from people whose judgment is usually better.

One of the chief early symptoms of a manic episode is decreased need for sleep, so that in many cases the individual may not sleep at all for 3 or 4 days at a time. A "hunger" for social interchange may be manifested by frequent and inappropriate phone calls to distant acquaintances, particularly during late-night periods when social stimulation is minimal. Hypergraphia (excessive writing) and a fascination with music and playing musical instruments are frequently noted. A significant increase in alcohol consumption (particularly beer or wine) is common. Whether this represents an attempt at self-medication or poor impulse control is unclear. Manic patients may have a tendency also to wear bright colors and unusual combinations of eccentric attire or may exhibit an attitude of carelessness about clothes or makeup. Public disrobing is also common.

*In order to avoid redundancy, *DSM-III-R* lists criteria for manic and major depressive episodes and their subclassifications and then offers criteria for major affective disorders and other specific affective disorders. This table follows the *DSM-III-R* outline but omits criteria for some subclassifications of episodes.
†Affective disorders are now called mood disorders in *DSM-III-R*.

Manic speech is characteristically rapid and discursive. Manic patients are difficult to interrupt and have difficulty not interrupting when others are speaking. The speech itself may involve rhyming, punning, and bizarre associations, but there are no pathognomonic elements. Manic patients are readily distractible and respond to both internal and external stimuli in a self-referential manner. More severe manic episodes and manic episodes observed later in the natural history of the disorder may be characterized by paranoia and irritability rather than euphoria and grandiosity. Anxiety and feelings of suspicion can cause the verbal output of such individuals to be markedly decreased, leading to erroneous diagnostic conclusions. Significant social aggression is rare, although acute mania and hypomania are common diagnoses in individuals with a psychiatric treatment history who commit violent crimes. In some cases, severe depression may occur concomitantly with the manic state or in abrupt alternation with the manic state. True delusions and auditory hallucinations may be present, giving rise to difficult problems of differential diagnosis. The content of the delusions or hallucinations is often consistent with the predominant mood (mood-congruent). A manic patient may, for example, hear a voice from God proclaiming him the new prophet, a hallucination congruent with the underlying grandiose mood. The usefulness of the distinction (congruent versus incongruent) is controversial, since it requires a highly subjective interpretation on the part of the assessor.

In severe cases, mania can present as a state of catatonia. In such cases, the individual appears "willfully" unresponsive, often assuming a fixed posture and appearing mute except for occasional shouts or guttural sounds. Less severe states may be characterized by primitive delusions, fecal smearing, and extremes of fearfulness and emotional lability.

Natural History

A. Manic Disorder: Now that the use of lithium carbonate in treatment has become widespread, the complete natural history of a manic episode is seldom observed. Speed of onset, severity, and duration of the manic episode vary greatly in different individuals, depending in part, apparently, upon genetic and other factors not clearly understood. Descriptions of past manic episodes are the best source of information about future episodes. Predictions about the future course of a patient experiencing a first manic episode are necessarily vague. In many individuals, the onset will be abrupt, occurring over a period of days or in some cases hours. The onset of the manic episode classically occurs in the early morning hours and is first noted either as early morning awakening or inability to fall asleep. Some patients experience a more protracted onset over a period of weeks. Increases in psychomotor activity, increased energy, and elevated mood are the most common early signs, with manic speech and thought disorder occurring later if at all. Not all individuals pass through the classic sequence of events or progress to the same level of severity.

There have been reports of manic individuals who have no complaints of sleep disturbance or obvious euphoria and who appear not to differ either in the natural course of the illness or in response to treatment.

It appears that in many cases manic episodes are self-limiting within days, weeks, or months. The variables that account for the wide reported ranges make assessments based on anything other than the individual's own past history unreliable. Chronic mania has been described and may remain stable at different levels of severity. Although lithium carbonate represents a dramatic advance in the treatment of bipolar disorders, 10–15% of manic patients respond inadequately to the medication and continue to present either episodically or chronically with classic signs of the disorder. Even with appropriate treatment, patients who present with rapidly alternating episodes of mania and depression are more likely to remain ill for an extended period of time than are purely manic patients. Bipolar patients experiencing their first episode of depression have approximately a 20% chance of remaining depressed for at least 1 year, a rate comparable to that of individuals with pure depression. In subsequent episodes, the cumulative risk for development of chronic refractory depression rises to 30%.

B. Bipolar Disorder: Although traditional textbooks have associated bipolar illness with a relatively late age at onset, current evidence indicates that the average age is 30 years, with a peak between 20 and 25 years. Onset after age 60 is rare. Bipolar illness with onset during adolescence is commonly mistaken for an adjustment disorder, a fact that may reflect historical diagnostic bias or diagnostic confusion arising from normal physical and psychologic developmental changes during this period. Behavioral disturbances expressed as truancy, promiscuity, reckless driving, and impulsiveness are less likely to be recognized as part of a major psychiatric syndrome during adolescence and more likely to be attributed to maturational crises.

Differential Diagnosis

Manic symptoms can occur in association with known organic disorders but should in such cases be diagnosed as organic affective syndrome (ie, "secondary mania") rather than as bipolar disorder. There appear to be no clinical characteristics that might distinguish the 2 diagnoses, and it is probable that future research will result in the shifting of many manic diagnoses from a primary to a secondary category. The list of known causal agents is a long one and includes drugs (eg, corticosteroids, levodopa, stimulants), metabolic disturbances (such as those associated with hemodialysis), infections, neoplastic diseases, and epilepsy (particularly partial complex seizures).

In manic patients presenting with prominent delusions and hallucinations, the differential diagnosis is likely to include schizophrenia, paranoid type. Both syndromes can present with identical clinical symptoms, which means that the diagnosis can only be based on the clinical course or on secondary features such as the presence of a family history of affective disorder, the level of premorbid adjustment, a history of manic symptoms, or a prior response to treatment. The diagnosis of schizoaffective disorder is available for cases in which the clinician is unable to choose between manic episode and schizophrenia. Unfortunately, there is at present no agreement on how this category should be defined or on its etiologic or prognostic relationship to schizophrenia or affective disorder. A diagnosis of schizoaffective disorder would be justified (for example) in a patient with clear evidence of a manic episode and a history of a mood-incongruent delusion or hallucination that persists after the affective symptoms subside. Recent evidence suggests that in many cases of schizoaffective disorder the prognosis and treatment response are more similar to those of bipolar disorder than of schizophrenia.

Prognosis

Emil Kraepelin, the German psychiatrist who coined the phrase "manic depression," wrote that bipolar illness, in contrast to schizophrenia, usually has a good prognosis. In Kraepelin's original sample of 459 patients, 45% had only one attack, and very few had more than 4 episodes. The average duration of a pharmacologically untreated manic episode was 7 months, but a wide range was reported. Although most later studies have validated Kraepelin's findings, particularly when the disorder is compared to schizophrenia, it would appear that the prognosis of bipolar illness is less favorable than originally reported. Up to 15% of patients respond inadequately to medication and must endure chronic or recurrent symptoms.

The phases of bipolar illness may differ in their responsiveness to treatment and in their effect on ultimate outcome. Some individuals, for example, experience complete remission of acute manic symptoms and prophylactic benefit from medication but continue to have unmodified or attenuated depressive episodes. The best predictor of cycle frequency and treatment response is the personal and family psychiatric history. Once the episode has resolved, the duration of the symptom-free interval varies greatly in different individuals. In contrast to Kraepelin's original impression, it is now clear that most patients who satisfy the criteria for bipolar disorder will experience another episode within 2–4 years. The complete cycle—ie, from manic to depressed to manic state—may be as short as 48 hours or so long that the concept of cyclicity becomes meaningless. Patients with bipolar disorder who experience rapid cycles—3 or more a year— respond less well to lithium than individuals with longer symptom-free intervals. The few available prospective studies of the course of bipolar illness indicate that for any given individual, the cycles become shorter as time goes on.

The prognosis thus depends on the frequency and duration of individual episodes and the response to medication. Since lithium is effective in moderating the severity of symptoms in most cases, there is always a strong possibility that recurrences represent failure of compliance with the drug regimen. Perhaps because of the quality of the mood experience, manic patients often utilize the psychologic defense mechanism of denial, admitting that problems may exist but attributing them to overwork or to job or family stress. Even patients who have enjoyed complete remission of symptoms and have a multigenerational family history of bipolar disorder may discount the effect of drug therapy and fail to take their daily medication. Many patients thus suffer needless recurrence of symptoms because they resist the diagnosis. Patients with mild bipolar episodes may be able to function adequately during a period in which they demonstrate most of the symptoms of a manic episode. In such cases, factors such as psychologic coping mechanisms, social supports, and socioeconomic status influence the outcome as much as response to medication.

Illustrative Case

A 27-year-old male graduate student in molecular biology was brought to the emergency room by his fiancée, who explained that over the preceding 2 weeks he had become increasingly irritable and suspicious and had undergone a "personality change." She noted that he had not slept at all for the past 3 nights and had become preoccupied by the belief that his research thesis would be regarded as the "new bible of the computer age." Fearing that his ideas might be stolen by government agents, he had constructed an elaborate mathematical code that would allow only him and his appointed "prophets" to understand the documented work. The patient was dressed in a mismatched 3-piece suit he claimed was a disguise that would enable him to elude agents assigned to follow him. Although during the initial stages of the interview the patient refused to speak, he suddenly observed that since the interviewing physician was on the faculty of the university, he might be better able to understand the meaning of his research than the resident physician who screened him at the admission desk. He also remarked that the interviewing physician's name contained a syllable similar in sound and spelling to the Latin word for "trust" and suggested that their meeting must have been preordained. Throughout the remainder of the interview, the patient paced around the room, interrupting his responses to questions with associations to the interviewer's style of dress, a paperweight on the desk, and a book whose title he misread.

The history obtained from the fiancée revealed that the patient had never had any symptoms similar to these but that for about 3 months during the past 12 months, the patient had felt too tired to go to class and spent much of the day sleeping. She recalled that the patient had an aunt who was hospitalized twice following the birth of her 2 children and that an older brother had been married 4 times and was "quite moody".

After some urging by his fiancée, the patient agreed to enter the hospital and began taking medication, which he called "thought pills." Neuroleptic medication resulted in marked amelioration of symptoms within 5 days. After 2 weeks of treatment with lithium, his suspiciousness and grandiose beliefs diminished significantly. With partial recovery, the patient was mildly depressed and embarrassed about his recent behavior, but he still seemed excessively concerned that his research was important enough so that it might, in the future, require protection from industrial spies.

Epidemiology

Multinational studies indicate that the lifetime risk of bipolar disorder is approximately 1–2%. The concordance rate for bipolar illness in monozygotic twins is approximately 65%; in dizygotic twins the rate is 15%. Bipolar illness occurs in relatives of bipolar patients much more frequently than in relatives of patients with major depression; the rates for depression alone are approximately the same. Adoption studies show that rates of illness clearly depend on the risk associated with biologic rather than adopted parents. In general, bipolar probands have more bipolar relatives and more relatives with affective disorder than unipolar probands. Since the old classification of "manic-depressive illness" is not synonymous with the *DSM-III* classification of bipolar illness, it is difficult to calculate the rates of bipolar disorder from studies of manic-depressive illness. The point prevalence of bipolar disorder—ie, the proportion of the population having the disorder at a given time—has not been specifically studied. Although these figures have some historical validity, definitive epidemiologic data must await the completion of multicenter collaborative studies now under way. Differences in diagnostic criteria have resulted in reports of markedly different indices of risk in different areas of the USA and between the USA and Great Britain.

Etiology & Pathogenesis

A. Biochemical Factors: Although many differences in biochemical indices have been described when bipolar patients are compared to normal control subjects, there is no agreement about which alterations have etiologic significance and which are secondary effects or epiphenomena. Since the "switch" from depression into mania (and vice versa) can occur in minutes, attempts have been made to identify biochemical changes that might be associated with the switch. Specific changes in brain monoamine neurotransmitter metabolism and receptor function appear to be the most likely mechanisms. Although now regarded as too simplistic, the catecholamine hypothesis suggested that catecholamine (most specifically norepinephrine) deficiency was associated with motor retardation and depression, while catecholamine excess could result in excitement and euphoria. Since all of the major neurotransmitter systems are functionally linked, it is not surprising that changes in other major neurotransmitter systems have also been documented. Increases in dopaminergic function and adrenergic-

cholinergic system imbalance have been reported during manic episodes. Trait-dependent alterations in platelet serotonin uptake, in cerebrospinal fluid levels of serotonin metabolites, and in endocrine response to serotoninergic agonists have also been found in patients with bipolar illness. Overall, however, there have been few biologic studies of *mania,* since the nature of the syndrome interferes with the necessary compliance with research procedures.

Electrolyte disturbances have also been found in bipolar disorders and may represent a defect of cellular membrane function. In general, sodium retention increases during depression, together with increased potassium and water excretion. The reverse is true during manic intervals. Others investigating the role of regulatory enzymes have reported alterations in monoamine oxidase (MAO) and catechol-O-methyltransferase (COMT) activity. A variety of neuroendocrine changes have also been reported for patients with bipolar disorder who are in the depressed phase. About half of both bipolar and unipolar depressed patients show evidence of any or all of the following during a severe depressive episode: increased adrenal glucocorticoid function, decreased thyroid-stimulating hormone response to thyrotropin-releasing hormone, decreased basal prolactin levels, and decreased growth hormone response to insulin challenge. Although several studies have also reported significant differences between bipolar patients in the depressed phase and patients with unipolar disorder, the findings are preliminary and must await confirmation.

Abnormalities in lithium-sodium transport and in the ratio of lithium level in erythrocytes to that in plasma occur in some patients with bipolar disorder and appear to be genetically transmitted. Several studies have also found a link between bipolar disorder and certain haplotypes of the major histocompatibility complex (MHC) on chromosome 6, but these findings remain controversial. Recently, using DNA markers, independent groups have shown associations to chromosome 11 and to the X chromosome in differing pedigrees. Genetic heterogeneity may account for these disparate findings.

B. Psychosocial Factors: There is no reliable evidence that psychosocial factors cause bipolar disorder, though such influences may precipitate manic or depressed bipolar states and may in fact be necessary for the expression of symptomatology in milder bipolar syndromes. A project deadline at work, for example, may result in decreased sleep and increased psychosocial stress, which in turn may trigger a mild manic episode in certain susceptible individuals. Retrospective analyses are unreliable, since every examined life contains historical matter that could account for behavioral changes. Recent research in biologic circadian rhythmicity indicates that subtle changes in the light-dark cycle (eg, seasonal variations) are a better predictor of risk.

Treatment

A. Biomedical Therapies: Treatment of bipolar disorder depends upon the specific form of behavioral disorder at presentation. Lithium carbonate is the treatment of choice for the acute manic state, even though 10–14 days may be required before full effect is achieved. A favorable response to lithium is reported in 80% of bipolar manic patients. In a substantial number of manic patients, remission may be incomplete and significant thought disorder found at follow-up. Complications are relatively infrequent, but a transient "rebound" depression following resolution of a manic state is not uncommon. Before lithium treatment is started, it is prudent to obtain baseline indices of thyroid and kidney function, electrolyte levels, and, in individuals over age 40, an electrocardiogram. For patients in the acute manic state, a lithium blood level of 1–1.5 meq/L is desirable. After an optimal response has been achieved, the dosage can be decreased. Maintenance lithium levels for prevention of manic or depressive episodes must be individualized but range from 0.5 to 1 meq/L. Overall response to lithium appears to improve as duration of treatment continues. (For a detailed discussion of the pharmacology of lithium, see Chapter 52.) The degree of psychomotor activation and the fragile structure of the treatment alliance in acute mania require that supplemental treatment with faster-acting neuroleptics be instituted in most cases. For patients who do not respond satisfactorily to lithium, the anticonvulsant drug carbamazepine may be tried; studies show that this drug has both acute antimanic and antidepressant effects on bipolar illness. Valproic acid, clonazepam, and the calcium channel antagonist verapamil have recently emerged as empirical alternatives to lithium, but these should not be considered agents of first choice. The cholinergic agonist lecithin has also been successfully used for mania, lending support to the hypothesis that the manic state is associated with a relative decrease in the ratio of cholinergic to adrenergic nervous system function.

B. Psychosocial Therapies: Some form of psychosocial intervention is almost always indicated in the treatment of bipolar disorder, although its nature and extent will necessarily depend upon the degree of disruption of family and financial situations, the baseline character of the individual, and the response to somatic treatment. The nature of the biologic contribution to the disorder (see also Chapter 11) makes it almost impossible to ascertain in advance what the individual's ongoing psychosocial needs might be after acute symptoms subside. Some patients with bipolar disorder have infrequent recurrences, experience long symptom-free intervals, and are able to lead productive lives. Others may have a particularly malignant form of the syndrome or may exhibit pathologic degrees of denial and lead turbulent lives calling for active psychosocial involvement by the therapist. Since there is a strong genetic component to bipolar illness, it may be impossible to determine to what extent the patient's problems are referable to the genetic contribution and what aspects reflect environmental and developmental experiences created by a primary disorder in parents and siblings. A number of social events frequently associated with bipolar episodes (divorce, alcoholism, loss of job or friends, etc) have long-term consequences that will affect the psychologic state of the individual and the prognosis even if the disorder is successfully controlled.

CYCLOTHYMIA

Symptoms & Signs

Cyclothymia is characterized by manic and depressive states not of sufficient severity or duration to meet the criteria for either major disorder (Table 30–1). Symptoms must persist for at least 2 years and have no psychotic component. Individuals meeting the criteria for this diagnosis may experience an exacerbation of depression or mania sufficient to warrant a change in diagnosis. Most clinicians presently consider cyclothymia to be an attenuated form of bipolar disorder rather than a personality disorder, as originally thought. Cyclothymia is common in outpatient psychiatric practice and may account for as much as 3–4% of an unselected clinic population.

Cyclothymic patients suffer from short cycles of depression and hypomania that can at times be as *severe* as what are observed in other disorders but which usually fail to meet the criteria for *duration*. It is often difficult to ascertain any regular pattern of mood switching, and patients will commonly describe mood changes that come and go spontaneously over the course of hours or days. A patient may feel perfectly well the night before and awake with significantly depressed mood. Because of the attenuated nature of manic symptoms, patients are more likely to present with complaints about the depressive phase. Studies of behavioral characteristics of these patients show that they are extroverted sociable individuals who appear self-assured, energetic, and often impulsive. At times this cheerful exuberance turns into irritability and extreme sensitivity to rejection or loss. Cyclothymic patients are frequently described as "stimulus-seeking," a characteristic that leads them to become involved in daring hobbies and results in checkered work and school careers. Promiscuity and drug abuse are also noted, as is a history of repeated romantic disasters. Although many of these characteristics are likely to lead to a socially maladaptive life-style, cyclothymic individuals often achieve substantial success and status in society. This may in part reflect a cultural bias that values "outgoing" personality characteristics, but it is also an outcome of a periodic increase in energies and enthusiasms that leads to accomplishments beyond the reach of more placid individuals.

Natural History

Close examination of the cyclothymic patient's personal history will usually reveal an age at onset of symptoms of early to late adolescence. There is some evidence that a higher percentage of such individuals are described as hyperactive during childhood. About a third of patients with this diagnosis will experience an intensification of symptoms during a 2-year follow-up, sufficient to meet the criteria for mania, hypomania, or major depression. The close relationship of cyclothymia to bipolar disorder is supported by the finding that treatment of the depressed phase with tricyclic antidepressants can result in pharmacologically induced hypomania in 40–50% of patients. There seems to be a higher risk for the natural development of formal depressive as opposed to manic episodes.

Differential Diagnosis

As mentioned previously, the main task in differential diagnosis is to determine the severity and duration of the altered mood state. A chaotic life history with poor interpersonal relationships often suggests a diagnosis of borderline personality. Many cyclothymic individuals experience difficulties in ego development and in achieving an integrated sense of self. These issues may come up more frequently in cyclothymia than in formal bipolar disorder, since the milder and more evanescent quality of cyclothymia will make it more difficult for patient and family, friends, and therapist to recognize the constitutional contribution. The deleterious effects on personality development of a constantly changing and autonomous mood state that colors, in random fashion, the critical developmental experiences of childhood and adolescence should be obvious.

Prognosis

Since the syndrome is more broadly defined than either bipolar disorder or major depression, estimates of prognosis depend on assessments of the quality, quantity, and frequency of mood change and the effect of such changes both on the patient and on his or her social and professional world. About 35% of such individuals will go on to develop more severe episodes over a period of several years. Longer follow-up studies are not available; thus, the lifetime prediction of risk is unknown. Approximately 60% of these patients improve when treated with lithium carbonate.

Illustrative Case

A 34-year-old divorced secretary sought psychotherapy because of her long history of unsatisfactory relationships with men. She was currently employed by an agency that provided temporary secretarial help and admitted that she had quit and been fired from several jobs because of inability to keep regular working hours. She stated that she did not really like secretarial work and hoped to return to fashion modeling, an occupation she had pursued several years previously with modest success. She reported that she encountered difficulties even then from failing to show up for assignments and, on 2 occasions, from going to an appointment after having had several drinks. Further questioning revealed sporadic recreational use of marihuana, cocaine, and amphetamines.

She attributed her difficulty in relationships with men to the fact that most of the men she had been attracted to were too career-oriented and "homebody" types. She acknowledged that several individuals with whom she had been close described her as "moody." She described her life as alternating between times when she felt "buzzed, like on speed" and other times when she felt "blank" and wanted to sleep most of the day. During these latter periods, she stated she felt somewhat better after drinking a bottle of wine but felt especially guilty about the fact that her life was "not going anywhere." The family history revealed a turbulent family environment created principally by an abusive father with a history of binge drinking. Clinical and laboratory evaluation disclosed no organic cause of the mood disorder. The patient was started in psychotherapy and was given a trial of lithium carbonate. Over the succeeding year, she obtained permanent employment and reported an increased sense of emotional stability.

Epidemiology

This disorder seems to be more prevalent than previously acknowledged. It is more common in women, and there is apt to be a family history of affective disorder and "affective spectrum" problems such as alcohol abuse and antisocial personality.

Etiology & Pathogenesis

A. Biochemical Factors: Very little is known about biochemical changes in cyclothymia. Most of the evidence has come from genetic studies linking the disorder to the major affective syndromes and from studies documenting a response to antimanic or antidepressant drug treatment.

B. Psychosocial Factors: Although the primary process responsible for sudden and recurrent mood change in cyclothymia is thought to be biologic and genetically transmitted, the psychosocial sequelae of such changes may over time emerge as the most significant aspect of the patient's discontent. This is particularly true for individuals with an early onset of the disorder. Persons who suffer recurrent unpredictable and intense affective upsets, seemingly unrelated to circumstance, develop major themes of loss and low self-esteem. A history of interpersonal conflicts and generalized anger is common, because the character of presentation is often subtle enough to escape the awareness of clinicians and the sympathy of friends.

Treatment

Biomedical treatment of cyclothymia should be empirically derived and should be offered only if the individual's functioning is significantly adversely affected. A trial of lithium carbonate may ameliorate manic symptoms and reduce the frequency of most cycles. Antidepressant medication may relieve depressive symptoms. (See Chapters 52 and 53.) Even with successful drug treatment, many patients with this disorder will benefit from psychotherapy that focuses on interpersonal relationships and self-image.

MAJOR DEPRESSION

Depression is one of the most prevalent medical disorders and has been recognized as a distinct pathologic entity from early Egyptian times. Common usage of the word "depression" stems principally from the attempts of the 19th century psychiatrist Emil Kraepelin to introduce a term that would have greater diagnostic specificity than "melancholia." The term "melancholia" had been used by physicians from the fourth century BC and encompassed a variety of behavioral disorders now viewed as discrete entities. Currently, the term melancholia denotes major depressive disorder with changes in endogenous or vegetative function, eg, disturbances of sleep, appetite, and libido.

Throughout most of this century, clinicians have attempted to subclassify the syndrome on the basis of symptoms and causes. Many of the subclassifications proved to be invalid or unreliable. For example, the distinction between depressions that were "reactive" and those that were nonreactive or endogenous—ie, not precipitated by psychosocial stress—has not proved to be of predictive value. Such judgments in any case are highly subjective and depend on how detailed a history is obtained and how much weight is assigned by the patient or clinician to the changes that routinely occur in life. Distinctions on the basis of age have likewise proved suspect, with recent research indicating that depression during the involutional period is qualitatively no different from that experienced during any other stage.

Symptoms & Signs

From a symptomatic perspective, 2 classic dichotomies continue to be of clinical utility in describing major depressive disorder. A variety of studies have distinguished depressed individuals with prominent psychomotor retardation and anhedonia from those who evidence psychomotor activation, guilt, anxiety, and, occasionally, delusional thinking. The number and severity of somatic symptoms generally increase along with the severity of depression. Separating major depressions according to whether they are endogenous or autonomous has not been found to be useful, either in predicting drug response or in improving assessments of general risk. Individuals may in fact show endogenous features in one episode and not in another.

The character of depressive symptoms depends to a large extent on the severity of the disorder. In the most severe cases, patients may present with an extensive paranoid or nihilistic delusional system and the experience of hallucinations, usually self-deprecatory in content and consonant with the underlying mood state. Because such individuals have more psychomotor disturbance and generally respond poorly to antidepressant medication, some investigators have considered psychotic depression as a separate entity and not simply a severe variant of major depression.

Depression occurs at any age and can present with primary symptoms that do not involve obvious mood change. Depression in children may be difficult to diagnose. Because of cognitive and linguistic developmental changes occurring in childhood, emotional states are experienced and projected differently. In old people, the most significant symptom may be a change in cognitive function. The term "pseudodementia" has been applied to a state clinically identical to irreversible senile dementia but which resolves with antidepressant treatment. Recent research questions the utility of this distinction, since an unremitting course and lack of pharmacologic response of senile dementia are far from unconfirmed. In "masked depression," a condition in which there is no apparent mood change, the course of illness, prognosis, and response to treatment are the same as those associated with classic major depression. This condition has been described in individuals suffering from anorexia nervosa, psychosomatic disorders, and chronic pain syndromes who respond to antidepressant medication.

Natural History

There is great variation in the clinical presentation and course of major depression. As the individual patient's history accumulates, recurrent episodes tend to develop a cyclic pattern of presentation, so that better judgments about the probable future course can be made.

Depression can occur at any age, but the average age at onset is about 40 years. In general, the earlier the age at onset, the more likely it is that there will be a recurrence. Symptoms develop either gradually over a period of many months or more dramatically over a shorter period, in many cases following a significant loss or episode of stress, although this is not necessary. If untreated, the depressive episode may resolve spontaneously over a period of weeks to months or may become chronic and remain essentially unchanged over a period of years. Although most patients with major depression respond well to somatic treatment, uncontrolled studies have revealed that recovery from major depressive disorder is not as good as once thought. Only about half of patients are completely recovered at 1-year follow-up. The prognosis worsens with increased severity of symptoms at onset, less acute onset, and occurrence of the acute episode superimposed on an underlying state of chronic depression. The risk of relapse after recovery from major depressive disorder is high for a short period—about 25% relapse within 12 weeks. For individuals with recurrent episodes, the question arises how soon another episode can be expected. The presence of a chronic underlying depression or a history of 3 or more depressive episodes significantly increases the risk of early relapse. In addition, there is evidence that the interval between episodes becomes shorter as the individual ages.

At least 20–30% of patients with major depression and no history of mania will experience a manic or hypomanic episode later in life. Factors positively correlated with eventual bipolar outcome include pharmacologic induction of mania, a history of postpartum depression, early onset (< 25 years), and symptoms of hypersomnia and psychomotor retardation.

Differential Diagnosis

Major depression occurs concomitantly with a number of different disease states, such as pancreatic and bronchogenic carcinoma, hypothyroidism, and Cushing's syndrome. As noted, depression and dementia, especially in the elderly, may be confused. However, patients with dementia may develop major depression as well. A diagnosis of organic affective syndrome with depression should be made in all of these secondary depressive disorders. The diagnosis of a major depressive episode depends on exclusion of specific organic causes. In some individuals, depression occurs in association with seasonal change, giving rise to the term "seasonal affective disorder." Such individuals have experienced improvement in mood through "phase advance" alteration of their sleep-wake cycle and through the administration of several hours daily of full-spectrum light, usually during morning hours. A regulatory disturbance of pineal gland function and melatonin secretion has been hypothesized in these patients, and the syndrome itself is seen as an evolutionary remnant of the mammalian hibernation cycle. In *DSM-III-R*, a seasonal pattern may be a specific diagnostic feature of *either* bipolar disorder or recurrent major depression.

Schizophrenia commonly presents with significant depressive symptoms, either during the acute phase or shortly following resolution of psychotic symptoms. In such cases, the diagnosis of depressive disorder not otherwise specified is added to the primary diagnosis. The differential diagnosis between major depression with psychosis and schizophrenia with depressive signs is exceedingly difficult and can best be made by considering aspects of the patient's premorbid history and a family history of psychiatric disorder. Because a diagnosis of schizophrenia requires a duration of at least 6 months, the data at onset is important.

In dysthymia and cyclothymia, aspects of the depressive syndrome may occur but are not of sufficient intensity or duration to meet the criteria for major depression. It should be remembered, however, that major depression can occur in these or other disorders as an independent, superimposed entity and should be recorded as such.

Patients with bipolar disorder, mixed type, may likewise exhibit features of severe depression but will also present manic symptoms.

Grief syndromes often present with behavioral and physiologic changes identical to those observed in major depression. "Major depression" should not be diagnosed until it is determined that the reaction is either too severe or too prolonged to be explained as simple bereavement.

Chronic personality disorders and substance use disorders may also be associated with depressive symptoms. Again, the diagnosis of major depression is made only if requirements of severity and duration are met.

Prognosis

In individual cases, estimates of the degree of recovery and the likelihood of staying well depend mostly upon the patient's age at onset, the number of previous episodes, and the response to somatic and psychosocial treatment. Many individuals have only one depressive episode in a lifetime. The likelihood of recurrence is dramatically increased with the onset of a second episode and continues to rise slightly with each additional episode, eventually reaching a statistical plateau. The prognosis is, of course, dramatically affected by the individual's response to treatment and by the response to maintenance antidepressant or lithium regimens. Specific assessments of prognosis in individual cases can be complicated by changes in psychosocial support and status that occur as predictable sequelae of recurrent depressive episodes. Patients who lose their jobs, drop out of school, or become divorced as a result of their behavior during an acute episode do not readily experience restitution of these losses with remission of depression and thus must deal with increasing psychologic stress in euthymic periods. In cases where suicidal preoccupation is recurrently noted in successive episodes and in those where profound delusional content is noted, the prognosis for recovery is generally poor.

Illustrative Case

The patient was a surgeon referred by an internist for evaluation of complaints of fatigue and hand tremor. During outpatient evaluation, the patient said that 4 months previously he began noticing a significant worsening of manual dexterity during surgery. He attributed his difficulties to a fine tremor that he demonstrated for the examiner. He felt guilty about several patients who had put their faith in him and had suffered for it. He was sure that people in the hospital were making disparaging comments about his condition, though he could offer no specific examples. He had become reluctant to schedule operations but at the same time said that his decreased income was mainly attributable to fewer referrals from colleagues and "the word getting out." Although this was the first occurrence of this kind, he felt that his whole career had been a sham and that his previous accomplishments were undeserved. He could see no medical or psychiatric solution to his difficulties and expressed an intention to retire, though he was only 47 years old and not financially able to do so.

Although the patient had full health and disability insurance coverage, he expressed great concern about the impending hardship to his family from medical expenses and his failure to earn a good income. This concern magnified even trivial expenditures; eg, he felt he could no longer buy a morning paper without jeopardizing his son's college education. He reported poor appetite and a weight loss of 15 lb in less than 2 months. He reluctantly acknowledged that he and his wife had not had sexual relations in 4 months because of his impotence. He was unable to read professional journals or popular reading matter. Direct questioning revealed early morning awakening, but he said this was not a problem. Despite a strong feeling that all of his troubles were due to the hand tremor, he agreed to enter the hospital for a trial of antidepressant medication. On the ward, he received a combination of drug treatment and individual and group therapy. After 10 days of drug treatment (imipramine, 200 mg orally daily), he began sleeping better and eating regularly. He continued to complain of depression but admitted to an increase in energy level, a decrease in tremulousness, and an ability to maintain an erection. A week later, he began to express an interest in returning to work and initiated plans for discharge.

Epidemiology

Although affective disorders are widely acknowledged to be common, their prevalence is difficult to determine because of differences in diagnostic procedures and criteria. Assessments of depressive symptoms—ie, intense, pervasive, and almost daily feelings of sadness or disappointment that affect normal functioning—show prevalence rates of 9–20%. (The relationship of such subjective assessments to the objective diagnosis of major depression is not known.) When more stringent criteria for major depression are used, prevalence of major depression is 3% for men and 4–9% for women. The lifetime risk is 8–12% for men and 20–26% for women. These figures also may be high, since they are largely dependent upon subjective evaluations of individuals who have not sought treatment. There has been a progressive increase in rates of depression in successive birth cohorts throughout this century as well as a progressively earlier age of onset. The majority of those affected are never diagnosed or appropriately treated.

Ill effects resulting from major depression may be severe. About 12–20% of persons experiencing an acute episode develop chronic depressive syndrome, and up to 15% of patients who have depression for more than 1 month commit suicide.

Etiology & Pathogenesis

A. Biochemical Factors: Genetic studies and studies on the effect of specific antidepressant drugs have led to the conclusion that most cases of recurrent major depression have some biologic basis. This does not mean, however, that psychologic factors have no role in symptom formation or in precipitation of episodes of depression of lesser severity.

Family and genetic studies indicate that the risk rate among first-degree relatives of individuals suffering from major depression (unipolar) is approximately 2–3 times the risk in the general population. This, it should be noted, is approximately half the rate reported among first-degree relatives of individuals suffering from *bipolar* illness. The concordance rate is about 11% for dizygotic twins and approaches 40% for monozygotic twins. Biologic parents of adopted probands have a much greater prevalence of mood disorder than adopting parents.

The most prominent hypotheses generated to ac-

count for the actual mechanism of the mood disorder focus upon regulatory disturbances in the monoamine neurotransmitter systems, particularly those involving norepinephrine and serotonin (5-hydroxytryptamine). More recently, it has also been hypothesized that depression is associated with alteration in acetylcholine-adrenergic balance and characterized by a relative cholinergic dominance. In addition, there are suggestions that dopamine is functionally decreased in some cases of major depression. Because the central nervous system monoamine neurotransmitter systems are widely distributed and involved in tonic regulation of autonomic functions, arousal, movement, sleep, aggression, and other vegetative functions, they are particularly well suited for their hypothesized role. Original reports suggesting that patients with endogenous depression experienced either decreased noradrenergic or serotoninergic activity now appear to be overly simplistic. All the monoamine neurotransmitter systems are interrelated and subject to compensatory adaptation to perturbation over time. In addition, the discovery that many neuropeptides and hormones may serve as neurotransmitters and neuromodulators in certain contexts has underscored the complexity of the neural regulation of mood (see Chapter 11).

Reports of biologic changes in major depression offer potential utility in diagnosis and assessment of treatment response. Foremost among these findings is that a significant number of patients have evidence of either increased or decreased noradrenergic function, as reflected by urinary levels of 3-methoxy-4-hydroxyphenylglycol (MHPG), the chief metabolite of central nervous system noradrenergic function. Other major studies have pointed to a decrease in serotoninergic activity in certain subgroups, as measured by levels of 5-hydroxyindoleacetic acid (5-HIAA), the principal metabolite of serotoninergic activity in the brain. Although these findings derive principally from investigations of the therapeutic effect of antidepressant medication, it has historically been difficult to reconcile the short time course of such changes with the usual 10- to 14-day lag in clinical response. Most current hypotheses of neurotransmitter function in altered mood states have focused on changes in receptor sensitivity and number rather than on changes in the amount of neurotransmitter available. Long-term antidepressant treatment has been found to be associated with reduced postsynaptic beta-adrenergic receptor sensitivity and enhanced postsynaptic serotoninergic and alpha-adrenergic receptor activity. Effects on presynaptic receptor sensitivity are more variable. In addition to direct measurement of neurotransmitter and metabolite levels in brain and peripheral fluids, there have been reports that monoamine oxidase (MAO) and catechol-O-methyltransferase (COMT), enzymes important in monoamine metabolism, are lower in depressed patients.

Several specific abnormalities in neuroendocrine regulation may represent evidence of either primary disturbance in hypothalamic-pituitary control or secondary alteration in neurotransmitter function in limbic sites. The most consistent finding is that many patients with severe depressive disorder have an excess secretion of cortisol from the adrenal cortex. This is not simply a stress-related phenomenon, because the actual number of secretory episodes is increased, principally in the early morning hours when the system is normally quiescent. Many cortisol hypersecretors also have levels of norepinephrine, MHPG, and epinephrine in plasma and urine that are several times higher than normal. The cause and meaning of this parallel activation are unclear. The **dexamethasone suppression test** has been used as a diagnostic test for major depressive disorder, although its use for this purpose is controversial. It seems to be more useful in monitoring the efficacy of treatment. Individuals whose tests fail to normalize have a poor prognosis despite symptomatic response. The test is most commonly performed by giving dexamethasone, 1 mg orally at 11:30 PM, and then measuring plasma cortisol levels at 8 AM, 4 PM, and 11 PM on the next day. "Nonsuppression" is most commonly defined as a cortisol level of greater than 5 μg/dL in any sample. In addition to alterations in the pituitary-adrenal axis, elevation in serum triiodothyronine and thyroxine have been reported, as has a significant blunting of the response of thyroid-stimulating hormone to an infusion of thyrotropin-releasing hormone. Reports of changes in growth hormone, prolactin, luteinizing hormone, and testosterone regulation in major depressive disorder are contradictory.

From a neurophysiologic perspective, the most replicable finding is that sleep in severe depression is characterized by decreased total sleep, decreased REM (rapid eye movement) latency (ie, sleep time from onset of sleep until the first epoch of REM sleep), increased REM density (ie, ratio of REM activity to REM time), and decreased stage 4 delta sleep. Sleep electroencephalography does not differentiate subgroups of depressed patients but may help predict a positive response to antidepressant medication.

B. Psychosocial Factors: Although psychosocial stress may play a role in precipitation of a major depressive episode and shape the particular constellation of symptoms noted, current research indicates that environmental factors as such do not cause severe depressive episodes. However, depressed individuals are often unable to accept the concept of biologic vulnerability and remain convinced that they "themselves" or changes in their environment are principally responsible for their mood state. Self-doubt, guilt, and an overriding sense of worthlessness will often lead to disruption in relationships with friends and family and to a withdrawal from work—actions that have understandable long-term effects on mood. Chronic depression and depressive personality traits may thus emerge as the psychologic and social precursors, concomitants, and sequelae of recurrent biologic depressive states. In general, personality disorder is more common among unipolar nonmelancholic depressed patients than among unipolar melancholic or bipolar depressed patients. Histrionic and hostile character traits

are often noted, as is a long history of difficulty in maintaining stable interpersonal relations. The presence of a personality disorder does not affect the symptom profile but does presage a worse outcome.

The observation that many patients with depression have similar distinctive personality traits led Freud and other psychoanalytic writers to see clinical depression as a psychologically reparative mechanism. The loss of a love object and the consequent psychic injury could only be overcome by self-punishment in which the internalized object was devalued. Freud maintained that ego development depended upon successful resolution of object loss. Through a process of narcissistic identification, the ego became the target of revengeful aggressive treatment intended for the original object. Depression thus emerges as the construct of guilt over anger toward an ambivalently perceived (loved, hated) object. Other psychoanalytic writers have elaborated and adapted Freud's views, focusing on depression as an ego response to helplessness rather than internalized anger. Such formulations are undoubtedly useful for conceptualizing the origin of milder depressive episodes in individuals who are still socially functional and for understanding symptom formation in more severe depressive states. However, biologic vulnerability is probably an essential prerequisite to the expressions of major depressive disorder.

More recently, investigators have laid stress on the cognitive distortions that dramatically prolong the morbid affective state. The most common cognitive distortions involve negative interpretation of experience, a negative evaluation of the self, and pessimism about the future. Thus, a reverberating loop is established in which a dysphoric affect can give rise to distorted perceptions that in turn exacerbate the dysphoria. This formulation is helpful in understanding the tenacity with which depressed patients seem to cling to the depressive experience even in the face of apparent reward, success, and support.

One cognitive theory based on animal studies is called "learned helplessness." In this formulation, individuals in stressful situations in which they are unable to prevent or alter an aversive stimulus (ie, physical or psychic pain) withdraw and make no further attempts to escape even when opportunities to improve the situation become available. Another theory postulates that a reduction in the rate of positive reinforcement is the principal cause of depression. Low self-esteem is a consequence of the inability of depressed patients to engage in successful goal-seeking behaviors and a resultant low rate of positive reinforcement.

Cognitive and behavioral approaches to the depressive syndrome seem to be more useful for conceptually understanding the psychosocial effects of the depressive state and for planning psychotherapy than for explaining the origin of such episodes. None of the psychosocial theories account for studies documenting a strong genetic influence in the development of major depression or for the dramatic response to antidepressant medication noted in most patients (70%). In certain circumstances, however, psychosocial factors may be necessary, if not sufficient, for the formal occurrence of major depression. An individual carrying a biologic predisposition for recurrent depressive episodes may successfully negotiate critical "vulnerable" periods during times of little conflict or stress.

Treatment

A. Biomedical Therapies: A trial of antidepressant medication is indicated for most individuals with major depression, particularly if melancholic features are present (see p 340). Some clinicians prefer to delay such a trial until the patient's response to a course of brief psychotherapy is evaluated. A few individuals with major depression respond favorably to psychotherapy alone, although most controlled studies have shown that psychotherapy does not control acute symptoms. The wisdom of such a delay depends upon the assessment of severity and the estimated risk of prolonging morbidity. Most patients with depression are either undertreated or inappropriately treated. Benzodiazepines, which may exacerbate the problem, are prescribed much more often than tricyclic agents. Premature withdrawal of antidepressant medication and symptomatic relapse are also unfortunately common.

The drug of first choice is usually a tricyclic or tetracyclic agent, although new agents appear to be no more effective than those in longer use. Drug selection should be based upon the patient's general medical condition, the drug's side effects, and a personal or family history of therapeutic response to a specific agent. About 70% of patients with major depression respond favorably to antidepressant medication. Most cases of poor response are due either to the patient's failure to take the medication as prescribed or to inadequate dosage. Because the blood level from a given dosage varies as much as 30-fold in different individuals, it is useful in cases of nonresponse to measure plasma drug levels even in patients receiving maximal doses. The value of plasma levels is most clear with nortriptyline and desipramine. Although useful for titrating dosage into a general range, variations in blood levels within that range do not correlate well with clinical response.

Clear therapeutic benefit usually is noticed 10–14 days after starting treatment, although earlier and later responses are not uncommon. In general, objective signs of improvement (increased appetite, weight gain, improved sleep and affect, less agitation, increased purposeful activity) are noted before subjective improvement. A drug of a different class should be considered for patients whose symptoms do not improve after 6 weeks of medication with adequate blood levels. Patients with depression accompanied by delusions require more extended treatment periods (up to 8–9 weeks) and dosage levels higher than those for patients not experiencing delusions. Alternatively, another drug may be added, such as liothyronine, lithium, tryptophan, or MAO inhibitors. A trial of an MAO inhibitor alone might be considered at this point, as might a trial of lithium carbonate.

MAO inhibitors—isocarboxazid, phenelzine, tranylcypromine—can be drugs of first choice for individuals who present with prominent anxiety associated with depression or who complain specifically of fatigue, hypersomnia, and weight gain rather than weight loss. Although lithium does not have as specific an antidepressant effect as more traditional antidepressant agents, it may be the drug that helps in patients with clear periodicity of depressive recurrences and is a better prophylactic agent than traditional tricyclic agents.

It is not always clear how long maintenance treatment should be continued after acute symptoms have subsided. In general, a period of 4–6 months of antidepressant medication in decreased doses is necessary to prevent relapse. For individuals with a history of many depressive episodes, the maintenance period is extended to a year or more. There is preliminary evidence that response to the dexamethasone suppression test may indicate how long individuals should be treated. If a repeat dexamethasone suppression test also shows nonsuppression, relapse can be expected if medication is discontinued.

Patients with very severe depressions and prominent delusional features are relatively refractory to traditional antidepressant treatment. The response often can be enhanced by addition of an antipsychotic agent. Electroconvulsive therapy should be considered in such cases and in cases of nondelusional major depression resistant to drug therapy. Most controlled studies have shown that electroconvulsive therapy is at least as effective as antidepressant medication in the treatment of major depression and often produces a much faster recovery. There are few contraindications to the use of electroconvulsive therapy, and side effects are limited to memory loss for the period just before and after treatment.

B. Psychosocial Therapies: Psychotherapy is often indicated for major depression, particularly in improving social functioning following remission of acute symptoms. Controlled studies have indicated that the combination of psychotherapy and antidepressant medication is more effective than either used alone. It should be noted, however, that in most cases of major depression, drug therapy alone is significantly better than psychotherapy alone and may be all that is needed, particularly for individuals whose depression has been treated effectively with a brief course of medication in the past. Many psychotherapeutic approaches have been utilized, but therapies focused on the depressed patient's interpersonal functioning and cognitive distortions appear to be the most productive. Insight therapy is made difficult by the depressed patient's tendency to interpret therapeutic suggestions as criticism. Cognitive therapy is often didactic in nature and may profitably include "homework assignments" in which the patient is asked to critically examine and test erroneous assumptions deriving from the depressive experience. For example, a patient may say, "I fail at everything I do." Asking that patient to keep a log of daily tasks and document the outcome of each effort affords the therapist an effective means of challenging the patient's derogatory self-image. Testimony from others who are able to state that the tasks were performed satisfactorily can be sought if necessary (see Chapter 46).

Family and spouse involvement should not be neglected in treatment planning. This may take several forms, including education about the illness, emotional support, and consideration of interpersonal issues. Although prepubertal children with major depression who receive drug treatment usually show a return to normal functioning in areas such as school performance, ongoing deficits in peer and family relationships frequently continue and require specific intervention.

DYSTHYMIA

Symptoms & Signs

The term "dysthymia" was recently coined to denote in a specific operational way a group of patients formerly described as having "neurotic" or characterologic depressions. Clinicians have long observed that such individuals experience chronic feelings of inadequacy and self-denigration and express these feelings in a dramatic manner that defies all attempts at treatment. Such patients describe a loss of interest or pleasure in most activities of daily life but do not have symptoms severe enough to meet the criteria for major depressive episode. Depressed mood may be unremittent or separated by short periods of normal mood lasting no longer than a few weeks. Dysthymic patients have a tendency to overreact to the normal stresses of life with depressive mood. They are often described as manipulative and unwilling to engage in activities that might be expected to result in improvement in mood. Dysthymic patients have low self-confidence but can be quite demanding and complaining, blaming others for their failures as much as they blame themselves. Obsessional traits are common. As a result of such attitudes, dysthymic patients tend to lead limited social lives and have unstable relationships with others. Abuse of alcohol and other drugs is common in this group of patients.

Natural History

Dysthymic patients often complain of having felt depressed throughout life. A specific time of onset usually cannot be identified or is described as having occurred very early in childhood or adolescence, with a subsequent history of many therapeutic interventions. In some cases, dysthymia seems to date from a major depressive episode.

Individuals with a characterologic predisposition to depressive experience may also be subject to recurrences of major depressive episodes and thus have "double depression" at certain points in their lives. Poor self-esteem, hopelessness, and chronic anhedonia can be viewed as learned phenomena initiated and reinforced at critical junctures by the major depressive

event. Since depressive symptoms are usually mild or moderate in severity, morbidity associated with major depression, such as suicide, is less common. Relationships with family or friends may be adversely affected, as well as performance at school or at work. Dysthymic patients are voracious consumers of medical and mental health care resources, and a history of participation in self-help organizations can often be obtained.

Differential Diagnosis

Dysthymia is easily distinguished from major depression on the basis of severity and chronicity. Occasionally, individuals with dysthymia experience periods of superimposed major depression, and both diagnoses are warranted during such periods. The personality characteristics of individuals with dysthymia are such that an additional diagnosis of personality disorder may be warranted. Again, both diagnoses should be recorded regardless of the hypothesized causal relationship between the 2 diagnoses.

The essential feature of this diagnosis is the chronic nature of the depressed mood. Although normal individuals experience mood states similar to what is noted in dysthymia, their depressions are not as persistent or generally as severe as is the case in dysthymic disorder, and there is no ongoing interference with personal or social functioning.

Prognosis

A broad range of impairment is associated with dysthymia. In some cases, social function and job performance are only mildly affected, while others are characterized by recurrent suicidal preoccupation and inability to sustain adequate performance at school or at work. Since the disorder undoubtedly encompasses a heterogeneous group of individuals, the prognosis depends upon the response to psychotherapy, antidepressant medication, or both together.

Illustrative Case

A 34-year-old unmarried computer programmer was referred for evaluation of chronic depression. He stated that he had felt depressed his "whole life" and that previous psychiatric treatment had been of no benefit. The past history revealed that the patient, who had no siblings, had been socially isolated and shy and had avoided participation in athletics and social events during high school. He had a dependent relationship with his mother following the divorce of his parents when he was 4 years old. His college career was uneventful. When asked how he came to choose computer science as a major, the patient replied that it was more "logical" and "real" and did not require participation in small seminar sections, in which he felt he performed poorly.

The patient's chief complaint was that "life is meaningless." He complained of hypersomnia but admitted he often went to sleep a few hours after returning from work because "there is nothing else to do and television is bad." He had no hobbies and stated that he did not like to try things where "I'll look bad." He had been involved in 2 therapeutic relationships, one lasting 4 months and the other 2 years. He stated that he enjoyed the experience, particularly the longer relationship, but did not feel treatment "really changed anything." He denied ever having experienced any periods of increased energy but did admit that he could "think of being suicidal" if his life did not improve soon.

Epidemiology

Because the term has only recently come into use, the prevalence of dysthymia is not known. Although defined more specifically than the older term "depressive neurosis," the disorder is common in the practice of most clinicians. Dysthymia is somewhat more prevalent in women. Information regarding genetic transmission with familial occurrence of the disorder is lacking, although it is believed that there may be a subgroup of individuals with dysthymia who are experiencing an attenuated form of a biologically based major depressive disorder.

Etiology & Pathogenesis

Biologic and psychosocial theories of the causes of dysthymic disorder are similar to those discussed in the section on major depression, the chief distinction being that dysthymia presents as a less severe but more chronic syndrome. Because of this, social functioning is usually not markedly affected, and the specific nature of the mood disorder may go unrecognized. Over time, however, even mild depressive states can have an insidious effect on personality and character structure. The autonomous nature of the mood state is either denied or unrecognized; its acknowledged existence would arouse conflicts over the individual's growing sense of personal responsibility.

Treatment

Psychotherapy is the principal treatment resource for patients with dysthymia. Although most patients with dysthymia show no particular benefit from antidepressant medication, the diagnostic category undoubtedly includes individuals experiencing milder forms of major depressive disorder. Such individuals, even with chronic histories, may benefit from a trial of an antidepressant drug or lithium carbonate. The guidelines for assessing the potential utility of drug therapy are a contributory family history and a past history of poor response to other forms of treatment. The relative ease and efficiency with which such a trial can be undertaken usually outweigh concerns about risks of medications or the appropriateness of their use.

Although individual psychotherapy is the most common psychosocial treatment offered, many individuals with dysthymia will benefit from group therapy and from active investigation and restructuring of maladaptive social functioning.

Historically, the term "depressive neurosis" was used to identify a group of individuals whose depres-sive experience responded well to psychotherapy. Since the syndrome was not operationally defined, it is unclear what percentage of such individuals would now qualify as having dysthymic disorder.

In traditional psychodynamic therapy, analysis of the patient's emotional response to the therapist is a critical factor in resolution of the depressive experience. The patient's unrealistic expectations of abandonment, criticism, and devaluation by the therapist are revealed and explained as phenomena related to the depression. When the unrealistic nature of these expectations is understood, the patient may emerge from therapy feeling valued and able to form relationships without excessive fear of loss. The recognition and ventilation of anger accompanying such experiences is an important goal in therapy.

Psychotherapy with chronically depressed individuals is an emotionally draining process for the therapist, and recurrent examination of the therapist's own feelings toward the patient is required. Analysis of one's own anger, boredom, or frustration about some aspect of the patient's behavior can help to isolate the key issue in therapy and lead to symptomatic improvement. The patient's unrealistic and idealistic expectations of himself or herself may, for example, be transmitted to the therapist and give rise to overly optimistic expectations of progress in therapy. If the patient shows no subjective improvement over time, the therapist may inadvertently respond somewhat in the way significant individuals in the patient's life have responded. Interpretation of such personal experiences by the therapist can, in the proper context, be therapeutic.

"Short-term" focused psychotherapy and therapeutic programs that stress changes in interpersonal relationships and cognitive self-awareness are becoming more popular, in part because long-term analytic approaches to personality change are economically unfeasible. Family-centered approaches differ from individual methods in their direct focus on the "role of the sick member" in the family system rather than on the symptoms of the identified patient.

OTHER AFFECTIVE DISORDERS

1. BIPOLAR DISORDER NOT OTHERWISE SPECIFIED

Some individuals with bipolar disorder not otherwise specified experience episodes with manic features not severe enough or protracted enough to meet the criteria for a full manic episode. This syndrome is sometimes referred to as "bipolar II" and signifies a current complaint or history of major depressive episode coupled with a current complaint or history of hypomania. The mild form of mania is often socially acceptable and adaptive for the individual. Hypomanic individuals usually experience benefits from increased energy, decreased need for sleep, increased gregariousness, and greater creativity without the disabling consequences of grossly inappropriate social behavior or delusional preoccupation. Most hypomanic episodes do not call for pharmacologic treatment; however, in specific cases a trial of lithium carbonate may be advisable. The subtle nature of many hypomanic episodes results in frequent misdiagnosis. Patients and clinicians alike may see such episodes as "normal" and view only the depressive episodes as pathologic. Rarely, bipolar disorder not otherwise specified is used to refer to patients in whom a manic episode is superimposed on schizophrenia or delusional disorder.

2. DEPRESSIVE DISORDER NOT OTHERWISE SPECIFIED

Depressive disorder not otherwise specified is a diagnosis given to individuals whose depressive symptoms do not meet the criteria for severity or duration noted in the previously described categories. Individuals may experience occasional brief and mild episodes of depression not associated with psychosocial stress or may have dysthymia with periods of normal mood that last longer than several months. Because of the heterogeneous character of the diagnosis and its "by exclusion" feature, no meaningful data are available about prevalence, course, outcome, or treatment response.

Diagnostic problems may arise with depressed individuals whose mood change is either associated with or follows a psychotic process. The rationale for putting patients in this category rather than some other such as schizoaffective disorder (also poorly defined) is unclear (see Chapter 29).

Historically, the diagnosis of depressive disorder not otherwise specified has been most often used to denote individuals with mood disorder with prominent phobic and anxious features. Such individuals may respond to MAO inhibitor medication, though more research is needed.

SUMMARY

It is difficult to conceive of an area in psychiatry in which the clinician's attitude, knowledge, and skills are more severely tested than in the diagnosis and treatment of affective disorders. Knowledge in this area has been accumulating at such a rate that even the most diligent physician would be hard pressed to keep up with all of the new developments in the field. As reviewed in this chapter, there is considerable evidence for a biologic basis for most mood disorders. Data supporting this hypothesis have come from genetic, biochemical, psychopharmacologic, and neuroendocrinologic investigations, and the hope is that psychiatric diagnosis in this area will become a more objective process as these research efforts continue.

Although subgroups of affective disorders seem relatively distinct from one another as described, in clinical practice there is often considerable overlap between symptoms of different disorders as well as ambiguity about which class a given individual belongs in. With the present state of knowledge, predictions about course of illness and response to treatment for patients with mood disorders remain as much an art as a science. Use of the biopsychosocial model in the understanding of mood disorders illustrates the awesome complexity of central nervous system regulation of affect but holds out promise of successful methods of treatment on many different levels.

REFERENCES

Akiskal HS, Hirschfeld R, Yerevanian BI: The relationship of personality to affective disorders. *Arch Gen Psychiatry* 1983;**40**:801.

Akiskal HS et al: Bipolar outcome in the course of depressive illness. *J Affective Disord* 1983;**5**:115.

Andreasen NC et al: The validation of the concept of endogenous depression. *Arch Gen Psychiatry* 1986;**43**:246.

Belmaker R, Van Praag H (editors): *Mania: An Evolving Concept.* SP Medical & Scientific Books, 1980.

Casper RC et al: Somatic symptoms in primary affective disorder. *Arch Gen Psychiatry* 1985;**42**:1098.

Charney D, Menkes D, Heninger G: Receptor sensitivity and the mechanism of action of antidepressant treatment. *Arch Gen Psychiatry* 1981;**38**:1160.

Consensus Development Panel: Mood disorders: Pharmacologic prevention of recurrences. *Am J Psychiatry* 1985;**142**:469.

Coryell W: Hypomania. (Invited editorial.) *J Affective Disord* 1982;**4**:167.

Cytryn L et al: A developmental view of affective disturbances in the children of affectively ill parents. *Am J Psychiatry* 1984;**141**:219.

Davidson J et al: Atypical depression. *Arch Gen Psychiatry* 1982;**39**:527.

Harrow M et al: A longitudinal study of thought disorder in manic patients. *Arch Gen Psychiatry* 1986;**43**:781.

Howarth BG, Grace MGA: Depression, drugs, and delusions. *Arch Gen Psychiatry* 1985;**42**:1145.

Keller MB et al: Differential outcome of pure manic, mixed/cycling, and pure depressive episodes in patients with bipolar illness. *JAMA* 1986;**255**:3138.

Keller MB et al: Long-term outcome of episodes of major depression. *JAMA* 1984;**252**:788.

Kidman A: Neurochemical and cognitive aspects of depression. *Prog Neurobiol* 1985;**24**:187.

Klerman GL et al: Birth-cohort trends in rates of major depressive disorder among relatives of patients with affective disorder. *Arch Gen Psychiatry* 1985;**42**:689.

Malt U: Classification and diagnosis of depression. *Acta Psychiatr Scand [Suppl]* 1983;**No.302**:7.

Nelson JC et al: Drug-responsive symptoms in melancholia. *Arch Gen Psychiatry* 1984;**41**:663.

Post RM, Ballenger JC (editors): *Neurobiology of Mood Disorders*. 2 vols. Williams & Wilkins, 1984.

Prien RF, Kupfer DJ: Continuation drug therapy for major depressive episodes: How long should it be maintained? *Am J Psychiatry* 1986;**143**:18.

Rodin G, Voshart K: Depression in the medically ill: An overview. *Am J Psychiatry* 1986;**143**:696.

Schuckit MA: Genetic and clinical implications of alcoholism and affective disorder. *Am J Psychiatry* 1986;**143**:140.

Stavrakaki C, Vargo B: The relationship of anxiety and depression: A review of the literature. *Br J Psychiatry* 1986;**149**:7.

Weissman MM, Prusoff BA, Merikangas KR: Is delusional depression related to bipolar disorder? *Am J Psychiatry* 1984;**141**:892.

Anxiety Disorders **31**

John H. Greist, MD, & James W. Jefferson, MD

Anxiety and fear are ubiquitous emotions. The terms anxiety and fear have specific and scientific meanings, but common usage has made them interchangeable. For example, a phobia is a kind of anxiety that is also defined in *DSM-III-R* as a "persistent or irrational fear." **Fear** is defined as an emotional and physiologic response to a recognized external threat (eg, a runaway car or a sharp descent in an airplane). **Anxiety** is an unpleasant emotional state, the sources of which are less readily identified. It is frequently accompanied by physiologic symptoms that may lead to fatigue or even exhaustion. Because fear of recognized threats causes similar unpleasant mental tension and physical changes, patients discuss fear and anxiety interchangeably. Thus, there is little need to strive to differentiate anxiety from fear. However, distinguishing among different anxiety disorders is important, since accurate diagnosis is more likely to result in effective treatment and a better prognosis.

The intensity of anxiety has many gradations ranging from minor qualms to noticeable trembling and even complete **panic,** the most extreme form of anxiety.

The course of anxiety also varies, with peak severity being reached within a few seconds or more gradually over minutes, hours, or days. Duration also varies from a few seconds to hours or even days or months, although episodes of panic usually abate within 10 minutes and seldom last more than 30 minutes.

The signs and symptoms of anxiety are detailed in the diagnostic criteria for the anxiety disorders (Tables 31–1 and 31–8).

If anxiety arises unexpectedly ("out of the blue"), it is called **spontaneous anxiety** (or if very intense, **spontaneous panic).** When anxiety occurs predictably in specific situations, it is called **phobic** or **situational anxiety** (or when extreme, **phobic** or **situational panic). Anticipatory anxiety** (or **anticipatory panic)** is the term used to describe anxiety triggered by the mere thought of particular situations.

The boundary between normal and pathologic anxiety cannot be drawn with great precision or confidence. People sometimes seek treatment for anxiety that disappears spontaneously before they can be seen. Physicians sometimes delay treatment until disruption of functioning is obvious or suffering is severe. These differences are understandable in the context of present knowledge regarding anxiety, attitudinal differences of both patients and doctors about seeking and giving help, and the effectiveness of various treatments. When anxiety substantially impairs work style or social adjustment, most authorities agree that careful assessment is indicated and that treatment is likely to be worthwhile. Suffering itself is often justification for treatment, even if the person with anxiety can continue to function.

Anxiety commonly occurs as a manifestation of appropriate concern about medical and psychiatric disorders. Medical problems involving any body system can produce anxiety as a symptom. Drugs and dietary factors—particularly caffeine and alcohol—may also provoke anxiety.

Anxiety & Depression

At least three-fourths of patients with primary depression complain of feeling anxious, worried, or fearful. Extreme anxiety may occur in agitated depression in the form of anguished facial expressions; lip biting; picking at fingers, nails, or clothing; handwringing; constant pacing; and inability to sit quietly. Conversely, primary anxiety can be depressing in its own right. If anxiety persists, and particularly if it interferes with functioning, secondary depression is the rule rather than the exception. Some patients have both primary anxiety and primary depressive disorders. While most patients with anxiety or depression fall clearly into the respective *DSM-III-R* categories for anxiety or depression, differential diagnosis can be challenging and require several interviews, further evaluation, and trials of medications.

Theories of Anxiety

A. Genetic: Isaac Marks (1986) has provided an elegant summary of the genetics of fear and anxiety disorders:

> From protozoa to mammals, organisms have been selectively bred for genetic differences in defensive behaviour which are accompanied by differences in brain and other biological functions. Studies of twins indicate some genetic control of normal human fear from infancy onwards, of anxiety as a symptom and as a syndrome, and of phobic and obsessive compulsive phenomena. Anxiety disorders are more common among the relatives of affected probands than of controls, especially among female and first-degree relatives; alcoholism and secondary depression may also be overrepresented. Familial influences have been found for panic disorder, agoraphobia, and obsessive compulsive problems. Panic disorder

in depressed probands increases the risk to their relatives of phobia as well as of panic disorder, major depression, and alcoholism. The strongest family history of all anxiety disorders is seen in blood-injury phobia; even though it can be successfully treated by exposure, its roots may lie in a genetically determined specific autonomic susceptibility. Some genetic effects can be modified by environmental means.

B. Psychodynamic: Although Freud at first proposed a physiologic basis for anxiety, he later concluded that anxiety serves as a signal to the ego of the emergence of an unconscious conflict or impulse. His theory led to the development of psychoanalysis for the study and treatment of emotional disorders. According to psychoanalytic theory, anxiety is seen as an emotion of the ego (the part of our mental apparatus that balances the impulses and demands of our childlike id, the stern and punitive controls of our parentlike superego, and external reality). Anxiety is also seen as the key indication of hidden psychologic conflict. (See Chapters 3 and 5 for details.)

C. Learned: Behavioral therapists hold that anxiety is a learned response to some noxious stimulus. When a situation or stimulus provokes anxiety in a person who then avoids it, anxiety is diminished and the person learns to reduce anxiety by avoiding situations that provoke it. Generalized anxiety disorder may result from unpredictable positive and negative reinforcement—the person is uncertain which avoidance behaviors will be effective in reducing anxiety.

It is also possible to develop anxiety in response to generally positive or neutral stimuli if these are associated with a noxious or aversive stimulus. This conditioning process is held to be responsible for the avoidance of neutral or benign situations in which distressing anxiety (such as panic) has occurred. Pairing of a recurrent anxiety-inducing thought (such as "contamination") with a compulsive behavior (such as handwashing) that reduces anxiety is thought to explain the development of obsessive compulsive disorder. (For details on this theory, see Chapter 3; for details on treatment applications, see Chapter 46.)

D. Biochemical: When compared with normal controls, patients with anxiety disorders have significantly different physiologic functioning (eg, higher heart rate, higher blood lactate levels, and greater oxygen debt during moderate exercise). Patients with panic disorders are more sensitive to a number of substances (eg, caffeine, lactate, isoproterenol, epinephrine, yohimbine, and piperoxan). Many of these substances increase activity of the locus ceruleus, the midbrain nucleus which supplies about 70% of the norepinephrine neurons in the central nervous system. Human subjects given these substances report increased anxiety, and monkeys demonstrate fear behaviors similar to those they show when placed in a confrontational setting. Electrical stimulation of the locus ceruleus in monkeys produces a similar fear response, while its ablation reduces fear behaviors. Medications that inhibit locus ceruleus functioning also reduce fear responses in monkeys and anxiety in humans with anxiety disorders as well as in controls. Although α_2 agonists and beta-adrenergic receptor blockers have been shown to have some antianxiety properties, the heterocyclic and monoamine oxidase inhibitor antidepressants and benzodiazepine drugs, which down-regulate locus ceruleus (norepinephrine) function, are the most useful clinically.

The benzodiazepines have a second putative mode of action in that they potentiate gamma-aminobutyric acid (GABA), a widely distributed inhibitory neurotransmitter. Discovery of benzodiazepine receptors in the central nervous system led to a search for endogenous benzodiazepines, and these have now been found (see Chapter 10).

The evocative and modulatory roles of acetylcholine, histamine, dopamine, serotonin, and enkephalins in anxiety are also being studied.

The apparent biochemical basis of every behavior, thought, and feeling does not dictate that biochemical abnormalities must be treated with chemicals—brain chemistry can also be changed by behavioral, psychologic, and surgical interventions.

Epidemiology

In the recent National Institute of Mental Health Epidemiological Catchment Area (NIMH-ECA) Study (Meyers et al, 1984), anxiety disorders were more prevalent over the preceding 6 months than any other mental disorder (8.3% of the populations surveyed in their homes). Of those with anxiety disorders, only 23% were receiving treatment. Other studies have found similar or slightly lower rates of anxiety disorders. The lifetime incidence of anxiety disorders is uncertain but is probably in the range of 15–25%.

DSM-III-R Diagnosis

In *DSM-III-R,* panic disorder has assumed greater importance while agoraphobia has, with one exception, become a subcategory of panic disorder. This change reflects the commonly observed sequence in which panic produces anticipatory anxiety about the possible recurrence of panic in certain situations, which, in turn, leads to avoidance of those situations in a misguided attempt at self-treatment. The sequence of panic → anticipatory anxiety → avoidance is common, and treatments are often selected for their purported effectiveness for each component of the triad; however, not all agoraphobic persons experience anxiety of panic proportions.

The substantially reduced emphasis on hierarchic diagnosis in *DSM-III-R* is consistent with clinical observations that individuals often have 2 or more concomitant independent disorders that could not be diagnosed under *DSM-III* rules. Most other changes in the concept of anxiety disorders in *DSM-III-R* are minor and involve shifts in duration or number of symptoms or signs associated with a particular disorder.

Use of structured interviews (eg, the National Institute of Mental Health Diagnostic Interview Schedule [DIS], which can be administered directly to patients by a **computer interview,** or the Structured Clinical

Interview for *DSM-III* [SCID], which requires clinical judgment) can ensure that all relevant diagnostic items are considered and that diagnostic logic is faithfully followed. The substantial time required to conduct a structured interview is one argument in favor of using a direct patient-computer interview (Greist et al, 1984). An approach combining structured interviews and direct contact with patients will lead to the most accurate clinical diagnoses.

PANIC DISORDER

The emphasis on panic disorder in *DSM-III-R* as an etiologic factor in the development of agoraphobia is a reversal of the emphasis in *DSM-III*, which described "agoraphobia with panic attacks" as the most common phobic disorder. There is still substantial debate about the incidence and prevalence of panic episodes or attacks. The NIMH-ECA study found a 6-month prevalence of panic disorder of only 0.7%; the prevalence of agoraphobia was 2.8%. More than one-third of the population may have a paniclike episode during any given year, but fewer individuals develop panic disorder. According to *DSM-III-R*, a diagnosis of panic disorder requires either 4 panic attacks in a 4-week period or the development of fear, of at least 1 month's duration, of having another panic episode.

Symptoms & Signs

Table 31–1 lists *DSM-III-R* criteria for panic disorder. The distressing constellation of sudden and unpredicted episodes involving pronounced alteration of physiologic functions frequently leads to fears of death, "going crazy," or "doing something uncontrolled." Commonly, patients will experience 8 or 9 of the 13 symptoms. Panic attacks begin suddenly and usually abate within 5–10 minutes, rarely lasting 30 minutes or more. Patients may confuse panic with anticipatory anxiety early in the course of the disorder, although most become expert at distinguishing between the 2 as time passes. Moving about during a panic attack makes many individuals feel somewhat better, but avoidance of situations in which panic has occurred leads to the development of phobias.

Differential Diagnosis

Medical causes of anxiety should not be overlooked, nor should anxiety disorders be overinvestigated or treated as medical disorders. Most medical causes of anxiety symptoms are readily recognized if a careful history, physical examination, and indicated laboratory tests are performed.

Medical problems that may produce anxiety include those affecting the cardiovascular system (angina pectoris, acute myocardial infarction, arrhythmias, congestive heart failure, shock); respiratory problems (asthma, emphysema, pulmonary embolism); neurologic disorders (encephalopathy, seizure disorder, benign essential tremor, vertigo); hematologic and immunologic disorders (anemia, anaphylactic shock); and endocrine dysfunction (diabetes, hy-

Table 31–1. *DSM-III-R* diagnostic criteria for panic disorder.

Panic disorder:
A. At some time during the disturbance, one or more panic attacks (discrete periods of intense fear or discomfort) have occurred that were (1) unexpected, ie, did not occur immediately before or on exposure to a situation that almost always caused anxiety, and (2) not triggered by situations in which the person was the focus of others' attention.
B. Either 4 attacks, as defined in criterion A, have occurred within a 4-week period, or one or more attacks have been followed by a period of at least 1 month of persistent fear of having another attack.
C. At least 4 of the following symptoms developed during at least one of the attacks:
   (1) Shortness of breath (dyspnea) or smothering sensations.
   (2) Dizziness, unsteady feelings, or faintness.
   (3) Palpitations or accelerated heart rate (tachycardia).
   (4) Trembling or shaking.
   (5) Sweating.
   (6) Choking.
   (7) Nausea or abdominal distress.
   (8) Depersonalization or derealization.
   (9) Numbness or tingling sensations (paresthesias).
   (10) Flushes (hot flashes) or chills.
   (11) Chest pain or discomfort.
   (12) Fear of dying.
   (13) Fear of going crazy or of doing something uncontrolled.

Note: Attacks involving 4 or more symptoms are panic attacks; attacks involving fewer than 4 symptoms are limited symptom attacks (see Table 31–3).

D. During at least some of the attacks, at least 4 of the above symptoms developed suddenly and increased in intensity within 10 minutes of the beginning of the first symptom noticed in the attack.
E. It cannot be established that an organic factor initiated and maintained the disturbance, eg, amphetamine or caffeine intoxication, hyperthyroidism.

Note: Mitral valve prolapse may be an associated condition but does not preclude a diagnosis of panic disorder.

Panic disorder without agoraphobia:
A. Meets the criteria for panic disorder.
B. Absence of agoraphobia, as defined above.

Specify severity of panic attacks, as defined above.

pothyroidism, hyperthyroidism, parathyroid disease, Cushing's disease, pheochromocytoma).

Medications may also provoke anxiety symptoms. Antispasmodics, cold medicines, thyroid supplements, digitalis, stimulants, and—paradoxically—antianxiety and antidepressant medicines used to treat panic may all induce anxiety. Discontinuation of certain medications (eg, some blood pressure medicines, sleeping pills, and antianxiety drugs) may lead to withdrawal symptoms in which anxiety may be prominent. Caffeine, alcohol, and marihuana are frequent causes of anxiety symptoms, including panic.

Illustrative Case

A 30-year-old woman had experienced panic episodes since age 20. They usually began spontaneously, "out of the blue," although they often appeared in the context of anger or other emotional extremes of sadness or disappointment. She had awakened from sleep in panic on several occasions. Although she worried initially that the settings or circumstancess in which panic occurred might be causing the episodes, she later concluded that no reliable pattern could be detected. She neither smoked nor used alcohol and had discontinued use of caffeine because it made her feel jittery.

Attacks were characterized by rapid heart rate, sweating, nausea, chills, trembling, and a fear of doing something uncontrolled. Early severe episodes had included symptoms associated with hyperventilation, including "smothering," choking, chest discomfort, faintness, and paresthesias, but once she recognized their association with overbreathing, she was able to control them by learning to breathe "slow and shallow."

The patient reported increased frequency but not severity of panic attacks in the premenstruum.

Family history was positive for similar episodes from ages 25 through 45 in her mother and for depression on both sides of her family.

After each of her first few attacks, the patient sought treatment in an emergency room or from her primary care physician, who had carefully examined her and, finding "nothing wrong," attempted to reassure her that her symptoms were a manifestation of anxiety. She had briefly used a benzodiazepine prescribed by her physician but objected to the "drugged" feeling it produced. Panic ceased for one 3-year period and occurred less than once per month for another 3 years. She remained, however, worried that panic could recur at any time. For the 2 years before she sought treatment, panic attacks had occurred at least twice per month. Imipramine in gradually increasing doses (see below) was prescribed, and at levels of 100 mg/d, panic attacks ceased for 6 months. They resumed when the dose was decreased to 75 mg/d.

Epidemiology

The NIMH-ECA study found a 6-month prevalence of panic disorder of only 0.7%, whereas agoraphobia was present in 2.8%. More than one-third of individuals may experience a single episode of panic in any given year. A much smaller proportion will have repeated panic attacks, and less than 1 percent will develop panic disorder. The peak age of onset for spontaneous panic is between 15 and 25 years, and panic beginning after age 40 would suggest depression or possible medical causes. There is some genetic basis for panic disorder, although many who experience panic attacks come from families with no history of anxiety. Women have been thought to have panic disorder twice as commonly as men, but some of this difference may be due to cultural factors that permit women, more than men, to complain about and seek treatment for symptoms of panic or anxiety.

Etiology & Pathogenesis

The underlying pathophysiology of panic disorder

is far from clear. It is commonly held that panic disorder has a biochemical basis, but its precise characteristics have not been elucidated. Many authorities suspect that noradrenergic dysfunction, perhaps mediated through the locus ceruleus (Redmond, 1977), is involved, and drug treatments that alter this system have been shown to be of benefit. Panic appears pathogenetic for phobic complications of anticipatory anxiety and avoidance, which may persist after panic has abated. Further disability may be caused by overconcern that the physiologic changes associated with panic may signal a catastrophe.

There may be an association between early separation anxiety manifested by school avoidance and the later development of agoraphobia. The role of panic in this situation is unclear, however, since few children with separation anxiety experience spontaneous panic.

Treatment

Treatment is largely empirical, since etiologic factors have not been clearly established.

A. Psychologic Treatment: Many case reports and personal testimonials claim positive benefits from the many varieties of psychotherapy; no one type is clearly any more or less effective than another. In psychotherapy, as well as behavioral therapy and drug therapy, nonspecific factors common to any good patient-clinician relationship (eg, expectation of success, belief in treatment, reassurance, encouragement) probably account for much of the improvement in anxiety disorders achieved with psychotherapeutic approaches.

Cognitive therapy (see Chapter 46) that attempts to modify catastrophic negative thoughts that may accompany panic attacks shows considerable promise and is now the subject of controlled investigations. Thus, an attempt can be made to help a patient whose train of thought runs, "My heart just skipped a beat and my chest feels tight, so I must be having a heart attack and will surely die," to reinterpret these physiologic symptoms along a train of thought such as, "My heart just skipped a beat and my chest feels tight. These are familiar symptoms of panic. I can expect several other 'old friends' such as numbness and tingling of my fingers, feeling faint, sweating, shortness of breath, and trembling to appear soon. These are all symptoms of panic which I have been through many times before. Panic is unpleasant but not dangerous, and I know this attack will end soon." This reassignment of the physiologic components of panic from life-threatening to familiar and manageable may help a larger proportion of patients than other psychotherapies. It also includes elements of exposure therapy (see below).

B. Behavioral Therapy: There is growing evidence that panic attacks can be substantially reduced in frequency and severity by the use of exposure therapy (see Chapter 46). Agoraphobic patients who experience spontaneous panic report marked reduction in the frequency and severity of panic when given exposure therapy without medication. In some studies, panic attacks have stopped altogether in two-thirds of patients. When hyperventilation is a substantial component of panic, teaching patients techniques to control it is often helpful. The voluntary induction of hyperventilation can be coupled with both education and instruction in diaphragmatic breathing. Patients who experience only panic without anticipatory anxiety and avoidance can be exposed, in fantasy or imagination, to the physiologic aberrations associated with panic. Thus, they would be asked to imagine that the full constellation of panic symptoms is emerging just as it does during a panic attack and to continue that fantasy until associated anxiety dies down.

When panic attacks are accompanied by anticipatory anxiety and avoidance, exposure is the treatment of choice. Exposure can be simply taught in an office setting in as little as 5 minutes. The patient is instructed to "find and face the things you fear and remain in contact with them until your anxiety subsides." The therapist must reiterate the instruction as treatment progresses and monitor compliance with written records kept by the patient for mutually agreed-upon exposure tasks. Homework assignments constitute the bulk of exposure tasks, and enlistment of a family member or friend who can serve as co-therapist is often helpful. A self-help chapter in a book authored by Greist and coworkers (1986) has been shown to be as effective as sessions with a behavioral therapist in treating individuals with agoraphobia.

C. Drug Therapy: Medications are currently the cornerstone of treatment of panic disorder (see Chapter 54). Antidepressant medications have been shown to substantially reduce the frequency and severity of spontaneous panic attacks and often block them altogether. Studies show that antidepressants that have a greater effect on the noradrenergic system may be more useful in treating panic disorder than preferential serotonin reuptake-blocking antidepressants. Treatment with all classes of antianxiety agents should begin at low doses and be increased gradually when the current dose is ineffective. Thus, imipramine should be prescribed in one 25-mg bedtime dose with instructions to increase the dosage to 50 mg at bedtime on the day after the patient experiences another panic attack, and so on, as necessary, to the usual or maximum tolerable antidepressant dose range. Antidepressant medications are effective in the treatment of panic in that they ameliorate depression that may precipitate the emergence of panic. These drugs may also prevent the development of depression in the wake of the constricted life-style associated with anticipatory anxiety and avoidance.

Benzodiazepine antianxiety agents (eg, alprazolam) have also been shown to reduce the frequency and severity of both spontaneous and situational panic and have a faster onset of action than the antidepressants. Benzodiazepine antianxiety agents carry the risk of side effects and dependence. Relapse is the rule rather than the exception when these medications are withdrawn, although long-term use appears safe in most patients.

Beta-adrenergic blocking agents (eg, propranolol, metoprolol) are sometimes prescribed to help control heart rate, arrhythmia, sweating, and tremor. Although helpful for some patients, these agents are not generally as effective in the treatment of panic or anticipatory anxiety as antidepressant and antianxiety drugs.

Barbiturates, meprobamate, and antihistamines are less effective than antidepressant and antianxiety agents and are seldom used for that reason and because of the potential for abuse of barbiturates and meprobamate. Antipsychotics should not be used routinely for treatment of anxiety symptoms except in the context of psychosis.

A combination of medication and behavior therapy appears to be most helpful for many patients; when the 2 therapies are combined, relapse rates may be substantially lower upon withdrawal of medication.

AGORAPHOBIA

Symptoms & Signs

The diagnostic criteria for panic disorder with agoraphobia are listed in Table 31–2. Table 31–3 lists the diagnostic criteria for agoraphobia without a history of panic disorder. Agoraphobia is a fear of being caught in a situation from which a graceful and speedy escape to safety would be difficult or embarrassing if the patient felt discomfort (often in the form of panic). Situations likely to induce fear and avoidance include church and sporting events where the individual may be seated far from an aisle; eating out, especially at formal sit-down restaurants; appointments with dentists, doctors, or hairdressers; driving in situations where opportunities to pull over, stop, or get off the highway quickly may be infrequent (eg, turning left across oncoming traffic or traveling on interstate highways where exits are far apart). Being accompanied by a trusted family member or friend permits many agoraphobic individuals to increase the number of possibly

Table 31–2. *DSM-III-R* diagnostic criteria for panic disorder with agoraphobia.

A. Meets the criteria for panic disorder.
B. Agoraphobia: Fear of being in places or situations from which escape might be difficult (or embarrassing) or in which help might not be available in the event of a panic attack. (Include cases in which persistent avoidance behavior originated during an active phase of panic disorder, even if the person does not attribute the avoidance behavior to fear of having a panic attack.) As a result of this fear, the person either restricts travel or needs a companion when away from home or else endures agoraphobic situations despite intense anxiety. Common agoraphobic situations include being outside the home alone, being in a crowd or standing in a line, being on a bridge, and traveling in a bus, train, or car.

Specify current severity of agoraphobic avoidance.

Specify current severity of panic attacks.

Table 31–3. *DSM-III-R* diagnostic criteria for agoraphobia without history of panic disorder.

A. Agoraphobia: Fear of being in places or situations from which escape might be difficult (or embarrassing) or in which help might not be available in the event of suddenly developing a symptom(s) that could be incapacitating or extremely embarrassing. Examples include dizziness or falling, depersonalization or derealization, loss of bladder or bowel control, vomiting, or cardiac distress. As a result of this fear, the person either restricts travel or needs a companion when away from home or else endures agoraphobic situations despite intense anxiety. Common agoraphobic situations include being outside the home alone, being in a crowd or standing in a line, being on a bridge, and traveling in a bus, train, or car.

B. Has never met the criteria for panic disorder.

Specify with or without limited symptom attacks.

uncomfortable situations they can endure and to extend the range of their excursions.

For those who panic, fear of fainting during an attack is the most common fear after fear of panic itself. Hyperventilation with its attendant decreases in blood carbon dioxide, ionized calcium, and phosphorus produces paresthesias, light-headedness, visual changes, and feelings of unreality that contribute to the fear of fainting. Actual fainting, if it occurs at all during panic, must be exceedingly rare, since none of the patients seen by the authors has fainted during a panic attack.

By definition, phobias are irrational fears involving avoidance of objects or situations that are extremely unlikely to cause harm and that most people approach without discomfort. Agoraphobic patients lament their inability to face everyday situations and often become discouraged, depressed, and demoralized by the constriction in their lives occasioned by agoraphobia.

Differential Diagnosis

Avoidance or withdrawal can occur in depression, schizophrenic disorders, and paranoid disorders, some organic mental disorders, other anxiety disorders (eg, social or simple phobia, obsessive compulsive disorder, and posttraumatic stress disorder), and certain personality disorders. This avoidance occurs in the context of other symptoms and signs that usually clarify the underlying diagnosis. A few simple questions (also useful with other anxiety disorders) are likely to point to or away from a diagnosis of agoraphobia:

(1) Are there situations or things you avoid? What are they? (Agoraphobic patients are likely to describe situations in which they would feel caught or trapped.)

(2) What do you feel will happen if you cannot avoid (the situations described in Question 1)? (Expect agoraphobic patients to describe fears of panic, fainting, "going crazy," or dying.)

(3) Do your fears seem exaggerated or out of proportion? (Most agoraphobic patients clearly recognize the unreasonableness of their fears and frequently describe them with words such as dumb, stupid, crazy, goofy, irrational.)

(4) If you must face (avoided situations), how do you bring yourself to do it? (Agoraphobic patients usually describe anticipatory anxiety that leads to excuses to avoid the situation or frank refusal to proceed; frequent requests that others accompany them; or use of alcohol or other sedatives to decrease anxiety.)

(5) Have you ever had the experience of anxiety decreasing if you could not leave the uncomfortable situation for a long time? (Most agoraphobic patients have found themselves in such situations from time to time, and most reported a reduction in anxiety with this fortuitous exposure therapy.)

Since panic attacks and consequent agoraphobia may develop secondary to major depression, it is important to establish the sequence of symptoms and disorders in patients with both depression and agoraphobia. Agoraphobia secondary to depression often remits without additional measures as depression is treated.

Prognosis

Agoraphobia may remit spontaneously, particularly if panic attacks abate or if life circumstances force or encourage patients to go about their business. Typically, untreated agoraphobia runs a chronic and undulating course with periods of relative exacerbation and remission and with major incapacity associated with anticipatory anxiety and avoidance. It is common for individuals to avoid phobic situations because of anticipatory anxiety even if they have not experienced panic for years. Alcohol and other substance abuse becomes a problem for a small proportion of agoraphobic patients who derive initially beneficial antianxiety effects from these substances, rely increasingly upon them, and develop both psychologic and physiologic dependence.

Approximately 10% of agoraphobic patients have obsessive compulsive symptoms, although these are usually mild and rarely require treatment. Agoraphobia can have devastating effects on both the sufferers and their families. Roles within the family often change dramatically. For example, spouses work fewer hours after their partners develop the disorder, because of increased family responsibilities. Agoraphobia frequently leads to discouragement and complaints of tension, fatigue, obsessions, and depression.

With treatment, some individuals appear cured, and most make substantial gains, so that they are able to resume their previous occupational and social roles with minor residual anxiety. A very small number of agoraphobic patients fail to respond to available behavioral and drug treatments.

Illustrative Case

A 23-year-old woman who had experienced panic while driving on an expressway on 3 separate occasions became worried about driving on the expressway again; worrying about it brought on another panic attack. She stopped driving on the expressway but still experienced extreme anxiety in other situations, such as standing in a supermarket checkout line, sitting in church or under a hair dryer at the beauty parlor, where means of egress were not readily available. She became increasingly worried about panic attacks and avoided more and more settings where they might occur and leave her feeling helpless. She was able to continue working only because a trusted friend conveyed her to and from work.

After reading about agoraphobia in a magazine, she recognized her disorder and sought treatment. Careful history taking revealed that she had last experienced panic 3 months before coming to the clinic but worried about attacks almost constantly (anticipatory anxiety). Treatment was begun with exposure therapy, and she made rapid gains in the range of her activities while experiencing progressively less discomfort. Panic attacks did not recur either in the treatment setting or spontaneously, and at 1-year follow-up she had regained her full range of activities, although she still worried somewhat that panic attacks might recur.

Epidemiology

The NIMH-ECA study reported an overall 6-month prevalence of agoraphobia of 3.8% for women and 1.8% for men. Some of the higher prevalence in females may be culturally determined. Agoraphobia is the most common anxiety disorder seen in clinics specializing in treating patients with anxiety, and it is somewhat less common in people of higher income and education and in whites. The age of onset peaks in the early 20s, and onset after age 40 is uncommon.

Before agoraphobia begins, people who will develop the disorder and those who will not are similar in terms of social or marital status, marital and sexual adjustment, separation anxiety, dependency, and other personality characteristics. *After* agoraphobia occurs, many of these attributes change for the worse.

Etiology & Pathogenesis

There is growing evidence that an agoraphobic trait disorder may be inherited, although it is difficult, without studies of individuals adopted at birth, to distinguish inheritance from behaviors learned from parents or siblings with agoraphobia. In 2 studies, specific severe trauma preceded the onset of agoraphobia in only 3% and 8% of people, respectively. However, less severe life stress events were reportedly twice as common in agoraphobic patients as in controls. (This is also true for many other psychiatric and medical disorders.)

Commonly, panic leads to anticipatory anxiety of another panic in the same situation which, in turn, leads to avoidance of that situation. Many patients report this sequence, but others develop classic agoraphobic avoidance without ever experiencing panic. In some, panic occurs after entering agoraphobic situations (situational or phobic panic). The exact role of panic in the etiology of agoraphobia remains unresolved and is the subject of continuing study.

Treatment

A. Psychologic Treatment: The effectiveness of specific psychotherapies for treatment of agoraphobia has not been established. All therapies (including medications and behavioral therapy) should include nonspecific but important elements of education and support; this may partly explain the improvement sometimes seen with psychotherapy.

Freud probably suffered from agoraphobia and clearly recognized the ineffectiveness of psychoanalysis in treating phobias when he wrote: "One can hardly master a phobia if one waits till the patient lets the analysis influence him to give it up . . . one succeeds only when one can induce them through the influence of the analysis to . . . go into the street and to struggle with their anxiety while they make the attempt." (Freud, "Lines of Advance in Psychoanalysis," 1955.)

B. Behavioral Therapy: Exposure therapy is the single most effective treatment for agoraphobia with and without panic attacks. Panic, anticipatory anxiety, and avoidance are all reduced by this straightforward approach when it is systematically applied according to simple instructions that many patients can put into practice by themselves or with the help of a family member or friend. Patients can be given suggestions for "coping tactics" to be used when anxiety rises to disturbing levels. Over the past decade, the average number of contact hours spent with an experienced behavioral therapist in the successful treatment of agoraphobia has declined from nearly 20 to less than 4. Patients using exposure therapy develop a new attitude toward the fears they experience and the risks they are willing to take regarding those fears. This change often spreads to other aspects of their functioning, with beneficial results.

C. Drug Treatment: When panic is present, drug treatment is often indicated (see Panic Disorder, above). In the absence of panic, exposure therapy alone is usually sufficient. Some patients have pronounced anticipatory anxiety when they begin exposure therapy; such patients may be given antianxiety medications. The lowest effective dose should be used, since some individuals may fail to learn how to deal effectively with anxiety-causing stimuli while under the influence of anxiolytics. (This phenomenon is known as state-dependent learning, in which what is learned in the drugged state is forgotten in a state of normal consciousness.) There is also a small risk of dependence on anxiolytics (see Chapter 54).

SOCIAL PHOBIA

Symptoms & Signs

The *DSM-III-R* diagnostic criteria for social phobia are listed in Table 31–4. Individuals with social phobia have a persistent and recognizably irrational fear of embarrassment or humiliation when performing in social situations. All individuals with social phobia fear that their performance will be found wanting in some way and lead to embarrassment or humiliation.

Whereas some performance anxiety can provide people with an "edge," social phobia is performance

Table 31-4. *DSM-III-R* diagnostic criteria for social phobia.

A. A persistent fear of one or more situations (the social phobic situations) in which the person is exposed to possible scrutiny by others and fears that he or she may do something or act in a way that will be humiliating or embarrassing. Examples include being unable to continue talking while speaking in public, choking on food when eating in front of others, being unable to urinate in a public lavatory, experiencing hand trembling when writing in the presence of others, and saying foolish things or not being able to answer questions in social situations.

B. If an axis III or another axis I disorder is present, the fear in criterion A, above, is unrelated to it, eg, the fear is not of having a panic attack (panic disorder), stuttering (stuttering), trembling (Parkinson's disease), or exhibiting abnormal eating behavior (anorexia nervosa or bulimia nervosa).

C. During some phase of the disturbance, exposure to the specific phobic stimulus (or stimuli) almost invariably provokes an immediate anxiety response.

D. The phobic situation(s) is avoided or endured with intense anxiety.

E. The avoidant behavior interferes with occupational functioning or with usual social activities or relationships with others, or there is marked distress about having the fear.

F. The person recognizes that his or her fear is excessive or unreasonable.

Specify generalized type if the phobic situation is most social situations, and also consider the additional diagnosis of avoidant personality disorder.

anxiety of such great proportions that it interferes with performance.

Individuals asked to face their particular type of social phobia describe anticipatory anxiety and may experience situational panic indistinguishable from spontaneous panic. Avoidance is a common complication of social phobia.

Differential Diagnosis

Marked anxiety and avoidance of social situations may occur in schizophrenia, major depression, obsessive compulsive disorder, and paranoid and avoidant personality disorders. However, the reasons given for such avoidance and anxiety are closely tied to content appropriate for those specific disorders and seldom involve embarrassment or humiliation. For example, a patient who is paranoid may avoid social situations because of delusional fear of being harmed.

Prognosis

Mild social phobias seldom interfere with functioning but may consign sufferers to repeated discomfort when in their phobic situations. More severe social phobia frequently interferes substantially with functioning and causes great suffering. It is not uncommon for individuals with social phobia to change professions in order to avoid situations that raise performance anxiety.

Illustrative Case

A medical student ranking in the top 10% of his class sought treatment before making a decision to drop out of medical school during the first clinical rotation in his third year. He had always experienced extreme anxiety whenever called upon to speak in class and had successfully avoided such presentations through high school, college, and the first 2 years of medical school. He had taken pains to select a medical school where he thought formal oral presentations were not required. At the beginning of his junior year, he was informed that he would have to make a "medical advances" presentation 4 months later. Although he quickly developed the topic and was confident of his material, he felt that he could not face the ordeal of making the presentation. Anticipatory anxiety had already begun to mount to a level that interfered with his sleep and his performance on the wards.

The student reported that his father had similar anxiety and had given up a career in law for work as an accountant because of his anxiety in mock trials during law school.

Treatment was begun with a combination of exposure therapy (videotape feedback) and drug therapy (a beta-blocker). Within 2 weeks (4 exposure sessions), the student's anticipatory anxiety abated substantially, and he reported enjoyment of his newfound confidence and improved performance in public speaking. His presentation was a success, and he continued to feel and function well through the rest of medical school.

Epidemiology

Many individuals with social phobia were shy as children; however, most shy children do not develop social phobia. Age at onset is usually around puberty, with peak presentation for treatment in the 20s and few new cases emerging after age 30. Males are almost as likely as females to experience social phobia (the NIMH-ECA study 6-month prevalence is 1.3% for males and 1.7% for females).

Etiology & Pathogenesis

The specific cause of social phobia is unknown. A family history is often discovered, although the relative contributions of heredity and environment have not been determined. As with other phobias, avoidance in a misguided attempt at self-treatment probably increases severity of symptoms and perpetuates dysfunction (Greist and coworkers, 1980).

Treatment

A. Psychotherapy: Many individuals suffering from social and other phobias continue to receive analytic and other dynamic psychotherapies with the ambitious goal of uncovering and working through unconscious psychologic causes of the anxiety disorder. There is little research support for the effectiveness of these approaches for phobic disorders. Their continued use in the face of evidence supporting more effective treatments indicates that many clinicians find it difficult to abandon models learned while in training.

B. Behavioral Therapy: Exposure therapy with videotape feedback and with fantasy (for situations that are difficult to produce in real life) is helpful to many individuals with fear of public speaking and other forms of social phobia. At times, paradoxic exaggeration of the feared performance will *decrease* anxiety (eg, asking a patient with fear of writing illegibly to write more illegibly). Although many individuals with social phobias have become convinced that they cannot face their feared situation, a few exposure treatments usually reverse this misapprehension.

C. Drug Treatment: Beta-blocking drugs (see Chapter 54) are often helpful in decreasing such peripheral symptoms of anxiety as tremor, tachycardia, and sweating. They may be used in a single dose 1 hour or more before entering situations likely to invoke social phobia. Benzodiazepine antianxiety drugs are sometimes used in combination with beta-blockers. Monoamine oxidase inhibitor antidepressants (usually phenelzine) are thought by some authorities to be helpful in treating the fundamental insecurity experienced in conjunction with some kinds of social phobia, although they must be used regularly and require a diet low in tyramine.

Frequently, a combination of exposure therapy and beta-blocking drugs works well, and patients who have experienced years of disability are helped to substantially higher levels of functioning in a few weeks.

SIMPLE PHOBIA

Symptoms & Signs, Differential Diagnosis, & Prognosis

Simple phobia is something of a misnomer; while less incapacitating than agoraphobia or social phobia, simple phobias can have major effects on sufferers' lives. The terms specific phobia and single phobia convey the concept more clearly without diminishing the potential impact of this disorder.

The most common phobic objects or situations that invoke single phobias are snakes, spiders, heights, elevators and other small closed spaces, and flying. Fewer individuals seek treatment for single phobias than for agoraphobia and social phobia, both because many single phobias remit spontaneously and because it is easier to avoid a single phobic situation than the multiple situations often associated with agoraphobia and social phobia.

Flying phobia can cause significant morbidity for those who need to travel because of their work and substantial inconvenience for those who must use surface transportation to cover long distances. Occasionally, insect phobias reach such proportions that individuals remain indoors during the season when the feared insect is active (as with bees). Blood-injury phobia, while less common than some other single phobias, is of particular interest because it commonly causes fainting. While agoraphobic individuals often fear fainting but seldom if ever faint, individuals with blood-injury phobia actually faint owing to vasovagal syncope when exposed to their phobic stimulus.

Brought on by sight, experience or discussion of blood, operations, injuries, or even minor pain, blood-injury phobia can lead to long-term avoidance of visits to physicians and dentists as well as other situations that have induced fainting. The *DSM-III-R* diagnostic criteria for simple phobia are listed in Table 31–5.

Since individuals with single phobia can usually successfully avoid their feared object or situation ("I know where spiders hang out, so I stay away from those places"), few experience pervasive anxiety. When such individuals know they must face the source of their phobia, they develop anticipatory anxiety, and when they encounter that source, either intentionally or inadvertently, a situational panic indistinguishable from spontaneous panic often occurs.

Differential diagnosis is seldom a problem because of the specific nature of the phobia in an individual with either no other psychologic disturbance or a disturbance that stands independently. Some flying phobia is actually agoraphobia in which the individual fears confinement in the plane's cabin without means of ready egress.

Illustrative Case

A 32-year-old man presented for treatment because he had fainted every time he had had blood drawn since age 12. This experience led to fearful avoidance of doctors and venipuncture in this otherwise healthy and physically fit individual. He was worried because he avoided routine health monitoring and might find it difficult to seek care for acute medical problems. He also reported embarrassment about his inability to have blood drawn without fainting unless recumbent. His mother and maternal grandfather also experienced fainting with minor pain.

Epidemiology, Etiology, Pathogenesis, & Treatment

Single phobias are the most common anxiety disorders. Peak onset is in childhood (fears of strangers, large animals, snakes, the dark, and injury are very common), and a rapid and spontaneous resolution of

Table 31–5. *DSM-III-R* diagnostic criteria for simple phobia.

A. A persistent fear of a circumscribed stimulus (object or situation), other than fear of having a panic attack (as in panic disorder), or of humiliation or embarrassment in certain social situations (as in social phobia).
B. During some phase of the disturbance, exposure to the specific phobic stimulus (or stimuli) almost invariably provokes an immediate anxiety response.
C. The object or situation is avoided or endured with intense anxiety.
D. The fear or the avoidant behavior significantly interferes with the person's normal routine or with usual social activities or relationships with others, or there is marked distress about having the fear.
E. The person recognizes that his or her fear is excessive or unreasonable.
F. The phobic stimulus is unrelated to the content of the obsessions of obsessive compulsive disorder or the trauma of posttraumatic stress disorder.

most of these phobias is the rule, probably because of development maturation and natural exposure. In the past, many of these fears had actual survival value for comparatively defenseless small children and would not have been diagnosed as phobias. Their atavistic persistence leads to their definition as phobias. The vast majority of such fears abate without formal treatment; it is a fascinating research question to try to define characteristics that perpetuate single phobias in phobic individuals. The NIMH-ECA study found that 4.3% of males and 7% of females met *DSM-III* diagnostic criteria for simple phobia. That learning plays a part in some single phobias is most dramatically illustrated by epidemic anxiety (or mass hysteria), such as widespread fainting in schoolgirls (see Chapter 60) after one of their number has fainted, and by the somatic delusion held by victims of koro, who fear that the penis will retract into the abdomen (see Chapter 15).

Treatment of single phobia with exposure therapy is highly successful. Spider phobia, for example, can often be alleviated in a single 2-hour session. One or 2 "booster" sessions are a prudent follow-up procedure. Patients with flying phobia can be successfully treated in one or 2 flights in a small plane in which an experienced pilot repeatedly exposes patients to specific phobic stimuli (eg, takeoffs and landings, particular maneuvers, turbulence) until anxiety diminishes to comfortable levels. Blood-injury phobia should first be treated with the patient recumbent; patients seldom faint when recumbent even if bradycardia occurs. The patient's pulse rate should be monitored. Gradual exposure at a rate that does not produce bradycardia is the preferred treatment technique for blood-injury phobia. Most individuals can be treated in one or two 2-hour sessions in a blood-drawing facility.

OBSESSIVE COMPULSIVE DISORDER

Of all the anxiety disorders, obsessive compulsive disorder is the most difficult to treat. Cleanliness, orderliness, punctuality, and diligence are traits that enhance functioning; in a few individuals, however, they increasingly consume hours spent in excessive cleaning, tidying, worry about punctuality, and extremes of diligence that seem unbelievable, all in an attempt to relieve unbearable anxiety.

Symptoms & Signs

Obsessions are repetitive, intrusive thoughts, images, ruminations, or impulses. Some individuals experience obsessions that focus briefly on a single object. Treatment is usually sought when an individual suffers persistent obsessions involving many topics. Obsessions commonly focus on harming others, acquiring or spreading contamination, doubt about having performed routine tasks properly, and transgressing social norms (eg, swearing in public or making unacceptable sexual overtures).

Compulsive rituals are repetitive and sometimes stereotypic acts usually performed reluctantly. The acts may be sensible in the abstract, but the frequency and duration of their repetition make them repugnant and inconvenient, even incapacitating. Attempts are usually made to resist rituals, although children and those who have been performing rituals for years may not resist. If prevented from carrying out a ritual, obsessive compulsive individuals usually become anxious. Rituals are usually preceded by obsessions, but obsessions do not always lead to rituals. Rituals of cleaning, repeating, checking, tidying, hoarding, and avoiding may consume almost every waking hour. See Table 31–6 for the *DSM-III-R* diagnostic criteria for obsessive compulsive disorder.

Differential Diagnosis

A classic picture of obsessive compulsive disorder can emerge as a secondary complication of major depression. Obsessions alone may appear in the context of either depression or schizophrenia, and the distinction between obsessions and delusions can be difficult. There is a tendency to overdiagnose delusions and un-

Table 31–6. *DSM-III-R* diagnostic criteria for obsessive compulsive disorder (or obsessive compulsive neurosis).

A. Either obsessions or compulsions:

Obsessions: (1), (2), (3), and (4):

(1) Recurrent and persistent ideas, thoughts, impulses, or images that are experienced, at least initially, as intrusive and senseless, eg, a parent's having repeated impulses to kill a loved child, a religious person's having recurrent blasphemous thoughts.
(2) The person attempts to ignore or suppress such thoughts or impulses or to neutralize them with some other thought or action.
(3) The person recognizes that the obsessions are the product of his or her own mind, not imposed from without (as in thought disorder).
(4) If another axis I disorder is present, the content of the obsession is unrelated to it, ie, the ideas, thoughts, impulses, or images are not about food in the presence of an eating disorder, about drugs in the presence of a psychoactive substance use disorder, or guilty thoughts in the presence of a major depression.

Compulsions: (1), (2), and (3):

(1) Repetitive, purposeful, and intentional behavior performed in response to an obsession, or according to certain rules or in a stereotyped fashion.
(2) The behavior is designed to neutralize or to prevent discomfort or some dreaded event or situation; however, either the activity is not connected in a realistic way with what it is designed to neutralize or prevent, or it is clearly excessive.
(3) The individual recognizes that his or her behavior is excessive or unreasonable (this may not be true for young children; it may no longer be true for people whose obsessions have evolved into overvalued ideas).

B. The obsessions or compulsions cause marked distress, are time-consuming (take more than an hour a day), or significantly interfere with the person's normal routine, occupational functioning, or usual social activities or relationships with others.

derdiagnose obsessions. Other attributes of schizophrenia are usually absent in patients with obsessive compulsive disorder, although some of these patients also suffer from schizotypal personality disorder, which worsens the prognosis.

Obsessive compulsive disorder can usually be differentiated from phobias in the following ways:

(1) Phobic individuals are more fearful about confronting the feared object than are obsessive compulsive individuals, who are usually more concerned about the rituals they will face because of contact with the feared object.

(2) The fears of phobic individuals are usually less complex than those of obsessive compulsive individuals. Phobic fears are more typically focal (for example, fear of fainting while having blood drawn) than those of obsessive compulsive individuals (there are myriad ways one can become contaminated or spread contamination).

(3) Anxiety of phobic individuals is usually greater than that exhibited by obsessive compulsive individuals when both confront the things they fear.

So-called "compulsive" behaviors such as gambling, drinking, eating, and paraphilic sexual behavior are not true compulsions because they provide pleasure (see Chapters 34 and 38).

Prognosis

Dysfunction is defined in terms of the amount of time consumed by obsessions and rituals, interference with functioning, control over obsessions and rituals, and the amount of suffering endured. The disorder usually lasts for decades once it has begun and runs an undulating course, worsening if the individual becomes depressed and temporarily improving if the individual can successfully avoid obsessions that provoke rituals. However, such relief is usually short-lived, as new obsessions and corresponding rituals replace those that have disappeared. At its worst, obsessive compulsive disorder can consume the individual and interfere in a major way with family functioning.

Illustrative Case

A 31-year-old registered nurse noted gradual onset of fears that she would contaminate needles or intravenous apparatus 10 years before she sought treatment. Nine years before treatment, she changed from inpatient to outpatient nursing because of constant doubt about her skill in safely performing common nursing tasks. For intramuscular injections, she would aspirate 2 or 3 times before injecting medication to ensure that the needle was not in a blood vessel. Cleaning instruments was an ordeal because she often repeated the procedure to ensure sterility and still felt anxious about the possibility of contamination. She repeatedly asked for reassurance from physicians regarding the safety of air bubbles in syringes. At this point, her worries were confined to work. As her anxiety and uncertainty in outpatient work increased, she left clinical medicine and became a claims adjuster in an insurance

company. Her quest for accuracy and certainty led to checking and rechecking of coding, which interfered substantially with the quantity of work performed and produced feelings of guilt about not working to her full potential.

As years passed, her concerns spread to the home setting and her person. She worried that she had become soiled by urine and feces, and this led to rituals of repeatedly washing her body and clothing. The latter then became impossible because she felt that she might have put feces, instead of soap, into the washing machine. This "grotesque" thought continued until she was treated with a combination of exposure therapy (she no longer permitted herself to wear gloves or use tissues when touching the telephone, doorknobs, etc) and response prevention, in which she was asked to delay her washing and checking rituals for 3 hours after exposure sessions. With these behavioral treatments, her symptoms diminished rapidly and dramatically, so that she eventually experienced little interference with everyday activities. Common heterocyclic antidepressants had not modified her anxiety or rituals at all, but clomipramine (in the USA, investigational use only), administered after improvement due to behavior therapy had stabilized, yielded further worthwhile gains.

Epidemiology

In one-third of obsessive compulsive individuals, onset of the disorder occurs by the age of 15. A secondary peak of incidence occurs during the third decade of life. Once established, obsessive compulsive disorder is likely to persist throughout life with varying degrees of severity. Men are only slightly less likely to suffer this disorder than women. Six-month prevalence of obsessive compulsive disorder in the NIMH-ECA study was approximately 1.5%, and the lifetime prevalence was 2.5%.

Etiology & Pathogenesis

Obsessive compulsive disorder clusters in families and appears to have a partly hereditary basis.

Once an obsessive thought intrudes, the forces maintaining its recurrence are uncertain. Efforts to demonstrate meaningful linkages between obsessions and unconscious conflict have failed to yield useful treatment techniques or to persuade many psychiatrists that such hypotheses have anything to do with the cause or pathogenesis of the disorder. A more credible behavioral explanation is that once the anxiety or discomfort associated with obsessive thought begins, sufferers gain at least temporary partial relief by performing rituals that are tied in a quasilogical way to their obsessions. However, the rituals must be performed to great excess.

The biochemical and anatomic bases of obsessive compulsive disorder have not been fully defined, but exploratory research suggests that they may involve dysfunction of serotonin neurotransmission in the orbital gyri (in the left gyrus more than in the right) and in the caudate nuclei.

Treatment

A. Behavioral Therapy: Behavioral therapy employing exposure therapy and prevention of the obsessive compulsive response yields a 60–80% reduction in symptoms for the three-fourths of patients who are able to comply with treatment instructions. Gains range from symptom reduction to enhanced functioning in work and social situations and correspondingly reduced suffering. Family members are often included as co-therapists to help patients respond suitably when exposed to stimuli that usually lead to obsessive compulsive behavior. They are instructed to praise the patient when appropriate and to refrain from giving the patient counterproductive reassurance. Many obsessive compulsive individuals become "reassurance junkies" in their quest for certainty; the reassurance they seek can be viewed as a form of avoidance of the anxiety associated with uncertainty. Behavioral therapy for these patients essentially involves asking them to run the same risks of contamination, uncertainty, and doubt that confront everyone and to stop performing rituals as an excessively costly and ineffective method of gaining transient and illusory certainty.

B. Drug Therapy:

1. Antidepressants–Most antidepressants do not appear to have specific anti-obsessive compulsive properties, but several studies have shown that clomipramine has anti-obsessive compulsive effects independent of its antidepressant properties. Other serotonin reuptake-blocking agents have also shown promise.

2. Anxiolytics–Antianxiety medications have a limited role in the long-term treatment of obsessive compulsive disorder but are sometimes helpful in the management of acute anxiety.

3. Antipsychotic drugs–Antipsychotic medications are unlikely to be beneficial but may be given a brief trial if other treatments with documented effectiveness have failed.

C. Other Treatment:

1. Electroconvulsive therapy–Electroconvulsive therapy is sometimes helpful in individuals with depression of psychotic proportions, but it is seldom necessary for patients with less severe depression who are likely to respond to antidepressant medications.

2. Psychotherapy–Some obsessive compulsive patients are still treated with dynamic psychotherapy, often for many years, without manifest relief or improvement in functioning. Psychotherapists often point to "intrapsychic" benefits in patients who remain as troubled with obsessions and rituals as when therapy began. While unfortunate, this example of difficulty in changing treatment methods in the face of strong evidence supporting an effective alternative approach has long been recognized (Kuhn, 1962).

3. Psychosurgery–Stereotactic limbic leukotomy (Kelly, 1980) has been shown to be of some benefit in more than 80% of obsessive compulsive patients who have failed to benefit from other treatments.

POSTTRAUMATIC STRESS DISORDER

Symptoms & Signs

The *DSM-III-R* diagnostic criteria for posttraumatic stress disorder are presented in Table 31–7. Many people experience a psychologically traumatic stressor "outside the range of usual human experience," but few develop posttraumatic stress disorder. Many of those subjected to psychologically traumatic stressors reexperience them in dreams or memory with associated unpleasant feelings; changes in affect and reexperiencing of trauma usually diminish in frequency and intensity (just as recall of pleasant events does) and are not in themselves signs of posttraumatic stress disorder.

A diagnosis of posttraumatic stress disorder requires the presence of substantial disruption in functioning or suffering associated with reexperiencing the trauma; persistent symptoms of arousal; and signs of numbing or avoidance.

A diagnosis of posttraumatic stress disorder cannot be made unless symptoms persist for at least 1 month; delayed onset should be specified if symptoms became apparent more than 6 months after the trauma.

Differential Diagnosis

Most of the time, the human capacity for recall and associated affect does not provoke substantial dysfunction or suffering and should not be diagnosed as posttraumatic stress disorder.

Adjustment disorders involve "a maladaptive reaction to an identifiable psychosocial stressor" but involve a broader range of less extreme human experiences (eg, the nonviolent death of a relative) and may result in a few of the symptoms found in posttraumatic stress disorder (eg, symptoms of arousal, numbing, or avoidance). Intense reexperiencing is less common with adjustment disorders.

Prognosis

Acute posttraumatic stress disorder usually responds well to simple measures if they are promptly applied. Full recovery is the rule rather than the exception. Chronic posttraumatic stress disorder, however, is more difficult to treat and may last for decades while causing varying degrees of disability.

Illustrative Case

Four years before seeking treatment, a highly successful truck driver with a 21-year history of accident-free driving had been involved in a 2-truck accident in which the other driver was trapped and burned to death despite the patient's effort to free him. In addition to burns received in the rescue attempt, he also suffered a concussion, bruises, and a scalp laceration. While still in the hospital immediately after the accident, the man had nightmares involving repetition of the incident. He became wary about falling asleep, was reluctant to discuss the accident with his family or authorities, and claimed he could not remember much of what hap-

A. The person has experienced an event that is outside the range of usual human experience and that would be markedly distressing to almost anyone, eg, serious threat to one's life or physical integrity; serious threat or harm to one's children, spouse, or other close relatives or friends; sudden destruction of one's home or community; or seeing another person who has recently been, or is being, seriously injured or killed as the result of an accident or physical violence.

B. The traumatic event is persistently reexperienced in at least one of the following ways:
   (1) Recurrent and intrusive distressing recollections of the event (in young children, repetitive play in which themes or aspects of the trauma are expressed).
   (2) Recurrent distressing dreams of the event.
   (3) Sudden acting or feeling as if the traumatic event were recurring (includes a sense of reliving the experience, illusions, hallucinations, and dissociative [flashback] episodes, even those that occur upon awakening or when intoxicated).
   (4) Intense psychologic distress at exposure to events that symbolize or resemble an aspect of the traumatic event, including anniversaries of the trauma.

C. Persistent avoidance of stimuli associated with the trauma or numbing of general responsiveness (not present before the trauma), as indicated by at least 3 of the following:
   (1) Efforts to avoid activities or situations that arouse recollections of the trauma.
   (2) Efforts to avoid activities or situations that arouse recollections of the trauma.
   (3) Inability to recall an important aspect of the trauma (psychogenic amnesia).
   (4) Markedly diminished interest in significant activities (in young children, loss of recently acquired developmental skills such as toilet training or language skills).
   (5) Feeling of detachment or estrangement from others.
   (6) Restricted range of affect, eg, unable to have loving feelings.
   (7) Sense of a foreshortened future, eg, child does not expect to have a career, marriage, children, or a long life.

D. Persistent symptoms of increased arousal (not present before the trauma), as indicated by at least 2 of the following:
   (1) Difficulty falling or staying asleep.
   (2) Irritability or outbursts of anger.
   (3) Difficulty concentrating.
   (4) Hypervigilance.
   (5) Exaggerated startle response.
   (6) Physiologic reactivity upon exposure to events that symbolize or resemble an aspect of the traumatic event (eg, a woman who was raped in an elevator breaks out in a sweat when entering an elevator).

E. Duration of the disturbance (symptoms in criteria B, C, and D) of at least 1 month.

Specify delayed onset if the onset of symptoms was at least 6 months after the trauma.

pened. The patient seemed markedly distant to close family members and expressed the worry that there was not much one could count on in life. Irritability was noted by all, and he appeared to have difficulty concentrating.

Because of the circumstances of the accident, he was not permitted to resume work as a truck driver for more than 9 months until administrative hearings con-

cluded that he had not been at fault. During that interval, his condition remained largely as described, although his nightmares became less frequent and the quality of his relationship with his family improved. When he was allowed to resume work, he felt extreme apprehension and could not bring himself to drive again because of fear that another accident would result. He was also fearful about driving or riding in a car, and he specifically stated that he had "seen what trucks can do." Tricyclic antidepressant medication decreased the frequency of nightmares and improved sleep but had little effect on his anxiety and avoidance. Previous psychotherapy had not been helpful, and exposure therapy did little to ease his distress.

Epidemiology

Since a psychologically traumatic experience is a prerequisite for posttraumatic stress disorder, incidence and prevalence figures would ideally be related to several different types of trauma. However, no uniform classification of trauma has been agreed upon. The prevalence of posttraumatic stress disorder-like phenomena is demonstrated by an 80% incidence of acute posttraumatic syndrome in survivors of the Buffalo Creek flood disaster and a 57% prevalence after 1 year in survivors of the Cocoanut Grove fire; it should be remembered that diagnostic criteria have changed and that some diagnoses were based on unstructured interviews.

A survey of 2500 St. Louis citizens conducted as part of the NIMH-ECA study found a lifetime prevalence of 1% in both sexes. Fifteen percent of subjects in the study had at least one symptom of posttraumatic stress disorder. Of those exposed to psychologic trauma "outside the range of usual human experience," 4% satisfied *DSM-III* criteria for the disorder and 20% experienced some symptoms of the disorder. In a group of 15 Vietnam combat veterans who were wounded, 20% fully satisfied *DSM-III* criteria and 60% had one or more combat-related symptoms (Helzer, in press).

Etiology & Pathogenesis

Since different individuals experiencing the same trauma respond differently, the cause and pathogenesis of posttraumatic stress disorder involve many factors. The relative contributions of genetic endowment, physical development, psychologic maturity, social support, cultural expectations, past experience with trauma, and the nature of the trauma itself are unclear. Psychologically, failure to integrate a traumatic experience into a person's life experiences may lead to a pattern of alternating reexperiencing of the traumatic event and defensive numbing when the reexperiencing itself proves traumatic (Horowitz, 1976).

Treatment

A. Acute Posttraumatic Stress Disorder: Excellent evidence gathered in military conflicts from World War II onward indicates that individuals suffering from incapacitating acute posttraumatic stress disorder are highly likely to recover fully if they are treated as follows: As symptoms and signs of posttraumatic stress disorder emerge in combat and are recognized by fellow soldiers, the affected individuals are removed from the front line and sent to the nearest aid station. There, they are kept in uniform, given food, encouraged to talk about their experiences, and told that their reaction is normal for the trauma they have experienced. They are expected to perform such duties as they are capable of, are not permitted to assume the role of a patient, and are returned to the front line within 24–72 hours. Sedation is unnecessary and may be counterproductive because of the suggestion of a "sick role" and possible induction of state-dependent learning. The Israeli experience in the 1973 Yom Kippur War found these techniques effective in restoring soldiers to combat fitness and preventing development of chronic posttraumatic disorder. This approach appears to include important elements of graduated exposure.

The implications of war experience for acute posttraumatic stress syndromes in civilians are obvious and confirm the old aphorism: "You must climb right back on the horse that throws you."

B. Chronic or Delayed Posttraumatic Stress Disorder: There are no effective treatments for chronic posttraumatic stress disorder. However, some of its manifestations may be treated symptomatically. Exposure in fantasy or, when it may be done with safety, in real life (eg, asking a woman who has been raped to revisit the site of the rape) has been shown to be helpful to some, but not all, patients. For others, exposure seems a form of reexperiencing which they (and some therapists) view as too distressing and possibly sensitizing. Other behavioral therapists experienced in working with patients suffering from posttraumatic stress disorder maintain that exposure is effective for most patients unless they are markedly depressed. Exposure is most helpful for the phobic avoidance and anxiety symptoms associated with this disorder.

Medications are often helpful in relieving dysphoric and depressive symptoms associated with chronic posttraumatic stress disorder. In particular, sleep disturbance and nightmares are often alleviated with heterocyclic or monoamine oxidase inhibitor antidepressant medications. Antianxiety medications may be of benefit as well, although the risk of dependence must be kept in mind. Beta-blocking agents may be helpful if tremor is a major problem.

Psychotherapy aimed at integration of the traumatic experience into the patient's sense of self may be helpful. Such therapy should first employ techniques of catharsis and abreaction, which may properly be viewed as a form of exposure in fantasy. If these brief psychotherapeutic approaches prove ineffective, more extensive exploration of the meanings of the trauma may be undertaken, although evidence for the effectiveness of long-term psychotherapy is scanty.

GENERALIZED ANXIETY DISORDER

Symptoms & Signs

The *DSM-III-R* diagnostic criteria for generalized anxiety disorder are listed in Table 31–8. This diagnosis has been made less frequently in the USA since panic disorder was included in *DSM-III*. In Great Britain and Europe, where panic is usually viewed as extreme anxiety and not as a categorically discrete disorder, a diagnosis of generalized anxiety disorder is more common.

Differential Diagnosis

Several of the symptoms of generalized anxiety

Table 31–8. *DSM-III-R* diagnostic criteria for generalized anxiety disorder.

A. Unrealistic or excessive anxiety and worry (apprehensive expectation) about 2 or more life circumstances, eg, worry about possible misfortune to one's child (who is in no danger), and worry about finances (for no good reason) for a period of 6 months or longer during which the person has been bothered more days than not by these concerns. In children and adolescents, this may take the form of anxiety and worry about academic, athletic, and social performance.

B. If another axis I disorder is present, the focus of the anxiety and worry in criterion A is unrelated to it, eg, the anxiety or worry is not about having a panic attack (as in panic disorder), being embarrassed in public (as in social phobia), being contaminated (as in obsessive compulsive disorder), or gaining weight (as in anorexia nervosa).

C. The disturbance does not occur only during the course of a mood disorder or a psychotic disorder.

D. At least 6 of the following 18 symptoms are often present when anxious (do not include symptoms present only during panic attacks):

Motor tension

(1) Trembling, twitching, or feeling shaky.
(2) Muscle tension, aches, or soreness.
(3) Restlessness.
(4) Easy fatigability.

Autonomic hyperactivity

(5) Shortness of breath or smothering sensations.
(6) Palpitations or accelerated heart rate (tachycardia).
(7) Sweating or cold, clammy hands.
(8) Dry mouth.
(9) Dizziness or light-headedness.
(10) Nausea, diarrhea, or other abdominal distress.
(11) Flushes (hot flashes) or chills.
(12) Frequent urination.
(13) Trouble swallowing or "lump in throat."

Vigilance and scanning

(14) Feeling keyed up or on edge.
(15) Exaggerated startle response.
(16) Difficulty concentrating or "mind going blank" because of anxiety.
(17) Trouble falling or staying asleep.
(18) Irritability.

E. It cannot be established that an organic factor initiated and maintained the disturbance, eg, hyperthyroidism, caffeine intoxication.

disorder are commonly present in mild depression (sometimes called dysphoria or dysthymia). Generalized anxiety disorder usually causes less dysfunction than other anxiety disorders (except simple phobia). Caffeine intoxication and withdrawal from central nervous system depressant substances can mimic generalized anxiety disorder. Because of the substantial overlap in motor tension and autonomic hyperactivity symptoms with those of panic disorder, careful attention to the possibility of panic is essential in distinguishing between generalized anxiety disorder and panic disorder.

Epidemiology

The NIMH-ECA study did not diagnose generalized anxiety disorder, but it is thought to be quite common, affecting approximately 5% of the population and with a female-to-male ratio of approximately 2:1.

Etiology & Pathogenesis

As with all of the anxiety disorders, many factors are probably involved in the etiology and pathogenesis of generalized anxiety disorder.

A. Biochemical Theories: The up- and down-regulation of noradrenergic function mediated largely through the locus ceruleus (Redmond, 1977), and demonstration of brain benzodiazepine receptors (Squires and Braestrup, 1977) and their interaction with GABA (Paul and coworkers, 1980), have stimulated research on the role played by the GABA-benzodiazepine and noradrenergic-locus ceruleus systems. The GABA-benzodiazepine system may be more active in generalized anxiety disorder, while the noradrenergic-locus ceruleus system is more often implicated in the etiology of panic.

B. Behavioral Theories: Successful avoidance of noxious stimuli (unconditioned stimulus) that reduces discomfort or trauma (unconditioned response) is usually reinforced in both humans and other species (Kandel, 1983). When avoidance in humans produces unpredictable results, avoidance becomes unreliable and generalized anxiety is thought to develop (see Chapter 1).

C. Psychologic Theories: A state of general anxiety is thought by many dynamic psychotherapists to reflect an unconscious conflict about dangerous emotions, behaviors, or states (eg, anger, depression, injury or death, sexual arousal, hunger, and anxiety itself). Another theory holds that some individuals with generalized anxiety disorder may seek anxiety-provoking stimuli and maintain themselves in situations likely to evoke high anxiety in order to achieve mastery over anxiety, gain relief through the eventual cessation of such anxiety states, or avoid an even less enjoyable affective state such as anger or boredom.

Prognosis

Generalized anxiety disorder persists for at least 6 months and, commonly, for many years. Untreated, it usually waxes and wanes in response to common stressors and unspecified factors. With treatment (eg, an-

tianxiety medication), symptoms are reduced but usually reemerge when treatment is stopped.

Illustrative Case

For as long as he could remember, a 53-year-old male had "worried" about things that never came to pass; their possible occurrence had little foundation in reality, and if they did occur, they were unlikely to be of serious consequence. He described himself as always feeling tense and restless, sometimes trembling or being on edge, and feeling irritable and easily fatigued. He had trouble falling and staying asleep because of "worries." At times of peak worry, he described symptoms of autonomic distress, including dry mouth, sweating, tachycardia, urinary frequency, and diarrhea. These symptoms were present most days to a greater or lesser degree and never worsened suddenly.

He had engaged in 2 courses of psychotherapy, each lasting more than 1 year, as well as "relaxation training" and biofeedback. None of these treatments had led to meaningful reduction in symptoms. When benzodiazepines became available, his family physician began treatment with diazepam, which proved remarkably effective over the following 20 years at a dose of 15 mg/d. The patient never increased the dosage, and on repeated occasions, when he or his doctor had attempted to withdraw the medication, symptoms returned.

Treatment

A. Drug Treatment: Benzodiazepine antianxiety drugs (see Chapter 54) are effective in reducing or alleviating symptoms of generalized anxiety in many patients. Return of symptoms is common when benzodiazepines are discontinued. Sedation is the major side effect, and there is a potential for physiologic dependence that is greatest in those who have abused alcohol and other sedative drugs. Despite this potential, the incidence of benzodiazepine abuse is quite low, and many patients find these agents effective for generalized anxiety disorder and do not take more than the prescribed dosage.

Buspirone, a nonbenzodiazepine antianxiety agent, may complement benzodiazepines in the treatment of generalized anxiety disorder. Apparently, it does not have sedative effects, it does not interact with alcohol, and it does not lead to dependence. Its exact strengths and limitations are currently being defined by wide-scale use.

Beta-adrenergic blocking agents and antihistamines have limited roles in the treatment of symptoms associated with generalized anxiety. Barbiturates and meprobamate have been superseded by benzodiazepines, buspirone, and, to a lesser degree, beta-blockers and antihistamines.

B. Behavioral Therapy: Behavioral therapy has not been shown to be of particular benefit in the treatment of generalized anxiety disorder because it is difficult to specify situations or stimuli to which the individual should be exposed. Relaxation and biofeedback are commonly advocated, but their efficacy has not been validated in controlled studies of clinically significant generalized anxiety disorder.

C. Psychotherapy: For decades, dynamic psychotherapy was the treatment of choice for generalized anxiety. Unfortunately, evidence from controlled studies supporting the efficacy of this approach is limited at best.

Cognitive therapy is being evaluated in the treatment of generalized anxiety disorder and has shown some promise (Woodward and coworkers, 1980).

Summary

Anxiety is a common emotion with adaptive value

for most individuals most of the time. For some, anxiety is so intense or lasts so long that it becomes maladaptive and is properly diagnosed as a disorder. Treatment of anxiety disorders has improved substantially over the last 2 decades, with behavioral therapy and drug therapy forming the foundations of effective treatment. Classification is becoming more refined, and understanding of the epidemiologic, genetic, developmental, psychologic, behavioral, biochemical, and environmental aspects of anxiety is growing steadily (Marks, 1987).

REFERENCES

Baxter LR et al: Local cerebral glucose metabolic rates in obsessive-compulsive disorder. *Arch Gen Psychiatry* 1987;**44:** 211.

Charney DS et al: Drug treatment of panic disorder: The comparative efficacy of imipramine, alprazolam, and trazodone. *J Clin Psychiatry* 1986;**47:**580.

Freud S: Lines of advance in psychoanalysis. In: *Standard Edition of the Complete Psychological Works of Sigmund Freud.* Vol 17. Hogarth Press, 1955.

Greist JH, Jefferson JW, Marks IM: *Anxiety and Its Treatment: Help is Available.* Washington, DC, American Psychiatric Press, 1986. [Also available as a Warner paperback, 1986.]

Greist JH et al: Avoidance versus confrontation of fear. *Behav Res Ther* 1980;**11:**1.

Greist JH et al: Using computers: Psychiatric diagnosis: What role for the computer? *Hosp Community Psychiatry* 1984;**35:**1089.

Horowitz MJ: *Stress Response Syndromes.* Jason Aronson, 1976.

Jenike MA, Baer L, Minichiello WE (editor): *Obsessive-Compulsive Disorders: Theory and Management.* PSG Publishing Co., 1986.

Kandel ER: From metapsychology to molecular biology: Explorations into the nature of anxiety. *Am J Psychiatry* 1983;**140:**1277.

Kelly D: *Anxiety and Emotions: Physiological Basis and Treatment.* Thomas, 1980.

Kuhn TS: *The Structure of Scientific Revolutions.* Univ of Chicago Press, 1962.

Marks IM: *Fears, Phobias and Rituals: The Nature of Anxiety and Panic Disorder.* Oxford Univ Press, 1987.

Marks IM: Genetics of fear and anxiety disorders. *Br J Psychiatry* 1986;**149:**406.

Myers JK et al: Six-month prevalence of psychiatric disorders in three communities. *Arch Gen Psychiatry.* 1984;**41:**959.

Paul SM, Skolnich P, Gallager DW: Receptors for the age of anxiety: Pharmacology of the benzodiazepines. *Science* 1980;**207:**274.

Redmond EE: Alterations in the function of the nucleus locus coeruleus: A possible model for studies of anxiety. Pages 293–306 in: *Animal Models in Psychiatry and Neurology.* Hanin I, Usie E (editors). Pergamon Press, 1977.

Squires RF, Braestrup C: Benzodiazepine receptors in rat brain. *Nature* 1977;**266:**732.

Woodward RP, Jones RB: Cognitive restructuring treatment: A controlled trial with anxious patients. *Behav Res Ther* 1980;**18:**401.

Somatoform Disorders

32

Stephen D. Purcell, MD

As the name implies, the essential feature of the category of psychiatric disturbances termed the somatoform disorders is the presence of symptoms that sugggest physical disorder. In order to establish a diagnosis of any one of the somatoform disorders, however, there must be no demonstrable physical findings or known physiologic mechanisms that might account for the symptoms *and* there must be positive evidence—or a strong presumption—that the symptoms have a psychologic origin.

There are 7 subtypes of somatoform disorders: somatization disorder, conversion disorder, somatoform pain disorder, hypochondriasis, body dysmorphic disorder, undifferentiated somatoform disorder, and somatoform disorder not otherwise specified. In each type, though the symptoms are physical, the specific pathophysiologic processes involved are not demonstrable or explicable on the basis of laboratory or other physical diagnostic procedures.

It is now well documented that a large proportion of patients in general medical outpatient clinics and private medical offices do not have organic disease requiring medical treatment. It is likely that many of these patients have somatoform disorders, but they do not perceive themselves as having a psychiatric problem and thus do not seek treatment from psychiatrists. It is especially important, then, that nonpsychiatrist physicians be familiar with these disorders so they can be recognized and treated appropriately.

SOMATIZATION DISORDER

Historically, somatization disorder has been known as both hysteria and Briquet's syndrome.

Symptoms & Signs

According to *DSM-III-R,* somatization disorder is characterized by multiple physical symptoms that recur over a period of several years and are either unrelated to an identifiable physical disorder or grossly in excess of physical findings. A diagnosis of somatization disorder cannot be made unless symptoms occur in contexts other than panic attacks and unless symptoms have been severe enough to drive the patient to attempt self-medication with drugs other than aspirin, to seek medical attention, or to make life-style changes. The symptoms are often part of a compli-

cated medical history and may be vaguely defined or presented in a dramatic or exaggerated manner. People with this disorder have usually seen many physicians, sometimes simultaneously. Anxiety and depressed mood are common associated symptoms. When mental health care is sought by people with these disorders, it is usually because of these symptoms and not because the physical symptoms are believed to have a psychologic basis. Histrionic personality disorder and, less frequently, antisocial personality disorder are sometimes present in addition to somatization disorder; and concurrent occupational, interpersonal, and marital difficulties are common. The hallucination of hearing one's name called (without impairment of reality testing) has been reported in association with this syndrome. Otherwise, however, "psychoticlike" symptomatology does not occur. The most common complaints are of being "sickly," with pain, psychosexual symptoms, and symptoms associated with the neurologic, gastrointestinal, cardiopulmonary, and female reproductive systems (Table 32–1).

Natural History

The pattern of multiple, recurrent physical symptoms begins most often during the teen years but (by definition) always before age 30. In women, menstrual problems may signal the onset of this disorder, but a wide variety of symptoms may be observed in both sexes. Somatization disorder is a chronic disorder, and spontaneous remission occurs rarely; fluctuations in the number and severity of symptoms do occur, but it is unusual for a year to pass without medical attention being sought.

The impact on the lives of people who have this disorder should not be underestimated. Symptoms may be quite severe and persistent to the point of being incapacitating or disruptive to occupational and interpersonal relationships. Because of the continuing search for medical care from different physicians, there is a risk of iatrogenic complications. Physicians who fail to perceive the psychologic basis of the patient's physical complaints may perform unnecessary surgical procedures or prescribe medications aimed at treating physiologic abnormalities—each procedure or treatment with its own set of adverse reactions or complications. There is also a risk of substance use disorder from prescribed analgesics or antianxiety agents. Because of associated depressive thoughts or moods, suicidal threats and attempts occur; when suicide results, it is usually in association with substance abuse.

Differential Diagnosis

The differential diagnosis of somatization disorder obviously includes physical disorders that present with vague or multiple somatic symptoms. These include multiple sclerosis, systemic lupus erythematosus, hyperparathyroidism, and porphyria. In addition, a recent study has shown an association between Briquet's syndrome and polycystic ovary disease (Orenstein and coworkers, 1986). It is important to remember that somatization disorder begins before age 30 and, conversely, that the onset of multiple physical symptoms later in life usually represents physical disease. Schizophrenia with multiple somatic delusions and major depression with somatic symptoms may occasionally require differentiation from somatization disorder. In panic disorder, physical symptoms may oc-

cur, but only in association with panic attacks. Conversion disorder involves certain physical symptoms that occur in the absence of the full clinical picture of somatization disorder. Factitious disorder with physical symptoms is distinguished by the presence of voluntary control of the symptoms. Somatization disorder, which does not involve any demonstrable physiologic abnormality, should not be confused with psychologic factors affecting physical condition, in which psychologic factors contribute to the onset or exacerbation of a physical disorder. These last-mentioned disorders have been called "psychosomatic" or "psychophysiologic" in the past and include such disorders as peptic ulcer disease, rheumatoid arthritis, regional enteritis, and ulcerative colitis.

Prognosis

Without treatment, the prognosis is poor. Spontaneous remission is rare, and a lifelong pattern of seeking medical attention develops with its attendant interference with other aspects of the patient's life and with iatrogenic complications.

Table 32–1. *DSM-III-R* diagnostic criteria for somatization disorder.

A. A history of many physical complaints or a belief that one is sickly, beginning before the age of 30 and persisting for several years.
B. At least 13 symptoms from the list below. To count a symptom as significant, the following criteria must be met:
  (1) No organic pathology or pathophysiologic mechanism (eg, a physical disorder or the effects of an injury, medication, drugs, or alcohol) to account for the symptom or, when there is related organic pathology, the complaint or resulting social or occupational impairment is grossly in excess of what would be expected from the physical findings.
  (2) Has not occurred only during a panic attack.
  (3) Has caused the person to take medicine (other than over-the-counter pain medication), see a doctor, or alter life-style.
Gastrointestinal symptoms: (1) vomiting (other than during pregnancy); (2) abdominal pain (other than when menstruating); (3) nausea (other than motion sickness); (4) bloating (gassy); (5) diarrhea; (6) intolerance of (gets sick on) several different foods.
Pain symptoms: (7) pain in extremities; (8) back pain; (9) joint pain; (10) pain during urination; (11) other pain (excluding headaches).
Cardiopulmonary symptoms: (12) shortness of breath when not exerting oneself; (13) palpitations; (14) chest pain; (15) dizziness.
Conversion or pseudoneurologic symptoms: (16) amnesia; (17) difficulty swallowing; (18) loss of voice; (19) deafness; (20) double vision; (21) blurred vision; (22) blindness; (23) fainting or loss of consciousness; (24) seizure or convulsion; (25) trouble walking; (26) paralysis or muscle weakness; (27) urinary retention or difficulty urinating.
Sexual symptoms for the major part of the person's life after opportunities for sexual activity: (28) burning sensation in sexual organs or rectum (other than during intercourse); (29) sexual indifference; (30) pain during intercourse; (31) impotence.
Female reproductive symptoms judged by the person to occur more frequently or severely than in most women:
  (32) painful menstruation; (33) irregular menstrual periods; (34) excessive menstrual bleeding; (35) vomiting throughout pregnancy.
Note: Symptoms 1, 7, 12, 16, 17, 28, and 32 may be used to screen for the disorder. The presence of 2 or more of these items suggests a high likelihood of the disorder.

Illustrative Case

A 36-year-old divorced woman who worked as a salesclerk entered the hospital emergency room at 2:00 AM complaining loudly that something was wrong with her stomach. She was tearful and agitated, with arms held tightly across her abdomen. She stated that shortly after her evening meal she began to feel nauseated and "bloated" and that she vomited some undigested food. Within minutes of vomiting she began to feel a dull pain in her periumbilical area that gradually became sharper and spread throughout her entire abdomen; when the pain became "unbearable," she decided to come to the emergency room.

As the patient calmed down and became more comfortable, she stated that she had had many similar episodes of abdominal discomfort over the past 15 years but that no doctor had been able to determine the cause. At the age of 18 she had had severe salpingitis requiring removal of the left oviduct, and 2 years later, because of persistent abdominal pain, the right ovary was removed. When she was 22, she underwent cholecystectomy, and over the next 10 years she had 3 abdominal surgical procedures to correct "adhesions" causing abdominal pain. At various times, she said, physicians had told her that she had "an ulcer" or "colitis," but despite a variety of medical treatments her symptoms had persisted. On further questioning, she also admitted to sporadic episodes of dizziness, chest pain that awakened her from sleep, chronic dysuria, occasional urinary retention requiring catheterization, and chronic low back pain. As she finished relating her history, she commented that "only someone with a poor constitution could be sick for this long." She admitted taking diazepam (10 mg) 4 times a day for "nerves," phenobarbital (30 mg) 4 times a day for her gastric symptoms, and "some pain pills whenever I need them"—each medication prescribed by a different physician.

Except for voluntary guarding on palpation of the abdomen and the old abdominal surgical scars, physical examination was normal.

Epidemiology

Somatization disorder is estimated to occur in 1–3% of women but seems to be truly rare in men (Cloninger and coworkers, 1986). There is a strong familial tendency. Antisocial personality disorder and alcohol abuse are more common in such families.

Etiology & Pathogenesis

The specific cause of this disorder is unknown, but it is presumed to be psychologic in origin. Although the increased incidence among family members suggests a genetic basis, there is no conclusive evidence of that, and no biochemical theories have been adduced to explain the disorder.

Most psychiatrists believe that psychologic factors play a major role in the genesis of somatization disorder, but there is no consensus about their exact nature. Pathologic identification with a parent, immature efforts to deal with dependency needs, and maladaptive resolution of intrapsychic conflict have all been proposed as mechanisms by which symptoms similar to those seen in somatization disorder are produced.

Treatment

In a review of the treatment of somatization disorder, Ochitill (1982) concludes that because of diagnostic confusion and therapeutic controversy, there is no standard effective treatment. Neither biologic nor behavioral treatments have had practical success, and psychotherapy remains the usual therapeutic approach. However, patients usually do not see any relationship between their symptoms and psychologic factors, and the psychologically based treatments—individual or group psychotherapies—are usually not helpful. Most patients refuse psychotherapy, and the literature suggests that psychotherapy is not successful when it is used. Thus, the nonpsychiatrist physician often has the only opportunity to engage the patient in a beneficial relationship. The physician must be sensitive to the psychologic and social needs and problems of the patient and able to tolerate the patient's "incurable" chronic complaints. A useful management objective in such cases would be to prevent multiple medical consultations and unnecessary somatic treatments with associated costs and iatrogenic complications. In selected cases, when the physician can detect some psychologic thinking (insight) or motivation to change, psychiatric consultation may be indicated.

CONVERSION DISORDER

Historically, conversion disorder also has been known as hysterical neurosis, conversion type.

Symptoms & Signs

Conversion disorder is characterized chiefly by loss or alteration of physical functioning that suggests physical disorder but which instead is apparently an expression of psychologic conflict or need. The symptom is not under voluntary control and cannot be explained by any physical disorder or known pathophysiologic mechanism.

Conversion symptoms suggesting neurologic disease of the sensory or motor systems are most common: paresis, paralysis, aphonia, seizures, blindness, anesthesia. Occasionally, the autonomic nervous system or the endocrine system may be involved, as with vomiting or pseudocyesis.

By definition, the diagnosis of conversion disorder is not made when the physical alteration is limited to pain or to a disturbance in sexual functioning—in which case the diagnoses of somatoform pain disorder or sexual dysfunction, respectively, are made. This diagnosis is also precluded when the conversion symptom occurs as one component of somatization disorder (Table 32–2).

Natural History

Conversion disorder may begin at any age but is most likely to make its first appearance in adolescence or early adulthood. There may be only one episode, or episodes may recur over a lifetime. The natural history of the disorder cannot be described with certainty at present, but the onset seems to be most often abrupt and in the context of psychosocial stress; though variable, the duration is probably most often short, and resolution is rapid. In some instances, the "conversion symptom" is later found to be the first manifestation of a neurologic disorder, in which case either the initial diagnosis of conversion disorder was incorrect or the neurologic disorder "predisposed" to the development of the conversion symptom. Occasionally, a patient with a chronic neurologic disorder (eg, multiple sclerosis) may develop symptoms (eg, paraplegia) without physical evidence of active disease. It is as if the patient "learned" the conversion symptom from previous experience with neurologic illness.

As with the physical symptoms occurring in somatization disorder, the symptoms of conversion disorder

---

Table 32–2. *DSM-III-R* diagnostic criteria for conversion disorder (or hysterical neurosis, conversion type.)

A. A loss of, or alteration in, physical functioning suggesting a physical disorder.
B. Psychologic factors are judged to be etiologically related to the symptom because of a temporal relationship between a psychosocial stressor that is apparently related to a psychologic conflict or need, and initiation or exacerbation of the symptom.
C. The person is not conscious of intentionally producing the symptom.
D. The symptom is not a culturally sanctioned response pattern and cannot, after appropriate investigation, be explained by a known physical disorder.
E. The symptom is not limited to pain or to a disturbance in sexual functioning.

Specify: single episode or recurrent.

can be extremely disruptive and can place the individual at risk for the costs and complications of unnecessary medical or surgical treatment. Actual physical problems may result from the conversion symptoms, eg, contractures or disuse atrophy associated with conversion paralysis. A number of factors have been noted to predispose to the development of conversion disorder, including an antecedent physical disorder, exposure to others with physical symptoms, severe psychosocial stress, and histrionic and dependent personality disorders.

Differential Diagnosis

The differential diagnosis includes physical disease and is especially difficult when the underlying disease is one that characteristically presents with vague neurologic symptoms, such as multiple sclerosis. A diagnosis of conversion disorder is suggested when the physical symptom does not conform to an actual known physical disorder or does not correspond to the anatomy of the nervous system. An example of this situation would be normal pupillary and electroencephalographic responses to light in someone with "blindness"; another example is "stocking-glove anesthesia," in which numbness in a foot or hand is complete and sharply delimited at the wrist or ankle rather than conforming to the distribution of sensory nerves. Even when a physical disorder cannot be identified, the diagnosis of conversion disorder should not be made unless there is also evidence that the symptom serves a psychologic function. Conversion symptoms may occur as one component of somatization disorder or schizophrenia, and when this occurs, the diagnosis of conversion disorder is not made. Hypochondriasis involves physical symptoms but without any loss or distortion of bodily function. In both factitious disorder and malingering, physical symptoms are under voluntary control, whereas in conversion disorder they are not.

Prognosis

There are no good data on the natural history of conversion disorder, nor have there been large-scale systematic studies characterizing response to treatment. It is believed that many conversion symptoms may resolve over a period of days to months without treatment and, conversely, that some conversion symptoms may persist for years in spite of intense efforts at treatment. The prognosis seems to be highly variable, probably has little to do with the specific symptom involved, and is seemingly dependent on the interplay of the individual's psychologic makeup, the social environment, and the response to the symptom by people who are important to the patient.

Illustrative Case

A 21-year-old college student telephoned her physician and, later the same day, appeared (with her mother) at his office with the complaint that she had awakened from sleep 2 days earlier with total numbness and paralysis in both legs. She said she had no

idea what was the matter but that she was incapable of caring for herself and had summoned her mother from another state to come and take care of her.

The patient had a history of good physical and mental health except for an episode of bilateral hip pain at age 14 that had resolved spontaneously. For the past 2 years she had shared an apartment with her boyfriend, but after a prolonged series of arguments he had moved out on the day preceding the onset of her symptoms.

On examination, the patient appeared slightly tense but in no acute distress. She stated that she knew she should seek medical help for the paralysis, but her main worry was how she was going to "support" herself without her boyfriend's contributions to the household expenses. She was completely unable to move either leg, and there was total anesthesia and lack of response to painful stimuli (pinprick) in both legs up to the inguinal ligament bilaterally, where sensation abruptly resumed. All deep tendon reflexes and both plantar reflexes were normal, as was the rest of the physical examination.

Epidemiology

There are no firm data on the prevalence or sex distribution of conversion disorder. In the 19th century, the disorder was apparently much more common than it is now and was seen predominantly in women. Cases seen today usually appear in nonpsychiatric settings such as in neurology clinics and among military personnel. Some believe that one particular converison symptom, **globus hystericus** (impaired swallowing caused by a sensation of a lump in the throat), is more common in women.

Etiology & Pathogenesis

Conversion disorder is unusual in the *DSM-III-R* classification, because a presumed cause (relationship to psychologic conflicts or needs) is incorporated into the definition, and it is unique because specific psychologic mechanisms to account for the disorder are proposed in the concepts of primary and secondary gain. An unacceptable sexual or aggressive drive is denied expression and repressed and thus becomes unconscious. The mental energy associated with the drive, which would normally push the drive into conscious experience, is converted into a somatic symptom. This allows the individual to remain unaware of the drive and at the same time permits symbolic expression of it. Protection from experiencing the drive is a **primary gain.** The symptom itself elicits from others responses that gratify needs which were not involved in the original symptom production—eg, sympathy and attention, which may gratify dependency needs. This gratification is referred to as a **secondary gain.** The source of the symptom, in other words, is primary gain; once established, both primary gain and secondary gain serve to maintain the symptom.

Historical Note

The story of the discovery of the psychologic

mechanisms responsible for conversion symptoms is worthy of a brief digression here.

What are now called conversion symptoms were recognized in women by the ancient Greeks and Romans and were explained by them as resulting from a wandering of the uterus from its normal anatomic position into various other parts of the body, which were adversely affected. The term "hysteria," which in the past was used synonymously with conversion disorder, is derived from the Greek word for uterus. In the Middle Ages, conversion phenomena were given various supernatural and religious interpretations. By the late 19th century, conversion symptoms (called hysteria then) had become a legitimate focus of medical and scientific investigation, and there were 2 prominent and opposing European schools of thought regarding their origin. One theory, whose major proponent was Jean-Martin Charcot, was that conversion symptoms were a manifestation of degenerative neurologic disease. The other theory held that conversion symptoms derived from psychologic factors, some of which were unconscious, and Hyppolyte Bernheim most strongly represented this point of view.

Although he studied with Charcot and was committed to understanding hysteria as a neurologic disease, Pierre Janet also made significant contributions to understanding the psychology of conversion symptoms. Specifically, Janet proposed the psychologic mechanism of **dissociation,** by which selected mental contents could be removed from consciousness (dissociated from experience) but continue to produce motor and sensory effects. This mechanism was thought to be illustrated by posthypnotic suggestion, in which a directive given to a subject in a hypnotic trance would be carried out after return to the normal waking state of conciousness without any memory by the subject of having received the directive.

Sigmund Freud, at that time a neurologist interested in hysteria, worked with both Charcot and Bernheim. He observed the use of hypnosis in treating conversion symptoms and returned to his own practice of neurology to use the new technique in treating his own patients. Freud was especially interested in the psychologic theories of hysteria, and his psychologic theorizing was given an important boost by an accidental discovery made by a colleague, Josef Breuer. Breuer was treating a woman with hysteria ("Anna O"), who in a hypnotic trance produced memories of previously unconscious traumatic events that appeared to be directly and causally related to the hysterical symptoms. Furthermore, the expression of these memories and the associated emotions caused the symptoms to disappear. Drawing on the concept of the psychologic mechanism of dissociation and these new observations, Freud proposed that emotions associated with the traumatic event were morally unacceptable to the woman and, because of this, the emotions were forced (repressed) into her unconscious. The mental energy associated with these emotions and denied expression was then "converted" into a somatic symptom that symbolically represented the traumatic event. In these early formulations, it was emotions associated with the sexual drive that were subjected to dissociation and "conversion." Subsequent observations have shown that the aggressive drive also is subject to these same processes; therefore, both sexually and aggressively based conflicts may underlie conversion symptoms.

Treatment

During World War II, the use of pentobarbital was common in the treatment of soldiers who developed conversion symptoms as a result of traumatic combat experiences. Sometimes called narcosynthesis, the intravenous use of a barbiturate to place the patient in a trancelike state of complete relaxation was combined with direct encouragement of the patient to remember traumatic events and emotions associated with the onset of the conversion symptom. An emotionally intense reliving of the traumatic experience often occurred which, when accepted and remembered by the patient, caused the symptom to disappear. This method of treatment is uncommonly used today.

Given our present understanding of the origin of conversion disorder, only psychotherapy would be expected to provide lasting benefit. Some patients are effectively treated with psychoanalytically oriented individual psychotherapy, but the appropriateness of this type of treatment has less to do with the conversion symptom per se than with the suitability of the patient. Only a minority of patients with conversion disorder are well suited for psychotherapy aimed at achieving insight. For most patients, individual or group supportive psychotherapy aimed at changing the patient's psychosocial environment is indicated. Environmental manipulation should include adjustments to alleviate the stress that initially precipitated the conversion symptom as well as interventions with important people in the patient's life who may be maintaining the symptom by providing secondary gain.

Successes have been reported with behavior therapy. The role of hypnosis is controversial. It is used most often when rapid relief of symptoms is indicated.

There is no evidence for the effectiveness of any somatic therapy in the treatment of conversion disorder.

SOMATOFORM PAIN DISORDER

Symptoms & Signs

Somatoform pain disorder is essentially the same as conversion disorder except that the symptom involved is limited to physical pain. Because of the relative frequency of this symptom and the special clinical problems associated with the management of pain, separate diagnostic categories are indicated.

Somatoform pain disorder is diagnosed when the major complaint is preoccupation with pain of at least 6 months' duration in the absence of, or grossly in excess of, explanatory physical findings (Table 32–3). In contrast to conversion disorder, there is no evidence of a psychologic factor that might be causing the pain.

Table 32–3. *DSM-III-R* diagnostic criteria for somatoform pain disorder.

A. Preoccupation with pain for at least 6 months.
B. Either (1) or (2):
   (1) Appropriate evaluation uncovers no organic "pathology" or pathophysiologic mechanism (eg, a physical disorder or the effects of injury) to account for the pain.
   (2) When there is related organic pathology, the complaint of pain or resulting social or occupational impairment is grossly in excess of what would be expected from the physical findings.

This change from *DSM-III* reflects a move away from inferred psychologic factors and theory.

Natural History

Patients with somatoform pain disorder typically make repeated visits to doctors for diagnosis or pain relief. Many physicians may be consulted successively or simultaneously, and there is an obvious risk of substance use disorder involving prescribed analgesics. Complaints of anxiety or depression are common but are not the predominant symptom, and there is an increased incidence of conversion symptoms. Histrionic personality disorder is an uncommon associated disorder.

This disorder may begin at any age but usually starts in adolescence and young adulthood. It seems to begin suddenly and increases in severity over days to weeks. It may resolve spontaneously or with treatment or may become chronic despite treatment. Severe symptoms may seriously disrupt overall function and expose the individual to iatrogenic complications of medical or surgical treatment.

Differential Diagnosis

Differential diagnosis includes painful physical disorders, such as atherosclerotic coronary artery disease and lumbar disk disease. The dramatic presentation of physical pain out of proportion to physical findings is not sufficient for the diagnosis, since the manner of expressing pain may reflect individual personality traits or cultural factors. Futhermore, pain that shows temporary improvement with placebo medications or suggestion should not be judged to be of psychologic origin, since these phenomena also occur with pain due to physical disease. Complaints of pain in somatization disorder, major depression, and schizophrenia rarely dominate the clinical picture, and the diagnosis of somatoform pain disorder is not made if the pain is judged to be due to any other mental disorder. In malingering, pain is under voluntary control, and that is not the case in somatoform pain disorder.

Prognosis

There are no good data on the prognosis of somatoform pain disorder. Clinical experience suggests a variable course with chronicity as a frequent characteristic.

Illustrative Case

A 32-year-old unemployed college graduate ar-rived at the emergency room frightened and breathless, complaining of severe substernal chest pain that he characterized as an unbearable "tightness." Except for slight tachycardia, his vital signs and electrocardiogram were normal. Despite reassurance from the physician, he continued to complain of severe pain and demanded "a shot of Demerol." After a time the physician ordered 75 mg of meperidine intramuscularly, after which the patient felt "a little better."

A telephone call to the family physician elicited the following information: There was a strong family history of heart disease, and the patient's father had died suddenly of acute myocardial infarction in his son's presence 4 years earlier. The patient's first episode of chest pain occurred 1 year later, when he was awakened from sleep the night before he was due to appear in court to testify in a legal proceeding contesting his father's will. Since that time he had had bouts of chest pain, usually requiring narcotic analgesia for relief, about twice a month and occasionally as often as 3–4 times a week. Thorough physical evaluation, including coronary angiography, revealed no organic disease.

Epidemiology

The prevalence of somatoform pain disorder is not known, but the disorder seems to be common in general medical practice. It is more common in women than in men. Familial distribution has not been reported. However, there is an increased familial incidence of painful injuries and illnesses, suggesting that some symptomatology may be learned or may result from identification with an ill family member.

Etiology & Pathogenesis

The pain is thought to be of psychologic origin. The specific psychologic mechanisms involved in pain production are unknown and are probably multiple and variable. It has been proposed that the pain of somatoform pain disorder is a conversion symptom produced by the same mechanisms responsible for the symptoms of conversion disorder. A psychologic cause is indicated by the following: (1) a temporal relationship exists between a presumed environmental stimulus (stressor) and pain; (2) the pain enables the person to avoid a noxious activity; or (3) the pain enables the person to obtain added support from the environment. It has also been observed that in certain cases the psychologic mechanism appears to be identification, where the individual takes on the attributes (symptoms) of an emotionally significant other person, such as a parent. Pinsky (1978) has proposed that people with somatoform pain disorder have less capacity to directly experience and verbalize emotions; the implication is that emotions are more or less directly translated into physical pain (by unknown mechanisms) rather than being expressed in other ways.

Treatment

In recent years, there has been considerable interest and progress in the treatment of chronic pain. Studies have shown that a multidisciplinary approach (neurologists, internists, and anesthesiologists in addition to psychiatrists) to management in an inpatient setting, which includes treatment with tricyclic antidepressants, can be effective in achieving pain relief and improving depressive symptoms. It is difficult to explain the benefit derived from treatment with antidepressants or the relationship between chronic pain and depression. Because the studies were done on patients with a variety of chronic pain syndromes and not necessarily somatoform pain disorder, it is impossible to generalize about the implications for treatment of the narrowly defined group of patients under consideration here.

There are increasing numbers of multidisciplinary treatment centers for patients with chronic pain, and referral to one of these centers may be appropriate when that is possible. Specialized treatment methods often include group, milieu, and behavioral approaches to the problem and are aimed at "replacing pain-related behavior with normal activity" (Brena and Chapman, 1983) rather than pain alleviation. When specialized treatment resources are not available, the physician should attempt to establish a supportive relationship with the patient that helps to prevent unnecessary medical and surgical procedures and treatments. When drugs are used in treatment, sedative and antianxiety agents should be avoided, and the use of opiates has no place in the treatment of patients with this disorder. Most patients should be given a trial of tricyclic antidepressant medication in the dosages used to treat a major depressive episode. Probably only a few patients will benefit from individual psychotherapy, but with a very small subset of patients who seem to possess characteristics predicting good responses to psychotherapy, direct or indirect psychiatric consultation is indicated for the purpose of deciding whether a trial of individual psychotherapy should be offered.

HYPOCHONDRIASIS

Hypochondriasis was formerly called hypochondriacal neurosis. A "hypochondriac" is a person who complains about minor physical problems, worrying unrealistically about serious illness, and persistently seeks professional care and consumes multiple over-the-counter remedies. This use of the term includes elements of somatization disorder and hypochondriasis.

Symptoms & Signs

The chief manifestation of hypochondriasis is the fear of having (or the belief that one has) a serious physical disease. This fear is based upon actual benign symptoms or signs or normal physiologic sensations, and it exists despite the absence of evidence of physical disorder to account for the belief—although there may in fact be a coexistent physical disorder. The misinterpretation of symptoms is quite natural. In hypochondriasis, however, the fear of having a serious disease persists despite medical reassurance, and it interferes with social or occupational function.

A person with hypochondriasis may interpret normal functions (heartbeat, peristalsis) or minor abnormalities (tension headache, viral respiratory infection) as evidence of serious disease. The fear of serious disease usually involves multiple organ systems simultaneously or in succession, though in some individuals the fear will center on a single organ system, such as in "cardiac neurosis," in which the unrealistic fear is of heart disease (Table 32–4).

Natural History

Anxiety, depression, and compulsive personality traits are commonly associated with hypochondriasis. When asked about their state of health, hypochondriacal patients usually respond at great length, often expressing frustration with physicians and the inadequate medical care they have received.

This disorder usually begins in adolescence but may not begin until the fourth decade in men and the fifth decade in women. It is usually chronic but marked by fluctuation in the intensity with which the belief is held and in the degree of disruption of social and occupational functioning. As with the other somatoform disorders, disruption of the patient's life may be marked (eg, the patient may take to bed and adopt an invalid life-style). The tendency to seek treatment from different physicians involves an increased risk of unnecessary medical or surgical treatments and their associated costs and complications.

Differential Diagnosis

The differential diagnosis of course includes actual serious physical disease. Occasionally, hypochondriasis will require differentiation from schizophrenia or major depression with somatic delusions. In these cases, although the final diagnosis will be based on specific diagnostic criteria, the belief that physical dis-

Table 32–4. *DSM-III-R* diagnostic criteria for hypochondriasis (or hypochondriacal neurosis).

A. Preoccupation with the fear of having, or the belief that one has, a serious disease, based on the person's interpretation of physical signs or sensations as evidence of physical illness.

B. Appropriate physical evaluation does not support the diagnosis of any physical disorder that can account for the physical signs or sensations or the person's unwarranted interpretation of them, and the symptoms in criterion A are not just symptoms of panic attacks.

C. The fear of having, or belief that one has, a disease persists despite medical reassurance.

D. Duration of the disturbance is at least 6 months.

E. The belief in criterion A is not of delusional intensity, as in delusional disorder somatic subtype (ie, the person can acknowledge the possibility that his or her fear of having, or belief that he or she has, a serious disease, is unfounded).

ease exists does not have the rigidly fixed quality of a true delusion, in that the person with hypochondriasis will usually entertain the possibility that the feared disease does not exist. Differentiation from somatization disorder is usually on multiple physical symptoms rather than on the fear of having a specific disease.

Prognosis

Hypochondriasis is considered by most psychiatrists to be a chronic disorder with a very poor prognosis.

Illustrative Case

A 28-year-old salesman sought a medical appointment for "a complete physical examination." He stated that several months ago he had consulted another physician but now was looking for a doctor who could "get to the bottom" of his problems. He expressed some anger because the other physician had refused to perform tests the patient thought were indicated, and he hoped the new doctor would be more helpful.

When asked what was troubling him, the patient said he was sure he had cancer—probably cancer of the stomach. He reported that 4 or 5 years ago he began to have occasional burning sensations in his upper abdomen after meals. He saw several doctors then, all of whom performed multiple diagnostic procedures and pronounced him healthy except for mild indigestion. He began to scrupulously monitor his diet, keeping records of the frequency and intensity of his gastric symptoms. Gradually he began to "suspect the worst" (cancer) and again saw several different physicians, hoping that his cancer could be diagnosed and treated. He began to feel tired at the end of the workday and occasionally thought he felt "swollen glands" in his neck, which suggested that his cancer might be spreading. He cut back on the amount of work he was doing ("to rest more") and broke off a relationship with a woman.

Recently the patient became angry when his last physician refused to repeat diagnostic procedures already done and instead requested records from other physicians. He then made the startling admission that unless the cancer could be diagnosed this time, "I guess I'll have to give up the idea that I have it. But I feel like I do."

Epidemiology

Hypochondriasis is common in general medical practice and seems to occur with equal frequency in men and women. It is not known if there is an increased incidence among family members.

Etiology & Pathogenesis

Hypochondriasis is believed to have its origin in maladaptive attempts to cope with unmet psychologic needs or unconscious psychologic conflicts, but there is no agreement about the specific psychologic mechanisms involved. Some feel the hypochondriacal patient merely shows an excessive self-concern; others suggest that hypochondriasis represents a physical expression of low self-esteem (sick, weak, defective); and still others have proposed that this way of viewing oneself protects the individual from awareness of destructive impulses toward others (seeing oneself as being damaged rather than as wishing to damage others). Some writers have recently proposed that these symptoms result from serious deficits in the ability of a patient to maintain a "sense of the self" (as well integrated or "put together") and that hypochondriacal symptoms must be viewed as one manifestation of this underlying problem.

Treatment

Psychotherapy appears to be useful for only a few hypochondriacal patients. Most are resistant to the idea of psychiatric treatment, and it should probably be offered only to highly motivated, insightful patients who will readily accept the recommendation. There is no evidence that somatic treatments are effective.

Since people with hypochondriasis usually present to nonpsychiatrist physicians and are opposed to psychiatric treatment, the general medical practitioner has the best opportunity to be of help. In order to benefit a hypochondriacal patient, the physician must give up the idea of cure in the usual sense of relieving symptoms. The physician must be able to accept the patient's fears and complaints as manifestations of a chronic psychiatric disorder that serve an important (if poorly understood) psychologic function and which will continue indefinitely. With this approach, the physician may be able to avoid becoming frustrated, angry, or hopeless and will maintain a sensitivity to the patient's social and psychologic needs and problems. The possibility exists that as a consequence of this supportive doctor-patient relationship, there will be a reduction in the patient's anxiety, which may result in a lessening of the fears of disease and improved social and occupational functioning. The physician should have fixed, regular appointments of unvarying duration with the hypochondriacal patient and should continue to respond in appropriate ways to physical complaints or true disease while avoiding unnecessary diagnostic or therapeutic procedures. This approach at least prevents "doctor-shopping" by the patient and reduces the risk of iatrogenic complications.

BODY DYSMORPHIC DISORDER

Body dysmorphic disorder is a disturbance characterized by preoccupation with an imagined defect in one's physical appearance that is out of proportion to any actual physical characteristic or abnormality. By definition, this preoccupation is not of delusional proportions; ie, it is not a conviction but an overvalued idea. The diagnosis of body dysmorphic disorder is not made when the preoccupation occurs as a component of anorexia nervosa. The etiology of this disorder is presumed to be psychologic. Although scientific data on its treatment are not yet available, some patients with this disorder may benefit from psychotherapeutic approaches.

UNDIFFERENTIATED SOMATOFORM DISORDER

The diagnosis of undifferentiated somatoform disorder is made when the predominant disturbance is of multiple physical complaints such as pain, fatigue, and loss of appetite of at least 6 months' duration. As with other somatoform disorders, no organic findings or known pathophysiologic mechanisms account for the symptoms, or complaints are grossly in excess of physical findings. If symptoms occur only in the course of another somatoform disorder, a sexual dysfunction, an affective (mood) disorder, an anxiety disorder, a sleep disorder, or a psychotic disorder, the diagnosis of undifferentiated somatoform disorder is not made.

SOMATOFORM DISORDER NOT OTHERWISE SPECIFIED

Cases that do not meet the diagnostic criteria for any specific somatoform disorder or adjustment disorder with physical complaints are categorized by *DSM-III-R* as somatoform disorder not otherwise specified. Examples include (1) an illness involving nonpsychotic hypochondriacal symptoms of less than 6 months' duration, or (2) an illness involving non-stress-related physical complaints of less than 6 months' duration.

SUMMARY

The somatoform disorders are a group of psychiatric syndromes characterized by physical symptoms suggesting the presence of a physical disorder. There must be no physical findings or demonstrable pathophysiology to account for the symptoms, and there must be direct or strong presumptive evidence of psychologic origin. People with these disorders usually do not perceive themselves as psychiatrically disturbed and therefore frequently present to nonpsychiatrist medical practitioners for treatment. It is important that physicians be knowledgeable about these syndromes in order to avoid unnecessary and potentially harmful diagnostic and therapeutic interventions and to minimize secondary gain in the context of the medical treatment or in the patient's other relationships. At present, there are no specific treatments for most of these disorders, although a variety of psychotherapeutic treatments have been effective in a few cases.

REFERENCES

Brena SF, Chapman SL: *Management of Patients With Chronic Pain*. Spectrum Publications, 1983.

Breuer J, Freud S: Studies on hysteria (1895). In: *Standard Edition of the Complete Psychological Works of Sigmund Freud*. Vol 2. Hogarth Press, 1955.

Cloninger C et al: A prospective follow-up and family study of somatization in men and women. *Am J Psychiatry* 1986; **143:**873.

Greist JH, Jefferson JW, Spitzer RC (editors): *Treatment of Mental Disorders*. Oxford Univ Press, 1982.

Kaplan HI, Freedman AM, Sadock BJ (editors): *Comprehensive Textbook of Psychiatry/IV*, 4th ed. Williams & Wilkins, 1985.

Ochitill H: Somatoform disorders. Chap 8, pp 266–308, in: *Treatment of Mental Disorders*. Griest JH, Jefferson JW, Spitzer RC (editors). Oxford Univ Press, 1982.

Orenstein H et al: Polysymptomatic complaints and Briquet's syndrome in polycystic ovary disease. *Am J Psychiatry* 1986;**143:**768.

Pinsky JJ: Chronic intractable benign pain: A syndrome and its treatment with intensive short-term group psychotherapy. *J Human Stress* 1978;**4:**17.

33

Dissociative Disorders

Stephen D. Purcell, MD

The dissociative disorders are a group of psychiatric syndromes characterized by a sudden, temporary disruption of some aspect of consciousness, identity, or motor behavior. There are 6 types: **psychogenic amnesia,** an alteration of the memory function of consciousness; **multiple personality disorder,** a disturbance in personal identity; **psychogenic fugue,** characterized by disturbances in both identity and motor behavior; **depersonalization disorder,** a more limited disruption of identity in which perception of one's own reality is disturbed; **possession/trance disorder,** marked by disturbances in either the attention function of consciousness or identity; and **dissociative disorder not otherwise specified,** a residual category.

The functions of memory, personal identity, and motor behavior are crucial for the integrated operation of the complex set of mental and behavioral activities we call personality. Thus, although these syndromes are statistically quite rare, when they do occur they may present very dramatic clinical pictures of severe disturbance of normal personality functioning. These disorders are presumed to share the mental mechanism of dissociation (discussed in Chapter 32) in their pathogenesis.

PSYCHOGENIC AMNESIA

Symptoms & Signs

Psychogenic amnesia (Table 33–1) is characterized by a sudden onset of a single episode of inability to recall important personal data. The memory disturbance is not due to organic mental disorder (see Chapters 10, 24, and 25) and is too severe to be ordinary forgetfulness. There is no associated major disturbance of motor behavior. An individual with psychogenic amnesia is usually aware of the memory deficit but may show indifference to it, and during an amnestic episode, the person may demonstrate disorientation, perplexity, and purposeless wandering.

Four different types of memory disturbance are identified, and any one may occur in this disorder. The most common type is "localized" amnesia, inability to recall *everything* occurring within a brief period (hours to days) surrounding a given event. "Generalized" amnesia is inability to recall anything that has happened during the individual's lifetime. Both localized and generalized amnesia may be "selective"—ie, the memory loss (whether circumscribed in time or ex-

Table 33–1. *DSM-III-R* diagnostic criteria for psychogenic amnesia.

A. The predominant disturbance is an episode of sudden inability to recall important personal information that is too extensive to be explained by ordinary forgetfulnes.
B. The disturbance is not due to multiple personality disorder or to an organic mental disorder (eg, blackouts during alcohol intoxication).

tending over the entire lifetime) may be for some events but not all. "Continuous" amnesia is an unusual memory disturbance in which all events subsequent to a specific time (up to and including the present) are forgotten, so that the individual is unable to form new memories even though apparently alert and aware.

Natural History

An episode of psychogenic amnesia typically begins following a life event that causes severe psychologic stress in the affected individual. The precipitating event is often an extraordinary one and severely stressful, eg, something that threatens the patient's life or in which injury or death of others is witnessed. At other times the precipitating event may be only moderately stressful but experienced as extremely threatening because of idiosyncratic personality traits, eg, participation in an extramarital affair in spite of strong moral disapproval of such behavior. The onset and termination of the episodes are usually sudden, followed by complete recovery. Recurrences are unusual.

Differential Diagnosis

The differential diagnosis includes organic mental disorder, in which memory loss is sometimes one feature. In organic mental disorder, the disturbance in memory is usually more severe for recent events than for remote ones, and there is no temporal association with psychologic stress. Memory return in organic mental disorder is gradual and usually incomplete if it occurs at all. A circumscribed memory loss is common in substance-induced intoxication (eg, "alcoholic blackouts"), but the ingested substance and absence of full return of memory are distinguishing features. A deficit limited to short-term memory (not immediate recall) is characteristic of alcohol amnestic disorder, also called Korsakoff's disease, and does not occur in psychogenic amnesia. Alcohol amnestic disorder occurs in the context of heavy and prolonged alcohol abuse, often follows an episode of Wernicke's encephalopathy, and is not associated with psychologic stress. Postconcussion amnesia follows head injury and if necessary can be distinguished from psychogenic amnesia through the use of hypnosis or amobarbital interview techniques. Under the influence of hypnosis or amobarbital, return of memory is strongly suggestive of emotional origin. Psychogenic fugue may include amnesia but is distinguished from psychogenic amnesia by the additional features of travel to a new locale and assumption of a new identity. Malingering involving feigned amnesia may be difficult to distinguish from psychogenic amnesia, but the motivation (secondary gain) is usually obvious. Hypnosis or amobarbital interview will usually make the diagnosis of malingering also.

Illustrative Case

A 25-year-old woman was admitted to the orthopedic service of a general hospital for treatment of a fractured femur, sustained when the car she was driving left the road and struck a utility pole. Her only child, a 2-year-old daughter, was killed in the crash, and the ambulance attendant reported that when he arrived at the scene, the patient was sitting quietly in the car holding her daughter's body and appearing slightly dazed.

There was no evidence of head injury, and the neurologic examination was normal. It was apparent to the hospital staff that the patient was suffering from amnesia. She spoke freely of some portions of her past life but did not remember the accident. During a psychiatric interview the next day, she seemed only vaguely disturbed by recent events and made no mention of her daughter's death. Close questioning by the psychiatrist demonstrated that she had no memory of her daughter or of most events subsequent to a vacation trip with her husband about $2\frac{1}{2}$ years ago. In a later discussion with the husband about this trip, the psychiatrist learned that it was then the patient first suspected she was pregnant.

Epidemiology

Psychogenic amnesia is rare, though it occurs more frequently in conditions of war or as a sequela of natural disaster. Adolescent and young adult women appear to be most commonly affected. There is no known familial tendency.

Etiology & Pathogenesis

Although efforts have been made to explain dissociative amnesia (and other dissociative phenomena) on the basis of neurophysiologic dysfunction, most psychiatrists believe that psychologic theories of psychogenic amnesia have the most credibility and usefulness.

In Chapter 32 (Somatoform Disorders), it was proposed that a morally unacceptable sexual or aggressive drive could be actively repressed and relegated to the unconscious. This same mechanism is the basis for our current understanding of psychogenic amnesia. In the case of amnesia, it is proposed that the memory of a painful event (along with the associated emotions) is repressed as a protective mechanism. In some cases, escape can be achieved by selective disruption of memory; in others, a much more far-reaching disturbance is required.

The concepts of primary and secondary gain, discussed in Chapter 32, also contribute to our understanding of psychogenic amnesia. The primary gain is protection from painful emotional experience. Responses of others may provide gratification of other psychologic needs (secondary gain) and thus serve to maintain the amnesia after it is established. Examples of secondary gain are the soldier who develops amnesia on the battlefield and is sent home or to a hospital in a rear area, and the dependent wife who develops amnesia upon her husband's sudden death so that she is cared for by sympathetic friends and relatives.

The great majority of people experiencing severe psychosocial stress do not develop dissociative disorder. Most are able to cope psychologically with emotional responses in ways that permit adaptive functioning. People who do develop dissociative disorders often have chronic underlying psychiatric problems. A severe personality disorder or an organic mental disorder may prevent a normal adaptive response.

Treatment & Prognosis

Many cases of psychogenic amnesia resolve spontaneously when the individual is removed from the stressful situation.

Intravenous administration of intermediate- and short-acting barbiturates has been used in the treatment of psychogenic amnesia. The amobarbital interview can be useful in differentiating psychogenic amnesia from other types of amnesia, and in some cases therapeutic benefit (symptom relief) also occurs. A patient who under the influence of a barbiturate can recall "forgotten" events and come to terms emotionally with the painful memories (ie, abreact) may be able to retain the memories later in a drug-free state. Most clinicians recommend psychotherapy also to reinforce adjustment to the psychologic impact of retrieved memories and the emotions associated with them.

Psychotherapy has also been used as primary treatment for patients with psychogenic amnesia. When relief of symptoms is the main goal of treatment, techniques of persuasion (directly encouraging remembering) and directed association (urging the patient to ruminate freely about events surrounding the amnestic period), gently applied in a supportive manner, have been helpful. Hypnosis, to facilitate recall and abreaction, has been effective in treating some cases and may be used in combination with psychotherapy. (The reader is referred to Nemiah's [1980] discussion of the case of "Barbara M" for an excellent example of the combined use of psychotherapy and hypnosis in the treatment of psychogenic amnesia.)

If the patient is found to have some underlying psychiatric disorder when the episode of amnesia resolves, treatment of the amnesia should be followed by further psychiatric assessment and appropriate treatment. In the case of an underlying personality disorder, psychoanalysis or long-term insight-oriented psychotherapy might be indicated.

MULTIPLE PERSONALITY DISORDER

Symptoms & Signs

Despite increased public awareness of this illness because of movies such as *The Three Faces of Eve* and *Sybil,* multiple personality disorder is rare. It is characterized by the existence of 2 or more personalities within a single individual (Table 33–2). Clinically, only one of the personalities is "present" at any given moment, and one of them is dominant most of the time over the course of the disorder. Each personality is well integrated and is a complex aggregate of unique memories, behavior patterns, and social relationships that control each individual's functioning during its dominant intervals. The transition from one personality to another is sudden, often dramatic, and usually precipitated by stress.

The various personalities are almost always quite discrepant and often seem to be opposites—eg, a shy, socially withdrawn, faithful husband may become a gregarious womanizer and heavy drinker. The original personality usually has no knowledge of the other personality or personalities, but when there are 2 or more subpersonalities, they are usually aware of each other's existence to some degree. When a given personality is dominant and interacting with the environment, the other personalities may not perceive all that is happening.

Natural History

One of the existing personalities may function reasonably well and alternate with another that does not. Studies of individuals with this disorder have shown that various subpersonalities may have measurably different physiologic and psychologic attributes such as pulse and blood pressure. A subpersonality may even have a specific, separate mental disorder: Somatoform disorders and psychologic factors affecting physical condition are apparently common diagnoses in people with multiple personality. Most often, the various subpersonalities have different names, but they may be unnamed and may be of a different sex, race, and age.

Table 33–2. *DSM-III-R* diagnostic criteria for multiple personality disorder.

A. The existence within the person of 2 or more distinct personalities or personality states (each with its own relatively enduring pattern of perceiving, relating to, and thinking about the environment and self).
B. At least 2 of these personalities or personality states recurrently take full control of the person's behavior.

Multiple personality disorder may begin at any age but usually not before adolescence. It seems to be related to physical abuse and other types of severe emotional trauma in childhood. The degree of functional impairment is variable, but it is usually at least moderate and may be severe. In contrast to other dissociative disorders, it tends to be more chronic, with only incomplete recovery.

Differential Diagnosis

The differential diagnosis of multiple personality disorder includes schizophrenic disorders, in which an individual may report delusions of multiple personality or auditory hallucinations when another personality speaks. The distinction is based on the presence of distinguishing features of the schizophrenic disorders and the absence of subpersonalities that are complex and well-integrated units of unique behavior patterns and social relationships. Malingering may also present a diagnostic problem, but as in the differential diagnosis of the other dissociative disorders, the malingerer's symptoms will serve a recognizable goal and the true nature of the symptoms will be disclosed under hypnosis or during an amobarbital interview. Psychogenic amnesia and psychogenic fugue have similar characteristics but are distinguished, in part, by the repeated shifts of identity and the "interloper's" awareness of the existence of the original identity in multiple personality disorder.

Illustrative Case

A 21-year-old single woman who lived with her parents and attended a local college had been reared in a family that strictly adhered to the teachings of a fundamentalist religious denomination that prohibited drinking and dancing and forbade intercourse for any reason other than procreation. She was a good student but had no close friends and few social acquaintances. She lived a quiet life.

Acting on the advice of their minister, the patient's parents brought her to a psychiatrist after she told them she was pregnant but did not know how it had happened. (The fact of pregnancy was verified by the family physician.) In interviews with the psychiatrist, she seemed to be a painfully shy, soft-spoken, moralistic young woman who evidenced great remorse and apparently genuine perplexity about how her pregnancy had occurred. The psychiatrist asked for the patient's cooperation using hypnosis. The patient agreed and was easily hypnotized; in the hypnotic state, she demonstrated an entirely new personality. She insisted on being called "Dominique" and interacted with the psychiatrist in a provocative and flirtatious manner. She spoke loudly and used clichés and profanity in describing to the psychiatrist her recent escapades as Dominique. She told about slipping out of the house at night, consuming large quantities of alcohol, and having intercourse with men she picked up. When brought out of her hypnotized state, she was her usual self and had no memory of "Dominique."

Epidemiology

Little information is available about the incidence and distribution of multiple personality disorder. The illness is most common in late adolescent and young adult women. There is no known familial occurrence.

Etiology & Pathogenesis

The cause of multiple personality disorder is poorly understood. Because it is less often precipitated by stressful life events and has a more chronic course than the other dissociative disorders, it has been proposed that internal psychologic conflicts play a more important role in the pathogenesis. In some cases, the various personalities seem to represent expressions of or defenses against certain psychologic drives (eg, aggression, sexual desire), and it appears that the individual has developed entirely separate personalities that center around gratification of the impulse or compliance with prohibitions against it. In the same individual, one identity may be highly expressive and sexually promiscuous and another very inhibited, excessively moral, and sexually abstinent.

Treatment & Prognosis

Some success has been achieved with intensive, long-term psychotherapy directed toward uncovering the underlying psychologic conflicts, providing the patient with insight into these conflicts, and synthesizing the various identities into one integrated personality. However, too few cases have been reported upon which to base any valid generalizations about treatment and prognosis.

PSYCHOGENIC FUGUE

Symptoms & Signs

Psychogenic fugue (Table 33–3) is characterized by sudden, unexpected "flights" from home or workplace and assumption of a new identity. It is as if the patient is running away from something but is unaware of fleeing. There is inability to recall one's past, and when the episode resolves, there is inability to remember events of the fugue state. Although apparent disorientation and perplexity may occur, this disorder cannot be diagnosed in the presence of organic mental disorder.

The moving about that is part of psychogenic fugue is purposeful, in contrast to the confused wanderings that may be seen in psychogenic amnesia. In a typical case, the fugue consists of brief, purposeful journeying during which contacts with other people are mini-

Table 33–3. *DSM-III-R* diagnostic criteria for psychogenic fugue.

A. Sudden unexpected travel away from one's home or customary place of work, with inability to recall one's past.

B. Assumption of a new identity (partial or complete).

C. The disturbance is not due to multiple personality disorder or to an organic mental disorder (eg, partial complex seizures in temporal lobe epilepsy).

mal and in which the new identity is simple and incompletely developed. In rare cases, the assumed identity is quite elaborate, and the individual may take a new name and residence and engage in complex interpersonal relations or occupational activities so that the presence of a mental disorder is not suspected. When a new, complex identity is established, it is often characterized by more gregarious and uninhibited social behavior than was the patient's style before.

Natural History

There is evidence that heavy alcohol abuse may predispose to development of psychogenic fugue, but other predisposing factors have not been identified. The course of this disorder is similar to that described for psychogenic amnesia: An episode most often begins in the context of severe psychosocial stress and typically is of a brief duration (hours to days). Occasionally, an episode may last for months and involve complex social activity. Recovery is usually spontaneous, rapid, and complete, and recurrences are rare.

Although in most cases functional impairment is not severe or long-lasting, the degree of disruption or distress is variable. Violent behavior may occur, but this is not typical.

Differential Diagnosis

The differential diagnosis includes organic mental disorders, although the distinction is not usually difficult. Unexpected wandering from home is unusual in organic mental disorder, and when it does occur it usually has an aimless quality. The memory disturbance of psychogenic fugue may be similar to what occurs in psychogenic amnesia, but the latter does not involve purposeful travel or the assumption of a new personal identity. Complex partial seizures may be associated with a brief journey, but there is no assumption of a new identity and usually no psychosocial precipitating episode. Malingering, which involves an apparent inability to remember one's identity, is difficult to distinguish from psychogenic fugue, but as is the case with all instances of malingering, a practical motive can usually be discerned. Hypnosis or amobarbital interview techniques might be a useful adjunct in distinguishing malingering from psychogenic fugue.

Illustrative Case

A 32-year-old married schoolteacher and minor town official, after learning of his wife's sexual involvement with another man, left home for work and just disappeared. Two months later, an acquaintance stopped for a meal in a small restaurant in the next state and saw him washing dishes behind the counter. The patient claimed not to know the friend and did not respond to his own name. The friend informed the local police, who found that the patient was unable to remember anything about his life prior to the preceding 2 months. He claimed he had found himself in the town 2 months ago not knowing who he was or how he had gotten there and that he invented a name for himself, moved into a rooming house, and took a job as a dish-washer, hoping he would remember who he was. His employer described him as a quiet and secretive man who nonetheless had been a reliable worker.

Epidemiology

Accurate prevalence rates are not available, but psychogenic fugue is rare and occurs most often under conditions of war, natural disaster, or intense personal crisis. No information is available regarding sex distribution or familial patterns of occurrence.

Etiology & Pathogenesis

Psychogenic fugue is thought to be related to some disorder of personality development. Because of severe anxiety or other unpleasant emotional experience (resulting from a traumatic life experience or internal conflict), certain aspects of the personality are psychologically put aside, "dissociated" from the usual complex organization of ideas, memories, emotions, and behavior patterns comprising the personality. The dissociated aspects of the personality are then *repressed* and thus unconscious. The underlying motivation is escape from painful emotional experience. A new identity is substituted. Leaving home might be "necessary" to make the new identity believable to oneself and others.

People who develop psychogenic fugue may have underlying emotional or mental abnormalities, including organic mental disorders, which make them especially vulnerable to psychologic stress. These abnormalities also require that they resort to the extreme psychologic maneuver of change in personal identity to deal with the stress rather than reacting in normally adaptive ways. The reasons for these underlying problems are thought to lie in early personality development.

Treatment & Prognosis

Recovery is usually rapid, spontaneous, and complete, and no specific treatment is required other than supportive care. Depending on the circumstances, environmental manipulation or supportive psychotherapy might play a role in ameliorating factors related to stress or in helping the patient adapt to stress in the future. If the episode is prolonged, psychotherapeutic techniques such as gentle encouragement or directed association may be helpful, either alone or in combination with other techniques, such as hypnosis or amobarbital interviews, which are also aimed at facilitating recall of the previous identity.

DEPERSONALIZATION DISORDER

Symptoms & Signs

Historically, the symptoms of depersonalization and derealization have been recognized as part of the clinical picture of a wide variety of mental disorders. Common to both of these symptoms is a temporary disturbance in the subjective experience of reality, so that the usual quality of familiarity associated with perception is replaced by a sense of estrangement or unreality. In the case of **depersonalization,** the disturbance is in the perception of oneself; in **derealization,** the alteration is in the perception of the external environment. In depersonalization disorder, the major symptom is that of depersonalization, but as presently defined, the disorder may include the symptom of derealization as well.

Depersonalization disorder is defined in *DSM-III-R* as the occurrence of one or more episodes of depersonalization, not due to any other mental disorder, that causes marked distress (Table 33–4). The major feature is sudden temporary loss of the sense of one's own reality, manifested as an experience of being detached from one's body or mental processes or feeling as though one were an outside observer of one's body or mental processes. Patients may also describe feeling as though they were mechanical or as though they were in a dream. Reality testing remains intact, but various feelings of self-estrangement or beliefs that the body's physical characteristics have changed may accompany the episode. Various types of automatism or sensory anesthesias may also occur.

Derealization typically involves the perception that objects in the external world have changed in size or shape, or the subjective feeling that other people are automated, mechanical, somehow inhuman, or dead.

All of these distorted perceptions are experienced as being unpleasant and undesired and may be accompanied by anxiety, dizziness, a fear of becoming insane, feelings of depression, obsessive thoughts, or disturbances in the subjective experience of time.

Natural History

The onset of an episode of depersonalization is usually sudden, and resolution is gradual. The duration of the episode is usually brief, lasting a period of minutes, but complete disappearance of the symptom may take hours.

Differential Diagnosis

When episodes of depersonalization occur as part

Table 33–4. *DSM-III-R* diagnostic criteria for depersonalization disorder (or depersonalization neurosis).

A. Persistent or recurrent experiences of depersonalization as indicated by either (1) or (2):
  (1) An experience of feeling detached from and as if one is an outside observer of one's mental processes or body.
  (2) An experience of feeling like an automaton or as if in a dream.
B. During the depersonalization experience, reality testing remains intact.
C. The depersonalization is sufficiently severe and persistent to cause marked distress.
D. The depersonalization experience is the predominant disturbance, not a symptom of another disorder, such as schizophrenia, panic disorder, or agoraphobia without history of panic disorder, but with limited symptom attacks of depersonalization or temporal lobe epilepsy.

of another mental disorder, the frequency or intensity of episodes usually parallels the severity of other symptoms occurring as part of the primary disorder. The course of depersonalization disorder as defined here is usually chronic, with exacerbations and remissions.

Mild episodes of depersonalization may occur in people without any mental disorder; the diagnosis of depersonalization disorder is not made, even if episodes are recurrent, unless the symptom causes social or occupational dysfunction. Episodes of depersonalization may also occur in the presence of a variety of mental disorders; examples include schizophrenia, affective disorders, organic mental disorders, anxiety disorders, personality disorders, and epilepsy. In such cases, the diagnosis of depersonalization disorder is not made.

Illustrative Case

A 35-year-old lawyer telephoned a psychiatrist and asked for an appointment, saying, "I don't know what's the matter with me, but I'm afraid I'm going crazy." At the first appointment, he explained that for several years he had been having strange "attacks" about once a month. The "attacks" generally occurred during the course of his work, and on 2 recent occasions he had had to leave the courtroom in the midst of a legal procedure "to get control" of himself. He explained that an "attack" usually was heralded by a sudden feeling of nervousness and awareness that his heart was pounding. This was followed by the experience that all objects in his visual field had diminished to about half their normal size and by the perception that people's actions (his own and others) had lost their usual fluid quality and took on a mechanical, jerky character, "as in silent movies." These symptoms occasionally would be accompanied by the experience that he had become someone else ("I don't know who, but not myself"). On the day he telephoned the psychiatrist, an "attack" had begun while he was driving his car, and the usual symptoms were accompanied by the perception that his arms had become detached from his body and continued to steer the car "on their own."

Epidemiology

There is no information on the prevalence, sex ratio, or possible patterns of familial distribution of depersonalization disorder.

Etiology & Pathogenesis

Empirical observations have led some investigators to propose that the phenomenon of depersonalization (as distinct from depersonalization disorder) has a neurophysiologic basis. Patients with brain tumors and epilepsy have reported depersonalization episodes in association with their neurologic disorder. Electrical stimulation of the temporal lobe cortex has been reported to produce depersonalization phenomena, and some psychotomimetic drugs (eg, LSD) produce various distortions of reality (including the sense of reality in the perception of the self) in some individuals.

Explanations emphasizing psychic conflict and disturbances of ego structure have been offered within the framework of psychoanalytic theory, but they have been incomplete and unsatisfactory. Experiencing the self as "not real" would offer protection or escape from (ie, function as a defense against) anxiety or some unpleasant emotional state resulting from internal psychologic conflict. For example, individuals with strong internal prohibitions against aggressive feelings might, when threatened with aggressive impulses, perceive themselves as not "real" and thus in a sense negate the knowledge that they "really" have aggressive impulses.

Attempts to explain depersonalization in terms of constructs regarding the structure of the ego are beyond the scope of this discussion.

Treatment & Prognosis

Little is known about the treatment of depersonalization disorder. Pharmacotherapy with dextroamphetamine or amobarbital has been used, with inconclusive results. Both supportive and insight-oriented psychotherapeutic techniques have been attempted, again with variable success. Evaluation of treatment is complicated by the fact that much of the work has been with patients who experienced depersonalization phenomena in association with a variety of other psychiatric disorders and not with depersonalization disorder as defined here.

POSSESSION/TRANCE DISORDER

Possession/trance disorder has been introduced in *DSM-III-R,* but its natural history, epidemiology, and treatment have not been studied scientifically. The etiology is presumed to be similar to that of the other dissociative disorders—it reflects maladaptive attempts to deal psychologically with internal psychologic conflict or to escape severe emotional pain. Possession/trance disorder is characterized either by a trance (ie, an altered state of consciousness with markedly diminished or selectively focused responsiveness to environmental stimuli) or by possession (ie, the belief that one has been taken over by a spirit or another person). By definition, this disorder occurs outside a culturally sanctioned context (eg, a religious ceremony). A diagnosis of possession/trance disorder cannot be made when symptoms and signs occur as a component of physical disorders such as temporal lobe epilepsy or in the course of psychoactive substance-induced organic mental disorder, multiple personality disorder, brief reactive psychosis, or a psychotic disorder.

DISSOCIATIVE DISORDER NOT OTHERWISE SPECIFIED

The *DSM-III-R* category of dissociative disorder not otherwise specified is reserved for those disorders in which the predominant feature is a dissociative symptom that does not meet the specific diagnostic criteria of the dissociative disorders discussed above. Examples of such symptoms include derealization in the absence of depersonalization and dissociative states resulting from coercive persuasion (brainwashing).

SUMMARY

The dissociative disorders are a group of distinct psychiatric syndromes characterized by severe disturbances in one or more of the personality functions of consciousness, personal identity, or motor behavior. The primary disturbance in psychogenic amnesia is of memory; in multiple personality and depersonaliza-tion disorders, it is of identity; in possession/trance disorder, consciousness or identity is disturbed; and in psychogenic fugue, both identity and motor behavior are affected. As a group, the dissociative disorders are rare, but psychogenic amnesia occurs frequently enough so that most physicians will encounter it at some time during their careers. Although depersonalization disorder is apparently unusual, depersonalization phenomena are common among normal people as well as among people with other psychiatric disorders. The causes of the various dissociative disorders are not clearly or specifically defined, but psychologic theories of causation are widely accepted. The treatment of dissociative disorders is poorly understood and not always effective, and except when resolution of symptoms is spontaneous, referral of patients to a psychiatrist is indicated.

REFERENCES

Combs G Jr, Ludwig AM: Dissociative disorders. Chap 9, pp 266–308, in: *Treatment of Mental Disorders*. Greist JM, Jefferson JW, Spitzer RC (editors). Oxford Univ Press, 1982.

Dysken MW: Clinical usefulness of sodium amobarbital interviewing. *Arch Gen Psychiatry* 1979;**36:**789.

Greist JM, Jefferson JW, Spitzer RC (editors): *Treatment of Mental Disorders*. Oxford Univ Press, 1982.

Kaplan, HI, Freedman AM, Sadock BJ (editors). *Comprehensive Textbook of Psychiatry/IV,* 4th ed. Williams & Wilkins, 1985.

Disorders of Impulse Control

34

Geoffrey K. Booth, MD

Despite their familiarity to the lay public in novels and films as an almost folkloric paradigm of "madness," the impulse control disorders have received little attention in the psychiatric literature during the past 50 years. Four disorders are discussed in this chapter: pathologic gambling, kleptomania (compulsive stealing), pyromania (compulsive fire setting), and trichotillomania (compulsive hair pulling). *DSM-III* included 2 other disorders, intermittent explosive disorder and isolated explosive disorder, which have now been incorporated into a fifth additional category, impulse control disorders not otherwise specified. This category includes atypical impulse control disorders or idiosyncratic, nonspecific irresistible impulses, eg, oniomania (compulsive buying) and dromomania (compulsive wandering or running away). Impulsive behaviors that are either overtly sexual or related to the compulsive ingestion or craving for alcohol or other drugs are classified as paraphilias (Chapter 38) and substance use disorders (Chapters 25 and 26), respectively. Bulimia (impulsive eating) is characterized as an eating disorder (Chapter 39).

All of the disorders in this category share 3 characteristics that help to differentiate them from other phenomena labeled "compulsive," "addictive," or "irresistible." *First,* there is inability to resist an impulse or temptation to do something that is considered harmful to oneself or others. Individuals with an impulse control disorder know either that the act is considered *wrong* by society or that it is potentially harmful to themselves or to others. The impulse may or may not be consciously resisted, and the act may or may not be premeditated. *Second,* there is a sense of increasing tension before the individual commits the act. Many patients describe this mounting tension as restlessness, discomfort, "pressure," or bursts of energy. They may describe a feeling they have that the tension can be relieved only by performing the act. *Third,* there is an experience of excitement or gratification at the time the act is committed. The sense of release from tension is perceived as pleasurable, but there may be a feeling of remorse or regret shortly afterward. The act itself is **ego-syntonic;** ie, it gratifies a conscious wish at the moment. This is in contrast to the compulsion of the obsessive compulsive patient, who perceives the compulsive act as **ego-dystonic** ("bad" or "sick") but does it anyway to avoid an unpleasant sensation (usually anxiety). The neurotic individual is usually uncomfortable and embarrassed by the act while performing it, whereas the individual with an impulse disorder experiences a need or desire that must be satisfied immediately regardless of the consequences.

Because the impulse control disorders involve actions and thus are essentially disorders of behavior as opposed to disorders of thought or cognition, they are regarded as symptoms of other underlying conditions. The individuals seldom know why they do what they do or why it is pleasurable. Many authors have commented on the similarities of these behaviors to sexual excitement and orgasmic release; others have noted that most of the acts have adverse or even destructive consequences for the doer. Psychoanalytic theories help explain many of the underlying conflicts and motivations that produce the behavior. The dynamic theories will be discussed in the sections that follow, but some ideas that pertain to this group of behaviors as a whole are discussed below.

Freud postulated that a major role of the mental apparatus was to discharge tension and to achieve a low-energy, resting state. Release of tension is pleasurable. In the primitive (infantile) state, excitation is quickly discharged through action (musculoskeletal or autonomic-visceral). Gradually, by a process of maturation and learning from the continuing impact of the external environment, the "quick-discharging" primitive mode of the primary process becomes subservient to the reality principle and the mode it governs, secondary process (logical thought). As the maturing organism becomes aware of the consequences of its actions and its capacity to do harm, it learns to delay gratification and to seek other ways of discharging tension and attaining pleasure. Disorders of impulse control can be viewed as temporary lapses in ego control or the control exerted by the reality principle. Such lapses are usually stereotyped and situation-specific. People with impulse control disorders usually function well enough in other areas of their lives. Many are stable individuals with no serious disorders of thought or cognition. Although other behavior disorders are occasionally associated with some impulse control disorders, the problem for many of these individuals consists solely in a socially unacceptable discharge of tension that is momentarily gratifying but which causes misery and remorse later.

PATHOLOGIC GAMBLING

Symptoms & Signs

Pathologic gambling is easily distinguished from "social" gambling. The impulse-disordered gambler has increasing difficulty in resisting the impulse to risk sums of money in games of chance despite the consequences of losing. There tends to be a preoccupation with gambling for its own sake that intensifies when the individual is under stress. Impulsive gamblers may gamble alone rather than in the company of friends and may try to conceal their gambling (and their losses) from their families and others. The more they lose, the more they gamble. Unlike social gamblers, who usually gamble with friends at parties or at resort casinos, allow themselves a fixed amount of "playing money," and stop when that amount is gone, the pathologic gambler makes excuses to get away from family and friends to gamble and is unable to confine losses to a budgeted amount, ie, cannot stop once the stake has vanished in a run of bad luck. Characteristically, the pathologic gambler borrows money and fails to repay creditors. Such individuals continue to pawn items or to encumber their estates until they are bankrupt or destitute. Out of desperation, they may resort to forgery, tax evasion, and (though rarely) theft or embezzlement to get money for gambling or to pay gambling debts. In such instances, however, there is usually a conscious intent to replace the stolen or misappropriated money or property "with my winnings." In contrast to other criminal behavior committed by sociopathic individuals, the impulse-disordered gambler uses money obtained in such illicit ways solely to pay off debts or to indulge in more gambling. Classically, the pathologic gambler experiences a buildup of intolerable tension when a betting opportunity presents itself. Many individuals describe a physical sensation of restlessness and anticipation that can only be relieved by placing a bet. During a game or a race, the tension is amplified. Whether the pathologic gambler wins or loses, there is typically an immediate urge to place another bet until all the money is gone or until the impulse is temporarily quelled by a run of winning chances, which confers a heightened sense of self-esteem or security.

Natural History

Gambling and other forms of risk taking usually begin in adolescence, but it is rare for betting to become compulsive until young adulthood. Gambling is often a feature of adolescent group behavior in much the same way drinking is. All gambling behavior is affected in a general way by cultural mores and specific social settings, but according to *DSM-III*, there are certain associated and perhaps predisposing factors for the development of pathologic gambling: loss of a parent by death, separation, or divorce before age 15 years; marked harshness or inconsistency of parental discipline during childhood; exposure to gambling activities of family members or friends during adolescence; little emphasis in the family on budgeting, financial restraint, planning, or security; and a high degree of materialism in the family and an emphasis on money and possessions as symbols of success.

The typical pathologic gambler is a man who acquired some familiarity with games of chance in adolescence and who actually has had some successes, winning modest sums. He comes from a family where gambling is at least condoned or where an adult is a compulsive gambler or alcoholic. In the far rarer case of the female compulsive gambler, it is not uncommon to find an alcoholic female family member or another woman in the family who gambles.

The problem gambler usually begins compulsive gambling during young adult life, usually during a period of stress. The stresses involved are usually job-related, but occasionally the problem begins when a marriage or other significant relationship falls apart. Problem gambling often follows a period of betting successes. A pattern is usually established in which the gambler begins to make stupid mistakes and take greater risks ("long shots") to recoup. The individual eventually enters a "down and out" phase or a "point of no return."

Although generalizations about personality types may be misleading, the typical gambler is often described as jovial, extroverted, brash, and energetic. Many gamblers show narcissistic and grandiose traits and difficulties with intimacy, empathy, and trust.

Pathologic gambling tends to become a hidden feature of other levels and areas of the gambler's life. The family is almost always involved, but the gambling also affects employers, customers, creditors, distant relatives, and financial institutions. In its final stages, compulsive gambling becomes a true "systems problem." It is common for those close to pathologic gamblers to protect them, pay their debts, lie for them, and make excuses. Gambling often increases during periods of marital discord or family strife and remits when communication is good among family members. Self-esteem also plays a role, as evidenced by the fact that the gambling behavior of some individuals tends to subside while they are receiving positive reinforcement in other areas of their lives.

Differential Diagnosis

The most common phenomena confused with impulse-disordered gambling are (1) risk taking and poor judgment associated with a manic or hypomanic episode; (2) gambling associated with an antisocial personality disorder; and (3) a form of "social gambling" as defined above that may become temporarily heavy as a response to some stressful event.

Gambling during a manic episode may be accompanied by grandiosity, irrationality, and (occasionally) delusional ideation or rationalizations about winning or losing. This behavior during mania rarely serves the goal of tension release but is usually part of a general frenetic spree that includes other behaviors indicative of poor judgment, irrationality, and an increased energy level. It is not uncommon for pathologic gamblers to have mood swings, occasionally toward a hypomanic pole, but this almost always follows a winning streak and is usually short-lived. In antisocial personality disorder, gambling is associated with criminal behavior, a poor work history, and a history of conflicts with the law and of unstable, opportunistic relationships with other people. Criminal behavior by a true impulsive gambler is almost always for the purpose of obtaining money for gambling or for paying bookies and loan sharks. Gambling to excess may occur as a response to life stress by individuals who do not have true impulse control disorders, usually as part of "acting-out" behavior that may include reckless driving, heavy drinking, fistfights, and sexual adventures. Although pathologic gambling is associated epidemiologically with alcoholism among family members, episodic gambling, physical fighting, and antisocial acts related to drinking are usually symptomatic of substance use disorder and not typical of the true impulse gambler.

Prognosis

Pathologic gambling is a chronic disorder that waxes and wanes. It may be incapacitating and may cause severe financial hardship for the individual and the family. Spontaneous permanent cessation of gambling occurs, but how often is not known. The disorder responds to individual therapy and to group therapy and peer support systems such as Gamblers Anonymous.

Illustrative Case

A 37-year-old man, arrested for embezzling from a small company of which he was an officer, stated that he fully intended to return the money to his partners with the winnings he was "sure to have" because of "a very good inside tip on a horse race." He was embarrassed and remorseful, though this was not the first time his need for gambling money had caused him legal trouble. At age 26 years, he had been arrested for credit card fraud and for issuing bad checks. Recently he had obtained money from his mother-in-law by telling her that he wanted to take his wife on a trip and had instead used the money to pay gambling debts. Because of the embezzlement charge, he lost his position in the business and was forced to surrender a business license. His wife was quite concerned about him but tended to minimize his gambling as a "needed release" from the pressures of work. His parents, however, had had enough, refused to lend him any more money, and were demanding that he surrender his car to them as collateral for unpaid obligations.

The patient was anxious, tearful, and preoccupied during the first interview; he bit his nails and occasionally paced about the room. He said that he knew his gambling was excessive but that some day he would "really make a killing." He believed that his worst problems now were the criminal charge for embezzlement and his unpaid debts.

Epidemiology

Men whose fathers and women whose mothers have the disorder are at greatest risk. According to Schubin (1977), there are about 1 million pathologic gamblers in the USA, most of them men.

Etiology & Pathogenesis

As is true also of other impulse disorders, pathologic gambling is believed to be a manifestation of some underlying psychologic conflict. Although efforts have been made to relate impulsive gambling to some neurophysiologic dysfunction (eg, epilepsy, subcortical lesions, minimal brain dysfunction), the prevailing view is that it is an expression of unconscious conflicts. Different writers have different ideas about what these conflicts might be, and there is disagreement over whether the gambling behavior is indicative of the same conflicts at the same general level of psychosexual maturation for all individuals.

Fenichel (1945) and Freud both hypothesized that the gambler's conflicts were centered on masturbation. According to Fenichel, gambling and masturbation are a kind of play. Both derive motive force from a build-up of tension that is released through repetitive actions or the anticipation of them. Bergler (1943) wrote about the gambler's unconscious need to lose, based on unconscious guilt, usually because of unconscious aggression toward a mother who blocked the child's search for gratification in genital manipulation. Gambling behavior is also strongly affected by its context in the patient's life. The behavior itself eventually takes on a certain currency in the individual's dealings with others, so that the person is known as an individual who likes to "have a bet down," who "will bet on anything," etc. In a secondary way, gambling may become symbolic of being "naughty" or powerful. It may be a source of self-esteem or a self-reinforcing part of a person's sense of identity. Gambling, as an almost archetypal intermittent reinforcement model (sometimes you win, sometimes you lose), is "addictive" behavior in its own right.

Treatment

Because of its ego-syntonic and self-reinforcing nature, pathologic gambling is often not perceived as "mental illness" by the afflicted individual. Treatment usually begins when significant people in the patient's life define the behavior as a problem. Occasionally, a gambler in a "down and out" position will seek help voluntarily, without urging from others, but even in such cases with the secret intent to return to the casino as soon as the current crisis is past. Individual insight-oriented therapy has had moderate success with motivated patients, and other techniques have recently been found to be more effective. The similarities between compulsive gambling and alcoholism have suggested treatment based on peer pressure, public confession, and the availability of other reformed gamblers to help individuals resist the urge to gamble. Gamblers Anonymous, founded in 1957, was modeled on Alcoholics Anonymous. Most large cities have a chapter as well as the gambling analogs of Al-Anon and Al-Ateen (support groups for the spouses and children of pathologic gamblers). Facilities for the inpatient treatment of compulsive gambling exist, where milieu therapy and peer groups are emphasized, followed by extended individual psychotherapy on an outpatient basis.

KLEPTOMANIA

Symptoms & Signs

The essential feature of kleptomania is the recurrent inability to resist the impulse to steal. The objects taken are usually of little or no obvious value to the individual. The "kleptomaniac" steals purely for the sake of stealing. The booty may later be given away, abandoned, or even surreptitiously returned. Usually the individual has money to pay for the merchandise, and sometimes the theft occurs during a shopping trip for other items that are paid for in the normal way. Items taken may be symbolic of some unconscious conflict, but just as often they are not. Impulsive stealing is a response to increasing tension, and the individual experiences a sense of relief and gratification at the time. The thief almost always knows that the act is wrong but simply cannot resist the force of mounting tension. Some individuals later feel remorse or shame and if apprehended experience depression and self-denigration. Others never show remorse or depression. The act of stealing is always done alone and usually without extensive forethought. Contrary to popular belief, kleptomaniacs do not want to be caught. The act is done in pursuit of the pleasure associated with the relief of tension. The impulse to steal often renders the person inattentive to the possibility or consequences of being caught.

Natural History

Kleptomania is a chronic, waxing and waning disorder. It usually begins in adolescence, but the onset may be at any time during adult life. It is often associated with other emotional disturbances such as eating disorders, pyromania (in women), or chronic depression. The symptoms tend to reappear during times of stress, especially separations, losses, or terminations of significant relationships. Spontaneous remission or "burnout" of the disorder is reported, but it is not known how often it occurs. Kleptomania is amenable to treatment, especially if the afflicted individual is motivated for change. There is evidence that childhood kleptomania can be successfully treated by individual therapy and work with families.

Differential Diagnosis

By far the most common behavior that is confused with true kleptomania is ordinary stealing. The common thief steals merchandise for its value or utility and not to discharge tension created by an irresistible impulse. Many thieves may feign kleptomania, but it usually becomes obvious that their intent was to steal a specific item for its value. Evidence of premeditation or advance planning should exclude the diagnosis of kleptomania except in rare instances. Kleptomaniacs may ruminate for days about the *act* of stealing but do not set out on planned forays to steal specific objects. In the mania of bipolar affective disorder, there may be episodes of impulsive shoplifting, but these do not have the characteristic quality of building tension and gratification. When shoplifting occurs in association with mania or a schizophrenic process, other stigmas of the diagnosis are usually apparent (eg, grandiosity, increased energy level, command hallucinations, poor reality testing). Theft is a common feature of antisocial personality disorder, but there is usually a history of conflicts with the law, a poor work history, and poor interpersonal relationships. Stealing that fits neither the criteria for kleptomania nor the general picture of antisocial personality disorder is usually classified as a conduct disorder.

Patients with organic mental disorder occasionally take things that do not belong to them. In such cases, there is usually evidence of nonspecific impulsiveness (temper tantrums, impulsive exhibitionism, inappropriate interactions with strangers). Other evidence of dementia usually exists, and people close to the individual are aware of a personality change. Khan and Martin (1977) have shown an association of classic kleptomania with progressive cortical atrophy.

Prognosis

The prognosis for patients with kleptomania is good. Treatment is usually successful, and since kleptomania does not seriously impair job performance or the capacity for relationships with others, the typical patient brings to treatment many psychologic and social resources.

Illustrative Case

An attractive and well-educated 44-year-old woman, recently divorced from her third husband, received a great deal of money and property by way of settlement. Shortly after the divorce, she experienced an impulse to walk into a popular department store and take inexpensive clothing and costume jewelry. She had had these feelings off and on since about age 16 years, and in her 20s she had been arrested twice for shoplifting. She worried about getting caught but made no special plans to avoid discovery. She felt such relief and pleasure as she left the store with the merchandise that she was tempted to repeat the behavior. She would start ruminating and fantasizing about stealing something several days before she actually entered the store. She would sometimes try to avoid the department store but would then experience increasing tension and irritability. When interviewed about her problem, she showed embarrassment and discomfort and tried to change the subject by telling of her accomplishments. She claimed that all of her marriages had failed because her husbands had never really understood her. She saw them as being less intelligent than she and less "aesthetically aware." She described herself as an "extremely gifted" and sensitive woman and said that as a child she had often felt misunderstood and unwanted by her busy and successful parents. It came to light later during treatment that her marriages had ended because of her frequent infidelities and "pathologic lying."

Epidemiology

True kleptomania is very rare. The literature describes the disorder as being more common in women, but there is little evidence on which to base any statements about prevalence, familial distribution, or sex ratio. Arieff and Bowie (1947) reported that in a sample of apprehended shoplifters, 3.8% were considered to be suffering from kleptomania.

Etiology & Pathogenesis

In the 18th century, kleptomania was considered a **monomania,** a disorder of a specific area of mental functioning that rendered its victims susceptible to acting on powerful impulses. At that time, the disorder was seen as a distinct entity whose causes had innate origins. Over the past 200 years, the disorder has been viewed as the behavioral manifestation of some underlying psychologic conflict. *DSM-III* classifies kleptomania as a distinct entity, but most writers have assumed a psychologic cause. Abraham (1953) observed that a central concern for many kleptomaniacs was a feeling of being neglected, injured, or unwanted. They reported childhood memories of abandonment (real or imagined) and a sense of lovelessness and deprivation. Stekel (1924) equated kleptomania with frustrated infantile sexuality. Alexander and Healy (1935) again focused attention on the kleptomaniac's dependency, neediness, and sense of deprivation and a need to deny these feelings. Fenichel (1945) saw taking objects belonging to others as symbolic of recouped self-esteem and affection. Other authors have noted the association of impulsive stealing with bulimia and anorexia nervosa (Bruch, 1973; King, 1963). Most dynamic theories of the causes of kleptomania center either on stealing as an attempt to obtain nourishment, esteem, and love or as a sexual equivalent—a quest for a penis in a woman or as a defense against castration anxiety in men. Some writers have developed theories in which both mechanisms play a role.

Treatment

Individual psychodynamic (insight-oriented) psychotherapy has been the most successful method of treatment of kleptomania. Insight-oriented therapy has been most helpful with patients who feel guilt and shame and are thus motivated to change their behavior. Behavior therapy, including systematic desensitization, aversive conditioning, avoidance of opportunities to succumb to temptation, and resolution of tension-engendering interaction with others, has been successful in some cases even when patients have not been strongly motivated for change.

PYROMANIA

Symptoms & Signs

Pyromania is the inability to resist the impulse to set fires. Pyromaniacs have a pathologic fascination with setting fires and seeing things burn. They experience overwhelming impulses to light fires and derive intense pleasure as the flames leap up. They may make elaborate plans to set the fire, but unlike other arsonists, their sole motive is self-gratification—not insurance proceeds, revenge, or sabotage. They are aware that their behavior is destructive and potentially life-threatening, but they cannot resist the impulse. They usually fear punishment and may take steps to avoid being caught, though many pyromaniacs are callously indifferent to consequences. For some pyromaniacs, part of the impulse gratification derives from the power and destructiveness of the fire.

Natural History

Most adult pyromaniacs have a history of fire setting in childhood. They report seemingly lifelong fascination with fires, firefighting equipment, and fire fighters. Many fire setters have a history of sounding false alarms and watching fire fighters rush to the scene. They tell how as children they wanted to follow fire engines to the scene of a fire. Pyromaniacs are often among the onlookers at neighborhood fires and may become volunteer fire fighters. This disorder is much more common among men, though cases involving women have been reported. In males there is an association with low intelligence, learning disabilities, hyperkinesis and enuresis in childhood, and poor impulse control in other areas (eg, outbursts of temper, recklessness, and fascination with high speed). Female fire setters usually begin their careers later than boys do. They do not usually set fires with the intent to be destructive or to bring out the fire engines. Pyromania in women is associated with sexual promiscuity and petty theft, which may actually be kleptomania. The strength of the impulse to set fires may wax and wane over time, but without treatment, the patient is always at risk of giving in to it. Most pyromaniacs are directed to psychiatric treatment through the court system.

Differential Diagnosis

Pyromaniacs do not commit arson for financial gain, personal revenge, or other motives of that sort. Arson by an individual with an antisocial personality disorder usually serves some end other than release of tension. Although many antisocial individuals have a history of fire setting as well as enuresis and cruelty to animals during childhood, their adult careers usually involve chronic conflicts with authority, a poor work record, and exploitative relationships with significant others. None of these adult traits are typical of the pyromaniac.

Children are often fascinated by fire and play with matches, but such behavior during childhood is less frequent, dramatic, and pernicious than what is reported in the childhood histories of pyromaniacs. Many schizophrenic patients set fires, usually in response to internal stimuli. These acts can be differentiated from pyromania by the lack of true gratification and release after the act. Although many pathologic fire setters have a history of minimal brain dysfunction or subnormal intelligence, their fire-setting behavior is usually different from that of demented individuals. Patients with organic mental disorder may set fires because of poor judgment and failure to appreciate the consequences of the act. Many fire setters drink heavily, and both the drinking and the fire setting are indicative of poor impulse control, primitive urges to seek gratification, and attempts to bolster self-esteem.

Prognosis

The treatment of pyromania is difficult because of denial, associated drinking problems, poor insight, and (occasionally) limited intelligence. The treatment of fire setting in children has been far more encouraging, and complete remission is not an unrealistic therapeutic goal. Most adult pyromaniacs are eventually confined in mental hospitals or in prison. Only limited success has been reported in the treatment of institutionalized patients.

Illustrative Case

An 11-year-old boy who was repeating the fifth grade had been fascinated with fires since age 8 years. In the third grade, he was sent home from school twice for setting off false fire alarms. Neighbors complained that he had been seen setting brush fires in a lot behind his house and that appeals to the boy's mother—a working divorcee—had done no good. The most recent episode of fire setting motivated the mother to bring her son to a child guidance clinic. While alone in the house because his mother had a date with a man she had been seeing for several months, he became restless and irritable, turned on the gas burners in the kitchen, and began setting fire to paper napkins. He became increasingly excited and eventually carried a burning cloth towel into the living room, where he set the drapes on fire. Neighbors called the fire department. The boy ran from the house but eventually returned to watch the fire fighters extinguish the blaze.

In the interview, the patient was outgoing and pleasant, appearing younger than age 11 years, but afraid of being punished by his mother's boyfriend. Apart from fire setting, there was no history of impulsiveness or other discipline problems. The patient had wet the bed until age 7 years. The school report said he was a bit slow academically but an obedient and compliant child who worked and played well with others. The only notable problems at school were short bursts of temper during games at recess.

Epidemiology

The disorder is reportedly quite rare, is probably more common in men than in women, and tends to be associated with a history of enuresis and learning disabilities.

Etiology & Pathogenesis

As in the case of other impulse disorders, pyromania has long been considered a symptom of underlying psychologic conflict. Recent writers have noted the coincidence of learning disabilities and brain dysfunction among this population as perhaps indicating some type of neurophysiologic dysfunction, but most discussions of etiology have assumed a predominantly psychologic cause. In general, 3 major psychologic issues appear in the psychoanalytic literature in connection with impulsive fire setting: (1) an association between fire setting and sexual gratification, which is frequently linked to urination and sadism; (2) concerns about inferiority, impotence, and annihilation; and (3) unconscious anger toward a parent figure.

Psychoanalysts have observed that any mucous membrane has the potential to become eroticized; ie, sexual sensations can be generated by stimulation of mucous membranes anywhere they occur. (An example is the eroticization occasionally reported at colostomy and ileostomy sites.) Stimulation of the urethral mucosa by the passage of urine or with matches or other objects inserted through the meatus is experienced by some individuals as sexually exciting. This phenomenon of **urethral eroticism** may play a role in pyromania. Several authors have described patients who have masturbated after setting fires. Some pyromaniacs describe the gratification they experience as "orgasmic."

Lewis and Yarnell (1951) found other motives for impulsive fire setting. Many individuals in their study showed evidence of poor self-esteem and a craving for power and prestige. These authors saw the pyromaniac's act as a vehicle for exercising power by creating commotion at the scene of the fire, for identifying with powerful fire fighters, and for relieving frustration and venting anger derived from an internalized sense of social and sexual inferiority. Stekel (1924) and others have noted the association of fire setting, especially in children and adolescents, with anger directed toward one or both parents. A higher than expected number of fire setters come from broken homes or single-parent families. Fire setting by a child often begins when a parent remarries or when a child perceives that one parent is being emotionally or sexually unfaithful to the other parent. Thinly veiled sadistic impulses directed against the offending parent or his or her new consort may be acted out as fire setting.

Treatment

In adults, insight-oriented individual psychotherapy to explore the meaning the patient attributes to the impulsive act has had mixed results. Behavior therapy techniques have been used with moderate success. Group therapy and family therapy have been quite successful with children.

TRICHOTILLOMANIA

Symptoms & Signs

Trichotillomania (compulsive hair pulling) is relatively rare but more common in both adult and pediatric populations than was once thought. Most practicing dermatologists see one or 2 cases a year. The disorder is usually associated with children but can (less often) be found in adolescents and adults. It tends to be predominantly a disorder of girls and women and can include hair pulling at different sites on the body (eg, eyebrows, eyelashes) as well as the scalp.

On clinical examination, the scalp of the patient with trichotillomania has the appearance of alopecia areata, a disorder with which it is often confused. There are ill-defined patches of denuded scalp with much evidence of short broken hairs around areas completely devoid of hair. Severe cases show almost total loss of scalp hair. Early in the disorder, the hair follicles are not disturbed, and there is evidence of new hair growth within older bald patches. In longstanding trichotillomania with severe and constant local irritation, new hair growth may be significantly compromised, and bald patches may be permanent.

The disfigurement caused by constant hair pulling is often a source of embarrassment for the patient, who nevertheless continues to experience periods of profound mounting tension and is compelled to relieve it by pulling out hair. Especially among adults and adolescents, hair pulling is often done in solitude, and steps are taken to conceal the behavior and its results. Secrecy is usually less common in younger children. In older populations, hair pulling is often accompanied by depressive symptoms, but the behavior still conforms to the pattern of mounting tension and then relief when the hair is pulled out. In rare instances, both adults and children may eat the hair they have pulled and thus present with a trichobezoar, or concretion of hair, in the stomach or intestine. Depending on the size of the bezoar, and if complications develop, the patient may be forced to seek medical or surgical treatment.

Natural History

Trichotillomania is usually a life-long habit pattern originating in childhood. The onset is usually between 4 and 10 years of age, although onset in adolescence is also common. Cases have been reported in one-year-old children. Onset in late adulthood (age > 45 years) is rare and suggestive of some other coincidental disorder, eg, neurologic disease, psychosis, or metabolic disturbance. Spontaneous remissions do occur in all age groups, but in the untreated patient, a life-long habit pattern of susceptibility to episodes of hair pulling in times of intense stress becomes established. When trichotillomania in the pediatric patient is complicated by (or perhaps engendered by) family strife or turmoil at home, the prognosis usually improves after the disturbance has abated. For adult patients, the overall prognosis is fair to poor; trichotillomania is a difficult disorder to treat, and patients with this disorder have not responded well to most forms of psychodynamically oriented psychotherapy.

Differential Diagnosis

The differential diagnosis of trichotillomania requires attention to its dermatologic aspects first; then, if compulsive hair pulling is suspected, psychiatric diagnosis should be considered.

The bald patches in trichotillomania resemble those in alopecia areata, but new hair growth and active follicles in affected regions and broken, partly pulled hairs are evidence of trauma as a cause of the baldness of trichotillomania. Another disorder that should be ruled out is tinea capitis, in which fungal elements are seen on slides fixed with potassium hydroxide; usually, there is also evidence of excoriation. Various other dermatologic disorders can usually be differentiated from compulsive hair pulling by a careful history and interviews with parents and family members.

The psychiatric differential diagnosis includes all of the childhood and adult psychotic disorders. In trichotillomania (as in all impulse control disorders), patients function well in all other aspects of their lives and show few if any symptoms other than hair pulling. Autistic and schizophrenic children and adults who pull their hair show other signs of mental illness such as auditory hallucinations, bizarre behavior, and poor job, school, and interpersonal functioning. They seldom conform to the pattern of mounting tension that is relieved when hair is pulled. In adults, trichotillomania is sometimes seen as a complication of depressive disorders. In most cases, hair pulling occurs in the context of dysphoric feelings, sleep and appetite disturbances, and a subjective sense of sadness. Sometimes the depressive symptoms are less well defined, but trichotillomania subsides with adequate pharmacologic and psychologic treatment of depression—in these cases there may or may not be a history of compulsive hair pulling.

Prognosis

Trichotillomania is difficult to treat, especially in older individuals. Historically, patients have not responded well to psychoanalytically oriented therapy. Most successful treatments involve behavior therapy, hypnotherapy, and family therapy interventions. Patients with a depressive disorder may respond well to monoamine oxidase inhibitors. Drugs such as clomipramine and amitriptyline have been moderately helpful for both depressive concomitants to the disorder in adults and the obsessive-compulsive nature of the hair pulling itself.

Illustrative Case

A young mother brought her 4 ½-year-old daughter to a pediatrician after she noticed 2 bald patches on the sides of the child's scalp. The child denied that anything was wrong and seemed embarrassed about the fuss her mother was making. The doctor ascertained that the mother was a recent divorcee who had taken a job as a dispatcher for the local police department. She worked long hours and frequently left her daughter at a reputable child care center on days when preschool was not in session. In the recent past, there had been a fairly dramatic drop in the amount of time that mother and daughter spent together. The child was bright, personable, and functioned well in preschool. The pediatrician examined the child and then gently asked about hair pulling. She gave the child a doll and asked her to "make the doll-baby have bare spots." The little girl pulled on the doll's hair and indicated that the pulling should result in "bare spots." The child admitted to the doctor that she had impulses to pull her own hair because it "felt good." The doctor was reassuring but referred the patient to a behavioral therapist experienced in play therapy and family counseling.

Epidemiology

Trichotillomania is more common in females than males, with a ratio of 5:1 to 2.5:1 depending on the studies cited. Pediatric cases are more common than those of adult onset; the disorder tends to be resistant to treatment and to remit and recur throughout the young life of the patient. Spontaneous remission occurs quite commonly in middle-aged and geriatric populations. Hair pulling that is not an irresistible impulse is found in older populations as part of dementias, psychoses, or neuroendocrine disorders.

Etiology & Pathogenesis

Little has been written recently about the causes and psychodynamic underpinnings of this behavior. Galski, in a summary of his findings in a case study of trichotillomania, posits that hair pulling tends to begin early in life in response to the parent-child relationship:

Specifically, the trichotillomanic's mother sets the stage for the emergence of this symptom by extending the child's dependence upon her as the primary need-gratifier beyond early childhood into latency, adolescence, and adulthood. As a result, the child is not gradually propelled to participate in new and more complex learning experiences that ultimately lead to a sense of mastery and independent functioning in the environment. Important developmental stimuli are not presented at the appropriate times and the child is not exposed to certain types of interactions at the optimal times, so that some very important ego functions do not develop, or develop minimally, or in a distorted manner. Simply, the mother cannot "let go" of her child, apparently deriving gratification of her own needs through infantilization of the child; as a result, the child develops a limited or illusory sense of self sufficiency. Continuation of such an unhealthy symbiotic relationship, however, is found in many forms of psychopathology and the fact that it also underlies trichotillomania may partially account for hair pulling as a symptom associated with such a wide range of nosological categories. It is the main contention of this study, however, that the quality of the parent-child relationship impairs the ego development and causes failure

of the trichotillomanic patient to establish object constancy. Without the establishment of object constancy an individual requires visible evidence that the object/person capable of gratifying basic security needs is present or available. In trichotillomania the hair seems to symbolize the need-gratifying object/person who is lost when the hair is pulled out and, more importantly, regained when it is eaten or restored. It appears to be this latter component of trichotillomania, ie, reincorporation of the need-gratifying object/person, which reassures the patient that infantile needs can be gratified and security can be reestablished. Unfortunately, the trichotillomanic is driven to repeatedly and compulsively remove hair so that it can be regained temporarily, since object constancy is never really established.

Treatment

Behavioral therapy has been the most successful method of treatment of trichotillomania. Self-destructive behaviors are discouraged through either "attention-reflection," in which the patient is made acutely aware of the behavior in question, the circumstances in which the behavior may occur, and coincident behaviors that may intensify the urge; aversive conditioning, in which unpleasant experiences are paired with the hair pulling urge; and reinforcement of alternative behaviors such as clenching one's fist when the urge takes over. Hypnotherapy has been moderately helpful in stopping the behavior. Drug therapies have included clomipramine (not yet available in the USA) and amitriptyline, which seem to have sedating, antidepressant, and anticompulsive effects. These drugs are not usually indicated for children. Family therapy has proved helpful with children and families in conflict when turmoil at home seems to be causing or complicating the condition.

IMPULSE CONTROL DISORDERS NOT OTHERWISE SPECIFIED

This category of impulse control disorders comprises rare disorders that nevertheless conform to the pattern of mounting tension, a destructive or bizarre act, and a sense of gratification after the act is committed. These disorders have been classified in older psychiatric literature as "morbid impulses" or "monomanias." They include such rare disorders as dromomania (an impulse to wander) and hair cutting and braid snipping. These phenomena are generally considered to be manifestations of an underlying psychologic conflict that is often sexual in nature. The usual treatment is insight-oriented psychotherapy.

CONCLUSION

Impulse control disorders are disorders of behavior that result from inability to resist an impulse, drive, or temptation. All of these disorders are characterized by increasing tension before the act is committed and feelings of relief and gratification when the deed is done. All of the behaviors described in this chapter are ego-syntonic when the act is committed, though individuals may show remorse or guilt later. Individuals with impulse control disorders are often productive, seemingly well-adjusted members of society and often quite skillful in keeping their peculiar behaviors secret.

The following characteristics are important in diagnosis:

(1) The degree to which the impulsive acts are performed in response to increasing tension, an irresistible urge, and gratification upon completion.

(2) The absence of disordered thinking, affect, or cognition.

(3) The absence of obvious, conscious secondary gain or motives other than pure release of tension.

(4) The presence of generally good psychosocial functioning in most areas of the individual's life.

The following illustrative case describes a patient whose presentation is complicated by multiple impulse control problems. The case illustrates how the principles outlined above might be applied to the differential diagnosis of a patient with "kleptomania."

Illustrative case. A 29-year-old unemployed man was brought for psychiatric examination after he was apprehended for shoplifting. He had stolen a transistor radio and some batteries. When stopped by a store security officer, he sheepishly admitted that he was a "kleptomaniac."

The patient reported that recently he and his girlfriend had been having conflicts. He was sure she was being unfaithful to him and telling secrets to their acquaintances. About 4 months after they had first met, the girlfriend told him that she did not want to move in with him until they were better acquainted. He became enraged, broke furniture in her apartment, threw turpentine on her car upholstery, and set a trash bin on fire. He went on a drinking binge that ended when he drank down a bottle of cold medicine as a suicidal gesture. He was hospitalized briefly and released to outpatient psychiatric follow-up. He attended one outpatient session but failed to keep other appointments. He told his girlfriend that psychotherapy was "useless and boring." He was dependent on his girlfriend for most of his support. He took odd jobs where he could find them and washed cars, mowed lawns, and occasionally sold illicit street drugs. Acquaintances characterized him as quick-tempered, unpredictable, impulsive, and "dramatic." His family considered him emotionally unstable and "a lost soul." As a child, he had been an average student. He was moody, short-tempered, and a "loner." He had been enuretic until age 10 years. He had been married twice since high school, and both relationships ended in divorce owing chiefly to his suspiciousness, unpredictable behavior, shoplifting, and impulsiveness. During his second marriage, he was arrested for car theft and for assaulting a police officer. His second wife once discovered a cache of goods he had shoplifted. When she confronted him, he explained that he was going to sell the goods and that he would use some of the money to take her on a trip. When she threatened to notify the police, he became wildly enraged and beat her severely. Her filing for divorce caused him to attempt suicide by cutting his wrists.

During the interview, the patient was obsequious and melodramatic. He stated that he knew he needed help and that he was "very sick," as evidenced by his compulsion to steal things. He discussed what he called his "identity crisis" and reported that at times he was not sure who he was or "why I am on this planet." He stated that he was 2 people: a good and happy person who was never angry or mean, and a "dark person" who was evil and hateful. He said that his moods changed abruptly depending on which person was "out." He said that he disliked being alone and being bored and that he stole things to "get attention."

The patient in the illustrative case presented above demonstrates several behaviors similar to those discussed in this chapter. He identifies himself as a "kleptomaniac," and he does in fact shoplift with some regularity. He has outbursts of rage that result in assault or destruction of property. On at least one occasion he set a fire, and his history is positive for enuresis. When we apply strict diagnostic criteria to the facts, however, we see that his manifold impulse problems are not typical of the disorders described in this chapter.

(1) His shoplifting, intermittent explosions, and fire setting do not conform to a pattern of mounting tensions and subsequent gratification.

(2) He shows evidence of possible disordered thinking and feeling states. He may have paranoid tendencies (girlfriend telling secrets), identity confusion (2 people: good and bad), and sustained dysphoria and anger.

(3) Much of his behavior is the result of clear precipitants (usually abandonment by a significant person) and has elements of revenge and other ulterior motives (selling his cache of stolen goods for money).

(4) His impulsive behavior is not an isolated aberration in the context of an otherwise well-adjusted personality structure. He is a troubled, self-destructive man who has difficulty with jobs and relationships.

Despite the presence of several examples of impulsive behavior, this patient should not be diagnosed as suffering from an impulse control disorder as described in this chapter. Given his disturbances of mood, self-image, impulsiveness, and interpersonal relationships, a diagnosis of borderline personality disorder may be more appropriate.

REFERENCES

Abraham K: Manifestations of the female castration complex. In: *Selected Papers on Psychoanalysis*. Bryan D, Strachey A (editors). Basic Books, 1953.

Alexander F, Healy W: *Roots of Crime*. Knopf, 1935.

Arieff A, Bowie C: Some psychiatric aspects of shoplifting. *J Clin Psychopathol* 1947;**8:**565.

Bach-y-Rita G et al: Episodic dyscontrol. *Am J Psychiatry* 1971;**127:**1473.

Bergler E: The gambler: A misunderstood neurotic. *J Criminal Psychopathol* 1943;**4.**

Bergler E: *The Psychology of Gambling*. Hill & Wang, 1957.

Bruch H: *Eating Disorders*. Basic Books, 1973.

Cossidente A, Sarti MG: Psychiatric syndromes with dermatologic expression. *Clin Dermatol* 1984;**2:**201.

Dahlquist LM, Kalfus GR: A novel approach to assessment in the treatment of childhood trichotillomania. *J Behav Ther Exp Psychiatry* 1984;**15:**47.

Dalton K: Cyclical criminal acts in premenstrual syndrome. *Lancet* 1980;**2:**1070.

Fenichel O: *The Psychoanalytic Theory of Neurosis*. Norton, 1945.

Freud S: Civilization and its discontents (1930). In: *Standard Edition of the Complete Psychological Works of Sigmund Freud*. Vol 21. Hogarth Press, 1961.

Freud S: Formulations on the two principles of mental functioning (1911). In: *Standard Edition of the Complete Psychological Works of Sigmund Freud*. Vol 12. Hogarth Press, 1958.

Galski TJ: The adjunctive use of hypnosis in the treatment of trichotillomania: A case report. *Am J Clin Hypn* 1981;**23:**198.

Gambling: Crave or craze? (Editorial.) *Lancet* 1982;**1:**434.

Gruber AR, Heck ET, Minitzer E: Children who set fires: Some background and behavioral characteristics. *Am J Orthopsychiatry* 1981;**51:**484.

Jones FD: Therapy for firesetters. (Correspondence.) *Am J Psychiatry* 1981;**138:**261.

Kaplan HI, Freedman AM, Sadock BJ (editors): *Comprehensive Textbook of Psychiatry/IV*, 4th ed. Vol 2. Williams & Wilkins, 1985.

Khan K, Martin IC: Kleptomania as a presenting feature of cortical atrophy. *Acta Psychiatr Scand* 1977;**56:**168.

King A: Primary and secondary anorexia syndromes. *Br J Psychiatry* 1963;**109:**470.

Krishnan KR, Davidson JR, Guajardo C: Trichotillomania—A review. *Compr Psychiatry* 1985;**26:**123.

Krishnan RR, Davidson J, Miller R: MAO inhibitor therapy in trichotillomania associated with depression: Case report. *J Clin Psychiatry* 1984;**45:**267.

Lant JE, Early JP, Pillow WE: Family aspects of trichotillomania. *J Psychiatr Nurs* 1980;**8:**32.

Lester D: The treatment of compulsive gambling. *Int J Addict* 1980;**15:**201.

Lewis NDC, Yarnell H: *Pathological Firesetting (Pyromania)*. Nervous and Mental Disease Monographs, 1951.

Lowenstein LF: The diagnosis of child arsonists. *Acta Paedopsychiatr (Basel)* 1981;**47:**151.

Lutzker JR, Lamazor EA: Behavioral pediatrics: Research, treatment, recommendations. *Prog Behav Modif* 1985; **19:**217.

Medansky RS, Handler RM: Dermatopsychosomatics: Classification, physiology, and therapeutic approaches. *J Am Acad Dermatol* 1981;**5:**125.

Monroe RR: Episodic behavioral disorder. In: *American Handbook of Psychiatry*, 2nd ed. Arieti S, Brady E (editors). Basic Books, 1974.

Moskowitz JA: Lithium and lady luck: Use of lithium carbonate in compulsive gambling. *NY State J Med* 1980;**80:**785.

Rosenbaum MS: Treating hair pulling in a 7-year-old male: Modified habit reversal for use in pediatric settings. *J Dev Behav Pediatr* 1982;**3:**241.

Schubin S: The compulsive gambler: An interview with Robert L. Custer. *Today Psychiatry* 1977;**4:**1.

Snyder S: Trichotillomania treated with amytriptylene. *J Nerv Ment Dis* 1980;**168:**505.

Stekel W: *Peculiarities of Behavior*. Liverwright, 1924.

Stevens MJ: Behavioral treatment of trichotillomania. *Psychol Rep* 1984;**55:**987.

Tabatabai SE, Salari-Lak M: Alopecia in dolls! *Cutis* 1981; **28:**206.

Wray I, Dickerson MG: Cessation of high frequency gambling and "withdrawal" symptoms. *Br J Addict* 1981;**76:**401.

Adjustment Disorder

35

Kathryn N. DeWitt, PhD

Other chapters in this text describe psychiatric disorders that seriously impair psychologic functioning and are characterized by identifiable symptom patterns. Although these disorders are important subjects of psychiatric research and teaching, they do not include the emotional problems of a great many individuals who seek help. The patients whose problems comprise the subject matter of this chapter lack some or all of the specific symptoms characteristic of the disorders discussed in other chapters. Adjustment disorder is generally associated with difficult life experiences, but the suffering or dysfunction that results is out of proportion to the degree of stress.

The category of adjustment disorder serves 3 important functions: (1) It draws attention to people who need professional help; (2) it provides a way of collecting data that might be used to devise subcategories of illness, should that prove useful in the future; and (3) it describes specific procedures for identifying these patients and for distinguishing them from those with other mental disorders or those experiencing normal responses to the problems of life. Patients with "problems in living" but no mental disorder are classified by use of "V" codes (see below and Chapter 23).

Establishing a Diagnosis of Adjustment Disorder

DSM-III-R characterizes adjustment disorder as "a reaction to an identifiable psychosocial stressor or multiple stressors that occurs within three months of the onset of the stressors." The reaction may take the form of "impairment in occupational (including school) functioning or in usual social activities or relationships with others" or "symptoms that are in excess of a normal and expectable reaction to the stressors." The disturbance may not have persisted for longer than 6 months. The diagnosis of adjustment disorder is not used when symptoms conform to the specific criteria for another mental disorder, excluding personality disorder or developmental disorder, nor is it used when current distress represents but one instance of a general pattern of overreaction to stressors. For this reason, adjustment disorder has come to be known as a diagnosis of exclusion.

Four major decision-making processes are involved in the diagnosis of adjustment disorder: (1) establishing a relationship to a psychosocial stressor, (2) evaluating the level and duration of disturbance, (3) ruling out other mental disorders (excluding personal-

ity disorder or developmental disorder), and (4) evaluating the context of the patient's total personality.

A. Establishing a Relationship to a Psychosocial Stressor:

Illustrative case. A 17-year-old high school girl was caught shoplifting an expensive pair of earrings. When apprehended, she seemed surprised and somewhat dazed. In court, she pleaded guilty and told the judge that she really did not know what made her take the earrings, especially since her father would have bought them for her if she had asked him to. Since the girl had no history of arrests, she was given a suspended sentence and referred to a court-appointed psychiatrist for adolescent group counseling.

In the initial evaluation, the psychiatrist learned that the girl's arrest for shoplifting was the latest and most serious of a series of incidents in which she had gotten into trouble for doing something she knew was wrong. Her grades had been falling for most of the past semester, and her friends and teachers had remarked that she did not seem to be herself lately. In describing her home life, she revealed that her parents had been separated for about 3 months and that it now looked as though they would obtain a divorce, since her father wanted to remarry. The girl denied being upset about her parents' marital troubles, saying, "Who they sleep with is their business." She said she was not aware of feeling especially anxious or depressed but that she was "kinda spaced out" much of the time. She had also gained 15 lb over the previous 3 months.

Before a diagnosis of adjustment disorder can be assigned, the clinician must determine whether the patient's current problem is causally related to a psychosocial stressor. Stressors may be one-time events, such as the loss of a job or death of a relative, or they may be ongoing situations or conditions, such as marital discord, involvement in a lawsuit, or accident-induced disability. They may be expected life changes, such as menopause or retirement, or unexpected catastrophes, such as natural disasters or rare diseases. They may be single or multiple, recurrent or continuous, individually experienced or culturally shared.

In occasional cases, a patient or someone who knows the patient may make a causal connection between the stressor and the disturbance. In other cases, patients may be unaware of the connection or even deny it when asked, as was true of the girl in the illustrative case presented above. The clinician should note whether the current disturbance represents a change in functioning that coincided with the occurrence of the stressor. The patient's problems may have begun within minutes or hours after the onset of stress or may have been delayed. The *DSM-III-R* diagnostic criteria for adjustment disorder require that the dysfunction be evident within 3 months after occurrence of the stressor and persist for no longer than 6 months.

Clinicians may also seek a logical connection between the particular kind of stressor and the form or content of the patient's disturbance. In some cases, the patient may report being consciously preoccupied with the stressor. For example, the girl in the illustrative case presented above might have responded to questions about her poor grades by saying that worry about whether she would ever again be close to her father made it impossible to concentrate on her homework. In other cases, the connection between the symptoms and the stressor may be obscure. In the case of the same girl, the clinician might conjecture that her escalating misconduct represented an increasingly desperate attempt to regain the attention of her "lost" father. In more ambiguous circumstances, discerning a connection may depend on the creativity and clinical experience of the clinician, and these may introduce an element of unreliability into the diagnosis. A diagnosis of adjustment disorder is applicable only to patients whose current disturbance is clearly linked to a specific event, as would appear to be the case with the 17-year-old girl, since her misconduct, weight gain, and falling grades began soon after her parents separated and were not characteristic of her style of functioning before the event.

B. Evaluating the Level and Duration of Disturbance: The second decision-making process in the diagnosis of adjustment disorder is evaluation of the patient's specific signs and symptoms. A diagnosis of adjustment disorder is warranted only if the following circumstances apply: (1) The patient's symptoms are more severe than would be expected in the absence of some mental disorder; (2) the disturbance does not meet the criteria established for other mental disorders; and (3) the duration of symptoms does not exceed 6 months. A diagnosis of adjustment disorder is used for patients whose responses to a stressor are more severe than normally expected but somehow nonspecific or incomplete.

Clinicians must rely on experience in discriminating between stress reactions not associated with a mental disorder and those that might be part of an adjustment disorder. Since stressors vary in number, kind, and time of occurrence, only general guidelines can be provided. *DSM-III-R* indicates that the clinician should compare the patient's response with that of "an 'average' person in similar circumstances and with similar sociocultural values." However, "the severity of the reaction is not completely predictable from the severity of the stressor. Individuals who are particularly vulnerable may have a more severe form of the disorder following only a mild or moderate

stressor, whereas others may have only a mild form of the disorder in response to a marked and continuing stressor." The seriousness of a stressor is evaluated in terms of how much change it has caused, how central it has been to the person's life, how expected it was, whether it was a negative or a positive event, and whether it was shared or not.

The diagnosis of adjustment disorder is considered when a person's stress response is stronger or lasts longer than most other people's. Patients whose reactions exceed expectable limits often are an object of concern to those around them, so that patients may come to the physician's office accompanied by a friend or relative, or they may come alone but make a point of having done so at another's urging. Other people may have become irritated and impatient with the patient's behavior, and patients may report being criticized at work or at home for "taking it so hard" or "not being over it by now." Patients' responses often fail to meet others' expectations and in this way bring the patient to the attention of others.

The reactions of others may help the clinician determine whether or not the patient's response to stress may be diagnosed as adjustment disorder. Responses not indicative of mental disorder are eliminated from further diagnostic consideration but may be assigned a V code (see below) to identify the condition that was the focus of medical attention. Responses indicative of some mental disorder by virtue of inappropriate severity or duration are examined more closely so that a specific diagnosis may be assigned. In the illustrative case discussed above, the current disturbance appears to exceed the normal reaction expected of a 17-year-old responding to her parents' separation. Her symptoms are interfering with her functioning at school, have caused concern among her friends and teachers, and have brought her to the attention of legal authorities.

C. Ruling Out Other Mental Disorders (Excluding Personality and Developmental Disorders):

Illustrative case. A 64-year-old retired teacher came to an internist, seeking help for a feeling of constant exhaustion. She said that her troubles had begun months earlier with the death of her husband from kidney disease. She had thought then that her troubles were due to sadness at her loss, but now that they had lasted unchanged for nearly 6 months, she wondered whether she had "high blood pressure or low blood sugar or some such." She could not understand why she was constantly tired, since her sleeping patterns had not changed and she had continued her regular pattern of daily walks for exercise. The patient and her husband were both accomplished bridge players, and she had a reputation as an excellent cook, yet neither playing cards nor cooking was pleasurable any more. She still had a good appetite and attended her bridge club regularly, but her lack of enthusiasm was frequently commented on by other club members. The patient admitted that much of the time she felt that she would be better off if she had died with her husband, although she would not do anything to hurt herself. She found that she was able to get around and take care of herself, but life did not seem to have the meaning that it used to.

Physical examination and laboratory tests failed to show evidence of any physical disorder. The physician concluded that the symptoms were of psychologic origin.

Patients are not given a diagnosis of adjustment disorder if their stress response includes a specific, identifiable feature that meets the criteria for some other mental disorder. Patients for whom a diagnosis of adjustment disorder is inappropriate include those whose disturbances are organically caused, psychotic in nature, or limited to psychosexual problems, amnesia, loss of integration of consciousness, or loss of identity. Also eliminated are those whose current disturbances are a single instance of a continuing psychosexual, substance abuse, or impulse control problem; similarly excluded are manic episodes, panic attacks, or phobic avoidance. It should be noted that many of these excluded diagnostic categories are defined in part as an untoward reaction to a psychosocial stressor; examples include brief reactive psychosis, somatoform pain disorder, conversion disorders, psychogenic amnesia, psychogenic fugue, depersonalization disorder, and separation anxiety. However, each of these diagnoses has additional specific distinguishing features that differentiate it from the nonspecific category of adjustment disorder.

Patients with adjustment disorder complain of disturbances of mood (either anxiety or depression) and impaired social and occupational functioning (withdrawal, misconduct, inhibition). The disturbances are more severe or complicated than normally expected but not severe or complex enough to warrant a diagnosis of some other mental disorder characterized by inappropriate responses to problems encountered in everyday life. Patients with adjustment disorder usually satisfy some but not all of the criteria for generalized anxiety disorder, posttraumatic stress disorder, major

depressive disorder, dysthymia, cyclothymia, conduct disorder, or avoidant disorder. For example, the 17-year-old girl demonstrated misconduct, but since her difficulties were not "repetitive and persistent," the diagnosis of conduct disorder was not appropriate.

In the second illustrative case, the symptoms of fatigue, loss of pleasure in formerly satisfying activities, and passive death wishes characterize the spectrum of depressive disorders, and 5 diagnoses might be considered. As set forth in Table 35–1, they include uncomplicated bereavement, adjustment disorder, major depressive disorder, dysthymia, and posttraumatic stress disorder. The patient's symptoms exceed the normal reaction to the death of a spouse. They began soon after her husband's death and continued unchanged for 6 months; they also caused concern to her and those around her. Therefore, "uncomplicated bereavement" would be eliminated as a diagnostic consideration, and, by extension, the presence of a mental disorder would be confirmed. The duration of symptoms is insufficient for a diagnosis of dysthymia which requires that symptoms be continually present for at least 2 years. The death of the patient's husband from kidney disease does not meet the criteria for posttraumatic stress disorder, since that diagnosis requires that the precipitating stress be one that is beyond the range of usual human experience. A diagnosis of major depressive disorder is inappropriate, because the patient demonstrates only 3 of the 8 major symptoms. The diagnosis of adjustment disorder is thus reached by a process of exclusion.

D. Evaluating the Context of the Patient's Total Personality:

Illustrative case. A 56-year-old steelworker was brought by his daughter to a family practitioner. The daughter explained that although her father had always been considered "difficult at best," lately he had been "nearly impossible," and she was beginning to be concerned about his health. She reported that her father was known for saying things such as, "I wouldn't trust him as far as I could throw him." He usually kept to himself and was especially touchy about being swin-

Table 35–1. Differential diagnosis of depressed mood in bereavement.

	Type of Death	Duration of Symptoms	Type of Symptoms
Uncomplicated bereavement	Any type.	2–3 months; longer by social custom or relationship to deceased.	Limited to those normally expected.
Adjustment disorder	Any type.	Begin within 3 months; may be longer than normally expected; may not persist beyond 6 months.	Either impaired social or occupational functioning or symptoms in excess of those normally expected.
Major depressive disorder	Any type.	Every day for at least 2 weeks.	Dysphoric mood plus 4 out of 8 major symptoms (see Table 30–1).
Dysthymia	Any type.	Continually present for 2 years, with remissions of 2 months or less.	Depressive mood, but symptoms not severe enough for major depression; 3 out of 13 key symptoms present (see Table 30–1).
Posttraumatic stress disorder	Outside the range of usual experience.	Immediate or delayed; duration not specified.	Reexperiencing of trauma; numbing of responsiveness plus 2 out of 6 additional symptoms (see Table 31–7).

dled or taken advantage of. For the past 4 months, the father's suspicions had become almost frantic. He spent every waking moment worrying about some possible harm until he collapsed into a state bordering on exhaustion.

The patient indeed seemed haggard and exhausted, though hyperalert during the interview and nervously scanning the room as they talked. He nearly jumped off the examining table when a nurse knocked and entered the room. When asked to explain how he perceived "what the trouble was," the patient replied that he had merely come "to get my daughter off my back." He said that although he was very tired, he could not let up, because he knew that "guys from work had it in for me." He further explained that he had been out of work for 4 months since the local plant had closed and that previously he could "keep those bums in their place" because of his seniority but that now he was less able to defend himself and had to be constantly on the alert.

The patient was in touch with reality. His fears about his coworkers had the flavor of self-fulfilling prophecy and were not out of the realm of possibility, given his usual behavior in social situations. He showed no signs of abnormal thought patterns and was oriented as to time and place. He refused physical examinations and tests. In the absence of additional clinical information, the physician concluded that the patient's symptoms were probably due to psychologic causes.

The clinician must assess the patient's personality style to determine whether the current maladaptive response stands out as a unique and striking episode or whether it is simply one aspect of a consistently maladaptive pattern of relating to and thinking about the environment and oneself, as occurs in personality disorder. Against the background of the patient's total personality, a current emotional flare-up may be seen as an example of a general tendency to "make mountains out of molehills" that is typical of many personality disorders. In general, a diagnosis of adjustment disorder is made if no diagnosis of personality disorder or developmental disorder alone can account for all of the symptoms and signs; if symptoms of the current stress response are atypical for a preexisting personality disorder (eg, persistent, uncontrollable crying spells in compulsive personality disorder); or if current symptoms represent a dramatic worsening of a central feature in a preexisting personality disorder.

Of the patients discussed here, the symptoms of neither the 17-year-old student nor the retired teacher met the criteria for any of the personality disorders. Both patients were capable of warm personal relationships, and each had a well-developed sense of self. In contrast, the steelworker's usual manner of relating to his inner and outer world was compatible with a diagnosis of paranoid personality disorder. His current symptoms of exhaustion, extreme suspiciousness, and hypervigilance were judged to be a stress-related exacerbation of a long-standing and stable dysfunctional

personality style. Since the patient did not have symptoms that would lead to a diagnosis of organic delusional syndrome, paranoia, or paranoid schizophrenia, diagnoses of adjustment disorder and paranoid personality disorder were made.

Types of Adjustment Disorder

DSM-III-R describes 9 main symptom patterns in adjustment disorder and assigns a code to each. The codes and their corresponding symptoms are set forth in Table 35–2.

Of the illustrative cases discussed above, the stealing and school misbehavior of the student warrant a diagnosis of adjustment disorder with disturbance of conduct. Although the patient's overeating points to the possibility of an anxious or depressive emotional component, she denies any conscious experience of these mood disturbances, and a diagnosis of mixed disturbance of emotions and conduct is therefore inappropriate. The diagnosis of the older woman is the most straightforward; adjustment disorder with depressed mood is the appropriate diagnosis, since all of her symptoms (exhaustion, loss of pleasure, death wishes) lie within the spectrum of depression. The steelworker's predominant symptoms of excessive vigilance against possible attack justify a diagnosis of adjustment disorder with anxious mood.

V Codes for Conditions Not Attributable to Mental Disorder

DSM-III-R includes 13 V codes for "conditions that are a focus of attention or treatment but are not attributable to any of the mental disorders noted previously." These codes were adapted from a longer listing of similar conditions in *ICD-9-CM* (World Health Organization's *International Classification of Diseases, Injuries, and Causes of Death,* 9th ed., with clinical modification codes [CM]) and include such categories as malingering, adult antisocial behavior, noncompliance with medical treatment, and marital problems. The reactions of some patients in whom a diagnosis of adjustment disorder is being considered may fall within the limits of a normal and expectable response to a stressful life event; these patients would be assigned an appropriate V code to show the reason for their contact with a health facility. A V code may also be used when information is insufficient to deter-

Table 35–2. Types of adjustment disorder.

Code	Predominant Symptom Pattern
309.00	Depressed mood
309.24	Anxious mood
309.28	Mixed emotional features
309.30	Disturbance of conduct
309.40	Mixed disturbance of emotions and conduct
309.23	Work (or academic) inhibition
309.82	Physical complaints
309.83	Withdrawal
309.90	Adjustment disorder not otherwise specified

mine whether a mental disorder is present or when the focus of treatment is not related to a coexisting mental disorder, eg, treatment of an uncomplicated marital problem in a person with simple phobia.

The patients in each of the illustrative cases presented above might have been assigned a diagnosis with a V code if their symptoms had been within normal and expectable limits. The diagnosis for the retired teacher might have been uncomplicated bereavement if her symptoms had not exceeded those of the *DSM-III-R* description for such bereavement. The diagnosis in the case of the high school student might have been childhood and adolescent antisocial behavior, which describes isolated antisocial acts of children and adolescents. A diagnosis of phase of life problem or other life circumstance problem might have been assigned to the steelworker had his symptoms been those normally associated with developmental or circumstantial changes such as beginning school, changing jobs, or obtaining a divorce.

Natural History

A. Course and Outcome: Empirical data show that the course and outcome of adjustment disorder are less severe and disabling than those of other major psychiatric disorders. A large study of navy personnel ranging in age from adolescence to middle age who were assigned a *DSM-II* diagnosis of transient situational disturbance showed that the problems of persons with this diagnosis tended to be less severe with regard to chronicity, length of treatment, and disposition than those of other major psychiatric disorders (Looney and Gunderson, 1978). The course of an episode of transient situational disturbance was found to be roughly one-half as long as that of neurotic disturbances and one-fourth the length of psychotic episodes (15 days versus 29 days and 65 days); about one and one-half times as many patients with transient situational disturbance returned to their previous level of functioning compared to neurotic patients (90% versus 66%); and the ratios for patients with transient situational disturbance compared to patients with personality disorder (2:1) and psychoses (3:1) were even higher.

During follow-up 3–4 years later, only one in 4 persons who had received a diagnosis of transient situational disturbance was found to have recurrent psychiatric problems requiring treatment. Among those who did later develop disorders, personality disorders were found to be the most common type (47%), with neurotic disorders (25%), additional episodes of transient situational disturbance (21%), and psychotic disorders (7%) following in order of frequency of occurrence.

B. Differential Course and Outcome in Adolescents and Adults: A study at the University of Iowa (Andreasen and Wasek, 1980; Andreasen and Hoenk, 1982) found important differences in the expression of adjustment disorder in adolescents and in adults. In this study, adolescents showed more serious disturbance than did adults with regard to symptoms, required length of treatment, and duration of symp-

toms before diagnosis. Adolescents also differed from adults with regard to their main presenting symptoms. The diagnosis of adjustment disorder with disturbance of conduct was 3 times more likely to be used in adolescents than in adults (77% versus 25%); adults were more likely than adolescents to report depressive symptoms (87% versus 64%). Although adults were more likely to report thoughts of suicide than were adolescents (36% versus 29%), nearly all adolescents who did report such thoughts were likely to attempt suicide (25% of the sample, or 86% of those reporting such thoughts, versus 17% and 47% for adults).

Prognosis

The patient's age has been found to be one of the most significant predictors of the outcome of adjustment disorder. In the University of Iowa sample, about twice as many adolescents as adults experienced an episode of some confirmed psychiatric disorder during a 5-year follow-up period (56% versus 29%). The findings of both the University of Iowa and the navy studies showed that regardless of their age group, patients with behavior problems were more likely to develop an illness later diagnosed as antisocial personality disorder. The navy study also found that after treatment, patients with multiple psychiatric disorders were less likely to return to their previous level of functioning.

In summary, available empirical evidence does indicate that adjustment disorder is less severe than other disorders with regard to both course and outcome. However, for some patients, especially adolescents, an episode of adjustment disorder may be characterized by distress that is not self-limited and may be recurrent.

Epidemiology

A. General Prevalence: Adjustment disorder is thought to be common, although few empirical data on its prevalence are available. The scarcity of information may be due in part to the short time the diagnosis has been used as currently defined. The definition of situationally induced disorders has been substantially revised; eg, the shift from the category of transient situational disturbance in *DSM-II* to adjustment disorder in *DSM-III* has changed the defining characteristics as well; the new definition requires that the stress be overwhelming, that the symptoms be transient, and that the diagnosis not be used in conjunction with any other axis I disorder. The changes in the definition make earlier data on stress-induced disorders of questionable value in establishing epidemiology.

The limited data available support the view that adjustment disorder is common in the psychiatric population, especially among adolescents. The diagnosis was used in roughly 20% of cases classified in *DSM-III* field trials. About 10% of adults and 30% of adolescents in this sample were assigned a diagnosis of adjustment disorder. Additional data from a large sample at the University of Iowa Hospitals and Clinics show that a diagnosis of adjustment disorder was used in about 5% of newly diagnosed psychiatric inpatients and an assumed "appreciably higher" percentage of outpatients.

No data are available on the prevalence of adjustment disorder in the general population.

B. Differential Prevalence in Adolescents and Adults: The diagnosis of adjustment disorder is frequently made in adolescents. It is not clear whether the disorder is actually more common during adolescence or whether there are other reasons why the diagnostic category is more commonly used in patients in that age group.

Adolescence has been described by theoreticians such as Anna Freud (1958) as a time of turmoil during which the adolescent must struggle to master challenging requirements of adult functioning within a context of heightened conflict caused by surging sexual and physical development. This viewpoint remains popular in spite of arguments and evidence to the contrary (see Chapters 6 and 7). Those who believe that significant distress is a common response to physiologic and cultural events that normally occur during adolescence may therefore automatically classify cases of adolescent psychologic disturbance as examples of adjustment disorder. In some cases, patients with more severe psychologic disturbances may be misdiagnosed.

Frequent use of the diagnosis of adjustment disorder during adolescence may simply reflect its function as a provisional diagnosis. A crucial requirement of many alternative diagnoses is that the observed disturbance be long-standing and persistent; however, many psychiatric problems begin or first appear during adolescence and persist from then on. The ambiguous picture may force the diagnostician to use the category of adjustment disorder as a nonspecific provisional diagnosis until the long-range clinical picture is clarified.

Researchers who have studied the use of this diagnosis have found that some clinicians overuse the category because they are concerned about the adverse effects of applying pejorative psychiatric labels such as alcoholism or antisocial personality disorder to young people; overusing the diagnosis of adjustment disorder is perceived as less harmful than stigmatizing people for life as having had some more ominous diagnosis.

Careful epidemiologic studies should eliminate such diagnostic inaccuracies, so that a more valid estimate of the prevalence of adjustment disorder can be made. Meanwhile, the diagnosis should be used with discretion; in an adolescent, there should be strong evidence that current problems are related to some specific event or to some identifiable aspect of the adolescent experience. When the diagnosis is unclear after careful assessment, a diagnosis of atypical psychosis or unspecified mental disorder (nonpsychotic) should be used instead.

Etiology & Pathogenesis

A. Presumed Causal Mechanism: Stress-related disorders are a disruption of the normal process of adaptation to stressful life experiences. Models of normal adaptation to stressful events, such as death of a loved one, assault, or accident, have been developed by Lindemann (1944), Pollock (1977), and Horowitz (1976), among others. In the Horowitz model of adaptation (see Chapter 5), the person experiencing stress passes through regular stages of response to a painful life change. In the stage of **outcry** (the first stage), the person protests that what has happened cannot be true. This brief stage is followed by stages of **intrusion** and **denial,** during which the person is either painfully aware of or oblivious to the new reality. During the stage of **working through** the event, the person steadily becomes better able to integrate the change. The **completion** stage (the final stage) is marked by function at or above the prestress level.

In adjustment disorder and other stress-related disorders, this process of adaptation to stress does not proceed to completion. The presumed cause is **psychic overload,** ie, a level of intrapsychic strain that exceeds the individual's ability to cope and may therefore disrupt normal functioning and cause psychologic or somatic symptoms.

The pattern of disruption of adaptation may take many forms. Some persons become caught in a seemingly endless stage of denial; they act as if the stressful event had never occurred, avoid all reminders of the stress, and remain emotionally numb or isolated. In other people, intrusive symptoms predominate; individuals become so painfully aware of the stressor that they are unable to sleep or control the flood of incoming emotions and images associated with the event. Still others oscillate between symptoms of intrusion and denial, with no overall change in their psychologic assimilation of the stressor. Any of these cognitive-emotional patterns may be accompanied by difficulties in interpersonal relationships. In all patients, it is the persistence of unwanted emotions and images and the feeling of being powerless to stop them that distinguish dysfunctional from normal adaptational responses.

B. Contributing Factors: Several models have been developed to explain why some people can handle stress and even grow as a result of the experience, whereas others develop distress of psychopathologic proportions. Most comprehensive models take into account the interaction of the stressor, the situation, and the person.

1. Stressors–Stressors are of 2 general types: **Shock-type stressors** are time-limited events; **continuous stressors** are ongoing situations. Most descriptions of adaptation to stress concentrate on shock-type stressors. However, results of the University of Iowa study found that continuous stressors were more commonly cited than shock-type stressors as precipitating causes of psychiatric disorders. Adults usually developed adjustment disorder in conjunction with continuous stressors such as ongoing problems in marriage, finances, work, or school; in adolescents, stressors were more likely to be problems with school, parental rejection, or the parents' marital problems. Shock-type stressors such as death of a loved one or moving to a new area were less commonly cited precipitating factors.

Research on shock-type stressors shows that the degree of undesirable change they cause is the most significant aspect of their ability to cause strain. Other characteristics that influence the amount of strain produced by a stressor include whether the event was sudden or anticipated, whether it was central or peripheral to the life of the individual, and whether it was culturally shared or experienced in social isolation. The characteristics of continuous stressors that cause strain have not been as clearly defined.

2. Situational context–The situational context of a stressor is instrumental in determining whether an individual's response to stress will be functional or dysfunctional. The availability of material and social supports or handicaps can mitigate or exacerbate the strains of adaptation. Pertinent factors in the individual's material environment include personal and general economic conditions, occupational and recreational opportunities, and weather conditions. Factors in the social environment include the availability of social supports such as family, friends, neighbors, and cultural or religious support groups. These extrapersonal elements create a supportive or nonsupportive climate for adaptation.

3. Intrapersonal factors–Intrapersonal factors are considered to be the most crucial in determining whether or not the response to stress will be normal or dysfunctional. There is no clear correlation between the severity of the stressor and the severity of stress response and between the level of situational adversity and the severity of response; ie, not all persons with roughly similar stressors and environmental circumstances develop similar dysfunctional responses to stress. Some are vulnerable to even minor stressful events, whereas others show an amazing resilience in the face of the most traumatic experiences.

Intrapersonal vulnerability to stressful life experiences may be general or specific. General factors include limitations in social skills and in adaptive capacities such as intelligence, flexibility, and range of coping strategies. The presence of chronic disorders such as organic mental disorder, mental retardation, psychotic disorder, or personality disorder is thought to limit the general adaptive capacity of an individual. Vulnerability to specific types of stressful events or circumstances may arise from relevant life traumas, unresolved conflicts, or developmental issues; eg, research has shown that women who experience loss of the mother in infancy are more likely to develop serious depressive episodes in response to adult losses than are women who did not have this experience. People who have unresolved conflicts about expressing aggressive impulses respond to physical assault with a mixture of phobic and counterphobic activities, ie, alternately avoiding and provoking fights with people who are similar to their assailants. Individuals who lack the capacity to make choices based on their own wishes and feelings rather than those of others may respond to the lack of structure in retirement with a help-less sense of directionless floundering. Each of these general and specific intrapersonal factors combines with extrapersonal factors and characteristics of the stressor to produce the individual's stress response.

Treatment

A. Controversy About Treatment: The *DSM-III-R* definition of adjustment disorder has engendered controversy about the advisability of treatment. On the one hand, the disorder is expected to eventually remit after the stressor ceases or, if the stressor persists, when a new level of adaptation is achieved, and it may not persist for longer than 6 months. This postulated spontaneous remission has led some to argue that treatment is unnecessary and wasteful of time, effort, and money. Others have suggested that treatment may actually have adverse effects; ie, it may interfere with normal coping processes and result in worsening symptoms and delayed resolution of the problem.

On the other hand, adjustment disorder is also defined as a maladaptive response to stress that includes exaggerated symptoms and social or occupational impairment. Those who recommend treatment are responding to those features which mark a response to stress as abnormal rather than normal and which thereby warrant a diagnosis of mental disorder. Clinicians who favor treatment point to the excessive symptoms and suggest that these must be brought within manageable limits before the patient can cope positively with the stress. They also point out that many types of adjustment disorder are so labeled because duration of symptoms may have exceeded the usual point of spontaneous remission. Such longer-lasting disturbances sustain themselves and require some means of interrupting the downward spiral if potentially serious effects on work and social relationships are to be avoided.

Proponents of crisis intervention theory, such as Caplan (1964) and Langsley and Kaplan (1968), offer additional arguments in favor of treatment. They maintain that a crisis caused by a particular situation (as occurs in adjustment disorder) offers an ideal opportunity for psychosocial treatment that goes beyond immediate remedies to act as a catalyst for positive change in coping strategies. Persons who develop inappropriate responses in times of stress are thought to have some general or specific vulnerability to stress. Since, by definition, the normal coping strategies of such people are in a state of disarray during stress, clinicians argue that it should be possible to influence the eventual reorganization of their impulses and defenses so as to favor increased positive adaptation.

B. General Recommendations: The general recommendation for treatment of adjustment disorder is time-limited treatment with scheduled periodic reassessments to determine the need for continued treatment. The primary goals of such treatment are to relieve symptoms and assist patients in achieving a level of adaptation that at least equals their level of functioning before the stressful event. A secondary goal is to foster positive change whenever possible—especially in areas still vulnerable to recurrent stress-related disorders.

C. Psychosocial Treatment Methods: Mental health professionals most commonly recommend some form of psychosocial treatment for patients with adjustment disorder. In the University of Iowa sample, 70% of adults and 85% of adolescents participated in psychosocial treatment. Common psychosocial treatment methods include individual psychotherapy, behavior therapy, family therapy, and support group experiences.

The rationale for the widespread use of psychosocial treatments for adjustment disorder arises from common assumptions about the cause of the disorder. Since adjustment disorder is generally thought to arise from vulnerabilities in the patient's psychosocial functioning, treatment measures are designed to have an impact on whatever habits, conflicts, developmental inadequacies, or disturbing social symptoms are thought to be the source of the patient's problem. It is therefore assumed that this type of treatment holds the greatest promise for preventing recurrent disorders.

1. Individual psychotherapy–The most common psychosocial treatment for adjustment disorder is some form of individual psychotherapy. Fifty percent of adolescents and 60% of adults in the University of Iowa sample participated in individual psychotherapy. The brief psychodynamic psychotherapy developed by Horowitz and Kaltreider (1980) is a good example of the typical approach to individual psychotherapy. In this approach, the patient's problems are seen to result from the meanings assigned by the individual to the stressful event and expressed by activation of unresolved conflicts; previously latent negative self-images; earlier traumatic experiences; and developmental inadequacies. The goal of treatment is to remove these blocks to adaptation so that normal developmental processes can resume. Common psychodynamic techniques of supportive or expressive psychotherapy are used to discover these meanings and to make needed remedial adjustments. Special emphasis is placed on clarifying links between the current stressor and earlier experiences. The relationship with the therapist may be examined for clues to relevant issues, and the patient and therapist may talk openly about the similarity between the parental relationship and the therapeutic relationship. Treatment tries to counteract maladaptive styles of responding to stressful situations, whether these reactions be overcontrolled (ie, not admitting any emotional impact) or undercontrolled (ie, being overwhelmed by the thoughts or feelings related to stressful events).

2. Family therapy–The second most common form of psychosocial treatment for adjustment disorder is family therapy (see Chapter 48). Twenty percent of adolescents and 5% of adults in the University of Iowa sample participated in family therapy. In this approach, the focus of diagnosis and treatment is shifted from the individual to the system of relationships in which the individual is involved. The problems of the person identified as the patient are symptomatic of a disordered or disrupted social network that both affects and is affected by all of its members. Treatment is designed to alter the functioning of the social network, and when possible, all relevant family members are included in treatment sessions. Techniques vary widely but are usually characterized as more active and directive than those used in psychodynamic approaches. Therapists may make comments, give directions, or assign tasks designed to promote clear communication between family members, especially about family rules or interaction patterns that cause problems. Family therapy has become increasingly popular over the last 3 decades. Since it is specifically intended to treat problems that affect the entire family, its use should be seriously considered in adjustment disorder associated with stressful developmental milestones in the lives of either adults (birth of a child, mid-life transition, retirement) or children (beginning school, coping with adolescence, leaving home). It is also helpful in situations such as family bereavements and marital problems (separation, divorce).

3. Behavior therapy–Behavior therapy is usually conducted on an individual, one-on-one basis but differs significantly in theory and technique from individual psychodynamic psychotherapy. In behavior therapy, the patient's problems are seen as the result of habitually dysfunctional patterns of responding to situations. The goal of treatment is to replace ineffective adaptive response patterns with successful ones. The diagnostic process focuses on identifying the responses that cause problems and the conditions within the person or environment that both trigger and sustain these responses. Once these response patterns have been identified, modeling (with the patient following the therapist's behavioral example), coaching, didactic presentations, and carefully designed reinforcement schedules are used to alter them. Treatment is sometimes provided on an inpatient basis, so that better control may be obtained over the patient's behavior and its consequences. Behavior therapy has usually been considered most appropriate for problems of impulse control, which may occur in adjustment disorder with disturbance of conduct. It is probably for this reason that this approach was used for 10% of adolescents in the University of Iowa sample.

4. Self-help groups–Group psychotherapy has not been commonly used for adjustment disorder; the University of Iowa sample does not even list group psychotherapy among the offered treatments. However, self-help groups, in which people who have experienced similar stressful life events come together without a professional facilitator, are increasing in popularity. This fact has alerted mental health professionals to the demand for and benefit of such groups. Group experiences with or without a professional facilitator provide a context in which members may consider and compare their responses to similar life experiences. Group members often gain reassurance from discovering that many of their frightening emotional experiences are common and therefore not "crazy," as they had feared. Members also benefit from having an arena in which they can talk about painful topics without worrying about being a burden to family and friends. Within the group, members exchange advice, share coping strategies, and provide support and encouragement. Some self-help groups also provide new social networks to replace those lost through events such as death or divorce. The one problem with group psychotherapy and self-help groups is availability; it is sometimes difficult to locate or organize groups of people with a background of similar stressful events. Community service agencies may be a good source of information on ongoing groups and may be willing to assist in attempts to form new support groups.

D. Biomedical Treatment Methods: Medication may be the most commonly used treatment for adjustment disorder, since self-medication with alcohol, caffeine, over-the-counter medications, and street drugs is undoubtedly widespread. Treatment of symptoms of depression and anxiety (headaches, appetite and sleep disturbances, gastrointestinal complaints) with drugs prescribed by physicians (especially sedatives and antianxiety and antidepressant medications) is common also. In contrast to over-the-counter and street drugs, prescription drugs have the potential advantage of being carefully chosen and continually monitored.

Mental health professionals usually do not treat adjustment disorder with medication, however. Only 15% of adolescents and 30% of adults in the University of Iowa sample received medication, either as the sole form of treatment or in combination with psychosocial treatments. Reasons for not using medication include concerns that their effect is temporary (that they will last only as long as the prescribed treatment period); that alleviating symptoms only masks the real problem or interferes with the motivation to find a real, lasting solution; and that patients may develop either psychologic or physiologic dependence.

The reluctance of mental health professionals to use medication for adjustment disorder is shown by the fact that although 50% of adults and 25% of adolescents in the University of Iowa sample reported 4 or more symptoms of depression, only 9% of adults and 7% of adolescents were given antidepressant medication. In general, concerns about side effects and the length of time required to achieve effective results with antidepressants persuade most clinicians that their use should be limited to patients with major depressive disorder. Klerman and Weissman (1981) have argued that this assumption should be reexamined and that data should be collected about the effectiveness of antidepressant medication in treatment of adjustment disorders.

When used, medications are generally considered only adjuncts to treatment or as backup treatment when psychologic treatment methods are either unavailable or unacceptable to the patient. Medications are used as adjunctive treatment when patients feel that their symptoms are out of control. In these patients, medications are used to bring distress within tolerable limits, so that the patient's coping strategies may be effectively mobilized. Whenever medications are used, the clinician should prescribe the lowest effective dosage and the shortest possible duration, together with frequent monitoring of efficacy and side effects.

SUMMARY

Adjustment disorder is one of the more common psychologic disorders for which patients seek professional help, especially among general practitioners. For this reason, all clinicians should have a good working knowledge of the 4 decision-making procedures used to diagnose adjustment disorder. These include (1) establishing a relationship to a psychosocial stressor; (2) evaluating the level and duration of disturbance; (3) ruling out other mental disorders (excluding personality or developmental disorder); and (4) evaluating the context of the patient's total personality. Patients with adjustment disorder demonstrate inadequate or incomplete adaptation to life stresses. The treatment of choice is a brief psychosocial treatment designed to enhance the patient's ability to cope with and adapt to the stressful incident. When patients feel that their symptoms are out of control, special psychosocial techniques or appropriate medications may be used to alleviate symptoms to the point that the patient can attempt to cope with the stressful situation.

REFERENCES

Andreasen NC, Hoenk PR: The predictive value of adjustment disorders: A follow-up study. *Am J Psychiatry* 1982;**139:** 584.

Andreasen NC, Wasek P: Adjustment disorders in adolescents and adults. *Arch Gen Psychiatry* 1980;**37:**1166.

Caplan G: *Principles of Preventive Psychiatry.* Basic Books, 1964.

Freud A: Adolescence. *Psychoanal Study Child* 1958;**13:**255.

Horowitz MJ: *Stress Response Syndromes.* Jason Aronson, 1976.

Horowitz MJ, Kaltreider N: Psychotherapy of stress response syndromes. Pages 162–183 in: *Specialized Techniques in Individual Psychotherapy.* Karasu T, Bellak L (editors). Brunner/Mazel, 1980.

Klerman GL, Weissman MM: Affective responses to stressful life events. Program of the National Institute of Mental Health Conference on Prevention of Stress-Related Psychiatric Disorders, University of California at San Francisco, December 1981.

Langsley D, Kaplan D: *The Treatment of Families in Crisis.* Grune & Stratton, 1968.

Lindemann E: Symptomatology and management of acute grief. *Am J Psychiatry* 1944;**101**:141.

Looney JG, Gunderson EK: Transient situational disturbances: Course and outcome. *Am J Psychiatry* 1978;**135**:660.

Pollock GH: The ghost that will not go away: Specificity theory today. *J Am Acad Psychoanal* 1977;**5**:421.

Pollock GH: The psychosomatic specificity concept: Its evaluation and reevaluation. *Ann Psychoanal* 1977;**5**:141.

Personality Disorders

36

Charles R. Marmar, MD

Patients with personality disorder are common both in medical and in psychiatric practice. Such people frequently make pressing demands for treatment of their numerous complaints while at the same time resisting appropriate treatment recommendations. Their lack of cooperation may cause resentment and possibly even alienation and burnout in the health care professionals who treat them. Although this chapter focuses on the difficulties encountered by health care professionals in caring for patients with personality (character) disorders, the problems caused by such individuals may be set against the broader perspective of society at large, where they are among the most disruptive elements in political, corporate, and professional positions of leadership. The frequently overriding needs of such individuals for self-aggrandizement, their diminished capacity for understanding and respecting the needs of others, and their mistrust and emotional instability lead to maladaptive behavior, including manipulation and exploitation of others. Such individuals are limited in their capacity to participate in mutual give-and-take with another person.

In this chapter, each major personality disorder is discussed from 2 perspectives, that of formal psychiatric nosology and that of management of the medically or surgically ill patient with an impaired personality.

Medical illness may have a recurrent, predictable psychologic meaning for patients with specific personality disorders. Hidden motives (covert agendas) in the patient's relationship with the physician may lead to problems of overutilization or underutilization of the health care system, substance abuse, and potential negative reactions in the physician. This chapter presents coping strategies for the physician that may increase the chances of patient compliance with medical or surgical treatment and minimize medical complications and interpersonal problems involved in the care of such patients.

Characteristics of Personality Disorders

DSM-III defines **personality traits** as "enduring patterns of perceiving, relating to, and thinking about the environment and oneself . . . exhibited in a wide range of important social and personal contexts." It is only when these patterns are "inflexible and maladaptive and cause either significant impairment in social or occupational functioning or subjective distress" that they constitute **personality disorders.** Such personality disturbances can be recognized by adolescence or earlier and commonly continue through adulthood; the pathologic characteristics have their precursors in early developmental disturbances and remain as enduring qualities of a person. A diagnosis of personality disorder is not appropriate if the disturbance in functioning is episodic, since the symptoms of personality disorder should represent the person's *stable* characteristics and social functioning.

Because elements of character disorders appear early in life, childhood and adolescent disorders correlate strongly with adult personality disorders. For example, a child with conduct disorder frequently presents as an adult with antisocial personality disorder. Similarly, schizoid disorder of childhood or adolescence is linked to schizoid personality disorder of adulthood; avoidant disorder of childhood or adolescence may become avoidant personality disorder of adulthood; oppositional disorder of childhood may become passive-aggressive personality disorder of adulthood; and identity disorder of childhood may become borderline personality disorder in adulthood.

Because individuals with personality disorders exhibit recurrent maladaptive strategies in their interpersonal relationships, they may be markedly dissatisfied with the impact of their behavior on others and with their inability to function effectively. The resulting distress is prevalent in personality disorders, contrary to earlier conceptualizations, which asserted that these patients were free from distress. Anxiety and depression are especially common, and "disturbances of mood, frequently involving depression or anxiety, are common and may even be the individual's chief complaint."

Substantial evidence suggests that individuals with personality disorders—which by definition are long-standing and at times lifelong disturbances in functioning—are at greater risk for various other psychiatric disorders, with symptomatic flare-ups occurring during occupational or personal stresses or developmental milestones (adolescence, mid-life crisis, aging, etc).

DIFFERENTIATION BETWEEN PERSONALITY DISORDERS & OTHER PSYCHIATRIC DISORDERS

Differentiation of Personality Disorders From Neurotic Disorders

Because anxiety and depression are common both in personality disorders and in neurotic disorders, these symptoms cannot be used as differential diagnostic criteria; however, other factors are useful in making a differential diagnosis. Individuals with personality disorders have **alloplastic** defenses and react to stress by attempting to change the *external* environment. For example, such patients often deal with a potential disappointment by threatening to retaliate and in that way manipulate another person to gratify rather than disappoint them. In contrast, patients with neurotic disorders have **autoplastic** defenses and react to stress by changing their *internal* psychologic processes. For example, neurotic patients might rationalize that a disappointment is of no great importance.

Another distinguishing factor is the difference in self-awareness manifested in patients with the 2 types of disorders. In patients with personality disorders, character deficits are frequently perceived by the patient as **ego-syntonic,** ie, acceptable, unobjectionable, and part of the self. For example, patients with such a disorder disavow personal responsibility for hurting another person, have difficulty in appreciating the pain they have inflicted on another, and attribute blame to another person. In contrast, personal shortcomings in individuals with neurotic disorders are perceived by the patient as **ego-dystonic,** ie, unacceptable, objectionable, and alien to the self. Patients with neurotic disorders blame and chastise themselves for disappointing or hurting a valued person through their shortcomings.

Differentiation of Personality Disorders From Psychotic Disorders

Although there may be severe disturbances in social and occupational functioning in individuals with personality disorders, persistent psychotic features such as formal thought disorder (as manifested by loosening of associations), delusions, and hallucinations are absent. Transient psychotic states, or "micropsychotic episodes," in people with severe borderline personality disorders are important exceptions (see below). The quality of the psychotic disturbance in borderline personality disorder is different from that in schizophreniform psychoses; episodes are short-lived, directly related to a given situation, and usually self-limited, and they normally do not require hospitalization or medication. (See Chapter 29 for discussion of brief reactive psychoses.)

Differentiation of Personality Disorders From Organic Mental Disorders

Individuals with uncomplicated personality disorders have a clear sensorium; are oriented as to time, place, and person; and show normal intellectual functioning, so that memory for recent or remote events, fund of general knowledge, ability to perform calculations, and so on are within normal limits. Individuals with personality disorders may of course develop organic mental syndromes later in life and in certain cases may be at greater risk for such disorders (eg, through sustained alcohol or substance abuse). Multiple diagnoses are warranted in such patients.

GROUPING OF PERSONALITY DISORDERS

DSM-III groups the personality disorders into 3 clusters:

Cluster 1 – Paranoid, schizoid, and schizotypal personality disorders. Individuals seem **odd** or **eccentric.**

Cluster 2 – Histrionic, narcissistic, antisocial, and borderline personality disorders. Individuals are **dramatic, erratic,** and **labile.**

Cluster 3 – Avoidant, dependent, compulsive, and passive-aggressive personality disorders. Individuals seem **fearful, inhibited,** and **anxious.**

PARANOID PERSONALITY DISORDER

Systoms & Signs

The diagnostic criteria for paranoid personality disorder are summarized in Table 36–1.

According to *DSM-III-R* the essential features of paranoid personality disorder include "a pervasive and unwarranted tendency . . . to interpret the actions of people as deliberately demeaning or threatening . . . ." These symptoms and signs are characteristic of the patient's long-term functioning and are not episodic in character or limited to particular episodes of illness. They are also associated with significant impairment in work and personal relationships. Patients are hostile, stubborn, and defensive, and they avoid intimacy. They are rigid and uncompromising, interested primarily in inanimate objects rather than human relations, extremely sensitive to rank, and disinterested in the arts and aesthetics.

Natural History & Prognosis

Systematic data are not yet available on this disorder.

Differential Diagnosis

In paranoid schizophrenia and paranoid disorders, there are persistent psychotic symptoms, including delusions and hallucinations, that are not features of paranoid personality disorder. Individuals with para-

Table 36–1. *DSM-III-R* diagnostic criteria for paranoid personality disorder (coded on axis II).

The diagnostic criteria for the personality disorder refer to behaviors or traits that are characteristic of the person's recent (past year) and long-term functioning (generally since adolescence or early adulthood). The constellation of behaviors or traits causes either significant impairment in social or occupational functioning or subjective distress. Behaviors or traits limited to episodes of illness are not considered in making a diagnosis of personality disorder.

A. A pervasive and unwarranted tendency, beginning by early adulthood and present in a variety of contexts, to interpret the actions of people as deliberately demeaning or threatening, as indicated by at least 4 of the following:
   (1) Expects, without sufficient basis, to be exploited or harmed by others.
   (2) Questions, without justification, the loyalty or trustworthiness of friends or associates.
   (3) Reads hidden demeaning or threatening meanings into benign remarks or events, eg, suspects that a neighbor put out trash early to cause annoyance.
   (4) Bears grudges or is unforgiving of insults or slights.
   (5) Is reluctant to confide in others because of unwarranted fear that the information will be used against him or her.
   (6) Is easily slighted and quick to react with anger or to counterattack.
   (7) Questions, without justification, fidelity of spouse or sexual partner.
B. Does not occur exclusively during the course of schizophrenia or a delusional disorder.

noid personality disorder may develop paranoid psychoses, however, at which time an additional diagnosis is justified.

Illustrative Case

A 52-year-old man was referred for psychiatric evaluation after a medical workup revealed no basis for his persistent headaches. The headaches had begun 6 months earlier, at about the same time that he became preoccupied with the possibility that his supervisor wanted to fire him. They had an argument about the vacation schedule, and he felt that he was being taken advantage of unfairly, since coworkers with less seniority had more favorable schedules. After the argument, he had seen his supervisor joking with one of the other mechanics and had assumed that he was the object of their derision.

Although emotionally distant, the patient had been a loyal, serious, hardworking, and productive employee and had stayed at the same company for the past 18 years. Although he could always be counted on to do a good job, he tended to be excluded by other workers, who found him unable to relax and make jokes. He had been married for 25 years to a school librarian and described his marriage as satisfactory: "She's always there, but she doesn't make a lot of demands on me." They had decided not to have children, because "they're disruptive, unpredictable, demanding, take whatever they can get out of you, and then go off on their own."

In the interview, the patient appeared tense and vig-

ilant, and he seemed to search for verbal or nonverbal clues indicating that the interviewer did not have his best interests at heart. When the interviewer suggested that he might have provoked his supervisor, he snapped back irritably that the interviewer, like most people, misunderstood him. The patient was understandable and goal-directed in his thinking, and there was no evidence of well-formed delusions or hallucinatory experiences. He admitted that he might be overreacting to the altercation with his supervisor. He noted that this had happened several times before and that in each instance he had been later reassured that he was a valued employee.

Epidemiology

Paranoid personality disorder is more commonly diagnosed in men than in women. A familial pattern has been suggested (see below). The relationship of paranoid personality disorder to paranoid schizophrenia and paranoid disorder is uncertain.

Etiology & Pathogenesis

The specific causes of paranoid personality disorder are not known. However, genetic predisposition may play a role, and if a patient has paranoid personality disorder, the chances are good that someone in the family has a paranoid disorder. Early childhood deprivation or child abuse alone or in concert with genetic susceptibility may lead to a paranoid sense of mistrust.

Treatment

An honest, respectful attitude is important in psychotherapeutic treatment of the patient with paranoid personality disorder. The therapist must pay attention to the degree of closeness shown toward the patient, since too much intimacy, warmth, and empathy may be seen as an intrusive attempt at control. Deep psychologic interpretations tend to increase feelings of suspicion rather than clarify conflicts about warded-off feelings or intentions. The therapist can reduce the chances of being perceived as yet another enemy by insisting on prompt and repeated examination of the patient's distorted image of the therapist (reality testing) in a firm but noncritical way.

The therapist should readily acknowledge and confirm any errors, feeling of irritation, or lapse in consideration, because patients with paranoid personality disorder will interpret denials of such behavior as proof of covert persecutory intentions. A tactful and polite but not overly elaborate apology by the therapist can do much to restore the patient's trust.

Paranoid Personality Disorder in Medical Practice

The paranoid patient's underlying mistrust, hypersensitivity to slights, fear of dependency, and underlying sense of shame and vulnerability are heightened during illness or even with the threat of illness. A trusting relationship between the physician and the patient is essential to ensure compliance with surgical or pharmacologic treatments. A low-key and friendly but not overly intimate attitude on the part of the physician effectively counters the paranoid patient's dual expectations of being disregarded as worthless on the one hand and being intruded upon on the other. In the first few visits, the therapist can ask the patient about previous doctor-patient relationships, especially about both the helpful and the irritating elements. It is worthwhile to inquire whether the patient has ever abruptly terminated treatment with another physician because of actual or fantasied injury or betrayal. Such an inquiry is valuable with any patient but may be particularly informative in establishing an effective working relationship with a paranoid patient, since the physician can avoid the pitfalls encountered in the patient's previous relationships with health care professionals.

A physician who is being berated by a paranoid patient and who can acknowledge—without being defensive or attacking or encouraging the patient's distorted view—that the patient's pain and fear aroused by aspects of the physician-patient relationship are real is creating an invaluable opportunity to provide an atmosphere in which the patient can feel safe in working toward clarification of past difficulties. For example, a patient who developed unanticipated side effects from an antibiotic threatened to discontinue the medication until the physician explained that although the side effects were real, they were not potentially lethal, as the patient had feared, and that the physician had not deliberately withheld information about the toxicity of the drug. For paranoid patients, the primary problem in the doctor-patient relationship is frequently not any actual failure in treatment but rather the patient's subjectively distorted image of the physician as an individual with malevolent intentions toward the patient, a fear that proves "justified" when difficulties occur in diagnosis or treatment.

In discussion of the hostile, suspicious, and recalcitrant patient in medical practice, Dennis Farrell offers the following case (personal communication) as an example of the need to provide clear explanations of all procedures undertaken by the medical staff in treating such patients.

Illustrative case. A 42-year-old man with paranoid personality disorder who had presented at a medical clinic for treatment had a history of changing doctors and of not complying with prescribed medical regimens. The patient scowled when he was handed a prescription for medication, and the medical student assigned to work with the patient noted the patient's reaction aloud. The patient muttered a comment about "cheap medication," and the student asked him to explain the remark. It appeared that when the dosage of the patient's medication had recently been changed, the patient had not received an adequate explanation and had merely been told that he was receiving the same medication. The patient concluded that the doctors had decided to give him some cheap, second-rate medicine because he was a clinic patient. To the patient's way of thinking, there was no good reason why the same medication should look different except that

it was in some way inferior. When the medical student expressed genuine interest in the patient and offered a clear explanation of why the dosage had been changed, the patient felt comfortable in taking the medication as prescribed.

SCHIZOID PERSONALITY DISORDER

Symptoms & Signs

The diagnostic criteria for schizoid personality disorder are presented in Table 36–2.

According to *DSM-III-R* the disorder is characterized by "a pervasive pattern of indifference to social relationships and restricted range of emotional experience and expression . . . ." Patients have difficulty in expressing hostility. They are excessively self-absorbed and detached, and they engage in daydreaming. Their work performance is generally better than their ability to participate in interpersonal relationships.

Natural History & Prognosis

Onset is in early childhood. Prospective studies indicate that the majority of shy children do not go on to develop schizoid personality disorder. However, once the pattern is established, it tends to be stable during adolescence and throughout adulthood.

Differential Diagnosis

Schizoid personality disorder must be differentiated from schizotypal personality disorder, in which

---

Table 36–2. *DSM-III-R* diagnostic criteria for schizoid personality disorder (coded on axis II).

The diagnostic criteria for the personality disorders refer to behavioirs or traits that are characteristic of the person's recent (past year) and long-term functioning (generally since adolescence or early adulthood). The constellation of behaviors or traits causes either significant impairment in social or occupational functioning or subjective distress. Behaviors or traits limited to episodes of illness are not considered in making a diagnosis of personality disorder.

A. A pervasive pattern of indifference to social relationships and a restricted range of emotional experience and expression, beginning by early adulthood and present in a variety of contexts, as indicated by at least 4 of the following:

  (1) Neither desires nor enjoys close relationships, including being part of a family.

  (2) Almost always chooses solitary activities.

  (3) Rarely, if ever, claims or appears to experience strong emotions, such as anger and joy.

  (4) Indicates little if any desire to have sexual experiences with another person (age being taken into account).

  (5) Is indifferent to the praise and criticism of others.

  (6) Has no close friends or confidants (or only one) other than first-degree relatives.

  (7) Displays constricted affect, eg, is aloof, cold, rarely reciprocates gestures or facial expressions, such as smiles or nods.

B. Does not occur exclusively during the course of schizophrenia or a delusional disorder.

there are eccentricities of communication and behavior and in which a positive family history of schizophrenia occurs more frequently. Schizoid personality disorder must also be differentiated from avoidant personality disorder, in which there is social withdrawal despite a desire for acceptance; this withdrawal in the avoidant personality is due to an exquisite sensitivity to rejection. People with schizoid personality disorder do not directly experience or acknowledge a wish for closeness.

Illustrative Case

A 32-year-old assistant professor of philosophy presented for psychiatric evaluation, primarily to satisfy a request from his aging parents. They were worried about their son's impoverished social life and wanted to see him happily married so they could die in peace, knowing that their son would not be alone in the world. He was not overtly dissatisfied with his life and found gratification in his theoretical writings and occasional intellectual debates with colleagues. He did not seem to feel the loneliness that troubled his parents. He said that it was not a matter of wishing to be included in the company of others or feeling shy about forming an attachment but that he simply had no wish to be close to others.

When the patient was not working, he spent his evenings and weekends refining a mathematically elaborate system for winning at blackjack. In testing this theory, he always visited the casinos alone. He said that as a child he had preferred to read about politics and religion rather than participate in sports or associate with other children, and he felt that he had been a loner all his life.

In the interview, the patient appeared timid. He was unable to sustain eye contact, and he provided circumscribed, emotionally barren responses to questions. He fidgeted and appeared to be counting the minutes until he could leave the room. When asked if he resented being asked to come to the interview to relieve his parents' anxieties, he answered in the affirmative, but without any apparent feeling. The interviewer found it difficult to empathize with the patient's position, since he seemed so remote and uninvolved in the discussion.

Epidemiology

There is little evidence linking schizoid personality disorder to schizophrenia, in contrast to schizotypal personality disorder, which is considered part of the spectrum of schizophrenic disorders. The prevalence of schizoid personality disorder has not been established.

Etiology & Pathogenesis

It is not clear whether there is a genetic predisposition to development of schizoid personality disorder. Important psychologic factors include a cold, unempathic, emotionally impoverished childhood, as shown by retrospective (not prospective) studies.

Treatment

Long-term psychotherapy has been useful in selected cases. The course of therapy involves gradual development of trust. If this can be achieved, the patient may share long-standing fantasies of imaginary friendships and may reveal fears of depending on others. Patients are encouraged to examine the unrealistic nature of their fears and fantasies and to form actual relationships. Successful psychotherapy will produce gradual change.

Group psychotherapy may be helpful. A prolonged period of silent withdrawal may often be followed by gradual involvement in the group process. It is important for the group leader to protect the schizoid patient from criticism by other members for not participating verbally in the early affiliative phase of the group.

Schizoid Personality Disorder in Medical Practice

The person with schizoid personality disorder sustains a fragile emotional equilibrium by avoiding intimate personal contact and thereby minimizing conflict that is poorly tolerated. Illness is not only a threat to personal integrity but also requires that the patient seek treatment from a health care team made up of people who may seem to impose a demand for dependent involvement that is hard for this type of patient to accept. For this reason, the patient may delay seeking help until symptoms become severe. Once treatment has started, the patient frequently appears detached, as though unappreciative of the help being offered. Such individuals may dissociate the tolerable, technical aspects of treatment from its frightening interpersonal context.

The physician should appreciate the need for privacy in a person with schizoid personality disorder and should maintain a low-key approach that focuses on the technical elements of treatment. Such a focus will enable the patient to feel the physician's concern and caring and know that caretakers will not press beyond comfortable limits. The patient should be encouraged to maintain daily routines so that a sense of "life as usual" can counteract the worry that illness will shatter the patient's efforts to remain detached and uninvolved. Knowledge of the patient's usual pattern of functioning will counteract any tendency on the part of the health care team to become personally overinvolved or be too zealously concerned with providing social supports for the patient.

SCHIZOTYPAL PERSONALITY DISORDER

Symptoms & Signs

The diagnostic criteria for schizotypal personality disorder are set forth in Table 36-3.

According to *DSM-III-R*, the disorder is characterized by "deficits in interpersonal relatedness and peculiarities of ideation, appearance, and behavior . . . ."

The patient suffers from anxiety, depression, and

Table 36–3. *DSM-III-R* diagnostic criteria for schizotypal personality disorder (coded on axis II).

The diagnostic criteria for the personality disorders refer to behavior or traits that are characteristic of the person's recent (past year) and long-term functioning (generally since adolescence or early adulthood). The constellation of behaviors or traits causes either significant impairment in social or occupational functioning or subjective distress. Behaviors or traits limited to episodes of illness are not considered in making a diagnosis of personality disorder.

A. A pervasive pattern of deficits in interpersonal relatedness and peculiarities of ideation, appearance, and behavior, beginning by early adulthood and present in a variety of contexts, as indicated by at least 5 of the following:

  (1) Ideas of reference (excluding delusions of reference).

  (2) Excessive social anxiety, eg, extreme discomfort in social situations involving unfamiliar people.

  (3) Odd beliefs or magical thinking, influencing behavior and inconsistent with subcultural norms, eg, superstitiousness, belief in clairvoyance, telepathy, or "sixth sense," "others can feel my feelings" (in children and adolescents, bizarre fantasies or preoccupations).

  (4) Unusual perceptual experiences, eg, illusions, sensing the presence of a force or person not actually present (eg, "I felt as if my dead mother were in the room with me").

  (5) Odd or eccentric behavior or appearance, eg, unkempt, unusual mannerisms, talks to self.

  (6) No close friends or confidants (or only one) other than first-degree relatives.

  (7) Odd speech (without loosening of associations or incoherence), eg, speech that is impoverished, digressive, vague, or inappropriately abstract.

  (8) Inappropriate or constricted affect, eg, silly, aloof, rarely reciprocates gestures or facial expressions, such as smiles or nods.

  (9) Suspiciousness or paranoid ideation.

B. Does not occur exclusively during the course of schizophrenia or a pervasive developmental disorder.

other dysphoric mood states. If features of borderline personality disorder are present, both diagnoses may be assigned. Reactive psychoses and eccentric convictions occur. The patient also demonstrates magical thinking, as illustrated by superstition and by a belief in clairvoyance and telepathy.

Natural History & Prognosis

Systematic data are not yet available on this disorder.

Differential Diagnosis

The differential diagnosis should include schizoid personality disorder, in which behavioral and communicative oddities do not occur; and schizophrenia, in which formal thought disorder occurs.

Illustrative Case

A 34-year-old single woman presented at a community mental health center complaining of feelings of detachment and unreality. She said she felt cut off from her environment, as though she were looking out at the world through "semitransparent gauze." She also complained that when she was walking in the evening, moving shadows cast by the wind blowing through the trees created the frightening illusion of a potential assailant. She momentarily visualized a menacing figure, only to realize it was merely an illusion. This experience occurred repeatedly.

The patient had supported herself over the past few years by tea leaf and palm reading and other forms of fortune-telling. She said that this choice of occupation followed from her long-standing belief that she possessed special powers. During adolescence, she had claimed to be clairvoyant. She was regarded as either odd or fascinating by her acquaintances. She was deeply superstitious and preoccupied with numbers, colors, and dates. For example, she only traveled on airplanes when the day of the month, the flight number, and the scheduled arrival time were even numbers.

The patient's relationships usually involved superficial acquaintances, primarily people who shared her superstitious belief systems. She spent long periods daydreaming and fantasizing that she was a beautiful woman who would achieve great prominence by foretelling important world events. Such daydreams usually occurred after she experienced insults or slights.

At the interview, the patient was colorfully dressed in a juxtaposition of clashing, gypsylike styles that gave her a patchwork, disheveled appearance. Although she showed no frank disorder of speech such as incoherence or gross loosening of associations, her language was stilted, and she used inappropriately formal and technical terms in a disjunctive fashion that made her speech difficult to follow. There was no evidence of delusions or hallucinations. When she was asked about a family history of mental disorder, she replied that an older sister had undergone several psychiatric hospitalizations and was currently receiving antipsychotic drugs.

Epidemiology

The incidence of schizophrenia is increased in first-degree relatives of individuals with schizotypal personality disorder.

Etiology & Pathogenesis

Schizotypal personality disorder shares a genetic relationship with schizophrenia, as shown by family, twin, and adoption studies, which have demonstrated that these disorders occur more often in genetically related family members than in unrelated individuals.

Treatment

The physician must exercise tact when exploring idiosyncratic belief systems during psychotherapy. Antipsychotic medication is useful in patients with pronounced psychotic manifestations, particularly during stress.

Schizotypal Personality Disorder in Medical Practice

The problems encountered in management of the schizotypal patient and the management approaches are similar to those used for schizoid patients, as described above. The physician must also be able to help the patient with reality testing and differentiating fantasy from fact. In this respect, management techniques are similar to those used for patients with paranoid and borderline personality disorders and patients with psychotic disorders. Occasionally, the physician may consider the use of antipsychotic medications if the patient becomes frankly psychotic. If psychosis persists, the possibility of a coexisting mental disorder must be considered, and psychiatric consultation is indicated.

HISTRIONIC PERSONALITY DISORDER

Symptoms & Signs

Table 36–4 lists the diagnostic criteria for histrionic personality disorder.

DSM-III-R states that the essential feature of this disorder is "a pervasive pattern of excessive emotionality and attention seeking . . . ."

Patients with histrionic personality disorder experience reactive dysphoria in the face of loss or rejection as well as difficulty with linear, analytic thought, although they are often creative and imaginative. Patients are impressionable, suggestible, and intuitive; ie, they "play hunches" instead of thinking decisions through methodically. There is a tendency toward somatization, and homosexuality may be associated with this disorder in some cases.

Natural History & Prognosis

Systematic data are not yet available on this disorder.

Differential Diagnosis

Histrionic personality disorder must be differentiated from somatization disorder, borderline personality disorder, and narcissistic personality disorder. These 3 disorders may coexist in some combination with histrionic personality disorder, in which case all relevant diagnoses may be assigned.

Illustrative Case

A 32-year-old single professional photographer sought psychiatric treatment because of repetitive disappointments in her love relationships. She had achieved considerable success in her career over the last few years but was unmotivated to work after the recent breakup of an affair with an older man, one of the teachers at an art institute she had attended. The affair had begun when he was unhappily married, and during the course of the relationship, he had left his wife. After the separation, the patient grew disenchanted as she began to note his unattractive character traits. Instead of becoming more available to her emotionally, he became preoccupied with work, and she felt left out. In her own words, "His work became his mistress, and I felt like the other woman, abandoned, except for diversionary relief when he needed some entertainment."

The patient went on to describe several other disappointing love relationships that had occurred over the past few years and seemed unaware that she repeatedly chose powerful and attractive but self-absorbed men. She was the youngest of 3 daughters. Her father was an architect and her mother an interior decorator. Her older sister had a congenital heart defect; in the patient's view, "She got all the attention. My achievements were taken for granted, but a big deal was made out of everything she could do."

At the interview, the patient appeared attractive and chic. Her manner of relating to the interviewer was dramatically intense as she gestured widely and maintained unwavering eye contact. She showed labile emotional shifts from sadness to shame to anger as she reviewed aspects of her love relationship. Her thinking was organized and coherent but vague and highly emotional, with sparse detail in her descriptions of the difficulties in her relationships.

Epidemiology

Histrionic personality disorder is more common in women than in men, and there is an increased familial incidence.

Table 36–4. *DSM-III-R* diagnostic criteria for histrionic personality disorder (coded on axis II).

The diagnostic criteria for the personality disorders refer to behaviors or traits that are characteristic of the person's recent (past year) and long-term functioning (generally since adolescence or early adulthood). The constellation of behaviors or traits causes either significant impairment in social or occupational functioning or subjective distress. Behaviors or traits limited to episodes of illness are not considered in making a diagnosis of personality disorder.

A pervasive pattern of excessive emotionality and attention-seeking, beginning by early adulthood and present in a variety of contexts, as indicated by at least 4 of the following:

(1) Constantly seeks or demands reassurance, approval, or praise.

(2) Is inappropriately sexually seductive in appearance or behavior.

(3) Is overly concerned with physical attractiveness.

(4) Expresses emotion with inappropriate exaggeration, eg, embraces casual acquaintances with excessive ardor, uncontrollable sobbing on minor sentimental occasions, has temper tantrums.

(5) Is uncomfortable in situations in which he or she is not the center of attention.

(6) Displays rapidly shifting and shallow expression of emotions.

(7) Is self-centered, actions being directed toward obtaining immediate satisfaction; has no tolerance for the frustration of delayed gratification.

(8) Has a style of speech that is excessively impressionistic and lacking in detail, eg, when asked to describe mother, can be no more specific than, "She was a beautiful person."

Etiology & Pathogenesis

The causes of histrionic personality disorder are mainly psychologic; in better-functioning patients, these are typically unresolved oedipal problems. The more immature, dependent (so-called oral) hysteric has a history of disturbance early in life in attachments and separation.

Treatment

Long-term psychoanalytic psychotherapy is the treatment of choice and should focus on developing the patient's insight into the reasons for repetitive difficulties in sustaining love relationships and on promoting autonomous self-expression. The therapist should also help the patient think more clearly and systematically, so that information processing and decision making are not distorted by vagueness or failure to attend to relevant details.

Histrionic Personality Disorder in Medical Practice

For people with histrionic personalities, self-esteem is heavily centered in perception of their body image, with physical prowess and attractiveness being prized attributes. Although all people have some concerns about physical beauty and power, these elements figure prominently in the psychology of histrionic personalities, and this central role creates specific emotional vulnerabilities during illness. Men with histrionic personality disorder may, when physically ill, display hypermasculine ("macho") behavior to counteract their perception of themselves as weak. Such counterphobic behavior may worsen the course of illness. Such men may act in an overtly seductive fashion toward female physicians and other members of the health care team. Women with histrionic personality disorder may attempt to reaffirm their sense of self-worth by exhibiting dependent and coquettish behavior in an attempt to evoke reassuring admiration from their male physicians. Patients of both sexes may attempt to draw the physician into a rescuing, admiring role in order to ward off anxiety associated with the threat to self-esteem that is posed by the illness.

The physician must be able to provide maximal emotional support and interest in order to lessen the patient's anxiety but at the same time must avoid entering into a close personal relationship that might be misinterpreted as sexual. The physician must also avoid fostering magical expectations of cure. The physician should adopt a kindly but objective stance and should periodically provide a clear explanation of the disorder and plans for treatment so as to foster trust and firmly counteract the patient's denial of illness. This must be done without returning seductive or regressively dependent overtures. Such patients tend to fluctuate between a state of overwhelming anxiety about the potential loss of capacities (intrusions or flooding of affect) and a state of numbing and apparent disregard (*la belle indifférence*). A flexible approach combining support or tactful confrontation as appropriate will help the patient gain a realistic understanding of the disorder and cooperate with treatment. The patient's capacity for overly dramatic expression and the shifting focus of somatic distress raise the risk that the physician will dismiss the complaints as those of a hypochondriac or even as the conscious manipulations of a malingerer. The histrionic patient will challenge the physician's diagnostic acumen, since serious illness, conversion symptoms, and dramatization of minor somatic disturbances may coexist or evolve sequentially within the same individual.

Leigh and Reiser (1980) illustrate the difficulty that a patient with histrionic personality disorder has in coping with physical illness.

Illustrative case. A 59-year-old married businessman had severe chest pain and was admitted to the intensive care unit after an electrocardiogram and serum enzyme determinations confirmed that he had suffered a massive myocardial infarction. Absolute bed rest was prescribed in order to minimize the threat of further myocardial damage. The patient prided himself on his physical prowess, and when his physician empathically commented on how frightening the attack must have been for him, the patient replied, "No. I didn't get frightened at nothing—nothing scares me. All I did was holler up to my wife. I've got a bull voice—you know what I mean: I can't help myself. You understand. I got a powerful chest, so it comes out strong."

The patient presented a problem in management, because in an effort to ward off the anxiety associated with his illness, he persuaded himself that a daily exercise program would hasten his rehabilitation, and despite the admonitions of the intensive care unit staff, he began repeatedly lifting up his bed in order to improve his circulation. He told one of the nurses, "My doctor thinks I had a heart attack. All I need is to get my strength back, which I lost from being in here too long." His denial and counterphobic behavior precipitated a burst of cardiac arrhythmias that required urgent medical treatment and subsequent psychiatric consultation.

Appropriate psychologic management of this patient would include a review of the events leading up to his admission to the hospital, tactful confrontation of his defensive need to appear invincible, and step-by-step efforts to help him gradually accept his real vulnerabilities while countering his fear of being a "cardiac cripple." The physician's admiration of the patient's efforts to cope more adaptively would help restore the patient's sense of self-esteem and safety.

NARCISSISTIC PERSONALITY DISORDER

Symptoms & Signs

The diagnostic criteria for narcissistic personality disorder are listed in Table 36–5.

Narcissistic personality disorder is characterized

Table 36–5. *DSM-III-R* diagnostic criteria for narcissistic personality disorder (coded on axis II).

The diagnostic criteria for the personality disorders refer to behaviors or traits that are characteristic of the person's recent (past year) and long-term functioning (generally since adolescence or early adulthood). The constellation of behaviors or traits causes either significant impairment in social or occupational functioning or subjective distress. Behaviors or traits limited to episodes of illness are not considered in making a diagnosis of personality disorder.

A pervasive pattern of grandiosity (in fantasy or behavior), lack of empathy, and hypersensitivity to the evaluation of others, beginning by early adulthood and present in a variety of contexts, as indicated by at least 5 of the following:

(1) Reacts to criticism with feelings of rage, shame, or humiliation (even if not expressed).

(2) Is interpersonally exploitative: takes advantage of others to achieve his or her own ends.

(3) Has a grandiose sense of self-importance, eg, exaggerates achievements and talents, expects to be noticed as "special" without appropriate achievement.

(4) Believes that his or her problems are unique and can be understood only by other special people.

(5) Is preoccupied with fantasies of unlimited success, power, brilliance, beauty, or ideal love.

(6) Has a sense of entitlement: unreasonable expectation of especially favorable treatment, eg, assumes that he or she does not have to wait in line when others must do so.

(7) Requires constant attention and admiration, eg, keeps fishing for compliments.

(8) Lack of empathy: inability to recognize and experience how others feel, eg, annoyance and surpise when a friend who is seriously ill cancels a date.

(9) Is preoccupied with feelings of envy.

by *DSM-III-R* as "a pervasive pattern of grandiosity . . . lack of empathy, and hypersensitivity to evaluation by others . . . ."

Brief reactive psychoses may occur; in psychodynamic theory, these represent fragmentation of a coherent sense of self under psychosocial stress. This fragmentation is experienced as a loss of the sense of continuity of oneself as worthwhile and lovable in the face of a current disappointment, criticism, or rejection. Depression is common, as is chronic intense envy. Defensive self-delusion or lying to oneself by distorting the facts so that a feeling of self-importance is preserved ("sliding of meanings") is also seen. The patient may pretend to have certain feelings in order to impress others.

Natural History & Prognosis

Systematic data are not yet available on this disorder.

Illustrative Case

A 38-year-old recently divorced and infrequently employed actor who was the father of an 8-month-old sought help because of depression. He had left his wife and son 6 weeks earlier because he could no longer tolerate his wife's "slavish devotion to our baby boy; I may as well not exist as far as she's concerned." He complained that since his wife had become pregnant—and especially over the last months of caring for their

child—she was disinclined to admire his acting abilities and less interested than before in sympathizing with his envy of actors who obtained better and more frequent employment.

The patient had had a relatively lucrative minor role in a television comedy series but was "written out" after he antagonized the director. In his view, "Most of the directors are jerks. They're so busy kowtowing to the producers, they've lost whatever artistic talents they ever had." He admitted that in private moments, he felt ashamed of his career setbacks, was enraged by his own limitations, and was at times suicidally distraught.

The patient was the eldest child and only son of a materially successful but emotionally withholding, punitive, and sniping father who, in the patient's view, magnified his son's slightest imperfections. The patient described his mother as an indulgent and admiring woman who frequently made excuses for him. His 2 younger sisters were competent in their professions, and their success was a source of shame and guilt for him.

The patient had experienced a rapid turnover in friendships, since he initially idealized people and then impulsively trashed the relationships when he was frustrated or disappointed. Before his marriage he had fancied himself as a Don Juan, saying, "I had women on a string, but after a while I couldn't stand their vanity and pettiness."

In the interview, the patient presented as an expensively dressed, well-groomed, and handsome man who tried to project a smooth, self-assured facade. There was, however, a palpable undercurrent of insecurity, loneliness, and depression. His distraught feelings had a quality of caricature to them that was evident to the interviewer. He presented himself as though he were a colleague rather than a patient, and he provided his own formulations for his psychologic difficulties in an effort to save face. Although there were no gross abnormalities of thinking or perception, he presented an apparently distorted account of his role in his marital and occupational difficulties and cast himself in a better light than was warranted. He found an external power to blame, which lent a quality of self-delusion to his version of his interpersonal difficulties.

Epidemiology

The prevalence of narcissistic personality disorder is unknown, although it is apparently common in outpatient psychiatric and medical practice.

Etiology & Pathogenesis

In normal psychologic development, all very young children have an exaggerated sense of their own importance as well as an idealized view of parental figures as protective, powerful, and immortal. These immature, idealized views of the self and others are modified as children learn to face gradual, tolerable disappointments with the empathic support of their caretakers. The result of this process is that healthy adults can accept their own realistic limitations, tolerate criticism and setbacks, and still maintain an overall positive self-regard. In contrast, the early life experiences of individuals with narcissistic personality disorder were described by Kohut (1971) as marked by premature, repeated, and intense injuries to self-esteem as well as by radical disillusionment in parental figures, rather than gradual and tolerable disappointments in themselves and important caretakers. The long-term sequelae in adulthood are characteristic disturbances in self-esteem, with alternating idealization and devaluation of others that is accompanied by alternating grandiose and inferior images of the self.

Treatment

Long-term psychoanalytic psychotherapy and psychoanalysis have been attempted with these patients, although their use has been controversial. The goal is to increase the patient's capacity to tolerate disappointments, to appreciate the needs of others, and to develop healthy self-esteem.

Narcissistic Personality Disorder in Medical Practice

Narcissistic patients try to sustain an image of perfection and personal invincibility for themselves and attempt to project that impression to others as well. Physical illness may shatter this illusion, and a patient may lose the feeling of safety inherent in a cohesive sense of self. This loss precipitates a panicky sensation that "my world is falling to pieces," and the patient feels a sense of personal fragmentation. The narcissistic individual shares with the histrionic personality a concern about loss of admiration and approval, but the person with narcissistic personality disorder shows a more disturbed response to illness. The histrionic patient's idealization of the physician stands in contrast to the narcissistic patient's frequent contemptuous disregard for the physician, who is denigrated in a defensive effort to maintain a sense of superiority and mastery over illness. Only the most senior physician in a prestigious institution is deemed worthy of respect as the frightened patient seeks an external reflection of his or her own fragile grandeur in the doctor. More junior members of the health care team may be the targets of derision as the patient seeks to establish hierarchic dominance in order to counter the shame and fear triggered by illness.

Health care professionals must convey a feeling of respect and acknowledge the patient's sense of self-importance so that the patient can reestablish a coherent sense of self, but they must at the same time avoid reinforcing either pathologic grandiosity (which may contribute to denial of illness) or weakness (which frightens the patient). An initial approach of support followed by step-by-step confrontation of the patient's vulnerabilities may enable the patient to deal with the implications of illness with feelings of greater subjective strength. The increased self-confidence may reduce the patient's need to attack the health care team in a misguided effort at psychologic self-preservation

and eases the pressure to provide perfect care, since the patient's antagonistic feeling of entitlement (defined by *DSM-III-R* as an "unreasonable expectation of especially favorable treatment") is reduced.

The following case shows the difficulty encountered in medical management of the narcissistic personality.

Illustrative case. A partner in a prestigious law firm was admitted to the specialized endocrine service of a teaching hospital for investigation of inflammation of the thyroid gland. The patient had sought consultation with the chief of the endocrine service after seeing the endocrinologist's recent research findings reported on network television and characterized as a glamorous, high-technology innovation. The patient recalled thinking at the time, "Finally, here is a doctor who can understand the complexities of my illness!"

When the patient arrived at the endocrine service, he was greeted by the junior resident, who introduced himself and explained that he would be responsible for the patient's day-to-day care, while the chief of the service would consult on major diagnostic and treatment issues. The lawyer flew into a rage and shouted, "No damn wet-behind-the-ears student doctor is going to lay a hand on me!"

The resident attempted to calm the patient and agreed to ask the chief of the service to mediate the dispute. When the chief arrived and was informed of the situation, his previous experience in dealing with influential patients enabled him to grasp the nature of the lawyer's narcissistic rage, the underlying sense of entitlement and fear that motivated it, and the embarrassment of the resident who was the unwitting target of the tirade. He welcomed the patient and apologized for not being able to meet him at the time of admission. He introduced the resident as "one of our brightest young colleagues, who has the potential to make a creative contribution in his own right" and continued, "He and I will work closely together to get to the bottom of your problems."

The lawyer was reassured by this respectful apology and the statement of confidence in the junior resident. The chief of the service had in effect transferred his reputation for excellence to his younger colleague ("passed the baton") and had thereby imbued the resident with the charismatic healing qualities the narcissistic patient needed in order to feel the trust necessary for a successful therapeutic relationship with the health care team.

ANTISOCIAL PERSONALITY DISORDER

Symptoms & Signs

The diagnostic criteria for antisocial personality disorder are set forth in Table 36–6.

DSM-III-R states that this disorder is characterized by a history of chronic antisocial behavior that begins

Table 36–6. *DSM-III-R* diagnostic criteria for antisocial personality disorder (coded on axis II).

The diagnostic criteria for the personality disorders refer to behaviors or traits that are characteristic of the person's recent (past year) and long-term functioning (generally since adolescence or early adulthood). The constellation of behaviors or traits causes either significant impairment in social or occupational functioning or subjective distress. Behaviors or traits limited to episodes of illness are not considered in making a diagnosis of personality disorder.

A. Current age at least 18.

B. Evidence of conduct disorder with onset before age 15, as indicated by a history of 3 or more of the following:
  (1) Was often truant.
  (2) Ran away from home overnight at least twice while living in parental or parental surrogate home (or once without returning).
  (3) Often initiated physical fights.
  (4) Used a weapon in more than one fight.
  (5) Forced someone into sexual activity with him or her.
  (6) Was physically cruel to animals.
  (7) Was physically cruel to other people.
  (8) Deliberately destroyed others' property (other than fire-setting).
  (9) Deliberately engaged in fire-setting.
  (10) Often lied (other than to avoid physical or sexual abuse).
  (11) Has stolen without confrontation of a victim on more than one occasion (including forgery).
  (12) Has stolen with confrontation of a victim (eg, mugging, purse-snatching, extortion, armed robbery).

C. A pattern of irresponsible and antisocial behavior since the age of 15, as indicated by at least 4 of the following:
  (1) Is unable to sustain consistent work behavior, as indicated by any of the following (including similar behavior in academic settings if the person is a student): (a) significant unemployment for 6 months or more within 5 years when expected to work and work was available; (b) repeated absences from work unexplained by illness in self or family; (c) abandonment of several jobs without realistic plans for others.
  (2) Fails to conform to social norms with respect to lawful behavior, as indicated by repeatedly performing antisocial acts that are grounds for arrest (whether arrested or not), eg, destroying property, harassing others, stealing, pursuing an illegal occupation.
  (3) Is irritable and aggressive, as indicated by repeated physical fights or assaults (not required by one's job or to defend someone or oneself), including spouse- or child-beating.
  (4) Repeatedly fails to honor financial obligations, as indicated by defaulting on debts or failing to provide child support for other dependents on a regular basis.
  (5) Fails to plan ahead, or is impulsive, as indicated by one or both of the following: (a) traveling from place to place without prearranged job or clear goal for the period of travel or clear idea about when the travel will terminate; (b) lack of a fixed address for 1 month or more.
  (6) Has no regard for the truth, as indicated by repeated lying, use of aliases, or "conning" others for personal profit or pleasure.
  (7) Is reckless regarding his or her own or others' personal safety, as indicated by driving while intoxicated or recurrent speeding.
  (8) If a parent or guardian, lacks ability to function as a responsible parent, as indicated by one or more of the following: (a) malnutrition of child; (b) child's illness resulting from lack of minimal hygiene; (c) failure to obtain medical care for a seriously ill child; (d) child's dependence on neighbors or non-resident relatives for food or shelter; (e) failure to arrange for a caretaker for young child when parent is away from home; (f) repeated squandering, on personal items, of money required for household necessities.
  (9) Has never sustained a totally monogamous relationship for more than 1 year.
  (10) Lacks remorse (feels justified in having hurt, mistreated, or stolen from another).

D. Antisocial behavior does not occur exclusively during the course of schizophrenia or manic episodes.

---

before the age of 15 and "a pattern of irresponsible and antisocial behavior since the age of 15," as indicated by poor job performance, academic failure, participation in a wide variety of illegal activities, recklessness, and impulsive behavior.

The patient with antisocial personality disorder also experiences a feeling of subjective dysphoria, characterized by tension, depression, inability to tolerate boredom, and a feeling of being victimized. There is also a diminished capacity for intimacy.

Natural History & Prognosis

Antisocial personality disorder tends to remit with time. After 21 years of age, the remission rate is about 2% of all patients each year. As destructive social behavior diminishes, patients tend to develop hypochondriacal and depressive disorders.

Differential Diagnosis

If characteristic features of antisocial personality disorder are present but the person is younger than 18 years of age, a diagnosis of conduct disorder is appropriate. When criminal behavior is present without other features of antisocial personality disorder, the appropriate diagnosis is adult antisocial behavior, usually without the precursory signs seen in adolescents with conduct disorders.

Illustrative Case

A 21-year-old divorced independent trucker was referred for pretrial psychiatric evaluation after being charged with interstate transportation of stolen property. He had a history of repeated criminal offenses, prison terms, and psychiatric disturbance during childhood and adolescence. He had been apprehended 4 weeks earlier when a random road inspection revealed stolen automobile parts hidden among cartons of groceries.

The patient had been working for a national grocery chain, which had hired him after he was felt to have successfully completed a vocational rehabilitation program in which he participated while on probation from a prior offense. He had managed to persuade his employers of his intention to "go straight" despite his history of erratic and impulsive behavior in other work situations.

About 8 months before his latest arrest, the patient

had suddenly abandoned his wife when he learned from an acquaintance that she sometimes flirted with customers at the sandwich shop where she worked.

The patient was the second in a family of 4 boys. His alcoholic father was episodically violent toward him when drunk, and his mother was absent long hours while she worked to support the family.

During childhood, the patient had been evaluated and briefly treated in a community mental health center after he had been caught setting fire to an abandoned warehouse. During adolescence, he had received counseling from a school psychologist because of a consistent pattern of antisocial behavior, including car theft, joyriding, drunk driving, driving with a suspended license, truancy, and stealing money from his mother. While he was growing up, he had no close friendships, although he was a peripheral member of a hot-rod gang. Though sexually active from a young age and proud of his sexual prowess, he was mistrustful of women and became easily bored with the same partner.

In the interview, the patient appeared nonchalant and composed, with an apparent equanimity that was incongruent with the seriousness of his situation. He made eye contact with the interviewer but appeared to be looking through the interviewer rather than at him. There was an unspoken but clearly communicated disregard for the interviewer's authority. There were no major disturbances in thought, perception, or mood, with the exception of a lack of remorse or anxiety when he was confronted with his lifelong pattern of destructive behavior and the seriousness of the charges presently lodged against him.

Epidemiology

Onset of antisocial personality disorder is before age 15, frequently around puberty in girls and quite early in childhood for boys. The disorder is more prevalent in men, with incidence being about 3% for men and 1% for women. Prevalence is increased in lower socioeconomic groups. Family histories are often positive for antisocial personality disorder, with increased incidence in the fathers of both male and female patients with this disorder. Evidence suggests that this familial occurrence is due to both genetic and environmental causes; the relative contribution of each factor is unknown. Antisocial personality disorder may be diagnosed in as many as 75% of prison inmates.

Etiology & Pathogenesis

A. Genetic and Biologic Factors: Robins (1966) found an increased incidence of sociopathic characteristics and alcoholism in the fathers of individuals with antisocial personality disorder. Schulsinger (1972) reports findings of twin studies and adoption studies that support the hypothesis of a genetic component in this disorder. At present, there is no evidence that organic brain damage contributes to antisocial personality disorder. Earlier findings of electroencephalographic abnormalities, such as those

reported by Kiloh and Osselton (1966), are probably attributable to adolescent substance abuse.

B. Psychologic Factors: Bowlby (1944) correlated antisocial personality disorder with maternal deprivation in the child's first 5 years of life. Glueck and Glueck (1968) reported that the mothers of children who developed this personality disorder show a lack of consistent discipline, lack of affection, and an increased incidence of alcoholism and impulsiveness. These qualities contribute to failure to create a cohesive home environment with consistent structure and behavioral boundaries. In the prospective study, children found to be at risk by age 6 frequently showed features of antisocial personality at 18 years.

Antisocial Personality Disorder in Medical Practice

The relationship between a physician and a patient with antisocial personality disorder is characterized by mutual feelings of suspicion and, at times, hostility. The antisocial person's mistrust of the physician stems from unwarranted generalizations about physicians that are based in part on early abusive experiences at the hands of parental caretakers, especially during the formative periods of childhood and adolescence. The physician's mistrust of the antisocial patient may well be grounded in unpleasant personal experience. Persons with antisocial personality disorder may feign physical symptoms in order to obtain narcotic analgesics for substance abuse. They may attempt to defraud third-party health care payment sources in seeking reimbursement for services not rendered or may be delinquent in payment for services they have actually received. Unfortunately, individuals with antisocial personalities are at least as vulnerable to physical illness as any other type of patient and are in fact at higher risk for illnesses associated with substance abuse and stress, because of their chronic unstable interpersonal and occupational adjustments. The physician is therefore challenged to find a way to create an effective therapeutic alliance. A firm, no-nonsense approach that is not punitive but conveys a streetwise awareness of the patient's potential for manipulation will encouraage respect without aggravating the patient's hostility against authority.

Illustrative case. A 25-year-old man presented for an initial visit to a local general practitioner and complained of recurrent backache. He said that he had tried many analgesics in the past and found that they either were ineffective or caused intolerable side effects, with the exception of high doses of codeine. Physical examination revealed significant disease of the lumbosacral spine secondary to a congenital defect in the alignment of the vertebrae.

Alerted by the patient's specific request for a potentially addictive narcotic that also had high resale value in the illicit drug market, the physician inquired further into the patient's work and occupational history. A typical unstable pattern of impulsive and manipulative interpersonal relations was identified, including an irregular work history and other features characteristic of antisocial personality disorder. A respectful but appropriately tough tone of inquiry into the patient's previous use of analgesics revealed a history of morphine addiction following lower back surgery. Denial of the patient's request for codeine led to an angry outburst, with the patient declining alternative treatment. Several months later, however, the patient reappeared with legitimate complaints of upper respiratory tract infection. He told the physician, "I came back to see you again because I figure you're nobody's fool, but you're not going to lecture me about how I should live my life either."

BORDERLINE PERSONALITY DISORDER

Symptoms & Signs

Table 36–7 sets forth the diagnostic criteria for borderline personality disorder.

As described by *DSM-III-R*, borderline personality disorder is characterized by "instability of mood, interpersonal relationships, and self-image . . . ."

The patient with borderline personality disorder is

Table 36–7. *DSM-III-R* diagnostic criteria for borderline personality disorder (coded on axis II).

The diagnostic criteria for the personality disorders refer to behaviors or traits that are characteristic of the person's recent (past year) and long-term functioning (generally since adolescence or early adulthood). The constellation of behaviors or traits causes either significant impairment in social or occupational functioning or subjective distress. Behaviors or traits limited to episodes of illness are not considered in making a diagnosis of personality disorder.

A pervasive pattern of instability of mood, interpersonal relationships, and self-image; beginning by early adulthood and present in a variety of contexts, as indicated by at least 5 of the following:

(1) A pattern of unstable and intense interpersonal relationships characterized by alternating between extremes of overidealization and devaluation.

(2) Impulsivity in at least 2 areas that are potentially self-damaging, eg, spending, sex, substance use, shoplifting, reckless driving, binge eating. (Do not include suicidal or self-mutilating behavior covered in criterion [5].)

(3) Affective instability: marked shifts from baseline mood to depression, irritability, or anxiety, usually lasting a few hours and only rarely more than a few days.

(4) Inappropriate, intense anger or lack of control of anger, eg, frequent displays of temper, constant anger, recurrent physical fights.

(5) Recurrent suicidal threats, gestures, or behavior, or self-mutilating behavior.

(6) Marked and persistent identity disturbance manifested by uncertainty about at least 2 of the following: self-image, sexual orientation, long-term goals or career choice, type of friends desired, preferred values.

(7) Chronic feelings of emptiness or boredom.

(8) Frantic efforts to avoid real or imagined abandonment. (Do not include suicidal or self-mutilating behavior covered in criterion [5].)

vulnerable to development of transient reactive psychoses (micropsychotic episodes) and may be chronically depressed. The patient alternates between the wish for closeness and the need for distance. Borderline personality disorder may coexist with schizotypal, histrionic, narcissistic, or antisocial personality disorder.

Natural History & Prognosis

Follow-up studies by Werble (1970) and by Carpenter and coworkers (1977) suggest that the clinical picture in patients with borderline personality disorder is chronically unstable but that the disorder does not deteriorate into schizophrenia. In both studies, symptoms were present over long periods, and patients experienced major disturbances in social functioning and enjoyed little satisfaction from their low quality of life. These individuals were unlikely to marry. The patients in the 2 studies were suffering from a severe form of the borderline disorder; the prognosis is better for individuals with higher levels of functioning.

Differential Diagnosis

If an individual with characteristics of borderline personality disorder is under 18 years of age, the appropriate diagnosis is identity disorder.

Borderline personality disorder must be differentiated from cyclothymic disorder, in which there are hypomanic periods.

Illustrative Case

A 25-year-old single graduate student was brought to a crisis clinic by her girlfriend, who had become worried after the patient expressed a wish to commit suicide. Two weeks earlier, the patient's boyfriend had left for a summer vacation trip to Europe. The vacation had initially been planned as a joint trip, but the patient had persuaded her boyfriend to go alone so they could have a period of independence from each other. She was worried that they were becoming psychologically enmeshed and "like Siamese twins," a view that threatened her chronically fragile sense of separateness and autonomy. In the 2 weeks since his departure, she had grown progressively more distraught and had felt a panicky sense of abandonment, emptiness, and loss of all positive feelings and memories of her relationship with her boyfriend, all of which contributed to a sense of unreality about her life. She considered taking an overdose of drugs, because "nothing else would numb the pain I feel." She had also harbored an increasing sense of rage at being left behind, because "he didn't understand that I was only testing his loyalty when I told him to go alone."

The patient's current relationship, like her previous love relationships, had been characterized by periods of intense intimate contact alternating with flights into independence. She felt she could not achieve a comfortable compromise that would enable her to feel close to another person yet preserve a sense of her own separateness. Although she was a gifted student, she had enrolled in 3 widely different graduate programs after having made abrupt shifts in her career training just when she was nearing completion of any one program. Her academic interests were scattered over the fine arts, social sciences, and business. She was by her own description a "chameleon" who had no strong preferences of her own. She was powerfully influenced by charismatic teachers whose value systems and career goals she would make her own in an effort to counter her inner sense of emptiness and lack of direction.

The patient was an only child whose mother became bedridden with rheumatoid arthritis when the patient was between 18 and 30 months of age. Her mother made a partial recovery but struggled with physical pain and depression during subsequent relapses. Her parents were divorced when the patient was 9 years of age, and her father subsequently maintained only a distant relationship with the family. After her parents' divorce, the patient felt even more responsible for the health and happiness of her mother than she had before. She was made to feel guilty for placing her own social and intellectual needs ahead of those of her mother. In her view, "Every step I took toward becoming my own person was a step closer to destroying my mother."

In the interview, she was an appealing young woman who seemed distraught and somewhat disheveled and physically exhausted. In describing her separation from her boyfriend, she oscillated between uncontrollable sobbing and furious rage but was able to regain her composure in responding to the structuring and supportive remarks of the interviewer. There was no evidence of delusions or hallucinations. Her sensorium was clear, though she reported a subjective sense of disorientation and unreality that she attributed to the change in her world as a result of her boyfriend's absence.

Epidemiology

No direct studies of the prevalence of borderline personality disorder have been performed, though it is believed to be common. In the Stirling County (Nova Scotia, Canada) study (see Chapter 13), Leighton and coworkers (1963) found that 1.7% of the sample met the diagnostic criteria for emotionally unstable personality, a diagnosis with criteria similar to those of borderline personality disorder. The same study noted that the diagnosis was made more frequently in women than in men by a 2:1 ratio.

Etiology & Pathogenesis

A. Genetic and Biologic Factors: Kernberg (1975) and Klein (1977) have suggested that patients with borderline personality disorder have a "constitutionally based" inability to regulate affects, especially anger. There may be a relationship between borderline personality and depressive illness, which is prevalent in first-degree relatives of patients with borderline personality disorder.

B. Psychologic Factors: Kernberg hypothesized an arrest in normal psychologic development,

with failure to integrate ambivalent feelings originally aroused against the primary caretaker but later occurring in other close relationships as well. The primitive defenses ordinarily relinquished in early childhood are prolonged into adulthood, and patients tend to have distorted appraisals of others, who are perceived as virtual caricatures that are either "all-good" or "all-bad." This all-or-nothing thinking extends to an exaggerated view of physical symptoms as well, so that the patient tends to feel that he or she is either completely well or deathly ill. The threat of physical illness is exaggerated to terrifying proportions.

Mahler (1971) and Masterson (1972) have hypothesized that borderline personality disorder results after a disturbance occurring in children between 16 and 25 months of age during the rapprochement subphase of separation-individuation. In this phase, the child practices independent behavior and returns to the primary caretaker for approval, admiration, and emotional "refueling." The critical, rejecting parent or the suffocating, smothering parent interferes with optimal progression of attachment-separation sequences.

Treatment

A. Psychologic Treatment Measures: Controversy exists about which of the 2 dominant psychologic approaches is more effective in the treatment of borderline personality disorder. Long-term psychoanalytic psychotherapy with some supportive modifications tries to develop trust early in treatment and progresses to deeper exploration with time. The other approach is long-term, more reality-oriented supportive psychotherapy that does not focus on unconscious fantasies and attempts instead to provide structure and prevent the deterioration or overstimulation sometimes seen in more insight-oriented approaches.

B. Drug Treatment Measures: Klein (1977) advocates the use of monoamine oxidase inhibitors for patients with borderline personality disorder who are sensitive to rejection. These patients experience intensely unpleasant affects, particularly anxiety and depression, when they feel rejected. The use of other antidepressant and antianxiety agents may become necessary at certain times. During brief reactive psychoses, low doses of antipsychotic drugs may be useful, but they are usually not essential adjuncts to the treatment regimen, since such episodes are most often self-limiting and of short duration.

Borderline Personality Disorder in Medical Practice

Persons with borderline personality disorder have marked difficulty in differentiating reality from fantasy, so that a minor health problem may be perceived as a life-threatening event. Loss of perspective and miscommunication with the physician may occur as a result. Such patients frequently delay in presenting for medical treatment. They fear the worst with regard to the diagnosis, and they mistrust physicians because of their previous experiences with unreliable caretakers. Some patients may have a subconscious need to suffer in order to expiate guilty feelings. Once they have delivered themselves to the health care team, these patients ward off their catastrophic fear of being damaged by imperfect caretakers by imagining them as "all-good." If any problems occur, patients switch abruptly to an "all-bad" image of medical personnel; the omnipotent rescuer becomes the persecutory invader. The patient may bolt from treatment and attempt to resurrect an idealized relationship with a new doctor, only to be painfully disillusioned later. Patients with borderline personality disorder may interpret any "intellectual" errors in diagnosis or treatment on the part of the health care team on an emotional level. They see themselves as having been rejected, callously disregarded, and abandoned to struggle with their illnesses alone because they are unworthy of the time and interest of their physicians.

The physician should provide clear, nontechnical answers to questions to counter any elaborate fantasies about the dangers of the illness or its treatment. Honest but not overly dramatic information should be provided about the course of the illness and potential side effects of treatment. The physician should be careful to avoid encouraging the patient to idealize the physician and should not be drawn into the patient's denigration of other physicians. More frequent periodic checkups may reassure the patient of the physician's empathy and interest and may provide closer monitoring of illness; they also reduce the chances that the patient will create a frightening mental scenario out of proportion to any genuine threat. Although the physician should offer reassurance, this should not be premature, since it may deprive the patient of an opportunity to spell out these fearful expectations about the illness and may deny the physician a chance to clarify the often idiosyncratic and unexpected nuances of the patient's beliefs about the illness. The physician's tolerance of the patient's episodic angry outbursts demonstrates to the patient that the physician cannot be destroyed by the patient's strong negative feelings and that the physician will not retaliate by leaving the patient to a self-fulfilling prophecy of abandonment.

Illustrative case. A 29-year-old man was admitted to the chest service of a community hospital for investigation of an undiagnosed lesion found during routine annual physical examination. The night before a scheduled biopsy, the patient had a nightmare in which he was lying on the operating table surrounded by medical personnel. The 2 surgeons who were attending him appeared kindly at first, but as the dream progressed, their expressions grew more threatening. He finally awoke when the surgeons were transformed into vampirelike creatures. When the nursing staff arrived at the patient's bedside after the nightmare, he was extremely agitated. He was hyperventilating, complained of a pounding headache, and shouted that he was going to die. After the nurses encouraged him to talk about his fears, he said that he was convinced he had lung cancer that had spread to his brain, and he felt that his severe headache supported this self-diagnosis.

The nurses explained that he probably had a tension headache because of anxiety about the biopsy, and they showed him a relaxation exercise that relieved his headache and enabled him to gain a more realistic perspective on his situation. The biopsy revealed a benign fibrous cyst that was treated without complication.

AVOIDANT PERSONALITY DISORDER

Symptoms & Signs

Table 36–8 sets forth the diagnostic criteria for avoidant personality disorder.

Features of the disorder, as outlined by *DSM-III-R*, include social discomfort, hypersensitivity to criticism and rejection, and timidity.

The patient with avoidant personality disorder also experiences depression, anxiety, and anger for failing to develop social relations.

Natural History & Prognosis

The prognosis in avoidant personality disorder is unknown.

Differential Diagnosis

Avoidant personality disorder must be differentiated from schizoid personality disorder, social phobia, and avoidant disorder of childhood or adolescence (when the disorder occurs before age 18).

Table 36–8. *DSM-III-R* diagnostic criteria for avoidant personality disorder (coded on axis II).

The diagnostic criteria for the personality disorders refer to behaviors or traits that are characteristic of the person's recent (past year) and long-term functioning (generally since adolescence or early adulthood). The constellation of behaviors or traits causes either significant impairment in social or occupational functioning or subjective distress. Behaviors or traits limited to episodes of illness are not considered in making a diagnosis of personality disorder.

A pervasive pattern of social discomfort, fear of negative evaluation, and timidity, beginning by early adulthood and present in a variety of contexts, as indicated by at least 4 of the following:

(1) Is easily hurt by criticism or disapproval.
(2) Has no close friends or confidants (or only one) other than first-degree relatives.
(3) Is unwilling to get involved with people unless certain of being liked.
(4) Avoids social or occupational activities that involve significant interpersonal contact, eg, refuses a promotion that will increase social demands.
(5) Is reticent in social situations because of a fear of saying something inappropriate or foolish, or of being unable to answer a question.
(6) Fears being embarrassed by blushing, crying, or showing signs of anxiety in front of other people.
(7) Exaggerates the potential difficulties, physical dangers, or risks involved in doing something ordinary but outside his or her usual routine, eg, may cancel social plans because she anticipates being exhausted by the effort of getting there.

Illustrative Case

A 34-year-old single professional musician sought psychiatric treatment to deal with chronic feelings of insecurity, inferiority, and shyness. Although she was a gifted and sensitive musician, success in her career had not been matched by parallel gratifications in her social life. She came for treatment several weeks after a man in her orchestral group had moved to a different city. She was particularly fond of this man though reticent about approaching him on other than a superficial, chatty basis. She had fantasized their falling in love and was disheartened when he moved away before a deeper relationship could develop.

The disappointment she experienced in this potential relationship was a recurring pattern for the patient. She very much wanted to fall in love and be married but felt that any attractive, intelligent, and caring man would reject her. She was an esteemed member of her musical group but was perceived as someone who kept to herself, lived on the periphery of the group, and gave the impression of being a loner—all despite her wish to be one of the "in" group.

The patient described herself as having been a shy, insecure child and adolescent. Her role among her peers at school had closely paralleled her present position in the social structure of the orchestra. She had always felt that she was on the outside looking in, wanting to become involved but frightened that she would not be accepted. She had often daydreamed about artistic and social successes.

The patient was the eldest daughter of professional parents. Her father had been a tax attorney who died suddenly when the patient was 6 years old. Her mother was a music teacher who was herself highly intelligent, shy, and sensitive, and the patient identified with her.

In the interview, the patient appeared to be a soft-spoken, articulate woman who seemed embarrassed by her situation and gave a low-key presentation of herself. She displayed no oddities of speech or behavior. Her mood was sad when she talked about her disappointment in the fantasied love relationship, but signs of a major depressive disorder were absent.

Epidemiology

The prevalence of avoidant personality disorder is unknown, and there are no clear data available on the sex ratio and familial pattern.

Etiology & Pathogenesis

A complex interaction of early childhood environmental experiences and innate temperament plays a role in the occurrence of avoidant personality disorder, but definitive studies concerning the cause have not yet been conducted. Avoidant disorder of childhood and adolescence is said to predict avoidant personality disorder of adulthood.

Treatment

Psychoanalytic psychotherapy is useful in selected patients with avoidant personality disorder. The thera-
pist must expend considerable effort in establishing an effective therapeutic alliance, since their exquisite sensitivity to rejection often causes these patients to abandon treatment abruptly. Assertiveness training and training in general social skills may also be helpful. Group therapy may desensitize the patient to the exaggerated threat of rejection.

Avoidant Personality Disorder in Medical Practice

When a person with avoidant personality disorder falls ill, preexisting shyness and insecurity may intensify. Since the person is already sensitive to social rejection, he or she may feel further stigmatized by the illness and uncomfortable about asking for help and attention from the physician. Embarrassment about being scrutinized during physical examination may also contribute to downplay of symptoms and delay in seeking help.

Tact and timing—especially in history taking and physical examination—are of the utmost importance in establishing the gradual deepening of trust and rapport required to form a satisfactory working relationship with these patients. This approach encourages the patient with avoidant personality disorder to disclose physical symptoms frankly and without undue embarrassment. The physician needs to steer a middle course between inadvertently cooperating with the patient to minimize complaints and possibly missing the diagnosis on the one hand and adopting an overly intrusive approach that may threaten the patient's sense of privacy and modesty and perhaps contribute to noncompliance on the other. A low-key approach that emphasizes the physician's friendliness and availability and includes prompt return of phone calls, respect for punctuality at appointments, and periodic reassurance of the physician's personal interest and commitment will counter the patient's normal inclination to see himself or herself as unimportant or undeserving of the physician's attention.

Illustrative case. A 23-year-old woman sought consultation with a dermatologist because of an extensive reaction following exposure to poison oak. The patient had delayed seeking help by persuading herself that she was overreacting and using a variety of home remedies that failed to stop the spread of the rash. When she finally requested an appointment, the receptionist inquired about the urgency of the problem in order to appropriately schedule the appointment. The patient replied, "Well, uh, it's not that bad, but it's sort of uncomfortable; I also have a mild fever."

The alert receptionist recognized the tentative quality of this response and brought the physician to the telephone. After more detailed inquiry into the severity of symptoms, an immediate appointment was arranged, and examination revealed a moderately severe allergic reaction with superimposed bacterial infection. The dermatologist took the time to explore the patient's ambivalence about seeking consultation without at the same time making her feel that she was being criticized. He explained the necessity for close follow-up examination in a low-key, friendly manner devoid of arrogance or pretense. He appeared genuinely unhurried and not overly burdened by the pressures of his practice, and he gave an impression of accessibility that was conveyed more through nonverbal communication than in anything he said. His manner of relating to the patient contradicted her stereotype of the doctor as one of the busy professionals who have better things to do with their time than "pander to my self-indulgent concerns." This new view of physicians made it more comfortable for her to comply with the recommendations for follow-up visits and easier for her to think about seeking consultation for future problems.

DEPENDENT PERSONALITY DISORDER

Symptoms & Signs

The diagnostic criteria for dependent personality disorder are listed in Table 36–9.

Dependent personality disorder, according to *DSM-III-R*, is characterized by "a pervasive pattern of dependent and submissive behavior . . . ."

The person with dependent personality disorder may be anxious and depressed and may experience intense discomfort when alone for more than a short time. The patient is often intensely preoccupied with the possibility of abandonment. Dependent personality disorder may coexist with another personality disorder such as schizotypal, histrionic, narcissistic, or avoidant personality disorder.

Natural History & Prognosis

The prognosis in dependent personality disorder is unknown.

Differential Diagnosis

Dependent personality disorder must be differentiated from histrionic and avoidant personality disorder as well as the more severe personality disorders, including narcissistic, borderline, and schizotypal personality disorder.

Illustrative Case

A 32-year-old married postal worker presented for psychiatric evaluation because she was considerably upset after receiving a job promotion. She had earlier refused several promotions because she had not wanted to assume the responsibility for supervising others. She was now being forced either to accept a promotion or to leave her position. She desperately wished to maintain her present rank, despite the fact that she had an excellent work record and was regarded by management as a good candidate for the supervisory position.

The patient's husband was an ambitious and domineering man who "ruled the roost" in the family, just as her father had done when she was growing up. She was aware that she suppressed her own needs in favor of meeting those of her husband, and though she was occasionally frustrated because of this, she admired his strength of character and felt relieved to know that someone was in control.

The patient was the youngest child in her family and had 2 older brothers who had enjoyed fussing over their baby sister and of whom she said, "To them I was a real live doll to play with." When she was growing up, she had been hesitant to compete academically and had felt socially stigmatized as the "square" in her peer group.

During the interview, the patient seemed to be quiet, passive, and deferential and appeared younger than her stated age. She cooperated enthusiastically during the interview and in fact seemed eager to anticipate the interviewer's questions in an effort to appear likable. There were no abnormalities of thought, perception, or sensorial functioning. Although she seemed mildly anxious, her symptoms did not meet the diagnostic criteria for anxiety disorder.

Epidemiology

In the Midtown Manhattan Study, Langner and Michael (1963) found that 2.5% of the patients in their sample had passive-dependent traits, such as those seen in dependent personality disorder. The diagnosis of passive-dependent personality disorder is made more frequently in women than in men, and it is more common in the youngest child of a family.

Table 36–9. *DSM-III-R* diagnostic criteria for dependent personality disorder (coded on axis II).

The diagnostic criteria for the personality disorders refer to behaviors or traits that are characteristic of the person's recent (past year) and long-term functioning (generally since adolescence or early adulthood). The constellation of behaviors or traits causes either significant impairment in social or occupational functioning or subjective distress. Behaviors or traits limited to episodes of illness are not considered in making a diagnosis of personality disorder.

A pervasive pattern of dependent and submissive behavior, beginning by early adulthood and present in a variety of contexts, as indicated by at least 5 of the following:

(1) Is unable to make everyday decisions without an excessive amount of advice or reassurance from others.
(2) Allows others to make most of his or her important decisions, eg, where to live, what job to take.
(3) Agrees with people even when he or she believes they are wrong, because of fear of being rejected.
(4) Has difficulty initiating projects or doing things on his or her own.
(5) Volunteers to do things that are unpleasant or demeaning in order to get other people to like him or her.
(6) Feels uncomfortable or helpless when alone, or goes to great lengths to avoid being alone.
(7) Feels devastated or helpless when close relationships end.
(8) Is frequently preoccupied with fears of being abandoned.
(9) Is easily hurt by criticism or disapproval.

Etiology & Pathogenesis

A. Genetic Factors: Gottesman (1963) found that the presence of submissiveness or dominance was more highly correlated in identical twins than in fraternal twins, which supports the hypothesis that dependent personality disorder has a genetic component.

B. Psychologic Factors: A disturbance at the oral stage of psychosexual development is believed to occur in patients who later develop dependent personality disorder; it takes the form of maternal deprivation rather than overgratification during early attachment (see Chapter 6).

Treatment

Long-term psychoanalytic psychotherapy is the treatment of choice and should focus on the patient's exaggerated fears of damaging others or oneself by pursuing autonomy and becoming one's own person.

Dependent Personality Disorder in Medical Practice

Patients with dependent personality disorder may make a dramatic appeal for caretaking, with urgent and inappropriate demands for immediate attention to their medical complaints, which have an exaggerated quality. If they fail to receive a prompt response, they may erupt in angry outbursts that threaten important emotional ties, including that with the physician. Since illness provides secondary gains in the form of caretaking and attention, such patients tend to be passive participants in the healing partnership rather than seeking active solutions. The well-known oral characteristics of dependent persons may be expressed in food, alcohol, and drug problems. The physician must be especially alert to the possibility of abuse of sedatives, hypnotics, tranquilizers, and analgesics. Patients with dependent personality disorder are overly compliant in their acceptance of medical treatment and may search for gratification of their unmet dependence needs by seeking unnecessary procedures while minimizing the associated hazards.

To patients with dependent personality disorder, physical illness represents the wish for the continuous soothing ministrations of the physician and also embodies a fear of abandonment. Being physically ill, with its considerable discomforts, may be equated with a lack of love or interest, and patients blame "bad" caretakers for their distress. The physician should provide reassurance and convey an impression of being available and accessible to the patient but should be careful to explain clearly and firmly the realistic limits of such availability. The physician can provide help in other ways, eg, coordinating support services and instituting flexible appointment scheduling, in which the patient assumes some responsibility for establishing the timing of appointments. Physicians treating these patients must guard against "burnout" and the hostile rejection that may be aroused by these patients' strong dependence needs. The patient's exaggerated compliance with the treatment regimen may lead to overutilization of medical

care systems and is another item that health care professionals need to be aware of. Others members of the health care team, including nurses and physical therapists, may play an important role in communicating the physician's interest and concern and in alleviating physical discomfort, so that the burden of meeting dependence needs is distributed throughout the team rather than being focused exclusively on any one member.

Illustrative case. A 45-year-old man was admitted to the hospital for surgical repair of damaged cartilage in his left knee. On the evening of admission, the resident on the surgical service completed the preoperative physical examination and noted the following in the chart: "Except for the damaged medial meniscus in the left knee, the patient is in remarkably good health. He does, however, present a psychologic management problem. He has made frequent requests for analgesics and bristled with irritation when I was called away to the emergency room before I could complete the physical examination. When I returned, the nurse assigned to his care remarked that the patient acted as though this were a Hilton Hotel and that he regarded his pain and anxiety as the only concerns of the hospital staff."

The resident held a meeting with the nurse, the physical therapist, and other members of the health care team in order to prevent further development of hostile reactions on the part of the staff toward this patient and to develop a management strategy. They agreed to meet the patient's requests for attention within realistic limits but decided that the burden of care would be distributed across the entire team. They also decided that a premedical school student summer volunteer should be assigned to the patient. This decision proved mutually rewarding, since it alleviated the patient's anxiety about being alone at a time when he felt vulnerable and provided the student volunteer with a glimpse of the way patients may react to illness.

COMPULSIVE PERSONALITY DISORDER

Symptoms & Signs

Table 36–10 lists the diagnostic criteria for compulsive personality disorder.

DSM-III-R states that the patient with this disorder shows a "pervasive pattern of perfectionism and inflexibility . . . ."

Patients with compulsive personality disorder experience distress associated with indecisiveness and difficulty in expressing tender feelings. They are generally depressed and feel suppressed anger about feeling controlled by others, and they demonstrate extreme sensitivity to social criticism and excessively conscientious, moralistic, scrupulous, and judgmental behavior.

Natural History & Prognosis

Full-blown axis I obsessive compulsive distur-

Table 36–10. *DSM-III-R* diagnostic criteria for compulsive personality disorder (coded on axis II).

The diagnostic criteria for the personality disorders refer to behaviors or traits that are characteristic of the person's recent (past year) and long-term functioning (generally since adolescence or early adulthood). The constellation of behaviors or traits causes either significant impairment in social or occupational functioning or subjective distress. Behaviors or traits limited to episodes of illness are not considered in making a diagnosis of personality disorder.

A pervasive pattern of perfectionism and inflexibility, beginning by early adulthood and present in a variety of contexts, as indicated by at least 5 of the following:

(1) Perfectionism that interferes with task completion, eg, inability to complete a project because own overly strict standards are not met.
(2) Preoccupation with details, rules, lists, order, organization, or schedules to the extent that the major point of the activity is lost.
(3) Unreasonable insistence that others submit to exactly his or her way of doing things, or unreasonable reluctance to allow others to do things because of the conviction that they will not do them correctly.
(4) Excessive devotion to work and productivity to the exclusion of leisure activities and friendships (not accounted for by obvious economic necessity).
(5) Indecisiveness: decision-making is either avoided, postponed, or protracted, eg, the person cannot get assignments done on time because of ruminating about priorities (do not include if indecisiveness is due to excessive need for advice or reassurance from others).
(6) Overconscientiousness, scrupulousness, and inflexibility about matters of morality, ethics, or values (not accounted for by cultural or religious identification).
(7) Restricted expression of affection.
(8) Lack of generosity in giving time, money, or gifts when no personal gain is likely to result.
(9) Inability to discard worn-out or worthless objects even when they have no sentimental value.

bances may break out periodically and remit. Kringlen (1965) noted the presence of characteristics of compulsive personality disorder in 72% of individuals who developed symptoms of obsessive compulsive disorder. Despite the compulsive individual's worry about the loss of impulse control, the incidence of sexual or aggressive behavior that is out of control is not higher in individuals with compulsive personality disorder than it is in the normal population. The risk of major depressive episodes appears to be increased during mid-life crisis.

Differential Diagnosis

Compulsive personality disorder must be distinguished from obsessive compulsive disorder, in which the patient experiences obsessive thoughts (eg, intrusive, unwanted impulses to shout obscenities or handle feces in an ordinarily controlled, moralistic, and meticulous person) or compulsive behavior (eg, repeated checking and rechecking of door locks) (see Chapter 31). The 2 disorders may coexist, in which case both diagnoses are warranted. Compulsive personality disorder must also be differentiated from schizoid and paranoid personality disorders. Obsessive traits (often seen in persons successfully engaged in professional careers) must be distinguished from full-blown compulsive personality disorder (which is maladaptive and interferes with normal functioning).

Illustrative Case

A 43-year-old senior vice president in an accounting firm sought psychiatric treatment because of a chronic sense of personal dissatisfaction. He had risen rapidly to the highest management level in his firm, but he derived no internal sense of pride and satisfaction. Reporting on this chronic feeling of dissatisfaction, he said, "When I successfully complete a project, it is a reprieve from my fearful expectations; when I experience a setback, it confirms my worst fears."

The patient's wife was a caring and competent woman who was a special education teacher. They had 2 children. The wife was a lively, articulate, and emotionally spontaneous person who had complained in the past about her husband's emotional remoteness and lack of adventuresome spirit. He felt great affection for his wife and children but was afraid to commit himself emotionally to these relationships, saying, "What if I allow myself to give and receive the love that I crave, and then something happens to them? I would be devastated."

The patient was the eldest son of 2 professional parents. While growing up, he had been extremely well provided for materially but had felt a lack of warmth and intimacy at home. His primary involvement with his family had centered around performance, and he felt pressured to succeed in school and sports. He felt that the family had placed little value on the quiet unstructured times of just enjoying one another's company. He had excelled in school but felt driven, and he had feared that his competitive strivings alienated him from his peers. In addition, he had felt stigmatized when he was left out of social activities during adolescence.

At the interview, the patient was dressed conservatively in somber tones and was meticulously groomed. He was reserved, emotionally distant from the interviewer, and provided a carefully detailed account of his unhappiness. His manner was that of a colleague consulting with another professional about a third person's difficulties rather than that of a patient visiting a doctor. There was no evidence of delusions, hallucinations, or disturbance in consciousness. His thinking was characterized by marked intellectualization and rationalization, a tendency to veer away from emotion-laden topics, and preoccupation with details to the exclusion of understanding the overall issues. Although he said that he felt a chronic sense of unhappiness in his life, he denied the presence of vegetative or other specific symptoms of depression.

Epidemiology

Although compulsive personality disorder is frequently diagnosed in men and is believed to be common, especially in the oldest children of a family, its prevalence is unknown.

Etiology & Pathogenesis

A. Genetic Factors: Twin and adoption studies have demonstrated that there is a genetic contribution to compulsive personality disorder.

B. Psychologic Factors: According to Freud, compulsive personality disorder is caused by arrest at the anal level of psychosexual development that results in repetitive power struggles with authority figures, dominance-submission conflicts, and emotional withholding (see Chapters 3 and 6). According to Erikson, disturbance in the stage of development characterized by the issue of autonomy versus shame and self-doubt predisposes to development of compulsive personality disorder (see Chapter 7). Family life is characterized by constrained emotions, and members are often criticized and socially ostracized if they express anger.

Treatment

Insight-oriented psychoanalytic psychotherapy is the treatment of choice. The focus must be on feelings rather than thoughts and would emphasize the clarification of the defenses of isolation of affect (intellectualized distancing from emotions) and displacement of hostility.

Group and behavioral therapy may be helpful in developing skills in achieving intimacy.

Compulsive Personality Disorder in Medical Practice

When they are confronted with physical illness, individuals with compulsive personality disorder are particularly troubled by the sense of loss of control over bodily functions. Feelings of shame and vulnerability for being in a weakened condition are typical. The patient also feels angry about the disruption of routines and is fearful of relinquishing control to the health care team. There may be exaggerated worries about submitting to authority figures. Under pressure from the many emotional aspects of the illness, the patient may be apprehensive about the possibility of giving way to emotional outbursts. The patient will attempt to ward off these anxieties by redoubling efforts at composure and presenting a precisely detailed, orderly account of progression of symptoms in an emotionally detached manner.

A scientific approach on the part of the physician—as conveyed in thorough history taking and careful diagnostic workups—is reassuring and fosters the trust necessary for an effective therapeutic alliance. A well-articulated account of the disease process and treatment alternatives reassures the patient that someone is in control and that the doctor respects the patient's capacities to participate as an informed partner in the healing process. The reassurance provides a foundation upon which the patient can begin to reconstruct a sense of order in everyday life.

Patients with compulsive personality disorder are not reassured by vague impressionistic overviews of their prognosis. Patients feel most comfortable when the doctor provides documentary evidence in the form of specific laboratory test results, eg, electrocardiograms or x-rays, or cites actual reports from the literature when presenting statistics about risk factors.

The healing process may be promoted by harnessing patients' innate thoroughness through encouraging such self-monitoring activities as measurement of fluid intake and output and weight fluctuations and control of graduated exercise programs. When feasible, patients can take over management of more routine procedures, such as changing their surgical dressings. Meticulous adherence to treatment protocols will restore morale as patients regain a sense of mastery and dignity in taking charge of their lives. The physician must remain alert to the possibility that compulsive patients may wish to carry this self-healing process too far and cross the boundaries of their competence while stubbornly resisting the expertise offered by the health care team.

Illustrative case. A 47-year-old woman who was an executive in a large accounting firm developed symptoms of unexpected weight loss and dizziness. Measurement of fasting blood glucose levels and urinalysis confirmed the diagnosis of adult-onset diabetes. The patient reacted to this news by conducting an extensive search of the literature on diabetes and by requesting that her internist refer her to an endocrinologist for further evaluation. The internist, who had known the patient for a long time, was empathically aware of how emotionally out of control the patient felt and promptly referred the patient to an endocrinologist, who confirmed the diagnosis and provided a detailed description of the nature and expectable course of the illness and alternative treatment strategies. The patient was reassured by the consensus of opinion shown by the 2 trusted experts and agreed to work with her internist in developing a treatment plan.

Although the patient was initially jolted into a state of panicky confusion by what she termed the "internal rebellion of my body," she regained a sense of order and predictability as she became an active partner in the healing process. Through a program of strict dietary control, weight loss, and exercise (which the patient meticulously pursued), she was able to bring her metabolic status within normal limits and thus avoided the need for exogenous insulin. In a 1-year follow-up appointment with the endocrinologist, the patient was complimented on her courageously disciplined response to the illness. When she was asked what had been most helpful in assisting her to cope with the problem, she replied, "Both you and my regular doctor had faith in my capacity to understand the illness and make informed choices about treatment, and you both supported my resolve to fight back. When I first became ill, I felt like a rudderless ship tossed about in dangerous waters. You were like a safe harbor, but even more important, you helped me regain the confidence that I could sail again on my own power."

PASSIVE-AGGRESSIVE PERSONALITY DISORDER

Symptoms & Signs

Table 36–11 sets forth diagnostic criteria for passive-aggressive personality disorder.

According to *DSM-III-R,* this disorder is characterized by "passive resistance to demands for adequate social and occupational performance . . . ."

People with passive-aggressive personality disorder may experience a feeling of dependence and lack of self-confidence as well as a chronic sense of pessimism. They often fail to connect their passive-resistant behavior with their feelings of resentfulness and hostility toward others.

Natural History & Prognosis

In a follow-up study of 100 inpatients with severe symptoms of passive-aggressive disorder, Small and coworkers (1970) found that of the 73 former patients located, 12% were free of symptoms and 79% had persistent difficulties. At the time of follow-up, 44% were employed full-time. A number of patients attempted suicide, although only one person succeeded. About 38% of patients were later rehospitalized. The prognosis is much better for people with milder forms of this personality disorder, for whom outpatient rather than inpatient care is the treatment of choice.

Differential Diagnosis

The differential diagnosis of passive-aggressive personality disorder includes dependent and avoidant personality disorder. In some cases, the patient may

Table 36–11. *DSM-III-R* diagnostic criteria for passive-aggressive personality disorder (coded on axis II).

The diagnostic criteria for the personality disorders refer to behaviors or traits that are characteristic of the person's recent (past year) and long-term functioning (generally since adolescence or early adulthood). The constellation of behaviors or traits causes either significant impairment in social or occupational functioning or subjective distress. Behaviors or traits limited to episodes of illness are not considered in making a diagnosis of personality disorder.

A pervasive pattern of passive resistance to demands for adequate social and occupational performance, beginning by early adulthood and present in a variety of contexts, as indicated by at least 5 of the following:

(1) Procrastinates, ie, puts off things that need to be done so that deadlines are not met.

(2) Becomes sulky, irritable, or argumentative when asked to do something he or she does not want to do.

(3) Seems to work deliberately slowly or to do a bad job on tasks that he or she really does not want to do.

(4) Protests, without justification, that others make unreasonable demands on him or her.

(5) Avoids obligations by claiming to have "forgotten."

(6) Believes that he or she is doing a much better job than others think he or she is doing.

(7) Resents useful suggestions from others concerning how he or she could be more productive.

(8) Obstructs the efforts of others by failing to do his or her share of the work.

(9) Unreasonably criticizes or scorns people in positions of authority.

---

meet the criteria for both compulsive and passive-aggressive personality disorder.

Illustrative Case

A 47-year-old man reluctantly sought psychiatric treatment when progressve financial and marital difficulties led to insomnia. Despite his reputation as a capable housing contractor, he had repeatedly been unable to meet his deadlines with both homeowners and subcontractors. He would often forget important appointments, drag his heels on commitments, and make excuses for being behind schedule, while inwardly feeling, "I'll do it in my own sweet time." His wife was threatening to leave him because she was unable to obtain his help around the house; she felt that she had to ask him 10 times to do anything, and even when he complied, he made only a half-hearted effort.

The patient was the youngest son in his family and had 2 older brothers who, he recalled with some bitterness, had teased and bullied him. He described his father as "the head honcho of the house," who had been more interested in maintaining peace and quiet than in being emotionally close to his sons. He felt his mother had been more caring but overinvolved in his life: "She had to know about every nook and cranny of my life and couldn't tolerate my keeping any secrets from her." As an adolescent he had enjoyed sports but had been prone to outbursts of righteous indignation when he felt he was being treated unfairly. He had been a good student but had been episodically disruptive in the classroom, particularly with strict male teachers. As an adult he had several close friends, but these relationships were strained because of his stubborn refusal to compromise on social plans and his chronic tardiness.

The patient arrived 20 minutes late for the interview and said that traffic had been heavy across town, when in actuality he was familiar with the traffic patterns and simply had not allowed enough time to ensure his prompt arrival. He indicated that he made the appointment reluctantly and only because of his wife's nagging complaints about his uncooperativeness at home. He provided little spontaneous information during the interview, so that the psychiatrist had great difficulty in obtaining useful data. The patient denied that he was in any way "testing" the psychiatrist when the latter tactfully confronted him about his provocative, obstructionist style. Mental status examination revealed no disorder of sensorium, thought organization, or perception, and though the patient's mood was irritable, he did not demonstrate any features of a major affective disorder.

Epidemiology

In the Stirling County (Nova Scotia, Canada) study, Leighton and coworkers (1963) found that in a community sample, about 1% of the total population showed passive-aggressive or passive-dependent behavior patterns. The sex ratio and familial pattern of passive-aggressive personality disorder are not known.

Etiology & Pathogenesis

Prospective studies of passive-aggressive personality disorder are lacking. Psychodynamic and learning theories both hypothesize a pattern of parental punishment of the child's assertion and aggression that results in a style of pseudopoliteness hiding resentment that can then only be covertly expressed.

Treatment

A study by Small and coworkers (1970) found that supportive psychotherapy was effective. The treatment of choice in most patients in insight-oriented (expressive) psychotherapy with a goal of gradually converting passive-aggressive behavior to more successful assertive behavior. The insight-oriented approach involves examination of the patient's covert expressions of hostility, first in the context of current repeatedly maladaptive social and occupational relationships and then in the patient's relationship with the therapist. Drug treatment is rarely used. When it is indicated, it is used mainly during periods of severe anxiety and depression.

Passive-Aggressive Personality Disorder in Medical Practice

Individuals with passive-aggressive personality disorder may be a source of considerable irritation to physicians, since they tend to make a dramatic display of their suffering while at the same time only minimally acknowledging the actual help they are receiving and exaggerating their continuing discomfort. Such patients derive secondary gains from remaining ill; eg, they have a means of punishing the envied and resented authority figures in their life, including physicians. They may attempt to place the responsibility for getting well on the physician's shoulders while they themselves subtly fail to cooperate with the treatment procedures. Such patients tend to forget appointments and be late in paying their accounts, and the physician finds little reward in treating them. The physician may then feel a sense of resentfulness and guilty responsibility, since the patient seems neither to improve nor to cooperate with the help offered but still seems to require the physician's attention.

The physician should take the time to acknowledge and empathize with the suffering of these patients before steering the conversation toward specific treatment recommendations. Such patients will then feel understood rather than forced into giving up their suffering before they are prepared to do so. Information is often presented to the patient more effectively in the form of questions rather than statements, such as "What will happen to you if you don't take your medication?" or "What do you think would be a fair fee for this treatment?" This approach encourages the patient's cooperation rather than inviting rebelliousness. If physicians understand that these patients have an investment in illness as a means of passively gaining control, they in turn need not feel weak or guilty because patients do not seem to improve.

Physicians should be alert to subtle forms of non-compliance; eg, patients may deliberately ask for information about treatment procedures so that they may later blame the physician for difficulties in treatment. A nonpunitive but frank discussion about the ways in which patients subtly undermine their own well-being may prevent such passive-aggressive patterns.

SELF-DEFEATING PERSONALITY DISORDER

Symptoms & Signs

Table 36–12 lists the diagnostic criteria for self-defeating personality disorder.

This disorder, which represents a new addition to the personality disorder section in *DSM-III-R*, is characterized by a pattern of recurrent self-defeating behavior in work and interpersonal relationships. Individuals with self-defeating personality disorder complain that others exploit, abuse, or otherwise take

Table 36–12. *DSM-III-R* diagnostic criteria for self-defeating personality disorder (coded on axis II).

The diagnostic criteria for the personality disorders refer to behaviors or traits that are characteristic of the person's recent (past year) and long-term functioning (generally since adolescence or early adulthood). The constellation of behaviors or traits causes either significant impairment in social or occupational functioning or subjective distress. Behaviors or traits limited to episodes of illness are not considered in making a diagnosis of personality disorder.

A. A pervasive pattern of self-defeating behavior, beginning by early adulthood and present in a variety of contexts. The person may often avoid or undermine pleasurable experiences, be drawn to situations or relationships in which he or she will suffer, and prevent others from helping him or her, as indicated by at least 5 of the following:
  (1) Chooses people and situations that lead to disappointment, failure, or mistreatment even when better options are clearly available.
  (2) Rejects or renders ineffective the attempts of others to help.
  (3) Following positive personal events (eg, new achievement), responds with depression, guilt, or a behavior that produces pain (eg, an accident).
  (4) Incites angry or rejecting responses from others and then feels hurt, defeated, or humiliated (eg, makes fun of spouse in public, provoking an angry retort, then feels devastated).
  (5) Rejects opportunities for pleasure, or is reluctant to acknowledge enjoying himself or herself (despite having adequate social skills and the capacity for pleasure).
  (6) Fails to accomplish tasks crucial to his or her personal objectives despite demonstrated ability to do so, eg, helps fellow students write papers but is unable to write her own papers.
  (7) Is uninterested in or rejects people who consistently treat him or her well, eg, is unattracted to caring sexual partners.
  (8) Engages in excessive self-sacrifice that is unsolicited by the intended recipients of the sacrifice.
B. The behaviors in criterion A do not occur exclusively in response to, or in anticipation of, being physically, sexually, or psychologically abused.
C. The behaviors in criterion A do not occur only when the person is depressed.

advantage of them and are often unaware of their own contribution to their misfortunes, which may include repeatedly choosing inappropriate friends, lovers, or colleagues or provoking others to mistreat them. Individuals with this disorder see themselves as self-sacrificing and complain bitterly when their needs are not met. However, the supportive nurturant overtures of others are often overtly or covertly rejected.

Because such individuals both wittingly and unwittingly choose situations likely to be unrewarding and sabotage more promising situations, they experience more failures than successes. When success is attained, it is frequently met with an attitude of exaggerated worry and skepticism and viewed as an aberration rather than as progress toward positive self-esteem or healthy optimism.

Natural History & Prognosis

Systematic data are not yet available on this disorder. There is, however, a strong clinical consensus that individuals with this disorder show stable long-term maladjustment patterns in work and interpersonal relationships. These self-defeating patterns have an inertial quality—setbacks feed upon themselves, and internal negative models of the self are validated by repeated disappointments in life experiences. Because of the predominance of failures over successes in the lives of these individuals, they are at increased risk for major depressive episodes.

Differential Diagnosis

The differential diagnosis of self-defeating personality disorder includes chronic dysthymia and major depressive episode in partial remission. Self-defeating personality disorder and affective disorders may coexist and require combined treatment strategies. Individuals with this personality disorder sometimes share overlapping features with narcissistic, borderline, and passive-aggressive personality disorders.

Illustrative Case

A 38-year-old man sought psychiatric treatment because of depression and loneliness following the breakup of a love relationship. He had been involved for 8 months with an attractive, intelligent, and caring woman. The breakdown of this relationship was particularly painful to him because the woman, unlike most women with whom he had been involved, had been genuinely committed to deepening the relationship. His earlier pattern had been to involve himself with self-absorbed, emotionally aloof partners who "trashed him in favor of someone more interesting."

He initially portrayed his current disappointment as yet another confirmation of his view that the world would victimize him and was not aware of having provoked the separation by repeatedly frustrating his lover's efforts to show him affection.

In the interview, he presented himself as a downtrodden victim who seemed impervious to help and who seemed convinced in advance that treatment would be of no value. The mental status examination revealed no disorder of sensorium, thought organization, or perception. Although his mood was both sad and irritable, he did not demonstrate the prototypical features of major depressive episode.

Epidemiology

The incidence and prevalence of this disorder are unknown, although it is assumed to be common.

Etiology & Pathogenesis

Psychodynamic theorists emphasize an unconscious need for self-punishment related to real or imagined transgressions against parental and sibling figures during childhood. Learning theorists emphasize the low frequency of rewarding life experiences. Cognitive theorists point out the importance of pathogenic schemas, ie, irrational, enduring beliefs about the self as a helpless victim unable to effect positive changes in one's life.

Treatment

Long-term multimodal treatments that combine identification of self-defeating patterns, alleviation of unconscious guilt, revision of pathologic beliefs about the self, and formation of more rewarding interpersonal relationships gradually alter maladaptive patterns. Antidepressant drug treatment with tricyclics or monoamine oxidase inhibitors is indicated when a major depressive episode complicates the course of the disorder.

Self-Defeating Personality Disorder in Medical Practice

Patients with self-defeating personality disorder present a special treatment challenge for the physician. Such patients frequently have an unconscious need to defeat the physician's efforts to effect a cure. Often, they overreact to minor side effects of treatment, discontinue treatment against medical advice, or develop symptom substitution. It is difficult to recruit the patient's active cooperation. When treatment is successful, such individuals frequently place themselves at risk for relapse by neglecting nutritional and exercise needs, abusing alcohol and drugs, or not complying with rehabilitation programs.

When treating self-defeating patients, it is useful for the physician to maintain the perspective that the course will be long-term and often complicated. The physician should resist the patient's witting or unwitting invitation to perform miracles only to be defeated by the patient's compulsive need to undermine help when it is offered. The physician should also anticipate the patient's difficulty in cooperating with treatment. Referral for psychiatric treatment, although initially met with reluctance, may later be accepted as the patients gradually gain insight into their own role in self-defeating patterns.

PATIENTS WITH MIXED PERSONALITY DISORDERS

The descriptions provided above present the personality disorders as discrete diagnostic entities so as to point out the distinctive characteristics of each disorder and thereby provide some framework around which to organize clinical observations. As is also sometimes the case in medical patients, psychiatric patients may show features of more than one disorder simultaneously, so that careful management using a skillful synthesis of the approaches described for each separate disorder is imperative, eg, for a patient with mixed compulsive and narcissistic personality disorder or one with mixed histrionic and borderline personality disorder. The problem is analogous to that encountered in medical management of multisystem disease, eg, coexisting diabetes and hepatitis. In the case of combined personality disorders, the physician must avoid minimizing or overemphasizing any one element at the expense of a balanced "systems" approach.

MANAGEMENT OF THE "HATEFUL" PATIENT

A common theme in this chapter is the resentment that may be aroused in physicians and other caretakers by certain patients with personality disorder. Groves (1978) describes the 4 types of patients with personality disorder who are most likely to evoke an attitude of dislike or even hatred in their physicians: dependent clingers, entitled demanders, manipulative help rejectors, and self-destructive deniers. The similarity of these 4 diagnostic categories to specific personality disorders described in *DSM-III* is readily apparent. The dependent clinger corresponds to dependent personality disorder; the entitled demander is the same as narcissistic personality disorder; the manipulative help rejector equals passive-aggressive or borderline personality disorder; and the self-destructive denier corresponds to histrionic or borderline personality disorder.

Groves frankly acknowledges the dislike that physicians often feel for certain patients. Although conscious recognition and acceptance of negative feelings toward a patient run counter to the idea of the physician as an unfailingly kind and generous healer of the sick, the denial of such feelings when they really exist can only lead to further disturbances in management of the patient. Recognizing feelings of resentment is an important cornerstone in developing an appropriate management strategy that will create a strong working alliance between the physician and the patient in order to facilitate healing.

REFERENCES

Bowlby J: Forty-four juvenile thieves. *Int J Psychoanal* 1944; **25**:19.

Carpenter WT, Gunderson JG, Strauss JS: Considerations of the borderline syndrome: A longitudinal comparative study of borderline and schizophrenic patients. In: *Borderline Personality Disorders: The Concept, the Syndrome, the Patient*. Hartocollis P (editor). Internat Univ Press, 1977.

Freud S: Three essays on the theory of sexuality (1905). In: *Standard Edition of the Complete Psychological Works of Sigmund Freud*. Vol 7. Hogarth Press, 1964.

Glueck S, Glueck E: *Delinquents and Nondelinquents in Perspective*. Harvard Univ Press, 1968.

Gottesman II: Heritability of personality: A demonstration. *Psychol Monogr* 1963;**77**:1.

Groves JE: Taking care of the hateful patient. *N Engl J Med* 1978;**298**:883.

Horowitz MJ: Sliding meanings: A defense against threat in narcissistic personalities. *Int J Psychoanal Psychother* 1975; **4**:167.

Kahana R, Bibring G: Personality types in medical management. In: *Psychiatry and Medical Practice in the General Hospital*. Zinberg N (editor). Internat Univ Press, 1964.

Kernberg O: *Borderline Conditions and Pathological Narcissism*. Jason Aronson, 1975.

Kiloh L, Osselton JW: *Clinical Electroencephalography*. Butterworths, 1966.

Klein D: Psychopharmacological treatment and delineation of borderline disorders. In: *Borderline Personality Disorders: The Concept, the Syndrome, the Patient*. Hartocollis P (editor). Internat Univ Press, 1977.

Kohut M: *The Analysis of the Self*. Internat Univ Press, 1971.

Kringlen E: Obsessional neurotics. *Br J Psychiatry* 1965;**111**: 709.

Langner TS, Michael ST: *Life Stress and Mental Health*. Free Press, 1963.

Leigh H, Reiser MF: *The Patient: Biological, Psychological, and Social Dimensions of Medical Practice*. Plenum Press, 1980.

Leighton DC et al: Psychiatric findings of the Stirling County study. *Am J Psychiatry* 1963;**119**:1021.

Mahler MS: A study of the separation-individuation process and its possible application to borderline phenomena in the psychoanalytic situation. *Psychoanal Study Child* 1971;**26**:403.

Masterson JF: *Treatment of the Borderline Adolescent: A Developmental Approach*. Wiley, 1972.

Robins LN: *Deviant Children Grown Up: A Sociological and Psychiatric Study of Sociopathic Personality*. Williams & Wilkins, 1966.

Schulsinger F: Psychopathy, heredity, and environment. *Int J Ment Health* 1972;**1**:190.

Small F et al: Passive-aggressive personality disorder: A search for a syndrome. *Am J Psychiatry* 1970;**126**:973.

Werble B: Second follow-up study of borderline patients. *Arch Gen Psychiatry* 1970;**23**:307.

Sexual Dysfunction

37

Evalyn S. Gendel, MD, & Emmett J. Bonner, PhD

Sexual dysfunctions are defined in *DSM-III-R* as follows: sexual desire disorders (including hypoactive sexual desire and sexual aversion); sexual arousal disorders (including female sexual arousal disorder and male erectile disorder); orgasm disorders (including inhibited female orgasm, inhibited male orgasm, and premature ejaculation); sexual pain disorders (including functional dyspareunia and functional vaginismus); sexual dysfunction not otherwise specified; and other sexual disorders not otherwise specified. After a general discussion of sexual dysfunctions, each of these entities will be discussed in a separate section.

The sexual dysfunctions are the most common of sexual disorders. Gender identity disorders, paraphilias, and other sexual disorders are discussed in Chapter 38.

Early Recognition of Sexual Dysfunction

Sexuality is an important component of physical, intellectual, psychologic, and social well-being. The central role of sexual behavior—how it affects and is affected by health and illness—was emphasized in *Education and Treatment in Human Sexuality: The Training of Health Professionals,* a report published by the World Health Organization in 1976.

Physicians have the opportunity to assess sexual dysfunction in the course of a routine history and examination of patients. A simple sexual history taken at some appropriate time during the office visit signifies to the patient that sexuality is as important as any other physical or psychologic function. By taking such a history as a routine matter, medical students and physicians can help prevent sexual dysfunction, become more aware of paraphilias, and find cases of gender identity disorders. Since most patients do not present with sexual complaints, the responsibility rests with the physician to elicit and identify complaints as primary unexpressed problems, as possible early clues to organic mental and physical disorders, and as complications of general medical conditions.

Although all but a few of the medical schools in the USA teach some aspects of human sexuality, it is unfortunate that sexual history taking is not a skill in which physicians are expected to excel. Students who become interested in sexual factors in diagnosis and treatment may not be encouraged to sustain their interest unless other physicians on the medical service agree that sexuality is an important factor in health.

Many students and physicians are uncomfortable with patients' questions about sexuality and feel uneasy about broaching the subject themselves. In some cases, they feel that such questions are an intrusion on the patient's privacy, even though they realize that bowel patterns, sleep disturbances, drinking and drug habits, and reproductive status are also private matters. In other cases, they believe that the patient's sexual concerns are not of medical significance or that their own ability to treat such concerns is limited; thus, they ignore or dismiss the patient's concerns.

Physicians must recognize not only the role of sexuality in health and illness but also their own feelings about patients' sexual problems, since this is a first step in learning to be more effective in caring for patients with sexual complaints.

Patients expect their physicians to be authorities on sexual matters, but they frequently are unable to express their concerns to the physician for fear of being criticized or misunderstood. Although there are no longitudinal, controlled research studies of most sexual dysfunctions, it is estimated that 60–80% are psychogenic in origin. These data reflect the fact that medical causes of sexual dysfunction are now diagnosed more frequently because more reliable diagnostic procedures are available. Many of these dysfunctions are never identified unless the patient introduces the subject or presents with the complaint. Surveys of practicing physicians conducted over the past decade show that only 10% of patients will initiate a discussion of sexual problems if the physician does not; but over 50% will describe a sexual concern if the physician provides an opportunity for discussion. These concerns frequently provide the first clue to other diagnostic considerations or are recognized as the major problem in an otherwise elusive diagnosis.

A common situation involves the male patient with repeated though episodic inability to achieve or maintain an erection. He reports to his family physician that he has not "felt like himself" but does not describe any specific symptoms. Physical examination reveals no abnormalities, but a sexual history is not taken. The patient is reassured that he is "quite healthy and there are no physical problems." This reassurance is puzzling. If he is well, why is he having this difficulty? In a subsequent office visit, the patient may describe his problem to the physician, who may refer him to a urologist. The urologist may also find the patient physically well. The patient will generally develop more severe symptoms affecting his sexual activities and relationships as well as other aspects of his life, and eventually the family physician or a specialist may refer him for psychotherapy or for marriage or sexual counseling. By this time, however, the problem is usually more difficult to treat. This example illustrates the important role of the primary physician in early detection of sexual dysfunction. The primary-care physician can often provide satisfactory initial treatment or appropriate referral (or both), which would implement early recovery and prevention of the more severe, less easily treated problems.

Sexual Response Cycle

A. Sexual Instincts and Learned Behavior: Procreation via sexual activity is an adaptive response developed through biologic evolution that gives the species a high potential for survival. Sexual behavior, however, is learned behavior and is influenced by familial patterns, sociocultural factors (public media, community institutions, and the social milieu), and individual experiences and patterns of development as well as by choice. This is in contrast to sexual behavior in other mammalian species, which is under instinctual control with timing governed by the estrous cycle of the female.

Even though sexual behavior and attitudes toward sex vary greatly among individuals, the desire for sexual pleasure is thought to be strong in most men and women. Although there are no data from longitudinal group studies on the quality and intensity of sexual desire or on the quality of sexual activity, clinical experience indicates that the intensity of desire and the degree of satisfaction vary throughout an individual's life. The factors that influence these variations are dependent on the relationship to a particular sexual partner or to different partners; changing sexual fantasies at different periods of growth and development—youth to old age; emotional mood and physical and mental well-being; and varying influences on self-image and self-esteem.

B. Phases of the Sexual Response Cycle: The biophysiologic events in the sexual response cycle have been described by Dickinson (1949), Masters and Johnson (1966), and Kaplan (1974), with elaborations by them and others. However, 4 basic phases are generally recognized:

1. Appetitive or desire phase—In this phase, one or more stimuli (eg, visual, olfactory, tactile, fantasied) engender a desire to engage in sexual activity.

2. Excitement or arousal phase—This phase includes the individual's feelings of sexual pleasure and accompanying physiologic changes. The major change in both men and women is pelvic vasocongestion with accompanying myotonia. In men, this results in penile tumescence, stimulation of Cowper's gland, drawing of the scrotum and testicles closer to the body, and penile erection. In women, pelvic congestion and myotonia result in engorgement of the vessels of the external genitalia and the vaginal lining; sweating (transudate production) of the vagina, which pro-

duces lubrication; increased tension of the pubococcygeal muscle surrounding the vaginal orifice; development of the orgasmic platform; increased sensitivity and enlargement of the clitoris; and "ballooning" of the inner two-thirds of the vagina. Breast tissue frequently engorges, with accompanying nipple erection and sensitivity.

3. Orgasmic phase—In both men and women, generalized muscle tension is followed by muscle contractions, resulting in involuntary pelvic thrusting and heightened sexual sensations. With the release of muscle tension, there are rhythmic contractions of the pelvic and perineal muscles. In women, contractions occur in the lower third of the vagina and in the uterus, which has been elevated in relation to the other pelvic structures (orgasmic platform). In men, contractions of the prostate, seminal vesicles, and urethra propel seminal and prostatic fluids to the exterior while the bladder sphincter closes.

4. Resolution phase—In both sexes, vasocongestion and myotonia become less intense, and there is general body relaxation. Men experience a physiologic refractory period before erection and orgasm can occur again. Vasocongestion and myotonia subside less quickly in women, and the clitoral and perineal tissues are sensitive enough to respond almost immediately to continued stimulation.

Symptoms & Signs

Most sexual dysfunctions are related to disturbances in one or more phases of the sexual response cycle. The disturbance may be physiologic or psychologic. For example, a man who feels strong desire for a partner (psychologic) may find that he is not being aroused, as evidenced by an absent or partial erection (physiologic). Similarly, a woman who is sexually aroused by her partner and responding physiologically may be unable to reach orgasm as she begins to worry about losing control.

Diagnosis of sexual dysfunction requires that the dysfunction be the central factor in the clinical course, even though it may not be the chief complaint. The dysfunction is usually chronic and perceived by the patient as a change in the sense of sexual pleasure as well as in performance. It is rare for a patient to have symptoms of inhibition or lessening of pleasure without a dysfunction being present; it is also rare for a dysfunction to be present without the patient exhibiting distress. Symptoms may be lifelong or of recent onset; they may be constant or may be present only at certain times (eg, "facultative"—with one partner but not with others); and they may be manifested as complete or partial sexual disability.

Patients may have no serious psychologic disturbances or symptoms, but they may exhibit vague complaints of anxiety, guilt, or shame associated with the problem. Their concerns are often focused on fear of not pleasing a partner or inability to feel confident about their sexual "technique." Men and women often describe a sense of "not doing it right," which contributes to further concerns about their sexual capabilities. This "spectatoring" (self-monitoring) exacerbates the symptoms.

Most sexual dysfunctions are not associated with impairment in occupational functioning, although patients may report that their job creativity has suffered or that the quality of life has been impaired. The major complications occur in relationships with partners and often affect relationships with others as well.

Patients without partners can be treated for dysfunction. With couples, successful involvement of the partner in treatment is important in conducting therapy and can help prevent further complications.

Natural History

The general course of these conditions is variable, depending on whether they are chronic or recently acquired; persistent, episodic, or partner-specific; and complicated by other forms of dysfunction. The following discussion of sexual dysfunction demonstrates that although psychogenic disorders may have similar orgins, their manifestations and response to treatment differ.

Differential Diagnosis

Many patients are concerned about whether they are "sexually normal." Questions often asked are whether sexual intercourse is as spontaneous and natural or as frequent as it "should" be for persons of the same age and marital status. The physician who suspects that such questions may be a clue to a sexual problem that should be explored must use the sexual history to distinguish patients who need further investigation from those who only need sensible information about intimate matters.

When an organic disorder (eg, physical reaction to medication) may have contributed to the sexual dysfunction, both diagnoses should be used, with the organic disorder described on *DSM-III-R* axis III (see Chapter 23 for further information about *DSM-III-R* procedures).

When symptoms are due primarily to a mental disorder, the diagnosis of sexual dysfunction should be avoided; the axis I mental disorder classification should be used. However, if sexual dysfunction developed first and was the cause of the resulting mental disorder, the axis I diagnosis of sexual dysfunction should be used.

If a personality disorder coexists or is an etiologic factor in sexual dysfunction, the sexual dysfunction should be diagnosed on axis I and the personality disorder on axis II. A V-code condition (eg, marital problem, interpersonal conflict, or life crisis) is frequently the featured cause of sexual dysfunction and should be noted as part of the axis I sexual dysfunction diagnosis (see Chapter 35).

When the clinician believes that there has been inadequate sexual stimulation—inadequate either in focus, intensity, or duration—the diagnosis of sexual dysfunction is not appropriate. The clinician is dependent on the patient's description of the details of sexual interactions. The physician's skill at open-ended, non-

judgmental history taking is paramount to this process.

Epidemiology

The overall incidence of sexual problems is fairly equal in men and women. At one time, it was believed that more women than men sought treatment, but this no longer appears to be the case, according to recent surveys.

Sexual dysfunction may have its onset at any time. The most common period appears to be from 20 to 40 years of age—the time when long-term relationships are usually established. However, current data show that increasing numbers of people in their 40s, 50s, and 60s are seeking treatment of sexual problems.

Etiology & Pathogenesis

Etiologic factors common to most sexual dysfunctions will be described here. Factors involved in specific types of dysfunction are discussed in subsequent sections.

In both men and women, the cause of sexual dysfunction is usually multifactorial. Some sexual problems have their basis in experiences and circumstances far removed from the patient's current life situation. Most problems, however, have more immediate causes and arise after an extended relatively satisfactory period of sexual function. Patients usually postpone seeking help for 3–12 years, believing that the problem will be resolved when changes occur in activities (work, studies), relationships (pregnancy, marriage), or other aspects of their lives. They often believe there must be a medical problem and are usually willing to submit to physical examinations and tests so that a cause may be found and a "cure" instituted. It is only after these avenues have been explored that the patient arrives at the conclusion that there is some other cause.

A. Sociocultural Factors: Family customs, traditions, and attitudes may be incongruent with the patient's present situation.

1. Sexual attitudes and values–The attitudes formed in early life may interfere with the ability to enjoy current behavior. For example, parents may instill the attitude that "sex is dirty" by associating it with elimination of body wastes or by scolding or punishment for masturbation, which often produces guilt without modifying the behavior. The attitude that display of passion is "animalistic" and the family's reinforcement of the "double standard" of behavior for men and women are other common examples.

2. Religious beliefs–Some religious sects or denominations try to impose restrictions on sexual activity—eg, by preaching that sex is only for procreation and that pleasure is somehow wicked.

3. Trauma in early adolescence–Examples include sexual awkwardness due to ignorance about sexuality and lack of experience; hasty sexual encounters in anxiety-provoking situations during adolescence; and incest or sexual abuse or assault (more common than previously believed).

B. Intrapsychic Conflicts:

1. Anxiety—Anxiety is probably the most common etiologic factor and, regardless of its source, interrupts feelings of pleasure accompanying the cycle of sexual response.

a. Performance anxiety—This form of anxiety is usually self-imposed, and expectations or standards of performance are often based on something the individual has heard, seen, or read, such as exaggerated accounts of what constitutes sexual adequacy in popular fiction, magazine articles, and movies. Sexual adequacy becomes equated with the partner's approval rather than with the personal attainment of joy, satisfaction, intimacy, and love.

b. Performance pressure—There may be pressure from either the male or the female partner to reach orgasm. This occurs both in heterosexual and in homosexual relationships. Men may feel an obligation to achieve and maintain erection almost on demand, or this "duty" may be self-imposed. Women may feel an obligation to reach orgasm during intercourse or to attain multiple orgasms.

2. "Spectatoring"—The following may erect barriers to erotic feelings: monitoring one's own sexual expertise or reactions to pleasure; intellectualizing the sexual experience; imagining how one appears to others during lovemaking (eg, to the partner, the parents, or the children); and imagining that one's lovemaking is being heard or observed by neighbors or other people. Some patients will say, "I was mentally critiquing my own lovemaking."

3. Fear—There may be fear of abandonment because of some sexual or personal flaw, fear of loss of self-control during sexual excitement or orgasm, fear of displeasing a partner, or fear of unwanted pregnancy or sexually transmitted disease (eg, AIDS). In couples being treated for infertility, there may be fear of missing opportunities for conception.

4. Guilt—Guilt can be related to enjoyment of activity, choice of partner, or engaging in "forbidden" or "sinful" sexual activity. The list of origins of guilt for patients is extensive.

5. Self-hatred—The individual may feel unworthy of being loved or of experiencing pleasure.

6. Depression—Depression focused on life situations or events (eg, job, increased home or office responsibilities, illness in the family) may interfere with sexual activity.

7. Denial—An individual engaging in sexual activity may refuse to consider the activity as sexual behavior.

C. Interpersonal or Relationship Factors:
These factors frequently incorporate many other etiologic factors.

1. Anger—Anger may be either passive or active. Hostility toward the partner can be expressed by creating pressure and tension before sexual activity; choosing an inappropriate time to initiate sexual activity (especially when the time is known to be irritating to the partner); making oneself physically or psychologically repulsive to the partner (eg, deliberate lack of cleanliness, avoidance of physical contact, verbal attacks on family members or on the partner in the presence of others); or finding excuses to frustrate the partner's sexual desires (eg, claiming exhaustion, feigning physical illness, preferring to watch television or finish a book).

2. Lack of trust—Partners may feel that something they do sexually or otherwise will be used against them. Lack of trust may also result from repeatedly being asked to engage in sexual activities known by one partner to be unpleasant to the other (eg, oral-genital stimulation).

3. Power struggles—Many satisfactory relationships are marred by each partner wanting to be "in control." Passive resistance to partners' wishes occurs. Devices are used to gain or maintain power, including threats to withhold money, a vacation, etc, if sexual demands are not met; threats to end the relationship or marriage; and threats of suicide or violence to a partner.

4. Lack of communication with the partner about sex—Failure to communicate what is pleasurable is often the result of unrealistic expectations: "If you really cared about me, you would know what I like." Failure to disclose what is desired or preferred establishes an unsatisfying pattern of sexual activity, and this pattern can last for many years. This type of communication problem—labeled "mind reading" by many clinicians—is a habit many couples develop in other aspects of their lives. Fearful of being hurt or of wounding the other person's ego, each attempts to decide what the other partner wants.

5. Development of a "sex manual mentality"—This is the belief that there is a specific recipe for sexual behavior and that following it step-by-step will lead to sexual gratification. (This may be considered a type of "spectatoring.") The partners are convinced that if their sex life is unsatisfactory it must be because they have failed to learn the "right way" to make love.

D. Educational and Cognitive Factors:

1. Early learning experiences—Sources of information about sexuality (parents, other adults, peers) may convey biased attitudes or misrepresent "facts." These early learning experiences appear to strongly influence later sexual behavior.

2. Sexual ignorance—For example, failure to engage in erotic stimulation may be due to ignorance of its role in mature sexual activity.

3. Belief in sexual myths—

a. Sex role expectations—Stereotypical assumptions are that men are the initiators of sexual activity, are more experienced, and are easily angered if not allowed to maintain full control of the situation; and that women are submissive, need not enjoy sexual activity in order to participate, and are solely responsible for contraception. These assumptions are widely held and are a frequent major problem in sexual dysfunction.

b. Myths about age and appearance—There is a myth that old, disabled, or unattractive people are incapable of or uninterested in sexual activity or cannot find partners. People who believe they fit any of these categories or people who meet and are attracted to others who fit the stereotype may avoid sexual activity for fear of being thought "abnormal."

c. Myths about proper sexual activity— People often have strong opinions about what constitutes improper sexual activity (eg, taboos against manual genital stimulation or sexual activity during menstruation).

d. Myths about sexual prowess— Examples include the belief that penile size (generally in the flaccid state) is indicative of sexual potency or prowess; the belief that women with small breasts lack femininity or are unable to nurse infants; and the belief that ejaculatory capacity will be diminished at some particular age. Myths about masturbation are that it impairs sexual competence, is indicative of homosexual tendencies, or causes mental illness, among others.

E. Iatrogenic Factors: Lief (1981) and others have reported several instances in which comments, jokes, and casual notice given to sexual problems by physicians were adverse factors in psychosexual dysfunction. For example, an internist's remark to a diabetic patient—that he should realize that 50% of diabetics become impotent—was not accompanied by explanation; the patient developed sexual problems as he tried to deal with this prediction. In some cases, the physician provides unrealistic reassurances that the problem will pass but offers no suggestions, and the patient assumes that nothing can be done if the problem does not resolve itself. In other cases, a superficial solution to a complex problem is offered. For example, when a 25-year-old woman complained of failure to experience orgasm with her husband, the physician gave her a book about female masturbation and told her she would no longer be abnormal if she read it and practiced what it suggested.

Levels of Intervention & Treatment

Although approaches to treatment of sexual dysfunction vary widely among clinicians, some general principles are applicable.

Sex therapy is generally characterized as follows: (1) short-term, eg, 5–20 visits approximately 1–2 weeks apart; (2) focused on the sexual problem; (3) directed to present and future goals, ie, not requiring retrospective analysis except to the extent the therapy suggests its usefulness; (4) action-oriented, ie, involving the individual or couple in assignments to be carried out at home; and (5) incorporating behavioral and psychodynamic approaches. Therapy can be instituted with patients without partners, homosexual or heterosexual, but appears to be most effective when a partner also participates. The approaches discussed below involve therapy for couples; however, specific suggestions for home assignments can be adapted for treatment of patients without partners.

Sex therapy is not always indicated or necessary. The clinician may diagnose and treat dysfunction long before intensive sex therapy is needed.

A. Ruling Out Organic Disease: Many patients with sexual dysfunction have had a physical examination before they seek or are referred for therapy. There is usually a strong feeling on their part that some physical problem exists and can be readily "cured"; thus, they prefer to believe in an organic rather than a psychologic cause.

The clinician must verify or repeat the physical examination. In some cases, a review of the patient's previous medical records will suffice. In patients of either sex, laboratory reports of blood glucose levels, thyroid and liver function, and hormone levels should be normal. A history of current alcohol or drug use—prescribed, over-the-counter, and recreational—should be elicited.

B. Assessing a Contributing Physical Illness: Occasionally, there is a preexisting chronic medical condition (eg, arthritis) or a postsurgical condition (eg, following appendectomy or radical mastectomy) that does not interfere with sexual response but may contribute to the current behavior. (The presence of a contributing physical condition should be recorded on *DSM-III-R* axis III.)

C. Eliciting Discussion and Educating the Patient: The clinician should assist the patient in understanding the relationship between physiologic and psychologic components of dysfunction. While the history is being taken, the physician can encourage the patient ("give permission") to talk openly about sex and can also give educational feedback in a nonjudgmental manner about the patient's fears, anxieties, or items of misinformation. For an individual or couple, this session is often the first step in the therapeutic process. For a few, it may be the only session required. Many patients have never had the opportunity to discuss with a health professional what they are experiencing sexually with their partner. Partners who hear each other's perceptions of their problem in these circumstances often develop enough confidence to continue to explore the problem on their own. If the barrier of silence is broken and anger is sufficiently reduced, patients may feel less anxious about the situation. By the end of the second session, many couples wonder aloud, "Why couldn't we have done this on our own when our problem first began?" Couples or individuals with this attitude generally require only a short course of therapy.

D. Setting the Parameters of Therapy: Once patients have described the problems and their goals, they need to know what therapy will be like. Negative images and sensational images of sex therapy abound. A forthright explanation should be made about their active participation in therapy sessions and home assignments or exercises. They should also be informed of the ground rules, which will often seem mechanical but at the same time will make them feel emotionally vulnerable. The therapist should provide an overview which can be expanded as necessary during therapy and which allows the patients to recognize and take responsibility for much of their treatment.

E. Suggesting Forms of Therapy: Making specific suggestions for "homework" consisting of verbalization of sexual needs and physical expression of closeness actively involves the patients in their own care.

1. Sensate focusing exercises–These are structured 1-hour exercises, with 3–4 sessions assigned between office visits. The purpose of the exercises is to help the couple recognize that sexual activity is not limited to sexual intercourse and that "pleasuring"—ie, stimulating the partner, which gives pleasure to oneself as well as the partner, and receiving stimulation—can be enjoyable without being regarded as foreplay or a preliminary to intercourse.

Early assignments are devoted to stimulating nongenital parts of each other's bodies, with emphasis on "nondemand" pleasuring—ie, pleasuring to explore one's own feelings about the experience rather than to please the partner. Later assignments incorporate caressing breasts and genitals, but sexual intercourse is prohibited for the period of the exercise. Partners need only concentrate on tactile sensations and on verbalizing what feels best. The partners should be told how they can sabotage the process by not arranging for sufficient time to carry out assignments and by going through the motions but evading the spirit of the assignment.

Sexual arousal and intercourse are not the goals of these exercises. The partners are instructed to refrain from intercourse even if aroused and to continue to enjoy the sensations and physiologic relaxation. Caresses (relaxing, affectionate touching) should be used rather than massage or sexual stimulators such as vibrators. Explaining to the partners how touching produces physiologic responses is useful to their understanding of the treatment process.

Some therapists prohibit intercourse during the early weeks of treatment, others only during assignments. Patients may be told that they can indulge in orgasmic experiences, including intercourse, at times other than their assignment if they mutually desire to do so. In cases in which erectile or orgasmic problems are due to performance anxiety, these nondemand pleasuring exercises relieve the pressure to "succeed" and allow patients to experience their own sensations without concentrating on pleasing the partner.

2. Systematic sensitization or desensitization–In cases of premature ejaculation, the patient is taught to recognize (through sensate focusing exercises) when orgasm or ejaculation is about to become inevitable. If he has a partner, he can show her how he stimulates himself by masturbation or she can provide manual stimulation to be stopped at a signal from him when orgasm becomes imminent. The process is then resumed, and in this way a **start-stop sensitization cycle** is established. When some degree of control has been gained, the partners should then try intravaginal containment, usually with the man supine. Rhythmic movements are gradually increased until the man gives the signal to stop. After a pause, the movements are resumed and stopped again, etc, as the partners learn how to prolong the pleasure of intercourse while containing the urge to ejaculate.

This start-stop technique has almost entirely replaced the older squeeze technique, which required learning one inhibiting mechanism and later learning natural control. The squeeze technique consists of squeezing the corona and frenulum of the penis to "hold back" ejaculation at the moment of inevitability. This can be done by the man but works best when done by a partner, who places a thumb on the frenulum and the first and second fingers just above and below the coronal ridge on the opposite side. Pressure is applied for about 4 seconds and abruptly released. The pressure is always applied in front-to-back manner, never from side-to-side. Pinching is avoided by using the pads of the fingers (not the fingernails). The man should try to concentrate on the exciting sensations rather than divert his attention with nonsexual thoughts.

Similar desensitizing and sensitizing techniques can be used in treating orgasmic problems in women. With progressive stimulation of clitoral and other genital areas by a partner, arousal is experienced without demand or pressure for intercourse. Gradual sensitization occurs until the woman can guide the course of stimulation and penetration.

For women with problems in initiating sexual activity, a series of exercises can be assigned to help the woman feel more in control and help the male partner feel less responsible for all aspects of expressing sexual desire. Sex role expectations—which may have inhibited interpersonal as well as sexual communication—are most likely to be overcome in this manner.

3. Therapy sessions following homework assignments–Sexual dysfunctions usually affect and are affected by other aspects of the patient's lifestyle. Important life events often precipitate dysfunctions, while ongoing daily pressures, lack of interpersonal communication, and family and business pressures prolong and exacerbate them. Consequently, couples who have developed poor patterns of relating (either caused by sexual problems or exaggerated by them) are often angry, resentful, distrusting, and guilty about each other's behavior. The dysfunction is often seen as "her" or "his" problem or as only "my" problem. These perceptions must be explored early in therapy. Individuals without partners often perceive themselves as abnormal, deviant, unattractive, or unworthy of love and affection, and they are determined to overcome their sexual problems before becoming involved with anyone again.

The couple or individual must make a good faith commitment of time and effort to the sex therapy process. Partners do not have to be permanently committed to each other but must be willing to cooperate in treatment. The therapist observes their style of relating to each other and assists them in interpreting their behavior. Home exercises or assignments become the behavioral vehicle for a progressive integration of the partners' ideas of their own sexual functioning, anatomy, and physiology. They learn to develop nonverbal and verbal ways of communicating about sexual matters and become more aware of their own sensuality. The goals are to reduce anxiety, to eliminate or modify destructive or other maladaptive styles of relating, and to make decisions about what they would like to change. "Not having time" for assignments is often a form of resistance. Patients may feel that they should cancel an appointment because they have not done their homework. But doing the homework will not "cure" the problem, and patients need to be reminded that homework is only one aspect of this combination of psychodynamic and behavioral treatment.

HYPOACTIVE SEXUAL DESIRE

Symptoms & Signs

Hypoactive sexual desire can occur in men and women at any age. As shown in Table 37–1, one of the *DSM-III-R* diagnostic criteria is the persistent absence or deficiency of sexual fantasies and desire. The current life situation of the patient—and, more significantly, the history of events preceding the patient's first awareness of lack of desire—must be reviewed. Age, general health, the quality and frequency of sexual activity in the past, and the partner's responses may contribute to the problem. The problem is seldom presented as a medical complaint unless the patient has reason to be concerned about the partner's distress.

Some patients (both men and women) indicate that they have always had low levels of sexual desire, but the *absence* of desire is perceived by them as a different and disturbing circumstance. Some men have had difficulty with erection or with premature ejaculation. In the course of trying to correct the symptom, usually with a partner, the condition becomes worse, so that sexual encounters tend to then be avoided.

Etiology

Hypoactive sexual desire may be due to a combination of any number of factors listed in the general section on etiology (see p 427). The most common causes, however, are relationship and interpersonal factors and life stresses affecting the partners.

There are often other contributory organic factors, as in the patient with myocardial infarction who receives only vague or no information from the cardiologist or family physician about sexual activity. Because of uncertainty about the amount of exertion associated with intercourse, such patients may avoid initiating

Table 37 – 1. *DSM-III-R* diagnostic criteria for hypoactive sexual desire.

A. Persistently or recurrently deficient or absent sexual fantasies and desire for sexual activity. The judgment of deficiency or absence is made by the clinician, taking into account factors that affect sexual functioning, such as age, sex, and the context of the person's life.

B. Does not occur exclusively during the course of another axis I disorder (other than a sexual dysfunction), such as major depression.

sexual activity with their partners. The partner may have similar fears and thus avoid initiating intercourse or responding to sexual overtures. A pattern of fear, avoidance, frustration, anger, and lack of communication may develop and continue for months or years before one or both partners decide that something must be done. Since myocardial infarction as such has no adverse implications for sexual function, psychogenic factors are the cause of inhibited sexual desire in patients who have recovered and are back to work.

Illustrative Case

A couple in their early 30s had been married 10 years. Their only child was 5 years old. Since the child's birth, the frequency of intercourse had steadily decreased. The husband reported that he had lost all interest in sex after 8 years of marriage, and the couple had not had intercourse in the 18 months before treatment was sought.

The wife at first believed that the decrease in sexual activity was due to their preoccupation with caring for their daughter, especially in the first 6–8 months. During their few times together, the wife thought sexual activity was highly satisfactory, whereas the husband recalled that he participated only because she seemed so amorous. When he became aware of his relative unresponsiveness, he blamed increased responsibilities, an increased office work load, and resulting "exhaustion." This made no sense to her, since he seemed to find time to run 5 miles 4 times a week, entertain clients, and do other things.

The wife's own family life and her sexual experiences before her marriage had been healthy and joyful. She and her 2 siblings were close to their parents but encouraged to develop as individuals. Sexual topics were openly discussed, and the parents had always had their "private" time, which the children respected. The children had learned that sexuality was a natural and necessary expression of life and love.

The husband's family had never discussed sexual issues, nor had there been many open displays of affection or any indications that the parents were sexually active. He recalled hearing his mother resist his father's hugging by saying "not in front of the children."

During the pregnancy, the husband was fearful about sex because he imagined that the fetus was aware of their lovemaking, and this inhibited his responses to his wife's increased sexual sensitivity during that period. After delivery, she seemed to him more like a mother than a lover, even though her level of sexual awareness and desire did not change. When she began to initiate sexual activity and become more sexually aggressive, he became more withdrawn, dwelling on thoughts of his parents' seemingly sexless existence, which he believed was his own destiny. He began to concentrate more on success in his work, personal competitiveness, and maintaining fitness— virtues he had early learned to hold in high regard.

Treatment was directed toward helping the couple understand their different attitudes toward sex in general and particularly toward sexual activity between parents. Since they loved each other and their daughter, they responded well to a psychodynamic and behavioral therapeutic approach. Involving both partners in active therapy (assigned exercises to be done at home: communication, nongenital caressing, scheduling time to be together) helped to modify the husband's avoidance behavior. They felt their relationship was more intimate and their sexual satisfaction greater than in the 5 years preceding the birth of their daughter.

Treatment

The treatment method, as described in the above case and outlined on p 429, must be tailored to the patients' particular problems and to their willingness to try the assignments even if they are not sure they fully accept them. The major objective of graduated behavioral treatment is to reestablish the patients' ability to become involved in sexual contact and, through increased verbal feedback, to begin to experience sexual excitement. Patients with inhibited sexual desire have not lost their capacity to become sexually excited. The desire phase of the sexual response cycle has been affected, but the potential for arousal has not.

The chances for successful therapy are reduced if there is little "glue" in the marriage—if pregnancy, for instance, is repugnant to the wife or if the partners have become hostile and combative or involved in affairs. If both partners still have a hope and need for realized gains from their investment in the relationship, the chances for success are good.

SEXUAL AVERSION DISORDER

Sexual aversion disorder is characterized by extreme avoidance of genital contact with a sexual partner over a long period of time. It must be differentiated (1) from the sexual aversion that may be associated with an axis I disorder such as obsessive compulsive disorder or a major depressive episode and (2) from hypoactive sexual desire, which is a common presenting sexual disorder (sexual aversion disorder is rare). The *DSM-III-R* diagnostic criteria for sexual aversion disorder are listed in Table 37–2.

Symptoms & Signs

Individuals with sexual aversion disorder experi-

Table 37 – 2. *DSM-III-R* diagnostic criteria for sexual aversion disorder.

A. Persistent or recurrent extreme aversion to, and avoidance of, all or almost all, genital sexual contact with a sexual partner.
B. Does not occur exclusively during the course of another axis I disorder (other than a sexual dysfunction), such as obsessive compulsive disorder or major depression.

ence uncontrollable, overwhelming anxiety at even the thought of sexual activity. There is a phobic nature to their reaction, which may be accompanied by sweating, palpitations, and nausea and other somatic paniclike responses, while in others, there may be no outward manifestation of their intense distress.

Sexual aversion does not imply that sexual dysfunction is also present. Both men and women with this diagnosis are capable of experiencing orgasm on the rare occasions when they grudgingly participate in sexual activity to preserve a relationship. However, the conflict that frequently develops between partners because of the disorder may cause so much distress that the patient may lose the ability to respond.

Distress occurs in anticipation of any gesture that may be interpreted as preliminary to a sexual encounter with a partner, such as holding hands, hugging, or touching. Simply undressing or being nude in the presence of a partner may be threatening. Patients are likely to want sexual intercourse or other orgasmic experience without any preliminary fondling or caressing. As in other phobias, the anxiety is just as intense when anticipating the feared activity as it is when actually participating in it. Self-stimulation without a partner present does not provoke the same level of anxiety; this indicates that the libido is relatively intact.

Patients frequently have a history of an earlier period in their lives when sexual activity was not associated with phobic repsonses. There may be brief periods of lessened anxiety (often associated with a celebration such as a birthday or anniversary).

Etiology

Masters and Johnson reported on 116 cases between 1972 and 1977 and attempted to categorize some etiologic factors. These were much the same as those causing sexual dysfunction, eg, negative parental attitudes toward sexuality during the developing years; inadequate emotional support or insensitivity to sexual concerns of a child by the family; restrictive or punitive reactions to sexual behavior; and sexual abuse. Some early adolescent loss of self-esteem may be evident, but, overall, these patients are more frequently achievers on the job or in school. In some cases, the patient may be responding to an overzealous or perfectionist partner who perceives sexual activity as a performance that must meet certain standards.

Differential Diagnosis

The diagnosis requires a careful history taking. Consistency of the phobic reaction is a critical component for establishing the disorder. Both males and females may develop the disorder, but it is more frequent in females. The phobic reactions are not usually associated with other phobias or panic reactions. Sexual aversion in males is frequently associated with global lifelong anxiety about sexual identity or orientation. For example, men who consider themselves homosexual because they do not relate sexually to women but who have not had sexual contact with men (self-classification by exclusion) are often placed in this category.

Treatment

Treatment consists of desensitization to sexual panic and phobic reactions through modified nongenital sensate focusing exercises (see above). The partner's activity must be adapted to the pace at which the patient feels comfortable. Exercises that provoke the least anxiety must be chosen. For example, the first assignment might be to hold hands and then progress to touching arms and shoulders (rather than assigning nongenital touching or caressing of the entire body). If the patient experiences phobic reactions, the exercise should be stopped and should be resumed only after the patient has been reassured by the partner that sexual contact is not the goal. Within this structure, the patient guides the activity over several weeks to a level that does not precipitate panic symptoms. Partners frequently improve their ability to talk about sexual problems. The goal is to decrease the level of anxiety and use insights developed to lessen the phobic reactions.

Illustrative Case

A 27-year-old woman, a master teacher of retarded children, had been living for 6 years with a partner she met in college. She was a virgin when they became sexual partners and did not find the initial sexual experience traumatic in any way. However, within 6–8 weeks she became highly anxious by midday in anticipation of the evening, which usually ended in prolonged lovemaking. At first, she thought she might have some temporary illness that was causing the paniclike feelings or that stress of work was simply "turning her off." Neither of these explanations seemed realistic to her, but she did not want her partner to feel rejected and felt that excuses were necessary until the problem resolved itself. Instead, her anxiety increased, and she began to avoid undressing when her partner was near, wore a full-length, long-sleeved nightgown to bed, and read until her partner went to sleep. After several months, she was able to tell him about her unexpected, frightening anxiety. He was supportive and nondemanding about sex for months at a time, assuming, as she did, that the phase would pass. Eventually, she would feel guilty and would ask for sexual intercourse with the provision that they "get right to it," that she did not have to remove the nightgown, and that he did not fondle or caress her or expect to be touched by her. When he followed her guidelines, she would become distressed and anxious after intercourse and blame him for causing her guilt feelings for becoming sexually involved. During intercourse, she reached orgasm and was highly aroused but felt sad about her responsiveness.

Her partner became less supportive and demanded that she seek help to overcome her problem. Her first therapist made a diagnosis of frigidity and suggested that she might have no capacity for sexual pleasure despite her description of momentary orgasmic pleasure. She discontinued the therapy after 3 months, greatly discouraged and more anxious than before about any discussion of sex or sexual activity. In addition, she felt deficient and inadequate.

The partner suggested that they seek therapy as a couple. After an assessment visit, they were referred for sex therapy. The woman's early history revealed that although she loved her father, she had always hated his description of her to relatives and friends as "my sexy little girl." She reported no sexual abuse. She related that her mother, who was a social worker, had a fixation on the "loose sexual behavior" of the pregnant teenagers in her caseload. Over time, she realized that some of these early messages about sexuality might have surfaced once she became sexually active and might have contributed to the evolution of the aversive behavior. There were further problems related to the dynamics of the relationship over this period, as well as other complicating factors. On several occasions, the couple stopped therapy when the desensitization process no longer seemed to reduce her anxiety. However, the couple and the therapist remained in contact via telephone, and the couple returned to therapy and appeared to proceed well with a continued psychodynamic/behavioral approach.

SEXUAL AROUSAL DISORDERS

Symptoms & Signs

Sexual arousal disorders, formerly termed impotence in men and frigidity in women, can occur at any age. In the past, the problem was thought to be more prevalent in older couples, but clinical experience reported from many sex therapy centers does not bear this out.

Although patients have no change in their level of sexual desire, they report recurrent and persistent decrease or loss of sexual arousal during sexual activity. The interference with function is at the second phase of the sexual response cycle (see p 426). In men, this results in inability to attain or maintain an erection to completion of intercourse. In women, the complaint is inability to feel sexual sensation, with accompanying partial or complete lack of lubrication sufficient for satisfactory intercourse. The *DSM-III-R* diagnostic criteria are outlined in Table 37–3.

Two major patterns may develop: (1) The first occurrence of problems with erection or lubrication may be dismissed as a matter of no importance. The partners may decide to increase the intensity of sexual stimulation, talk more openly about their sexual needs, and, in general, be supportive and exploratory. If continued attempts to overcome the difficulty produce no results, either partner may worry that the other partner has simply lost interest. Couples who go to doctors with such problems are most likely to be referred for psychologic counseling, because of their expressed desire to remain sexually active. (2) At the first occurrence of the problem, one or both partners may respond with disappointment, anger, fear, and intense anxiety. All sexual activity may cease at this

Table 37 – 3. *DSM-III-R* diagnostic criteria for sexual arousal disorders.

Female sexual arousal disorder:
A. Either (1) or (2):
  (1) Persistent or recurrent partial or complete failure in a female to attain or maintain the lubrication-swelling response of sexual excitement until completion of the sexual activity.
  (2) Persistent or recurrent lack of a subjective sense of sexual excitement and pleasure in a female during sexual activity.
B. Does not occur exclusively during the course of another axis I disorder (other than a sexual dysfunction), such as major depression.

Male erectile disorder:
A. Either (1) or (2):
  (1) Persistent or recurrent partial or complete failure in a male to attain or maintain erection until completion of the sexual activity.
  (2) Persistent or recurrent lack of a subjective sense of sexual excitement and pleasure in a male during sexual activity.
B. Does not occur during the course of another axis I disorder (other than a sexual dysfunction), such as major depression.

point, and there may be no attempt at increased stimulation. Communication about sexual concerns may also cease, for fear of causing further anger or rejection. The couple may avoid the problem for months or even years before seeking help.

Between these 2 major patterns, gradations of distress are commonly reported.

Etiology

One or more of the factors listed in the section on etiology (see p 427) are usually present. The most common cause is performance anxiety, precipitated sometimes by the first episode of "failure." In such cases, the woman often assumes that her partner finds her unattractive or has become involved with someone else. The man assumes that his partner believes he has lost his sex drive and regards him as foolish or weak. He is fearful of losing her and feels more pressure to "perform." The point at which the partners are unable to express their fears to each other is often the time when they decide to seek help.

Many men believe that sexual prowess begins to decline at a particular age. This notion is sometimes reinforced by physicians, especially if the patient is over 55. The same feelings occur in women who once were easily aroused but suddenly find themselves unresponsive though their desire level remains high. If they are postmenopausal, they may be told by a physician not to expect the same arousal levels they had in the past.

Illustrative case

The patients, both in their late 50s, had been married 25 years and reported having had a fulfilling sex life. About a year before seeking treatment, the husband found that he did not respond to their lovemaking in his usual way. At first, he believed his inability to maintain an erection was due to simple fatigue. The

next time they made love, he lost his erection at the moment of penetration. He proceeded to stimulate his wife manually and orally to orgasm, but he did not become aroused (as he once did) by her responsiveness. Her unsuccessful attempts to stimulate him genitally made him impatient and angry. He sometimes experienced an ejaculation with no erection or sensation of orgasm, and this bothered and embarrassed him even more. He became reluctant to make any sexual overtures for a few days, though he and his wife "cuddled" at night before going to sleep.

During the next few months, the husband's anxiety and fear increased. He still felt a strong desire for his wife, but he could not achieve arousal. When partial erection was achieved, he would immediately attempt intercourse and then lose the erection entirely. He became frustrated and depressed each time this happened and began to worry whether the next attempt would also be unsuccessful. A cycle of negative expectations exacerbated the condition. The wife was concerned about her husband's health and persuaded him to have a thorough checkup. The examination showed nothing abnormal, and her sincere concern then began to irritate him, so that he reproved her for meddling in "his" problem. She began to wait for him to initiate lovemaking and no longer tried to excite him. Their frequent quarreling affected their older children (aged 20 and 23). The husband became less attentive at work and believed that, at age 56, he was probably just "old before his time."

As the patients described their history to the therapist, they were able to perceive the cycle of anger and anxiety that over the years had finally caused them to feel hostile and alienated.

The therapist urged the patients to discuss the positive things they wanted for their future and to describe how they envisioned sexual activity as part of that picture. Both expressed a desire to reintroduce sexual satisfaction and personal closeness into their lives. The husband began to recognize that performance goals for attaining erection and penetration prevented him from relaxing and enjoying sexual play. Both expressed the feeling that sexual encounters had begun to seem like work, and the more they worked or tried for the results the husband wanted, the more difficult sexual contact became. The wife admitted that in the beginning, she felt she was being rejected but could not understand why. Later, when she was able to voice these fears, her husband assured her that they were unfounded and that the problem was his.

To help the patients interrupt the goal-oriented sexual performance cycle, the therapist suggested structured 1-hour pleasuring sessions at home. In these sessions, intercourse was prohibited, whether or not the husband had a partial or complete erection. The patients were also encouraged to explore each other's feelings, deliberately recall their best sexual experiences together, and talk to each other about their assignments. Later assignments included taking turns initiating sexual pleasuring and becoming reacquainted with their own and their partner's sensuality.

Treatment

Therapy is discussed in the illustrative case above. For further details, see the section beginning on p 429.

INHIBITED FEMALE ORGASM

Symptoms & Signs

As shown in Table 37–4, this disorder is characterized by recurrent or persistent inhibition of female orgasm after a normal sexual excitement phase during sexual activity. Since some women are able to experience orgasm during noncoital clitoral stimulation but not during coitus in the absence of manual clitoral stimulation, clinical judgments about whether this response represents a sexual dysfunction are based on a thorough description of sexual behavior patterns and often require a trial of therapy.

A more accurate diagnosis can be made if the problem is further classified as (1) **primary anorgasmia (preorgasmia),** in which the patient has never had an orgasm either through coitus or through autoerotic activity; or (2) **secondary (situational) anorgasmia,** in which the patient has reached orgasm but can no longer do so or can only experience orgasm in specific situations (eg, through autoerotic stimulation or with certain partners).

Etiology

Primary anorgasmia is most commonly due to sociocultural factors that result in misunderstandings about the body, such as being taught to believe that the genital area is "dirty" or that "sinful" sexual desires will occur if a girl touches or examines her genitals. In one case, a woman reported that her mother gave her a separate washcloth to use for washing herself "down there."

In both primary and secondary anorgasmia, psychic factors may be fear of loss of control if genital stimulation and sexual excitement are permitted or guilt feelings about sexual pleasure. There is often a combination of factors, including fear of pregnancy and problems in interpersonal relationships. Sexual abuse, assault, or incest in the early years is being recognized more frequently as a cause of inhibited female orgasm.

Illustrative Case

The patients were both in their mid 30s, had been married for 14 years, and had 2 children. The husband had suggested that his wife have a gynecologic checkup to determine if something physical was preventing orgasmic response. The gynecologist found no organic disorder and suggested consultation with the family physician. The physician recommended a sex therapist. The patients then wondered whether they really wanted to disclose their sexual problem to more people. Neither partner was interested in forming new relationships, but they were not sure how committed they still were to the marriage. Thus, both were considerably distressed and angry when they entered the therapist's office. The husband said he had agreed to attend the therapy session for his wife's sake and because they had been told by the physician that the problem could only be dealt with if both parties sought therapy together.

The wife said that during most of the years of their marriage, her major satisfaction from lovemaking was from the physical closeness it required. It was only at those times that she felt loved. She had had orgasms during these years, including during pregnancy and after the birth of each child. However, during the past 3 years, she felt that sexual activity had become mechanical; that they spent very little time together other than while having intercourse; and that her husband seemed anxious to have it over with quickly. She was left without orgasm and had been afraid for almost a year to tell him this was the case. He expressed surprise on hearing this, saying he had assumed that the brevity of their times together was due to lack of interest on her part. The wife felt that her husband was still enjoying intercourse and reaching orgasm and did not care whether she did or not. Her growing resentment led to frequent refusals to engage in any type of lovemaking, with retaliatory responses from him. Within the last year, they could barely remember how many times they made love; she thought it was 3 times, and he thought it had been twice.

Treatment included behavioral and educational exercises, but the emphasis was on interpersonal factors. The patients initially resisted the exercises, but over a 7-month period, with frequent interruption, they were able to understand the problem more fully and to cooperate in therapy.

Treatment

Both partners should work together and attend therapy sessions together, since sexual dysfunction is usually not only one person's problem. Success depends on the partners' agreement to strive together to achieve the goal of pleasure and satisfaction for both.

Women without partners often want to learn to attain orgasm. They have never been able to reach orgasm through fantasy and usually have never masturbated to orgasm.

Table 37–4. *DSM-III-R* diagnostic criteria for inhibited female orgasm.

A. Persistent or recurrent delay in, or absence of, orgasm in a female following a normal sexual excitement phase during sexual activity that the clinician judges to be adequate in focus, intensity, and duration. Some females are able to experience orgasm during noncoital clitoral stimulation but are unable to experience it during coitus in the absence of manual clitoral stimulation. In most of these females, this represents a normal variation of the female response and does not justify the diagnosis of inhibited female orgasm. However, in some of these females, this does represent a psychologic inhibition that justifies the diagnosis. This difficult judgment is assisted by a thorough sexual evaluation, which may even require a trial of treatment.

B. Does not occur exclusively during the course of another axis I disorder (other than a sexual dysfunction), such as major depression.

The therapeutic approach to **primary anorgasmia** includes (1) discussing the patient's feelings about sexual pleasure; (2) discussing any myths or unfounded beliefs she might have about sexual intercourse and other sexual activity; and (3) helping her to see herself as a sexual person through therapy sessions and home assignments in which she appraises her nude body and gradually initiates manual stimulation of the mons, clitoris, and other perineal structures. Therapy sessions must be continued in conjunction with these assignments, since they are important for obtaining an adequate sexual history, including early childhood sexual experiences, sources of sexual information, and the patient's assessment of these and other factors. Behavioral assignments should not be offered in the absence of such therapy sessions.

The goals of treatment for **secondary anorgasmia** are to reduce the fear of loss of control or of intimacy or closeness; to increase communication between the partners; and to utilize nondemand pleasuring exercises (see p 430) to improve stimulation and communication. If premature ejaculation is a problem for the male partner, it may be contributing to the overall dysfunction. Both issues should be addressed in therapy.

INHIBITED MALE ORGASM

Symptoms & Signs

Inhibition of orgasm is recurrent or persistent and is manifested by a delay in or absence of orgasm and ejaculation following an adequate phase of sexual excitement. *DSM-III-R* diagnostic criteria are set forth in Table 37–5.

Etiology

There are few organic factors that affect orgasmic response to the point of inhibition; almost all cases of orgasmic inhibition in males are of psychogenic origin.

The most common etiologic factors are authoritative family patterns and the antisex bias of religious orthodoxy (eg, parental regulation of dating and other sexual behavior; inculcation of attitudes that sex is sinful, the genitals unclean, and masturbation destructive and evil). Other causes include rejection of the partner or spouse, episodes of homosexual activity, fear of pregnancy, and a broad spectrum of psychosocial problems.

Table 37–5. *DSM-III-R* diagnostic criteria for inhibited male orgasm.

A. Persistent or recurrent delay in, or absence of, orgasm in a male following a normal sexual excitement phase during sexual activity that the clinician, taking into account the person's age, judges to be adequate in focus, intensity, and duration.
B. Does not occur exclusively during the course of another axis I disorder (other than a sexual dysfunction), such as major depression.

Illustrative Case

The patients had been married for 5 years and had wanted to have a child since they were first married. When they married, both were 20 years old and both were virgins. Both had come from families in which discussions of sex were prohibited. At the same time, there were explicit taboos against premarital sexual experimentation and masturbation, and sexual intercourse was held to be for procreation only. The husband had had a strict religious education and a brief period of preparation for the ministry.

The patients described the first 2 years of their married life as being sexually satisfying even though the husband was unable to ejaculate intravaginally during intercourse. The wife was orgasmic, and the husband was able to achieve ejaculation extravaginally only after prolonged manual stimulation. His wife had never attempted oral stimulation, although he had at times suggested they try. They told the therapist that neither of them was experienced enough to be overly concerned at the time. When they decided they wanted children, they went to a gynecologist, described the problem, and the wife underwent artificial insemination, which resulted in pregnancy and delivery. However, during the workup for insemination, they recognized they were involved in an abnormal situation—delay in and absence of orgasm for the husband. The physician had made some suggestions for changes in their sexual patterns, but they were uneasy about his ideas and never tried them. Eventually, they began to feel that the husband should be able to achieve intravaginal ejaculation. But the more he tried, the more anxious he became. His wife began to accuse him of deliberately "holding back." During the 6 months prior to seeking therapy, the couple had become increasingly uncomfortable and dissatisfied with their sexual activity, and they had abstained from sexual intercourse for 3 months.

Treatment consisted chiefly of helping the patients reestablish their trust in each other. Behavioral treatment initially consisted of nondemand pleasuring sessions, with a ban on intercourse. In subsequent home assignments, the wife agreed to continue manual stimulation for extended periods to the point of orgasm for her husband. Both partners then watched the ejaculation occur close to but outside the vagina. Insertion of the penis at the point of ejaculation finally occurred after manual and oral stimulation, and this gave the husband enough confidence so that he began to achieve intravaginal ejaculation.

Treatment

Careful explanation to both partners about the likely causes of this dysfunction is required. After the sexual history is taken, factors that seem specifically applicable to the couple's situation should be discussed. For example, if the woman wants to have children but there has been no mutual agreement about that, she may see the dysfunction as the partner's way of preventing conception. It is important to help her understand that his inability to ejaculate intravaginally is not deliberate and is not a defect in his physical or sexual capacity. Since the woman frequently plays an important role in the treatment of this problem, helping the couple overcome initial hostilities is necessary early in treatment.

Since men with this disorder generally have no difficulty achieving or maintaining an erection for long periods during coitus, their partners may sometimes be asked why they perceive inhibited intravaginal ejaculation as a problem. The fact is that they do, and the clinician's attention should be directed toward the ejaculatory problem, which is usually primary—ie, the man has never been able to ejaculate intravaginally and has difficulty reaching orgasm through masturbation or partner stimulation. Many men with this dysfunction claim they have not masturbated since they were adolescents. Although the patient himself is distressed by his inability to achieve orgasm, the partner usually cannot help feeling that he wishes to withhold part of himself and that she is being rejected.

Behavioral therapy consists of progressive stimulation, beginning with nondemand sensate focusing and pleasuring (see p 430), and is similar to that used in management of inhibited sexual desire (impotence). Therapy helps implement the man's awareness of his own tactile sensations and improves the communication between partners by removing the pressure to perform. The woman is asked to take the leading role in manually stimulating the penis, taking instructions from her partner about how to do it and how long to continue. The man then watches while ejaculation occurs close to her vaginal orifice. In subsequent attempts, the woman inserts the penis so that ejaculation occurs intravaginally. Once this has been accomplished, the partners generally become highly encouraged and gradually establish confidence that intravaginal intercourse and ejaculation will occur. A prominent feature of treatment is the emphasis on effective patterns of communication, both verbal and nonverbal. If the patients cannot respond to such consensual activity because of unresolved issues concerning intimacy, referral for in-depth individual psychotherapy may be beneficial.

PREMATURE EJACULATION

Symptoms & Signs

Premature ejaculation, which is one of the most common sexual dysfunctions in men, is difficult to define clinically. Generally, in addition to the *DSM-III-R* criteria set forth in Table 37–6, it is defined in terms of the couple's interaction: The ejaculation occurs before the man wishes it *and* before the woman has reached orgasm. If the woman reaches orgasm quickly, even with a man who considers that his ejaculation occurs too early, ejaculation is by definition not premature. The clearest cases are those in which ejaculation occurs before, during, or shortly after intromission.

Table 37–6. *DSM-III-R* diagnostic criteria for premature ejaculation.

Persistent or recurrent ejaculation with minimal sexual stimulation or before, upon, or shortly after penetration and before the person wishes it. The clinician must take into account factors that affect duration of the excitement phase, such as age, novelty of the sexual partner or situation, and frequency of sexual activity.

Etiology

The cause of premature ejaculation is not known. Although ejaculation is a reflex phenomenon governed by the autonomic and central nervous systems and probably by changes in endocrine activity as well, it is assumed that the major element in control over ejaculation is learned behavior. The pattern of control is believed to be established early in life, beginning with the onset of masturbation, when ejaculation most often occurs quickly and in secrecy. This pattern may carry over into the first sexual experiences, in which the same conditions may exist. Some families or peer groups may foster the idea that it is "manly" to be able to ejaculate quickly, and such early learning experiences may result in a reflex pattern that is not easy to alter.

Illustrative Case

The patients were in their mid 40s and had been married for 18 years before seeking therapy for what they described as sexual problems throughout their married life. Despite these problems, they were an affectionate and loving couple who shared interests in each other's professional lives. They had 2 teenage children.

The wife explained that although she was not satisfied sexually during intercourse in the early years of their marriage, she had not wanted to discuss this with her husband for fear it would be damaging to his ego. She thought the problem would eventually correct itself. She reached orgasm by masturbating when her husband fell asleep after intercourse. She explained that later she had partial success in "catching up"—ie, she learned to reach climax sooner but never before he did.

In the course of the therapeutic sessions, the wife admitted that part of her reason for withholding comments from her husband about their sexual life was that everything else was going so well. She feared that if she talked about "sex," her spouse might become defensive or hurt and might leave her and the children. Before marriage, she had once been rejected by a lover, but she had not experienced serious feelings of abandonment, because she had support from family and friends.

Two years after the birth of their second child, the wife began to resent her silence about the problem, which she felt was a result of her husband's not stimulating her adequately either before or after his own quick orgasm. In their first direct confrontation about her frustration and anger, the husband responded explosively because he had not been told sooner. Anger at himself and his wife caused him to ejaculate even more rapidly, sometimes before penetration. He then began having difficulty having an erection. They began avoiding sexual contact altogether, concentrating on their work, social schedules, and children. They agreed to seek assistance but delayed doing so for over 2 years.

By the time help was sought, the sexual problem was beginning to interfere with other aspects of the relationship. However, during their discussion of the problem, the therapist noticed how they were often able to laugh together. They were given initial nondemand pleasuring assignments, progressing to the start-stop sensitization method (see p 430). During therapy sessions, each partner was able to define the series of attitudes and behavior that contributed to the problem: He had at first not realized that a problem existed, and she did not complain. He later realized she was less responsive but did not want to explore the issue. She had tired of dealing with "his problem." Their confrontation had not been helpful. He had experienced severe anxiety that exaggerated the problem and more recently had begun to lose erections. Hearing about each other's experiences in the therapist's office helped them understand the communication problem caused by their defensive positions. They progressed rapidly in therapy, chiefly because of the relative lack of conflict in most of the other areas of their lives. Encouraged by the therapist, they used their ability to cooperate and eventually were successful in postponing ejaculation to the satisfaction of both.

Treatment

Although the above case was unusual in that the couple's general living pattern had endured despite the resentments surrounding their sexual unhappiness, their delay in seeking therapy was not unusual. Sexual activity is of low priority for some couples, and many believe premature ejaculation is an "inborn" response that cannot be changed.

The broad principles of sex therapy described for other conditions (see p 429) apply also to the management of premature ejaculation. The optimal approach is to work with both partners, since the problem also distresses the woman and can cause anxiety as well as sexual frustration. The common pattern is that the woman begins to feel resentful and hostile toward her partner over a perceived lack of true intimacy in their sexual relationship. The man is concerned about these same issues, which often lower his self-esteem or cause increased anxiety. Helping the couple understand that premature ejaculation is not deliberate "selfishness" on the man's part and not a "sexual defect" is a first step. Open discussion and education should encourage the partners to cooperate in nonthreatening ways to achieve mutual sexual satisfaction.

A common traditional method of treating men with this condition was to have them concentrate on nonsexual activities (multiplication tables, etc) during sexual intercourse. This had the adverse effect of distracting the patient's attention from pleasurable sensations and control and usually resulted in even quicker orgasm. This would reinforce the woman's belief that the man was not truly concerned about her sexual gratification. The current treatment of choice consists of the sensate focusing and start-stop behavioral approach (see p 430), combined with psychodynamic therapy. The couple should be told that during the beginning phases of treatment, premature ejaculation will frequently occur despite the man's best efforts to indicate when stimulation should be stopped. The partners should be allowed to feel they have not "failed" and that, over time, they will be able to accomplish these behavioral tasks.

Patients who attribute their inability to maintain long-term relationships to premature ejaculation are often determined to "cure" their condition before they enter into another relationship. Such a patient should be advised to determine by masturbation the "point of no return" before ejaculation, then stop manual stimulation, and proceed in somewhat the same way as with a partner. Achievement of more and more control will establish a feeling of confidence. The patient should be advised, however, that the condition may recur when a new relationship is established. Men who consider masturbation an adolescent activity or who have inhibitions about it for other reasons may be unwilling to cooperate in this form of therapy. The factors influencing these beliefs should at least be discussed (not necessarily altered), and with the help of films and reading materials, many patients come to understand their condition in ways that may help them as they begin new relationships.

FUNCTIONAL DYSPAREUNIA

Symptoms & Signs

DSM-III-R defines functional dyspareunia as coitus associated with recurrent and persistent genital pain in either sex (Table 37–7).

This sexual dysfunction is rare in men; although pain may occur episodically, especially at the point of intromission and at the time of ejaculation, it is usually not persistent and thus does not meet the *DSM-III-R* criteria. Our discussion here will address the problem as it relates to women.

Etiology

About 15% of cases of dyspareunia in women are caused by organic pelvic disorders. These should al-

Table 37–7. *DSM-III-R* diagnostic criteria for functional dyspareunia.

A. Recurrent or persistent genital pain in either a male or a female before, during, or after sexual intercourse.
B. The disturbance is not caused exclusively by lack of lubrication or by vaginismus.

ways be considered in the initial assessment of the patient before functional dyspareunia is diagnosed.

In most cases, a major etiologic factor is inadequate vaginal lubrication, caused by anxiety and apprehension on the part of the woman; tension about her sexual "performance" during intercourse; anticipation of pain (a reaction to previous experiences); or fear, guilt, and anger (self-directed, centered on the partner, or both). Penile insertion can often be accomplished comfortably in the early stages of excitement with the aid of an artificial lubricant. However, if the woman's anxiety or stress continues during penile thrusting, vaginal lubrication may cease, and continued thrusting causes pain.

Illustrative Case

A couple in their 30s had been married almost 3 years. During her early dating years, the wife had found intercourse to be an anxiety-provoking experience, frequently accompanied by pain. She was ashamed to admit this discomfort to her partners and believed they considered her unresponsive and "cold." She would frequently terminate a relationship rather than discuss her distress, even with partners she thought might understand. Before she met her husband, therefore, she had very little sexual contact.

The patients dated for 6 months before marriage. During this time, each felt that the other was the "right" person. Both became sexually aroused, but there was no pressure for intercourse. She told him she had had problems in the past that she thought resulted from not trusting herself or her partners during sexual excitement. When they got married, neither was prepared for the pain she experienced whenever intercourse continued for more than a brief period. She would urge him to reach orgasm, and when he did so she became angry because she could not. The husband began to feel that "pain" was an excuse to end intercourse quickly, and he accused his wife of being uninterested in sex. She reacted by ridiculing his techniques of lovemaking. Their bitterness and disappointment in themselves and in each other had caused them to consider divorce. A recent gynecologic examination had revealed no pelvic disorders. The gynecologist, sensing her distress even though she did not describe the problem, was able to obtain a thorough history of the problem.

The wife's parents had always encouraged their children to discuss any subject, including sex, pregnancy, and dating behavior. The patient had vivid memories of discussions about labor pain during childbirth. She had said she would want to be put to sleep during delivery if she were to have a child, and her mother had explained that new concepts in obstetrics no longer permitted such treatment—that it was necessary to endure the discomfort of labor to be a "good" mother. The patient told the physician that she did not know there were various methods of delivery and had never discussed her friends' pregnancies with them, since she did not want to hear "the gory details." The physician then elaborated on the cyclic process in which fear inhibits sexual excitement and responsiveness, which in turn generates more fear, so that feelings of inadequacy as a sexual partner exacerbate the problem. The patient began to recognize that her perceptions of labor and delivery might have contributed to the fear of pain during intercourse. At the physician's suggestion, she attended some prenatal classes and spoke with a number of women and their partners.

The wife began to understand the anxiety that caused her to "turn off" before she became aroused. She recognized that she was reluctant to use birth control because she "knew" none of the methods worked, which further convinced her at some low level of consciousness that pregnancy was the inevitable result of coitus.

The patients responded well to educational sessions. They both attended a prenatal class, so that the wife could share with her husband her new understanding of childbirth. She was eager to show him that she now understood how restricted her sexual perspective had been. They both understood how she had associated intercourse with the pain of delivery. Therapy also included exercises in which the wife initiated and guided the pace and rhythm of intercourse, which she felt gave her more control.

Treatment

Many women who have had a gynecologic examination and have been advised to seek therapy for a sexual problem will delay doing so until the interpersonal problems in their marriages become worse. A patient who has delayed seeking therapy may say that her physician did not show concern for her problem and indicated it was "all in her mind." Thus, when treatment is sought, it is often with a feeling of defensiveness at the start.

In addition to obtaining a detailed sexual history and describing the general process of treatment, the therapist should reassure the patient that her concern about the problem is justified. As part of the therapeutic plan, the couple and the therapist should examine what the patient thinks is happening at the time of sexual intercourse. Sensate focusing with nondemand pleasuring (see p 430) keeps the couple in close physical contact and increases their confidence. Although it is tempting to advise the use of artificial lubricants or saliva, such temporary symptomatic measures do not lead to spontaneous lubrication from the vaginal walls. Progression to partial penetration controlled by the woman is accomplished with mutual cooperation and concentration on increasing pleasure. Behavioral and relearning assignments must be accompanied by therapy sessions in which the partners describe their progress and the therapist continues to assess their general interaction.

FUNCTIONAL VAGINISMUS

Symptoms & Signs

Functional vaginismus is characterized by recur-

Table 37–8. *DSM-III-R* diagnostic criteria for functional vaginismus.

A. Recurrent or persistent involuntary spasm of the musculature of the outer third of the vagina that interferes with coitus.
B. The disturbance is not caused exclusively by a physical disorder and is not due to another axis I disorder.

rent and persistent involuntary spasms of the muscles of the outer third of the vagina that interfere with coitus (Table 37–8). In **primary vaginismus,** the woman has never experienced genital sexual activity without vaginismus. In **secondary vaginismus,** which is more common, the involuntary spasms and pain develop after periods of problem-free genital sexual functioning.

Most young women experience minor spasms and moderate vaginal pain when they first attempt to insert a tampon at the time of menarche, but this experience seldom leads to chronic vaginismus. The condition may become established, however, if the initial discomfort upon inserting a tampon or on inserting a finger during masturbation is associated with a type of fear that some women describe as close to panic. The fear is associated with images of injury, harm, or irreparable damage to the internal organs. Some women report a history of difficulty with pelvic examinations even when a small speculum or one-finger examination is used; these women are most likely to experience recurrent vaginismus during sexual contact.

Etiology

Vaginismus is now recognized to be a conditioned response, but it was once considered to be a hysterical or conversion symptom due to a specific intrapsychic conflict. Such clinical formulations are in agreement with the psychoanalytic theory of sexual development, and there are other plausible psychodynamic hypotheses also, all of which emphasize the patient's unconscious hatred of men; but even though many patients have been treated by psychodynamic methods and marital therapy, successful treatment based on these concepts has not been reported.

Functional vaginismus may be caused by a wide variety of psychologic and social factors, such as strict religious upbringing, the psychologic effects of rape, and sexual myths and misinformation. There may be anticipation of pain, due to other conflicts associated with shame, guilt, and anxiety about sex. In most cases, there is no clear-cut traumatic or psychic conflict.

Since functional vaginismus is by definition not due to organic causes, it is often regarded as the least common female sexual dysfunction. The true incidence is not definitely known, however.

Illustrative Case

A young couple married for 3 years had never accomplished vaginal penetration. When they were first married and the condition became apparent, the wife had a gynecologic examination, which showed no structural problems. When attempts at penetration continued to fail, they tried oral and manual stimulation, which they both found to be highly enjoyable and which resulted in orgasm for both. Although they were pleased with this "outercourse" aspect of their lovemaking, they were disappointed that they had not been able to achieve vaginal penetration.

The wife underwent psychiatric examination and gained some insight into the influence of her strict Christian fundamentalist upbringing. She was found to have some anxiety and feelings of guilt about most types of sexual behavior, although she found "outercourse" enjoyable. She was told by the psychiatrist, however, that she showed no signs of a psychopathologic disorder. He suggested another gynecologic examination, which again showed no abnormal findings. She then discussed her sexual history with her family physician, who recommended that the couple see a sex therapist.

During the first session with the therapist, the patient reported that her first attempt (as a teenager) to insert a menstrual tampon had been extremely painful and embarrassing, since the tampon had become "caught halfway" in the vaginal opening. The pain occurred as the tip of the tampon was pushed through a tight vaginal opening by the patient. She had been afraid to do anything to remove the tampon until finally, an older schoolmate was able to help. The patient remembered becoming angry at her mother over this experience and blamed her mother for not having explained about the onset of menstruation or about menstrual care. A bitter fight with her mother ensued during which the mother accused her daughter of simulating pain from the tampon to divert attention from the fact that she had been masturbating. She told the daughter she was sinful and would become a whore. This was the only time the girl and her mother ever talked about sex. The patient never again mentioned sex to her mother, and she never forgot what her mother had said. When the husband heard this story, he left his chair to embrace and comfort his wife. The therapist gave highly supportive encouragement to this spontaneous show of affection and assured the young people that their love for each other would be an asset in treatment. The couple responded well to the home assignments and progressed rapidly to the anticipated resolution of their problem.

Treatment

Behavioral treatment at home is usually successful in functional vaginismus and consists of having the patient insert plastic or metal dilators of increasing size—or her own or her partner's fingers—into the introitus. The goal of therapy is to prevent the reflex reaction of vaginismus. As the patient learns about the perineal structures and begins to recognize that she can control her responses, she relaxes the pubococcygeal muscles and the surrounding pelvic musculature. The patient must understand that dilators are used to help relax muscles, not to stretch the vagina. This should be stressed to dispel the patient's fears that she has an abnormally small vagina. Use of Kegel exercises (alternating contraction and relaxation of the pubococcygeal muscles) also helps teach voluntary control of responses during intercourse.

Some therapists prefer that the woman first use dilators without assistance from her partner and then demonstrate to him what she has learned. She and her partner may then progress to use of the penis, placed against the vaginal orifice without penetration. The amount of movement and depth of penetration are controlled by the woman.

The most successful approach to therapy is to engage the partner in the process from the outset, so that his reactions to the problem can also be discussed. Couples frequently develop mutual hostility and anger related to the unconsummated sexual act, and many are unable to achieve sufficient alternative genital stimulation and thus become increasingly resentful and accusatory. The man often feels rejected, angry, and guilty and may attribute the problem to the woman's desire to control the situation. Awareness of the involuntary nature of vaginismus and a better understanding of the problem help resolve these feelings. Interpersonal and intrapsychic factors should be dealt with as they arise during treatment, and the therapist should be flexible in the choices of therapeutic approach.

SEXUAL DYSFUNCTION NOT OTHERWISE SPECIFIED

Sexual dysfunctions that cannot be classified as one of the specific dysfunctions outlined in the above sections are considered in this category. Examples given in *DSM-III-R* are (1) the lack of erotic sensations or the presence of complete anesthesia despite normal physiologic components of sexual excitement and orgasm; (2) a "female analogue of Premature Ejaculation"; and (3) genital pain during masturbation. Although the specific cause and pathogenetic mechanism of the second are not known, some combination of the factors discussed on p 427 is usually present. Postcoital headache is an uncommon dysfunction that not only causes physical discomfort but may also become a source of tension between sexual partners. The therapist must determine that the pain is genuine and has no organic cause. Genital pain during masturbation requires differential diagnosis to rule out Peyronie's disease, pelvic varicosities, and other medical disorders. A woman who has an orgasmic response almost immediately on penetration may find this response to be a problem if it is her only orgasm and if the man is disturbed to know that his partner is experiencing no further pleasure as he continues thrusting to orgasm. The physician can usually help the woman and her partner discuss and understand their own reactions and develop a system of communication that eliminates speculation about each other's feelings.

REFERENCES

Annon JS: *Behavioral Treatment of Sexual Problems: Brief Therapy.* Harper & Row, 1976.

Butler RN, Lewis MS: *Love and Sex After Sixty.* Harper & Row, 1976.

Caird W, Wincze JP: *Sex Therapy: A Behavioral Approach.* Harper & Row, 1977.

Dickinson RL: *Atlas of Human Sex Anatomy,* 2nd ed. Williams & Wilkins, 1949.

Green R (editor): *Human Sexuality: A Health Providers' Text,* 2nd ed. Williams & Wilkins, 1979.

Group for the Advancement of Psychiatry: *Assessment of Sexual Function: A Guide to Interviewing.* Group for the Advancement of Psychiatry, 1973.

Kaplan H: *Disorders of Sexual Desire.* Brunner/Mazel, 1979.

Kaplan H: *The New Sex Therapy: Active Treatment of Sexual Dysfunctions.* Brunner/Mazel, 1974.

Kolodny RC, Masters WH, Johnson VE: *Textbook of Sexual Medicine.* Little, Brown, 1979.

Lieblum SR, Pervin LA (editors): *Principles and Practice of Sex Therapy.* Guilford Press, 1980.

Lief H (editor): *Sexual Problems in Medical Practice.* American Medical Association, 1981.

LoPiccolo J, LoPiccolo L (editors): *Handbook of Sex Therapy.* Plenum Press, 1978.

Marmor J: *Homosexual Behavior: A Modern Reappraisal.* Basic Books, 1980.

Masters WH, Johnson VE: *Human Sexual Inadequacy.* Little, Brown, 1970.

Masters WH, Johnson VE: *Human Sexual Response.* Little, Brown, 1966.

Meyer JK (editor): *Clinical Management of Sexual Disorders.* Williams & Wilkins, 1976.

Money J, Musaph H (editors): *Handbook of Sexology.* Elsevier, 1977.

Munjack DJ, Oziel LJ: *Sexual Medicine and Counseling in Office Practice.* Little, Brown, 1980.

Sadock BJ, Kaplan HI, Freedman AM (editors): *The Sexual Experience.* Williams & Wilkins, 1976.

Sandler M, Gessa GL (editors): *Sexual Behavior: Pharmacology and Biochemistry.* Raven Press, 1975.

Woods NF: *Human Sexuality in Health and Illness,* 2nd ed. Mosby, 1979.

World Health Organization: *Education and Treatment in Human Sexuality: The Training of Health Professionals.* Technical Report No. 572. US Government Printing Office, 1976.

38

Gender Identity Disorders
Paraphilias

Evalyn S. Gendel, MD, & Emmett J. Bonner, PhD

This chapter discusses gender identity disorders, paraphilias, and sexual disorders not classified elsewhere in *DSM-III-R*. The separate grouping of these disorders does not imply that they are less significant to medical practice than the sexual dysfunctions discussed in Chapter 37 but only that they probably occur less frequently and that less is known about their precise prevalence, causes, treatment, and outcome.

Classification

Classification of these disorders is as follows:

A. Gender Identity Disorders:
1. Transsexualism
2. Gender identity disorder of childhood
3. Atypical gender identity disorder

B. Paraphilias:
1. Fetishism
2. Transvestic fetishism
3. Zoophilia
4. Pedophilia
5. Exhibitionism
6. Voyeurism
7. Sexual masochism
8. Sexual sadism
9. Frotteurism
10. Atypical paraphilia

C. Other Psychosexual Disroders:
1. Ego-dystonic homosexuality*
2. Sexual disorders not elsewhere classified.

GENDER IDENTITY DISORDERS

Gender identity disorders are disturbances in the development of the individual's sense of masculinity or femininity. Certain characteristics of personality and behavior tend to cluster around the concept of masculinity or femininity as a result of parental and social approval of those characteristics as befitting members of a given sex.

A practical way to examine sexuality is to think of it in terms of a sexual system that includes both prenatal and postnatal factors. Prenatal components of the system consist of chromosomal patterns, sexual differentiation of the external and internal genitals, and male and female hormonal patterns. Postnatal factors include parental and social approval of those characteristics which cluster around the concept of masculinity and femininity appropriate to members of a given sex. Postnatal factors exert the major impact on sexuality.

Definitions

A. Biologic Sex: The chromosomal factor of sex (genotype) and physical appearance of the genitals (sex phenotype). The latter is also called **anatomic sex.**

B. Core Gender Identity: The sense of being male or female. This identification generally occurs before age 18 months and is irreversibly established by age 3 years.

C. Gender Identity: Feelings of masculinity or femininity; the sense of knowing to which sex one belongs and defining oneself as male or female.

D. Gender Role: The expression of gender identity toward oneself and others. It may be further defined as "everything that one says and does, including sexual arousal, to indicate to others or to the self the degree to which one is male or female." Money and Ehrhardt (1972) have said that "gender identity is the private experience of gender role, and gender role is the public expression of gender identity."

Gender identity disorders occur when a person experiences an incongruity between anatomic sex and gender identity. The individual has a strong desire to be a member of the opposite sex, which is not the same as feeling inadequate in behaving appropriately for one's gender role. The main forces creating gender identity are a feeling that psychologic gender agrees with anatomic gender and that gender is congruous with what culture defines as acceptable behavior for that gender. True gender disorders are rare. It is im-

---

*Ego-dystonic homosexuality has been a controversial *DSM-III* classification; it has been dropped from *DSM-III-R*. The condition has not been precisely defined and does not have easily discernible signs and symptoms. Information about incidence and prevalence is unavailable. Some clinicians argue that all psychiatric conditions are ego-dystonic. Since homosexuality is not a mental disorder, it cannot of itself be ego-dystonic.

portant to stress that congenital sexual anomalies should not be confused with gender identity disorders.

What distinguishes the congenital sexual anomalies from the gender identity disorders is that they are primarily physical rather than psychologic. At birth, a diagnosis of hermaphroditism can be made because the infant displays the attributes of both sexes; ie, both male and female external sex organs are present, accompanied by both testicular and ovarian tissue internally. Generally, the physical morphology of either male or female predominates. A decision must be made before 18 months of age to surgically correct the anomalous genitals according to the predominant features, even though they may not be consistent with any internal differentiation. In pseudohermaphroditism, the gonads may be of one sex rather than mixed, but external genitals are ambiguous. A decision about surgical correction must also be made in these cases, consistent with what is most surgically appropriate. When surgery has been performed before the critical age and if the rearing of the child is consistent with the established sex, conflict or confusion in gender identity does not develop. Most of the patients are sterile, however, because of the differences and mixtures of internal sexual morphology.

Some infants with ambiguous genitals do not receive surgical management and are nurtured and reared as male or female according to what the parents think is proper. The child thus adopts characteristics of that sex. At puberty, if secondary sexual development is the opposite of the sex of rearing, it becomes apparent that a mistake has been made, and surgical correction may be necessary. Surgery at this point usually does not alter gender identification but may make patients feel more at ease about the difference between their biologic sex and their gender identity.

TRANSSEXUALISM

Symptoms & Signs

DSM-III-R characterizes transsexualism as "a persistent discomfort and sense of inappropriateness about one's assigned sex in a person who has reached puberty. In addition, there is a persistent wish to be rid of one's genitals and live as a member of the other sex." Transsexualism may be further characterized as "asexual" when no sexual activity with a partner has been experienced; "homosexual" or "heterosexual" if sexual activity with a partner has occurred; or "unspecified" when the history provides no clear record of sexual activity with a partner.

Natural History

The onset of transsexualism often occurs during childhood, with the full syndrome becoming evident at adolescence. Onset may also occur in adulthood even after the individual has married and had children. Some clinicians feel that these different times of onset represent different types of transsexualism: primary and secondary. Transsexualism creates social and oc-

cupational problems, especially since the individual tries to live as a member of the other sex. Many patients suffer from depression, and suicide attempts are common because of confusion about sexual orientation, social isolation, and the experience of being labeled deviant.

Differential Diagnosis

Differential diagnosis stresses the *persistence* of the desire to be rid of the genitals and to be a member of the other sex. Transsexualism must be distinguished from effeminate homosexuality, in which the individual may look like a woman and affect feminine mannerisms but has no desire to *be* a woman. Transsexualism can be differentiated from physical intersexuality (characterized by abnormal sexual structures), since the genitals are normal for the biologic sex of the transsexual. What continues to puzzle investigators is that although transsexuals are reared in congruence with their biologic sex, dysphoria develops despite this consistency.

Atypical gender disorder must also be ruled out. In this condition, the person experiences transitory stress that may precipitate a wish to be the other sex; the desire disappears when the stress is relieved. For instance, men undergoing severe midlife crisis may feel that they would be more effective as women and could in that way escape male responsibilities and sexual expectations, which they believe they have failed to meet.

In schizophrenia, there may be delusions of belonging to the other sex, but patients do not wish to become the other sex by alteration of their genital anatomy.

In transvestic fetishism, the desire for cross-dressing in women's clothes occurs, but the transvestite does not wish to be rid of the genitals and become a person of the other gender.

Prognosis

The course of transsexualism is chronic and unremitting. The ultimate desire is for surgical reassignment of sex, and this is frequently attained. The long-range effects of these procedures are currently under study. Patients and surgeons agree on the usefulness of surgery for those who achieve success in becoming a member of the opposite sex, and many centers consider the surgery to be essential for the patient's future effective functioning. Some patients live successfully as members of the opposite sex without surgery. Relationships are established in which both partners agree that a sex-change operation is not necessary.

Illustrative Case

A 28-year-old male-to-female transsexual presented for routine physical examination after living as a woman for 5 years. Although no transsexual surgery had been performed, the patient's name, driver's license, and voter registration had been legally changed, and the patient had complete identification, with photographs, as a woman. (The patient will be referred to as "she" throughout the case description.)

The patient had been employed for the past 3 years as a computer programming consultant with a large electronics firm at a junior managerial level. She had a college degree in engineering (graduating third in her class), and she had attended night school to earn a business degree as well. Hormone therapy had been started during the last year of college, and cross-dressing on a constant basis had begun 1 year later.

On physical examination, the patient showed well-formed breasts, which she stated had developed slowly at first with hormone treatment but were now "the way I like them." Vital signs were normal, as were her reflexes. She had no structural abnormalities of the penis or scrotum, although both were small and soft. Pubic hair distribution was of the female pattern. She had little body hair, and what growth there was on the lower legs was soft and bleached to appear inconspicuous. Facial hair—which the patient stated had been abundant enough to require daily shaving at age 18 years—was almost nonexistent following nearly complete electrolysis and shaving of the few remaining scanty growth areas. The thyroid cartilage was palpable but not noticeable. The skin over the patient's entire body was supple and smooth.

The patient indicated that she had had a few voice lessons from an acting coach in college and had a pleasant, moderately low pitched, well-modulated speaking voice. She had long, ash-blonde hair and had never needed a wig, although she stated that she had practiced with one before she let her hair grow after she left college. She learned principles of makeup from the college theater group and had modified them to match her own skin tones, so that her makeup was neither unusual nor dramatic. Her mannerisms and body language were feminine, and her choice in clothing and accessories was traditional but stylish.

The patient had been married for the past 2 years to a heterosexual man who suppported her desire to undergo surgery for genital sex change but wanted her to be able to afford the best plastic surgery program.

The patient had already met the strict criteria for surgical candidates by living as a woman in the community for 2 or more years; maintaining adequate social, emotional, and vocational stability; and being free of a history of drug or alcohol abuse, severe depression, or suicidal ideation. Although the patient had begun heavy drinking during high school, drinking had been limited to weekends only by the time the patient entered college. When hormone therapy began, the physician had warned the patient that alcohol would interfere with treatment.

The patient stated that she had known since she was about 8 years old that she was uncomfortable with her biologic sex but that she only remembered hoping that the penis would disappear; she also remembered feeling joyful and at ease with girls and girls' games in school. Her parents, particularly her father, had wanted the patient to enter therapy to help with what the father believed were homosexual tendencies. In the course of working with the therapist for 2 years,

the family had been assured that the child was probably not homosexual, and the patient had been referred to a gender dysphoria clinic in Texas at age 14 years. Although a definitive diagnosis of transsexualism had not been made, the family and patient had been told of the possibilities.

A program had been suggested that followed a theory which is still being tested—namely, to encourage participation in male sports activities and male companionship and to observe progress in these areas. The patient remembered having enjoyed and excelled in basketball and cross-country running programs and indicated that she always knew she had been "a tomboy." In high school and college, therefore, the patient had been well liked by male teammates and had had numerous women friends not only because of an athletic image but also because of an ability to relate well to the women with regard to their own interests.

The patient recalled this period as exhilarating, disturbing, and frequently depressing because of having tried to satisfy everyone's desires but her own. The patient had liked the sports but not the association with men (as a man) and had longed to join the women openly in their activities and political groups as a woman rather than as a "sympathetic" male. In retrospect, the patient felt that the early drinking sprees in college had centered around feelings of ambiguity and indecision about how to become female. The patient had tried to discuss the issue with family members, but they had become more and more withdrawn as they had realized the seriousness of the patient's intent. During the last 2 years of college, they had become resentful and angry that the patient would be "ruining" her life and chances for a career in engineering and would be deliberately hurting herself emotionally. The patient had not been able to make the family understand her desperate feelings about changing sex.

The patient had not seen family members since the change in sexual identity. Good friends of the parents had been the patient's main link to the family. They had been helpful as people to whom the patient could turn when cross-dressing started, and they had assisted with early struggles to move out in public. They had gone out with the patient to dinner and entertainments and had supplied the nonprofessional character references needed when the patient had been seeking her first job and later when she applied for the position she held at the time of the physical examination.

The patient had met her husband at work as a colleague. They had dated, and the patient had realized that their involvement fulfilled all of her desires to relate to a man as a woman would. She had taken the risk of telling him her situation before they became sexually involved. Although he had read about transsexuals, he had not been prepared to fall in love with such a person. Their strong feelings for each other had led to a short period of living together and learning ways of sexual expression satisfying to both. Their marriage was gratifying and exciting. The patient was eligible for surgery if she wished it and whenever they decided to proceed. The patient gave this history of herself when she presented for routine physical examination and for reevaluation of her oral hormone dosage. She had not needed supplemental hormone injections for over 2 years.

The case presented above illustrates a common (though infrequently reported) history for a transsexual. Severe depression, suicide attempts, and drug and alcohol abuse are features of the early years of many transsexual patients who are moving toward a transition. Once they recognize that they must and can meet the stringent criteria for surgery, they usually stop such behavior. However, those who have had little supportive help or who have had to resort to prostitution or petty crimes to live become increasingly harassed and frustrated. Because they are a visible group to police and mental health authorities, they frequently are thought of as "typical" transsexuals. Others have been exploited by physicians who have provided hormones at exorbitant cost but who have never given such patients a thorough physical, mental, or laboratory assessment. Unscrupulous or merely uninformed surgeons have complied with demands for surgery without requiring psychologic and physical evaluation or adopting the criteria employed by established gender dysphoria centers.

Medical personnel will see transsexual patients more frequently as their numbers increase, and they should be aware of the need for empathy and understanding. Patients who are "women" in gender identity need to be protected, for example, from being hospitalized in men's wards. When such patients are on a women's ward, the staff must be careful to avoid subjecting them to unnecessary exposure. Humiliating and painful experiences in such situations often keep these patients from seeking needed medical care.

Epidemiology

Transsexualism is rare and is more common among men than women. Estimates of prevalence are one in 100,000 men and one in 130,000 women. Sex reassignment clinics in the USA report that the ratio of men to women seeking surgery ranges from 2:1 to 8:1, though the rate of requests for female-to-male reassignment is increasing. One recent estimate is that 30,000–60,000 people annually in the USA are requesting sex reassignment surgery.

Etiology & Pathogenesis

The cause of transsexualism is not known. Most investigators agree that some disturbance in the parent-child relationship may exist, although no consistent pattern has been recognized. Some authorities propose that there may be prenatal estrogen and androgen levels which influence neurologic changes (pituitary and other brain areas) that may favor the development of transsexualism. Others have suggested that chromosomal abnormalities may be involved. The information is inconclusive, however, because there have been no in-depth studies of either of these hypotheses. Chromosomal abnormalities, for example, generally produce physical abnormalities, as suggested on p 442. In a major study of transsexuals, Pauly (1974) demonstrated that 95% of patients for whom chromosomal and birth anomaly data were available showed none of these abnormalities.

Other theories propose that transsexualism is a severe defense mechanism against an early identity conflict or that unconscious parental reinforcement of cross-sexual behavior created the problem.

Treatment

Psychotherapy has not been successful in the management of transsexualism. Few individuals ask for it in any case. Transsexuals may have other psychologic problems (eg, depression, guilt and low self-esteem, alcoholism, and suicidal ideation) that may be helped by psychotherapy.

Not all individuals who request sex reassignment surgery are suitable candidates. Most clinicians have established criteria that require a 2-year period of living as a member of the other sex. Patients must demonstrate that they can function successfully in social situations and at work, and they must develop a supportive network of friends. During this period, the individual may receive hormone therapy (estrogen or testosterone). The person must be told that some changes that occur with administration of hormones are irreversible and also that the nature of the changes cannot be predicted with certainty. Assessment of general psychologic health, coping abilities, and social adjustment is made during the waiting period.

GENDER IDENTITY DISORDER OF CHILDHOOD

Symptoms & Signs

Gender identity disorder of childhood is characterized by *DSM-III-R* as "persistent and intense distress in a child about his or her anatomic sex and the desire to be, or insistence that he or she is, of the other sex." These children consistently repudiate their own anatomic attributes: Girls usually have male peer groups, enjoy sports and rough-and-tumble play, and are not interested in dolls or traditional girls' toys. Boys are preoccupied with stereotypically female activities, and they enjoy dressing in women's clothes, playing with dolls, and participating in girls' games. They avoid contact sports and imitate feminine behavior. These symptoms may occur as early as age 4 years.

Gender identity disorder of childhood is not simply a failure to fit cultural stereotypes associated with a particular sex and is not associated with physical abnormalities of the sex organs. Onset is prepubertal. Girls express a desire to be a boy or insist that they are boys. They are persistently unhappy about or deny that they are anatomically female. Typical verbal and emotional assertions are "I will grow up to become a man," "I cannot become pregnant," "I will not develop breasts," "I have no vagina," or "I will grow a penis."

For boys, there is a desire to be a girl or insistence that they are girls. They either repudiate male anatomic structures or make at least one of the following assertions: "I will grow up to become a woman," "My penis and testes are disgusting and will disappear," or "It would be better not to have a penis and testes." They are preoccupied with stereotypically feminine activities, as shown by a preference for either cross-dressing or simulation of feminine attire or by a compelling desire to participate in the games and pastimes of girls.

Natural History & Prognosis

As stated above, symptoms of gender conflict may occur as early as age 4 years. As children with gender identity disorder become older—and as peer pressure and ridicule increase—they may give up overt behavior of the other sex, but the identity conflict continues. During adolescence, some individuals discover that they have a homosexual orientation. For others, the childhood disorder may merge with transsexualism.

Illustrative Case

A 10-year-old boy had enjoyed wearing girls' clothing and jewelry since age 4 years. He used his mother's cosmetics to make up like a woman. He imitated feminine gestures and affected a feminine gait. He liked to help his mother cook and clean, and she enjoyed his company and "cute" behavior. Because he was teased by other boys for being a "sissy," he avoided boys and played almost exclusively with girls. On several occasions, he stated that he would grow up to be a woman and bear children, and on one occasion his mother gave him a pillow so that he could dress as a pregnant woman.

The boy was brought into psychotherapy when his mother realized that his predominant fantasy play was a caricature of adult women. He had become increasingly estranged from his father, who had always been remote and refused to meet the therapist or participate in the therapy. During the course of psychotherapy, the mother recognized her role in being overprotective and in unconsciously encouraging the feminine behavior. Role playing, behavior modification, and individual psychotherapy enabled the boy to develop a consistent sexual identity as a male by the time puberty began at age 14 years.

Epidemiology & Differential Diagnosis

Gender identity disorder of childhood is rare. No information is available on the sex ratio of occurrence. Gender identity disorder of childhood must be distinguished from childhood tomboyism in girls and effeminacy in boys, in which children make no references to changing their genital anatomy.

Etiology & Pathogenesis

The cause of gender identity disorder of childhood is unknown. Some authors suggest that in boys the condition results from intense, excessive, and pro-longed physical and emotional closeness between the infant and the mother and relative absence of the father. In addition, all of the theories about adult transsexualism are applied to both genders in the childhood disorder.

Another theory suggests that unavailability of the mother to a daughter in early infancy may be a contributing cause of the disorder in girls.

Treatment

Treatment must involve the entire family, since the family may be the source of the problem. One or both parents may feel threatened about psychotherapy, deny that they could have contributed to the situation, and refuse to participate. Intensive psychotherapy with the child may be necessary, especially if the condition is a result of early intrapsychic conflict (eg, if the mother was unavailable to her daughter, who repudiates her mother by repudiating her sex). If the condition is a learned response (eg, if a mother subtly encourages feminine behavior in her son), group therapy and behavior modification techniques may be beneficial.

Because of the increasing acceptance of alternative patterns of living and the recognition of cultural biases in sex role stereotyping, patients must be carefully evaluated to determine if a true psychologic disorder exists before therapy is begun.

GENDER IDENTITY DISORDER OF ADOLESCENCE & ADULTHOOD, NONTRANSSEXUAL TYPE

Symptoms & Signs

As in other gender identity disorders this condition is characterized by a "persistent or recurrent discomfort and sense of inappropriateness about one's assigned sex." It occurs in people who have attained puberty and is associated with persistent or recurrent cross-dressing.

Differential Diagnosis

This disorder can be distinguished from transvestic fetishism by the fact that cross-dressing in this disorder does not produce sexual excitement. Transsexualism should be ruled out by the lack of "persistent preoccupation (for at least 2 years)" with the wish to be rid of one's genitals and secondary sex characteristics and the wish to acquire those of the other sex.

Etiology

The cause of this gender identity disorder is unknown. The history of sexual orientation may include asexual, homosexual, or heterosexual behaviors and does not appear to be predictive of occurrence.

Epidemiology

This disorder is rare and no information about sex ratios is available.

Treatment

Clinicians do not agree on the appropriate method of treatment or whether therapy is desirable or effective.

ATYPICAL GENDER IDENTITY DISORDER

Some patients may have a gender identity dysfunction that is not classifiable as a specific gender identity disorder. These patients should not be confused with men and women who have mannerisms of the other sex (masculine women and feminine men) but have no doubt about their gender and do not want to change it. They are not said to have a gender identity disorder, and they do not need therapy. If they are sufficiently troubled or uncomfortable, they may seek training to develop gender-appropriate mannerisms, but this is not usual.

PARAPHILIAS

The concept of normality in human sexual behavior is impossible to define, since accurate statistics on the frequency of different types of sexual behavior are not available. In recognition of these difficulties, the pejorative labels "perversions," "deviations," and "aberrations" have been abandoned in favor of the term "paraphilias" (derived from Greek words meaning "along side of " and "love").

Symptoms & Signs

The paraphilias represent patterns of erotic arousal that are different from the typical pattern of mutual sexual arousal with a human partner of the opposite or same sex. The typical feature of the paraphilias, according to *DSM-III-R*, is "recurrent intense sexual urges and sexually arousing fantasies generally involving either (1) nonhuman objects, (2) the suffering or humiliation of oneself or one's partner (not merely simulated), or (3) children or other nonconsenting persons."

These behaviors also occur among the general population to some degree, and couples will occasionally describe their erotic activities as incorporating some of these features. The imagery and acts may range from "playful and harmless" with a consenting partner to "noxious and injurious" with a nonconsenting partner. Clothing fetishism is considered a minor problem, whereas sadistic lust murder is of course a most serious crime.

For the paraphiliac patient, the imagery is persistent, and the fantasies evoked are necessary for erotic arousal, for relief from nonerotic tension, and for sexual excitement and orgasm. The fantasies may or may not be acted upon, but they are distinguished by their consistency. The occasional employment of fantasy or objects in sexual activity between consenting partners is therefore excluded. An individual may incorporate several paraphilias at one time. A paraphilia may coexist with some other mental disorder and is not a symptom of the other disorder.

Many people with paraphilias feel no distress, whereas others admit to feelings of shame, guilt, and depression. Paraphilia represents an "impairment in the capacity for reciprocal affectionate sexual activity." It may produce sexual dysfunction, and social and sexual relationships may suffer. Personality disturbances are common, and behavior associated with paraphilia may take over an individual's life and completely disrupt it because of social condemnation and violations of the law.

Epidemiology

Paraphilias are rare. They occur mostly in men, with very few cases reported in women.

Etiology

Except for some cases of transvestic fetishism, most authorities agree that the cause of paraphilias is unknown.

Treatment

The treatment pattern is the same for all paraphilias. The general goals of therapy as described by Lief (1981) are to "increase heterosexual responsiveness and decrease paraphiliac behavior," "establish a rewarding sexual relationship," and "control undesirable sexual behavior." Several types of therapy have been successful in achieving these aims. Group therapy and marital therapy have been used, but individual psychodynamic psychotherapy and behavior therapy are the most commonly used types of psychotherapy.

One of the goals of psychotherapy is to discover the pattern of thoughts, feelings, and behavior that precedes the paraphiliac behavior in order to control it. For example, drinking is common before many instances of paraphiliac behavior. Other goals are to eliminate the anxiety or depression that accompanies the behavior and to help increase the patient's capacity for a better sexual relationship with a committed partner.

Behavior therapy usually consists of conditioning procedures carried out during office visits as well as assigned tasks to be done at home. Systematic desensitization using operant conditioning techniques is frequently helpful when controlled fantasy and guided imagery are used. Aversive techniques using drugs or electric shock have been used, but the reported results have not been consistent.

Recently, Abel and coworkers (1980) published a list of treatment recommendations for paraphilias. Not all of the recommendations must be used in treating each patient. The authors stress use of follow-up to provide reinforcement after therapy is concluded. Their goals are as follows:

(1) To decrease deviant sexual arousal.

(2) To develop adequate heterosexual arousal.

(3) To develop skills for social interaction with members of the opposite sex.

(4) To provide training in assertiveness.

(5) To provide training in empathy.

(6) To attain sexual knowledge.

(7) To treat sexual dysfunction within the marital unit.

Many patients with paraphilia are deficient in basic social skills. As they become more competent, their paraphiliac behavior tends to occur less frequently or may disappear. However, the person may sometimes need assistance in adapting to rather than changing the deviant behavior, because to try to change would cause the patient more intense psychologic suffering than the deviant behavior. Whenever possible, therapy should involve the spouse or other committed partner to facilitate change or adaptation.

DSM-III-R lists 9 specific paraphilias and an additional category. These are discussed in the following sections.

FETISHISM

Symptoms & Signs

Fetishism is defined by *DSM-III-R* as "recurrent, intense, sexual urges and sexually arousing fantasies, of at least 6 months' duration, involving the use of nonliving objects (fetishes)." These objects do not include female clothing used in cross-dressing or objects specifically designed to be sexually stimulating (eg, vibrators). Sexual arousal may involve the object alone or may be incorporated into activities involving a human partner. Most fetishes are articles of clothing.

Natural History & Prognosis

Fetishism may be considered a "safe" behavior by the individual, because it avoids the dangers of interacting with another person. The condition tends to be chronic, and relationship problems are common. As seen in the illustrative case discussed below, individuals with fetishes rarely present for treatment except to discuss interpersonal problems related to their paraphilia.

Differential Diagnosis

Many articles of clothing may be sexually arousing in certain circumstances, but a differential diagnosis of fetishism requires that nonhuman objects be "persistently preferred or required" to achieve sexual excitement. The occasional use of some object to enhance sexual enjoyment is not fetishism.

Illustrative Case

A 39-year-old man was brought to the physician for consultation by a good friend who felt he needed help. (The patient did not agree.) The patient said he experienced intense sexual excitement and frequently masturbated after seeing pictures of high-heeled, backless shoes that were popular during the late 1950s, when he was about 14 years old. He began buying shoes or picking up his mother's or sister's discarded single shoes and using them as a means of sexual arousal. He cleaned and packaged them and hid them in the house until he went to college. Away from home, he continued adding to his collection, which was stored in suitcases when it was not being used. On several occasions, he had had satisfactory intercourse with women, but only if shoes from his collection were visible to him at the time. He gradually stopped having intercourse because of fear of discovery and the feeling that sex was better without a partner.

The patient was now a successful businessman with a beautiful home and a "special" room for his 1200 unpaired shoes, collected from all over the world. He had shown this collection to his old friend, whom he had not seen in several years. The friend was fascinated not only by the patient's revelation about his sexuality but also by the elaborate secret panel that led from the library into the chandeliered "collection" room.

The patient did not "mind" having the psychiatric consultation, but he and the therapist agreed that since he was experiencing no psychologic symptoms or significant distress, no further visits seemed appropriate.

Etiology & Pathogenesis

The cause of fetishism is unknown. Some authorities think that the disorder commonly originates during association with some person with whom the individual was intimately involved during childhood, usually a significant, caring relative, teacher, or housekeeper. There is some inconclusive evidence of abnormal electrical activity in the temporal lobes during fetishistic behavior.

Treatment

Treatment is rarely useful or desirable.

TRANSVESTIC FETISHISM

Symptoms & Signs

Transvestic fetishism is defined in *DSM-III-R* as "recurrent, intense, sexual urges and sexually arousing fantasies, of at least 6 months' duration, involving cross-dressing (in a heterosexual male)." Cross-dressing usually involves more than one article of clothing and may involve being completely dressed as a woman. Intermittent incidents tend to become frequent or habitual.

Natural History & Prognosis

Transvestic fetishism usually begins in childhood or early adolescence. It tends to move from partial to complete cross-dressing and from occasional to frequent, habitual incidents. This pattern may produce anxiety, depression, or guilt feelings, and the depression may lead to suicide attempts. Married patients are frequently unable to maintain stable marital relationships, and divorce is common. The behavior begins as a secret and private activity and progresses to going out in public dressed as a woman. Such behavior may cause further marital or family distress as well as danger to a patient living in an area where going out in public dressed as a woman is against the law. The publicity or shame surrounding arrest may cause major emotional trauma and ultimately lead the individual to seek treatment. Some transvestites find that their condition has evolved to transsexualism or has disguised true transsexualism from the beginning. In such patients, an assessment of the problem and a possible new diagnosis must be considered.

Differential Diagnosis

Transvestic fetishism must be distinguished from transsexualism. Transsexuals wish to lose their genitals and live as members of the other sex; they receive no sexual excitement from dressing as a woman. Transvestites consider themselves to be basically male. They become sexually excited, at least at first, from cross-dressing. Transvestites report sexual frustration when there is interference with cross-dressing. Sexual arousal that is caused only by the female clothing used in cross-dressing rules out a diagnosis of fetishism.

Illustrative Case

A 40-year-old accountant came to therapy after his wife discovered him masturbating while he was wearing a bra, garter belt, black net stockings, and high-heeled shoes. After this incident, he admitted to his wife that he had been cross-dressing and masturbating episodically ever since adolescence. As a teenager, he had put on some of his sister's clothes and had become erotically aroused. He reported periods of trying to stop the practice by throwing away the outfits he kept hidden in the garage, but he always started again. His wife became upset and threatened to divorce him if he did not seek help.

The patient gave a history of growing up in a home with a passive, quiet father and a gregarious, generous mother. He had had little sexual experience before his marriage. He was attracted to his wife because of her moral principles and self-control. They had what they described as an ordinary sex life with no evidence of sexual dysfunction. They continued to have intercourse during his periods of cross-dressing. They had 2 children.

The therapist asked to see the couple together. Although she was angry with her husband and anxious about his behavior, the wife agreed to couples therapy. After a few sessions, the therapist recognized that he was taking the wife's "side" and was ignoring the patient's needs. At that time, the therapist recommended that the wife be seen separately by another therapist, and she agreed to do this if it would help maintain the marriage.

During therapy, the husband's cross-dressing occurred less frequently, although it could not be elim-

inated. The wife's anxiety and anger were lessened by the support of her own therapist, and she became more accepting, if not approving, of her husband's behavior.

Epidemiology

Although transvestic fetishism may occur among women, there are no reported cases of women who become sexually aroused by dressing as a man.

Etiology & Pathogenesis

The cause of transvestic fetishism is not known, but the case histories often include instances of punishment or humiliation by a parent or family member in which the child is forced to dress in girl's clothes. The punishment may have been initiated by the mother, an older sister, some other female relative, or, less often, the father. Such incidents often create enough tension in the child so that he masturbates while being punished, and the pattern of excitement begins. Negative family attitudes about masturbation, together with episodes of forced cross-dressing, further exaggerate the reaction the child experiences. Precipitating incidents may also include ridicule of a child who experiments in "dressing up" and who is then punished.

Treatment

Few transvestites seek help unless forced to do so by a spouse or legal authorities. Most are defensive about the activity and claim that it not only causes them no trouble but is quite enjoyable. In fact, few transvestites are appropriate candidates for psychotherapy. Those who are may seek counseling for relationship problems or may be recommended for treatment of episodic depression, guilt, anxiety, masochistic injury, or arrest for inappropriate public behavior. Some drugs such as medroxyprogesterone acetate have been used experimentally to treat transvestism, but their effectiveness is not known.

ZOOPHILIA

DSM-III defines zoophilia as "the use of animals as a repeatedly preferred or exclusive method of achieving sexual excitement." The disorder is rare, and it is now classified under "paraphilia not otherwise specified" in *DSM-III-R*.

As in all paraphilias, the differential diagnosis stresses the repetitive and preferred aspects of the object of sexual arousal. Isolated instances of sexual experimentation with animals do not represent zoophilia, and the disorder is not related to unavailability of human partners.

In some patients, early sexual arousal by humans may have occurred, but as time passes, the animal becomes the most powerful sexual stimulus.

The cause is unknown, but the preferred animal contact is usually one the individual was involved with during childhood, eg, a house pet or farm animal.

The goals of treatment are to encourage sexual fantasies about humans, help develop social skills with men and women, and reorient the patient to sources of human sexual stimulation. Combined behavioral techniques and psychotherapy are used.

PEDOPHILIA

Symptoms & Signs

The essential feature of pedophilia (literally "love of children") is defined by *DSM-III-R* as "recurrent, intense, sexual urges and sexually arousing fantasies, of at least 6 months' duration, involving sexual activity with a prepubescent child." The age difference between the parties has been established as at least 10 years unless the individual is in late adolescence, in which case it is the judgment of the clinician that determines whether the behavior may be diagnosed as pedophilia or not.

Natural History, Etiology, & Pathogenesis

The cause of pedophilia is unknown, but increasing numbers of patients have a history of being sexually abused as children by family members.

Pedophilia usually begins in middle age. Low self-esteem following marital and other relationship problems is frequently responsible for the first episodes of pedophilia. As isolation, fear, and depression increase, the patient turns to children for sexual gratification, because they give the pedophile a sense of security and mastery.

Differential Diagnosis

Differential diagnosis is based on the chronic and exclusive preference for children as objects of sexual desire. Mental retardation, organic personality syndrome, alcohol intoxication, or schizophrenia may be associated with low impulse control and isolated instances of sexual activity with children, but these are not chronic or exclusive activities and do not represent pedophilia. Sexual exhibitionism, for instance, may be directed toward children, but there is no overt sexual activity as there is in pedophilia.

Prognosis

The adult is usually married, and as pedophilia tends to be chronic, sexual and marital problems are frequent. Recidivism is high, with poor success rates following repeated attempts at therapy.

Epidemiology

Pedophilia is rarely reported in women, though it is thought to occur.

Recent reports indicate that increasing numbers of men in their 30s and 40s prefer sexual activity with children of the opposite sex. This occurs twice as often as a preference for children of the same sex. About 11% of pedophiliac patients are strangers to their victims; the rest are known to the children. About 15% of cases involve incest.

Treatment

The goal of therapy is to assist the patient in redirecting the object of desire toward mature partners.

EXHIBITIONISM

The essential feature of this disorder, as defined by *DSM-III-R,* is "recurrent, intense, sexual urges and sexually arousing fantasies, of at least 6 months' duration, involving the exposure of one's genitals to a stranger."

Exhibitionism has been thought to be a disorder only of men, with the victims being exclusively women. However, there have been isolated reports of female genital exhibitionism. The onset may be at any time from adolescence to middle age but most commonly occurs in the mid 20s.

The diagnosis of exhibitionism is made only if the individual achieves sexual excitement from the act of exposure but does not seek sexual activity with the stranger. Excitement may lead to masturbation, but commonly the person is unable to achieve an erection even by masturbation. Repeated exposure of the genitals in order to shock or attract attention but without a goal of sexual arousal is not exhibitionism, although it may be a manifestation of some other disorder. If exposure precedes sexual activity with a child, it is classified as pedophilia.

Exhibitionism becomes less of a problem after age 40 years, but before that, the recidivism rate is high. The typical exhibitionist is married and employed and shows no signs of severe psychiatric disturbance. Exhibitionists generally have shy and dependent personalities and are not likely to engage in other paraphiliac behaviors.

VOYEURISM

DSM-III-R states that voyeurism is the "recurrent, intense, sexual urges and sexually arousing fantasies, of at least 6 months' duration, involving the act of observing unsuspecting people, usually strangers, who are either naked, in the act of disrobing, or engaging in sexual activity." During observation of others, the individual masturbates, but no sexual activity with the person or persons being observed is sought. Voyeurism usually begins in early adulthood and tends to be chronic.

The diagnosis of voyeurism can be made only if the person views an unsuspecting individual in order to obtain sexual excitement but does not want to engage in sexual activity with that person. Other forms of sexual arousal, such as viewing pornography when the subjects know they will be seen, using nudity and disrobing when the person is not a stranger or unsuspecting, or inviting a third party to watch sexual activity for the purpose of erotic stimulation, are not voyeuristic behaviors.

SEXUAL MASOCHISM

The essential feature in making a *DSM-III-R* diagnosis of sexual masochism is "recurrent, intense, sexual urges and sexually arousing fantasies, of at least 6 months' duration, involving the act (real, not simulated) of being humiliated, beaten, bound, or otherwise made to suffer." The person exclusively prefers to be "humiliated, bound, beaten, or otherwise made to suffer" for the purpose of sexual excitement. Masochistic individuals intentionally participate in acts that cause physical harm or may be life-threatening to them in order to produce sexual excitement. Masochistic fantasies may begin in childhood, but activities with partners usually begin in early adulthood.

A diagnosis of sexual masochism is made only if the individual engages in acts, not just fantasies. Masochistic fantasies are commonly verbalized for the purposes of sexual arousal by many individuals, but they are rarely acted on. True masochistic behavior is repetitive and intentional. Experimentation with certain acts or unintentional suffering does not constitute masochism. Masochistic personality traits are also excluded, since sexual excitement is not associated with the masochistic personality disorders.

Masochism may be chronic and may lead to a need to increase the potential for self-harm and to increase the severity of the acts even to the point of death. For most masochistic patients, the activities remain at a nondestructive level for long periods. Since degrees of sexual sadism and masochism appear to exist in all people, disagreement about the clinical boundaries between what is normal and abnormal is common. Patients whose partners suffer no obvious distress seldom need or seek treatment.

SEXUAL SADISM

As defined in *DSM-III-R*, sadism is "recurrent, intense, sexual urges and sexually arousing fantasies, of at least 6 months' duration, involving acts (real, not simulated) in which the psychologic or physical suffering (including humiliation) of the victim is sexually exciting." The cause is not known. There are essentially 3 manifestations of sadistic behavior. If the partner is nonconsenting, it is the "repeated and intentionally inflicted psychological or physical suffering" that characterizes sexual sadism. If the partner is consenting, the essential feature is that the "repeatedly preferred or exclusive mode of achieving sexual excitement combines humiliation with simulated or mildly injurious bodily suffering." Also with a consenting partner, "bodily injury that is extensive, permanent, or possibly mortal is inflicted in order to achieve sexual excitement." Although sadistic fantasies may occur earlier, activities do not usually begin until young adulthood.

Sadism is sometimes combined with rape or lust murder. However, not all rapists are sadists, and some men cannot commit rape if they see signs of suffering in the victim. Rape is usually an act of hostile aggression and not a response to sexual excitement.

Sadism is chronic and may persist until the individual is apprehended, when nonconsenting partners are involved. Some individuals engage in milder forms of sadism and do not feel a need to increase the severity of suffering. However, others develop a need to increase the partner's suffering, or they lose their own capacity for control and so increase the severity of the suffering they inflict. The result may be rape, torture, or murder. Psychotherapy for these individuals is generally ineffective.

FROTTEURISM

Symptoms & Signs

"Touching or rubbing against a nonconsenting person" accompanied by "recurrent intense sexual urges and sexually arousing fantasies" over a period of at least 6 months is the diagnostic criterion for frotteurism. The rubbing generally involves movement of the penis against the buttocks of a woman when both people are fully clothed. This behavior occurs most commonly on crowded buses or subway trains. The female victim may not be aware of what is happening.

Natural History & Prognosis

Frotteurism is thought to be a male phenomenon and is considered rare. The touching, not the coercive nature of the behavior, produces sexual excitement. Some authorities hold that this behavior does not go beyond the rubbing or touching. Others suggest that in some circumstances it may lead to assault or rape.

Etiology

The cause of frotteurism is obscure.

Treatment

The goal of therapy, if the person requests it, is to redirect the locus of sexual stimulation to consenting partners.

ATYPICAL PARAPHILIA

Atypical paraphilias are rare types of abnormal sexual behavior, including sexual excitement produced by feces (coprophilia), urinating on a sexual partner (urophilia), being urinated on or thinking about urine (urolagnia), rubbing against strangers (frotteurism), self-administered enemas (klismaphilia), filthy surroundings (mysophilia), sexual activity with a corpse (necrophilia), and obscene telephone calls (telephone scatologia).

There is little information on the prevalence of these paraphilias or on other behavioral characteristics of the individuals involved. Some of these activities are noted in patients with other kinds of paraphilias. Isolated case reports are the major source of data. Although obscene telephone calls are frequently reported, few of the people making the offensive calls are caught and made available for examination.

OTHER PSYCHOSEXUAL DISORDERS

EGO-DYSTONIC HOMOSEXUALITY

Ego-dystonic homosexuality has been dropped from *DSM-III-R*.

SEXUAL DISORDERS NOT ELSEWHERE CLASSIFIED

Sexual disorders not elsewhere classified by *DSM-III-R* are those that cannot be classified in any of the specific categories. In rare instances, this category may be used concurrently with one of the specific di-

agnoses when both are necessary to explain or describe the clinical disturbance. Examples include (1) "marked feelings of inadequacy concerning body habitus, size and shape of sex organs, sexual performance, or other traits related to self-imposed standards of masculinity or femininity; (2) distress about a pattern of repeated sexual conquests or other forms of nonparaphilic sexual addiction involving a succession of people who exist only as things to be used; and (3) persistent and marked distress about one's sexual orientation."

These conditions are uncommon, but their true prevalence is unknown, since many people never seek treatment.

The cause is usually a combination of a number of psychosocial factors and so-called learned behaviors—culturally accepted behavioral norms exaggerated to an unacceptable degree—but no specific causative factor has been identified. Because of the idiopathic nature of these conditions, no preferred treatment has been established. Underlying psychologic disturbance is often disclosed when patients seek treatment.

REFERENCES

Abel GG et al: Aggressive behavior and sex. *Psychiatr Clin North Am* 1980;**3**:133.

Allen C: *A Textbook of Psychosexual Disorders*. Oxford Univ Press, 1969.

Bancroft J: *Deviant Sexual Behavior*. Clarendon Press, 1974.

Bancroft J: *Human Sexuality and Its Problems*. Churchill Livingstone, 1983.

Benjamin H: *The Transsexual Phenomenon*. Julian Press, 1966.

Bullough V: *Sexual Variance in Society and History*. Wiley, 1976.

Chalkey AJ, Powell GE: The clinical description of 48 cases of sexual fetishism. *Br J Psychiatry* 1983;**142**:292.

Chesser E: *Human Aspects of Sexual Deviation*. Jerrolds Publishing, 1971.

Gebhard PH et al: *Sex Offenders: An Analysis of Types*. Harper & Row, 1965.

Green R, Money J (editors): *Transsexualism and Sex Reassignment*. Johns Hopkins Univ Press, 1969.

Kiell N: *Varieties of Sexual Experience*. Internat Univ Press, 1976.

Lester D: *Unusual Sexual Behavior: The Standard Deviations*. Thomas, 1975.

Lief H (editor): *Sex Problems in Medical Practice*. American Medical Association, 1981.

Mohr JW, Turner RE, Jerry MB: *Pedophilia and Exhibitionism*. Univ of Toronto Press, 1964.

Money J, Ehrhardt A: *Man and Woman, Boy and Girl*. Johns Hopkins Univ Press, 1972.

Pariser SF, Levine SB, Gardner ML (editors): *Clinical Sexuality*. Marcel Dekker, 1983.

Parker T: *The Twisting Lane: The Hidden World of Sex Offenders*. Hutchinson & Company, 1972.

Pauly IB: Female transsexualism. *Arch Sex Behav* 1974;**3**:509.

Qualls CB, Wincze JP, Barlow DH (editors): *The Prevention of Sexual Disorders*. Plenum Press, 1978.

Stoller RJ: *Perversion: The Erotic Form of Hatred*. Pantheon Books, 1975.

Stroller RJ: *Sex and Gender*. Vol 2: *The Transsexual Experiment*. Aronson, 1976.

Tollison CD, Adams HE: *Sexual Disorders: Treatment, Theory and Reasearch*. Gardner Press, 1979.

Tripp CA: *The Homosexual Matrix*. McGraw-Hill, 1975.

Weinberg G: *Society and the Healthy Homosexual*. Doubleday Anchor, 1973.

Eating Disorders

39

Kim Norman, MD

DSM-III-R distinguishes 4 main categories of eating disorders: anorexia nervosa, bulimia, pica, and rumination disorder of infancy. Although all 4 are classified as disorders usually first evidenced in infancy, childhood, or adolescence, only rumination disorder of infancy is primarily limited to that age group. Anorexia nervosa and bulimia, which typically appear first in adolescence, may have their onset in childhood and adulthood also. Pica, the persistent eating of nonnutritive substances, is predominantly a childhood disorder but may begin during pregnancy.

Eating disorders that cannot be diagnosed using the criteria for specific ones are classified in *DSM-III-R* as eating disorder not otherwise specified. Persons with this type of disorder may be of average weight and may engage in vomiting or laxative abuse—but not binges—for weight control, or they may be of low weight and may exhibit abnormal attitudes toward eating or abnormal eating behavior but do not otherwise meet the criteria for anorexia nervosa.

Simple obesity is not included in *DSM-III-R* because it is not characteristically associated with any distinct psychologic or behavioral syndrome. A discussion of obesity is included in this chapter because it is perceived as a major public health problem and because it is best approached therapeutically using the biopsychosocial model.

People with eating disorders are not easily categorized into rigidly defined groups, and the diagnostic criteria for each category are necessarily somewhat arbitrary. Clinicians may encounter individuals who present with some or all of the symptoms associated with various diagnostic groups. The illness may vary in intensity over time, change pattern, and even change from one syndrome to another. The "eating disorders" may therefore be viewed as a collection of signs and symptoms afflicting a heterogeneous group of individuals, some of whom share distinct though overlapping psychologic, biologic, and sociocultural characteristics.

ANOREXIA NERVOSA

Anorexia nervosa is a complex disorder manifested by physiologic, behavioral, and psychologic changes and characterized by morbid fear of fatness, gross distortion of body image, and unrelenting pursuit of thinness. The name is actually a misnomer, since true anorexia (loss of appetite) does not usually occur until late in the course. Although it typically begins in adolescence, the average age at onset is between 10 and 30 years.

Symptoms & Signs

Individuals with anorexia nervosa go to incredible extremes in order to lose weight. They begin by drastically reducing caloric intake, with virtually complete avoidance of high-carbohydrate and fat-containing foods. They exercise incessantly—walking, running, swimming, cycling, dancing, and performing calisthenics. Hyperactivity is dramatic and persists even when weight loss has resulted in cachexia. Some patients alternate fasting with bulimia—episodes of uncontrolled gorging without awareness of hunger or satiation. Such eating binges are often followed by self-induced vomiting. Huge quantities of laxatives are commonly consumed. Diet pills and diuretics may also be abused in the effort to lose weight.

The eating behaviors of anorexics are often peculiar and may be bizarre. The diet may be exceedingly monotonous or highly eccentric. They may hoard large quantities or hide small amounts of food around the house. Although they eat very little, they are obsessively preoccupied with food and cooking. Food portions are carefully measured, and small meals may be eaten over many hours. Food is usually stored, prepared, served, eaten, and disposed of in specific, ritualistic fashion. Indeed, almost all types of behavior in which the patient engages may be highly ritualized, with each step taken or not taken, each bite swallowed or refused, each calisthenic completed or not as if it had profound consequences for the future well-being of the patient and those the patient cares most about. Patients with anorexia nervosa are usually highly secretive and often lie in order to protect the privacy of their eating behaviors. Kleptomania and stealing are sometimes associated with this disorder, especially among individuals who also have episodes of bulimia.

Although the features of anorexia nervosa described above can occur in individuals with a variety of premorbid personality structures and traits, a fairly consistent profile of emotional and psychologic manifestations common to all patients with this disorder has been described. Clinicians generally agree that the unrelenting pursuit of thinness manifests an underlying psychologic struggle to maintain a sense of personal autonomy and self-control. On the surface, patients are stubbornly defiant and fiercely independent. They insist they are happy, fully aware of their condition, and completely capable of taking care of themselves. But underneath they are stricken with a paralyzing sense of helplessness and ineffectiveness, with control over eating and body size the only mechanisms through which a sense of autonomy and mastery can be sustained. This important insight into the psychology of anorexia nervosa was first emphasized by Bruch (1962), who also described 2 other essential features of this disorder: a characteristic misperception of internal body cues, with inability to recognize manifestations of nutritional deprivation as the most pronounced example; and a disturbance of body image, so that patients may see themselves as fat even when exceedingly thin. These cognitive and perceptual distortions accentuate the sense of personal ineffectiveness and reinforce the need to continue the pursuit of thinness in order to maintain a sense of control.

The lack of confidence in basic self-control is compounded by feelings of personal mistrust. Patients fear they will give in to overwhelming impulses and, so far as eating is concerned, gorge themselves into obesity. Individuals with anorexia nervosa also tend to view themselves in terms of absolutes and polar opposites. Behavior is either all good or all bad; a decision is either completely right or completely wrong; and one is either absolutely in control or totally out of control. Thus, patients may respond to the gain of an ounce with the same horror as if they had gained 100 pounds. Self-mistrust and the tendency to view the world in absolutes reinforce the exaggerated need to maintain rigid control over what is and is not eaten.

Patients with anorexia nervosa often express fear about becoming adults, since that would mean taking responsibility for interpersonal and sexual relationships. They are often frightened of sexuality and usually avoid sexual encounters. When they do engage in sexual activity, it is usually without enjoyment.

Depressive symptoms are commonly associated with anorexia nervosa. These include dysphoric mood, crying spells, sleep disturbances (ie, insomnia or hypersomnia), and, occasionally, suicidal behavior. Low self-esteem is also characteristic, with many individuals claiming that thinness and the ability to lose weight are the only things they like about themselves.

Other psychiatric symptoms frequently associated with anorexia nervosa include obessive compulsive or histrionic traits, anxiety, perfectionism, and hypochondriasis.

Many of the symptoms described above are not exclusive to anorexia nervosa but are identical to those observed in individuals subjected to enforced starvation. Bizarre eating habits such as prolonging simple meals over many hours, mixing together foods that are ordinarily unrelated, episodic binges, hoarding food, stealing food, and even rummaging through garbage cans for food have been observed in individuals experimentally subjected to semistarvation as well as among victims of famine and prisoners of concentra-tion camps. Like patients with anorexia nervosa, victims of enforced starvation are often obsessed with food and cooking; irritable; emotionally labile; and depressed. They tend to withdraw socially, lose interest in sexual activity, and have sleep disturbances.

Both anorexics and famine victims show difficulty in making decisions and impairment of ability to concentrate. These symptoms are especially important in anorexia nervosa, since they increase the patient's feeling of personal ineffectiveness and fear of being out of control and thus add urgency to the need to fast in order to maintain a semblance of self-mastery.

It is, of course, the original decision and unrelenting determination *not* to eat rather than the consequences of nutritional deprivation that chiefly distinguish anorexia nervosa from starvation. However, the effects of starvation can reinforce the underlying feelings of helplessness that led to the decision to starve in the first place, and this tends to perpetuate the syndrome. Thus, the most important first step in treatment is to restore nutritional balance and normal eating habits in order to counteract the effects of starvation.

A weight loss of at least 15% of the baseline or ideal body weight is necessary to establish the diagnosis of anorexia nervosa. In addition to weight loss, a number of physical signs of anorexia nervosa can be attributed to weight loss, malnutrition, and generalized stress. Amenorrhea or oligomenorrhea, independent of weight loss and often preceding initial weight loss, is always present in women. Anorexia nervosa with premenarcheal onset often results in short stature and delayed breast development. Prolonged amenorrhea in women with anorexia nervosa may lead to the development of osteoporosis. Patients frequently complain of epigastric distress, and gastric emptying time is indeed prolonged. Vomiting, constipation, cold intolerance, headache, polyuria, and sleep disturbances are also commonly reported. Autophonia is sometimes noted. In addition to emaciation, physical findings may include edema, lanugo, low blood pressure, bradycardia, arrhythmias, diminished cardiac mass, and infantile uterus. Males with anorexia frequently have hemorrhoids and experience loss of libido. Low testosterone levels associated with emaciation often do not return to normal after weight gain (Brotman and coworkers, 1985).

Laboratory findings include abnormalities of vasopressin secretion, prepubertal plasma levels of follicle-stimulating hormone and luteinizing hormone, and a diminished response to gonadotropin-releasing hormone. Estrogen is at postmenopausal levels. There is abolition or reversal of the normal circadian rhythm of plasma cortisol; the metabolic clearance rate of cortisol is reduced; and there is incomplete suppression of adrenocorticotropin and cortisol by dexamethasone. There is diminished growth hormone response to insulin-induced hypoglycemia, arginine stimulation, and levodopa. Glucose tolerance test curves may be flat. Plasma levels of triiodothyronine (T_3) are reduced, and levels of plasma reverse T_3 may be elevated. In severe cases, the glomerular filtration rate may be reduced. Hematologic abnormalities may include leukopenia with a relative lymphocytosis, thrombocytopenia, and anemia. Bone marrow aspiration reveals hypocellularity, with large amounts of gelatinous acid mucopolysaccharide. The erythrocyte sedimentation rate is low, and plasma fibrinogen levels are reduced. Hypercarotenemia and hypercholesterolemia are common findings. Self-induced vomiting may produce a metabolic hypokalemia alkalosis. Electroencephalographic patterns may be abnormal, and the electrocardiogram may show flat or inverted T waves, S–T depression, and increased intervals.

Natural History

The onset of anorexia nervosa often follows new life situations in which the patient feels inadequate or unable to cope. Such changes may be biologic, such as the onset of puberty; psychologic, such as the stages of adolescence; or social, as in entering high school or college. The onset of anorexia nervosa may also follow the breakup of a relationship or the death of a relative or friend.

Typically, anorexia nervosa begins in individuals who are at normal weight or slightly to moderately overweight. Dieting is initially supported, even actively encouraged, by family and friends as well as in many cases by dance teachers and sports coaches. The patient is thus praised for the initial weight loss and takes pleasure in the achievement. Once the original weight reduction goal is attained, however, a new one is immediately set. Ostensibly, this is for "insurance" to offset future weight gains, but weight loss in the pursuit of thinness soon becomes an objective in itself.

Patients usually come to medical attention not because of weight loss but because of complaints such as amenorrhea, edema, constipation, or abdominal pain. They may complain of specific "food allergies" and ask for aids in dieting such as diet pills or diuretics. Patients may also present as medical emergencies, since the complications of dieting or vomiting, such as dehydration and fluid and electrolyte imbalance, may be severe. The patient may be brought in by the parents, who become worried when weight loss is extreme or are alarmed by bizarre eating habits and personality changes.

The course of anorexia nervosa is variable. There may be a single episode with complete recovery, or multiple episodes spanning many years. A single episode may also be chronic and unremitting. Complete or partial recovery may occur spontaneously in some cases or may follow treatment. Both single episodes and fluctuating courses may progress to death.

Differential Diagnosis

Anorexia nervosa must be distinguished from weight loss due to medical illnesses such as neoplasms, tuberculosis, hypothalamic disease, and primary endocrinopathies (anterior pituitary insufficiency, Addison's disease, hyperthyroidism, and diabetes mellitus). These can generally be diagnosed on the basis of thorough histories, physical examina-

tions, and laboratory studies. Patients with these medical illnesses do not present with the dread of fatness, unrelenting pursuit of thinness, and hyperactivity that characterize anorexia nervosa.

Weight loss frequently occurs in patients with depressive disorders or certain schizophrenic disorders characterized by peculiar eating habits prompted by delusions about food. Patients with other disorders also lack preoccupations with caloric intake, obsessions with body shape and size, and hyperactivity. Patients with somatization disorder may manifest weight fluctuations, vomiting, and peculiar food habits, but weight loss is usually not severe, and amenorrhea for longer than 3 months is unusual.

In order to establish the diagnosis of anorexia nervosa, patients should satisfy the *DSM-III-R* diagnostic criteria listed in Table 39–1.

Prognosis

There is marked variability in the prognosis for patients with anorexia nervosa. About 40% are completely recovered at follow-up, and 30% are improved; but 20% remain unimproved or severely impaired. The mortality rate for this disorder is as high as 22% in some studies, with suicide reported in 2–5% of chronic cases.

The presence of nonanorexic psychiatric impairments such as depression, anxiety, and agoraphobia is common at follow-up.

Indicators of a favorable prognosis include a good premorbid level of psychosocial adjustment, early age at onset, less extreme weight loss, and less denial of illness at presentation. Unfavorable prognostic factors include poor premorbid level of psychosocial adjustment, low socioeconomic status, extreme weight loss, greater denial of illness, and the presence of bulimia, vomiting, and laxative abuse. These indicators are all relative, since no single feature or set of factors can reliably predict the prognosis for any given individual.

Complete recovery in less than 2 years is unusual. The recovery rate is positively correlated with length of time at follow-up, ie, the more time that passes before follow-up, the greater the likelihood of finding re-

Table 39–1. *DSM-III-R* diagnostic criteria for anorexia nervosa.

A. Refusal to maintain body weight over a minimal normal weight for age and height, eg, weight loss leading to maintenance of body weight 15% below that expected; or failure to make expected weight gain during period of growth, leading to body weight 15% below that expected.
B. Intense fear of gaining weight or becoming fat, even though underweight.
C. Disturbance in the way in which one's body weight, size, or shape is experienced, eg, the person claims to "feel fat" even when emaciated, believes that one area of the body is "too fat" even when obviously underweight.
D. In females, absence of at least 3 consecutive menstrual cycles when otherwise expected to occur (primary or secondary amenorrhea). (A woman is considered to have amenorrhea if her periods occur only following hormone, eg, estrogen, administration.)

covery. Thus, clinicians will do well to remember the words of William Gull (1874), who described anorexia nervosa and wrote as follows: "As regards prognosis, none of these cases, however exhausted, are really hopeless while life exists."

Illustrative Case

The patient was 16 years old when she developed anorexia nervosa. Although never overweight, she had always been diet- and exercise-conscious, especially since menarche at age 13. She remembered wishing that the bodily changes taking place were under volitional control. She also remembered being happy with things the way they were. She was an excellent student, noted for her meticulous study habits and cooperative attitude. She was shy socially and declined invitations to go out on dates. She always had a few girlfriends but preferred to study and exercise alone.

Her parents had been reared in the Warsaw ghetto and as teenagers survived imprisonment in a Nazi concentration camp. Her father was a successful businessman who worked long hours and went on frequent business trips. Her mother was a homemaker who had devoted her life to her children and to "keeping the family together."

The patient's parents reacted to her weight loss with anger, horror, and surprise. They were angry because she refused to eat and rejected their efforts to help. They were horrified because she physically resembled a Holocaust victim. The patient had an older sister who was sexually promiscuous and had experimented with drugs and was viewed by her parents as the "troublemaker" in the family. Her parents were surprised because she had always been "the good girl."

The patient lost 30% of her ideal body weight and was cachectic when admitted to a medical ward for nutritional management. She insisted she could gain weight on her own and appeared to be eating all of the food on the trays at mealtimes. She was frequently observed performing calisthenics, including pull-ups on the orthopedic bar attached to her bed.

Despite her apparent increased caloric intake and continuous efforts by nursing staff to restrict her physical activity, the patient failed to gain weight in the hospital. After 3 weeks, she had even lost a few pounds.

Psychiatric consultation was obtained because of divided opinion among the staff about how to respond to the patient. Half of the treatment staff saw the patient as a sweet and innocent young girl who seemed confused and misunderstood. They believed that she simply needed more attention and emotional support in her struggle for autonomy. The other half perceived her as demanding and manipulative and were convinced she was disposing of the food she claimed to be eating or perhaps secretly vomiting after meals and then lying about it in order to avoid taking responsibility for her behavior. This group argued that total parenteral nutrition was necessary. The psychiatric consultant noted that such disagreements are common among medical personnel trying to help patients with anorexia nervosa. Since such patients typically have conflicts about autonomy and independence—wanting to be taken care of but fearing being overly controlled by parental figures and simultaneously wishing to be independent but fearing being overwhelmed by feelings of loneliness and isolation if parental figures are not involved enough—it was not surprising that a treatment staff responding to her emotional confusion would be divided along similar lines.

The patient was transferred to a psychiatric ward, where she was treated according to a behavior modification protocol based on the principles of operant conditioning. (See Chapters 3 and 46 for information on the theories and techniques of behavior modification.) She rapidly gained weight, saying, however, that she realized this was the only way she could "survive the ordeal" and win release from the hospital. She also reported that she was able to gain weight in the hospital because other people were in control. She said that since she had no choice but to eat (patients were tube-fed if they refused to eat everything on the plate), she was able to avoid the anxiety and guilt she associated with conflicts about eating and her need to feel in absolute control of herself and her impulses.

After discharge from the hospital, the patient rapidly lost the weight she had gained and was readmitted to the psychiatric ward in less than 6 months. Although she had been on the thin side of normal weight at discharge, she hated the way she looked and felt and continued to see herself as fat even though she was in fact emaciated on readmission. She made an interesting slip of the tongue on readmission, saying, "I know you see me as incredibly thin, but I really don't feel emancipated." She also complained that while in the hospital before, she had had no opportunity to practice maintaining her weight on her own after reaching her weight goal on the behavior modification protocol.

During her second hospitalization, the patient was more responsive to intensive individual psychotherapy. She felt supported in her efforts to attain a sense of personal autonomy and identified her rigid control over eating and body size as actually a false autonomy, because she was actually unable to choose to behave any other way. She recognized her tendency to divide staff members into "all good" and "all bad" caretakers and related this to her tendency to view people generally in this way and to difficulties in tolerating and sorting out mixed feelings. She listened to feedback from staff members who perceived her behavior as demanding and manipulative. She insightfully described her behavior as simple "contact seeking," with her argumentativeness helping her maintain a "safe distance" and preserving her fledgling sense of independence.

The patient also revealed for the first time intense feelings of anger toward her parents, especially her mother, whom she said she "simultaneously loved and hated." She described wishes to be exactly like her mother but felt "smothered" and "suffocated" by her. She wanted desperately to be separate and independent from her mother but felt "empty," "alone," and even "nonexistent" when she imagined being on her own. One might infer that her anorexia nervosa represented an attempt to resolve those conflicts. By starving herself to a state of cachexia, she could identify with her mother, who as a teenager was imprisoned in a German concentration camp, and keep her mother, who was frantic about her weight loss, overly involved with her. Her behavior also enabled her to maintain a sense of separateness—by willfully caricaturing her mother, whose psychology was so deeply affected by her concentration camp experiences; by rejecting in a hostile way her mother's attempts to feed and nurture her; and by reversing the process of physical maturation that was developing in the direction of an adult feminine figure like her mother's.

As therapy progressed, the patient also reported a preoccupation with death and described a number of rituals she engaged in for reassurance. For example, every night before going to bed she did a standing broad jump. As long as she could jump more than 5 feet, she "knew" she would not die in her sleep. Other rituals involved calisthenics and the preparation of food, all performed to protect against "something dreadful happening." In this context, her self-starvation and consequent reversal of physical maturation could be seen as an attempt to remain a child, which would allay anxiety about growing old and dying. These specific fears—of growing old and dying—were explicitly revealed by the patient in the course of her therapy.

Family therapy was also more productive during the second hospitalization. The parents acknowledged for the first time that there were tensions in the marriage, and they were able to discuss their conflicts openly. Both parents felt supported and even looked forward to the sessions. Her mother talked at length about how much she missed her own parents, who perished in the Holocaust, and recognized that she compensated for these feelings by being overly involved with her children. The patient felt relieved and much less worried about her parents, because she perceived them as happier and stronger. An unexpected benefit of the family therapy involved the older sister, who, with each session, expressed her feelings toward her parents and the patient, both positive and negative, with increasing openness. She eventually was able to give up her delinquent behavior.

The patient again regained her lost weight and remained in the hospital an extra 4 weeks to "practice" maintaining it. At follow-up 6 months later, she continued to express considerable anxiety about food and eating but was successfully maintaining her weight within 10% of ideal.

Epidemiology

The incidence of anorexia nervosa has increased dramatically in recent years. In their study in Monroe County, New York, Jones and coworkers (1980) reported a 400% increase in the number of new cases of severe anorexia nervosa among females aged 15–24, comparing the period 1970–1976 to 1960–1969. In Zurich, the incidence of anorexia nervosa increased from 0.38 per 100,000 between 1956 and 1958 to 1.12 per 100,000 between 1973 and 1975 (Willi and Grossman, 1983). A British study by Crisp and coworkers (1976) surveyed 9 populations of London schoolgirls. Among girls attending private schools, the prevalence was one severe case in 200 girls; considering girls 16 and older, the prevalence was one in 100. Willi and Grossman argued that since the reported severity of symptoms and the length of time between onset of symptoms and admission to hospitals have remained the same, the increased incidence is real and not simply the result of increased recognition. While it is impossible to design a retrospective study to conclusively confirm that view, it is the consensus of practitioners that the real incidence is in fact increasing.

Anorexia nervosa tends to occur in middle- and upper-class families. The risk is increased among sisters of patients with anorexia nervosa (6.6%), and several cases have been reported in twins.

Etiology & Pathogenesis

A. Biologic Factors: The number of hormonal changes in anorexia nervosa, as outlined above, suggest a hypothalamic-endocrine origin. These findings, together with the recognition that appetite, thermoregulation, and neuroendocrine function are under hypothalamic control, have led some investigators to hypothesize that anorexia nervosa is caused by a disorder of the hypothalamus. However, the changes all appear to be secondary to the effects of starvation, weight loss, malnutrition, and stress, and no evidence of primary hypothalamic dysfunction has been adduced in any of the cases.

Although there is an increased risk for the disorder in biologic siblings of patients with anorexia nervosa, twin and adoptive sibling studies have demonstrated no clear pattern of genetic transmission. Concordant and discordant identical twin pairs have been reported in approximately equal numbers. In addition, the fact that anorexia nervosa tends to occur chiefly in individuals of the upper and middle socioeconomic classes tends to refute an exclusive biologic origin. However, because the physiologic changes in anorexia nervosa (primary or secondary) definitely contribute to its pathogenesis, one must view the clinical features as resulting from interacting biologic and psychologic factors.

Anorexia nervosa has been diagnosed in at least 12 females with Turner's syndrome. However, because patients with Turner's syndrome frequently have the same psychologic characteristics commonly seen in chromosomally normal individuals who develop anorexia nervosa, these factors are just as likely to be responsible for the association as any of the biologic consequences of this chromosomal disorder. Here, too, the interplay of both biologic and psychologic factors may be responsible for the clinical presentation of anorexia nervosa.

There is a high incidence of depression among relatives of patients with anorexia nervosa and among the patients themselves, as revealed during follow-up interviews. These findings have led some authors to postulate that anorexia nervosa may represent a variant of biologically based, genetically transmitted affective illness (Swift and coworkers, 1986).

B. Psychosocial Factors: Because anorexia nervosa occurs predominantly in middle- and upper-class families, it is hypothesized that the disorder represents an exaggeration or caricature of class values emphasizing achievement and a thin, youthful appearance as primary virtues. These values may be more characteristic of the richer classes because low-calorie, high-nutrition foods, beauty aids, and leisure time for exercise are all expensive and not readily accessible to the poor.

A number of psychologic theories have been proposed to account for anorexia nervosa. Classic psychoanalysts have emphasized the avoidance of sexuality. They view self-starvation as a rejection of the wish to be pregnant and refusal of food as a behavioral response to fantasies of oral impregnation. Amenorrhea has been viewed as a symbolic manifestation of the wish to be pregnant. More recently, theorists have stressed impairment in the mother-child relationship as the primary cause. Such theorists view the characteristic struggle for autonomy as a manifestation of the failure to master conflicts associated with the process of separation and individuation. (See Chapters 6 and 7 for a discussion of these conflicts.) The cognitive and perceptual deficits associated with anorexia nervosa, such as the distortion of body image, may also arise from impairments in early childhood development. For example, repeated invalidation of a child's perceptions by overly intrusive parents who "know too well" what a child thinks, feels, and needs can result in development of a sense of personal mistrust characteristic of patients with this disorder.

In recent years, family systems theorists have argued that anorexia nervosa is the result of dysfunctional family interactions. The child who develops anorexia nervosa is seen as serving the function of maintaining the status quo, allowing the family to remain enmeshed, overinvolved, rigid, overprotective, and unable to handle conflicts openly. The child's illness may also provide the vehicle with which parents are able to seek fulfillment of their own unresolved dependency needs. (See Chapter 48 for a discussion of family dynamics.)

The abundance of theories reflects the multidimensional nature of this disorder. No single theory offers a satisfactory explanation of the origin of anorexia nervosa. Each has contributed a valuable perspective on treating this puzzling and life-threatening disorder.

Treatment

The initial goal of treatment is to counteract the effects of starvation by promoting weight gain and restoring normal nutritional balance. In mild cases, this may be accomplished on an outpatient basis; in moderate to severe cases, an initial period of hospitalization is usually required.

Weight gain may be accomplished by hyperalimentation or total parenteral nutrition. However, because of the risks of intravenous feedings, most programs utilize behavior modification protocols based on the principles of operant conditioning. While behavior modification may be effective in promoting initial weight gain, most outcome studies have concluded that behavior modification alone is not sufficient treatment. Lasting recovery occurs only when such methods are used in conjunction with psychotherapy that addresses the underlying psychologic conflicts. Clinicians should also be advised that too rapid weight gain may cause dangerous gastric dilatation or precipitate congestive heart failure.

Drug therapy may be useful in at least some cases. Some clinicians have considered the perceptual and body image disturbances characteristic of anorexia nervosa to be manifestations of psychosis, and chlorpromazine and similar drugs have facilitated weight gain in some patients. However, it is not clear whether the benefits of such medications are due to their antipsychotic or their sedative effects. Antidepressants have also helped some patients, thus supporting the argument that a subgroup of patients with anorexia nervosa may have a primary affective illness (Bond and coworkers, 1986). Cyproheptadine, an appetite stimulator and serotonin antagonist, has proved helpful in the treatment of a subgroup of anorexic patients with especially severe symptoms and a history of birth trauma.

Although psychoanalysis has not been generally effective in the treatment of anorexia nervosa, psychodynamically oriented psychotherapies that provide support to the patient and focus on issues relating to the struggle for autonomy and personal control are often successful. Family therapies, which view the symptoms of anorexia nervosa in the context of family structure and dysfunction, are also effective, especially in the treatment of children, teenagers, and adults still living at home.

In order to effectively treat anorexia nervosa, the biologic, psychologic, and behavioral changes must all be addressed. Effective treatment programs should not be welded to any single approach. Clinicians should be familiar with various methods of treatment and use them singly or in combination as called for.

BULIMIA

Bulimia is the episodic, uncontrolled binge eating of large quantities of food over a short period of time. It was originally described in the late 1950s as a pattern of behavior in some obese individuals. In the 1960s and early 1970s, it was recognized as a commonly associated feature of anorexia nervosa. Recently, it has been identified as a distinct disorder that occurs in persons of normal weight who are not obese and do not have anorexia nervosa.

Symptoms & Signs

The essential feature of bulimia is the episodic, uncontrolled gorging of large quantities of food in short periods of time. Patients are aware of their disordered eating habits and distinguish eating binges from simple overeating. They are usually unaware of hunger during binges and do not stop eating when satiated. They express fear about not being able to stop eating voluntarily and report that binges end only when nausea or abdominal pain becomes severe, when they are interrupted or fall asleep, or when they induce vomiting.

Binges are usually preceded by depressive moods in which the patient feels sad, lonely, empty, and isolated; or by anxiety states with overwhelming tension. These feelings are usually relieved during the binges, but afterward patients typically report a return of depressive mood with disparaging self-criticism and guilt feelings.

Binges usually occur in secret. They may last from a few minutes to several hours, typically less than 2 hours, with a median reported time of about 1 hour. Most binges are spontaneous, but some may be planned, especially as the disorder progresses to chronicity. The frequency of binges ranges from occasional (2 or 3 times a month) to many times a day. The quantity of food consumed varies but is always large. Bulimics report consumption of 3–27 times the recommended daily allowance for calories on binge days, and some claim to spend as much as $100 a day on binge foods. The food consumed is usually high in carbohydrates and of a texture that is easily swallowed. Patients often report eating the "junk foods" they ordinarily deny themselves but often eat whatever is available. Though high-carbohydrate foods are most commonly consumed, the nutritional content of binge foods varies. Although it is uncommon, some bulimics may eat huge quantities of vegetables, such as 7 lb of carrots at a single sitting.

Self-induced vomiting is very common but is not essential for the diagnosis. Some patients maintain normal weight by alternating binges with long periods of fasting, and many exercise excessively. Those who do vomit may use emetics such as ipecac syrup or induce vomiting by activating the gag reflex. Lesions on the back of the hand may be evidence of this. Many report that they no longer need chemical or mechanical stimulants to induce emesis, as they can simply vomit at will. Laxative abuse is commonly associated with bulimia, the use of diuretics is not unusual, and rumination may occur.

Patients with bulimia are usually self-conscious about their behavior and often go to great lengths to conceal it. They are very concerned about their physical appearance, and they fear becoming fat. Sexual adjustment may be disturbed, with behavior ranging from promiscuity to restricted sexual activity. A number of other symptoms related to poor impulse control are commonly associated with bulimia, such as alcoholism, drug abuse, stealing, self-mutilation, and suicidal gestures and attempts.

Most patients experience weight fluctuations, with weight typically ranging from slightly underweight to slightly overweight. Other symptoms associated with bulimia include edema of hands and feet, headache, sore throat, painless or painful swelling of parotid and salivary glands, erosion of tooth enamel and severe caries, feelings of fullness, abdominal pain, and lethargy and fatigue. Light-headedness, dizziness, syncope, and seizures may occur if vomiting is severe. Menstrual irregularities are common, but amenorrhea is usually not sustained.

Bulimia is usually not incapacitating except in extreme cases, where binge vomiting is a virtual full-time preoccupation. When vomiting is excessive, dehydration and electrolyte imbalances can occur and may result in medical emergencies. Deaths from gastric dilatation and rupture have been reported.

Natural History

Bulimia typically begins in adolescence or young adulthood in individuals consciously trying to stay slim. Some report a history of anorexia nervosa; others, of obesity. The onset often follows changes in living situations such as leaving home, starting college, changing jobs, or becoming involved in new relationships.

The course is usually chronic, and patients often engage in such behavior for years before seeking treatment. The chronicity of the illness may be punctuated by brief remissions in which the behavior is absent or the frequency and severity of the symptoms are reduced. Many report experiencing periods of relative improvement and other periods of worsening symptoms.

The natural history of bulimia may be affected in those who induce vomiting by the mechanism they use. Chemical emetics such as ipecac may cause death from poisoning (Friedman, 1984), and in one case ingestion of baking soda led to metabolic coma (Norman, 1984).

Diuretic and laxative use may exacerbate the hypokalemic alkalosis caused by excessive vomiting.

Differential Diagnosis

The *DSM-III-R* diagnostic criteria for bulimia are listed in Table 39–2.

If the patient also satisfies the diagnostic criteria for schizophrenia or anorexia nervosa, that should be the diagnosis. Severe weight loss does not occur in bulimia, and amenorrhea is unusual.

In diagnosing bulimia, it is necessary to rule out neurologic disease, such as epileptic-equivalent seizures, central nervous system tumors, Klüver-Bucy–like syndromes, and Kleine-Levin syndrome. Klüver-Bucy syndrome includes visual agnosia, compulsive licking and biting, exploration of objects by mouth, inability to ignore any stimulus, placidity, hypersexuality, and hyperphagia. This syndrome is very rare and

Table 39–2. *DSM-III-R* diagnostic criteria for bulimia.

A. Recurrent episodes of binge eating (rapid consumption of a large amount of food in a discrete period of time).
B. A feeling of lack of control over eating behavior during the eating binges.
C. The person regularly engages in either self-induced vomiting, use of laxatives or diuretics, strict dieting or fasting, or vigorous exercise in order to prevent weight gain.
D. A minimum average of 2 binge eating episodes a week for at least 3 months.
E. Persistent overconcern with body shape and weight.

unlikely to present a problem in differential diagnosis. Kleine-Levin syndrome occurs chiefly in males and is characterized by hyperphagia and periods of hypersomnia lasting 2–3 weeks.

Prognosis

The prognosis for bulimia is unknown, as there have been few controlled studies of this disorder. However, there are reports of a variety of successful treatment regimens, and clinicians report anecdotally that most of their patients with bulimia improve or recover completely. A number of deaths have occurred from dehydration and electrolyte imbalances caused by excessive vomiting, but the incidence is not known. There is an obvious need for controlled treatment and outcome studies for this disorder.

Illustrative Case

A 20-year-old woman sought outpatient treatment for her binge eating and vomiting behavior. Her symptoms began at age 17 when she was a college freshman. Although very bright and attractive, she worried about whether men would like her. Her weight was normal for height and age, but she decided to lose a few pounds in the spring in order to "be prepared for bathing suit season." She went on a diet together with her roommate, who suggested vomiting after meals.

The patient reported binging 3 or 4 times a week, usually in the evening and always when alone. She usually felt depressed and anxious when the urge to binge became overwhelming. She typically binged on breads and sweets. It was not unusual for her to eat a half-gallon of ice-cream, a box of cookies, and a loaf of bread during a binge, which typically lasted about 30–45 minutes. She felt relief from her depression and anxiety during binges and reported sensations of warmth, safety, security, and unconditional acceptance. She ended the binges when her stomach ached, at which time she induced vomiting mechanically. After vomiting, she felt guilty and angry at herself for giving in to her impulses and being out of control.

The patient was 5 feet 6 inches tall. Her weight had fluctuated between 110 and 150 lb since the onset of her bulimia. Although she weighed 122 lb at the start of treatment, she reported wishing she weighed 15–20 lb less. She took large doses of laxatives daily and occasionally used diuretics. She had taken amphetamines in the past and was worried about her increasing dependence on alcohol. She complained of spending up to $60 on a single binge and reported stealing food from grocery stores.

She described self-hatred as a result of her behavior and told of superficially cutting her wrists on 2 occasions that she characterized as "semisuicide attempts."

The patient decided to seek treatment after reading an article about the medical dangers of bulimia. She had been too embarrassed to discuss her symptoms and felt she might be the only person in the world with such a bizarre disorder. She was surprised by the article, which reported a high incidence of the disorder.

She entered individual psychotherapy and attended a support group for women with bulimia. Her symptoms improved during the first 6 months of treatment, with the frequency of binges dropping to once a week. After a year of therapy, she improved even further, with binges occurring only occasionally. She decided to continue in therapy, not only to better understand her eating disorder but also to work on long-standing problems related to low self-esteem and difficulty in social relationships.

Epidemiology

The prevalence of bulimia is unknown, and the few rigorous epidemiologic studies that have been attempted are complicated by the secretiveness and guilt associated with this syndrome, which may hamper accurate self-reporting. The syndrome is most common among adolescent girls and young women. However, 10% of reported cases are in men. Various surveys have reported the incidence of bulimia to range from 3 to 20% in college populations (Pyle, 1983, 1985). Although these figures vary greatly and include mild as well as severe cases, bulimia is becoming recognized as a common condition with an increasing incidence.

No familial pattern has yet been conclusively demonstrated in this disorder.

Etiology & Pathogenesis

The cause is not known. The episodic, uncontrolled nature of the eating behaviors has led some investigators to suggest that bulimia may be a variant of complex partial seizure disorder. However, the few electroencephalographic abnormalities reported in patients studied during the testing of this hypothesis did not correlate with treatment response to phenytoin. It has also been suggested that the presence of 14- and 6-per-second spikes in some patients with bulimia is evidence of a hypothalamic disorder. However, most investigators consider this electroencephalographic pattern a variant of normal and not likely to be of etiologic significance.

Psychodynamic theories emphasize the symbolic nature of eating binges as representing gratification of sexual and aggressive wishes. Self-deprecation and self-induced vomiting following binges may thus represent guilt-induced self-punishment for fantasized transgressions.

Psychologists have also noted that the binge-vomiting cycle may represent a ritual acceptance and taking in followed by a rejection of symbolic love objects.

Bulimia may thus represent an attempt to control the external environment. Patients with bulimia are noted to have low self-esteem, and the vomiting may represent a symbolic purging of bad aspects of the self. Patients with bulimia tend to have an overinvestment in body image and often have impaired object relationships that are recapitulated in their eating behaviors.

As with anorexia nervosa, cultural emphasis on thin, youthful appearance as a symbol of privileged social class may contribute to the increasing incidence of this disorder.

Treatment

There have been few treatment and outcome studies of bulimia, though many case reports have been published of successful treatment by individual and support-group therapies as well as with a variety of behavior modification techniques. The latter have included positive reinforcement, informational feedback, and progressive desensitization focusing on the thoughts and feelings prior to an episode of binge eating. There is a need for further clinical studies of this disorder.

Success has also been reported in some series with tricyclic and other heterocyclic antidepressants and with monoamine oxidase inhibitors. The use of anticonvulsant medication has not gained general acceptance and remains controversial.

PICA

Pica is the persistent ingestion of nonnutritive substances. Pica is the Latin word for "magpie," a bird remarkable for eating and carrying away a wide variety of things. More specific terms denote the specific substance eaten: geophagia (eating earth), amylophagia (eating large quantities of starch), trichophagia (eating hair), lithophagia (eating gravel or stone), and pagophagia (craving and ingesting large quantities of ice). Pica is most frequently a childhood disorder, but it may arise during pregnancy as well.

Symptoms & Signs

The essential feature of this disorder is persistent eating of nonnutritive substances. The practice is considered abnormal after 18 months of age. Pica is most frequently seen in children between 1 and 6 years of age but may occur in older mentally retarded children and in adults. Younger children tend to eat paint, plaster, string, hair, and cloth, whereas older children have greater access to and thus may ingest dirt, animal droppings, rocks, wood, papers, crayons, cigarette ends, and matches. Virtually any substance can be consumed.

There are no regularly associated features of pica, and symptoms vary with the substance eaten. Lead poisoning may occur in children who eat plaster and paint chips. Intestinal parasites may infect children who eat contaminated soil. Hair and stones may cause

intestinal obstruction. Severe cases of geophagia may result in life-threatening hyperkalemia.

Natural History

Pica in children usually disappears by adolescence. Pica with onset in pregnancy usually ends with the termination of pregnancy. The harmful effects of this disorder and thus its natural history are dependent on the quantity and composition of the substances ingested.

Differential Diagnosis

The *DSM-III-R* diagnostic criteria for pica are listed in Table 39–3. The second criterion lists several important differential diagnoses; others include iron deficiency anemia, which must be suspected with pagophagia.

Prognosis

The prognosis for pica depends largely on the medical complications that arise. The behavior itself is usually treatable by environmental manipulation, behavior modification, and correction of nutritional deficiencies if any.

Illustrative Case

A 4-year-old black boy was admitted to a community hospital for iron deficiency anemia and abdominal pain believed to be caused by persistent ingestion of dirt, paint chips, wood, crayons, and newspaper. He had had a similar hospitalization at age 2½ and an emergency room visit 6 months later following ingestion of household cleaning fluid.

The patient lived with his mother, father, and 2 younger sisters in a low-income housing project that was run down and badly in need of repair. The father worked at odd jobs and was rarely at home. Both parents were teenagers when the patient was born. They were described by hospital staff as immature, with strong dependency needs of their own. The mother had a history of ingesting dirt and starch during each of her pregnancies.

The anemia was corrected in the hospital by balanced nutrition with vitamin and mineral supplements. Abdominal pain also remitted. A behavior modification protocol with both positive and negative reinforcements was used to treat the abnormal eating behavior. The parents were instructed in these principles and thus became more involved with the patient on discharge. A visiting nurse went to the apartment at regular intervals and reported a dramatic reduction in the tendency to ingest nonnutritive substances at follow-up. The increased involvement by the parents ap-

---

Table 39–3. *DSM-III-R* diagnostic criteria for pica.

A. Repeated eating of a nonnutritive substance for at least 1 month.
B. Does not meet the criteria for either autistic disorder, schizophrenia, or Kleine-Levin syndrome.

peared to have a beneficial effect on the boy's general behavior, and the parents reported enjoying him more than before.

Epidemiology

Epidemiologic studies of pica have focused on selected groups of patients attending hospitals and clinics and thus may not accurately reflect the prevalence of this disorder in the population at large. A study in Georgia (O'Rourke and coworkers, 1967) reported geophagia in 55% of obstetric patients. Of 987 pregnant patients at a Chicago clinic, 34.6% reported eating starch (Keith and coworkers, 1968). A study of black families in rural Mississippi (Vermeer and Frate, 1979) reported geophagia in 57% of women and 16% of children. Such behavior was not reported in men. In a study of Boston children aged 1–6 years (Barltrop, 1966), 18.5% of the children interviewed and 32.1% of those studied by a questionnaire mailed to parents were affected by pica.

Studies reveal a slight preponderance of pica in black children compared to white children, and a few studies have found a slightly increased incidence in males.

Pica is more common in children whose mothers have had pica, and there is an increased incidence in the siblings of affected children.

Etiology

There are 2 main hypotheses regarding the cause of pica. The first suggests that specific nutritional deficiencies such as zinc and iron deficiencies cause the cravings for nonnutritional substances. The second emphasizes the role of psychosocial factors, particularly inadequate relationships with immature or unavailable parents and dilapidated, impoverished physical environments as causative factors. Proponents of the latter theory argue that children with pica may be arrested at oral stages of psychosexual development, with persistent eating of nonnutritious objects representing a search for fulfillment of unmet oral dependency needs.

Treatment

The treatment of lead poisoning associated with pica may be environmental, such as remodeling and repainting apartments where children eat plaster coated with lead-based paint.

As mentioned, pagophagia may be a symptom of iron deficiency. The correction of underlying mineral deficiency states has led to the resolution of pica in some children.

Several behavioral techniques have been effective in treating pica. Aversive therapies using mild electric shock, unpleasant noise, or emetic drugs have been used. Positive reinforcements, such as social recognition and affection or specific object rewards, have also been used with success. Positive reinforcement techniques are especially helpful when the parents are involved, thus giving children needed parental attention that may have been lacking before. Additional behav-

ioral techniques include behavior shaping and overcorrection procedures.

Visiting nurses and family counseling may also be helpful in treating this disorder.

RUMINATION DISORDER OF INFANCY

Rumination, or merycism, is a rare syndrome of infancy in which food after eating is returned to the mouth and either spit out or chewed and reswallowed. Although rumination is found primarily in infants, it also occurs in older children and adults. It has recently been identified as occurring in association with bulimia (Larocca and Della-Fera, 1986).

Symptoms & Signs

The essential feature of this disorder in infants is repeated regurgitation of food with weight loss or failure to thrive after a period of normal development. Partially digested food is returned to the mouth without nausea, retching, disgust, or gastrointestinal distress. The food is then spit out or chewed and reswallowed. Infants are often observed to assume a characteristic posture with arching of the back and head held back (opisthotonus). Sucking movements of the tongue are present, and the infant appears to gain pleasure from the activity. Regurgitation tends to occur when the infant is alone and stop when social contact is established.

A common complication is that the mother becomes discouraged by failure to feed her child successfully, withdraws emotionally, and understimulates the baby. The regurgitated material also has an offensive odor, which reinforces withdrawal by the mother and results in further understimulation of the infant.

Natural History

The disorder usually begins between 3 and 12 months of age. Mentally retarded children may develop the syndrome at later ages. Spontaneous remissions are thought to be common. However, severe malnutrition and failure to thrive may result, with delays in all developmental spheres. Some deaths have been reported.

Differential Diagnosis

Rumination disorder must be distinguished from congenital anomalies such as pyloric stenosis and infections of the gastrointestinal tract that cause regurgitation of food. Pyloric stenosis is usually associated with projectile vomiting and is evident before 3 months of age. Hiatal hernia may cause excessive regurgitation in infants. However, simple regurgitation can be distinguished from the rhythmic, seemingly pleasurable behavior of rumination. Hiatal hernia may coexist with rumination disorder, and the condition may improve with surgical repair of the hernia (Herbst and coworkers, 1971).

The *DSM-III-R* diagnostic criteria for rumination disorder of infancy are listed in Table 39-4.

Prognosis

Spontaneous remissions are thought to occur commonly, but severe malnutrition with developmental delays and failure to thrive is frequent. The mortality rate from malnutrition caused by this disorder has been estimated to be as high as 25%.

Illustrative Case

A 9-month-old girl was admitted to the hospital for treatment of pneumonia thought to be caused by aspiration of regurgitated food. She was underweight and behind in developmental milestones. It was learned that after 6 months of normal development, she began to regurgitate. Initially, this was occasional, but the frequency increased, and within a month, regurgitation occurred after every feeding. After each feeding, she was observed to arch her back and hold her head back. She seemed to facilitate regurgitation by rhythmically contracting her abdominal muscles and making sucking motions with her tongue. She seemed to enjoy the activity. Some of the food she brought up she spit out. The rest she chewed and reswallowed.

The mother was described by the hospital staff as an immature woman, emotionally deprived as a child, with strong unfulfilled dependency needs. Although the pregnancy was unplanned, she stated she had always wanted a baby. However, as the regurgitation became a pattern, she felt disgusted and alienated from the baby and found herself withdrawing emotionally.

In the hospital, regurgitation was noted to occur mostly when the baby was alone in a passive, self-occupied state. The behavior usually ceased whenever eye contact was established with a member of the hospital staff. A treatment program was devised in which the baby was held for most of the day and played with, especially after feeding. In the hospital, the rumination diminished and the baby gained weight.

On discharge, the parents agreed to ask the father's sister to move in to help care for the baby. Holding the baby much of the day in supine and upright positions and stimulating her socially with affection and age-appropriate play resulted in remission of symptoms. The baby continued to gain weight and caught up with normal developmental milestones. Her mother joined a support group for parents and disclosed that she withdrew from the baby out of fear that she would abuse her if she held her too long. She entered individual psychotherapy and talked at length about her own childhood. She expressed intense ambivalence toward her own mother. She had always felt neglected and unwanted as a child and both loved and hated her mother, whom she never seemed able to please. She felt great relief at having someone to talk with about these feelings. As her therapy progressed, she felt in much greater control of her impulses and learned to feed her baby with success.

Epidemiology

Rumination disorder of infancy is very rare; only 23 cases were reported in the American literature during 1954–1974. The sex incidence is equal. Although familial occurrence has been reported, a familial pattern for this disorder has not been established.

Etiology

Rumination disorder has been described in infants with hiatal hernia, and other physical anomalies such as autonomic nervous system dysfunction have been suggested as possible causes. Most clinicians, however, believe impaired parent-child interactions are responsible. In most cases the mother is immature and dependent, with a history of emotional deprivation in childhood. Marital conflict is a common historical feature, so that the mother may feel unable to give much attention to the baby at a time when sensory maturation is developing rapidly. Rumination occurs in isolation and does not occur when adequate stimulation is provided. What appears to be happening is that an infant who does not receive adequate gratification through visual, auditory, and tactile stimulation from the mother turns inward for stimulation and learns that it can get pleasure from rumination. Rumination thus apparently recreates gratifying early feeding experiences. Whether psychologically or biologically based, it has been proposed that the behavior is perpetuated because of "addiction" to endogenous opiates that may be stimulated during rumination (Chatoor and coworkers, 1984).

Treatment

Thickening the formula and mechanical devices to keep the mouth securely closed have not been successful. In 3 ruminating infants with hiatal hernia, one was treated successfully by feeding in the upright position and maintaining that position after feedings, and 2 recovered following surgical repair.

Aversive conditioning using mild electric shocks or squirts of lemon juice has also been successful.

Psychologic treatments are quite successful in this disorder. Treatment consists of providing an emotionally adequate mother substitute to help the infant form a trusting relationship with a caretaker, while the mother receives help with her own dependency needs until she can effectively take over. The mother substitute holds and stimulates the infant at times when it is most likely to ruminate. As rumination subsides, other developmentally appropriate stimulations are added. As in cases of failure to thrive, the mothers of these infants can learn appropriate techniques of feeding and stimulation, thus creating a healthy parent-child relationship that fosters normal growth and development.

Table 39-4. *DSM-III-R* diagnostic criteria for rumination disorder of infancy.

A. Repeated regurgitation without nausea or associated gastrointestinal illness for at least 1 month following a period of normal functioning.
B. Weight loss or failure to make expected weight gain.

OBESITY

Simple obesity is not included among the eating disorders in *DSM-III-R*. However, when there is evidence that psychologic factors play a substantial etiologic role in a specific case, this may be documented by noting "psychological factors affecting physical condition" in the diagnosis. A brief discussion of obesity is included in this chapter because effective treatment approaches must take into account biologic, psychologic, and sociocultural factors.

Symptoms & Signs

Despite the absence of clear-cut psychologic and behavioral profiles associated with the development of obesity, there is a subgroup of obese individuals who manifest emotionally based patterns of overeating. About 10% of obese individuals, usually women, display a night-eating syndrome characterized by anorexia in the morning and hyperphagia with insomnia during evenings. Such behavior is apparently precipitated by life stresses and tends to persist until the stresses are relieved. A smaller group of obese individuals (about 5%) are episodic binge eaters (see above). Such episodes tend to follow emotional stresses and may represent reactions to them.

Obese individuals with concomitant mental disorders may have severe disparagement of body image. They feel that their bodies are grotesque and that others view them with hostility and contempt. Such feelings may be reinforced by social attitudes, since fat people are often discriminated against and viewed by others as lazy, weak, self-destructive, and responsible for their condition. They also manifest low self-esteem and a negative self-concept. Ordinarily, obese persons with no coexisting mental disorder do not manifest disturbances of body image or self-concept.

Although many obese individuals tend to eat in response to emotional cues such as feelings of anxiety, fear, loneliness, boredom, and anger, so do many persons of normal weight. Obese individuals tend to chew less and eat more rapidly than other people, but both groups are strongly influenced by the eating behaviors of those around them.

Obese adults are usually physically less active than others, but this may be a consequence rather than a cause of obesity. Obese children are not less active than their normal-weight peers.

Dieting itself can be a significant biologic and psychosocial stress factor. Dieting may cause feelings of frustration, agitation, irritability, and heightened emotional reactivity in otherwise normal persons. Thus, some of the emotional features traditionally attributed to obese persons may be a consequence of attempts to lose weight by dieting rather than a cause of their condition. In contrast, the jovial image projected by some obese individuals may be a psychologic defense to gain acceptance by others.

Excess weight may cause low back pain, aggravation of osteoarthritis (particularly of the knees and ankles), and huge calluses on the feet and heels. Obesity may be associated with amenorrhea and other menstrual disturbances. The lower ratio of body surface area to body mass leads to impaired heat loss and increased sweating. Intertrigo in tissue folds, itching, and skin disorders are common. There is often mild to moderate swelling of hands and feet.

In massively obese persons, pressure of fatty tissue on the thorax combined with pressure of intra-abdominal fat on the diaphragm may reduce respiratory capacity and produce dyspnea on exertion. This condition may progress to the so-called **pickwickian syndrome,** characterized by hypoventilation with hypercapnia, hypoxia, and somnolence.

Obesity is associated with hypertension, hyperlipidemia, diabetes mellitus, carbohydrate intolerance, and renal and pulmonary disorders. Obese patients are at increased risk during surgery and anesthesia and in pregnancy. Obesity is also associated with increased risk of cardiovascular disease; however, it is not clear whether it is an independent risk factor or one resulting from associated hypertension, hyperlipidemia, and diabetes. It has also been suggested that certain health risks associated with obesity may be influenced by the pattern of distribution, as well as the total volume, of fat. Greater risks of cardiac disease, for example, may be associated with excessive accumulation of abdominal fat (Kopelman, 1984).

Natural History

Obesity can begin in childhood, adolescence, or adulthood. Amounts of body fat also increase with age even when weight remains constant. Obesity is usually a chronic and progressive condition.

Differential Diagnosis

By convention, obesity is defined as weight at least 20% above ideal weight listed in standard height and weight tables. Many investigators include measures of body fat, such as those taken with skin-fold calipers, in the diagnosis of obesity.

In assessing obesity, the clinician must rule out medical illnesses such as hypothyroidism.

Prognosis

The prognosis for losing excess weight and keeping it off is poor. In the late 1950s, it was reported that fewer than 5% of obese persons lose 40 lb or more, and even fewer maintain the loss. Although the prognosis for short-term weight loss has improved with the advent of new dieting and exercise strategies and the development of behavior modification programs, the long-term outlook remains poor. It is estimated that if an obese child does not achieve nearly normal weight by the end of adolescence, the odds against doing so later are 28:1. Morbidity and mortality rates for obese individuals are proportionate to the degree of obesity and the presence of associated risk factors such as hypertension and diabetes mellitus. Whereas mild obesity (overweight, but less than 30% above ideal weight) is not associated with an increased mortality rate, severe obesity (weight more than 50% above ideal weight) may increase the mortality risk by 90% compared to that of individuals of normal weight (Lew and Garfinkle, 1979).

Epidemiology

Estimates of the prevalence of obesity among adults in the USA range from 15 to 50%. The prevalence increases with age up to age 50, at which point it falls sharply in accordance with the increased mortality rate. Obesity is more common in women, especially after age 50, because of the higher mortality rate among obese men after that age. It has been estimated that about 25% of children are significantly overweight.

Social and cultural factors play a major role in the prevalence of obesity. Obesity is more common among ethnic groups during their first generation in this country. Gradually improving socioeconomic status reduces the prevalence from 24% to 5% between the first and fourth generations.

In general, the prevalence of obesity is higher among people of lower socioeconomic status. In a Manhattan study, obesity was present in 30% of poor women, 16% of middle-class women, and only 5% of wealthy and privileged women (Goldblatt and coworkers, 1965; Moore and coworkers, 1962). The differences were similar for men, but there were fewer obese men than women in each category (Stunkard, 1975; Stunkard and coworkers, 1972).

Ethnic and religious factors may also contribute to the development of obesity. A greater than 40% prevalence of obesity was found among Hungarian and Czech groups. Women with British or Italian ethnic backgrounds also tend to be overweight. Some studies have found a higher prevalence of obesity among Jews, followed by Roman Catholics and then Protestants.

Family studies of obesity show that 40% of adolescents studied at age 15 who had one obese parent were obese, while 80% of those with 2 obese parents were obese. This compares to only a 10% incidence of obesity among adolescents whose parents are of normal weight (Mayer, 1965a). Studies of monozygotic and dizygotic twins suggest genetic factors, but environmental influences are also present (Mayer, 1965b). Adoption studies have shown conflicting evidence for genetic transmission. Evidence for the heritability of somatotypes is stronger than for obesity (Seltzer and Mayer, 1964). This fact may be significant in that even a moderate degree of ectomorphic body habitus may protect against the development of obesity.

Etiology

Although there is great variability in weight among humans, individuals show remarkable consistency over time. Humans who agreed to increase their weights 20–25% for experimental purposes generally returned to their starting weights when allowed to eat freely. Such observations have led to the theory that there is a biologic set point for body weight in humans. In animal studies, lesions of the lateral and ventromedial hypothalamus cause hypophagia and hyperphagia, respectively. The animals will lose or gain weight but then maintain their new weight as if a new set point were created. If forced to gain or lose weight, these animals will adjust their intake and return to their new set points when allowed to eat freely. To the extent that the "set point theory" is applicable to humans, many obese individuals may be dieting in opposition to biologic factors that make dieting far more difficult than for other people.

Weight gain can occur by an increase in either the number or the size of fat cells. The fat cells of adults with juvenile-onset obesity may be of about the same size as those of normal-weight persons, but there may be up to 5 times as many. Persons with adult-onset obesity may have a normal number of larger than normal fat cells. In studies in which fat cell number and size were determined, individuals tended to stop losing weight when fat cell size returned to normal. Since fat cells once formed do not disappear, fat cell number may determine the lower limit of weight for persons who by dieting have worked to reduce cell size to normal. There are 2 periods of cellular proliferation in normal-weight children: birth to 2 years of age and 10–14 years of age. In obese children, the period may extend well past 2 years of age, with consequent hypercellularity of fat tissue early in life. Although this may be partly under genetic control, the cellular theory of obesity thus has important implications regarding nutritional practices and weight regulation for children.

The gene governing triglyceride metabolism has recently been identified and coded. Anomalies in this gene may result in some cases of obesity. It should also be noted that there are multiple central nervous system and peripheral chemical regulators of appetite, eg, neuropeptides and gastrointestinal hormones (bombesin, cholecystokinin, somatostatin, and substance P), and the endogenous opioids (serotonin, norepinephrine, and dopamine). (See Morley and Levine, 1985.)

Early psychoanalytic theories of obesity held that obese individuals had unresolved dependency needs and were fixated at the oral level of psychosexual development. The symptoms of obesity were viewed as depressive equivalents, attempts to regain "lost" or frustrated nurturance and care. Recent studies have failed to demonstrate an increased incidence of psychopathologic disorders in obese compared to normal-weight individuals. However, a subgroup of juvenile-onset obese subjects have gross disturbances in body image—ie, they view their bodies as hideous and loathsome and feel that others view them with contempt. They have a negative self-concept, are very self-conscious, and have impaired social functioning. Such experiences may contribute to the development and maintenance of obesity. Furthermore, since obese individuals are often discriminated against socially and are perhaps less often the object of sexual desire than normal-weight individuals, the maintenance of obesity may in some cases reflect an unconscious wish to remain isolated in order to avoid conflicts relating to sexuality or emotional intimacy.

Although there is no specific family constellation that predisposes to obesity, members of families lacking in warmth and love may use food and overeating as a "substitute for love." The mothers in such families are often lonely individuals whose own childhoods were marked by social, economic, or emotional deprivation. Such mothers may unconsciously wish to have fat children. Identification with their "well-fed, well-cared for" children may compensate for earlier deprivation. Such families may also equate physical size and the state of being "well fed" with physical and emotional strength. Obese children in such families may thus actually fear weight loss by concretely interpreting it as a loss of physical strength and emotional well-being.

The higher incidence of obesity among lower socioeconomic classes and certain ethnic groups is noted above. In some societies where food is scarce, obesity may be valued as a symbol of prosperity. In affluent countries such as the USA, value is instead placed on thinness, perhaps because foods low in calories but of high nutritional value are more expensive and unaffordable to the poor.

The definition of obesity may itself be culturally determined (Ritenbaugh, 1982). Since 1943, revisions in standard height and weight charts have steadily lowered the ideal weights for women. The ideal weight for an average 5-ft 4-in woman in 1943 was approximately 130 lb; in 1980 charts, it is under 120 lb. Ideal weights for men have also been lowered, though not as much, and in 1974 the ideal weight for an average 5-ft 10-in man was actually higher than the corresponding standard in 1943. These revisions have not been based on morbidity or mortality statistics but on measurements of the heights and weights of 25-year-old graduate students. Such standards do not take into account the fact that the percentage of body fat increases with age but instead reflect the fashion trends of the youthful, affluent college populations. For women, the steady decline in ideal weight reflects the upper-class emphasis on fashion model thinness as the standard of beauty. For men, there is greater acceptance of a wider variety of body types. Attractive men may be thin, eg, long-distance runners and basketball players; or bulky, eg, weight lifters and football players. This broader range of acceptability may account for the less consistent downward trend in ideal weights for men listed in standard charts.

If one accepts the 1980 standards for ideal weights and if obesity is defined as at least 20% above ideal, then the average American woman is by definition obese and the average American man is on the verge of obesity.

Treatment

Surgical procedures, such as intestinal bypass operations and gastric stapling, are effective in producing weight loss and in improving psychosocial functioning. These surgical procedures may also produce biologic change, perhaps by lowering the body weight set point (Stunkard and coworkers, 1986). However, risks of surgery and anesthesia, which are greater in obese individuals, plus the possibility of postoperative complications such as malabsorption syndromes following bypass procedures should limit the indications for these interventions to the treatment of massive and morbid obesity that has not responded to conservative management. Wiring the jaws shut to prevent the intake of solid food may help some individuals, especially when used in preparation for surgery. The use of intragastric balloons, a recently introduced noninvasive method of gastric restriction, appears promising but is still experimental.

Amphetamines were once widely prescribed as anorexigenic agents in the treatment of obesity. However, the high potential for abuse of amphetamines should preclude their use as diet aids. Furthermore, tolerance develops easily. Anorexigenic drugs with low abuse potential include diethylpropion (Tenuate, Tepanil), fenfluramine (Pondimin), and mazindol (Mazanor, Sanorex). Their effectiveness and side effects are comparable. The use of appetite suppressants alone is not currently recommended, since weight lost as a result of their use is usually rapidly regained. It can be argued that for these reasons, appetite suppressants that work directly on the central nervous system will always be problematic. Hope for the future probably lies with new drugs that regulate the peripheral conversion of food into fat.

Exercise regimens are recommended as part of most treatment plans. Exercise is helpful not only because of the increase in caloric expenditure but because physical activity (in otherwise sedentary individuals) is associated with decreased appetite and increased basal metabolism. This latter effect may offset the estimated 15–30% decrease in basal metabolic rate that occurs with caloric restriction and weight loss from dieting. Exercise also increases the proportion of weight loss from fat as opposed to lean body tissue. Exercise combined with low-calorie diets will result in weight loss; the difficulty, of course, is in motivating patients to comply with a disciplined regimen.

Support groups such as Overeaters Anonymous and Weight Watchers may be helpful in motivating some individuals to lose weight.

In recent years, behavior modification programs have been shown to be effective in reducing the high dropout rate associated with most weight reduction programs, especially when deposits of money are required and sums refunded with regular attendance or weight loss. Behavioral programs have been shown to be effective in the short run, but weight tends to be regained.

Although psychoanalysis and psychoanalytically oriented psychotherapy have not traditionally been regarded as being effective in the treatment of obesity, recent studies (Rand and Stunkard, 1983) suggest a more optimistic outlook. Of 84 men and women treated by 72 psychoanalysts, 72 had weight losses comparable to what was achieved by other methods even though only about 6% of obese persons who entered treatment did so because of their obesity. Analysts also reported dramatic improvements in body image perceptions in their patients. Whereas 40% of obese patients showed marked body image disturbances at the start of treatment, only 14% continued to have such problems at termination. This study suggests that psychoanalytic psychotherapy may be effective in some cases, especially for patients with disturbances of body image and self-concept.

SUMMARY

Food and eating may have a number of psychologic meanings. Eating may provide a source of pleasure and gratification; a means of diminishing anxiety, worry, and frustration; or an outlet for the expression of hostility. It may serve as a means of self-indulgence and may relieve feelings of loneliness and emptiness. Eating may serve to maintain the status quo and avoid maturity and as a substitute for or barrier against heterosexual involvement. Symbolically, food and eating may represent conflicts with the mother, a type of "alimentary orgasm," expression of sexual wishes, gratification of destructive or sadistic impulses, and an attempt to resolve underlying depression. Food and eating may represent penis envy or fantasies of oral impregnation; a means of possessing a "part-object" such as a penis or breast, of devouring an ambivalently loved object, or of feeling nurtured and loved; or an attempt to orally incorporate one's mother. This is merely a partial listing. Indeed, many clinicians agree that virtually any emotional conflict can be expressed behaviorally through food and eating.

Food is also important because of its role in social interactions. A mother's primary interactions with her infant involve food and eating. Difficulties in feeding because of a mother's immaturity, psychologic conflicts, or ambivalence toward her baby can result in severe impairments in the child's emotional and physical development, as observed in some cases of "failure to thrive" infants and those with rumination disorder. Conversely, a child who is difficult to feed because of allergies, excessive spitting up, or colic may cause the mother to feel frustrated and disappointed and prevent the development of a healthy mother-child relationship. Food may also be used in struggles for control by a mother who forcibly overfeeds her child or who gives or withholds food as a means of reward or punishment. The child may also use food as a means of rebelliousness and for establishing control by stubbornly refusing to eat what is put on the table. Such interactions may be important in the genesis of anorexia nervosa.

Food and eating as determinants of body size contribute significantly to body image and thus self-image. The social acceptibility of body size is culturally determined, and cultural pressures may therefore contribute to the development of eating disorders such as anorexia nervosa and bulimia.

Finally, biologic factors such as mineral deficiencies and pregnancy in pica and hypothalamic set points, somatotype, and the number of fat cells in obesity may be significant in the development of those disorders. The biologic consequences of malnutrition and fluid and electrolyte imbalances may perpetuate anorexia nervosa and bulimia once those syndromes have commenced.

Indeed, it is clear that any successful approach to the understanding, treatment, and prevention of eating disorders must include a thorough awareness of biologic, psychologic, and sociocultural determinants. Eating disorders thus provide a clinical paradigm for the application of the biopsychosocial model.

REFERENCES

Anorexia Nervosa

Bemis KM: Current approaches to the etiology and treatment of anorexia nervosa. *Psychol Bull* 1978;**85**:593.

Bond WS, Crabbe S, Sanders MC: Pharmacotherapy of eating disorders: A critical review. *Drug Intell Clin Pharm* 1986;**20**:659.

Brotman AW, Rigotti N, Herzog DB: Medical complications of eating disorders: Outpatient evaluation and management. *Compr Psychiatry* 1985;**26**:258.

Bruch H: *Eating Disorders: Obesity, Anorexia Nervosa, and the Person Within*. Basic Books, 1973.

Bruch H: *The Golden Cage*. Open Books, 1978.

Bruch H: Perceptual and conceptual disturbances in anorexia nervosa. *Psychosom Med* 1962;**24**:187.

Crisp AH, Palmer RL, Kalucy RS: How common is anorexia nervosa? A prevalence study. *Br J Psychiatry* 1976; **128**:549.

Falstein EI, Feinstein SC, Judas I: Anorexia nervosa in the male child. *Am J Orthopsychiatry* 1956;**26**:751.

Garner DM, Garfinkel PE: *Anorexia Nervosa: A Multidimensional Perspective*. Brunner/Mazel, 1982.

Gull WW: Anorexia nervosa. *Trans Clin Soc (Lond)* 1874; **7**:22.

Halmi KA: Psychosomatic illness review: Anorexia nervosa and bulimia. *Psychosomatics* 1983;**24**:111.

Herzog DB, Copeland PM: Eating disorders. *N Engl J Med* 1985;**313**:295.

Hsu LKG: Outcome of anorexia nervosa: A review of the literature (1954–1978). *Arch Gen Psychiatry* 1980;**37**: 1041.

Jones DJ et al: Epidemiology of anorexia nervosa in Monroe County, New York: 1960–1976. *Psychosom Med* 1980; **42**:551.

Keys A et al: *The Biology of Human Starvation*. Univ of Minnesota Press, 1950.

Minuchin S, Rosman BL, Baker L: *Psychosomatic Families: Anorexia Nervosa in Context*. Harvard Univ Press, 1978.

Mira M, Stewart P, Abraham S: Hormonal and biochemical abnormalities in women suffering from eating disorders. *Pediatrician* 1983;**12**:148.

Reatig N: Eating disorders: A bibliography. *Psychopharmacol Bull* 1986;**22**:523. [Major emphasis on psychopharmacology.]

Schiele BC, Brozek J: "Experimental neurosis" resulting from semi-starvation. *Psychosom Med* 1948;**10**:31.

Swift WJ, Andrews D, Barklarge NE: The relationship between affective disorder and eating disorders: A review of the literature. *Am J Psychiatry* 1986;**143**:290.

Theanders S: Anorexia nervosa: A psychiatric investigation of 94 female patients. *Acta Psychiatr Scand [Suppl]* 1970;**214**:1.

Theanders S: Outcome and prognosis in anorexia nervosa and bulimia: Some results of previous investigations, compared with those of a Swedish long-term study. *J Psychiatr Res* 1985;**19**:493.

Tolstrup K et al: Long-term outcome of 151 cases of anorexia nervosa: The Copenhagen Anorexia Follow-Up Study. *Acta Psychiatr Scand* 1985;**71**:380.

Toner BB, Garfinkel PE, Garner DM: Long-term follow up of anorexia nervosa. *Psychosom Med* 1986;**48**:520.

Vandereycken W, Van den Broucke S: Anorexia nervosa in males: A comparative study of 107 cases reported in the literature (1970 to 1980). *Acta Psychiatr Scand* 1984;**70**:447.

Willi J, Grossman S: Epidemiology of anorexia nervosa in a defined region of Switzerland. *Am J Psychiatry* 1983; **140**:564.

Bulimia

Abraham SF, Beaumont PJV: How patients describe bulimia or binge eating. *Psychol Med* 1982;**12**:625.

Boskind-Lodahl M, Sirlin J: The gorging-purging syndrome. *Psychol Today* (March) 1977;**10**:50.

Chernin K: *The Obsession: Reflections on the Tyranny of Slenderness*. Harper & Row, 1981.

Friedman EJ: Death from ipecac intoxication in a patient with anorexia nervosa. *Am J Psychiatry* 1984;**141**:702.

Gwirtsman H et al: Pharmacologic treatment of eating disorders (Symposium on Clinical Psychopharmacology II). *Psychiatr Clin North Am* 1984;**7**:863.

Herzog DB, Copeland PM: Eating disorders. *JAMA* 1985; **313**:295.

Masserman JH: Psychodynamisms in anorexia nervosa and neurotic vomiting. *Psychoanal Q* 1941;**10**:211.

Mira M, Stewart P, Abraham S: Hormonal and biochemical abnormalities in women suffering from eating disorders. *Pediatrician* 1983;**12**:148.

Mitchell JE et al: Electrolyte and other physiological abnormalities in patients with bulimia. *Psychol Med* 1983; **13**:273.

Norman KP: Unpublished case report. University of California, San Francisco, 1984.

Pyle RL: The epidemiology of eating disorders. *Pediatrician* 1983;**12**:102.

Reatig N: Eating disorders: A bibliography. *Psychopharmacol Bull* 1986;**22**:523. [Major emphasis on psychopharmacology.]

Russell G: Bulimia nervosa: An ominous variant of anorexia nervosa. *Psychol Med* 1979;**9**:429.

Pica

Barltrop D: The prevalence of pica. *Am J Dis Child* 1966; **112**:116.

Chisolm JJ, Kaplan E: Lead poisoning in childhood: Comprehensive management and presentation. *J Pediatr* 1968;**73**:942.

Keith L, Evenhouse H, Webster A: Amylophagia during pregnancy. *Obstet Gynecol* 1968;**32**:415.

Millican FK et al: The prevalence of ingestion and mouthing non-edible substances by children. *Clin Proc Child Hosp (Wash)* 1962;**18**:207.

Millican FK et al: Study of an oral fixation: Pica. *J Am Acad Child Psychiatry* 1968;**7**:79.

O'Rourke D et al: Geophagia during pregnancy. *Obstet Gynecol* 1967;**29**:581.

Singhi S, Singhi P, Adwani GB: Role of psychosocial stress in the cause of pica. *Clin Pediatr (Phila)* 1981;**20**:783.

Snowden CT: A nutritional basis for lead pica. *Physiol Behav* 1977;**18**:885.

Vermeer DE, Frate DA: Geophagia in rural Mississippi: Environmental and cultural contexts and nutritional implications. *Am J Clin Nutr* 1979;**32**:2129.

Rumination Disorder of Infancy

Bergman P, Escalona SK: Unusual sensitivities in young children. *Psychoanal Study Child* 1949;**3**:333.

Chatoor I, Dickson L, Einhorn A: Rumination: Etiology and treatment. *Pediatr Ann* 1984;**13**:924.

Escalona SK: Feeding disturbances in very young children. *Am J Orthopsychiatry* 1945;**15**:76.

Flanagan CH: Rumination in infancy: Past and present. *J Am Acad Child Psychiatry* 1977;**16**:140.

Fleisher DR: Infant rumination syndrome: Report of a case and review of the literature. *Am J Dis Child* 1979; **133**:266.

Herbst J, Friedland GW, Zboralske F: Hiatal hernia and "rumination" in infants and children. *J Pediatr* 1971; **78**:261.

Kanner L: Historical notes on rumination in man. *Med Life* 1936;**43**:27.

Larocca FEF, Della-Fera MA: Rumination: Its significance in adults with bulimia nervosa. *Psychosomatics* 1986; **27**:209.

Stein ML, Rausen AR, Blau A: Psychotherapy of an infant with rumination. *JAMA* 1959;**171**:2309.

Obesity

Blundell JE, Rogers PJ: Pharmacologic approaches to the understanding of obesity. *Psychiatr Clin North Am* 1978; **1**:629.

Brownell KD: Understanding and treating obesity. *J Consult Clin Psychol* 1982;**50**:820.

Goldblatt PB, Moore ME, Stunkard AJ: Social factors in obesity. *JAMA* 1965;**192**:1039.

Kaplan HJ, Kaplan HS: The psychosomatic concept of obesity. *J Nerv Ment Dis* 1957;**125**:181.

Keesey RE: Set points and body weight regulation. *Psychiatr Clin North Am* 1978;**1**:523.

Kopelman PG: Clinical complications of obesity. *Clin Endocrinol Metab* 1984;**13**:613.

Leon GR: Personality and behavioral correlates of obesity. In: *Psychological Aspects of Obesity*. Wolman B (editor). Van Nostrand Reinhold, 1982.

Lew EA, Garfinkle L: Variations in mortality by weight among 750,000 men and women. *J Chronic Dis* 1979; **32**:563.

Mayer J: Genetic factors in human obesity. *Postgrad Med* (April) 1965b;**37**:A-103.

Mayer J: Obesity in adolescence. *Med Clin North Am* 1965a; **49**:421.

Moore ME, Stunkard AJ, Srole L: Obesity, social class and mental illness. *JAMA* 1962;**181**:962.

Morley JE, Levine AS: Appetite regulation: Modern concepts offering food for thought. *Postgrad Med* 1985; **77**:42.

Rand CSW, Stunkard AJ: Obesity and psychoanalysis: Treatment and four-year follow-up. *Am J Psychiatry* 1983; **140**:1983.

Ritenbaugh C: Obesity as a culture-bound syndrome. *Cult Med Psychiatry* 1982;**6**:347.

Seltzer CC, Mayer J: Body build and obesity: Who are the obese? *JAMA* 1964;**189**:677.

Sjostrom L: The contribution of fat cells to the determination of body weight. *Psychiatr Clin North Am* 1978;**1**:493.

Stunkard AJ, Stinnett JL, Smoller JW: Psychological and social aspects of the surgical treatment of obesity. *Am J Psychiatry* 1986;**143**:417.

Stunkard AJ et al: Influence of social class on obesity and thinness in children. *JAMA* 1972;**221**:579.

Tan T-L, Handford HA, Soldatos CR: Current therapy of eating disorders. 2. Obesity. *Ration Drug Ther* 1984;**18**:1.

Wadden TA, Stunkard AJ: Social and psychological consequences of obesity. *Ann Intern Med* 1985;**103**:1062.

Wilson GT, Brownell KD: Behavior therapy for obesity: An evaluation of treatment outcome. *Adv Behav Res Ther* 1980;**3**:49.

40

Factitious Disorders

Stuart J. Eisendrath, MD

The term factitious means willfully produced. Factitious disorders are those in which the individual does something to produce the signs or symptoms of illness. The illness may be manifested chiefly by physical symptoms or chiefly by psychologic ones. The goal of illness production is to receive medical, surgical, or psychiatric care, though there may also be secondary motivations such as obtaining drugs or financial assistance.

Formal attention to these disorders in this century began with Asher, who in 1951 coined the term **Munchausen's syndrome** to denote the disorder observed in patients who traveled widely in England, presenting at hospitals and surgeries with plausible but dramatic stories of medical illness that resulted in numerous hospitalizations and operations. As the clinical history and diagnosis became clarified in these patients, it was discovered that they had sought and received medical care for its own sake rather than to be cured. Asher noted that the patients told elaborate tales, often in a quite entertaining manner, and therefore named the syndrome after Baron von Munchausen, an 18th century German soldier and raconteur known for his tall tales. Attempts to define these patients by the type of medical attention they pursued led to such coinages as "laparotomaphilia migrans." With further exploration, it appeared that no organ system was safe from these patients, so that different methods of categorization were developed. Nevertheless, terms such as "peregrinating problem patients," "hospital hoboes," and "surgical addiction" have been applied to this group.

Patients with Munchausen's syndrome have a history of repeated hospitalizations extending over years, so that they seem to have adopted the role of patient as a career. Reich and coworkers have found that these patients appear to represent a minority of those with factitious disorder with physical symptoms. Most patients do not have the Munchausen characteristics of sociopathy, imposture, peregrination, and marked resistance to treatment. They ususally have intermittent and mild physical illness (eg, factitious dermatitis). They generally do not seek invasive interventions and often have stable family and work roles. Their episodes of illness usually occur in reaction to a specific stressor.

Some patients display factitious psychologic symptoms in order to obtain psychiatric care. Others may display both physical and psychologic factitious symptoms, either alternately or concurrently.

FACTITIOUS DISORDER WITH PHYSICAL SYMPTOMS

Symptoms & Signs
(Table 40–1)

Any organ system will serve as a site of pain or other symptom for a patient with factitious illness, and histories compatible with virtually every known disease have been described by these patients. Laboratory abnormalities have also been produced, including anemia, hypokalemia, hematuria, hypoglycemia, coagulopathies, and hyperamylasuria. The choice of organ system is limited only by the patient's creativity and available resources. The means by which patients produce evidence of illness may be startling to the unsuspecting medical practitioner. One patient produced an elevated rectal temperature at will by alternately relaxing and contracting the anal sphincter to generate heat. Another patient would spit saliva into his urine sample so that the salivary amylase would elevate urinary amylase readings, thus producing spurious evidence of pancreatitis. Patients have injected insulin to produce hypoglycemia, and the spurious source was only detected by peptide studies.

A patient with Munchausen's syndrome may present to the emergency room with a classic history of myocardial infarction, bleeding ulcer, pulmonary embolism, etc. Upon admission, these patients are often loudly demanding of attention from the medical staff and may request high doses of narcotic analgesics. They are usually familiar with medical terms and procedures and may even suggest additional diagnostic tests to the attending physician. An important recur-

Table 40–1. *DSM-III-R* diagnostic criteria for chronic factitious illness with physical symptoms.

A. Intentional production or feigning of physical (but not psychologic) symptoms.
B. A psychologic need to assume the sick role, as evidenced by the absence of external incentives for the behavior, such as economic gain, better care, or physical well-being.
C. Does not occur exclusively during the course of another axis I disorder, such as schizophrenia.

ring symptom pattern is that these patients frequently request *invasive* diagnostic or therapeutic procedures. They often ask for surgery, saying, "I know that's the only thing that will help me."

These patients frequently travel from hospital to hospital, often over wide distances. Patients with Munchausen's syndrome who do this type of traveling, as well as having chronic factitious illness, are a subset of the broader category. Typical patients with chronic factitious illness do not travel unless forced to do so by rejection by a local hospital or physician. When traveling, these patients will often exhibit certain sociopathic characteristics such as lying without showing any feelings of guilt. They often take on the role of impostor, assuming the identity of a war hero, a lawyer, or even a doctor. They often let fall clues to the imposture, since part of what they are trying to achieve is to show how they have duped their admirers. When the imposture is discovered, they move on to repeat the pattern before a new group in a new hospital or city. Characteristically, these patients abuse narcotic analgesics and are strident in their demands for them. If the staff is reluctant to comply with their requests, they become angry and arrogant. If confronted with damaging documentation of their overuse of drugs or the possibility that their disease is factitious, these patients typically threaten litigation and leave the hospital against medical advice.

Detection of factitious illness is not usually difficult once the suspicion arises. A patient with bacterial abscesses has them only in areas accessible to self-inoculation. Unusual bacterial flora are noted on culture of the abscesses and indicate oral or fecal contamination. The major clue to detection lies in examination of the patient's background. In almost all cases, patients with factitious illness have worked in the health care field. When a patient with such a background presents with a chronic medical problem not fully explained by normal pathophysiologic mechanisms, one should consider the possibility of factitious disease.

The psychiatric symptoms of these patients are quite varied. Normal individuals, given sufficient emotional distress, might resort to factitious disease as a coping mechanism. Patients with borderline personality who tend to act impulsively and have difficulty tolerating anger or depression may briefly decompensate into psychosis. Borderline patients tend to view everybody, including the staff on the medical-surgical floor, as either "good people" or "bad people" and may struggle to escape from or defeat the bad ones. There is often controversy among the staff, with some taking the role of advocate for the patient and others acting with retaliatory anger.

Patients with factitious illness can produce illness at 3 levels. Certain individuals give only a history consistent with a known diagnosis without any supporting physical evidence; such patients may be considered to have factitious illness by virtue of their **factitious history.** The second level of enactment involves the **simulation of signs of illness.** An example would be the individual who pricks a finger with a pin and squeezes

a few drops of blood into a urine sample to give the appearance of hematuria and support a factitious history of renal stone. The most dangerous level of enactment involves those patients who actually produce **abnormal pathophysiologic states.** Individuals in this category take dicumarol, thyroid, or insulin and inject themselves with foreign substances. Patients who only give fictitious histories are easier to treat, and their periods of dysfunction appear to be more stress-related and time-limited. Patients who produce actual pathophysiologic abnormalities usually become chronic patients.

Natural History

Since only a few patients with chronic factitious illness with physical symptoms have had the benefit of careful psychologic study, the natural history of the disorder is unclear. Most patients have a deprived early childhood, and many have had hospitalizations during the first 5 years of life for some medical problem.

Children who stay home from school feigning illness are at risk for this disorder. Clinically significant factitious illness usually develops in the teen or early adult years.

Differential Diagnosis

Factitious disorder is an example of an abnormal illness-affirming behavior. Individuals with this behavior originate or amplify the idea that they are ill in order to achieve unconscious goals. Other examples of illness-affirming behaviors include hypochondriasis, somatization disorder, conversion disorders, somatoform pain disorders (psychalgia), and malingering. All of these must be included in the differential diagnosis of factitious disorder. The most important differential diagnostic problem is the true medical illness that is difficult to diagnose. The clinician must remember that even people with clear histories of factitious disorder do develop true medical or surgical disorders that must always be suitably investigated. Patients who perform self-destructive acts requiring medical care must also be distinguished. For example, the schizophrenic patient who performs some act of self-mutilation as part of a delusional psychosis certainly has produced the physical illness, but this differs from factitious disorders in that the goal of that individual's behavior was to act in accordance with the delusion (eg, to escape persecutory voices) and not to obtain medical care. Other behavior, such as persistent substance abuse or suicide attempts, also may cause the patient to receive medical attention. The primary goal, however, is usually not medical attention.

As shown in Table 40–2, in patients with hypochondriasis, somatization disorder, conversion disorders, and somatoform pain disorders, the production of illness-affirming symptoms or signs is entirely unconscious, as are the motivations of that behavior. These patients are not aware that they are exaggerating or focusing on normal bodily sensations. They are also unaware of the motivations for this behavior. An ob-

Table 40–2. Differential diagnosis of factitious disorder.

	Illness Production	Motivation
Hypochondriasis, somatization disorder, conversion reaction, somatoform pain disorder	Unconscious	Unconscious
Factitious disorder	Conscious	Unconscious
Malingering	Conscious	Conscious

server who is aware of the environmental situation might make psychodynamic inferences about the goal of such behavior. An example would be hysterical paralysis serving to avoid family conflict.

The malingerer, however, is aware of the conscious production of the signs or symptoms of a disease state, and the motive is known to the patient. For example, a soldier who claims illness in order to avoid an unpleasant duty assignment would be aware of why he was producing the signs or symptoms of illness.

The patient with factitious illness is aware that he or she produces the illness but does not know why. This is analogous to the phobic patient who consciously avoids the feared object but cannot explain why. Motivation for feigning illness is entirely unconscious, and an observer would be unaware of a reason for the behavior without resorting to some psychologic inference.

Prognosis

The prognosis for factitious disease with physical symptoms varies depending on the level of involvement. Patients with pathophysiologic states have a more serious prognosis than patients with other forms of the disorder, and occasionally a fatal outcome. It is difficult to assess the effectiveness of psychotherapy. Some patients are so fixed in the patient role that they are essentially untreatable. Perhaps, as Nadelson (1979) suggests, the most the physician can do for this type of patient is to refuse surgery and try not to do any further harm. Patients who intermittently resort to factitious symptoms when under stress are more likely to respond to psychotherapy.

Illustrative Case No. 1

A 30-year-old woman who worked as an x-ray technician was evaluated for skin lesions—superficial excoriations surrounded by normal skin, occurring over the inner thigh and pubic mound. A gynecologic assessment for spotty bleeding revealed similar vaginal lesions. Her symptoms had developed a few weeks after she underwent a total abdominal hysterectomy and bilateral salpingo-oophorectomy for a ruptured ectopic pregnancy—her first attempt at childbearing.

The dermatologist used skin patching to determine that the lesions were factitious and referred the patient for psychiatric consultation. The psychiatrist learned from the patient and her husband that she had suffered significant depressive symptoms since her surgery.

She noted that she "no longer felt like a whole woman" and had lost interest in sex. Her lesions were seen as an attempt to solve her problem by believing that "something's wrong down there." The vaginal bleeding was an attempt to produce a semblance of menstruation. She was referred for ongoing psychotherapy to help her deal with her sense of "lost womanhood."

Illustrative Case No. 2

A 30-year-old divorced registered nurse with a history of abdominal pain, nausea and vomiting, and hematemesis was admitted to a general hospital for evaluation. At the admissions desk she said, "I think I'll need surgery." She reported a 10-year history of peptic ulcer disease, for which she had been treated surgically. She had also had a cholecystectomy and several laparotomies for possible bowel obstruction. She described several episodes of septic shock for which no cause had ever been discovered. She had several surgery scars on her abdomen and numerous cutdown sites on her arms and legs. There was a tenderness to deep palpation in the epigastric region but no rebound tenderness. Stool was negative for occult blood. Endoscopy revealed modest gastric irritation, presumably secondary to bile reflux. Since one of her physicians felt there was a strong psychosocial component to her pain complaints, psychiatric consultation was obtained. The patient was at first angry about the consultation but agreed to participate. She complained to the psychiatrist that pain precluded intercourse with her boyfriend. In fact, the current pain had begun just when the relationship had become a sexual one.

The patient had worked off and on as a nurse for several years. She had also worked as a drug counselor. When the boyfriend was interviewed, it was learned that the patient herself had a history of abuse of barbiturates and narcotics. The family history disclosed that she had been raised by a cold, distant, and competitive mother who frequently criticized and humiliated her. The patient's father had raped her, according to her report, on 2 occasions when she was 12 and 13 years old. The patient felt guilty for perhaps having "unconsciously encouraged" her father's advances.

The consultant suggested psychotherapy and doubted that surgery would affect her pain complaints, since they seemed to serve an important psychologic function in relieving sexual guilt. Surgery was performed, however, and she did well until 6 days postoperatively, when she went into septic shock. One day prior to that event, the patient's boyfriend had brought in a diamond engagement ring for her. No cause was discovered for the patient's sepsis. Blood cultures yielded multiple organisms. In reviewing her earlier history of septic episodes and in exploring the similarity between the current episode of sepsis and the patient's previously reported episodes, the psychiatrist gently explored the possibility that she had played a role in the production of illness. After several sessions, she admitted she had injected urine intravenously because she felt guilty about her boyfriend being too nice to her. The patient was then referred for ongoing outpatient psychotherapy.

In psychotherapy, she revealed an extensive history of medical and surgical treatment for a variety of somatic complaints. She admitted that many of her symptoms were factitious but could not fully understand why she had committed the acts. Psychotherapy also revealed that the patient had numerous psychologic conflicts relating to her sexuality. She longed for a close sexual relationship with a man but felt guilty whenever the opportunity arose. This was directly linked to her interactions with her father. Encouraging her surgeons to operate was seen as an unconscious attempt to re-create her sexual relationship with her father, with the pain associated with surgery being her punishment. The sepsis was seen as a way of reducing guilt over the relationship with her boyfriend. This function had been performed by her pain symptoms upon admission. The injection of urine intravenously appeared to symbolize sexual penetration as well as an immediate punishment.

Admitting factitious illness and entering psychotherapy are unusual features of this case. It is not completely clear what allowed these features to develop, but the nonpunitive attitudes of the therapist and medical staff appeared to have been a major factor.

Epidemiology

Only a few studies have investigated the prevalence of factitious disease. Because of the nature of the disorder, factitious illness may be incorrectly diagnosed or not identified. The difficulty in identifying cases of factitious illness is even greater when the patient resorts to factitious symptoms rarely and intermittently. Factitious illness may also occur in patients who have documented organic illness, in which case diagnosis may be even more difficult. On the other hand, some individuals tend to be overreported in the medical literature as they go from hospital to hospital. Maur (1973) has reported one patient who had over 420 documented hospital admissions.

The best epidemiologic studies have been described in patients with fever of unknown origin. In a study at the National Institutes of Health, over 9% of such patients were diagnosed as having factitious fevers. A similar study at Stanford indicated factitious fever in 3% of such patients. It appears likely that factitious disorders are more often seen at tertiary-care centers where complex diagnostic problems are referred for evaluation.

This disorder appears to occur with equal frequency in men and women in some reports, but in several studies, females far outnumber males. In all studies, the health care field was the usual occupation of patients with factitious illness: nurses, ward clerks, physical therapists, x-ray technicians, and (less often) physicians. There are also a few reports of factitious disease occurring across generational boundaries; a mother of 2 children obtained the children's admissions by falsifying the results of the children's laboratory tests. Examples of "Munchausen's by proxy" appear to be extremely rare.

Etiology & Pathogenesis

The psychodynamic origin of adult factitious disorders is believed to lie in early childhood experiences. Emotional and sometimes physical deprivation in childhood is a common feature of the developmental history. The mother is often the major offender, with the father being passive or absent.

Early deprivation leads to a disturbance of self-image in these patients. Many authors have noted that patients with factitious disorders often have borderline personality characteristics. The borderline patient has a developmental difficulty during the separation-individuation (toddler) phase of childhood. When separation is not successfully achieved, the individual enters adult life with a poor self-image, feeling "needy" and dependent on others but expecting that needs will continue to be frustrated by authority figures.

The history often includes a period of hospitalization during early childhood when the patient's needs were met adequately by nurses and doctors who provided care and kindly ministrations. In other instances, a childhood hospitalization (and perhaps operation) was extremely frightening to a helpless and vulnerable toddler. Thus, childhood hospitalization may serve as a positive reinforcing experience or a major traumatic event. In still other instances, a patient's sense of vulnerability and helplessness is produced by the loss of a parent who was hospitalized.

The developmental history may uncover several major themes in a patient with factitious illness. The first involves the patient's sense of needing to be taken care of. The hospital provides a socially sanctioned way in which one can receive bodily ministrations and be an object of concern to symbolic parental figures, mainly doctors and nurses. Because of past experiences, however, the patient's desire to be taken care of is often accompanied by expectations of disappointment. Thus, these patients frequently present with a veneer of eager compliance over a hostile and wary underlying attitude.

Masochism is a second major theme. Anger over past deprivations often makes these individuals anxious and guilty. Such patients attempt to diminish guilt by being "punished" with invasive operations and diagnostic procedures. These painful interventions relieve guilt feelings while at the same time replaying early childhood experiences when the parents provided care as well as pain. Doctors and nurses thus represent parental figures of early childhood. Occasionally, these patients also develop positive feelings toward people in their lives, including their doctors and nurses. These positive feelings may have sexual features that cause just as much discomfort as their anger and hostility. Invasive and painful procedures may then serve to assuage feelings of guilt about positive responses as well as negative ones. Certain behaviors may then function as punishment for those feelings or as symbolic representation of the wishes involved with them. For example, a female patient who feels guilty about sexual arousal may invite a male physician to operate on her, an act that has both sexual and punitive symbolism.

A third major theme is mastery of an early trauma. Hospitalized children may feel extremely vulnerable. When repeating the experience as adults, they may hope to feel in control of the situation as they did not as children. This is sometimes what is happening when patients appear to be unconcerned about their clinical status while physicians feverishly perform diagnostic workups.

The patient with factitious illness may also utilize disease as a way of mastering a relationship with a parental figure. The feigned illness may provide retaliatory gratification. In effect, a patient can win victory over authority figures by showing that they are unable to control the symptoms. In accomplishing this, the patient ignores the fact that the victory is a Pyrrhic one. It is the patient who pays the price of disability and illness.

Patients with factitious illness commonly allow their fabrications and actions to be discovered. They may leave a syringe on the bedside table or let other patients see them performing their deceptive actions. By allowing themselves to be discovered, the patients show their contempt for the staff while at the same time provoking the staff to anger. The staff's first reaction may be to feel duped and deceived. When the staff does react angrily by confronting or immediately discharging the patient, the patient feels successful in having proved mistreatment by parental figures.

Treatment

Treatment is difficult, and there have been few reported successes. Treatment varies according to the level of enactment. The patient who occasionally simulates illness is more amenable to treatment than one who embarks on a career of illness and patienthood by creating actual disease states.

Treatment should begin with a psychiatric consultation after the factitious disorder has been identified by the primary physician. Two general approaches have been advocated. The primary physician may confront the patient in a nonpunitive manner: "We know you have been taking some anticoagulant medication, and we realize that you must be in great distress to have gone to such an extreme to get help. We'd like to help you learn different ways of dealing with your problems by having you meet with a psychiatrist." The psychiatrist is then brought in as the patient's ally rather than as a prosecuting attorney.

Some authors feel that patients who resort to chronic factitious illnesses are too fragile to survive confrontation, which would serve no other purpose than to humiliate patients and cause them to leave the hospital against medical advice. In such cases, a psychiatric consultant attempts to develop a supportive relationship with the patient without confrontation about the true origin of the feigned illness.

No matter which approach is used, the psychiatric consultant must allow the staff to ventilate their anger at having been deceived and duped by these patients. Since the physician treats the patient on the implicit foundation of honesty, it is natural for the physician to feel tricked when the factitious origin of the complaints is discovered. The psychiatric consultant can help inform the staff about the psychopathologic features of the patient's illness. This is important to keep the staff from acting out their anger. Operations and invasive diagnostic procedures should be avoided unless clearly indicated. If the staff does not act out of anger, the first step toward treating the patient has been accomplished—recognizing the factitious behavior as a psychopathologic symptom, not merely a hostile attack on the physician.

The patient may then be referred for inpatient or outpatient psychiatric management. It is usually well to involve the family, since valuable information can sometimes be obtained from family members. The family may also be helpful in setting behavioral limits once the patient leaves the hospital. Inpatient treatment provides a physically safe environment in which to explore pathologic patterns of behavior. Patients with factitious illness usually refuse inpatient treatment but may agree to outpatient psychotherapy. Some clinicians have suggested trials of antipsychotic agents or antidepressants, particularly when there is overt evidence of psychosis or depression, but there is no evidence that drugs are useful in uncomplicated factitious disorder. In any event, most factitious illness patients will resist psychotropic medications, so that treatment usually consists mostly of psychotherapy.

Management of this group of patients requires a skilled psychotherapist who is familiar with the disorder. Therapy is aimed at increasing the patient's autonomy and self-esteem while diminishing the sense of helplessness, vulnerability, and anger. When this is successful, the factitious symptoms become less and less useful until they are given up entirely.

FACTITIOUS DISORDER WITH PSYCHOLOGIC SYMPTOMS

Symptoms & Signs
(Table 40–3)

Patients with factitious disorder with psychologic symptoms often present with manifestations a lay person would regard as typical of psychiatric illness; there

---

Table 40–3. *DSM-III-R* diagnostic criteria for factitious disorder with psychologic symptoms.

A. Intentional production or feigning of psychologic (but not physical) symptoms.
B. A psychologic need to assume the sick role, as evidenced by the absence of external incentives for the behavior, such as economic gain, better care, or physical well-being.
C. Does not occur exclusively during the course of another axis I disorder, such as schizophrenia.

may be findings inconsistent with a specific disorder such as schizophrenia or affective illness. The term Ganser's syndrome ("balderdash syndrome") has been applied to some patients in this category. These patients give approximate answers to questions. For example, when asked what color snow is, such a patient will answer "red." Such answers indicate that the patient understood the meaning of the question. Patients with this disorder are often in situations of confinement, eg, in prison.

Patients with factitious psychiatric disorders may have some familiarity with psychiatric entities and present to psychiatric hospitals with plausible histories. The motive is the wish to assume the psychiatric patient's role. The unconscious motivations are similar to those of the patient with chronic factitious illness and physical symptoms. Gelenberg (1977) has described such a case. One difference when psychologic disorders are compared to physical ones is that verification of the diagnosis rests with the patient: Unless the patient admits falsifying the psychiatric history or there is conclusive psychologic diagnostic testing (requiring the patient's cooperation), it may be impossible to prove that the patient does not have a psychiatric disease. With factitious physical disorders, there is usually some objective evidence that does not rely on the patient's cooperation. The patient who feigns psychiatric factitious disorder often has a true psychiatric disorder (eg, borderline personality disorder) but not the one being feigned. It also appears that some patients can present with both factitious psychologic and factitious physical disorders at the same time or at different times.

Differential Diagnosis

The major differential diagnostic problem is malingering. Malingerers know their motivation, whereas the motivation for illness in patients with factitious disorder is unconscious and can only be arrived at by inference. Other differential diagnoses to be considered include brief reactive psychosis, schizophrenia, and organic psychosis. Occasionally, patients with borderline personality disorder may decompensate into psychosis for brief periods and may be difficult to differentiate from those with factitious disorder. The environmental context as well as an adequate history corroborated by family or friends usually clarifies the diagnosis.

Prognosis, Epidemiology, Etiology, & Treatment

Little is known about the incidence of factitious psychologic disorders. In one study (Pope and coworkers, 1982), 6.4% of patients admitted to a psychosis research ward were found to have factitious disorder. The causes, psychodynamics, and treatment are probably similar to those of patients with chronic factitious illnesses of a physical nature. Patients with factitious psychologic disorder typically come from emotionally depriving families. They are a bit closer to treatment, since they have presented themselves in a psychiatric setting to begin with. The only completed outcome study, however, suggests that patients with factitious psychologic disorders have a poorer prognosis than if they had a true major mental disorder. As Pope and coworkers (1982) have concluded, "It appears that acting crazy may bode more ill than being crazy." All of their patients had recurrent hospitalizations and poor social functioning.

Illustrative Case

A 40-year-old man presented to a psychiatric emergency service at a general hospital, complaining of severe depression. He described severe early morning awakening, loss of appetite, marked weight loss, and suicidal ideation. He was admitted to the inpatient psychiatric unit, where he told his attending psychiatrist that he had had similar episodes of depression in the past (in a distant state) that had responded to antidepressants and inpatient psychiatric treatment. He claimed he had no living relatives, that his wife had recently died of breast cancer, and that her death had precipitated the current episode of depression.

By chance, a new psychiatrist on the unit recognized the patient from another hospital in a nearby city. The psychiatrist told the staff that the patient was well known for feigning psychiatric illness. When not being observed by psychiatric staff, the patient showed no signs of clinical depression. The patient was known to have several brothers and sisters and had never been married. Confronted with this information, the patient's mood abruptly shifted from depression to defensive anger. He threatened litigation and signed out against medical advice. Since the patient was already receiving a disability pension, no apparent motivation for his behavior was determined during the hospitalization.

FACTITIOUS DISORDER WITH PHYSICAL & PSYCHOLOGIC SYMPTOMS

Merrin and coworkers have noted that some patients with factitious disorder display both physical and psychologic symptoms, either alternately or concurrently. Most commonly, these patients initially feign a physical disorder; when this is discovered, they then feign psychiatric symptoms. For example, a 34-year-old man was admitted to a coronary care unit to rule out myocardial infarction. When it became clear that he had had numerous similarly negative evaluations, he immediately claimed he was depressed because his wife and children had been killed in an automobile accident. Family members revealed that he had never been married. The treatment strategy for these individuals usually consists mostly of psychotherapy.

SUMMARY

Factitious disorders comprise a fascinating variety of self-destructive human behavior. The physician should regard such behavior as a sign of intrapsychic distress probably stemming from trauma or deprivation during childhood and should not react with anger or punitive rejection.

REFERENCES

Aduan RP et al: Factitious fever and self-induced infection. *Ann Intern Med* 1979;**90:**230.

Asher R: Munchausen's syndrome. *Lancet* 1951;**1:**339.

Bursten B: On Munchausen's syndrome. *Arch Gen Psychiatry* 1965;**13:**261.

Clarke E, Melnick SC: The Munchausen syndrome or the problem of hospital hoboes. *Am J Med* 1958;**25:**6.

Gavin H: *Feigned and Factitious Diseases.* Churchill, 1843.

Gelenberg AJ: Munchausen's syndrome with a psychiatric presentation. *Dis Nerv System* 1977;**38:**378.

Maur KV et al: Munchausen's syndrome: A thirty-year history of peregrination par excellence. *South Med J* 1973;**66:**629.

Merrin EL et al: Dual factitious disorder. *Gen Hosp Psychiatry* 1986;**8:**246.

Nadelson T: The Munchausen spectrum: Borderline character features. *Gen Hosp Psychiatry* 1979;**1:**11.

Perry JC, Klerman GL: Clinical features of the borderline personality disorder. *Am J Psychiatry* 1980;**137:**165.

Pope H, Jonas JM, Jones B: Factitious psychosis: Phenomenology, family history, and long-term outcome of nine patients. *Am J Psychiatry* 1982;**139:**1480.

Reich P, Gottfried LA: Factitious disorders in a teaching hospital. *Ann Intern Med* 1983;**99:**240.

Shafer N, Shafer R: Factitious diseases including Munchausen's syndrome. *NY State J Med* 1980;**80:**594.

Spiro H: Chronic factitious illness. *Arch Gen Psychiatry* 1968;**18:**569.

Mental Disorders of Childhood & Adolescence

41

Louis M. Flohr, MD, & Irving Philips, MD

The clinical manifestations and course of mental disorders of childhood and adolescence are varied. Many disorders discussed in the previous chapters first appear during childhood or adolescence and persist in adulthood. Other disorders are specific to childhood or adolescence; ie, they occur and resolve during this period. Because of the breadth of this field of study, it is not possible in a text such as this to review in detail each of the mental disorders suffered by children and teenagers. Therefore, a general approach to assessment is offered, and illustrative cases of disorders are presented with a review of essential features (symptoms, signs, and natural history). Comments on prognosis and treatment are made where appropriate.

The discussion of epidemiology in this chapter outlines special populations at higher risk of childhood mental disorders. Although these risk factors are suggestive of the etiology and pathogenesis of childhood mental disorders in general, the causes of the specific disorders are largely unknown. Many disorders are viewed as problems in psychosocial development (see Chapters 6 and 7). For disorders that also occur in adulthood (schizophrenic disorders, gender identity disorders, eating disorders), the reader is referred to earlier chapters for more detailed discussions of etiology, pathogenesis, and treatment. For more information on treatment, see Chapter 57.

EPIDEMIOLOGY

One-fourth of the United States population in 1983 (about 62 million people) were under the age of 18 years. Since the prevalence of psychiatric disorders in this population is estimated to be 10–15%, this means that at least 7 million children and adolescents were afflicted with psychiatric illness.

Groups at High Risk for Childhood Mental Disorders

According to the American Academy of Child Psychiatry (1983) and Steinhauer and Rae-Grant (1983), many young people with mental disorders come from the following high-risk groups:

A. Children From Low-Income Families: There are 10 million children from low-income families, and 16% live in poverty. Stressful living conditions contribute to childhood psychiatric problems, which often go unrecognized by parents struggling to provide for the family's physical needs. Economic restraints also keep low-income families from seeking health care.

B. Handicapped Children: Fewer than half of the 7 million handicapped children are considered adequately served by educational and rehabilitative programs. The incidence of emotional problems in disabled people is about 3 times that in the general population.

C. Foster Children: Over one-half million children live in foster care homes. Half of these children are subsequently moved to one or more other foster residences. While most professionals recognize that these children and their parents and foster parents need guidance and emotional support in adjusting to new living situations, special programs to provide such help where it is needed are almost nonexistent.

D. Institutionalized Mentally Retarded Children: The risk of psychiatric disorders is 3 times higher in mentally retarded children than in the general population. The risk is also higher in institutionalized than noninstitutionalized children. There are over 100,000 mentally retarded children in institutions—half of the population of such institutions.

E. Adolescents in Juvenile Dentention Facilities: Teenagers commit more than half of the serious crimes reported in the USA. On any given day, about 20,000 young people are detained by the United States juvenile court system for offenses ranging from joyriding to murder.

F. Children of High-Risk Mothers: Teenagers, pregnant women who abuse drugs or alcohol, and those who are malnourished tend to give birth to low-birth-weight and otherwise impaired infants. These infants are at risk for various central nervous system disorders and resultant learning and emotional problems. Pregnant young women are at high risk for emotional problems as well.

G. Single-Parent Children: About 9 million children (15% of all children) live in single-parent homes. In 40% of cases in which these children are 3 years of age or younger, the single parent works full-time. Of the single-parent families headed by a woman, 51.5% live below poverty level. These children and families are at added risk for emotional problems.

H. Children of Ethnic Minority Groups: Children in minority groups are more likely than those of the majority group to live in poverty and thus are at greater risk for both medical and psychiatric problems. There are about 12 million Mexican-American, black, Puerto Rican, and Native American children in the USA.

I. Children of Illegal Alien and Other Migrant Farm Workers: These children are at high risk for health problems of all types for a combination of reasons: poor housing, inadequate education, forced mobility, uncertain legal status, and their parents' low and unsteady incomes and long hours of exhausting work. Most of these children are underfed and medically neglected, and many are ineligible for publicly funded health and mental health services.

J. Children of Parents With Severe Psychiatric Disorders: Some mental illnesses have strong genetic components. The incidence of schizophrenia in children with one schizophrenic parent is almost 10%; when both parents are schizophrenic, it is 30–40%. More adult psychotic patients are living outside of institutions than in the past, and there has been an increased birth rate in this population. The genetic risk of mental illness, coupled with compromised parenting, places children of psychotic parents at even higher risk. Affective disorders also have a genetic component; however, these disorders are less severe and more readily treatable by current methods, so they represent a less alarming risk. Child abuse and alcoholism have both been shown to have a familial incidence.

K. Children With Chronic Physical Illness: About 5–20% of children have a chronic physical illness. With advances in medical technology that enable neonatologists to salvage more premature infants and severely ill children, the number of children with chronic congenital disorders may also increase. The incidence of developmental disorders and psychiatric problems in these children (and of emotional disturbances in their families) is higher than in the general population.

Other Correlates of Childhood Mental Disorders

A. Sex: The boy/girl ratio of mental disorders is 2–3:1. Conduct disorder, attention deficit disorder, schizophrenia, and autism are diagnosed with greater frequency in boys. Affective disorders occur equally in both sexes during childhood but are seen more often in girls during adolescence.

B. Age: Truancy, depressive episodes, bipolar affective disorder, schizophrenia, and suicide occur more frequently in adolescents than in children.

C. Socioeconomic Status: Low socioeconomic status is a characteristic of several of the high-risk groups outlined above. Rutter and colleagues (1976) studied childhood psychiatric disorders in populations from the middle-class Isle of Wight and a poor inner-city London borough and found that prevalence rates of all disorders were twice as high in the poor areas.

The disorders in children from poor areas had a greater tendency to begin in the early school years and run a chronic course. In their study in New York City, Langner and coworkers (1970) reported that the rates of mental impairment in children from high-, middle-, and low-income groups were 8%, 12%, and 21%, respectively.

D. School Influences: Studies by Rutter and Hersov (1977) confirmed that the type of secondary school a child attends makes a marked difference in academic achievement and in behavior. Children were extensively tested at age 10 to determine their presecondary school abilities and behavior characteristics. A comparison of these results with results during their secondary school careers demonstrated that certain schools, including some in the most economically disadvantaged areas, were more successful than others in promoting high academic achievement and reducing antisocial behavior, truancy, and dropout rates in their students. The significant variables appeared to be emphasis on an "academic atmosphere," student responsibility, and immediate rewards for effort.

THE DIAGNOSTIC PROCESS IN CHILD PSYCHIATRY

The evaluation of a child with emotional problems involves assessment of the child's family as well. As outlined in Table 41–1, a complete family history, including details of developmental, educational, emotional, and medical problems, should be elicited. The level of function is determined by psychologic, neurologic, and educational testing and by physical examination (see Chapters 18–20). Other special tests (eg, audiometry) may be indicated for children who exhibit speech and language problems or other defects in development.

Table 41–1. Outline for assessment and management of childhood and adolescent mental disorders.*

1. Identifying data (age, sex, source of referral, etc).
2. Chief complaint as indicated by the child, parents, and source of referral.
3. Patient's history and family history:
   a. Current and past emotional and educational problems.
   b. Current and past physical problems.
   c. Developmental milestones.
   d. Significant life events.
4. Assessment of the child (and family, if indicated):
   a. Physical examination.
   b. Mental status examination.
   c. Psychologic and educational testing.
   d. Other tests as indicated.
5. Assessment of other available data (medical and school records, etc).
6. Diagnosis and formulation of the problem (including provisional diagnosis and differential diagnosis).
7. Treatment plan.
8. Follow-up.

*See also Chapter 57.

Regardless of the duration of the diagnosis process—whether it be for a few visits or many—the clinician should try to establish a relationship with the child that fosters trust and self-expression. It is sometimes possible even in a time-limited relationship to judge the child's capacity for forming relationships and to determine what he or she is looking for in a relationship with an adult.

During the diagnostic process, the following questions are explored: What are the forces that shaped the child's and the family's development? How have they coped with problems in the past? What are the child's strengths? Where has development been blocked (eg, in learning, socialization, relationships with siblings or parents, self-image)? What can be done to facilitate the child's continuing development at an optimal pace?

In the remainder of this section, cases illustrating practical issues in evaluating children and their families will be presented and followed by discussions of these issues.

Illustrative Case No. 1

A. Problem for Assessment: Young child with school phobia (separation anxiety disorder).

B. Description: A 5-year-old boy who had been having tantrums and a "runny nose" every morning for 3 days was brought by his mother to the pediatric clinic, where he was first examined by a medical student. The patient had no fever or other signs of acute illness. The following developmental history was obtained: The boy was adopted at birth; developmental landmarks were normal; and immunizations were kept up to date. The parents were divorced 18 months before, and the father remarried a year later. The young boy spent every other weekend at his father's home with the father's new wife and 6- and 8-year-old stepdaughters.

The patient had started nursery school at age 4 and was now in kindergarten. Two weeks before the clinic visit, he began to be fearful about going to school. For the past 3 mornings, he had had tantrums and refused to board the school bus. His mother wondered whether this sudden change in behavior could be caused by a brain tumor or other serious medical problem, although she also realized that her divorce and later romantic involvement with another man might have something to do with the problem. In any case, she wanted a speedy resolution because she needed to return to her morning part-time job.

Since no abnormal results were found on physical and neurologic examination, the attending physician suggested (1) a telephone call to the kindergarten teacher; (2) one or more diagnostic playroom sessions with the child, allowing him to express his feelings through play; and (3) a meeting with both the father and the mother.

The findings were as follows: (1) The kindergarten teacher was puzzled by the change in her student and could not identify any reasons for it at school. (2) Although the patient left his mother reluctantly, in the playroom he became busily engaged in doll play. Among other things, he depicted a child being thrown out of the house and told, "This is not your house! Go find your own mommy!" (3) In the meeting with both parents, the father stated that his son's visits with him were viewed with some jealousy by his stepdaughters. When they discovered that the boy was adopted, they began to tease him about it, explaining to him that his "real mommy" gave him away. The parents agreed that the boy was probably worried that this would happen to him in subsequent visits. They decided to talk with him together several times at home and then report back to the clinic 2 weeks later. Upon their return visit, they related that their son was now satisfied that adoption meant he had a permanent home, and he was back in school again. He understood that his father moved out by his own free choice—not because of anything the child had done. Since the stepdaughters had been without a father for a long time and found it difficult not to tease their new brother when he visited, the parents decided to have him spend only one weekend a month at his father's home; during another weekend each month, the father would take him on an afternoon outing. At the 6-month follow-up visit, things were going fairly smoothly for the boy and his family.

C. Notes: This case demonstrates several points about childhood disorders and their assessment:

1. Primary-care health personnel are usually the first people to be asked for help by the distressed family. If they have adequate basic training in child development, primary-care physicians can often help families without referring them to specialists in child psychiatry.

2. When problems are clarified and family members begin actively communicating about them, resolution is often a natural result. In the above case, no advice was given by the practitioners. A plan of action grew out of the involvement of both parents in an attempt to understand their situation. There is always danger in giving premature advice: The advice may be "wrong" if given without complete understanding of the circumstances, as so often happens in rushed practice settings; and even if the advice is "right," there is little chance it will be accepted by parents who feel they have not been fully heard. In this boy's case, the parents were able to work out a solution after they understood the problem.

3. Children do not realize that they need psychologic help and thus do not ask for help directly. They usually present with a behavior problem (such as school phobia) that serves several purposes: It is momentarily adaptive because it helps them cope with immediate tensions (eg, staying home from school helped this boy control his fear of being locked out of the house), and it serves as a distress signal to alert adults to the problem.

4. In many cases, the child is not the only member of the family who needs help. The child's "cry for help" may in fact be an attempt to obtain help for or cope with problems of other members of the family—

eg, serious strife between parents or problems of a severely depressed parent or a disturbed older sibling. In the above case, the pediatrician's questions also brought out the serious lack of fathering suffered by the 2 girls in the father's new family.

5. Diagnostic playroom sessions facilitate the child's self-expression of the problem. Although only one session was needed to get an idea of this boy's fears, 3 or 4 sessions (at intervals of a few days to a week) are often necessary. A playroom separate from the examining room provides a relaxing atmosphere for the young child. If a separate room is not available, however, the following toys can be kept in the examining room to encourage self-expression by the child: dolls, a dollhouse with furniture, hand puppets, stuffed animals, toy guns, and crayons and paper. Children can tell remarkable stories in a brief time with this limited number of toys. For example, an 8-year-old depressed boy asked to draw a picture of "a family" produced a drawing of his father and mother with his younger sister between them; when asked where he was, he pointed to a small speck in the corner. (*Note:* It is better to ask a child to draw "a" family rather than "his or her" family, since children sometimes refuse to proceed when they feel confronted.) Children in playroom sessions should be told that they can play with all of the toys and say anything they want, but they cannot break objects or try to hurt themselves or the physician. Children with destructive impulses will test clinicians, sometimes repeatedly, to see if they mean what they say. Through their behavior, they are asking to be protected from these destructive impulses. The next case illustrates this point.

Illustrative Case No. 2

A. Problem for Assessment: Abused child with a conduct disorder of the undersocialized, aggressive type.

B. Description: A 7-year-old boy was physically abused and threatened with death or desertion by his severely disturbed mother. The court placed him in his grandparents' custody. In the second grade, he rapidly caught up to the academic level of achievement of his classmates; however, outside the structured classroom, his behavior was poor. He was not allowed in the school lunchroom during lunch hour because he provoked fights. His grandparents, both in their 60s, had their hands full and sought help with the child.

While in the clinic, the boy ran from the waiting room to the secretary's office and asked the secretary if he could kiss her. He seemed relieved when she refused. He held the doctor's hand on the way to his office and then ran over to the desk and swept some books and papers to the floor. The doctor, catching up with him, said, "Let's sit down and calm down. Then when you're ready we'll put things back on the table." While they were talking, the boy started to kick the doctor's leg, at first gently, then with increasing force. The doctor indicated to the patient that he was going to hold him so that he would not be able to hurt the doctor

or himself. He sat the boy on his lap and wrapped his legs around the boy's kicking feet while continuing to hold his hands. The patient settled down and began a stream of fantasy talk about situations he might encounter and violent ways in which he would defend himself. He included examples of how he could defend against the doctor, from whom he obviously expected violent retaliation. After about 5 minutes of this, the boy fell silent. The following discussion then ensued. *Patient:* "Aren't you going to do anything?" *Physician:* "Like what?" *Patient:* "Punish me!" *Physician:* "I'd rather have you fix the table with me, when you're ready." *Patient:* "I'm ready now." They put things back on the desk, and the child looked pleased.

During the next 3 visits, the boy acted out violent scenes with dolls and hand puppets. He got so wound up that 2 or 3 times he asked the doctor to hold him "until I'm ready to go on."

C. Notes: The physician should always be ready to prevent destructive or harmful actions. In this case, the physician's actions also prevented his becoming angry at the child. The gentle yet firm holding told the boy (as words never could) that he could safely speak "horrible thoughts" but that he would not be allowed to make himself feel guilty by engaging in destructive behavior. This enabled the physician to introduce the idea of the boy's making restitution ("fixing up the table") rather than suffering retribution from an angry adult. The cycle of destructive behavior and consequent self-blame for displeasing the adult was thereby avoided.

Illustrative Case No. 3

A. Problem for Assessment: Adolescent with physical concerns and emotional problems.

B. Description: A 15-year-old boy was in the 11th month of his 1-year probationary period for joyriding. As a condition of probation, he was regularly seeing a child psychiatrist. On this particular afternoon, he turned up at the pediatric clinic and asked to be examined for venereal disease. He wanted assurances that his visit would be kept confidential from his mother and psychiatrist. During his examination, he mentioned to the pediatrician that his probation would soon be over and then he could stop seeing his "shrink." As he said this, there was something in his voice that prompted the pediatrician to ask him, "And then what?" The adolescent replied, "Oh, I'll probably go back to the same gang and have some more fun." Thus alerted, the pediatrician asked more about the patient's life. He found out that he was living with his widowed mother and that his father had died 3 months before the joyriding incident. His psychiatrist was currently on a 2-week vacation, and the patient appeared to be fearful of ending his therapy. The following conversation ensued. *Physician:* "Do you want to know what I think? My guess is that it's tough for you to tell your psychiatrist that seeing him is useful and that you feel funny about quitting." *Patient:* "Well, he's only seeing me because the judge made me go." *Physician:* "Is that what he told you, or is that your idea?" *Patient:*

"My idea." *Physician:* "Why not ask him?" *Patient:* "Well, maybe."

The adolescent then hesitantly agreed to discuss his concerns about ending therapy with the psychiatrist; he was not ready to ask for his mother's help about anything. The conversation continued. *Physician:* "Before I examined you today, I agreed that your visit here would be confidential. But I think what we need is limited confidentiality . . . . I want your permission to call both your psychiatrist and your mother so I can recommend that you continue therapy even without being on probation. We don't have to tell them you came here because you were afraid you had VD." *Patient:* "That sounds OK to me."

C. Notes: Communication with adolescents requires sensitivity to their mixed sense of dependence and wish for independence. They may deny needing help, actively reject help, or seek help indirectly from their parents or other adults. Concerns about confidentiality are linked to their ideas of privacy and independence of thought and action. In this case, the pediatrician's unhurried manner and sensitivity allowed the adolescent boy, who had real doubts about his own effectiveness, to ask for backup help from a respected adult. By careful listening and questioning, the physician was also able to determine what the patient really wanted to remain confidential and what he wanted someone to communicate to his mother and psychiatrist. The physician did not confront the patient ("You just want me to do your talking for you. Why don't you take the responsibility for yourself?") but instead proceeded on the assumption that the boy would not be indirectly asking for help if he could handle his predicament alone. Although the patient came for only a "medical" checkup, the pediatrician felt free to ask questions about other areas of the adolescent's life. Most patients expect physicians to ask questions (ie, they consider it to be an expression of professional concern rather than prying), and adolescents in particular rely on their physicians to help them discover or express their real concerns.

CHILDHOOD PSYCHOPATHOLOGY

Most of the mental disorders of childhood and adolescence are viewed by child psychiatrists from a developmental perspective. Certain disorders are thought to arise from unresolved psychologic or family conflicts or unmastered tasks during specific stages in the process of growth and development, while others would result from the complex interplay of biologic and environmental forces. Some disorders (eg, autism in infancy) result in lifelong impairment, while others may be characteristic only of a particular period (eg, identity crisis of adolescence). Chapters 6 and 7 review normal human development. A developmental perspective on psychopathology does not permit us to describe and categorize all of the mental disorders seen in children and adolescents. Thus, a broader classification system, employing both the descriptive criteria outlined in *DSM-III* (1980) and *DSM-III-R* (1987) and the developmental categories outlined by the Group for the Advancement of Psychiatry (GAP, 1984), is used in this section.

Examples of typical cases seen in medical and psychiatric office practice illustrate the essential features of specific disorders. For the sake of clarity of organization, these are presented approximately in order of increasing severity, following the outline proposed by GAP in *Psychopathological Disorders in Childhood.* Examples will include the *DSM-III-R* diagnostic classification.

ADAPTIVE RESPONSES

Adaptive responses are the temporary and moderate behavioral changes seen in normal children responding to the forms of stress associated with normal growth and development. A clinician evaluating a child's behavior should always consider whether the child is exhibiting age-appropriate adaptive responses to stress. If this is the case, treatment is rarely required. Examples of adaptive responses are the **temporary regressions** of young children (eg, increased thumb-sucking at the time of weaning); the **stranger anxiety** of infants 6–12 months old ("8-month anxiety" was once a popular term); the **separation anxiety** of the toddler; the **"normal phobias"** of preschool children; the **compulsive ritualistic behaviors** of school-age children learning to work by rules and attempting to master earlier anxieties; and the **identity crisis of adolescence,** well within the reach of our adult recollections. Since adaptive responses are not considered disorders, there are no *DSM-III* classifications. Disconcerted parents of children with such problems usually respond well to an educational approach based on adequate assessment of the child's behavior in relation to his or her stage of development.

Illustrative Case No. 4

A. Diagnosis: Stranger anxiety as an adaptive response.

B. Description: A navy lieutenant and his wife consulted the pediatrician at the base hospital. The officer, who had just returned from a 3-month tour of duty, was concerned that his 9-month-old son acted frightened and cried whenever he approached him. This made the father feel unwelcome and rejected, and he wondered if there was something wrong with the child. The pediatrician explained to the parents that stranger anxiety was a natural response in the child's current stage of development; if the father had left for a similar period before or after this stage of development, the child's natural reaction would have been considerably less intense. The parents were relieved to hear this. On follow-up 2 weeks later, the parents reported a warming relationship between father and son.

Illustrative Case No. 5

A. Diagnosis: Separation anxiety as an adaptive response.

B. Description: A 2½-year-old girl "fussed" and cried each time her parents left her with a baby-sitter for the evening. Shortly after they left, she settled down and played well with the baby-sitter, who was an old friend of the family.

Illustrative Case No. 6

A. Diagnosis: "Normal phobias."

B. Description: Between 2 and 4 years of age, a boy developed fears of the dark basement, spider webs, bees, and the letter carrier. The parents noted that he was able to be comforted, and each of these fears passed within a few months.

Illustrative Case No. 7

A. Diagnosis: Adaptive responses in an adolescent identity crisis.

B. Description: At age 12, a girl began questioning her parents' way of looking at the world. She would argue with them about values and religion, burst into tears, and then go to her room. She criticized her parents' way of dressing and felt uncomfortable being seen in public with them. At the age of 14, the girl joined the fan club of a popular rock group. She was "in love" with the group's lead guitarist and cherished the autographed photo she received from him in response to her fervent love letter. She attended the band's concerts and enjoyed the sense of belonging she got from fan club activities. Her interest waned by age 16, and she said she found it hard to believe that she could have spent so much time on that "kid stuff." She began dating about this time and started to cautiously discuss some of her experiences with her mother.

C. Notes: During early adolescence, children need to question their identity and the family identity they have taken for granted throughout childhood. This is a natural but painful process, and temporarily belonging to a peer group can to some extent ease the anxiety caused by growing away from the family. As so many adolescents do, the girl in the above case practiced "being in love" with an unattainable distant figure until she was ready to begin dating. For details on adolescent identity formation, see Erikson's classic description in Chapter 7.

REACTIVE DISORDERS

Reactive disorders in children or adolescents are characterized by significant changes in mood or behavior or by the presence of physical symptoms and signs that occur in response to external stress. Although children may be consciously aware of both the distress and the external event causing it, their ability to express awareness is limited by their stage of cognitive development. *DSM-III* does not use the term "reactive disorders," but several disorders described in *DSM-III* as "adjustment disorders" fall into this category, as shown in the cases that follow.

Illustrative Case No. 8

A. Diagnosis:

1. GAP–Reactive depression.

2. DSM-III-R–Adjustment disorder with depressed mood.

B. Description: An 18-month-old girl was placed in her aunt's home for 2 weeks while her mother was hospitalized for surgery and her father was working out of town. The child's initial reaction to separation from her mother was a dramatic show of protest—several hours of crying and refusal to be picked up or comforted. This gave way to a phase of despair, characterized by exhaustion, extreme sadness, refusal to eat solids, and restlessness throughout the night. About 36 hours after her arrival at the aunt's house, she became more withdrawn and detached, showed little interest in people or toys, had a relatively expressionless face, and made almost no attempts at spontaneous communication. She sucked her thumb most of the day and rocked herself to sleep. The child brightened up after the fifth day, when her aunt brought her an old scarf that belonged to her mother. She clung to the scarf for the remainder of her 2-week stay, chewing and sucking on it as she went to sleep. The child at first seemed not to recognize her mother when she came to pick her up. Then she began to follow her mother around everywhere when they got home. She clung to her mother during the next 3 months and showed severe anxiety when her mother even mentioned going to the store.

C. Notes: This case illustrates the successive phases of protest, despair, detachment, and clinging. Although the phases of protest and despair appear brief from an adult perspective, a few days of desperation may seem very long to an infant, whose sense of time and urgency is vastly different from that of the older child or adult. Similar reactions occur when children are hospitalized. Problems may be prevented or alleviated by an increased number of parental visits and early recognition of reactive depression by hospital personnel. The parents should be cautioned not to react with rejection, anger, or guilt in response to the child's temporarily increased clinging, since this may serve to prolong or exacerbate the problem.

Adjustment disorders are discussed in Chapter 35.

Illustrative Case No. 9

A. Diagnosis:

1. GAP–Reactive depression with psychophysiologic concomitants.

2. DSM-III-R–Axis I, adjustment disorder with depressed mood; functional encopresis. Axis III, insulin-dependent diabetes mellitus.

B. Description: A 7-year-old boy had been aware of his parents' deteriorating marriage for about a year when he was told they were planning a divorce. Within a week, he had to be hospitalized to regain control of his insulin-dependent diabetes mellitus. While in the hospital, the boy began to show changes in mood and behavior. He cried and asked for his father at night, and he began to soil himself regularly, despite having been fully toilet trained since age 3 years. Because the encopresis continued, his parents consulted a child psychiatrist.

C. Notes: This boy's depression was manifested in multiple ways: (1) a psychophysiologic reaction, ie, the diabetes was exacerbated by emotional stress; (2) adjustment problems with depressive mood changes (see Chapter 35); and (3) regressive soiling. *DSM-III-R* diagnostic criteria for functional encopresis are set forth in Table 41–2.

DEVELOPMENTAL DEVIATIONS

This category includes lags, unevenness, and precocities in development—ie, the degree of maturation is not what is expected for a given age or stage of development. Developmental deviations are not necessarily of a fixed nature. They may resolve with the passage of time or be corrected with help from parents or others. The psychologic reaction of the child and others to the deviation may also influence the degree of impairment, as shown in some of the cases below. Sometimes the developmental deviation represents the premonitory stage of a specific long-term disorder that can be differentiated only on follow-up. Biologic factors are thought to contribute to many developmental deviations, particularly the specific developmental disorders listed in Table 41–3.

Illustrative Case No. 10

A. Diagnosis:

1. GAP–Delayed mastery of separation from the mother.

2. *DSM-III-R*–Axis I, separation anxiety disorder.

B. Description: A 6-year-old boy in the first grade began to whine and cling to his mother in the mornings before school. This behavior increased, and eventually he cried bitterly every morning and begged to be allowed to stay home from school. Since his mother had no close friends and was ambivalent about sending him off for an entire school day, the behavior was reinforced. The father, who had to leave home early each morning for work, was unable to help his wife see the child off to school.

Table 41–2. *DSM-III-R* diagnostic criteria for functional encopresis.

A. Repeated passage of feces into places not appropriate for that purpose (eg, clothing, floor), whether voluntary or involuntary. (The disorder may be overflow incontinence secondary to functional fecal retention.)
B. At least one such event a month for at least 6 months.
C. Chronologic and mental age of at least 4 years.
D. Not due to a physical disorder, such as aganglionic megacolon.

Table 41–3. *DSM-III-R* list of the specific developmental disorders (coded on axis II).

Academic skills disorders:
  Developmental arithmetic disorder
  Developmental expressive writing disorder
  Developmental reading disorder
Language and speech disorders:
  Developmental articulation disorder
  Developmental expressive language disorder
  Developmental receptive language disorder
  Cluttering
  Stuttering
Motor skills disorder:
  Developmental coordination disorder
Specific developmental disorder not otherwise specified
Developmental disorder not otherwise specified

C. Notes: *DSM-III-R* diagnostic criteria for separation anxiety disorder are outlined in Table 41–4.

Illustrative Case No. 11

A. Diagnosis:

1. GAP–Delayed toilet training.

2. *DSM-III-R*–Axis I, functional enuresis.

B. Description: A 6-year-old boy was brought to the clinic by his mother when the first-grade teacher

Table 41–4. *DSM-III-R* diagnostic criteria for separation anxiety disorder.

A. Excessive anxiety concerning separation from those to whom the child is attached, as evidenced by at least 3 of the following:
  (1) Unrealistic and persistent worry about possible harm befalling major attachment figures or fear that they will leave and not return.
  (2) Unrealistic and persistent worry that an untoward calamitous event will separate the child from a major attachment figure, eg, the child will be lost, kidnapped, killed, or be the victim of an accident.
  (3) Persistent reluctance or refusal to go to school in order to stay with major attachment figures or at home.
  (4) Persistent reluctance or refusal to go to sleep without being near a major attachment figure or to go to sleep away from home.
  (5) Persistent avoidance of being alone, including "clinging" to and "shadowing" major attachment figures.
  (6) Repeated nightmares involving the theme of separation.
  (7) Complaints of physical symptoms, eg, headaches, stomachaches, nausea, or vomiting, on many school days or on other occasions when anticipating separation from major attachment figures.
  (8) Recurrent signs or complaints of excessive distress in anticipation of separation from home or major attachment figures, eg, temper tantrums or crying, pleading with parents not to leave.
  (9) Recurrent signs of complaints of excessive distress when separated from home or major attachment figures, eg, wants to return home, needs to call parents when they are absent or when child is away from home.
B. Duration of disturbance of at least 2 weeks.
C. Onset before the age of 18.
D. Does not occur exclusively during the course of a pervasive developmental disorder, schizophrenia, or any other psychotic disorder.

urged her to find help for his lack of bladder control, which was making him an outcast in his class. The mother was only mildly disturbed by her son's primary enuresis, since her brother also had had occasional episodes of wetting until he was 8 years old.

C. Notes: See Table 41–5 for *DSM-III-R* criteria for functional enuresis.

Illustrative Case No. 12

A. Diagnosis:

1. GAP–Developmental deviation due to specific sensory deficit.

2. *DSM-III-R* – Axis I, adjustment disorder with depressed mood. Axis III, sensorineural deafness.

B. Description: An 8-year-old boy with congenital deafness and behavioral problems was brought to the pediatric clinic for evaluation. The sensorineural hearing loss was caused by maternal rubella infection during pregnancy. Although the child's deafness was suspected by his grandmother when he was 10 months old, diagnostic uncertainty and the parents' unrelenting search for a "cure" delayed a definitive diagnosis of deafness until age 4. He was then enrolled for the next 4 years in a school that used only "oralist" methods; the focus was on speech training and utilization of residual hearing with hearing aids. Since the boy was not allowed to use his meager repertoire of gestures to communicate and since he could hear almost nothing with a hearing aid, he did not benefit from the intensive program. He became more and more unhappy, frustrated, and anxious. Finally, at age 8, he began "skipping school." On 2 occasions, highway patrol officers found the boy walking alone at night. After thorough psychiatric, educational, audiologic, and psychologic evaluations (all done by professionals trained to use both sign language and speech with deaf children), the parents were advised to enroll the boy in a class that used "total communication" (both speech and sign language) and to learn sign language themselves. Six months later, his parents reported their pleasure at being able to communicate in simple sentences with him. His behavior problems subsided as he began to learn in school and found more satisfaction in communicating with his family.

PSYCHONEUROTIC DISORDERS

Psychoneurotic disorders originate from unconscious conflicts over the handling of sexual and ag-

Table 41–5. *DSM-III-R* diagnostic criteria for functional enuresis.

A. Repeated voiding of urine during the day or night into bed or clothes, whether involuntary or intentional.
B. At least 2 such events per month for children between the ages of 5 and 6 and at least one event per month for older children.
C. Chronologic age at least 5 and mental age at least 4.
D. Not due to a physical disorder, such as diabetes, urinary tract infection, or a seizure disorder.

---

gressive impulses. Although these conflicts are removed from awareness by repression, they remain active and unresolved. This aspect of psychoneurotic disorders distinguishes them from reactive disorders, in which children consciously experience a conflict between the environment and their own needs. Widespread personality disorganization is not seen in psychoneurotic disorders, although the symptoms can be dramatic, cause serious inconvenience, or markedly interfere with functioning. The patient usually functions adequately in other areas of life and finds the symptoms troublesome ("ego-dystonic").

Illustrative Case No. 13

A. Diagnosis:

1. GAP–Dissociative-type neurosis.

2. *DSM-III-R* – Axis I, psychogenic fugue.

B. Description: A 15-year-old girl disappeared from boarding school and was found 2 weeks later in a cheap hotel in a distant city. She did not know how she got to the hotel and did not remember anything about the previous 2 weeks. Another roomer at the hotel reported that the girl had been calling herself "Tootsie" and working as a prostitute. The history revealed that the girl was born when her mother was 16 and unmarried. She had never known her father. When she was 3 years old, her mother married an older man who adhered to strict fundamentalist Christian doctrine. Under his harsh discipline, the mother became a devout churchgoer. The girl and her younger sister were enrolled in a religious boarding school, where sexuality was mentioned only as an occasion of sin followed by divine retribution.

C. Notes: Psychogenic fugue is discussed in Chapter 33.

Illustrative Case No. 14

A. Diagnosis:

1. GAP–Obsessive compulsive neurosis.

2. *DSM-III-R* – Axis I, obsessive compulsive disorder. Axis II, compulsive personality traits.

B. Description: A 10-year-old girl developed a hand-washing ritual after her mother returned home from hospitalization for surgery. By the time she was brought to treatment, the girl was spending 2–3 hours a day washing her hands. During the interview, she was anxious but lucid and relatively cooperative, and it was clear that she wanted to be rid of her washing compulsion. The history revealed that the mother started toilet training the girl at age 10 months. The mother remembered feeling that she was in "competition" with her own sister, whose child was toilet trained by 14 months. The mother often used the threat of abandonment as a coercive measure during the toilet-training process. Similar psychologic pressure tactics were used during the early school years. The girl was expected to perform well socially and academically and thus became overly meticulous.

C. Notes: See Chapters 31 and 36 for discussions of obsessive compulsive disorders and personality types.

Illustrative Case No. 15

A. Diagnosis:

1. **GAP**—Phobic neurosis.

2. **DSM-III-R**—Axis I, panic disorder with agoraphobia.

B. Description: Within a 2-week period, a 7-year-old boy developed an incapacitating fear of going outdoors. Initially, he could go for rides in the family car if he ran from the house straight to the car. Eventually, he was unable to leave the house at all without severe anxiety. Cajoling, bribes, and force did not help. Psychiatric evaluation, performed in the home, revealed a cooperative and intelligent boy who was fully aware of his problem and wanted to be free of it.

C. Notes: Panic disorder with agoraphobia is discussed in Chapter 31.

Illustrative Case No. 16

A. Diagnosis:

1. **GAP**—Depressive neurosis.

2. **DSM-III-R**—Axis I, dysthymia.

B. Description: A 14-year-old girl was referred by the school principal to the child psychiatrist because of "skipping school, telling fantastic tales she appeared to believe, and behaving immaturely." She was a thin child who dressed and looked like a 10-year-old and showed no interest in dating. During the initial interview, she dropped candy wrappers all around her and behaved in a childish manner, yet she responded readily to reminders to pick up after herself. This history revealed that she was the oldest of 5 children born to a chronically depressed mother who had recently gone through a second divorce. The girl was the mother's chief helper in caring for her 1-year-old half brother, who preferred her to his mother.

In a joint interview, the girl and her mother described themselves and each other as having a tendency to giggle without reason and expressed concern that they might become "crazy, like grandmother." When interviewed alone, the girl was more somber and more willing to talk. She said her mother frequently announced that she was "fed up with housework" and threatened to leave the family. She invariably found herself taking care of the baby and the younger children while her mother stayed in bed in a depressed mood. During the past year (since the baby's birth), the mother's threats to leave had been more frequent, and the 14-year-old girl had been returning home from school worried that her mother might be gone. She described herself as often sad and worried about her mother's threats of leaving and about becoming "crazy" like her grandmother, who had left her own children. Throughout all this, she was unaware of any angry feelings in herself.

C. Notes: See also Chapter 30.

AFFECTIVE DISORDERS

DSM-III-R indicates that the mood (affective) disorders of childhood and adolescence have the same *es-*sential features as affective disorders in adults (see Chapter 30). For major depressive episode and dysthymia the *DSM-III-R* criteria include age-specific *associated* features found in children and adolescents. The predominant feature (presenting symptom) of depression in young children may be anxiety, while that in adolescents may be antisocial behavior. Suicidal ideation or suicidal behavior may be noted. The description of manic episode does not include age-specific associated features in children (reflecting the extremely low frequency of that diagnosis in childhood), but diagnosis can be used for children, of course, when it applies. Treatment of affective disorders usually includes psychotherapy and drug therapy—antidepressant medications for depression and lithium carbonate or antipsychotics for mania (see Chapters 52 and 53).

Illustrative Case No. 17

A. DSM-III-R Classification: Axis I, major depression, single episode.

B. Description: A 5-year-old girl's mother was admitted to a psychiatric hospital for the third time in less than a year. During the 2 previous hospitalizations, which lasted only 2–3 days, the mother's sister came to the home to care for the little girl. The third hospitalization was expected to last longer, so the girl was taken to the aunt's home. Beginning about a week after her mother's hospitalization, the girl became progressively more apathetic. She lost her appetite and desire to play and would sit in a corner for long periods, holding her doll and ignoring her aunt and uncle when they tried to interest her in food or play. She also slept more than usual. After 2 weeks of such behavior, the aunt took the child to her regular pediatrician. He noted that she had lost 3 lb and suspected a diagnosis of depression. She was referred to a child psychiatrist, who confirmed the diagnosis and treated her for major depression.

C. Notes: *DSM-III-R* diagnostic criteria for major depressive episode are listed in Table 30–1.

Illustrative Case No. 18

A. DSM-III-R Classification: Axis I, major depression, single episode.

B. Description: A 15-year-old boy was brought to the hospital emergency room by his mother and a classmate. He and his classmate had made a suicide pact, and the patient had fulfilled his part by trying to hang himself, as the rope burn on his neck attested. His frightened friend cut the rope and called the boy's mother.

When interviewed alone, the patient said he had been preoccupied for over a year with fears of becoming a homosexual, and he felt that he was "losing the battle against it." His mother remembered having noticed changes in her son's mood starting about a year before, but she and her husband tried to ignore his bad moods and "concentrate on the positive" (ie, enjoy his brief periods of being in a better mood). Behavioral changes they noted included the son's tendency to watch television late into the night; his "sitting and staring at his books" but falling behind in school work; and angry outbursts toward his parents, usually when he felt he was being "slighted" and his sister "favored." Yet because he managed to get by both in school and at home, he was able to hide his despair from caring adults. Psychiatric evaluation revealed major depression and no formal thought disorder.

C. Notes: In this case, early symptoms of depression were overt, but their severity was not detected by the parents. Although suicidal intent was discussed by the boy with his peers, there was no overtly suicidal or self-destructive behavior prior to the hanging incident. This is in contrast to the potentially self-destructive actions frequently seen in "masked" depression of childhood and adolescence (see below).

Illustrative Case No. 19

A. Diagnosis: "Masked" depression.

B. Description: A teenage girl was about to be dismissed from the third school in the past 2 years. Unless closely supervised, she skipped school whenever possible, got into mischief with friends, and was considered a "chronic liar." This time she had set a small fire at school.

The history revealed that her mother had had pulmonary edema during pregnancy and had developed acute renal failure while in labor for 72 hours. The girl had been delivered by emergency cesarean section, and her mother had suffered from chronic renal disease since that time. A kidney transplant had been rejected, and the mother's health continued to deteriorate while she was receiving hemodialysis. The responsibilities for child care were assumed by the father, who already had his hands full with his wife's medical care. The girl realized he was doing his best and frequently told him, "Don't blame my problems on Mom's illness."

By the time of the second interview, the school administrators had made their decision to expel the girl. She was then enrolled in a psychiatric day treatment program for adolescents, where she received individual, group, and milieu therapy in addition to a complete educational program. Her parents also began therapy. The mother was able to openly express feelings of sadness and anger, since this "weakness" could be attributed to her illness. However, the father and daughter had tried to be "strong" and had not openly expressed their feelings for 14 years, so it took them about 3 months in therapy before they could let down their guard enough to cry together. They eventually came to realize that expressions of sadness were not a sign of weakness. When the girl could admit to her feelings and express them openly, she no longer resorted to acting-out behavior. She continued outpatient therapy for another year "to make sure I don't skip anything important," and she kept the therapist's card for future reference "because I can't be sure how my mother's death will affect me."

C. Notes: While masked depression is not a diagnostic term recognized by GAP or *DSM-III*, it has clear utility in child psychiatry. Young people with masked depression protect themselves against the pain of their feelings by acting out in what sometimes appears to be a self-destructive or delinquent manner. This behavior is described as "pseudodelinquent" because it is secondary to depression and not part of an ingrained personality disturbance.

Illustrative Case No. 20

A. *DSM-III-R* Classification: Axis I, dysthymia.

B. Description: A 12-year-old boy was brought for evaluation by his mother, who was concerned about distinct changes in the boy's mood and behavior during the past 14 months. Until then, the boy had been easygoing and lovable and had gladly helped around the house. His attitude and behavior started to change about a month after his mother separated from her husband. He began by openly protesting and pleading against his parents' impending divorce. When he was unable to prevent the breakup, he became weepy for a few weeks and then turned surly and withdrawn. He was easily angered by his mother and was fearful and avoidant of his father, who was beginning to think that his wife was turning his son against him. Although the boy had been getting good grades, his school performance was deteriorating rapidly. During his first psychiatric interview, he admitted to fantasies of suicide.

C. Notes: For other examples of dysthymia, see illustrative cases 16 and 35. Table 30–1 outlines *DSM-III-R* criteria for dysthymia.

SUICIDAL IDEATION & BEHAVIOR

Depressed children often express suicidal thoughts, either consciously (verbally) or unconsciously (on projective testing). Although suicidal thoughts are reported frequently, especially in hospitalized children, suicidal behavior in children under age 12 is extremely rare. It is more common after that age, and suicide is one of the major causes of death in adolescents. Suicidal gestures (superficial attempts) are made more frequently by girls than by boys, whereas true suicide attempts are made more frequently by boys. Although the majority of suicidal adolescents are depressed, only about 25% of them meet the *DSM-III* diagnostic criteria for depressive illness; thus, the diagnosis of masked depression is useful for this age group.

PSYCHOTIC DISORDERS & PERVASIVE DEVELOPMENTAL DISORDERS

The child and adolescent section of *DSM-III-R* does not include classifications for schizophrenic disorders or other psychotic disorders. The various terms used to describe these disorders in children (eg, atypical ego development, childhood schizophrenia, infantile autism, disintegrative psychoses) caused much debate in the past, and these disorders are now categorized by *DSM-III-R* as pervasive developmental disorders. Those few preadolescents and the larger number of adolescents who develop full-blown adultlike schizophrenic disorders (with hallucinations, delusions, or both) are diagnosed on the basis of *DSM-III-R* criteria for adults. Table 41–6 outlines the newly proposed classification of developmental disorders (which include pervasive developmental disorders).

Psychotic disorders in individuals of all ages produce a widespread disorganization of the personality, with loss of reality testing and ego functions. When they occur in children, they result in pervasive deviations from the behavior expected for the child's age. Findings may include aloofness and inability to develop emotional relationships with others; preoccupation with inanimate objects; speech impairment, delay, absence, or loss (depending on age at onset); disturbances in sensory perception; bizarre or stereotyped behavior and movement patterns; marked resistance to change in environment or routine; unpredictable temper outbursts; panic attacks; seeming absence of a sense of personal identity; and blunted, uneven, or fragmented intellectual development. In some cases, intellectual function is unimpaired, with the disorder confined to areas of personality function.

The following 2 sections describe and discuss psychotic disturbances at different levels of development.

1. AUTISTIC DISORDER

Extensive efforts to date at phenomenologic description and involving neurophysiologic, biochemical, and psychodynamic research have not yielded easily distinguishable subgroups of the severe chronic psychoses of childhood currently subsumed under the heading of Pervasive Developmental Disorders (Rutter, 1985). The proposed classification shown in Table 41–7 reflects the variety of severe deviations that affect all areas of development. It is an operational classification, using descriptive terminology of observable events that should facilitate future research into this group of catastrophic illnesses.

Although the full-blown picture of autism may not appear until $2\frac{1}{2}$ or 3 years of age, a detailed developmental history usually reveals that characteristic signs developed during the first year of life, such as absence of social smiling at the parent, lack of anticipatory posture on being picked up, or lack of bodily molding when being held by the parent. The classic picture of infantile autism was first described by Leo Kanner in 1943 (see reference for Kanner, 1973). Current descriptions of autism include the following features: (1) onset before 30 months of age; (2) a state of self-absorbed aloneness (lack of affective contact with people) characterized by avoidance of eye contact, disinterest in complying with requests or pleasing adults, and lack of attachment to the mother; (3) a strong need for maintaining routines, with panic or tantrums when routines are interrupted; (4) delayed, absent, or noncommunicative speech; (5) sleeping and feeding problems, which may be severe; (6) stereotyped, repetitive, or bizarre motor patterns; and (7) in some cases, deviations in intellectual development, eg, limited or uneven development in one or more areas, often compromised by the child's impaired contact with reality.

Illustrative Case No. 21

A. *DSM-III-R* Classification: Axis I, autistic disorder, infantile onset (tentative diagnosis).

B. Description: A 2½-year-old boy who had never spoken a word or tried to communicate verbally was brought to the pediatric clinic for evaluation. The parents thought the child might be deaf, mute, or mentally retarded and were concerned about his eyesight as well.

During the examination, lack of eye contact with all adults was noted. The parents reported that the child was preoccupied with watching spinning objects and spent many hours watching his own hand movements in the air. His behavior in the examination room indicated that he could visually discriminate small objects, such as a piece of candy on a nearby table and the light switch on the far wall of the room. He ran to turn the switch on and off every time he could.

The developmental history and observation of this boy revealed that in addition to his muteness, he exhibited no communicative intent, unlike deaf or aphasic children who try to communicate with gestures or sounds. Inadequate development of attachment behavior (lack of social smiling and lack of preference for parents over strangers) also supported the diagnosis of primary autism. However, since deafness may coexist with autism, the boy was referred to a pediatric audiologist for evaluation. Several sessions with the audiologist were needed because of difficulty in gaining the boy's cooperation, but it eventually became clear that hearing was normal. He was then referred to a child psychiatric clinic for further diagnostic work and treatment planning.

C. Notes: As seen in Table 41–7, *DSM-III-R* proposes 36 months as the age cutoff for infantile autism.

After a relative decline between 3 and 6 years of age, the incidence of childhood-onset pervasive developmental disorders increases in children over age 6 (Kolvin, 1971), although they are seen in younger children also. Onset is preceded by normal development and may be gradual, with nonpsychotic symptoms (eg, phobias or obsessions) appearing first, followed by an increasingly psychotic picture. The

---

Table 41–6. Classification of developmental disorders.

A. Mental retardation (see Fig 41–1).
B. Pervasive developmental disorders (see Table 41–7).
C. Specific developmental disorders (see Table 41–3).

Table 41–7. *DSM-III-R* diagnostic criteria for pervasive developmental disorders (coded on axis II).

Autistic disorder:

At least 8 of the following 16 items are present, these to include at least 2 items from criterion A, one from criterion B, and one from criterion C.

Note: Consider a criterion to be met *only* if the behavior is abnormal for the person's developmental level.

A. Qualitative impairment in reciprocal social interaction as manifested by the following:

(The examples within parentheses are arranged so that those first mentioned are more likely to apply to younger or more handicapped, and the later ones to older, or less handicapped, persons with this disorder.)

  (1) Marked lack of awareness of the existence or feelings of others (eg, treats a person as if he or she were a piece of furniture; does not notice another person's distress; apparently has no concept of the need of others for privacy).

  (2) No or abnormal seeking of comfort at times of distress (eg, does not come for comfort even when ill, hurt, or tired; seeks comfort in a stereotyped way, eg, says "cheese, cheese, cheese" whenever hurt).

  (3) No or impaired imitation (eg, does not wave bye-bye; does not copy mother's domestic activities; mechanical imitation of others' actions out of context).

  (4) No or abnormal social play (eg, does not actively participate in simple games; prefers solitary play activities; involves other children in play only as "mechanical aids").

  (5) Gross impairment in ability to make peer friendships (eg, no interest in making peer friendships; despite interest in making friends, demonstrates lack of understanding of conventions of social interaction, for example, reads phone book to uninterested peer).

B. Qualitative impairment in verbal and nonverbal communication, and in imaginative activity, as manifested by the following:

(The numbered items are arranged so that those first listed are more likely to apply to younger or more handicapped, and the later ones to older or less handicapped, persons with this disorder.)

  (1) No mode of communication, such as communicative babbling, facial expression, gesture, mime, or spoken language.

  (2) Markedly abnormal nonverbal communication, as in the use of eye-to-eye gaze, facial expression, body posture, or gestures to initiate or modulate social interaction (eg, does not anticipate being held, stiffens when held, does not look at the person or smile when making a social approach, does not greet parents or visitors, has a fixed stare in social situations).

  (3) Absence of imaginative activity, such as playacting of adult roles, fantasy characters, or animals; lack of interest in stories about imaginary events.

  (4) Marked abnormalities in the production of speech, including volume, pitch, stress, rate, rhythm, and intonation (eg, monotonous tone, questionlike melody, or high pitch).

  (5) Marked abnormalities in the form or content of speech, including stereotyped and repetitive use of speech (eg, immediate echolalia or mechanical repetition of television commercial); use of "you" when "I" is meant (eg, using "You want cookie?" to mean "I want cookie"); idiosyncratic use of words or phrases (eg, "Go on green riding" to mean "I want to go on the swing"); or frequent irrelevant remarks (eg, starts talking about train schedules during a conversation about sports).

  (6) Marked impairment in the ability to initiate or sustain a conversation with others, despite adequate speech (eg, indulging in lengthy monologs on one subject regardless of interjections from others).

C. Markedly restricted repertoire of activities and interests, as manifested by the following:

  (1) Stereotyped body movements, eg, hand-flicking or -twisting, spinning, head-banging, complex whole-body movements.

  (2) Persistent preoccupation with parts of objects (eg, sniffing or smelling objects, repetitive feeling of texture of materials, spinning wheels of toy cars) or attachment to unusual objects (eg, insists on carrying around a piece of string).

  (3) Marked distress over changes in trivial aspects of environment, eg, when a vase is moved from usual position.

  (4) Unreasonable insistence on following routines in precise detail, eg, insisting that exactly the same route always be followed when shopping.

  (5) Markedly restricted range of interests and a preoccupation with one narrow interest, eg, interested only in lining up objects, in amassing facts about meteorology, or in pretending to be a fantasy character.

D. Onset during infancy or childhood.

Specify:

  Infantile onset (before 36 months of age).

  Childhood onset (after 36 months of age).

  Age at onset unknown or not otherwise specified.

Pervasive developmental disorder not otherwise specified:

The category should be used when there is a qualitative impairment in the development of reciprocal social interaction and of verbal and nonverbal communication skills, but the criteria for autistic disorder are not met. Some persons with this diagnosis will exhibit a markedly restricted repertoire of activities and interests, but others will not.

---

definition excludes delusions, hallucinations, incoherence, and marked loosening of associations. Antipsychotic medications are of little value, except in the treatment of specific symptoms (eg, psychotic agitation) for circumscribed periods of time.

Illustrative Case No. 22

A. DSM-III-R Classification: Axis I, autistic disorder (childhood onset).

B. Description: The developmental history of a 7-year-old girl brought to the pediatric clinic for evaluation of behavior problems indicated nothing unusual until age 5. She was considered shy but bright. Between 5 and $5\frac{1}{2}$ years of age, she changed remarkably.

Her speech became monotonous; she acted self-centered and frightened; and she began to have episodes of head banging and violent tantrums when routines were not followed. Her toilet habits, which consisted of occasional loss of bowel control, changed to frequent soiling and long periods of withholding feces. Retention of feces eventually resulted in megacolon.

The girl was admitted to a child psychiatric ward, and her parents began psychotherapy simultaneously. Although therapeutic trials of 3 different antipsychotic medications resulted in no improvement in the girl, she responded to psychotherapy. By age 8, she was attending regular first grade in a public school. Her speech still retained a sing-song quality, and she still occasionally soiled herself but no longer withheld feces.

2. ADOLESCENT SCHIZOPHRENIC DISORDERS

Although schizophrenic disorders often begin in adolescence and persist in adulthood, many adolescent psychotic episodes are of brief duration and respond well to antipsychotic medications. *DSM-III-R* diagnostic criteria for child and adolescent schizophrenic disorders are the same as those for adults (see Chapter 27). Schizophrenic disorders appear with increasing frequency after 9 years of age.

PSYCHOPHYSIOLOGIC DISORDERS

Psychophysiologic disorders are characterized by disturbances of *involuntary* body functions. The disturbances are precipitated or exacerbated by environmental and psychologic stress and may be mild or severe, transient or chronic. Any organ system may be involved, as shown in the following examples of disorders that may be psychophysiologic: ulcers, ulcerative colitis, arthritis, skin diseases, growth retardation, headaches, eating disorders, stereotyped movement disorders, stuttering, functional enuresis or encopresis, sleepwalking disorder, and sleep terror disorder. The target organ or organ system involved is thought to be determined by genetic factors.

In *DSM-III*, the term "psychophysiologic disorders" is not used. For some cases, the axis I classification is "psychological factors affecting physical condition," and the axis III classification is the physical condition. In other cases, a more specific diagnosis (eg, sleepwalking disorder) is used.

Psychophysiologic disorders should not be confused with conversion disorders, in which a *voluntarily* controlled body part becomes dysfunctional as a result of some psychologic state, eg, paralysis of one arm following a frightening murderous impulse (see Chapter 32).

Illustrative Case No. 23

A. *DSM-III-R* **Classification:** Axis I, psychologic factors affecting physical condition. Axis III, asthma.

B. Description: A 13-year-old girl had her first asthma attack in 2 years when she visited her divorced father during summer vacation. She had been a "croupy child" and had suffered multiple asthma attacks during childhood. Many of these attacks occurred at times when her parents were having a quarrel, and the attacks forced them to quit arguing with each other and provide or seek emergency help for the child. Her parents divorced when she was 10, and the asthma attacks stopped when she was 11 (shortly after menarche). Since she was attack-free for 2 years, her family thought she had outgrown her asthma.

Illustrative Case No. 24

A. *DSM-III-R* **Classification:** Axis I, adjustment disorder with depressed mood; Tourette's disorder. Axis II, developmental reading disorder.

B. Description: The mother of a girl with a 2-year history of behavioral and emotional problems had delayed taking her child for evaluation and treatment. By the time she decided to consult a child psychiatrist, the girl was 9 years old. The mother was worried about the child's problems but was preoccupied by an acrimonious property settlement controversy with her estranged husband. The mother indicated that her daughter had very few friends and received poor marks in school. She had recently been told that the girl had learning disabilities. When the psychiatrist asked about the girl's abnormal neck and facial movements (tics), the mother indicated that these had developed over a 2-year period, that the movements sometimes involved the entire body, and that they were occasionally accompanied by squeaks and grunts (vocal tics). The mother stated that the tics began about the time the marriage problems reached a peak. On further questioning, she also indicated that the tics had started a few months after the girl was sexually molested by a 12-year-old boy. During the interview, the child expressed her anger and sadness over the problems she was experiencing.

C. Notes: This case demonstrates the interaction of biomedical and psychosocial factors in the development of a childhood disorder. In most cases, Gilles de la Tourette's syndrome occurs without obvious psychologic stressors. Symptoms may wax and wane, and the involuntary grunting and barking vocal tics may be accompanied by coprolalia (explosively uttered vulgar language). The motor and vocal tics may be embarrassing or even socially incapacitating. Some ability to voluntarily suppress the tics for minutes to hours is considered a diagnostic sign of the disorder, as is the observation that psychologic and family changes result in remissions and exacerbations. Haloperidol frequently is effective in treating this unusual disorder.

Illustrative Case No. 25

A. *DSM-III-R* **Classification:** Axis I, sleepwalking disorder.

B. Description: A 12-year-old boy was taken to a pediatrician because he had experienced 4 episodes of walking in his sleep over the past 6 months. He was completely unaware of the first 3 episodes. In the fourth episode, he awakened to find himself sleeping on the floor of his younger brother's room; he became frightened because he had no idea how he got there. His mother said these episodes always occurred during the first 3 hours after the boy was in deep sleep.

C. Notes: See comments to the following case.

Illustrative Case No. 26

A. *DSM-III-R* **Classification:** Axis I, sleep terror disorder.

B. Description: About once a month or less often during the past year, an 8-year-old girl woke up her family by screaming during the night. When the parents came in, they would find their daughter deeply asleep yet in a state of panic and anxiety—sweating, breathing fast, eyes staring with dilated pupils (but not seeing her parents), and fingers picking at her pillow. She did not respond to their efforts to comfort her and seemed unable to physically escape from her terror.

C. Notes: Both sleepwalking disorder and sleep terror disorder arise during slow-wave sleep stages 3 and 4 rather than during rapid eye movement (REM) sleep (see Chapter 10). Sleepwalking appears to be a dissociative episode with amnesia, whereas sleep terror is more similar to a state of agitation in a delirious patient, with relative motor paralysis compared to the free movement of the sleepwalker. In both disorders, the electroencephalographic findings are normal, and the episode is not recalled as a dream or a nightmare. Treatment includes use of medications such as diazepam or antidepressants, which alter sleep stages 3 and 4.

DISRUPTIVE BEHAVIOR DISORDERS

This group of disorders includes oppositional defiant disorder (Table 41–8), conduct disorder (Table 41–9), and attention-deficit hyperactivity disorder (Table 41–10).

Illustrative Case No. 27

A. DSM-III-R Classification: Axis I, oppositional defiant disorder.

B. Description: An 8-year-old boy who was previously well-behaved "just went on a rampage," according to his mother. She explained that during the past 6 months, he refused to do his household chores,

---

Table 41–8. *DSM-III-R* diagnostic criteria for oppositional defiant disorder.

Note: Consider a criterion met only if the behavior is considerably more frequent than that of most people of the same mental age.
A. A disturbance of at least 6 months during which at least 5 of the following are present:
  (1) Often loses temper.
  (2) Often argues with adults.
  (3) Often actively defies or refuses adult requests or rules, eg, refuses to do chores at home.
  (4) Often deliberately does things that annoy other people, eg, grabs other children's hats.
  (5) Often blames others for his or her own mistakes.
  (6) Is often touchy or easily annoyed by others.
  (7) Is often angry and resentful.
  (8) Is often spiteful or vindictive.
  (9) Often swears or uses obscene language.
  Note: The above items are listed in descending order of discriminating power based on data from a national field trial of the *DSM-III-R* criteria for disruptive behavior disorders.
B. Does not meet the criteria for conduct disorder and does not occur exclusively during the course of a psychotic disorder, dysthymia, or a major depressive, hypomanic, or manic epi-sode.

Table 41–9. *DSM-III-R* diagnostic criteria for conduct disorder.

A. A disturbance of conduct lasting at least 6 months, during which at least 3 of the following have been present:
  (1) Has stolen without confrontation of a victim on more than one occasion (including forgery).
  (2) Has run away from home overnight at least twice while living in parental or parental surrogate home (or once without returning).
  (3) Often lies (other than to avoid physical or sexual abuse).
  (4) Has deliberately engaged in fire-setting.
  (5) Is often truant from school (for older person, absent from work).
  (6) Has broken into someone else's house, building, or car.
  (7) Has deliberately destroyed others' property (other than by fire-setting).
  (8) Has been physically cruel to animals.
  (9) Has forced someone into sexual activity with him or her.
  (10) Has used a weapon in more than one fight.
  (11) Often initiates physical fights.
  (12) Has stolen with confrontation of a victim (eg, mugging, purse-snatching, extortion, armed robbery).
  (13) Has been physically cruel to people.
Note: The above items are listed in descending order of discriminating power based on data from a national field trial of the *DSM-III-R* criteria for disruptive behavior disorders.
B. If 18 or older does not meet criteria for antisocial personality disorder.
Solitary aggressive type:
The essential feature is the predominance of aggressive physical behavior, usually toward both adults and peers, initiated by the person (not as a group activity).
Group type:
The essential feature is the predominance of conduct problems occurring mainly as a group activity with peers. Aggressive physical behavior may or may not be present.
Undifferentiated type:
This a subtype for children or adolescents with conduct disorder with a mixture of clinical features that cannot be classified as either solitary aggressive type or group type.

"talked back," and had tantrums when he did not get his way. The only explanation his mother could find was that after seriously considering marriage, she broke off a 2-year relationship with her boyfriend. Her attempts to talk with her son about this met with failure. ("No, Mom, that's dumb—I don't want to talk about it!")

C. Notes: Oppositional defiant disorder does not include breaking the rules of social interaction or infringement on the rights of others. Conduct disorders, by definition, do include such behavior (see below).

Illustrative Case No. 28

A. DSM-III-R Classification: Axis I, conduct disorder, socialized, nonaggressive.

B. Description: A 15-year-old girl was picked up by the police when she decided to "go into business for myself." She had been engaged in prostitution (and had a "manager") for over a year. She had run away from home several times but always returned. Although her mother was upset and worried about her daughter, she was afraid to ask authorities for help and thus allowed the daughter to come and go as she

Table 41 – 10. *DSM-III-R* diagnostic criteria for attention deficit hyperactivity disorder.

Note: Consider a criterion met only if the behavior is considerably more frequent than that of most people of the same mental age.

A. A disturbance of at least 6 months during which at least 8 of the following are present:

   (1) Often fidgets with hands or feet or squirms in seat (in adolescents, may be limited to subjective feelings or restlessness).
   (2) Has difficulty remaining seated when required to do so.
   (3) Is easily distracted by extraneous stimuli.
   (4) Has difficulty awaiting turn in games or group situations.
   (5) Often blurts out answers to questions before they have been completed.
   (6) Has difficulty following through on instructions from others (not due to oppositional behavior or failure of comprehension), eg, fails to finish chores.
   (7) Has difficulty sustaining attention in tasks or play activities.
   (8) Often shifts from one uncompleted activity to another.
   (9) Has difficulty playing quietly.
   (10) Often talks excessively.
   (11) Often interrupts or intrudes on others, eg, butts into other children's games.
   (12) Often does not seem to listen to what is being said to him or her.
   (13) Often loses things necessary for tasks or activities at school or at home (eg, toys, pencils, books, assignments).
   (14) Often engages in physically dangerous activities without considering possible consequences (not for the purpose of thrill-seeking), eg, runs into street without looking.

Note: The above items are listed in descending order of discriminating power based on data from a national field trial of the *DSM-III-R* criteria for disruptive behavior disorders.

B. Onset before the age of 7.

C. Does not meet the criteria for a pervasive developmental disorder.

wished. The girl had several friendships that had continued since childhood, and she was considered a good-hearted and generous friend.

   C. Notes: *DSM-III* classified 4 types of conduct disorder according to the presence or absence of antisocial aggression and the presence or absence of peer group social attachments that are based on psychologic ties rather than practical considerations: (1) undersocialized, aggressive; (2) undersocialized, nonaggressive; (3) socialized, aggressive; and (4) socialized, nonaggressive. This case demonstrates the fourth (and least deviant) type of conduct disorder. The proposed revision (from *DSM-III-R*) is shown in Table 41 – 9. It should be noted that conduct disorder is considered by many authors to be a diagnosis of dubious validity (Lewis, 1984).

Illustrative Case No. 29

   A. *DSM-III-R* Classification: Axis I, attention deficit disorder with hyperactivity.

   B. Description: A 5-year-old boy was referred to a pediatrician by his teacher during his second week in kindergarten because he was difficult to control and showed signs of impulsivity and inattention: (1) He

moved quickly from one activity to another, acted impulsively and sometimes too aggressively, was unable to wait his turn in games or group discussions, and generally needed a great deal of supervision. (2) He was easily distracted and had difficulty listening to what was being said to him or staying with school tasks or play activities.

   Although dismayed by her son's behavior in kindergarten, the mother said she expected such a problem, since he had also had problems in the several nursery schools he had attended. "He was even hyper before he was born," she explained. "Sometimes I thought he was doing somersaults in there. After he was born, his engine was always running; he even squirmed a lot in his sleep."

   C. Notes: There are 2 main categories of attention deficit disorder (Table 41 – 10): with and without hyperactivity. In the past, the disorder was often termed minimal brain damage, minimal brain dysfunction, hyperkinetic syndrome, etc. Impulsivity and inattention are hallmarks of attention deficit disorder of either category. The boy in this case also had hyperactivity, as described by his mother.

   In children with this disorder, the peak age for referral is 8 – 10 years. The disorder is most observable in situations that require self-application, as in the classroom, and thus the teacher is often the one to recommend evaluation. The parents may disagree with the teacher's report, since they may have fewer opportunities to see their child in this context. The clinician's observations of the child in a playroom diagnostic setting often do not correspond with the teacher's observations either. Results of structured psychologic and educational testing may support the diagnosis. Diagnosis is more difficult in children without hyperactivity. Those with hyperactivity usually have characteristic developmental histories.

   Adolescents or adults who once satisfied the diagnostic criteria of attention deficit hyperactivity disorder but have outgrown their hyperactivity often retain the impulsivity and inattention, and their occupational or social functioning is adversely affected.

   Treatment of attention deficit disorder in childhood includes family education about the disorder, drug therapy with methylphenidate or dextroamphetamine, psychotherapy, and remediation of coexisting learning disorders. Contrary to earlier beliefs and concerns, use of stimulants for attention deficit disorder is not associated with later drug abuse. However, it is still important to warn patients and their families of the side effects of stimulants and to institute periodic "drug holidays."

OTHER DISORDERS ORIGINATING IN CHILDHOOD

Illustrative Case No. 30

   A. *DSM-III-R* Classification: Axis I, reactive attachment disorder of infancy.

   B. Description: A 6-month-old boy was brought

to the pediatric clinic by his grandmother. She was visiting from out of town and was shocked to find her grandson so scrawny, apathetic, and unresponsive. The history was reviewed and the neglected infant immediately hospitalized for diagnostic studies, including observing the effect of adequate care and nutrition. The admitting diagnosis was failure to thrive. Results of physical and laboratory examinations were normal except for low weight, mild anemia, and apathy.

A social worker who visited the boy's home found his mother depressed, ineffectual, and terrorized by her alcoholic husband. The mother explained that she had her hands full with her 2 older children and with the 2 or 3 other children she "took in" for baby-sitting. She thought her son was too skinny because he was not a "big eater," but she indicated that he was a good baby.

Within days after admission to the hospital, the boy began to brighten up and to smile and look at people. His weight soon returned to normal, and he became a playful and assertive infant within a month. His mother found little time to visit him and said she was considering putting him up for adoption.

C. Notes: Diagnostic criteria for reactive attachment disorder are shown in Table 41–11. Although infants with this disorder are considered physically and emotionally starved, their longitudinal growth remains normal. After infancy, children with psychologic and family problems may fall behind their previous rate of growth in both height and weight. Some

Table 41–11. *DSM-III-R* diagnostic criteria for reactive attachment disorder.

A. Markedly disturbed social relatedness in most contexts, beginning before the age of 5, as evidenced by either (1) or (2):
  (1) Persistent failure to initiate or respond to most social interactions (eg, in infants, absence of visual tracking and reciprocal play, lack of vocal imitation or playfulness, apathy, little or no spontaneity; at later ages, lack of or little curiosity and social interest).
  (2) Indiscriminate sociability, eg, excessive familiarity with relative strangers by making requests and displaying affection.
B. The disturbance in A is not a symptom of either mental retardation or a pervasive developmental disorder, such as autistic disorder.
C. Grossly pathogenic care, as evidenced by at least one of the following:
  (1) Persistent disregard of the child's basic emotional needs for comfort, stimulation, and affection. *Examples:* Overly harsh punishment by caregiver; consistent neglect by caregiver.
  (2) Persistent disregard of the child's basic physical needs, including nutrition, adequate housing, and protection from physical danger and assault (including sexual abuse).
  (3) Repeated change of primary caregiver so that stable attachments are not possible, eg, frequent changes in foster parents.
D. There is a presumption that the care described in C is responsible for the disturbed behavior in A; this presumption is warranted if the disturbance in A began following the pathogenic care in C.
Note: If failure to thrive is present, code it on Axis III.

---

children with short stature also have abnormally low levels of growth hormone, apparently caused by significant emotional pressures. This disorder in childhood, called **psychosocial dwarfism,** is not listed in *DSM-III;* although mentioned in this section, psychosocial dwarfism could also be classified as a psychophysiologic disorder. Children with this disorder resume their normal rate of growth (and their growth hormone levels normalize) when the psychosocial causes of growth delay are corrected.

Illustrative Case No. 31

A. *DSM-III-R* **Classification:** Axis I, elective mutism.

B. Description: A 16-year-old girl whose mother had died a year before was living with her aunt and uncle and their 4 children. She had seen her father less and less frequently since her parents' divorce 3 years before. In her aunt's home, she saw herself as a stranger who had to earn her keep by baby-sitting and doing housework. She had always been studious, obedient, and somewhat shy, but now she simply refused to speak at school as well as at home. Her aunt took her to the pediatrician at the school's insistence. In response to the pediatrician's considerate and gentle questioning, to which the girl responded only by nodding or shaking her head, she indicated agreement that she was unhappy and that it was "easier not to talk." The pediatrician spoke with the aunt and uncle to emphasize the importance of immediate psychiatric referral.

CHILD MALTREATMENT

The spectrum of maltreatment of children ranges from nonorganic failure to thrive through child neglect to emotional, physical, and sexual abuse. Families at high risk for childhood mental disorders, described in the section on epidemiology (above), also are at greater risk for child maltreatment. In 1981, the National Center on Child Abuse and Neglect documented a physical abuse rate of 3.4 cases per 1000 children per year, an emotional abuse rate of 2.2 per 1000, and a sexual abuse rate of 0.7 per 1000. The incidence of educational neglect was 2.9 per 1000; of physical neglect, 1.7 per 1000; and of emotional neglect, 1 per 1000. These are underestimates, since some diagnoses are inevitably missed and many cases go unreported—especially cases of emotional abuse and neglect and educational neglect.

Even when there is a clear history, child protective services with limited budgets are able to intervene only in the worst cases of physical or sexual abuse. And even when help for the child is provided after abuse has occurred, it is too late then to prevent continuing negative interactions in the family and further abuse in the future.

1. NONORGANIC FAILURE TO THRIVE

Nonorganic failure to thrive is called "reactive attachment disorder of infancy" in *DSM-III-R*. (See Illustrative Case No. 30.) After exclusion of organic causes of height and weight retardation below the third percentile (head circumference is usually normal), the diagnosis is based on the family history and on observation of the child-parent relationship. Studies demonstrate a variety of maladaptive mother-child interactions—in most cases impaired mothering due to chronic depression, dependence, and poor day-to-day functioning. Fathers in these studies were often described as ineffectual with respect to the mother-child relationship.

The outcomes of hospitalization of infants with a diagnosis of nonorganic failure to thrive have been studied by Rutter (1985). The best results (ie, resumption of normal growth) are reported for infants whose mothers suffer from acute depression; 40% of infants with mothers suffering from chronic depression or chronic medical illnesses lost weight after discharge; and infants whose mothers were described as "extremely angry and hostile" had the worst outcomes. Long-term follow-up shows concordance between nonorganic failure to thrive and later child abuse and neglect, with 42% of children falling below the third percentile in height or weight.

Family involvement in treatment, or foster placement as needed, offers the best hope for a favorable long-term outcome.

2. CHILD NEGLECT

Inadequate or negligent parenting, which is to some extent culturally defined, implies indifference to a child's physical safety and well-being, schooling, or medical care, with concomitant emotional deprivation of the child. Even though about half of neglectful families studied live under conditions of poverty, one cannot equate low socioeconomic status with physical or emotional neglect, since most poor parents are properly attentive to their children's needs (Rutter, 1985). Neglectful parenting should be suspected when the mother or father of an emotionally disturbed child refuses to recognize that a problem exists or fails to seek help or take appropriate action to find a remedy. Many neglectful parents themselves grew up as deprived children, so that they never developed good judgment about the emotional needs of children.

Physical and emotional illnesses and drug and alcohol abuse are risk factors for child neglect.

3. PHYSICAL ABUSE

Ten percent of emergency room visits by children under 5 years of age are occasioned by physical abuse. The number of such incidents reported annually in the USA rose from 7000 in 1967 to over 200,000 in 1979 (Rudolph, 1982). The fatality rate resulting from physical abuse is variously estimated to be 5–25%; the average age at death is under 3 years; and the duration of exposure to physical abuse before the fatal outcome is a heartrending 1–3 years.

Physical abuse of children was first described as a pediatric entity by Kempe in 1962 and called by him the "battered child syndrome." The incidence of abuse is estimated to be 10 cases per 1000 live births per year (Steinhauer and Rae-Grant, 1983). Boys and girls are equally at risk overall, though the risk is greater for boys before age 12 and for girls during the teen years.

Most fatalities and serious injuries occur in children under age 3. Poverty, family dysfunction, and discriminatory underreporting have resulted in higher reported case rates among ethnic minority families, but child abuse occurs in all ethnic and socioeconomic groups. The underreporting of abuse and neglect in middle-class families is related to the way these families seek help. Since they tend to be referred to private therapists, they elude statistical reporting by government agencies.

Characteristics of Abusive Parents & Their Child Victims

The work of Kempe and Helfer (1972), amplified by Steinhauer and Rae-Grant (1983), has made it possible to characterize the abusive parent and the child victim in recognizable ways that are of help in case-finding and management.

A. The Parents: The parents commonly give an inadequate history of the incident and tend to be hostile or evasive, unconcerned about the child, and eager to establish their own innocence of wrongdoing. There may be an unexplained or fancifully explained delay in seeking treatment for the child, or a history of application to different hospitals in prior similar episodes. The parent may refuse hospitalization or diagnostic procedures for the child or may abruptly leave the child in the hospital after admission or even during the emergency room examination. If the child is admitted for observation and treatment, the parent may visit only infrequently or not at all and may show unconcern or relate poorly to the child during visits, thus provoking staff criticism. Lastly, the abusive parent is characteristically hard to reach by phone, changes residence frequently, has an unstable marital relationship, and has few friends or social resources.

B. The Child: The abused child characteristically has no explanation for its injury or gives a history contradictory to the parents' explanation—or parrots the mother's or father's obviously incongruous account of what happened. During the initial contact the child seems fearful, or passive and withdrawn, or hyperalert to the environment, looking to others and not to the parents for clues to how to behave. It responds to other adults indiscriminately, exhibits appeasing, smiling behavior, and shows obvious apprehension when other children cry. The workup of the child discloses injuries not mentioned in the history taken from the parent, including even multiple old fractures shown on radiographs. Developmental delays in gross motor function and speech and language skills are commonly present. There is general evidence of inadequate care, including dehydration and malnutrition, and the child typically gains weight in the hospital. There may be a history of ingestion of inappropriate food, drink, or drugs. Upon questioning, the child denies previous abuse or problems in the family. The child is viewed as "different" or "bad" by the family.

Contributing Factors

Factors contributing to child abuse are parental inadequacy resulting in low self-esteem and a wish to be "taken care of" by the child (role reversal); some "difference" in the child such as temperament; prematurity; a physical defect (cleft lip or palate, etc); and situational crises that provoke violent outbursts directed at the child as resident victim. Child abuse—like child neglect—often occurs in familial distribution from one generation to the next. Material abundance does not preclude attitudes of self-disparagement leading to physical abuse of children.

Treatment

When physical abuse of a child is suspected, the physician or other involved professional is apt to respond either by identifying with the child and directing anger toward the parents or, contrariwise, by identifying with the parent—who usually tries to deny or explain away the child's injuries, in some cases persuasively—and therefore denying the possibility of abuse. However, child abuse reporting laws require health care professionals to report all cases of suspected child neglect or abuse to local police officials, juvenile court officials, or the child protective agency of the county department of social services. Immunity against civil reprisal for groundless complaints is provided, and nonreporting is a criminal offense. The doctrines of confidentiality and privilege do not apply to reportable conditions.

Child abuse, once begun, becomes habitual and very difficult to stop despite repeated expressions of regret and the resolve to do better. It is therefore necessary to remove the child from the abusive environment during the peirod of assessment. Hospitalization is usually required to evaluate the extent of physical injuries and to begin the multidisciplinary team evaluation of the child and its family. The team should include a social worker, child psychiatrist, pediatrician, someone from the child protective agency, and, when necessary, a police officer. During the initial assessment phase, the child's siblings should be examined for evidence of injuries or neglect (Rudolph, 1982). Any person who has inflicted severe injuries on a child may be psychotic or suicidal and requires emergency psychiatric evaluation.

Because of the recurrent nature of child abuse, "crisis intervention" is not the answer. There must be an individualized long-term therapeutic program coordinated by the child psychiatrist, child protective agency, or child guidance clinic. Depending on the outcome of the multidisciplinary evaluation, the child may be permanently placed in a foster or adoptive family; may be removed from the family not permanently but for at least several months until the parents have proved they can offer a safe home; or may be returned to the family after assessment because a satisfactory rehabilitation plan is in place and there is a reasonable chance for successful reunion.

Assessment of Home Safety

Steinhauer and Rae-Grant (1983) have adapted guidelines from Kempe and Helfer (1972) as an aid to assessment of home safety when pondering the decision whether to return a child to its home or place it in foster care. It is of course a favorable sign if the parents have shown their willingness to accept help for the child and for themselves when it is needed. It must be clear also that help really is available at all times and that obstacles to seeking help are removed—eg, that there is a telephone in the home. Practical difficulties such as housing, food, employment, and illness should be in acceptable stages of resolution. It is a good sign if counseling has enabled the parents to accept an improved self-image and if they have developed some interests outside the home. Each spouse must be able to recognize when the other needs help and be willing to take necessary steps to obtain it. The parents must find the child "pleasing," with acknowledged needs of its own, and not "bad" and not "different" in unattractive ways. The parents' expectations of the child must be realistic. It is a very good sign if the parents consistently keep follow-up appointments for the child and themselves.

The Forensic Context of Child Abuse

Child neglect and abuse proceedings take place in juvenile or family court settings, where the people's burden of proof is not "beyond a reasonable doubt," as in criminal cases, but according to the civil standard of "the preponderance of the evidence." Even so, such proceedings are adversarial, and the parents' interests may be vigorously defended. For that reason alone, the need for unassailable documentation throughout the management of every case—including photographs and even videotaped child assessment sessions if possible—should be obvious.

Prognosis & Prevention

The prognosis for permanent cessation of child abuse is poor, even with protracted treatment. In the Rutter study, one-third to one-half of families abused the child victim again. One-fourth to one-half of children who are returned home without treatment beyond medical attention to injuries become victims subject to permanent injury or death.

In an attempt to ameliorate this grim prospect, Steinhauer and Rae-Grant (1983) have developed recommendations for social changes and professional safeguards aimed at prevention of physical abuse of children. Cultural as well as legal sanctions against the use of violence or force in child-rearing or in the schools are of first importance—sparing the rod to save the child. Social programs to eliminate poverty will ultimately benefit all children and remove from the home at least that stimulus for acts born of hopeless desperation. Adequate health care, social services, housing, and cultural and recreational facilities should be available to all citizens without exception. Family planning programs should include availability of abortion when appropriate to reduce the number of unwanted and rejected children. The same purpose without abortion can be served by family life education programs for young people preparing for sexual activity and perhaps marriage and parenthood. In the obstetrics unit in the hospital, the staff should be alert for evidence of rejecting behavior both before and after delivery. Child welfare and protective agencies should be adequately funded by an informed legislature and executive at the insistence of a concerned electorate. Lastly, physicians and other involved professionals should improve their cooperation in an effort to identify children at risk and act appropriately to prevent violence agianst children.

4. SEXUAL ABUSE

Definitions of child sexual abuse reflect cultural values and the professional orientation of the diagnostician. Mrazek (Rutter, 1985) perceives 4 types of child sexual maltreatment: exposure, molestation, sexual intercourse, and rape. Exposure includes pornography, the viewing of sexual acts, and exhibitionism. Molestation refers to fondling the child's genitals or asking the child to fondle the genitals of an adult. Sexual intercourse includes nonassaultive, often chronic vaginal, oral, or rectal intercourse. Rape is defined as assaultive, forced sexual intercourse. More than one type may be present in a single case. Incest is defined as sexual involvement with a relative whom the victim could not legally marry as an adult. The sexual abuser is usually an older sibling or parental figure (foster or adoptive parent). In 50–80% of cases, the abuser is known to the child or family (Steinhauer and Rae-Grant, 1983). The National Center on Child Abuse and Neglect (1981) estimates the incidence of child sexual abuse at 100,000 cases per year.

Various studies (Rutter, 1985) reveal that as many as 40% of adult women report at least one episode of sexual abuse during childhood; up to 6% were reported to the police. Most studies report a 10:1 ratio of girls to boys as victims.

Sexual assault of a child by a stranger is unrelated to family dysfunction, though children who develop protracted sexual relationships with adults outside the family do so in an attempt to satisfy unfulfilled emotional needs.

The most frequently reported form of incest occurs between father and daughter. Several studies have demonstrated that "incest is a family affair" (Stein-

hauer and Rae-Grant, 1983) in which many types of dysfunction, as well as the disinhibitory effects of drugs and alcohol, play a role. The family history often discloses incest in previous generations. The mother has often been described as rejecting her sexual role as wife, rejecting her daughter, and passively colluding with the perpetrating father. The father is typically described as authoritarian, immature, and sexually estranged from his wife. The other children in the family are often aware of the incest and may themselves be involved in incestuous behavior.

Clinical Findings

While extrafamilial sexual abuse is more willingly revealed by children, families fear the trauma of repeated questioning and the stress and humiliation of court appearances and publicity. Intrafamilial sexual abuse may never be disclosed, or not for years.

The child may present with symptoms or signs of medical, emotional, behavioral, or learning problems. Medical signs may consist of vaginal bleeding from trauma, recurrent urinary tract infections, proctitis, vaginitis, sexually transmitted diseases, pregnancy, and rectal or vaginal foreign bodies. Emotional or behavioral signs include psychosomatic illness, depression, attempted suicide, pseudomaturity, dissociative disorders, conversion disorders, shyness and avoidance of peer relationships, compulsive masturbation, precocious sexual behavior, adolescent prostitution, drug abuse, and running away from home. School-related difficulties include academic failure, frequent absences, poor peer relationships and avoidance of extracurricular activities, fearful or seductive behavior toward male teachers, and refusal to undress for physical education classes. The more of the above signs identified, the higher the likelihood that sexual abuse has occurred or is occurring.

Treatment

In cases of extrafamilial sexual abuse, the reactions of the average family may include self-doubt and questioning as well as outrage toward the perpetrator and protectiveness toward the child victim. Blaming the child victim or indifference to the event indicates serious family dysfunction. The effects of extrafamilial abuse on the child may be minimal (eg, after a brief episode of exhibitionism), requiring family discussion and reassurance that the perpetrator and not the child is "responsible" for what happened. At the other extreme, serious posttraumatic stress disorders can result from long-term or forcible abuse. Such posttraumatic stress disorders can be manifested by a wide variety of reactive psychologic symptoms superimposed on preexisting personality organization.

5. CONCLUSIONS

Child maltreatment brings into focus the multiple problems of dysfunctional families. Abusive or neglecting parental figures are suffering people who themselves need or deserve help, but they are also generators of misery. Dysfunctional families should be considered a high-priority public health problem. Measures that might prevent child maltreatment include training professionals to recognize and deal with real or suspected child abuse at least on a first-aid basis (Steinhauer and Rae-Grant, 1983); funding of child protection and victim assistance programs; systematic cooperation between medical, legal, child welfare, and law enforcement agencies; guidelines for interviewing and legal processing of abused children and families to reduce the sometimes catastrophic consequences of criminal court proceedings; and continuing education of professionals in related fields.

ORGANIC MENTAL DISORDERS

As in adults, organic mental disorders in children are characterized by (1) impairment of orientation, judgment, learning, memory, and other cognitive functions; and (2) lability of affect. Brain damage may be diffuse or focal and may result from trauma, tumor, metabolic abnormalities, drug toxicity, or other causes. Both acute and chronic brain syndromes are seen (see Chapter 24).

Ilustrative Case No. 32
A. *DSM-III-R* Classification: Axis I, barbiturate intoxication. Axis III, seizure disorder of unknown origin.

B. Description: A 7-year-old girl was falling behind in the second grade. Mental retardation was suggested because she had major motor seizures since the age of 4, and this implied "brain damage" to the family. During her yearly physical examination, her family doctor thought he detected mild nystagmus, a sign of barbiturate overdose. Since she was taking phenytoin and phenobarbital for her seizures, he ordered a blood test to determine drug levels. When the phenobarbital level was found to be elevated (above the therapeutic level), he instructed the parents to give her half of the usual dose. Within 2 months, the child's level of functioning in school returned to normal.

Illustrative Case No. 33
A. Diagnosis:
1. GAP–Chronic brain syndrome caused by drowning accident.
2. *DSM-III-R* –Axis I, delirium, followed by dementia. Axis II, mild mental retardation. Axis III, brain damage secondary to drowning accident.

B. Description: A 3-year-old girl wandered away from her mother and fell into a swimming pool. She was revived and spent 4 days in the intensive care unit in a state of delirium. She was hallucinating and confused and exhibited both stuporous and agitated states. Her condition showed some improvement within 2 weeks, and she was discharged from the hospital. However, her memory for recent events remained impaired; she cried and laughed at the slightest

provocation and had difficulty understanding statements and requests she once was able to understand. This evidence of persistent injury marked the onset of dementia.

At 5 years of age, the girl was enrolled in a special kindergarten class. She was impulsive and had difficulty attending to tasks long enough to learn to complete them. The parents were on the verge of divorce, as their depression and turmoil had continued since the child's accident. The family physician met with both parents twice and encouraged them to seek help for themselves and their daughter at a child psychiatric clinic. They accepted his advice, and at 6-month follow-up, the family physician noted a decrease in anxiety and better coping skills in all 3 family members. Although the child continued to require special class placement because of her mild chronic brain syndrome (dementia), her behavior was much improved at school and at home.

MENTAL RETARDATION

The American Association on Mental Deficiency (1977) defines mental retardation as "significantly subaverage intellectual functioning originating during the developmental period, accompanied by impairment in one or more of the following: maturation, learning, or social adjustment." The IQ test (see Chapter 20) is the standard measure of intelligence used, and mental retardation is defined by an IQ of less than 70 (ie, 2 standard deviations below the mean of 100). The classifications (mild, moderate, severe, and profound retardation) and IQ score distributions of mental retardation are shown in Fig 41–1.

The prevalence of mental retardation in the USA is estimated to be 3% of the general population. In 1983, there were 6 million mentally retarded people—twice the combined total of those who suffer from blindness, poliomyelitis, cerebral palsy, and rheumatic heart disease. The incidence of emotional disorders in mentally retarded individuals is also very high—ie, 3–5 times that in the general population. It is usually an emotional problem or a difficulty in adjustment that brings retarded people to the attention of society. For the vast majority of these individuals (the 85% who are mildly retarded and educable), difficulties begin during the school years. With adequate instruction in a supportive environment, these people can function in the general population and find a suitable vocation.

This section will present several illustrative cases, discuss some misconceptions about mental retardation, and outline causes and characteristics of mental retardation syndromes.

Illustrative Case No. 34
A. *DSM-III-R* Classification: Axis II, mild mental retardation.

B. Description: When a 10-year-old well-adjusted boy was noted by his teacher to be a slow learner, she requested evaluation and consultation

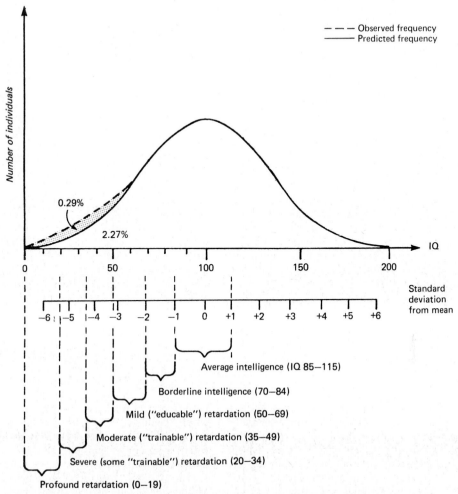

Figure 41–1. Distribution and classification of mental retardation. The shaded area denotes an increased incidence of 0.29% over the predicted frequency, resulting from organic causes of mental retardation. (Modified and reproduced, with permission, from Moser HW, Wolf PA: The nosology of mental retardation: Including the report of a survey of 1378 mentally retarded individuals at the Walter E. Fernald State School. In: *Nervous System*. Bergsma D [editor]. Part 6 of: *The Second Conference on the Clinical Delineation of Birth Defects*. Williams & Wilkins for the National Foundation–March of Dimes, Birth Defects Original Article Series 1971;7:117.)

from the school psychologist. Testing indicated that he had an IQ in the range of 63–69. His teacher continued to give him individually paced instruction in her class. A similar approach, with individual tutoring as needed, was followed when he reached high school. The placid boy enjoyed participation on the track team and was accepted by his peers. His family encouraged his interest in fishing, and at age 16, he began to learn about commercial fishing at a local firm. When he was subsequently hired by the firm, he told his family, "I may never make it to manager, but I'll always make a decent living." He later married and had 2 children.

Illustrative Case No. 35

A. Diagnosis:

1. GAP–Depression in a young child with mild mental retardation related to sociocultural deprivation.

2. DSM-III-R–Axis I, dysthymia. Axis II, mild mental retardation.

B. Description: The foster parent of an 8-year-old boy brought him to the pediatric clinic and requested that the child be given medication to "calm him down." The history revealed that the boy's biologic mother had been 17 years old at the time of conception. She did not want the baby but bowed to family pressure against abortion. She refused to let herself "get that fat look" and went on such a severe diet that she only gained 5 lb by the end of the full 9-month gestation period. Delivery was uncomplicated, and the boy weighed $4\frac{1}{2}$ lb. His young parents then married "to make things right." During the 2 chaotic years of the parents' unhappy marriage, the boy spent much of the time crying in his crib, attended only by baby-sitters. When his parents separated, he went to live with his grandmother. When he was 6, the grandmother had a stroke, and he was placed in a series of foster homes before the present one.

Examination revealed a sad-faced, hyperactive little boy overly eager to please. Doll play in the diagnostic play session showed a little boy scurrying about, doing chores, fixing things around the house—but knocking over the furniture and the other dolls. Psychologic testing showed depression with a negative self-image. The scores on IQ subtests all clustered around 65.

The child was seen in weekly play therapy sessions for the next 2 years. Although his behavior improved greatly, his IQ remained the same, perhaps reflecting permanent effects of fetal undernutrition and emotional deprivation during infancy. His improved emotional state subsequently enabled the child to perform up to his abilities in school, changing his prognosis from a potential social failure to a potentially satisfied and contributing member of society.

Illustrative Case No. 36

A. Diagnosis:

1. GAP–Anxiety reaction in an adolescent with moderate mental retardation.

2. *DSM-III-R* –Axis I, moderate mental retardation. Axis II, microcephaly.

B. Description: The neighbors of a moderately mentally retarded teenager (age 14) complained that he frightened their young daughter by asking her questions at the bus stop. The boy's parents were afraid that the next time this happened the police would be called and their son would be sent to a state institution for the retarded. They sought help from a child psychiatrist.

The history revealed that the boy was born with microcephaly after 8 months of gestation. He required assistance with breathing for 2 weeks in the neonatal intensive care unit. During infancy, he had multiple hospitalizations for respiratory problems. Between the ages of $2\frac{1}{2}$ and 8 years, he attended a day school for retarded children. From there, he went to public school and attended special classes for the trainable retarded. He was still enrolled in school at the time of evaluation.

Initial assessment showed a moderately retarded boy with odd-sounding nasal speech. When he felt anxious, he touched people's faces and clothes, asked many questions, and fidgeted. When he relaxed, he could sit still for longer periods. The parents reported that his anxiety level and inappropriate behavior had increased since puberty. They expressed their own worries about his sexual maturity and immature coping abilities: "What if he masturbates in public? What if he tries to kiss a little girl? How can we explain to him what he should and should not do?"

The parents agreed to counseling for themselves and their son to help them cope with this new period of adjustment. The boy continued in school and lived at home until he was 19 years old. He then moved to a group home for retarded young adults in a suburb of his hometown.

Misconceptions About Mental Retardation

Societal attitudes toward mentally retarded people have in the past varied—from reverence and awe to disdain and fear to unconcern and neglect. When state mental hospitals and state institutions for the retarded were built in the late 19th and early 20th centuries, large numbers of retarded people were institutionalized. Such isolation and labeling furthered the stereotyped view of the mentally retarded as a homogeneous group of subhuman, dangerous individuals who would commit crimes of all types, especially sex crimes, if allowed to roam free in the community. Another commonly held fear was that the retarded would have an abnormally high reproductive rate, thereby "polluting the genetic pool of society." This reflected the mistaken belief that mental retardation is uniformly inherited (when in fact only a small proportion of mentally retarded individuals have retarded parents). In California, these fears were kept alive by the Human Betterment Foundation of Pasadena, which was so active in the eugenics movement that by 1943 California could claim responsibility for 40% of all sterilizations performed in the USA. Large numbers of state hospital patients were sterilized, including delinquents and retarded and epileptic patients.

As scientific data accumulated, public opinion began to shift. Studies showed that the mentally retarded have no greater propensity to commit crimes than the general population and that their reproduction rate is actually somewhat lower than the general rate. Other common misconceptions still abound, including the idea that mentally retarded people are all alike. As the illustrative cases above demonstrate, retarded people are individuals with diverse characteristics. Although their chronic and frequently stigmatizing handicap imposes greater stress and thereby predisposes them and their families to a greater frequency of emotional difficulties, most of these difficulties are similar to those encountered by others. And, contrary to another popular misconception, many of these problems can be alleviated, with resulting improvement in social functioning.

Many aspects of mental retardation are currently under study, and advances have been made in the prevention of retardation (eg, through genetic counseling, amniocentesis, special diets for children with phenylketonuria) and in early detection and management of the disorder. In addition, the range of community services, facilities, and special programs has been expanded. Many adults with moderate retardation who would previously have been institutionalized are now able to live in group homes in the community with varying degrees of assistance, and many are able to work at simple jobs.

Classification of Mental Retardation Syndromes

Mental retardation syndromes are commonly classified on the basis of prenatal, perinatal, and postnatal causes.

A. Prenatal Causes: Prenatal causes have traditionally been categorized as chromosomal (sex chromosome abnormalities and autosomal anomalies), biochemical (metabolic abnormalities), environmental (acquired prenatal conditions), and of unknown origin. However, there is some overlap in these categories.

1. Sex chromosome abnormalities—These abnormalities, which range from the absence of a sex chromosome (XO) to the presence of multiple sex chromosomes (eg, XXXXY), are often accompanied by mental retardation. In **Turner's syndrome** (45,XO karyotype), findings include sterility and, occasionally, retardation. **Klinefelter's syndrome** (XXY) occurs in one in 1100 male births and is characterized by sterility, gynecomastia, and neurodevelopmental abnormalities. Findings in the **XYY chromosome complement syndrome** are controversial; some researchers have reported an increased incidence of retardation, tall stature, and delinquency, but these data have not been validated.

2. Autosomal anomalies—

a. Down's syndrome—The most frequent genetic disorder causing mental retardation is Down's syndrome, first described as "mongolism" in 1866. The incidence is one in 700 births, and about 10% of institutionalized retarded patients have Down's syndrome.

Three distinct chromosomal types of Down's syndrome have been identified: (1) The best-known type, **trisomy 21** (nearly 95% of cases), results when nondisjunction of chromosomes 21 occurs during meiosis. The complete descendant cell line has 3 chromosomes 21, or a total of 47 chromosomes in each cell of the body. The incidence is directly related to maternal age (and according to some research, paternal age). The risk of giving birth to an infant with trisomy 21 is less than 0.2% in women under 35 years of age; about 0.9% in those 35–40 years; 1.4% in those 40–45 years; and 2.5% in those over 45. (2) The second major form, the **translocation type,** is caused by fusion of 2 chromosomes, usually 21 and 15. The total number of chromosomes is 46 because the extra chromosome (or part of one) is fused to another. The abnormal chromosome can be found in an otherwise unaffected father, mother, or sibling. This type occurs at any maternal age; it is heritable; and, once present, subsequent pregnancies of the same parents are theoretically at an increased risk of about 33%, although empirically the risk is approximately 20%. For this reason, the parents of any child wih Down's syndrome should be given genetic counseling. (3) **Mosaicism,** the least frequent type of Down's syndrome, is caused by nondisjunction of chromosome 21 after fertilization during any of the early mitoses, which results in a "mosaic" of both normal and trisomic cell lines.

Down's syndrome has been extensively studied. Mental retardation, its cardinal feature, can be present to any degree—from profound retardation (IQ below 20) to borderline normal intelligence (IQ of 71–84). When the IQ scores of patients with Down's syndrome

are plotted on a graph, the scores form a normal distribution curve (gaussian curve) between 0 and 100, with the mean at the high end of the moderately retarded range (IQ of 35–49). Thus, while the characteristic clinical features of the syndrome (see below) make it easily diagnosable at birth, the future intellectual and social functioning cannot be predicted with certainty at that time. Appropriate medical support and immediate enrollment of the parents and child in an infant development program are recommended to ensure optimal early development.

Although the full syndrome description includes over a hundred features and numerous medical complications, it should be emphasized that only some of the features will be seen in any one individual and that the physician's approach to a given family must strike a properly informed note—neither too pessimistic nor too optimistic. Besides the chromosome findings and some degree of retardation, characteristic features include epicanthal folds, oblique palpebral fissures, high cheekbones (hence the term "mongolism"), a large and protruding tongue, microcephaly, anteroposterior flattening of the skull, broad and thick hands, shortened and rounded small ears, and hypotonic musculature. Many patients have a single transverse palmar ("simian") crease that was originally thought to be pathognomonic of the syndrome but is seen in many other retardation syndromes and in nonretarded people as well. Biochemical studies have revealed abnormal blood platelet levels of sodium and potassium, of the enzyme adenosine triphosphatase, and of the content and rate of uptake of serotonin into platelets. Patients with Down's syndrome are more susceptible to infections in childhood, have a 30–50% incidence of congenital heart defects, and have an increased incidence of cataracts, diabetes mellitus, seizures, thyroid disorders, and acute lymphocytic leukemia.

b. Trisomy 18 and trisomy 13—The incidence of trisomy 18 is one in 5000 live births, while that of trisomy 13 is one in 5000–10,000 live births. These retardation syndromes occur by the same genetic mechanisms as trisomy 21 but are associated with higher death rates both pre- and postnatally. Subsequent offspring of parents of children with these syndromes have an estimated 1% risk of having the syndrome.

c. Other genetic disorders—Many other disorders that can result in retardation are caused by an **autosomal dominant gene:** tuberous sclerosis and neurofibromatosis (see below); skull abnormalities (craniosynotosis, hypertelorism); connective tissue disorders (Marfan's syndrome); kidney disorders (nephrogenic diabetes insipidus); etc.

The severity and prognosis of **tuberous sclerosis (epiloia, Bourneville's disease)** are highly variable. Diagnosis is often made when hypomelanotic "ash leaf" patches (often mistaken for vitiligo) are found. Pringle's spots (resembling adenoma sebaceum) may be diffuse on the body and prominent over the malar area of the face. Multiple nodules of glial tissue are found throughout the brain, and retinal involvement and cardiorespiratory complications may occur. Mental retardation can be mild to profound, with or without psychotic symptoms. Mild forms of the disorder may present with skin lesions and epilepsy and often carry a good prognosis.

Skin and central nervous system lesions are also the hallmarks of **neurofibromatosis (Recklinghausen's disease).** Findings vary but may include small brown skin patches (café au lait spots) over the entire body, skin polyps, multiple benign tumors of the brain, and seizures. Mild to moderate retardation occurs in about 10% of patients.

About a third of the population carry an **autosomal recessive gene** for severe mental retardation; it is estimated that there are 114 such gene loci. Several maldevelopments of the skull and brain result from these: **anencephaly,** an absence of parts of the brain and skull, which is usually fatal; **hydranencephaly,** a disorder in which the cranium is filled with fluid instead of brain tissue; **porencephaly,** the presence of cavities or large fluid-filled cysts in the brain; **microcephaly,** abnormal smallness of the head; and **hydrocephalus,** a disorder in which an excess of cerebrospinal fluid causes increased intracranial pressure, destruction of brain tissue, and resulting neurologic problems. The latter 2 disorders may be due to a variety of different causes.

3. Metabolic abnormalities—These are caused primarily by endocrine disorders or by recessive gene abnormalities. Although the inborn errors of metabolism represent fewer than 10% of all known hereditary defects, they provide highly useful models for research into diagnosis, treatment, and prevention. The first described retardation syndrome due to a metabolic abnormality was **goitrous cretinism.** All forms of mental retardation were called cretinism until other syndromes began to be identified in the 19th century. Today the term refers to **hypothyroidism** and the resulting mental dullness, caused by various hypofunctions of the thyroid gland due to faulty hormone synthesis. Maternal hypothyroidism due to iodine deficiency in certain regions (endemic goiter) also results in hypothyroidism in infants.

a. Disorders of amino acid metabolism—The best-known example of the inborn metabolic errors is **phenylketonuria,** which has an incidence of one in 15,000. The disorder is due to a deficiency or defect in the liver enzyme phenylalanine hydroxylase, which gives rise to a series of biochemical abnormalities starting with accumulation of ingested phenylalanine (an essential amino acid) in the body. Most patients have severe mental retardation (some have normal intelligence), a small head and body, coarse features, and light complexion. Children with phenylketonuria exhibit the full range of disturbed behaviors associated with severe brain damage. Early diagnosis is essential, since brain damage can be prevented if a diet low in phenylalanine is started before 6 months of age; near normal intelligence is preserved if dietary treatment is begun by 3 months of age. Since phenylalanine is an essential amino acid, use of the special diet must be accompanied by regular follow-up evaluations. Many patients continue without mental impairment if the diet is stopped at 6 years of age, but some must remain on the diet for life. Women with phenylketonuria, regardless of their mental status, must take a low-phenylalanine diet if they intend to carry a pregnancy to term. Newborn testing for phenylketonuria is now required by law in most states.

Lesch-Nyhan syndrome is a rare disorder characterized by severe retardation and self-mutilation of the lips and fingers by biting. It is transmitted as an X-linked recessive trait, resulting in deficiency of the enzyme hypoxanthine-guanine phosphoribosyl-transferase. This deficiency produces a 20-fold increase in serum uric acid levels (5 times higher than in patients with gout). Thus, patients with Lesch-Nyhan syndrome also have gout and its complications (renal calculi, tophi) in addition to cerebral palsy, choreoathetosis, mental retardation, and the self-destructive biting that can only be partially controlled with firm physical restraints. Treatment for gout has no effect on the cerebral manifestations of this disorder.

b. Disorders of fat metabolism—These disorders include several genetically determined lipidoses that can be classified for convenience into 2 groups: (1) those resulting in accumulation of lipids in the central nervous system; and (2) those characterized by a decrease in central nervous system lipids, resulting in demyelination. (Enlargement of the liver and spleen is also seen in some lipid storage diseases.)

Tay-Sachs disease, the best-known example of the lipid storage diseases, is also called the *infantile* form of cerebromacular degeneration, in which the accumulation of lipids (gangliosides) produces a cherry-red spot on the retina in addition to the central nervous system degeneration. The disease begins at age 4–8 months and results in death by 2–4 years. The *late infantile* form, called **Bielschowsky-Jansky disease,** starts at 2–4 years of age and results in progressive dementia, with death in a few years. The *juvenile* form, **Spielmeyer-Vogt disease** (also termed Stock-Spielmeyer-Vogt syndrome and Batten-Mayou disease), usually begins with visual impairment at 5 or 6 years of age, progressing to blindness and mental deterioration over 10–15 years. The *late juvenile* form, **Kufs' disease,** is the rarest; it occurs after age 15. Although there is no treatment for Tay-Sachs disease, its occurrence is preventable by screening (through blood tests) for carriers of the recessive gene, which is found in about 4% of Eastern Europeans of Jewish ancestry.

Two other types of cerebromacular degeneration, both of autosomal recessive origin, occur primarily in Jewish children: **Niemann-Pick disease** is similar to Tay-Sachs disease except for the type of lipids that accumulate (sphingomyelins instead of gangliosides); it results in death by 4 years of age. **Gaucher's disease** has an acute infantile form, fatal in the first year of life, and an insidious form that occurs in adolescents and young adults and causes chronic physical handicaps. In Gaucher's disease, the accumulated lipids are glucocerebrosides.

There are several demyelinating lipid disorders, including **metachromatic leukodystrophy** and the **progressive leukoencephalopathies,** all of which result in neurologic degeneration.

c. Disorders of carbohydrate metabolism— Two major types bear mention here: (1) **Galactosemia** results from an inborn absence or deficiency of the enzyme galactose-1-phosphate uridyltransferase. This enzyme is necessary for the metabolism of galactose (found in milk), and its absence results in progressive mental deterioration, cataracts, and hepatic insufficiency. Normal development is possible if a galactose-free diet is started in early infancy. (2) There are many types of **glycogen storage diseases.** Type I is caused by a deficiency of the enzyme glucose-6-phosphatase, which results in accumulation of glycogen in the liver. Liver failure, mental retardation, and progressive deterioration in health follow. Type II, which causes death in infancy, is a defect in α-1,4-glucosidase (acid maltase).

4. Acquired prenatal conditions— Mental retardation may result from exposure of the fetus to (1) **toxic agents** (teratogenic medications; maternal drug abuse, including alcohol intake even in moderation); (2) **infectious diseases** such as rubella (preventable with immunization), toxoplasmosis, and cytomegalovirus inclusion disease (the most frequent viral cause of retardation) as well as other maternal diseases; and (3) maternal **malnutrition.**

B. Perinatal Causes: Causes of mental retardation associated with the birth process include prematurity; anoxia due to birth injuries or hemorrhage; brain damage from mechanical trauma; and infections (eg, herpes simplex) acquired by the infant during passage through the birth canal.

C. Postnatal Causes: This very large category includes traumatic, metabolic, infectious, toxic, and other causes of brain damage; accidents; hemorrhages (eg, from ruptured aneurysm, coagulation defects); hypothyroidism; encephalitis; meningitis; ingestion of lead or mercury; exposure to carbon monoxide, post-immunization encephalopathies (rabies, pertussis, smallpox); kernicterus from blood incompatibilities or other hemolytic diseases; etc.

Genetic Counseling & Prenatal Diagnosis

According to Rudolph (1982), "Genetic counseling is a multifaceted technique with medical, genetic, and psychological components and has as one of its principal objectives informed decision-making by patients . . . and families." The professional's goal is not to impose a policy of prevention of specific kinds of genetic disease on the parents but rather to provide them with information so they can understand their risks and make their own decisions.

In prenatal genetic diagnosis, techniques such as amniocentesis and ultrasonography are performed to determine whether the fetus is affected by genetic diseases for which it is thought to be at risk. In **amniocentesis,** about 15 mL of amniotic fluid is removed from the uterus after a local anesthetic is applied to the site of needle insertion. The procedure takes about 10 minutes. Most centers recommend that women under age 35 (some say under age 37) should not have amniocentesis unless a possibility of genetic disease is disclosed by genetic counseling. The procedure is performed between the 15th and 18th weeks of gestation, but results may not be available until up to 4 weeks later. Test results are negative in 95% of women over age 35. About 100 biochemical disorders and a large number of chromosomal problems are detectable.

Fetal visualization and biopsy are becoming increasingly useful for the detection of fetal abnormalities that are not associated with biochemical or chromosomal disorders. During the past 15 years, **ultrasonography** has replaced roentgenography as a means of visualizing uterine contents. Ultrasonography makes it possible to detect physical anomalies and intrauterine growth problems and to determine gestational age. **Fetoscopy** allows for direct fetal visualization and also makes possible sampling of fetal blood to detect hemoglobinopathies. **Chorionic villus biopsy** is a promising new technique that allows testing of fetal cells (without harm to the fetus) during the first trimester of pregnancy.

REFERENCES

American Academy of Child Psychiatry: *Child Psychiatry: A Plan for the Coming Decades.* American Academy of Child Psychiatry, 1983.

American Association on Mental Deficiency: *Manual on Terminology and Classification in Mental Retardation.* Grossman H (editor). American Association on Mental Deficiency, 1977.

American Psychiatric Association: *Diagnostic and Statistical Manual Disorders (DSM-III),* 3rd ed. American Psychiatric Association, 1980.

American Psychiatric Association: *Diagnostic and Statistical Manual of Mental Disorders (DSM-III-R),* 3rd ed. (Revised). American Psychiatric Association, 1987.

Anthony EJ: The behavioral disorders. In: *Carmichael's Manual of Child Psychology.* Mussen PH (editor). Wiley, 1970.

Erikson EH: *Childhood and Society.* Norton, 1962.

Fetal effects of maternal alcohol use. (Council report.) *JAMA* 1983;**249:**2517.

Fraiberg S: *Insights From the Blind.* Basic Books, 1977.

Group for the Advancement of Psychiatry (GAP), Committee on Child Psychiatry: *Psychopathological Disorders in Childhood.* Jason Aronson, 1974.

Helfer RE, Kempe CH: *The Battered Child.* Univ of Chicago Press, 1974.

Jersild AT, Markey FV, Jersild CL: *Children's Fears, Dreams,*

Wishes, Daydreams, Likes, Dislikes, Pleasant and Unpleasant. Columbia Univ Press, 1933.

Kanner L: *Child Psychiatry.* 4th ed. Thomas, 1972.

Kanner L: *Childhood Psychosis: Initial Studies and New Insights.* Winston/Wiley, 1973.

Kempe CH, Helfer RE: *Helping the Battered Child and His Family.* Lippincott, 1972.

Kempe CH, et al: The battered child syndrome. *JAMA* 1962;**181**:17.

Knobloch H, Pasamanick B: Mental subnormality. (3 parts.) *N Engl J Med* 1962;**266**:1045,1092,1155.

Kolvin I: Psychoses in childhood: A comparative study. Pages 7–26 in: *Infantile Autism: Concepts, Characteristics, and Treatment.* Rutter M (editor). Churchill Livingstone, 1971.

Lane H: *The Wild Boy of Aveyron.* Harvard Univ Press, 1976.

Langner TS et al: Children of the city: Affluence, poverty, and mental health. In: *Psychological Factors in Poverty.* Allen VL (editor). Markham, 1970.

Lewis DO et al: Conduct disorder and its synonyms: Diagnoses of dubious validity and usefulness. *Am J Psychiatry* 1984; **141**:514.

Marinelli RP, Dell Orto AE: *The Psychological and Social Impact of Physical Disability.* Springer, 1977.

McDermott JF, Harrison SI: *Psychiatric Treatment of the Child.* Jason Aronson, 1977.

Meadow KP: *Deafness and Child Development.* Univ of Calif Press, 1980.

Milunsky A: *The Prevention of Genetic Disease and Mental Retardation.* Saunders, 1975.

National Center on Child Abuse and Neglect: *Child Sexual Abuse: Incest, Assault, and Sexual Exploitation.* US Government Printing Office, Department of Health and Human Services Publication No. (OHDS) 81-30166, Washington DC, 1981.

Noshpitz JD (editor): *Basic Handbook of Child Psychiatry.* Basic Books, 1979.

Piaget J: *The Origins of Intelligence in Children.* Internat Univ Press, 1953.

Rudolph AM: *Pediatrics.* Appleton-Century-Crofts, 1982.

Rutter M, Hersov L: *Child Psychiatry: Modern Approaches,* 2nd ed. Blackwell, 1985.

Rutter M et al: Isle of Wight studies, 1964–1974. *Psychol Med* 1976;**6**:313.

Steinhauer PD, Rae-Grant Q: *Psychological Problems of the Child in the Family.* Basic Books, 1983.

Section IV. Treatment Modalities

Introduction to Psychiatric Treatment

42

Howard H. Goldman, MD, PhD

The biopsychosocial model provides a framework that is useful for thinking about psychiatric therapeutics and consistent with current understanding of the etiology and pathogenesis of the mental disorders. Biomedical and psychosocial factors in illness suggest biomedical and psychosocial treatments; biomedical and psychosocial problems need appropriate commensurate solutions. Specific interventions at the biologic, psychologic, and social levels are organized into mental health services and specialty practices that are further organized into the mental health services system (described in Chapter 13).

Earlier chapters have presented each of the mental disorders and included a discussion of treatment. Although specific treatments are discussed, details are not provided. Despite increased specificity of therapy in psychiatry, much treatment remains nonspecific: various discussion-oriented psychotherapies, behavioral interventions, social casework, and drug treatments targeted on problems, symptoms and signs (eg, anxiety), and syndromes (eg, major depression). The chapters in the final section of *Review of General Psychiatry* present the diversity of psychiatric treatments and specialized areas of psychiatric intervention.

The psychotherapies are presented first, beginning with psychoanalysis and long-term dynamic psychotherapy (Chapter 43), followed by brief dynamic psychotherapy (Chapter 44), existential approaches to therapy (Chapter 45), behavior and cognitive therapy (Chapter 46), and group, family, and marital therapy (Chapters 47–49). Chapter 50 discusses psychotherapy in patients with chronic medical conditions, and Chapter 51 presents material on behavioral medicine techniques in general medical practice.

Chapters 52–54 present details on psychopharmacologic approaches to treatment in psychiatry and general medicine. The drugs are grouped according to their target effects. Antipsychotic drugs (neuroleptics) and antimanic drugs are discussed together in Chapter 52. The antidepressant drugs are presented in Chapter 53 and the sedative-hypnotics and antianxiety drugs in Chapter 54. Some drugs are discussed twice because they have multiple effects. These chapters include material on drug chemistry as well as on their indications, contraindications, interactions, side effects, dosage and administration, and monitoring.

The final 6 chapters deal with special interventions in psychiatry. Chapters 55 and 56 are concerned with consultation/liaison psychiatry: Chapter 55 presents an overview of the theories of psychiatric consultation in community mental health practice; Chapter 56 deals with consultation/liaison psychiatry in the general hospital. Child psychiatry is discussed in Chapter 57; legal or forensic psychiatry in Chapter 58. Chapter 59 concerns psychiatric emergencies, focusing on suicide and violence. Occupational psychiatry and the problems of the workplace, retirement, and disability are discussed in Chapter 60.

MISCELLANEOUS TREATMENTS

There are several miscellaneous treatments not presented separately in the text but mentioned occasionally in other chapters. In general, they are controversial, either because of insufficient data on their efficacy, concerns about their safety, or evidence of their abuse. In the case of electroconvulsive therapy, public fear—heightened by abuses and past overuse of the therapy, as well as by its gothic associations with electric shocks and convulsions—has led to underutilization of this safe and effective treatment for major depressive disorder. A brief discussion of electroconvulsive therapy and other organic therapies is included below.

Electroconvulsive Therapy (ECT)*

Electroconvulsive therapy causes a central nervous system seizure (peripheral convulsion is not necessary) by means of electric current. The key objective is to exceed the seizure threshold, which can be accomplished by a variety of means. Electrical stimulation is more reliable and simpler than the use of chemical convulsants such as pentylenetetrazol (Metrazol) or hexafluorodiethyl ether (flurothyl; Indoklon). The mechanism of action is not known, but it is thought to involve major neurotransmitter responses at the cell membrane. Current insufficient to cause a grand mal seizure produces no therapeutic benefit and causes more postictal confusion.

Electroconvulsive therapy, which is effective in

---

* This section is contributed by James J. Brophy, MD.

70% of patients treated, is the most effective treatment for severe depression, particularly depression with psychotic ideation and agitation commonly seen in the involutional period. Comparative controlled studies of electroconvulsive therapy in severe depression show that it is slightly more effective than chemotherapy. It is also very effective in the manic disorders. It has not been shown to be helpful in chronic schizophrenic disorders, and it is generally not used in acute schizophrenic episodes unless drugs are not effective and it is urgent that the psychosis be controlled (eg, a catatonic stupor complicating an acute medical condition).

Before electroconvulsive therapy is administered, a history and physical examination are performed, along with indicated laboratory tests. Lateral spine films and an electroencephalogram are frequently done, particularly in elderly patients. Occasionally, the electroencephalogram will reveal a clinically silent intracranial lesion that may be a factor in the depression and is a contraindication to electroconvulsive therapy. The patient should not eat or drink for at least 8 hours before treatment. Dentures are removed prior to electroconvulsive therapy. An empty bladder is desirable because of incontinence resulting from the seizure. Atropine sulfate, 0.6–1 mg intramuscularly, is given for its vagolytic effect. A short-acting barbiturate such as methohexital, 40–70 mg, is given carefully intravenously (extravasation is irritating to tissues) to cause unconsciousness. Succinylcholine, 30–60 mg intravenously, will produce a flaccid paralysis, and the anesthesiologist can then administer 100% oxygen from the onset of unconsciousness until spontaneous respiration resumes. Succinylcholine is contraindicated if the patient is using echothiophate iodide for glaucoma, since the latter is absorbed in amounts sufficient to interfere with the hydrolysis of succinylcholine and can thus precipitate prolonged apnea. Chronic renal dialysis, excessive supported ventilation, and congenital pseudocholinesterase deficiency may also result in prolonged apnea. Patients taking lithium tend to have more confusion and memory disturbances after electroconvulsive therapy is given than patients who are not receiving this drug.

Placement of electrodes may be bitemporal or unilateral on the nondominant side. The latter is considered to produce less impairment of memory, although it may be slightly less effective and require more than the usual 9–12 treatments. Electroconvulsive therapy may be performed every few days (3 per week is usual), or all of the treatments may be given in 1–3 sessions under electroencephalographic monitoring of seizure activity (multiple monitored electroconvulsive therapy).

A seizure usually lasts 5–20 seconds, with a brief postictal state. The patient can resume activity in about 1 hour. The most common side effects are memory disturbance and headache. Memory loss or confusion is usually related to number and frequency of electroconvulsive therapy treatments. Some memory loss is occasionally permanent, but most memory faculties return to full capacity within several weeks. There have been reports that lithium administration concurrent with electroconvulsive therapy resulted in greater memory loss. Before anesthesia was used, spinal compression fractures and severe anticipatory anxiety were common.

An intracranial lesion is a positive contraindication. Other problems such as cardiac disorders are not major contraindications and must be evaluated in light of the severity of the medical problem versus the need for electroconvulsive therapy. Serious complications arising from electroconvulsive therapy occur in fewer than one in 1000 cases. Most of these problems are cardiovascular or respiratory in nature (eg, aspiration of gastric contents). Inadequate patient education and lack of acceptance of the technique are the biggest obstacles to the use of electroconvulsive therapy.

Other Organic Therapies

Psychosurgery has a limited place in selected cases of severe, unremitting anxiety and depression, obsessional nonpsychotic disorders, and, to a lesser degree, some of the schizophrenias. The stereotactic techniques now being used, including modified bifrontal tractotomy, are great improvements over the crude methods of the past. In the controversial area of **megavitamin treatment** for the schizophrenic patient, the overall therapeutic efficacy of nicotinic acid or nicotinamide as the sole or adjuvant medication is no better than that of an inactive placebo. **Acupuncture** and **electrosleep,** while currently of interest, are of unproved usefulness for any psychiatric conditions.

REFERENCES

Abrams R: Clinical prediction of electroconvulsive therapy response in depressed patients. *Psychopharmacol Bull* (April) 1982;**18**:48.

Abrams R: Electroconvulsive therapy and tricyclic antidepressants in the treatment of endogenous depression. *Psychopharmacol Bull* (April) 1982;**18**:73.

American Psychiatric Association: *Electroconvulsive Therapy.* Task Force Report No. 14. American Psychiatric Association, 1978.

Avery D, Winokur G: The efficacy of electroconvulsive therapy and antidepressants in depression. *Biol Psych* 1977;**112**:507.

Blaine JD: Assessing the effects of electroconvulsive therapy: Critical research issues. *Psychopharmacol Bull* (Jan) 1982;**18**:27.

Brophy JJ: Psychiatric disorders. Chapter 17 in: *Current Medical Diagnosis & Treatment 1988.* Schroeder S, Krupp MA, Tierney LM Jr (editors). Appleton & Lange, 1988.

Fink M: Predictors of outcome in convulsive therapy. *Psychopharmacol Bull* (April) 1982;**18**:50.

Freeman CP, Basson JV, Crighton A: Double-blind controlled trial of electroconvulsive therapy (ECT) and simulated electroconvulsive therapy in depressive illness. *Lancet* 1978; **1**:738.

Gangadhar BN et al: Comparison of electroconvulsive therapy with imipramine in endogenous depression: A double-blind study. *Br J Psychol* 1982;**141**:367.

Grahame-Smith DG, Green AR, Costain DW: Mechanism of the antidepressant action of electroconvulsive therapy. *Lancet* 1978;**1**:254.

Kendell RE: The present status of electroconvulsive therapy. *Br J Psychol* 1981;**139**:265.

Lerer B, Belmaker RH: Receptors and the mechanism action of electroconvulsive therapy. *Biol Psychol* 1982;**17**:497.

O'Connell RA: A review of the use of electroconvulsive therapy. *Hosp Community Psychiatry* 1982;**33**:469.

Small JG, Small IF: Electroconvulsive therapy update. *Psychopharmacol Bull* (Oct) 1981;**17**:29.

Squire LR, Slater PC: Electroconvulsive therapy and complaints of memory dysfunction: A prospective three-year follow-up study. *Br J Psychol* 1983;**142**:1.

Vlissides DN, Jenner FA: The response of endogenously and reactively depressed patients to electroconvulsive therapy. *Br J Psychol* 1982;**141**:239.

Weiner RD et al: Evaluation of the central nervous system risk of electroconvulsive therapy. *Psychopharmacol Bull* (Jan) 1982;**18**:29.

Welch CA et al: Efficacy of electroconvulsive therapy in the treatment of depression: Wave form and electrode placement considerations. *Psychopharmacol Bull* (Jan) 1982;**18**:31.

43 Psychoanalysis & Long-Term Dynamic Psychotherapy*

Robert S. Wallerstein, MD

Sigmund Freud said of psychoanalysis that it was 3 things:

(1) A theory of how the mind works. Psychoanalysis attempts to comprehend and explain the normal and the abnormal functioning of the human mind at all ages. Many of the central psychoanalytic concepts—the unconscious, psychic determinism, infantile sexuality and the theory of drives, the Oedipus complex, ambivalence, anxiety, the defense mechanisms, psychic conflict, the structure of the mind or of the psychic apparatus—form a body of scientific knowledge that has now become part of our intellectual heritage. (See Chapters 2 and 3.) In 1947, Ernst Kris summarized psychoanalysis as a theory of the mind most tersely: Psychoanalysis is *"nothing but* human behavior considered from the standpoint of conflict. It is the picture of the mind divided against itself with attendant anxiety and other dysphoric affects, with adaptive and maladaptive defensive and coping strategies, and with symptomatic behaviors when the defenses fail." However, psychoanalysis is more than a theory of the mind and behavior.

(2) An investigative or research method. The technique of free association by the patient (analysand) makes it possible for the analyst to gain access to the data and processes of mental life, conscious or otherwise and rational or not. The data thus retrieved are made coherent and intelligible according to the theory of psychoanalysis. As Otto Fenichel said in 1941, it is the phenomenal data of psychoanalysis that may be irrational; the method and the theory are rational.

(3) A specific form of therapy of mental illness. Psychoanalysis uses free association to obtain data in the form of thoughts, feelings, memories, fantasies, and dreams and then proceeds to order and comprehend them within the framework of psychoanalytic theory. Through interpretation of psychic data, leading to insight and "working through," the treatment process is carried progressively forward.

Dynamic psychotherapy—also called psychodynamic therapy, psychoanalytic psychotherapy, or psychoanalytically oriented psychotherapy—is intensive psychologic therapy based on psychoanalytic theory but without the specific technique of free association. A variety of techniques are employed, including interpretation, to treat patients not considered suitable candidates for psychoanalysis.

Both psychoanalysis and the psychoanalytic psychotherapies described in this chapter are "open-ended," ie, protracted therapies that may continue for many years. At the start of therapy, a pact is made between the analyst, or therapist, and the analysand, or patient, to explore the patient's psychologic problems for as long as necessary in order to achieve an acceptable result. This is in contrast to short-term or brief (time-limited) psychotherapy (described in Chapter 44), which usually consists of 12 or 20 weekly or twice-weekly sessions of 50 minutes each. The critical difference between psychoanalysis and short-term therapy is not only the difference in duration, important as that is, but also the fact that the patient in time-limited psychotherapy is conscious of the agreed termination date from the first session and knows that what is to be done must be achieved by that deadline. One consequence is that the patient may be tempted, consciously or not, to withhold painful areas from therapeutic scrutiny—to be "saved by the bell," as it were. If open-ended therapy is to be completed successfully, whatever is not talked about now or next week will come out later, because treatment continues until all of the relevant psychologic issues and problems are explored and resolved to the extent that is possible, however long it takes. Long-term and open-ended therapy is thus quite different in important ways from short-term (time-limited) therapy and not just the same kind of thing for more hours.

PSYCHOANALYSIS

Psychoanalysis is a process of examination in continuity of the internal working of the mind on a day-to-day basis. On each successive day, the analyst and the

---

* This chapter is an edited version of a more comprehensive and detailed treatment of the subject matter prepared by Dr Wallerstein for publication elsewhere. The editor is grateful for permission to adapt it for *Review of General Psychiatry*.–HHG.

patient can pick up where they left off and go from there. Ideally, this process would go forward 7 days a week for an hour each day. (This became the "50-minute hour" to allow analysts time between patients in which to order their thoughts, make notes, and get ready for the next patient.) However, because analysts and their patients want weekends for other things, the analytic work week is the traditional 5 working days, and Freud often complained of the "Monday crust"—the sealing over of open mental surfaces during the weekend, so that the first task on Monday would be to reestablish the continuity of daily exploration. Because of the limited availability of qualified analysts and the need to accommodate more patients, analyses are now conducted 4 days a week in some settings. Most analysts do not consider fewer than 4 days a week proper psychoanalysis, because the vital element of continuity does not survive longer or more frequent interruptions. Ideally, each session is scheduled at the same time each day so that the analysis can blend into the rhythm of the patient's life.

In classic psychoanalysis, the patient is recumbent on a couch with the analyst behind and out of the patient's line of vision. Intrusions, such as telephone calls, are avoided except in emergencies. The patient expressly undertakes to try to say whatever comes to mind no matter how seemingly remote, irrelevant, trivial, repugnant, anxiety-provoking, or shameful (the "fundamental rule"). The patient agrees to refrain from motor activity so that all available energy can be channeled into the effort to verbalize mental content. The analyst decides when and how to interject questions and comments; no attempt is made to sustain a conversational dialogue. The analyst must unswervingly focus attention on the effort to track the shifting subject matter of the patient's discourse and keep personal concerns, prejudices, values, and judgments out of the analytic field. The purpose is to gain and maintain full access to the contents of the patient's mind, conscious and unconscious, now and in the remote past and even to infancy if that can be achieved. Dreams, fantasies, wishes, fears, thoughts, and feelings of all kinds are discussed in the analysis. What is experienced by people practicing or undergoing psychotherapy is that "one thing leads to another." The patient focuses on his or her mental processes and free-associates in what is apparently a random manner. The analyst apprehends what the patient verbalizes by a counterpart process of "free-floating attention" without preconceptions about what is important or what the relationships are between various items of content.

It is within this "regressive" analytic process that the patient's mental life, including its conflictual matter, slowly begins to emerge around the figure of the analyst. Long-forgotten (repressed) feelings, traumas, and reaction patterns, along with active or discarded defensive or adaptive strategies, all eventually "come out again" in the interaction with the analyst, and what results is called the **transference.** The psychic past is reenacted in the analytic present. It is recognized and interpreted via the inappropriateness of the patient's present (transference) reactions and feelings to the reality of the ongoing interaction with the analyst. The complete revival of the past in the present is called the "regressive transference neurosis." Through the systematic interpretation of these complex transference phenomena, unresolved problems from the past are reworked, more adaptive solutions are found, and maladaptive, neurotic solutions are discarded. In the course of analysis, patients "rewrite" their autobiographies and along the way shed the neurotic symptoms and the problems that brought them to treatment in the first place.

Success in psychoanalysis relies essentially on skillful interpretation leading to enlarging insights. The analyst helps the patient see connections between unconscious wishes and beliefs and conscious speech and behavior. Slowly, patients begin to understand their own mental scheme of things. Symbolic meanings and mental connections begin to take on plausible configurations that "make sense." The insights gained are then "worked through" repeatedly as they reappear in other contexts as long as the analysis continues.

In a classic 1954 paper, Edward Bibring described 5 essential psychotherapeutic techniques: abreaction (catharsis), suggestion, manipulation, clarification, and interpretation. Different combinations of these techniques characterize the different psychoanalytically based psychotherapies. Within psychoanalysis proper, interpretation is the central technique, and the others are deployed only to enhance interpretation. There is a vast literature on the nature of interpretation: the issues of tact and timing in making interpretations; what makes interpretations "mutative" (ie, able to effect change); the special nature of interpretations of the transference relationship; interpretations in the here and now as opposed to reconstructive interpretations of past (including infantile) matter; and the role of interpretation and insight in relation to behavioral change. This essentially is what is involved in the proper conduct of psychoanalysis.

Indications & Contraindications

Psychoanalysis has been called the treatment of choice for that narrow middle band of patients who come for psychiatric evaluation who are sick enough to need it and well enough to tolerate it (Gill, 1951). Most psychiatric patients have symptoms or problems in living that can be resolved to their satisfaction with less intensive or less prolonged therapies than analysis (including expressive and supportive psychotherapies and crisis-oriented and brief dynamic therapies). Patients who do not need the thoroughgoing life and character reconstruction that psychoanalysis offers include those with acute reactive illnesses, situational maladjustments, and various circumscribed symptom-neurotic and character-neurotic states. There are also many psychiatric patients who come to psychotherapy—often needing psychoactive drug management also—whose illnesses are more severe and who cannot tolerate the anxiety-provoking stresses of psychoanalysis. For patients with fragile or vulnerable "ego strength" (including a tenuous hold on reality), an effort at psychoanalysis per se can be psychologically disorganizing, with dangers of regressive, even psychotic swings, severe acting out, flight from treatment, or suicidal pressures. Such patients, who are deemed too ill for psychoanalysis and who need to be treated by other dynamic (more supportive) psychotherapies, include borderline and narcissistic patients, those with character disorders, addictive disorders, severe sexual disorders, those with character neuroses, and even some with severe and refractory symptom neuroses.

Of the patients who come for psychiatric evaluation and treatment, then, a narrow middle band are good candidates for analysis. There is controversy within the field between those who advocate "narrowing" versus those who advocate "widening" the scope of indications for psychoanalysis. From the perspective of a proponent of "narrowing," about 5% of those who come to psychiatric evaluation are suitable candidates for psychoanalysis. These are patients with classic symptom neuroses and moderate character neuroses set within the context of a "strong ego organization"—ie, they are not only amenable to psychoanalysis but able to tolerate it as well.

A. Benefits: Given the limited role of psychoanalysis in the treatment of neurotic disorders, it is proper to question both its social value and its scientific importance. Psychoanalysis is valuable and important in 3 areas: research, education, and treatment. As a research investigative technique, psychoanalysis affords access to the innermost workings of the mind and to knowledge of psychologic development, character formation, and normal and abnormal mental processes. Knowledge about mental functioning derived from psychoanalytic research forms the basis of the theory of psychoanalysis as a comprehensive theory of the mind. Out of this theory have evolved the specific therapeutic applications of both psychoanalysis and the psychoanalytically based dynamic psychotherapies.

As an educational tool, the personal analysis of the therapist—required for those who seek certification as psychoanalytic practitioners and often sought by those who seek enhanced professional effectiveness as dynamic psychotherapists—is necessary to provide successive generations of clinicians best qualified to offer these therapeutic resources to patients who need them. As specific treatment for that small number of patients for whom it is indicated, psychoanalysis offers the best hope—not always realized—for the thoroughgoing resolution of neurotic problems and for fundamental character reconstruction. Since individuals in analysis are often in positions of responsibility, making decisions that affect others, the social value of the technique is apparent.

B. Limitations: Those who would widen the scope of indications for psychoanalysis feel that because the therapeutic goal of psychoanalysis is fundamental personality reorganization, the results when it succeeds are more complete and enduring than can be achieved with less ambitious forms of therapy. Over the years, psychoanalysis has therefore been extended and modified to treat broader categories of patients, including children and adolescents (Melanie Klein, Anna Freud)—an extension that has by now become the established discipline of child and adolescent analysis—groups (Henry Ezriel, S. R. Slavson), delinquents (August Aichhorn), patients with psychosomatic disorders (Franz Alexander and many others), overtly psychotic patients (Harry Stack Sullivan, Frieda Fromm-Reichmann), narcissistic characters (Heinz Kohut and others), and patients with borderline personality disorders (Otto Kernberg). The movement to extend the indications for analysis to more kinds of mental disorders was reviewed by Leo Stone in 1954 in a widely cited article on the widening scope of psychoanalysis. Anna Freud (1954), in discussing that paper, undertook to spearhead the opposed trend toward narrowing the indications for analysis back to classically neurotic adults and children. Glover in 1954 divided patients for whom psychoanalysis might be the treatment of choice into 3 categories that he called the ideally suitable, the moderately suitable, and those for whom psychoanalysis was the last hope but a forlorn one. The patients in the third category had severe personality disorders and were to be offered analysis as a "heroic measure"—this was in the days before adjunctive pharmacotherapy was available. The concept of intensive psychoanalytic treatment for patients much sicker than those seen in the usual outpatient psychoanalytic practice was a major rationale for the psychoanalytic sanatorium (such as the Menninger Foundation), where treatment could be conducted in a protected milieu with total life management.

PSYCHODYNAMIC PSYCHOTHERAPY

The psychoanalytically based dynamic psychotherapies other than formal psychoanalysis have been divided conceptually into 2 types: expressive and supportive. These methods of treatment are available for that much larger population of psychiatric patients who are not candidates for psychoanalysis proper. Psychodynamic psychotherapy is a peculiarly American creation, now practiced worldwide. It was developed between World Wars I and II and refined as a coherent body of theory and technique in the decade after World War II when psychoanalytic theory became the dominant psychologic perspective of American psychiatrists. The expressive and supportive dynamic psychotherapies arose in pragmatic response to the treatment needs of the vast majority of patients who were not suitable candidates for psychoanalysis proper.

The dynamic psychoanalytically based psychotherapies are of 2 types: (1) those whose treatment aim is **expressive,** ie, to uncover (or make conscious) psychologic conflict through analyzing the patient's defenses and resistances and in this way to resolve conflict through interpretation, insight, and change motivated by insight; and (2) those whose aim is **supportive,** ie, to diminish the force of external (situational) or internal (instinctual, drive-related) pressures by a variety of ego-strengthening techniques. Supportive therapies thus increase the patient's capacity to suppress mentally painful conflict and its dysphoric or symptomatic expression, thereby effecting behavioral change and symptomatic relief through means other than interpretation and insight.

As useful as this expressive-supportive division is for heuristic, prescriptive, and prognostic purposes, it is also a misleading oversimplification. All psychiatric treatment that helps patients is supportive even when most uncompromisingly expressive, as in psychoanalysis. What could be more *supportive* than an open-ended psychoanalysis offered daily for as long as necessary, in which the patient is encouraged to express any kind or amount of verbal content and where the entire enterprise consists of 2 people whose energies and intellect are focused exclusively on the problems and concerns of the one? Or, as Herbert Schlesinger (1969) has reminded us, any treatment, no matter how supportive in the sense of strengthening defenses and suppressing unwanted conflict and symptom expression, must also be *expressive* of some aspect of the patient's concerns. The important question, according to Schlesinger, is not expressive versus supportive but rather *expressive of what?*—and when, and how, in regard to the patient's mental and emotional life—and *supportive of what?*—and when, and how, in regard to that same mental and emotional life. Indeed, in every therapeutic decision to foster the expression of some aspect of mental conflict and distress in whatever way, there is a tacit decision to avoid (ie, suppress) some other aspect of mental conflict and distress.

Whatever one thinks of these arguments, at the practical level of ongoing psychotherapy there has always been a useful distinction between therapeutic interventions that have a preponderantly expressive effect and those that have a preponderantly supportive effect. Paul Dewald in his 1964 book has presented in a systematic way every aspect of the psychotherapeutic process: (1) The beginning of the process and the establishment of the therapeutic situation and the "therapeutic contract." (2) The patient's role and activity and (3) the therapist's role and activity in the therapeutic process. (4) The handling of the transference. (5) The handling of manifestations of resistance, regression, and psychic conflict. (6) The role of insight and working through in bringing about change. (7) The emotional involvements of the therapist (the "counter-transference"). (8) The adjuvant role of psychoactive drugs. (9) The process of natural termination. All of the foregoing are discussed by Dewald from the contrasting perspectives of expressive and supportive psychotherapeutic approaches to each of these issues.

Techniques & Patient Selection

The dynamic psychotherapies, expressive or supportive, are quite similar to each other in procedural form and greatly different from the formal structure of the psychoanalytic interview. The patient sits in a chair facing the therapist, with the expectation of feedback and reciprocal exchange. Unlike psychoanalysis, where the burden is on the patient to keep saying whatever comes to mind while the analyst chooses when and how to intervene, in psychotherapy the format is more like a conversational exchange. The patient in psychotherapy has made no commitment to try to say everything that comes to mind without editorial revision or censorship. The patient has agreed only to present problems and distress for consideration as he or she feels able and willing to do, and no "fundamental rule" is violated by a decision to withhold specific items of mental content, either temporarily or permanently.

The frequency of weekly sessions with the therapist is more flexible in the case of psychotherapy, ranging from one to 3 or 4 sessions a week but most often once or twice a week. Unless some form of time-limited therapy is elected, the duration is open-ended, as with psychoanalysis. Although in practice psychotherapy is usually briefer in duration than psychoanalysis (1–2 years versus 3–5 years), it can continue for just as long and may even (unlike psychoanalysis) continue for the life of the patient. Such "therapeutic lifers" have consciously undertaken, out of need, to continue a supportive relationship with the therapist similar to the lifelong medical maintenance regimens required by diabetic patients, cardiac patients, and others with chronic and incurable but manageable disorders. In terms of total hours spent in therapy, the dynamic psychotherapies consume usually 50–200 hours as against, in analysis, 600–1000 hours. The treatment hour usually is 50 minutes, but in some sustained, essentially supportive psychotherapies, especially with schizoid and other individuals fearful of interpersonal intimacy, sessions are in some instances curtailed to no more than 30 minutes each. In both expressive and supportive therapies, at times of acute crisis or emergency, sessions may be extended as long as necessary—up to 2 hours or more. Occasionally in the psychotherapies, emergency weekend or evening sessions are held. Supportive treatment sessions may be scheduled less frequently than once a week, and the time may come—if the patient is seeing the therapist only once a month—when the sessions should be characterized as follow-up visits or "reporting in" rather than a continuing psychotherapeutic process.

In the psychotherapies (again in contrast to psychoanalysis), there is greater use of adjuvant drug management, coordination of care with the patient's family physician, telephone contacts, and involvement of third parties (family, employers, teachers, etc). All of these kinds of extra-session activities are more frequent the more supportive and the less expressive the particular psychotherapy is intended to be. Within this overall common structure, then, how do the technical interventions differ between the more expressive and the more suppportive psychotherapies?

1. EXPRESSIVE PSYCHOTHERAPY

Essentially, in expressive psychotherapy, with the patient free to bring up problems and anxieties in his or her own way, the therapeutic emphasis is on interpretation and insight and the objective is to bring about beneficial change by resolution of as much psychic conflict as possible. This is accomplished by uncovering unconscious conflicts and, by understanding, achieving mastery. These are to some extent the techniques of psychoanalysis but without free association, dream analysis, or deep discovery of infantile sources of current pain.

Expressive psychotherapy is the treatment of choice for persons with enough ego strength, intelligence, and anxiety tolerance to participate in therapy and serious but relatively circumscribed neurotic conflicts and symptoms—ie, individuals who need help but not the greater commitment implied by a decision to enter analysis. If such patients will assume responsibility for their character traits and their problems in living and are willing to look introspectively at the irrational aspects of their interpersonal relationships, significant help and change can be effected without the full-scale reconstructive effort required to uncover the infantile developmental roots of the neurotic personality development. For example, the issue is whether a patient with severe marital problems can be helped to resolve the problems without the need to recreate the earlier prototype, the infantile conflicts with the mother, repressed behind the childhood amnesia. In psychoanalysis, the aim is to pursue conflicts back to their infantile roots so they can be carefully *analyzed;* the aim of analytically oriented expressive psychotherapy is to *recognize* (and only partially to analyze) those same conflicts and use that recognition in therapy. Insight is achieved but only to the "depth" of the problem being addressed—it never penetrates to the unconscious infantile origins of the patient's original conflicts.

Expressive therapy is indicated for patients with problems similar to those treated in psychoanalysis—patients with classic symptom neuroses (dysthymic disorder, anxiety disorders) and the character neuroses (personality disorders). **Character neuroses** that cause problems in living (eg, rigidly compulsive or chronically depressive characters) and **symptom neuroses** (eg, characterized by irrational compulsions or bouts of depression) can at times blend into each other, or one may give way to the other.

The distinction between those who need psychoanalysis and those who can be treated by less intensive therapy is well illustrated by the example of psychotherapeutic work with a patient suffering from posttraumatic stress disorder (see Chapter 31). The therapeutic work would be limited to a defined sector of the individual's life and problems and directed toward the stresses precipitating the breakdown and enough of their underlying causes to permit resolution of the current conflict. Thus, in the case of the survivor of an accident, grief-stricken over his companion's death and feeling guilty because he himself luckily survived, the events surrounding the death, ambivalent (love? hate?) feelings about the companion, and perhaps even a parallel between the adult friendship and the conflictual sibling relationships of childhood might all come within the scope of the expressive therapeutic work. Therapy in this example probably would not explore earlier conflicts in the infantile relationship with the parents.

However, expressive psychotherapy need not be confined in this way to a specific area of difficulty. Expressive psychotherapy would include concern with characterologic problems and symptoms and their maladaptive roles in the patient's life but with the object only of working at the level of the individual's willingness and capacity to assume responsibility for their modification in the present without the need for the concomitant uncovering of their infantile roots. Such treatment can be long-term and can undertake to explore and modify the entire range of the patient's life adjustments, attitudes, and reactions.

Conflict resolution and symptomatic relief in expressive psychotherapy are made possible by the relative "autonomy" of the conflict in the present from its earlier infantile prototype, though clearly a developmental line can be traced from the present-day neurotic problem to the original pathogenic conflict. Success depends on the ability of the patient and therapist to resolve the conflict in the "here and now," without needing to explore its roots in infancy or its development from earlier neurotic relationships. Such relative autonomy of conflict is common enough so that there is a very large population of psychoneurotic patients who can use expressive dynamic psychotherapy. Since it is received dogma among psychiatrists generally that expressive (uncovering, interpretive) treatment is "better" because it presumably leads to changes that are more stable and better able to withstand adverse environmental pressures, the therapeutic tendency is fostered among practitioners of dynamic psychotherapy to—in the words of a popular training aphorism—"be as expressive as you can be and as supportive as you have to be."

2. SUPPORTIVE PSYCHOTHERAPY

It is easier to agree on and expound the indications for techniques of expressive psychotherapy than to explain when supportive psychotherapy is called for and how it should be managed. Expressive psychotherapy can be likened to a foreshortened analysis, and most interested people understand something about analysis even if they do not agree on when it should be used. Supportive psychotherapy, on the other hand, employs all manner of techniques and can be used in the management of all classes of patients not candidates for analysis or expressive psychotherapy.

In the early days of psychoanalysis, that method of treatment was acclaimed as the first successful scientific psychotherapy, in contrast to all preexisting therapies, which were viewed only as different types of suggestion therapy and therefore inherently unpredictable and unstable. Hypnosis was the prototype of such suggestive therapies. This view was expressed by Freud many times and was underlined forcefully by Edward Glover in 1931. As employed by nonanalytically trained practitioners, supportive psychotherapy is often conducted by giving heavy doses of common-sense reassurance, to the extent that this too, along with suggestion, came to be considered a hallmark of the supportive approach. This perception is misleading and oversimplified. Explicit reassurance is seldom comforting to patients with problems severe enough to bring them to a therapist's consulting room in the first place. In such instances, the effort to give reassurance may only convince the patient that the therapist simply does not understand the nature of the difficulty or does not want to hear about it.

What, then, does supportive therapy actually consist of? One of the earliest efforts to explain supportive psychotherapy was that of Merton Gill (1951), who identified 3 kinds of interventions that he felt "strengthened the defenses," in contrast with expressive approaches that undertook to uncover and interpret defenses as a step toward eventual integration. These explicitly supportive interventions are (1) to consistently encourage adaptive (and discourage maladaptive) combinations of impulse and defense expression, both behaviorally and symptomatically; (2) to deliberately refrain from interpreting defenses and character configurations, no matter how rigid or maladaptive, that are deemed essential to maintain functioning; and (3) to partially uncover some aspect of neurotic conflict (eg, within a troubled marriage or work situation) in order to reduce inner conflict that might be creating unwanted symptoms (eg, anxiety, depression, phobic avoidances). In this way the balance of psychic forces is altered, rendering repression of the core of neurotic conflict easier to accomplish. An example would be not exploring in detail the origin of a troubled marital or work situation in earlier ingrained patterns of interpersonal difficulty.

Bearing in mind the 5 therapeutic techniques listed by Bibring—abreaction, suggestion, manipulation, clarification, and interpretation—psychoanalysis could be described as utilizing mostly interpretation, with other techniques employed only when necessary to facilitate and enhance interpretation. Expressive psychotherapy could be described as depending to a large extent on interpretation but using clarification also and the other techniques as well. And supportive psychotherapy could be described as using all 5 techniques in whatever proportions seem to be called for by the specific needs of the patient, interpretation included.

Techniques of Supportive Psychotherapy

The principal common therapeutic ingredient of supportive psychotherapy is the evocation and firm establishment of a positive dependent emotional attachment to the therapist. Within this bond, the patient's emotional needs and wishes are allowed to achieve varying degrees of overt or covert (symbolic) gratifiation. In supportive therapy, the meanings and sources of the bond between the patient and the therapist are for the most part not interpreted or "analyzed."

This dependent emotional attachment seems, in turn, to be an essential precondition to the proper functioning of various other supportive mechanisms. It is also the basis of the so-called "transference cure," the willingness and capacity of the patient to reach therapeutic goals, change behavior and modes of living, and give up symptoms as something being done "for the therapist"—as the quid pro quo for the emotional gratifications received within the benevolent dependent attachment. Upon this base, then, other supportive devices are employed as indicated by the clinical needs of particular patients. If the dependent need for continued emotional gratification cannot be transferred (see below) or somehow either terminated or made therapeutically sustaining, it can be incorporated into a continuing and even unending therapeutic relationship.

These chronic maintenance supportive therapies may be employed over long periods in the management of vulnerable patients whose hold on reality is tenuous. Patients with comparable dependent tendencies but greater psychologic resources (eg, a greater capacity to identify with the therapist) are often able to terminate treatment, perhaps after a period of "weaning" as first advocated by Alexander and French (1946). These are patients who can identify successfully with the therapist and the therapist's approach toward and mastery of conflict pressures and can thus learn to go forward on their own.

Intermediate between those patients who can be helped to achieve reasonable psychologic autonomy by identification with the therapist and those for whom continued (perhaps lifelong) therapy is necessary are those whose attachments and the emotional gratifications derived therefrom can be "transferred" within the patient's now improved life situation. The transfer is usually made to the spouse, and the success of transfer depends not only on the effectiveness of the psychotherapeutic work within ongoing treatment but also on the capacity and willingness of the spouse to carry the transferred emotional burden indefinitely. Obviously, some patients will be more fortunate than others in the matter of availability of someone willing and able to accept such a burden.

Another useful supportive mechanism is to foster the displacement of the neurotic behavior into the therapeutic relationship so that its ill effects can be ameliorated in the "real life" of the patient. A typical example would be to encourage an unduly dependent and submissive patient to be more assertive outside treatment by allowing greater (covert) submissiveness to the therapist, which is experienced by the patient as requiring the altered (more assertive) external behaviors as the price of continuation of the dependent gratifications within the treatment. The success of this maneuver depends upon life circumstance, the reinforcing positive feedback, and enhanced self-esteem. Beneficial change stabilizes when the new behaviors bring real reward and gratification rather than neurotically anticipated disaster.

What has just been described are varieties of the "transference cure," whereby the patient "does what the therapist wants" in exchange for the satisfaction of emotional needs. The "antitransference cure" occurs when the patient makes changes not "for the therapist" but "against the therapist," ie, in the face of what are perceived as the therapist's contrary expectations, usually as an act of triumph over the therapist in the overt or covert treatment struggle. Such "cures," of course, must somehow be buttressed against their potential instability by enduring, beneficial real-life consequences.

The **"corrective emotional experience"** is a concept Alexander and French have invoked almost as the all-explanatory construct to elucidate the mechanism of action of supportive psychotherapy. Basically, this consists of deliberately responding to the patient's expressed emotional needs in a way that is different from what he or she has been led by accumulated life experiences to expect, with the effect of jarring entrenched patterns of neurotic (ultimately self-defeating) interactions. The concept can in a sense be applied to the entire range of supportive therapeutic techniques, since everything that goes on in psychotherapy is intended to function in one sense or another as a corrective emotional experience. However, the term is more useful if it is restricted to treatments whose central mechanism consists of interaction with a kindly, understanding, reality-oriented therapist able to absorb the patient's onslaughts and importunities in a spirit of benevolent neutrality without becoming entangled in the kind of interacting neurotic relationships the patient has used to maintain a life of suffering in the years before treatment was sought.

Reality testing and reeducation are related but differ in subtle ways from the corrective emotional experience in the conduct of supportive psychotherapy. Reality testing and reeducation consist of helping the patient who has difficulties in this area to distinguish internally derived expectations and fantasy from the external reality of the situation. Again, broadly speaking, they have a role in any type of psychotherapy, including psychoanalysis, but directly educational efforts by the therapist are more characteristic of psychotherapy when the therapeutic emphasis is in greater part supportive. The therapist gives advice, explains, and instructs the patient about what kinds of behavior are tolerable and expected in the community. The therapist must do all this in a way the patient perceives as nonjudgmental and, to the extent that the therapeutic intervention is coercive, as guided solely by the patient's well-being and best interests.

No purpose is served by trying to make a clear distinction between such educational activities and the steady provision of a corrective emotional experience. In both instances, the patient is taught the techniques

of reality-oriented problem solving and reality-corrected emotional responses on the basis of the "borrowed strength" derived from psychologic identification with the therapist in the role of helper and healer. Again, the stabilization of progress during and after treatment depends on positive reinforcement from the environment along with some measure of transfer of the attachments to the spouse or other stable life companion.

Another form of supportive psychotherapy involves the kind of life manipulation required by very ill patients who come to hospital, residential care, and day hospital settings—eg, the alcoholic, the drug addict, the acting-out or suicidal patient. In such cases, a major aspect of treatment involves the planned disengagement, temporarily or even at times permanently, from noxious life situations. For other patients, the opposite is true—ie, success can only be achieved if psychotherapy is conducted while contact with the patient's accustomed environment is maintained. With these patients, if the usual interacting life situation cannot be properly maintained, for whatever reason, the chances for an optimal result diminish, at times sharply.

Still another helping mechanism that can play a major role in supportive psychotherapy has been called the "collusive bargain." The "bargain" the therapist makes with the patient is to exempt specific problems, symptoms, and areas of personality malfunction from therapeutic scrutiny—leaving more or less consequential islands of maintained psychopathology—in return for the patient's willingness to make substantial changes in other areas. This is similar to the "transference cure," in the sense that the patient makes changes "for the therapist" in return for a specific reward—the shielding from therapeutic interference of a particularly tenacious or rewarding symptom or behavior. The success of such a maneuver depends on the value of the symptom or behavior to the patient as well as the patient's ability to detach the symptom or behavior from other problems or symptoms, which patient and therapist can then set about dealing with. For example, a homosexual patient with conflicts about professional achievement may decide with a therapist to discuss the professional life issues and to ignore or de-emphasize the life-style issues. Since the symptom or behavior "allowed" to the patient in this compromise solution is experienced as at least in some ways rewarding or gratifying, these particular therapeutic outcomes have a built-in stability.

Another technique available to patients who need supportive therapy is transfer of the attachment or dependency either to fortunate life circumstances (wealth, social or cultural advantage can play such a role) or to alternative psychologic supports. These may be selected by the patients, sometimes with the concurrence of the therapist. Alcoholics Anonymous and similar self-help groups are examples. In turning to external material or alternative psychologic supports for continuing emotional dependencies and gratifications, patients can sometimes save a failing or stalled therapeutic situation; ie, they can stabilize even if they cannot always enhance their level of psychologic functioning.

It should be clear from the foregoing that there are many ways in which psychotherapy can support and maintain improved psychologic functioning and additionally that ways can be built in to maintain such improvement in stable and enduring fashion. These techniques can be combined in various ways to meet the needs of specific patients—to form a basis for therapeutic "trades"; to replace maladaptive impulse-defense configurations with more adaptive (healthy) ones; to decide what to talk about and explore; and to decide specifically what *not* to talk about. Success in these endeavors may improve the patient's life situation; may help in the transfer of emotional attachments or in undertaking or disengaging from ongoing life context; and may provide positive reinforcements that result in enhanced self-esteem and more comfortable and rewarding life experiences.

Given this great variety of techniques available for supportive psychotherapy, it should be obvious that a high degree of skill and long experience are required by the therapist. This is contrary to the common misconception that more skill in psychodynamics is required to conduct expressive psychotherapy and that the supportive psychotherapists dispense mostly common sense, good will, and kindly reassurance. Actually, neither kind of psychotherapy involves less knowledge or skill than the other, though supportive psychotherapy calls for greater flexibility and permits or even requires a wider deployment of "extras" in ragard to the 2-person treatment situation, such as the use of adjuvant psychoactive drug management, contacts with third parties (including other treating physicians), and telephone or other contacts with the patient outside of scheduled sessions.

Indications

Supportive psychotherapy is the treatment of choice for a more diverse range of patients than expressive psychotherapy. It is indicated for some patients "not sick enough" for analysis and for the great majority of very ill patients considered too sick for analysis or *any* intensive expressive approach. The first category includes many patients who may be caught up in disruptive responses (anxiety, depressed affect, rage) to traumatic or otherwise disturbing situations—some grief reactions, acute anxiety states, adjustment disorders, etc. In some cases, expressive-interpretive activity is also indicated, but often there may be just a need to slow up, to take stock, to reassess the clinical situation and the therapeutic options, and to reintegrate, over time, to the best of one's coping or mastery potential. Supportive therapy in such cases usually is of shorter duration than expressive psychotherapy or psychoanalysis.

A larger category of patients for whom supportive psychotherapy is indicated are those much sicker individuals who require sustaining psychotherapeutic relationships, perhaps for life, and who respond slowly to the therapist's best efforts. Stability of psychologic functioning at the best achievable level is often the modest therapeutic goal, though at times the hope for cure should be pursued because greater success is sometimes possible. This group includes most patients with psychosis or severe personality disorders, severe addictions, alcoholism, sexual disorders, and acting-out, delinquent, and antisocial characters. In almost all of these cases, some degree of expressive therapeutic work can usually be done, but with difficulty because these patients have poor impulse control and low tolerance for anxiety and are vulnerable to regressive (psychotic or suicidal) swings in psychologic functioning and integrity. The eruption of a florid psychotic state is a potential danger that often cannot be ignored. Attempts at "widening the scope" of expressive therapy (including psychoanalysis) in an effort to do something for these much sicker patients (see p 508) have met with poor results.

ADDITIONAL ISSUES & CONTROVERSIES

Space limitations do not permit more than brief statements about 4 related major issues in this field.

The Importance of Diagnosis, Formulation, & Assessment

Some theorists and practitioners argue that diagnostic formulations are unnecessary in psychiatry and may even be damaging, since the treatment approaches available are declared to be essentially nonspecific. Even more, some argue that diagnostic "labeling" actually hurts the patient by serving as a source of self-fulfilling negative prophecies. Against these views it is argued here that by education and reason the pejorative connotations can be avoided and that diagnostic assessment is vital because we do have different ways of treating patients: in hospitals, daycare centers, or other sources of intermediate care; with drugs and other somatic therapies; with behavior therapies; and with different kinds of psychotherapy (expressive and supportive, long- and short-term).

Special Training for Psychotherapists

The well-rounded psychiatric residency will develop the skills required for a general psychiatric practice, including training in psychodynamic theory and in expressive and supportive dynamic psychotherapy. The most important vehicle of this training is individual supervision, and many psychiatric graduates seek continued supervision on a personal basis during their first years of independent practice. Some also seek personal therapy for professional reasons either during or after residency training. Specific training in psychoanalysis is available at psychoanalytic institutes where it can be pursued for additional years as a part-time activity built into an ongoing life of professional practice.

Personal psychoanalysis is required for certification as a clinical psychoanalyst, as is of course the conduct of psychoanalysis under individual supervision. Persons trained as clinical psychoanalysts usually find their effectiveness as psychotherapists greatly enhanced.

Social Issues: Cost & Availability

Psychotherapy is expensive because of the long-term commitment required and because of the inadequate reimbursement policies of governmental and private third-party payors for mental health care. With psychoanalysis proper, where treatment is longest and third-party reimbursement proportionately least, this problem is greatest. This has exposed psychotherapy and particularly psychoanalysis to the charge of being elitist treatments reserved for privileged classes. The problem is only partly solved by the existence of psychiatric clinics in medical schools and general hospitals, where low-cost or free psychotherapy is available, as well as the availability of low-cost psycho-analysis at low-cost treatment centers sponsored by psychoanalytic institutes. This was a problem of great concern to Freud, who in 1918 expressed a hope that psychoanalytic treatment would be made freely available to all who needed it and could profit by it by a society that undertook to provide total health care for its citizens.

Other Schools & Paradigms

The discussion of psychotherapies in this chapter has been within the framework of psychoanalytic (psychodynamic) theories of mental functioning. Other kinds of psychotherapies have been developed within different theoretic models of how the mind works, such as the behavioral model based on a learning theory paradigm and the existentialist-humanist model based on a phenomenologic-existentialist view of mental life and function. The therapies that derive from these schools differ radically in concept and in practice from those described in this chapter, and they are discussed elsewhere in this book.

REFERENCES

Alexander F, French TM: *Psychoanalytic Therapy: Principles and Applications.* Ronald Press, 1946.

Bibring E: Psychoanalysis and the dynamic psychotherapies. *J Am Psychoanal Assoc* 1954;**2**:745.

Dewald PA: *Psychotherapy: A Dynamic Approach.* Basic Books, 1964.

Fenichel O: *Problems of Psychoanalytic Technique.* Psychoanalytic Quarterly, 1941.

Freud A: The widening scope of indications for psychoanalysis. (Discussion.) *J Am Psychoanal Assoc* 1954;**2**:607.

Freud S: Lines of advance in psychoanalytic therapy (1918). In: *Standard Edition of the Complete Psychological Works of Sigmund Freud.* Vol 17. Hogarth Press, 1955.

Gill MM: Ego psychology and psychotherapy. *Psychoanal Q* 1951;**20**:62.

Glover E: The indications for psychoanalysis. *J Ment Sci* 1954;**100**:393.

Glover E: The therapeutic effect of inexact interpretation: A contribution to the theory of suggestion. *Int J Psychoanal* 1931;**12**:397.

Kris E: The nature of psychoanalytic propositions and their validation. Pages 239–259 in: *Freedom and Experience: Essays Presented to Horace Kallen.* Hook S, Konvitz MR (editors). Cornell Univ Press, 1947.

Schlesinger HJ: Diagnosis and prescription for psychotherapy. *Bull Menninger Clin* 1969;**33**:269.

Stone L: The widening scope of indications for psychoanalysis. *J Am Psychoanal Assoc* 1954;**2**:567.

Wallerstein RS: *42 Lives in Treatment: A Study of Psychoanalysis and Psychotherapy.* Guilford Press, 1987.

Brief Dynamic Psychotherapy

44

Charles R. Marmar, MD

HISTORICAL TRENDS & RATIONALE FOR BRIEF DYNAMIC PSYCHOTHERAPY

In the decades since Freud's original writings on the technique of psychoanalysis, the trend among practitioners working in the tradition of psychodynamic psychotherapy has been toward increasing length of treatment. Whereas the earliest psychoanalyses were conducted over an 8- to 12-month period, the usual length of treatment in contemporary analysis is 4–6 years. Such longer-term analyses have as their goal not only remission of symptoms (eg, phobias, anxiety, depressed mood, conversion phenomena) and improvement in occupational and interpersonal functioning but also fundamental shifts in character organization, including increased capacity for the regulation of self-esteem, flexible pursuit of autonomous needs, and deepened capacity for empathy.

Although the field of psychodynamic psychotherapy as a whole has been moving toward longer courses of treatment, certain theoreticians have advocated briefer, more active, and more focused approaches to deal with carefully delineated areas of psychopathology. Ferenczi and Rank (1925) criticized long-term psychodynamic therapy, which they felt placed undue emphasis on oedipal problems as the cause of neurotic and character disorders in adults. **Oedipal problems** are conflicts over success in work and love relationships that reflect the anxiety originally associated with sexual longings toward the parent of the opposite sex and competitive strivings with the parent of the same sex for the affection of the parent of the opposite sex. Such conflicts are said to originate mainly in the oedipal period (age 3–5 years). Oedipal conflicts are distinct from conflicts over separation, which arise in the mother-child relationship and reach their greatest intensity between 6 and 36 months of age. Rank's interest in the physical separation of the infant from the mother at the moment of birth and later the psychologic emancipation of the child from the mother led to an emphasis on time-limited treatment, with a focus on the meanings of separation, a theoretical position reiterated in the contemporary work of James Mann (1973) (see below).

Alexander and French developed new techniques for time-limited psychoanalysis. They emphasized the therapeutic potential of the **corrective emotional experience,** or the reexperiencing (under more favorable circumstances) of a traumatic emotional situation from the past. Reexperiencing the trauma under the guidance of the therapist permits mastering of the anxiety in a setting of safety and enables the patient to gain a truer perspective on the traumatic situation. Alexander and French (1946) recommended that the therapist assume a particular role that might counteract the earlier trauma or interpersonal deficits. If, for example, a patient has repeatedly experienced painful relationships with critical, unappreciative, or abusive caretakers, the therapist might adopt a warm, empathic, and compassionate role to provide a compensatory experience.

Alexander challenged the prevailing assumption that there was a positive correlation between the length of treatment and the success of therapy. He argued that long-standing favorable changes could occur in more time-limited treatments and that reliving regressive experiences, as occurs in long-term analytic therapy, was not essential in resolving the patient's difficulties. He advocated countering such regressions by limiting the length of treatment, seeing patients less frequently, and sustaining a focus on current adaptive struggles rather than reconstructing childhood or adolescent trauma. He believed that the primary value of accurate formulation of early developmental conflicts or deficits lay not in facilitating the revival of the past but rather in guiding the therapist to provide a corrective emotional experience in the present.

Alexander's goal was to speed up the time course of psychoanalysis rather than to provide a specific set of technical guidelines for conducting brief, problem-focused dynamic psychotherapy. In contrast, contemporary schools of brief psychotherapy advocate a more restricted approach, with focus on a single problem or at most on several interrelated conflicts that have been purposely chosen to the exclusion of other possible issues. The theoretical writings of French are relevant in this regard. It was French (1958) who introduced the term **focal conflict,** which he defined as a wish or intention that conflicts with the person's enduring expectations and values. The conflict renders the person incapable of meeting his or her expectations, and the result is frustration, with use of various emotional defenses and compromises. For example, a person might wish to function as a more separate, independent person but fears that to pursue such autonomous aims would hurt other important people, who would be left out; the person would then compromise by resentfully stifling these strivings toward independence.

Choosing a specific focal conflict helps to organize the work in brief psychotherapy and focuses attention on an emotional problem of manageable proportions. This approach differs from that of long-term dynamic psychotherapy, in which multiple problems are addressed and the complex interplay of different levels of problems is included. Balint and coworkers (1972) provide an excellent example of the technique for limiting the approach in brief treatment to a selected sector of the personality and guarding against diffusion of effort.

Theoretical and clinical work in time-limited dynamic psychotherapy has proliferated in the last 2 decades. Shorter treatments have become especially salient in settings with strict cost-containment policies, eg, health maintenance organizations. General features of time-limited dynamic psychotherapy are discussed below, along with the contributions of major figures in the field of contemporary brief psychotherapy.

Features of Brief Dynamic Psychotherapy

A. Application of Psychoanalytic Principles: The principles of psychoanalytic psychotherapy are applied to the resolution of specific problems rather than to the entire range of personality functioning.

B. Selection Criteria: Specific selection criteria are designed to permit careful screening of prospective patients and selection of those for whom brief dynamic psychotherapy would be appropriate.

C. Primary Focus: A primary focus—typically a problem behavior or negative self-image that surfaces in the context of current difficulties in interpersonal relations—is chosen. The impact of brief treatment is potentially greater when the problem is a manifestation of long-standing characterologic difficulties that have been intensified by current life stresses. For example, a woman has had a long-standing tendency to spoil her own successes by conveying an attitude of haughty superiority toward her colleagues. She is aware that there is a defensive aspect to this behavior and that she is in fact anxious about her success, but she cannot restrain herself from repeating this pattern. A recent promotion has been particularly stressful psychologically, and she feels that the pattern is escalating and that she is in danger of losing what she has just gained. The focus of treatment for this patient would be the repetitive need to spoil success and the underlying relationship of this behavior to anxiety and guilt about being a powerful person.

D. Therapeutic Alliance: Because of the time limits on brief psychotherapy, the therapist must actively seek ways to facilitate the rapid establishment of a therapeutic alliance. Such a partnership creates a safe environment in which the patient feels understood and views the therapist as empathic, respectful, and nonjudgmental, all of which help to deepen rapport. Within this alliance, patients ideally are willing to reveal thoughts and feelings, reflect on the nature of personal problems, and explore their own contributions to these problems.

E. Working Through: Treatment includes a phase of working through that concentrates on the resolution of the focal conflict. This phase usually includes an opportunity for the patient to express feelings and ideas about current stressful interpersonal experiences and to identify subjectively distorted meanings of these events. Distortion may take the form of exaggerated self-depreciation or identification of current negative feelings about the self with difficulties in earlier relationships. The patient's relationship with the therapist is clarified, and ways in which the patient repeats various aspects of the focal conflict in the relationship with the therapist are pointed out. When possible, the patient's distorted reactions to the therapist are linked to similar reactions in important current interpersonal relationships and to related patterns in earlier developmental sequences.

F. Termination: The meaning that termination of therapy holds for the patient is carefully considered in brief dynamic psychotherapy. Because of the short overall duration of treatment, the patient may perceive termination as an abrupt loss of a valued supportive relationship. Although both parties have agreed that treatment should be brief, the patient often feels rejected, and the same negative self-images that brought the patient into treatment in the first place may be transiently intensified during termination. The loss of the therapist at termination is therefore another opportunity for the patient to master general problems in the area of separation and attachment.

Summary of Rationale & Features of Brief Dynamic Psychotherapy

Brief dynamic psychotherapy is indicated when a specific emotional problem can be identified and when the patient can tolerate exploration of that problem in a brief time frame. The goals of work are focused and more narrowly defined, as opposed to the more thorough but more diffusely defined longer-term dynamic therapies. Common to all brief therapies is a limited or fixed number of sessions, usually between 12 and 20 but sometimes extending to 30, although some flexibility exists in different approaches. The rationale for brief therapy is practical: Treatment seeks to be cost-effective and accessible to a broader segment of the population, since many people cannot make the commitment of time, money, and emotional energy required for more protracted treatment.

CONTEMPORARY SCHOOLS OF BRIEF DYNAMIC PSYCHOTHERAPY

DAVID MALAN & THE BRITISH SCHOOL

Beginning with the ground-breaking work of Balint and coworkers (1972) in the development of focal psychotherapy and evolving further through the efforts of David Malan (1963, 1976) at the Tavistock Clinic in London, the British have made major contributions to the theory, practice, and research evaluation of time-limited dynamic psychotherapy. The technical guidelines advocated by Malan and his collaborators are discussed below.

Selection Criteria

For Malan, the initial selection process is a crucial first step. The pretreatment interview begins with a careful psychiatric history and mental status examination in order to exclude individuals with a current or past history of serious psychiatric disorders (eg, schizophrenia, mania, major depressive episodes), suicide attempts, severe childhood trauma, and long-standing complex family and marital problems. The second component of the evaluation is a psychodynamic history focused on current and past major interpersonal relationships, with a search for recurrent patterns of conflict. The patient's capacity to form an open, trusting relationship with the interviewer is evaluated as well as the patient's response to some initial tentative interpretations of recurring difficulties in interpersonal relationships. The extent to which the patient is motivated to engage in psychotherapy is also determined.

Duration & Focus of Treatment

Malan recommends that a fixed time limit be determined at the outset of treatment. Experienced therapists conduct treatments extending over an average of 18 sessions, whereas a time limit of 30 sessions is recommended for trainee therapists.

Malan emphasizes work on the focal conflict in the context of important recurrent maladaptive patterns in relationships and points to 2 specific triangular configurations to be used in working on the focal conflict. The first triangle consists of the patient's aim or intention, the subjectively perceived threat that makes expression of the aim dangerous, and the efforts to ward off anxiety through the use of specific defenses. For example, a patient may intend to be more open in expressing emotions in close relationships but feels that this would not gain the respect of others, who would feel that the patient was being too sentimental or emotionally out of control. The patient then tries to ward off the potential anxiety about others' reactions by being intellectual and distant rather than emotional.

The second triangle is a triangle of persons and involves the identification of recurrent patterns of relationships in 3 contexts: (1) the relationship with the therapist (the transference relationship); (2) the patient's relationships in current interpersonal situations outside of therapy; and (3) the real or imagined relationships (both past and present) with parental figures or siblings. To continue with the patient used in the example in the previous paragraph, the person who feels blocked in expression of emotion is likely to act in a controlled, intellectualized manner both with the therapist and in current emotional and occupational relationships; such a person is also likely to have originally developed this pattern in relating to parental figures.

Treatment

A. Order of Interpretive Work: Malan's technique consists of carefully timing the work to make the patient aware of the triangular structure of the recurrent relationship patterns. The technical competence of the therapist conducting brief dynamic psychotherapy is therefore in part determined by the ability to formulate such triangular patterns quickly and accurately and pace subsequent interpretations at a level of awareness that is tolerable for a specific patient. Malan's recommendations for the order of interpretive work in brief dynamic psychotherapy are as follows:

1. The nature of the focal conflict is communicated to the patient before extensive connections are made among past, current, and transference relationships.

2. In interpreting the focal conflict, the therapist discusses the patient's defensive avoidance of the expression of aims before undertaking in-depth exploration of the aims themselves. For example, a patient who wants to be more direct in expressing anger but fears harming others in the process may be quiet and withdrawn when angry with friends. The therapist might point out that the patient became withdrawn in the same way after the therapist made a certain comment, and the therapist would then invite the patient to examine this behavior before directly asserting that the patient must be angry with the therapist.

3. The repetitive pattern of maladaptive interpersonal behavior is interpreted in its past, current, and transference aspects. The way in which this is done varies and depends on the patient's capacities to appreciate this pattern in different relationship contexts. Once it is clearly developed, the manifestation of the focal conflict in the patient's relationship with the therapist receives primary emphasis.

4. The analysis of the links between the way in which the patient relates to the therapist and the similar way the patient related to parental figures in the past is termed the **parent-transference linking interpretation.** Malan stresses the importance of this interpretation above all other possible interpretations that can be made in brief psychotherapy. The goal of treatment is first to examine the defensive aspects of this interpersonal relationship pattern and then to explore the patient's warded-off aims or intentions in these 2 different contexts.

B. Termination Phase: The loss of the therapist at the termination of brief psychotherapy has meanings for the patient that are explored for possible linkages to unresolved meanings of earlier losses, usually of parental figures. The focal conflict is frequently reactivated or intensified during the termination phase, so that there is yet another opportunity to work through the focal conflict. The parent-transference linking interpretation is emphasized in this phase as well, so that termination is viewed as a time to organize the therapeutic experience; this ordering of impressions helps to counteract the tendency toward diffusion of focus in brief psychotherapy.

PETER SIFNEOS: SHORT-TERM ANXIETY-PROVOKING PSYCHOTHERAPY

While Malan was formulating the technique of brief dynamic psychotherapy at the Tavistock Clinic, Peter Sifneos (1972) was articulating a similar approach based on his experience at Massachusetts General Hospital in Boston. Like Malan, Sifneos departed from the tradition of more supportive and anxiety-suppressive brief psychotherapies by advocating an exploratory, interpretive approach usually reserved for long-term psychoanalytic treatments. The objective of both theorists was to enable patients to make changes in their characters through resolution of certain key neurotic conflicts.

Selection Criteria

Sifneos's approach also emphasizes specific inclusion and exclusion criteria in order to select patients who can quickly engage in the therapeutic process and can tolerate the anxiety evoked by early and repeated interpretive work, in particular, frank examination of the transference reaction. Patients who are the most appropriate candidates for short-term anxiety-provoking psychotherapy have the following characteristics:

(1) Above average intelligence, as determined by the capacity for new learning.

(2) A history of at least one mutual, give-and-take relationship, with implied shared intimacy, emotional involvement, trust, and the capacity for ambivalent feelings.

(3) Ability to acknowledge and express a range of emotions, as directly observed in the patient's interaction with the evaluating therapist.

(4) A circumscribed chief complaint related to a limited area of interpersonal functioning.

(5) Motivation for change, which Sifneos regards as a multifaceted characteristic that includes the capacity and willingness to look for personal contributions to one's difficulties, an ability to appreciate that symptoms are psychologic in origin, the capacity to provide an open and honest account of feelings, a willingness to be actively involved in the therapeutic rela-

tionship, and a willingness to experiment with new ways of functioning. Sifneos stresses the importance of realistic rather than magical expectations about changes arising from therapy as well as the patient's willingness to make reasonable sacrifices with regard to schedule arrangements and payment of fees.

Treatment

Sifneos's approach incorporates 5 phases, as described below.

A. First Phase (Patient-Therapist Encounter): A therapeutic alliance is formed through mobilization of the patient's initial positive feelings toward the therapist as well as early exploration of the patient's apprehensions regarding treatment. In this phase, the therapist also arrives at a tentative psychodynamic hypothesis about the relationship of current symptomatic disturbances to long-standing character problems that cause conflicts in interpersonal relationships. This psychodynamic formulation draws on 2 main sources of information: a careful history of developmental relationships and observations of the patient's behavior with the therapist during treatment. The focus of treatment—an emotional problem which the patient is motivated to solve and which has relevance for both current interpersonal difficulties as well as basic (core) neurotic conflicts—is also determined during the first phase.

Occasionally, the therapist and the patient may not immediately agree on the focus, and further exploration is required until an acceptable compromise can be established. By the completion of the first phase of treatment, the therapist should be able to provide a written statement setting forth the minimally acceptable goals of treatment and including a prediction about the patient's chances of resolving the central neurotic problem.

B. Second Phase (Early Treatment): The therapist is careful to differentiate realistic goals from the patient's more immature wishes to be totally gratified in disavowing adult responsibility for dealing with problems. The therapist tactfully confronts the patient's idealized versions of what treatment will accomplish in order to encourage active problem solving and discourage the development of an overly dependent relationship.

C. Third Phase (Height of Treatment): In the third phase, the therapist relates the patient's past unresolved difficulties in interpersonal relationships to current emotional problems. As these patterns of conflict are explored, the patient frequently experiences moments of resistance (**transference resistances**) to the deeper understanding of these patterns, in part because of fearful expectations of the therapist's reactions or attitudes toward the patient.

These impediments to treatment are discussed so that the patient is allowed to see the irrational basis for these fears and so that exploration can then return to bolder elaboration of the focus. A cycle of events then typically occurs: Progress in understanding leads to resistance, followed first by interpretation of the fears underlying the resistance and then by further deepening of the work. The therapist asks anxiety-provoking questions in order to help the patient observe how he or she evades painful feelings as well as to demonstrate the reasons underlying this avoidance. Such confrontations may trigger the patient's anger toward the therapist, a response that is made more acceptable to the patient because of the prior establishment of a therapeutic alliance.

Sifneos has likened this emotional problem solving to the completion of a complex mathematical puzzle. He cautions against an overly intellectualized approach, however, and emphasizes that it is a learning experience that occurs within the context of an emotional exchange between the patient and the therapist.

D. Fourth Phase (Evidence of Change): In the fourth phase, the therapist determines when sufficient mastery and resolution of the problem have occurred, so that termination may be considered. The criteria for resolution include less anxiety during treatment sessions; relief of symptoms such as sleeplessness, phobias, or self-defeating behavior; adaptive changes in the interpersonal behavior associated with the focus; and evidence that the patient can begin to relate what has been learned to new social contexts by making appropriate changes in behavior. For example, after successful therapy, a patient who has stifled expression of independent wishes and actions in the presence of parental figures and who has sought treatment because this behavior has been carried over into the marital relationship will be able to define and assert needs not only with the spouse but also with important figures in the workplace or in social relationships.

E. Fifth Phase (Termination): Sifneos proposes that the exact termination date not be set until appropriate change has been demonstrated in the target behavior. At that point, the therapist addresses the natural ambivalence the patient feels at the thought of separating from the therapist. The disappointment of separating from a recently acquired helpful figure is set against the more realistic background of the gains achieved in treatment. The patient is encouraged to extrapolate this new knowledge to future challenges. The therapist in turn also experiences a resistance to termination that must be addressed, because as the therapist experiences growing concern for the patient, there will be a deepening curiosity about the origin of the patient's difficulties as well as anxiety and guilt in acknowledging that treatment is ending but has failed to address certain psychopathologic problems (specifically, those not related to the central focus). Therapists may have to struggle with the temptation to extend treatment. Sifneos believes that separation at termination is facilitated by a progressive, active, problem-solving posture on the part of the patient rather than a more regressive dependent attachment.

HABIB DAVANLOO: BROAD-FOCUSED SHORT-TERM DYNAMIC PSYCHOTHERAPY

Habib Davanloo's (1979, 1980) work, which incorporates some theoretical concepts from both Malan and Sifneos, has broadened both the scope of problems that can be addressed in brief psychotherapy and the extent of the resolution hoped for in treatment.

Selection Criteria

In this approach, selection criteria in time-limited therapy have been expanded to include patients with long-standing severe characterologic deficits (ie, personality disorders) that imply the existence of multiple interrelated conflicts that are not easily limited to a single focus. Davanloo considers neither severe problems nor long-standing difficulties as automatic criteria for excluding patients from treatment. Contrary to expectation, he reported some good outcomes in brief treatment of individuals with long-standing severe character problems and unexpected instances of poor outcome when mild character difficulties of more recent onset were the presenting complaint. Whereas Sifneos recommends his short-term anxiety-provoking psychotherapy for a rigorously selected 5–10% of psychiatric outpatients, Davanloo's broader selection criteria make it possible to treat about 30–35% of outpatients with psychiatric problems by broad-focused short-term therapy.

In 1979, Davanloo specified criteria for his approach to brief dynamic psychotherapy. These overlap the criteria of Malan and Sifneos (history of adequate interpersonal relationships, capacity to tolerate and express feelings, awareness that problems are psychologic in origin, and response to the therapist's initial interpretations). Davanloo emphasizes the need to confront the patient's way of avoiding real feelings by including such defensive behavior as vagueness, passivity, denial, or withdrawal. Such repetitive confrontation is often irritating to patients, who are encouraged to express the frustration and resentment they feel about this process. The ability to express that anger and to begin recognizing the pattern of not expressing feelings under frustrating circumstances reflects qualities indicating that the patient is a suitable candidate for broad-focused short-term therapy.

Duration of Treatment

Davanloo recommends a flexible number of treatment sessions. For well-functioning patients with circumscribed problems, 5–15 face-to-face sessions lasting an hour each are usually sufficient to deal with the presenting problem. For adequately functioning patients with several presenting problems, 15–25 sessions are recommended; about 20–30 sessions are recommended for patients with long-standing severe personality problems.

Treatment

A. Early and Middle Phases: As in other brief

dynamic psychotherapeutic approaches, the therapist assumes an active role and places high priority on the early and repeated interpretation of transference (ie, the ways in which the patient misperceives the therapist as a result of experiences in earlier relationships). For example, a patient with a harsh and critical mother was made to feel during her childhood that her anger toward her mother was not justified. The patient had therefore developed a pattern of suppressing her anger when frustrated and instead becoming moody and uncooperative, without clearly communicating what was upsetting her. Such a pattern is highly likely to recur during treatment, and when it does appear, the therapist will make the interpretation that the patient is feeling resentfully misunderstood, that she feels as though she is not justified in this anger, and that instead of expressing the feeling, she becomes moody and uncommunicative. After the pattern has been clarified, the therapist addresses the patient's unwarranted expectation that she will be punished for her behavior, and the patient gradually comes to trust more open expression of her frustration. This active, interpretive approach is recommended by Davanloo both to accelerate the understanding and resolution of emotional problems and to prevent patients from becoming excessively dependent on the therapist. Instead, patients are encouraged to rely on their own coping capacities in preparation for the termination of treatment.

In treatments that are going well, the patient gains considerable understanding into these recurrent ways of avoiding the expression of emotions and usually begins to experiment with more open demonstration of feelings by about the eighth session. This increased communicativeness occurs not only in the treatment setting but also in the patient's relationships with other important persons in everyday life. At the same time, anxiety and depression are lessened, partly because the patient feels an upsurge in morale as a result of participating in a helpful treatment relationship and partly because the patient is able to negotiate more appropriately for satisfaction of needs in interpersonal conflicts. At this point, termination of therapy may be contemplated.

B. Termination Phase: Although optimism about outcome characterizes all of the proponents of brief dynamic psychotherapy, Davanloo (1979) is especially sanguine in this regard. His criterion for consideration of termination is total cure:

> The therapy is not successful unless the patient is free of symptoms and all of his maladaptive behavior has changed. When this happens, termination is considered. In a successful outcome the patient almost universally refers to himself as a "free" person, a "new" person. Termination usually comes without difficulty.

While Davanloo's approach is promising—as are the approaches of Sifneos, Malan, and others working in the brief psychotherapy movement—much of the evidence for the effectiveness of these treatments rests in individual case reports. More systematic research is needed to substantiate claims of complete cures with these approaches.

Davanloo also recommends a flexible approach to the termination phase that takes into account the patient's level of functioning as well as the limited or extensive nature of the presenting problems. In well-functioning patients who are capable but hold themselves back in work and love relationships because of irrational fear of success, disengagement from treatment is uncomplicated, and patients do not ordinarily experience deep feelings of loss at termination. On the other hand, for those individuals who have sustained important losses in their lives, particularly during sensitive developmental periods in early childhood or adolescence, mourning the imminent departure of the therapist is an essential and helpful aspect of treatment. Because the patient knows when the relationship will end, there is an opportunity to explore the feelings about this loss, which stands in contrast to the more traumatic losses that occurred in earlier developmental periods. For patients with severe personality difficulties or those with multiple problems rather than a single focus, Davanloo recommends several additional sessions during the termination phase in order to help the patient negotiate a manageable separation.

JAMES MANN: TIME-LIMITED PSYCHOTHERAPY

James Mann's (1973) unique approach to brief dynamic psychotherapy places major theoretical and technical emphasis on the meaning of time—ie, the patient's difficulty in accepting the finiteness of time, in mastering separations, and in ultimately accepting his or her own mortality. As a result, the selection of patients, the development of the focus in brief treatment, the approach to working through emotional problems, and the handling of the termination phase are organized along a common theme that addresses the meanings of time for the patient. The termination phase assumes paramount importance, because it provides a living model of loss, separation, and the time-limited nature of attachments.

In his theoretical discussion, Mann differentiates 2 ways in which people experience time: (1) Categorical, or adult, time is governed by realistic understanding of the finite quality of time and is measured by the watch and the calendar; (2) existential, or child, time is governed by immature fantasies of timelessness and personal invincibility and goes beyond clock time. Because the development of a mature appreciation of time is a challenge for everyone, particularly for people with a history of difficulty in early separation experiences (who are forever waiting for the loved one's return), a child's perception of time is never entirely set aside, even in the most mature adults. Both kinds of time may be used simultaneously to evaluate an experience. Stressful life events may alter a person's perception of time from a realistic, adult appreciation of its finiteness to a more childlike experience of time and functioning (regression with stress). Alternatively, the same individual may simultaneously reflect different levels of adaptation to the finiteness of time, as shown in successful time management in one sphere (being prompt for meetings) with an adherence to more immature perceptions of time in another area of functioning (failing to plan for retirement as a denial of aging).

Selection Criteria

Ideal candidates for Mann's brief dynamic psychotherapy are young adults in developmental transition, ie, those who are moving from the late stages of adolescence into young adulthood. The prototype is a college student struggling simultaneously to handle separation from parents and to establish autonomous social, occupational, and sexual identities. Mann's approach stresses that the patient must have the ability to tolerate the frustration of the time limits inherent in this type of therapy. Above-average intelligence, a criterion emphasized by Sifneos, is seen as helpful though not essential in Mann's approach. Mann has suggested that his approach, which is both short-term and fixed in duration, may be appropriate for those with limited economic resources and educational background. Long-term exploratory psychotherapies are frequently both too costly and too ambiguously defined to serve the interests of this group of patients.

The exclusion criteria for Mann's time-limited approach include past or current psychotic disorders, serious alcohol or drug abuse, and borderline personality disorder. Patients with strong passive longings to be cared for, who are frequently reluctant to give up these feelings in favor of more independent behavior, are also excluded. Individuals in these groups frequently require long-term dynamic psychotherapy.

Duration & Focus of Treatment

Mann specifies a 12-session, once-weekly, time-limited treatment. The focus emerges after a process of gradual clarification, which may require several sessions, and the 12-session limit begins only after a focus has been mutually defined. Once the focus has been established, the time limit is fixed, and the date of termination is set in advance. If no workable focus can be specified during the preliminary interviews, the patient is referred for an appropriate alternative treatment.

Mann describes 4 basic conflicts that are a frequent focus in treatment: dependence versus independence, passivity versus activity, diminished versus adequate self-esteem, and unresolved versus resolved grief. Mann emphasizes the paramount importance of the elements of separation and individuation as they relate to the 4 central issues. For example, while activity-passivity struggles may involve anxiety about surpassing a rival, anxiety about aggressively dominating another, or anxiety about separating from a caretaker, Mann considers the latter to be the most important theme.

Treatment

A. Early Phase: Mann describes an initial "honeymoon" phase characterized by the patient's relief in feeling understood, particularly when the therapist is tactful in defining the problem that is the focus. The recommendation for brief rather than longer-term treatment stimulates hope for a rapid resolution of difficulties. The patient is intellectually aware of the time limit; at an emotional level, however, the patient longs for an open-ended and idealized reparative relationship with the therapist that will compensate for earlier disappointments and frustrations in formative relationships.

B. Middle Phase: The therapist's inevitable failure to meet all of the patient's expectations in the first few hours of treatment leads to disillusionment, which ushers in the middle phase of treatment, frequently at about the sixth session. The original presenting symptoms may intensify, as Mann (1973) explains:

> The characteristic feature of any middle point is that one more step, however small, signifies the point of no return. In the instance of time-limited psychotherapy, the patient must go on to a conclusion that he does not wish to confront. The confrontation that he needs to avoid and that he will actively seek to avoid is the same one that he suffered earlier in his life; namely, *separation without resolution from the meaningful, ambivalently experienced person.* Time sense and reality are coconspirators in repeating an existential trauma in the patient.

c. Termination Phase: With the inevitable approach of termination, a deepening sense of pessimism and disillusionment usually (not always) dominates the eighth through the tenth sessions. The patient is more or less aware of the threat of termination and struggles to guard against the emotional pain of the loss of a valued relationship only recently established. With surprising frequency, the patient seems to forget the termination date and believes there are more sessions left than are actually remaining. The therapist points out the patient's incorrect perceptions of time in the context of brief dynamic treatment. The patient's negative feelings toward the therapist at this stage frequently recapitulate negative feelings toward frustrating figures in earlier life. The important difference is that while facing an agreed upon termination date, the patient now has an opportunity to experience and master the emotions related to separation from the therapist and in so doing to develop a capacity to function more independently and deal more adaptively with the imperfect and time-limited nature of human experience. Feelings of anger at being abandoned, guilt for having angry feelings toward frustrating figures, sadness at the loss of a valued figure, and wishes for reunion can be examined in this phase.

KLERMAN & WEISSMAN: SHORT-TERM INTERPERSONAL PSYCHOTHERAPY

Klerman and Weissman have described a time-limited psychotherapeutic method specifically tailored to treat individuals with depression. The focus of this approach is on interpersonal behaviors that contribute to depressive states (Weissman and Klerman, 1973; Neu and coworkers, 1978). In contrast to the brief dynamic psychotherapies, little attention is directed toward the exploration of unconscious conflicts or the repetition of unresolved parent-child problems in the patient's relationship with the therapist (ie, there is minimal transference interpretation). Treatment is time-limited, averaging 14 sessions in one study. Weekly 50-minute sessions are provided for individuals with depression triggered and exacerbated by interpersonal problems.

Klerman and Weissman describe 7 types of technical interventions. The first is **nonjudgmental exploration,** which is particularly relevant early in treatment and denotes the support and encouragement given to the patient to discuss problems openly. The therapist's availability, empathy, and nonjudgmental attitude are essential in facilitating the patient's self-disclosure.

Elicitation of material, a second technique, involves active probing for new information. Such probing is common during early treatment but may be indicated whenever a more complete understanding of past or current difficulties is indicated. Next is **clarification,** or rephrasing of the patient's comments to point out inconsistencies and make covert communications more overt.

Additional techniques include **direct advice,** in which the therapist guides the patient toward more adaptive interpersonal behavior to increase the chances that others will be warmly receptive of the patient rather than critical or distant. **Decision analysis** explores alternative courses of action in order to broaden the patient's understanding of short-and long-range consequences of behavior toward others. **Development of awareness** is used to facilitate insight into the patient's interpersonal behavioral patterns and clarify ways in which the patient attempts to ward off or ignore these patterns.

This brief treatment approach is noteworthy both for its careful specification of treatment approaches in published manuals as well as for the attention paid to research on the effectiveness of the recommendations. The approach may be of particular interest to general practitioners and other nonpsychiatrist physicians, since extensive training in psychodynamic theory and technique is not required.

EFFECTIVENESS OF BRIEF DYNAMIC PSYCHOTHERAPY

Despite the methodologic difficulties encountered in assessing the outcome of various psychotherapies, major progress occurred in the 1970s. The most thorough research on the effectiveness of psychotherapy has been conducted by Smith and coworkers (1980), who reviewed and analyzed 375 studies. Since the average duration of treatment was 17 sessions, this report mainly considers the outcome of brief psychotherapy. In general, the average patient who received treatment was better off than 75% of those who either received no treatment or were on waiting lists for treatment and were used as controls. Effectiveness of treatment was assessed by several criteria, including improvement in symptoms, patient satisfaction, and decreased reliance on medication. The study indicated that the many different schools of psychotherapy were about equally helpful. Brief dynamic psychotherapy—along with brief behavioral, interpersonal, cognitive, and other approaches—is a treatment with well-documented effectiveness in relieving various psychologic symptoms, as described above.

The relative effectiveness of brief dynamic psychotherapy compared to long-term dynamic treatments has not been extensively studied. Although the general question of brief versus long-term treatment in the different approaches has been reviewed by Butcher and Kolotkin (1979) and by Luborsky and coworkers (1975), the former failed to find strong correlation between the efficacy of different therapies and the length of treatment. The negative finding may be due in part to currently limited abilities to reliably evaluate the types of personality changes that are more likely to occur in long-term treatment. Changes in psychologic symptoms and social functioning, on the other hand, are more easily determined. Definitive evaluation of the merits of brief versus long-term treatment awaits development of improved methods of assessing characterologic change.

Brief dynamic psychotherapy for outpatients with moderate to severe psychiatric conditions has been shown to be effective in alleviating symptoms and improving social functioning. Horowitz and coworkers (1984) have found that brief therapy is effective in treating posttraumatic stress disorders. They have also discussed the modification of the techniques of brief dynamic psychotherapy for patients with different personality disorders. Weissman and coworkers (1981) have studied the outcome of interpersonal psychotherapy and found that 14-session treatments have been effective in treating major depressive disorders. Very few negative effects of brief dynamic psychotherapy have been reported. Rather than becoming worse, patients for the most part either improve or (at worst) do not improve after brief dynamic psychotherapy. This method of treatment seems to be the most useful when a specific focus can be defined, when the problem is related to recent stressful life circumstances, and when the patient has the capacity to tolerate rapid engagement and confrontation, working through, and disengagement from the treatment process.

REFERENCES

Alexander F, French T: *Psychoanalytic Therapy: Principles and Applications*. Ronald Press, 1946.

Balint M, Ornstein PH, Balint E: *Focal Psychotherapy*. Lippincott, 1972.

Butcher NJ, Kolotkin RL: Evaluation of outcome in brief psychotherapy. *Psychiatr Clin North Am* 1979;**2:**157.

Davanloo H: Techniques of short-term psychotherapy. *Psychiatr Clin North Am* 1979;**2:**11.

Davanloo H (editor): *Short-Term Dynamic Therapy*. Vol 1. Jason Aronson, 1980.

Ferenczi S, Rank O: *The Development of Psychoanalysis*. Nervous and Mental Disease Publication Co., 1925.

French TM: *The Integrations of Behavior*. Vol 3. Univ of Chicago Press, 1958.

Horowitz MJ et al: Brief psychotherapy of bereavement reactions: The relationship of process to outcome. *Arch Gen Psychiatry* 1984;**41:**438.

Horowitz MJ et al: *Personality Styles and Brief Psychotherapy*. Basic Books, 1984.

Luborsky L, Singer B, Luborsky L: Comparative Studies of Psychotherapies. *Arch Gen Psychiatry* 1975;**32:**995.

Malan DH: *Frontiers of Brief Psychotherapy*. Plenum Press, 1976.

Malan DH: *A Study of Brief Psychotherapy*. Plenum Press, 1963.

Mann J: *Time-Limited Psychotherapy*. Harvard Univ Press, 1973.

Neu C, Prusoff B, Klerman G: Measuring the interventions used in short-term interpersonal psychotherapy of depression. *Am J Orthopsychiatry* 1978;**48:**629.

Sifneos PE: *Short-Term Psychotherapy and Emotional Crisis*. Harvard Univ Press, 1972.

Smith ML, Glass GV, Miller TI: *The Benefits of Psychotherapy*. Johns Hopkins Univ Press, 1980.

Weissman M, Klerman G: Psychotherapy with depressed women: An empirical study of content themes and reflection. *Br J Psychiatry* 1973;**123:**55.

Weissman M et al: Depressed outpatients: Results one year after treatment with drugs and/or interpersonal psychotherapy. *Arch Gen Psychiatry* 1981;**38:**51.

45

The Existential Approach in Psychiatry

Stephen J. Walsh, MD

The existential psychotherapeutic approach complements the biologic, psychodynamic, and social understanding of how and why a patient experiences emotional pain. It is a psychologic and philosophic construct which is useful in clinical psychiatry and medicine and which may help physicians make sense of much of the vast array of symptoms and behavior they regularly encounter. The existential perspective is based on a humanistic view of psychotherapy and utilizes insights from philosophy and literature as well as from clinical experience. (See Chapter 3.)

In common with other predominantly psychologic (as opposed to social, behavioral, or biologic) approaches to understanding human suffering and psychiatric illness, existential psychiatry views symptoms and maladaptive behavior as the product of unresolved inner conflicts arising from personal experience. The major distinguishing characteristic of existential psychotherapy is its emphasis on the "givens" of human existence, the "ultimate concerns" of human life. Yalom (1980:8) lists these as follows:

(1) Death: Awareness of the inevitability of death and of ceasing to exist conflicts with the wish to continue living.

(2) Freedom/responsibility: All human beings are "inescapably free" and must bear the ultimate responsibility for creating their lives and shaping their experience of the world. Despite inadequate data on which to base decisions, one must continually choose among attitudes or actions, forge an identity, and create a self-concept.

(3) Isolation/separateness: Each individual is separated from all others by an unbridgeable gap. This is true even in the most intimate of relationships. Each person thus stands alone in nature. This separation and isolation conflict with the desire for contact, union, and protection. This feeling of separateness and isolation is perceived most vividly by individuals going through the maturation process of adolescence and young adulthood and moving toward independence and self-reliance.

(4) Meaninglessness: People yearn for a sense of meaning and purpose around which to structure goals and realize values. But the universe has no meaning or purpose other than what each individual can personally create.

Many symptoms and maladaptive behavior patterns may result from conflicting and painful feelings flowing from a patient's experience of these existential truths. Psychiatric illness may be viewed as the result of ineffective defenses against the conscious direct experiencing of these painful thoughts and feelings. In contrast to the tenets of psychoanalytic theories, the most fundamental conflicts in existential psychotherapy are not necessarily the conflicts occurring earliest in life. The patient's history, developmental vulnerabilities, and genetic/biologic makeup are important in the way they affect the individual's experience and response to the existential "givens." Failure to confront death, freedom/responsibility, isolation/separateness, and meaninglessness directly and honestly will impair healthy emotional development.

The existential model does not exclude concerns about sources of anxiety and psychologic impairments discussed elsewhere in this text. Instead, it may be viewed as a shift of focus, with emphasis on and clarification of issues that are sometimes not dealt with explicitly in other types of psychotherapeutic approaches. In existential psychotherapy, the patient and the therapist identify the relevance of one or more of the existential "givens" to the presenting clinical problem and explore the specific difficulties created for the patient by these universal problems of human existence. In the process, patients acknowledge their feelings of fright in the face of these existential truths and learn not to find their anxiety incapacitating. Patients learn that other people share their fears and that there are constructive solutions to their dilemmas.

Talking with a supportive therapist who makes a commitment to stay with the patient enables the patient to express personal feelings in a safe environment, find individual solutions, and make decisions without feeling alone. During therapy, the patient can experiment with freedom and responsibility, discuss the meaning of life and the terror of death, and develop the potential for more pleasurable and independent living. As patients gain confidence in their ability to deal with existential "givens," they may leave therapy without feeling isolated or abandoned.

The following case illustrates some of the general concepts of existential psychotherapy.

Illustrative case. An attractive, single 28-year-old woman graduate student sought help for recurrent feelings of severe anxiety, depressed mood, thoughts of suicide, and an inability to express loving feelings in important relationships, with consequent feelings of alienation and isolation. A recent physical examination and medical history has revealed no somatic disorder. A psychiatric history and initial therapeutic inquiry revealed a pattern of relationships marked by conflict in which the fear of rejection, loss, and separation led her to distance herself from her partner, frustrating her need for love and intimacy. Fears of death as the ultimate separation were prominent, especially during occasional panic attacks.

Initial treatment with medication was not fully effective in controlling her panic attacks and anxiety. She continued to participate in psychotherapy and learned that an important long-term defense against anxiety was her covert belief in the existence of an ultimate male rescuer who would find her and take care of her. She fantasized that she would not have to assume responsibility for her life or feel burdened by the necessity of choice and freedom in creating her own identity and existence. Feelings of meaninglessness were pervasive in her work and studies, with little satisfaction in the exercise of her actual capabilities. Continuing psychotherapy focused on her immediate experience of the existential issues mentioned in the context of further exploration of childhood and adolescent events predisposing to her particular adult difficulties. In weekly therapy sessions over the next several months, she was able to confront directly her inner feelings and thinking patterns directly and to resolve many of her dilemmas, experiencing much less need for the distraction and ineffective functioning related to her symptoms.

This patient and her therapy can also be understood in terms of object relations theory, traditional psychoanalytic and developmental theories, or in the language of cognitive psychology. For many patients, however, the language and orientation of the existential approach may seem more immediate and more related to their actual experience. Several models of the mind may be useful, either concurrently or at different phases during the course of treatment. Whatever the complementary theoretic framework used, the conscious concerns and inner experience of the patient are the continual reference points for the existentially oriented psychiatrist.

The Defenses Against Death & Separateness

Many patients with hyperventilation syndrome, panic attacks, hypochondriasis, and somatization disorders also experience excessive anxiety about dying and being separate and isolated.

Illustrative case No. 1. An aging man used multiple somatic symptoms to maintain a connection with physicians and thereby to feel guarded against aging and death. He wanted to preserve a timeless boyhood by using doctors as parents to ward off his anxiety about death and isolation. As long as rescuers were present, he felt protected from death and from existential aloneness. His symptoms functioned to maintain his attachment to physician-rescuers.

Belief in an ultimate rescuer is seen in many patients with disturbed personality and behavioral patterns (severe passivity, dependency, masochism) and in some patients who feel especially vulnerable to loss and depression.

Another defense against death anxiety is the belief in personal uniqueness and invulnerability to death and isolation. Compulsive overworking may represent denial of the fear of mortality by continuing to advance into an endless future of career achievements. "Workaholics" may experience little immediate satisfaction and pleasure in working but tend to exaggerate the importance of their work. Weekends and vacations become anxious periods as awareness of time and of a shrinking future creeps in.

Illustrative case No. 2. A moderately obese workaholic patient in his mid 40s had a family history of early deaths from heart disease, a fact he unconsciously avoided by his compulsive work activity. In psychotherapy he was able to face his fears of death directly and let go of his defensive compulsiveness enough to lose weight, modify his diet, exercise more, and begin to experience more pleasure in his work.

A middle-aged male workaholic hospitalized in a coronary care unit after his first myocardial infarction may for a time be unable to understand why he must remain in the hospital and may even wonder how someone so important could have a heart attack.

Denial of life's finite limits and of one's separateness and the certainty of eventual death leads to restriction of general awareness and of the full richness of inner experience.

Illustrative case No. 3. A middle-aged woman entered psychotherapy after she was treated in an emergency room for hyperventilating during a panic attack. Her symptoms were later seen to be related to her conflicting feelings and fears of ending a bad marriage. She had the illusion that she had unlimited time to choose what she really needed and wanted in life. As she grew older, it became intolerable for her to remain in a painful (albeit protected) and constricting marriage. In twice-weekly psychotherapy sessions, she was able to confront, understand, and resolve her anxiety about being alone and isolated as a middle-aged single professional woman, and her symptoms abated. She was able to leave the marriage and subsequently advanced in her work and experienced pleasure in other relationships. She developed the ability to let go of less valuable commitments and trusted herself to embrace more creative opportunities.

Some patients deny death and aging by avoiding commitments or by compulsive sexuality. Acknowledging the fact of mortality frees an individual from psychologic bondage to the fear of death expressed as physical symptoms or maladaptive behavior.

Illustrative case No. 4. A 65-year-old married man with progressively disabling anginal pain sought psychologic treatment because of severe anxiety and somatic symptoms after his cardiologist recommended triple bypass surgery. The fear of dying during the procedure had evoked painful memories and symptoms of the severe anxiety he had felt as a lone radio operator on a South Pacific island mountaintop during World War II, when he had feared that his isolation from friendly forces would lead to his death. His current thoughts of being alone on an operating table for coronary artery surgery evoked similar severe anxiety and somatic symptoms. Several sessions of psychotherapy during which the patient confronted and talked about his death anxiety resulted in reduction of symptoms as well as a renewed sense of meaning and appreciation for his life.

Many patients confront existential issues vividly during severe illness, hospitalization, or major surgery. It may be helpful to engage the patient in sensitive psychotherapeutic discussion and exploration of the meanings and feelings evoked by these frightening situations. Existential concerns are real, concrete, accessible, and ubiquitous in both medical and psychiatric patients.

The Defenses Against Freedom & Responsibility

Psychotherapy with an existential orientation also focuses on how patients experience their freedom and to what extent they take responsibility for their own lives and behavior. Therapeutic change is less likely to occur when a patient cannot accept this responsibility or persists in blaming parents or others, external circumstances, or childhood experiences for personal distress. Existentialism is a philosophy of freedom, and the existentially oriented psychiatrist believes that individuals continually shape their experience of the self and the world, whatever the external conditions may be. The responsibility implied by this freedom may be deeply frightening, since it also ties in with the issues of separateness, isolation, death, and the absence of meaning in life. A patient who presents clinically with poorly defined complaints, a sense of aimlessness and meaninglessness, apparently searching for an authority to submit to or rebel against, may be struggling with the issues of freedom and responsibility. In contemporary society, these symptoms are made more severe by the decline of social institutions, such as the church, that once provided structure and meaning to the lives of many people.

Yalom (1980:223) lists several defenses patients may use to avoid experiencing their freedom and responsibility. These include compulsiveness (a practice that obliterates the experience of choice), displacement of responsibility to another, denial of responsibility (by playing "innocent victim" or by "losing con-

trol"), avoidance of autonomous behavior, and impaired decision making (deadening onself to wishing or feeling; abdicating choice; or attributing one's choices to other people, institutions, or external events). The most severely maladaptive defense against the anxiety caused by assuming responsibility for oneself is the denial of one's own feelings and the subsequent projection of those feelings onto another, as frequently occurs in paranoid patients.

Individuals' lives and experiences are shaped by their choices. Repeated failure to acknowledge this exercise of choice results in a sense of unremitting necessity, passivity, constriction of freedom, and feelings of obligation, with chronic resentment. Many patients are troubled by this dilemma, as in the case of paranoid patients who attribute their dysphoria to the "fact" of harassment or surveillance by others.

Illustrative case No. 1. A single man in his late 30s came from a family in which expression of negative feelings was not permitted. He had suppressed his own awareness of unpleasant feelings in order to feel more safe and secure within a family system in which individuals depended on each other in a paralyzing and destructive fashion. He was fearful of separation and rejection and therefore stifled his feelings and natural impulses toward emotional growth, maturity, and individuation. He developed paranoid symptoms during a disappointing love relationship, when suppressed hostility toward his family returned in the form of angry, fearful paranoid delusions and ideas of reference.

Avoidance of responsibility is often a major issue in patients with psychophysiologic and psychosomatic disorders, in which emotional distress may be experienced as disordered physiologic functioning and somatic symptoms. The patient may attribute such symptoms to external conditions and expect relief from external sources.

Illustrative case No. 2. After physical disorder was ruled out, a 35-year-old single man whose chief complaint was insomnia of 3 years' duration was referred for psychotherapy. He described a lifelong pattern of suppressing negative feelings and avoiding the experience of making free and responsible choices in directing his life. Fearing his freedom (with its inescapable responsibilities), he had contructed a view of himself as a victim of circumstances, "bad genes," and an unfortunate childhood, all of which he then felt powerless to alter. Chronic feelings of passivity and depression were prominent. He believed that any change that occurred in his life would be the doctor's full responsibility.

In habitually assuming the stance of a helpless victim, this patient had lost his sense of freedom and power to alter his life. Fearing rejection from others, he habitually chose to suppress feelings of resentment. The resentment was intensified in a love relationship that ended just before the onset of the insomnia. In this relationship, the patient had felt unable to express his needs or his negative feelings safely. In his job as administrator of a department in a retail store, he also had been unable to assert himself in a troubling relationship with the store manager. He felt resentful and victimized in both relationships and in his social relations in general. These feelings were expressed in angry ruminations and revenge fantasies that interfered with sleep.

During therapy, the patient came to understand the connection between the insomnia and his choice not to assert himself in important work and social relationships, with the resulting experience of himself as an angry, helpless (and sleepless) victim of others. His later decision to take responsibility for his own feelings and to express himself constructively toward others in more direct and honest ways led to clarification of his work and social relationships and created new options in each. Relief of the painful resentment and insomnia and enhanced feelings of control and self-direction followed his new assertiveness.

With patients such as the man described in the illustrative case above, psychotherapy must repeatedly seek to discover how they have played an active role in creating their dilemmas and distress and in constricting themselves emotionally. Until patients are able to acknowledge this, there can be little motivation or capacity for change. Secondary gains may be prominent in patients who avoid responsibility. In the case of this particular patient, guiding him to the painful awareness that he had created important elements of his own distress was important in his recovery and was accomplished without "blaming" him.

It is important for patients with *physical* illness to take responsibility for themselves as well. Encouraging patients to accept some responsibility for getting better gives them a feeling of power and assists them in appreciating those parts of their lives in which they are free to take more comfortable and less self-defeating attitudes toward conditions imposed by their illness. Taking responsibility is also important in the habit disorders, such as smoking or overeating. The existentially oriented physician explores the patient's capacities for choice and for exercise of the faculty of will, which is the bridge from insight and desire to action.

The Search for Meaning in Life

Both medical and psychiatric patients frequently report feeling a sense of meaninglessness, futility, or dissatisfaction with the incongruity between their goals and values and their current roles in family or work life. The resulting distress may generate mental and physical symptoms that must be carefully investigated so that major affective disorder or physical disorder may be ruled out. Patients may require assistance in discovering their own wants and needs or may need to be helped to become involved in daily concrete tasks and relationships in such a way that they experience more pleasure and meaning from them.

Illustrative case. A successful businessman in his mid 50s whose wife had died 2 years earlier was sleeping poorly, feeling less satisfaction with his work, and drinking excessively. Feelings of meaninglessness and apathy were pervasive. He complained of vague physical symptoms and fatigue of several months' duration. A medical screening evaluation revealed no evident physical disorder.

As the patient expressed and explored his thoughts and emotions with the psychiatrist, he discovered that he felt a continuing sadness about the loss of his wife. He also became aware of the extent to which his sense of meaning and purpose in life had been based on accumulating money for himself, his wife, and their 4 children, who were now grown and had left home. Since he had more than enough for his needs, working and making money were no longer sources of satisfaction to him. He had been raised on a farm as a member of a large poor family that out of necessity had valued thrift and hard work to ensure survival and self-esteem. Increased leisure time and plenty of money left him with a sense of diminished worth, since he was no longer needed as a provider.

Weekly psychotherapy sessions for 3 months helped this patient clarify his present conflicts and discover their origins. He was helped to reformulate his professional goals and to become more deeply involved in social activities. He developed a desire for more intimacy with his grown children and eventually clarified and resolved past misunderstandings in his relationships with them. Active engagement in these processes gave him a new sense of purpose and meaning.

The physician must help patients who describe having a sense of meaninglessness to look away from such feelings and involve themselves in work and personal relationships. A sense of meaning is a by-product of such engagement, and the physician should help remove obstacles to achieving a feeling of meaning and purpose in life.

SUMMARY

Existential psychotherapy is a psychodynamic approach focusing on the patient's ways of experiencing and responding to the major facts of human life, especially death, freedom/responsibility, isolation/separateness, and meaninglessness. These are intricately interwoven in everyday existence. The focus of existential psychotherapy is the in-depth exploration of the thought content, feelings, and processes of the patient's inner experience. This focus encourages patients to take responsibility for both the successes and the failures in their lives. The therapist explores the patients' experiences without prior assumptions, prejudices, or presuppositions. Patients are invited to talk, explore, and discover themselves as much as possible and are encouraged to spell out their concerns explicitly. As awareness and clarification of their experience increase and as patients grow to trust themselves more, they gain a greater sense of control, freedom, and choice.

Although an existential orientation in psychotherapy is relevant at some level to the concerns of all patients, it is more suitable in some contexts than others, and careful tailoring of the therapeutic approach to the needs of the individual is important. Within the context of the biopsychosocial model—and sometimes combined with pharmacologic approaches or those that focus on aspects of the patient's social environment such as family, marital, and work relationships—existentially oriented psychotherapy may be indicated for the anxiety disorders, dysthymic disorder, adjustment disorder, psychologic factors affecting a physical condition (eg, a patient with angina pectoris who experiences more severe and frequent chest pains because of unresolved anxiety about the possibility of death), and some somatoform disorders. In personality disorders, an existential approach is valuable in enhancing patients' understanding of their feelings and needs and the relationship of these feelings and needs to their habitually maladaptive social and occupational functioning. The existential psychotherapeutic approach is helpful in some schizoid, avoidant, histrionic, narcissistic, compulsive, dependent, passive-aggressive, and borderline personality disorders. The existential approach may have some value as part of the treatment of sexual disorders, some paranoid disorders, disorders of impulse control, eating and substance use disorders, schizotypal and paranoid personality disorders, the later resolving phases of the major affective disorders, and later phases of some schizophrenic disorders. Patients experiencing bereavement, life-stage problems, or noncompliance with medical treatment may also be helped by an existential approach. The existential approach is contraindicated—at least in the early, more disturbed phases—in the major affective disorders, the more severe schizophrenic disorders, organic mental disorders, and some paranoid disorders.

The existential approach is neither reductionistic nor dogmatic; rather than thrusting patients into diagnostic categories for purposes of treatment, it views each patient as different and unique, and it avoids rigid rules and formulas in its methodology. It is open to the understanding of whatever the patient is experiencing, is relevant to the most basic concerns of human existence, and gives a feeling of power and control to the patient. The existential approach enhances the dignity and value of the medical experience by helping patients become aware of their freedom and of their responsibility to manage their lives and to be conscious of the uniqueness of life's meanings for each person. It reminds patients of the power individuals have to create their own experience out of the conditions of life. To achieve these goals, the therapist becomes involved in the patient's inner world, focuses on the patient's specific concerns, and explores his or her experience of the existential givens—especially death, isolation, freedom, and meaninglessness—and tries to understand and empathize with the patient in a manner similar to Osler's advice to medical students: "The motto of each of you as you undertake the examination and treatment of a case should be: put yourself in his place. Realize so far as you can the mental state of the patient, enter into his feelings—scan gently his faults. The kindly word, the cheerful greeting, the sympathetic look—these the patient understands" (quoted in Havens, 1973).

REFERENCES

Bugental J: *Psychotherapy and Process: The Fundamentals of an Existential-Humanistic Approach*. Addison-Wesley, 1978.

Bugental J: *The Search for Authenticity*. Holt, Rinehart, & Winston, 1965.

Havens L: *Approaches to the Mind: Movement of the Psychiatric Schools From Sects Toward Science*. Little, Brown, 1973.

Kaplan HI, Freedman AM, Sadock BJ (editors): *Comprehensive Textbook of Psychiatry/IV*, 4th ed. Williams & Wilkins, 1985.

Niv MD: Schizophrenia: An existential approach. *Am J Psychoanal* 1980;**40:**43.

Niv MD: Symbols, symptoms, and delusions: An existential analysis. *Am J Psychoanal* 1981;**41:**239.

Osler W: *Aequanimitas, With Other Addresses to Medical Students, Nurses and Practitioners of Medicine*. Blakiston, 1952.

Phillips WM: Purpose in life, depression, and locus of control. *J Clin Psychol* 1980;**36:**661.

Rettig S: Existential dialectics in therapeutic groups. *Psychiatr Q* 1981;**53:**33.

Rynearson EK: Suicide internalized: An existential sequestrum. *Am J Psychiatry* 1981;**138:**84.

Yalom I: *Existential Psychotherapy*. Basic Books, 1980.

Behavior Therapy & Cognitive Therapy

46

Hanna Levenson, PhD, & Kenneth S. Pope, PhD

Approach Shared by Behavior & Cognitive Therapies

Although there are many types of behavior and cognitive therapies, they have in common several elements that form an underlying core and theoretical rationale (see also Chapter 3), and the approach of the behavior or cognitive therapist involves an implicit 5-step procedure:

(1) The individual is evaluated for "symptoms" of behavioral dysfunction, which may be noted by direct observation (eg, eating, stuttering, crying); by the individual's verbalization of thoughts and feelings (eg, suicidal thoughts, depression); and by clinical measurements (eg, blood pressure, heart rate). The behavioral-cognitive therapist does not conceptualize a problem in terms of a psychiatric diagnosis (eg, schizophrenia) but instead defines it in terms of specific behaviors that affect the individual's function (eg, hallucinating in public). Because it is not essential to use a "strictly medical" model in behavior or cognitive therapies, the individual seeking help is usually referred to as the *client* (not the patient).

(2) The therapist and client determine the goals of the treatment. These often focus on specific behaviors to be changed, ie, **target behaviors.**

(3) In addition to defining the problem in behavioral terms, the therapist assesses conditions that maintain or minimize these behaviors. Steps 1 and 3 are referred to as **behavioral analysis.** Careful documentation and quantification are of great importance in determining factors that influence or trigger the undesired behaviors and in evaluating the effectiveness of the interventions. Since clients are often unaware of sequences of events that lead to a specific type of behavior, direct observation of clients in their environments is sometimes a necessary part of behavioral analysis. Clients can often be trained in self-observation skills and in recording of events so that the behavioral analysis is more accurate. Data derived from the analysis are used by the therapist to formulate a clinical hypothesis about what stimulates (precedes) and what maintains (reinforces) the undesired actions, thoughts, feelings, or physiologic changes.

(4) Using methods supported by theories and findings from the literature, the clinician tests the hypothesis of cause and effect by altering the behavior or the environment (or both) and observing the effects of the alternation on the client's dysfunctional actions, thoughts, and feelings.

(5) From systematic observation and documentation of behavioral changes, the clinician either revises the hypothesis or continues with treatment until the goals of therapy are reached, ie, the target behaviors are changed. It is important to stress that behavior therapy is based on a way of thinking about people and problems and is not a set of techniques. Testing one hypothesis often leads to the development of another hypothesis, which in turn must be tested.

Other Characteristics Shared by Behavior & Cognitive Therapies

In addition to sharing the empirical, scientific approach outlined above, behavior and cognitive therapies have other characteristics in common:

(1) Therapy involves action as well as discussion. It is often directive, structured, and brief or time-limited.

(2) The client must be a responsible participant in the therapy and capable of achieving personal change.

(3) The present (here and now) determinants of behavior are emphasized rather than the historic (then and there) determinants.

(4) It is assumed that human behavior follows natural laws.

(5) It is assumed that people's behavior reflects their adaptation to the environment and not necessarily underlying pathologic disorders.

(6) It is assumed that behavior can be changed directly without changing personality dynamics.

(7) Paraprofessionals, lay people significant to the client, and even the clients themselves can carry out treatment.

(8) The treatment often involves "homework." Only in rare instances is treatment confined to 1 or 2 hours a week with the therapist. Exercise, rehearsal, practice, and other activities are generally carried out by the client between sessions.

Relationship of Behavior & Cognition to the Problem

A. Behavior: The behavioral system—what the client *does,* as well as the presumed causes, cues (stimuli), effects, and implications of that behavior—may be related to the client's problem in at least 3 major ways:

First, the behavior may *be* the problem. For example, one client may be striking his or her children, and another may be taking sedative-hypnotics and alcohol before going to sleep each night. The violence and abuse of alcohol and drugs constitute the problems that will be a focus of therapy. The client and therapist will work to eliminate these behaviors.

Second, behavior may *create or sustain* the problem. For example, a husband may tend to spend all his leisure time playing tennis with his friends. This results in an unhappy marriage and tension at home. His wife resents his frequent absences and refuses to have sex with him. His children feel abandoned, which makes him feel guilty and inadequate as a father. Although such behavior is not inherently pathologic, it can create or maintain the type of distress that brings people to therapy.

Third, behavior may be instrumental in *solving or treating* the problem. A woman who is extremely depressed may work with a therapist to devise a treatment plan that includes devoting at least 1 hour a day to running and other vigorous exercise. She is encouraged to engage in this behavior whether or not she feels depressed and regardless (within reason, of course) of the other tasks and obligations that fill her days. In this case, the behavior (running) may be essentially unrelated to the nature and causes of her problem (depression). Although it will most likely be important to deal with those causes more directly in other phases of the treatment plan, the psychologic and physiologic effects of running may bring some immediate relief from depression and may enable her to deal more effectively with the causes of depression.

B. Cognition: Cognitive perceptions and ideation may also be related to an identified problem in 3 ways. First, they may constitute the problem itself (eg, preoccupation with suicidal thoughts, obsessive thoughts about a former lover, hallucinations and delusions). Second, cognitions may cause, cue, or maintain the problem. For example, thinking about food may lead to overeating in an individual prone to overeating; thinking about previous failures in college examinations may lead to frustration and anxiety in test-taking situations. Finally, cognitions may serve to alleviate a problem. For example, covert self-instruction (see the section on self-talk, below) can help the client master new behaviors in formerly stressful situations. Identifying, analyzing, and eliminating excessively self-critical or self-defeating thoughts can help alleviate depression and low self-esteem. These processes can also help free clients to consider alternative ways of approaching challenges, disappointments, and new situations.

Historical Context

In his experiments on learned and unlearned (conditioned and unconditioned) behavior, Ivan Pavlov (1849–1936) trained dogs to salivate at the sound of a bell by repeatedly pairing a conditioned stimulus (bell) with an unconditioned stimulus (food powder) that naturally causes an unconditioned response (salivation). Similarly, John B. Watson (1878–1958) taught a 1-year-old boy to be afraid of a white rat by pairing the child's approach to the rat with a loud noise. The

boy then generalized his fear to other white furry objects. This study suggested the process whereby phobias might develop and gave impetus to later work on aversive conditioning and counterconditioning.

For their research using **classical conditioning,** Pavlov and Watson are credited with beginning the systematic study of the effects of environment on behavior. However, it is **operant (instrumental) conditioning** that has had the major effect on behavioral theory as applied to clinical problems. In the 1950s, behavioral modification began to attract attention, largely because of the work of B.F. Skinner (1904–   ). Skinner used operant conditioning principles—which hold that behavior is a function of its consequences (**reinforcers**)—to change the behaviors of psychotic patients in the wards of state hospitals. Techniques such as extinction and positive reinforcement, as well as programmatic efforts such as token economies (all described in subsequent sections), are examples of applied operant conditioning principles.

Throughout the 1950s and 1960s, behavior modification focused on stimulus (S) and response (R), while factors mediating the S-R connection were largely ignored. However, with the accumulation of empirical clinical data, it soon became clear that the variance in how one responded to a situation would not always be predicted by the stimulus that preceded it or the consequence that followed it.

In order to improve their ability to understand, predict, and control behavior, therapists and researchers (eg, Albert Bandura, Julian Rotter) began exploring cognitive variables such as expectancy (predictions of future happenings), attributions (inferred characteristics of people or events), and mental images (ideas). While traditional behavior therapy focused on observable stimulus-response (S-R) connections, cognitive behavior therapy took into account the importance of mediating factors within the organism (S-O-R). As pointed out by Turner and colleagues (1981) in the *Handbook of Clinical Behavior Therapy,* "the acceptance of the role of cognitive variables in behavior theory and therapy has been very slow and grudgingly given. From the very beginning of the behavior movement, cognitive behaviors and private events were viewed outside the realm of behaviors because they were not subject to direct observation, measurement, and manipulation." Since the 1970s, however, cognitive variables have been given a central role in the understanding of processes that influence behavior (eg, self-instruction, cognitive therapy for depression, imagery techniques).

Cognitive therapy—which is farther along on the continuum from behavior therapy to cognitive behaviorism—focuses more on the individual's interpretations of internal and external events and views them as crucial in understanding behavior. The purely cognitive view holds that dysfunctional thoughts may be influenced by dealing with the individual's thoughts directly.

Of recent interest to clinicians is the new field of behavioral medicine (see Chapter 51), which involves the use of behavioral and cognitive principles and techniques in the treatment of medical problems such as hypertension, weight reduction, obesity, and cancer.

TECHNIQUES

This section will briefly outline some of the many techniques that have been developed in the cognitive-behavioral area. Any attempt to classify these treatments into behavioral or cognitive categories is frustrating for all but the most naive, since the methods in the field have so intertwined behavioral and cognitive perspectives. We have, however, presented the 10 techniques in a progression from those relying more on observable behavior to those relying more on private and subjective cognitions.

Positive Reinforcement & Extinction

Reinforcement and extinction are discussed first, since they represent an early attempt to apply behavioral principles to treatment of seriously disturbed patients. It is a well-known learning principle that the probability a specific behavior will occur is increased when the behavior is followed by certain pleasurable consequences (reinforcers). For example, in a now classic study, it was demonstrated that certain verbal responses of a patient would be increased by an approving "mm-hm" from the therapist. When a behavior is no longer reinforced and is ignored, the probability of its occurring is decreased. For example, ignoring a paient's request for special treatment should lead to the elimination of these requests.

A clinical example from the literature will illustrate not only the effectiveness of positive reinforcement but also the care with which behavioral data are used for determining improvement.

Illustrative case. A 39-year-old woman with a diagnosis of schizophrenia exhibited self-destructive behaviors such as burning herself and her clothing with cigarettes at a baseline rate of once a day. Because she liked to smoke (ie, would frequently indulge in this behavior), hospital staff members were instructed to inspect the patient for burns every hour and to give the patient half of a cigarette (reinforcer) and praise her for her appearance (secondary social reinforcer) if she was found to be burn-free. If she burned herself during the hour, she received no further cigarettes that day. Burns decreased from one a day to one approximately every 4 days (0.24 burns a day), and during the last 2 weeks of her hospitalization she remained burn-free.

Among the learning theory concepts that are important in applying positive reinforcement and extinction are the concepts of shaping, prompting, and modeling. Since it may take some time for a specific behavior (eg, speech in a mute patient) to be elicited, the desired behavior must be **shaped** by the therapist's reinforcing successive approximations of the wanted behavior (eg, progressively rewarding lip movement, then vocalizations, then isolated words, and finally sentences). Desired behaviors may also be **prompted** (eg, shaping the lips of the patient) or **modeled** (eg, saying words in front of the patient).

In institutionalized settings such as inpatient psychiatric wards or prisons, behaviors can be reinforced indirectly by issuing tokens (secondary reinforcers) that can be "traded in" for primary reinforcers or for other reinforcers such as watching television. This **token economy** approach is based on the underlying premise that dysfunctional behavior exists because it has been reinforced. Even professional staff members inadvertently reinforce undesired behavior by attending to (and thereby reinforcing) unwanted behavior such as head banging or delusional speech. Token economies represent an effort to provide an environment that systematically reinforces the desired behavior and extinguishes self-defeating dysfunctional activities.

Tokens (such as poker chips or points) offer several advantages over direct reinforcers: (1) They are readily available and can be handed over immediately after the desired behavior. (2) Tokens may be saved and redeemed later when the desire arises for goods or services, so that satiation is not a problem. (3) The number of tokens issued for a specific behavior may be increased or decreased depending upon how consistently the new behaviors are evidenced.

The staff must be trained to recognize desired behavior, to administer tokens, and to ignore dysfunctional actions. They must consistently apply the reinforcement and extinction principles. One or 2 staff members who do not apply these principles reliably and readily can undermine the efforts of the others.

A study spanning a 6-year period including a postinstitutionalization follow-up indicated that 89% of the patients in a token economy unit had improved while on the ward, whereas improvement was seen in only 46% of patients receiving milieu therapy alone. Eighteen months following discharge, 92% of patients treated in the token economy unit and 71% of those treated in the milieu therapy unit were living in the community. A little-emphasized but important result of token economies is the improved morale and efficiency of the staff, who see progress and feel a sense of accomplishment with a difficult population.

Aversive Procedures

Much of our everyday behavior reflects avoidance of aversive consequences built into various components of our personal and institutional lives—disapproval from friends, failing grades, imprisonment, etc. The application of this principle to clinical problems is aversive therapy. Aversive procedures are useful clinically in 2 main sets of cases: when dysfunctional or inappropriate behavior is naturally reinforcing to the individual (eg, addictions, deviant sexual behavior) or when behavior is self-destructive and needs to be brought under control quickly.

There are 3 main aversive procedures: classical conditioning, punishment, and avoidance training. The aversive stimuli used clinically are numerous but usually involve electric shock, chemicals, or vivid descriptions of noxious scenes.

In **classical conditioning** procedures, the stimuli leading to unwanted behavior (eg, sight and smell of one's favorite alcoholic beverage) are paired with a noxious stimulus (eg, shock). After the unconditioned stimulus (shock) is repeatedly associated with the conditioned stimulus (alcohol), patients develop the same feeling toward the alcohol as they feel toward the shock (fear). Since learned responses are more generalizable in lifelike settings, clinicians have had barlike settings constructed in inpatient alcohol units. Here patients are exposed to the sights, sounds, and smells of a bar, but these stimuli are paired with shocks. The goal of such treatment is avoidance of bars by the patients once they have been discharged.

In **punishment** procedures, a specific behavior (eg, drinking alcohol) is followed by a noxious stimulus or punishment. In the bar setting just described, punishment was used as a component of the treatment. A patient who had poured a favorite alcoholic beverage received a strong electric shock to the little finger (punishment) when he or she started to take the drink. The shock continued until the patient spit out the alcohol (**negative reinforcement** or **escape conditioning**). Thus, the patient was punished for undesired behavior (drinking) and then reinforced for desired behavior (spitting out the alcohol).

Aversive procedures may become quite sophisticated and more advanced when they are used as part of an integrated program of behavioral change and when the noxious stimuli include verbal imagery techniques as well. For example, inpatient behavior treatment for alcoholism may include such components as "self-confrontation" and "discrimination training" for controlled drinking. The former consists of having patients view videotapes of their own drunken behavior. In the latter technique, electric shock is applied only when the drinking patient shows evidence of too-high alcohol levels.

In **avoidance training** procedures, patients can escape the noxious stimulus altogether if they avoid the undesired behavior. This is the theory behind the use of disulfiram (Antabuse). If the patient drinks even a small amount of alcohol while a dose of disulfiram is still in the body, severe nausea and vomiting will occur. The patient can avoid these unpleasant effects entirely by not drinking (see Chapter 26).

Aversive techniques have also been applied to other consumption behaviors such as cigarette smoking. One such technique is rapid smoking, in which cigarette smokers take a normal inhalation every 6 seconds until they are physiologically unable to continue because of the increased intake of nicotine and carbon monoxide. Clearly, such a technique is inappropriate for individuals with coronary or pulmonary diseases.

A risk-free alternative is focused smoking, in which subjects smoke at their normal rates but are sensitized by the clinician to focus on the aversive changes and discomforts associated with smoking—eg, burning throat, breathing difficulties, headaches. Use of rapid or focused smoking techniques has resulted in reported abstinence rates of 40–60% after 6 months.

The effectiveness of aversive principles for the treatment of self-destructive behaviors is also well documented. For example, Lovaas and Simmons (1969) reported a case in which a 16-year-old mentally retarded girl bit her hands (and had previously bitten them to the extent that one finger had to be amputated), ripped her nails out with her teeth, and severely banged her head. Five 1-second shocks following these behaviors eliminated the problem.

In general, aversive techniques are most effective when used in conjunction with other forms of treatment and with procedures that reinforce the patient for desired behavior. Aversive procedures have been shown to have little effect on patients who actively oppose treatment, because they do not generalize from the learning situation to the real world. However, regardless of the effectiveness of such techniques for voluntary, motivated subjects, one should consider ethical factors in using aversive techniques and keep in mind that aversive techniques are susceptible to greater and more harmful abuses than other procedures. Because of the potential for abuse, some states regulate the use of aversive procedures or even prohibit entirely their use with certain populations. For example, the District of Columbia prohibits the use of "aversive stimuli" for mentally retarded persons. The American Association on Mental Deficiency has recently issued a statement urging elimination of many of these techniques, including all which cause obvious physical pain and dehumanization (Rubenstein, 1987, personal communication). Similarly, some clinicians advocate that state licensing boards and professional societies approve and monitor the use of aversive techniques, especially in involuntarily institutionalized populations.

Systematic Desensitization

Both positive reinforcement and aversive procedures are used in an attempt to create links between patients' behavior and particular rewards or punishments. In this sense, patients become "sensitized."

However, people may become "sensitized" to a stimulus, and this link leads to pathologic, destructive, or unwanted behaviors. For example, the reaction of a very shy and insecure person to the "stimulus" of other people may be panic, and this reaction may lead the person to avoid other people as much as possible and become virtually incapacitated in the presence of others. A person who has grown up thinking sex is immoral, unclean, and forbidden may react to a sexual situation by becoming anxious and unable to function. A person who has been in a traumatic car accident may be overwhelmed with fear at the prospect of riding in a car again. In these cases, avoiding the stimuli (other people, sexual situations, and being in a car) can be positively reinforcing because it reduces panic, anxiety, and fear. The individuals are sensitized (in a defeating way) to the stimuli, and the problem is to help them become desensitized. To accomplish this goal, Wolpe (1958) developed a method of systematic desensitization.

In systematic desensitization, the strategy is to help the client create a state (ie, complete relaxation) that is incompatible with anxiety, fear, or tension and then to gradually introduce the stimulus. The incompatible state acts to inhibit the negative reactions. This part of the process is known as **reciprocal inhibition.** The connection between the stimulus and the anxiety is systematically weakened until complete desensitization occurs.

There are numerous ways to accomplish complete relaxation, but most are variations of the progressive relaxation procedure popularized by Jacobson (1938). Clients assume a comfortable, passive position in a quiet room. They are told to free their minds of all troublesome or anxiety-provoking thoughts and to become as comfortable as possible, beginning with relaxing their feet. First they tense all the foot muscles for several seconds (as is sometimes done in isometric exercises) and then let them go limp. This process not only helps them relax that part of the body but also helps them learn body signals relating to relaxation. They can feel the muscles release tension. They learn to identify the feeling of being without tension, which many people who are chronically tense have not experienced before. Once the feet are relaxed, the same process of tensing followed by relaxation is repeated for the calves and other parts of the body. This process may take some time to rehearse and learn. The next step is to begin desensitizing the stimulus, as illustrated below.

Illustrative case. The client was afraid of parties, formal dinners, and similar social situations. He worked with his therapist to construct a hierarchy of cues (stimuli) associated with fear: Most terrifying to the client was actually being at such a gathering; slightly less frightening, driving to the gathering; still less intimidating, dressing for the occasion; and least intimidating though still a problem, receiving an invitation in the mail.

After he was thoroughly relaxed, the client began by imagining the least frightening stimulus in his hierarchy. When he became tense, he repeated the relaxation process. After he could contemplate receiving an invitation without having an increased heart rate, sweaty palms, and thoughts of panic, he progressed to thoughts about the next stimulus, dressing for the party. Several sessions, each focusing on one stage of the hierarchy, were required before the client could run through the stimuli in his imagination without experiencing overwhelming anxiety.

The client then began to repeat the process, starting with the least threatening aspect, in real rather than imagined situations. Slowly and systematically, he became desensitized to the stimuli. He was finally able to attend and enjoy social gatherings.

It is not clear why systematic desensitization is effective, although Wolpe believes that the process of reciprocal inhibition is responsible. (See the following section on exposure treatment for a different explanation.) What does seem clear is that the technique works for many clients in relatively few sessions.

Exposure Treatment

Recent work indicates that overcoming avoidance behavior (eg, phobias, obsessive compulsive behavior) may depend not upon relaxation paired with progressively more anxiety-provoking scenes, as Wolpe suggests, but actual exposure to the feared stimulus. Exposure treatment involves exposure of clients to the stimuli that evoke discomfort until they become accustomed to them. The types of procedures vary, ranging from those evoking little anxiety (as in the slow, graded, imagined process of desensitization described earlier) to those immersing the client in the feared situation (process of flooding). A recent review of the literature by Marks (1978) revealed that there are at least 56 terms pertinent to treatments containing elements of exposure. For example, suddenly handing a snake to a person afraid of snakes and having the phobic individual hold it for a period of time is an illustration of **counterphobic treatment.** Asking clients to bring on an anxiety response (eg, "Can you make yourself have an anxiety attack?") is an example of **paradoxical intention.** Having them watch another person approach the phobic situation is called **participant modeling** or **contact desensitization.** And having them approach the phobic situation themselves in daily life is termed **self-observation** or **exposure homework.** A long, imagined exposure, usually experienced with much anxiety, is termed **implosion.**

Marks (1981) has done extensive work both in developing the theory and refining the clinical practice of exposure treatments. Based on past systematic research, he outlined the conditions most suitable for exposure therapy: agoraphobia, social phobias, illness phobias, simple ("specific") phobias, obsessive thoughts, compulsive rituals, and types of sexual dysfunction (see Chapters 31 and 37).

For treatment of agoraphobia, Marks suggests choosing to work on simple but important acitvities at first. Initially, a reassuring person should accompany the agoraphobic person into the feared situations (eg, driving on a freeway). Exposure can then be attempted alone but at less anxiety-provoking times (eg, not at rush hour). Prolonged exposures (1–2 hours) seem to be more effective than short exposures. The client is required to record behaviors in a diary. (See Marks's [1978] self-help book for clients, *Living With Fear*.)

Illustrative case. A married 40-year-old woman had been agoraphobic for 15 years. Lately, she had been unable to leave the house without her husband. She chose as her goal (target behavior) the ability to cross a busy street alone. Treatment began with crossing a street with the therapist. After they had done this several times, the therapist stood apart and then moved farther away as the client crossed the street. By the end of the first 1½-hour treatment session, the woman was able to cross the street alone. She felt pleased with her accomplishment and much calmer. She was given homework assignments consisting of crossing streets near her home. By the end of the eighth treatment, the woman was crossing streets and shopping alone without anxiety.

Recently, exposure therapy has been used to treat panic disorder (Gitlin et al, 1985). Using education about physiology and management of panic symptoms, relaxation, and exposure, 10 of 11 panic disorder clients became symptom-free. Interestingly, at follow-up, the factor most frequently mentioned by clients as helpful was the reassurance that resulted from education about the nature of panic attacks.

Although there is abundant evidence that exposure therapy is effective, it is not clear why it works—by habituation to the feared stimulus, expectancy of control, education, or learning to cope. It is also unclear why other methods of treating avoidance behavior (eg, antidepressant drugs or discussion-oriented therapies) are effective in reducing anxiety without using exposure techniques.

Covert Conditioning

Cautela (1972) developed the theory that many self-defeating behaviors are maintained, encouraged, or cued by elaborate chains of images (covert processes). For example, a man with a problem of overeating who overhears someone mention chocolate cake may have the following chain of thoughts: He remembers his last big meal, which was topped off by a huge, rich slice of German chocolate cake; he begins to think of his plans for an evening meeting and realizes that he has 2 hours before the meeting starts; he thinks of the restaurant down the street, which serves wonderful chocolate cake; he decides that waiting one more day to start his diet will make no real difference in the long run; etc.

In some cases, the imagery sequence leads to undesirable behavior, eg, overeating, nail biting, violence, or spending sprees. In others, it leads to a dysphoric mood, eg, depression resulting from distorted memories associated with guilt, panic when confronted with a new situation, or "falling apart" at seemingly minor inconveniences. Sometimes it may be the images themselves that are unwanted, eg, intrusive thoughts from a trauma once experienced, repetitive thoughts of having forgotten to turn off the bath water or lock the door before leaving home, or obsessive thoughts about a lost love.

Covert conditioning uses the principles of classical and operant conditioning to modify the chains of covert images. In one method, for example, thoughts that habitually lead to eating high-calorie foods may be paired with the startling and vivid aversive image of maggots crawling out of the cake or the painful image of the person undergoing triple bypass surgery for a heart attack brought on by overeating. In this manner, the individual is conditioned to respond to the disgusting or painful image rather than to the pleasurable image of biting into a piece of cake.

In Cautela's "self-control triad" method, 3 cognitive-behavioral techniques are used in sequence to enable clients to replace pathologic or self-defeating imagery with positive, adaptive, creative cognitive processes: First, clients are taught to recognize the onset of imagery sequences and to use clear and vivid **thought-stopping imagery** to alter them. As soon as the image occurs, the clients create a mental image of a huge red stop sign and imagine the word "stop" being shouted. Second, they use an abbreviated form of the **relaxation techniques** described above in the section on systematic desensitization. They begin deep breathing and covertly repeating the word "relax" when unwanted thoughts or mental images begin to emerge. Third, clients positively reinforce this self-control process by **imagining a pleasurable scene.** For example, the man with the problem of overeating might choose to imaging what he will look like after he has lost all his excess weight and can picture himself at the beach, being admired by everyone around him. It is important for the therapist to refrain from specifying what this pleasurable scene will be. Clients must instead be encouraged to identify and develop the scene themselves. These 3 methods are learned separately. After clients become adept at using them, the methods are used in sequence.

Covert Modeling

The behavioral research described earlier in this chapter and in other chapters focuses on how the behavior of individuals can be changed by the contingencies and other influences of the environment (by classical and operant conditioning and other principles of learning). In the last 2 decades, however, Bandura (1977) and others have shown how behavioral changes can be systematically brought about through **vicarious learning,** ie, through observing someone else (a model) perform a desired behavior. This process has gained widespread attention as a result of the controversy over research strongly suggesting that frequent viewing of violent scenes in the movies or on television increases one's tendency to engage in violent behavior.

Though the mechanisms of vicarious learning are not well understood, it seems likely that modeling affects the observer's cognitive processes as well as behavior. It may, for example, affect the covert imagery sequences described above in the section on covert conditioning. This reasoning led Kazdin (1977) and others to postulate that it may not be necessary to observe a "real" model for vicarious learning to occur; an imaginary model may be used, with the observation itself taking place on a covert, cognitive level.

Illustrative case. The client was insecure and had difficulty being assertive. She described her problem as follows: "People just walk all over me. I can never speak up. I have a piece of string for a backbone." The therapist asked her to give an example. She said she had purchased a videotape recorder, and when she got home, the machine worked poorly. She was afraid to take it back and "make a fuss," so she left it for several weeks in her living room, unable to use it.

The therapist asked her to imagine someone who meets her ideal of assertiveness and to describe how the model would act under the same circumstances. The client then imagined the model going to the store, making the same purchase, returning home, and finding that the machine did not function properly. The model promptly took the machine back to the store and said: "This recorder doesn't work as it's supposed to. Can you fix it quickly, or would it be better if you gave me a replacement?" The client then imagined all of the obstacles the customer might encounter in such a situation and "saw" her handling these situations confidently and effectively.

The client practiced this covert modeling technique and eventually learned to become more assertive.

There is evidence that covert modeling is more effective when the model and client are of the same sex, age, and social position; that use of several covert models is more effective than using only one; and that effectiveness is enhanced when the client elaborates on the description of any model or scene suggested by the therapist.

Self-Talk

It is common for children to repeat instructions to themselves as they attempt new tasks. For example, while crossing the street unaccompanied for the first time, a child may engage in a running monolog of the parents' instructions: "Stop at the corner. Wait for the light to change from red to green, and make sure the 'walk' sign is on. Now look both ways to make sure no traffic is coming." These instructions may be repeated aloud, in a whisper, or silently. Adults too may attempt to learn new tasks in this way, eg, in taking up golf or tennis or assembling a bicycle.

People may be taught to use such self-talk—in the form of evaluative statements, suggestions, reminders of sequential steps, and encouragement—to help them relax, to improve performance of cognitive and physical activities, to increase motivation, and to become more aware and alert. Such self-talk is obviously related to the processes of covert modeling (see above) and cognitive therapy (see below).

Various techniques may be used for teaching self-talk in therapy, but the general approach is demonstrated by Meichenbaum's (1977) program of self-talk for children, which has been successful in treatment of problems related to hyperactivity, aggression, disruption, and cheating. There are 5 basic steps after the problem has been identified and the behavior to be learned has been defined: (1) The child observes as an adult model performs the behavior. While the child is watching, the model describes the behavior aloud. (2) The child performs the same task while the model gives instructions. (3) The child performs the task while giving instructions aloud. (4) The child whispers the instructions while performing the task. (5) The child performs the task without audible speech.

Cognitive Therapy for Depression

The underlying premise of cognitive therapy is that effect and behavior are largely functions of how people construe (structure) their world. According to one cognitive theory, everyone has "filters" through which the world is interpreted (eg, seeing the glass half-full versus seeing it half-empty). When these constructs become distorted and dysfunctional, clients often experience helplessness, anxiety, and depression (depressogenic schemas). Beck and coworkers (1979) are the best-known investigators of cognitive therapy for depression. The goals of this cognitive therapy are (1) to make clients aware of their cognitive distortions through psychotherapy and (2) to effect change through correction of these distortions. Common distortions (errors in information processing) that make people depressed include selective abstractions (missing the significance of a total situation by selecting a detail out of context), arbitrary inferences (jumping to a conclusion with missing or contradictory evidence), overgeneralizations (unjustified generalizations on the basis of one incident), and magnifications (exaggerating or elaborating on specifics). (See the writings of Beck and coworkers [1979] for a detailed description of these common errors.)

The numerous strategies used in cognitive therapy are designed to help the client become aware of negative automatic thoughts (eg, "If I can't be perfect, then no one will love me"); to recognize connections between thoughts, affect, and behavior; and to replace distorted thoughts with more realistic and option-filled interpretations.

In a typical course of therapy for depression, clients are initially told how cognitive therapy works. They are then assigned "homework" such as keeping a schedule of activities to help them assess their present levels of functioning. In the next session, the relationship between thinking, behavior, and affect is demonstrated using specific experiences of the client. Later, the client is told how to recognize, monitor, and record emotions and situations associated with negative automatic thoughts (Table 46–1) and how to devise rational responses. These automatic thoughts and their underlying assumptions are then discussed in therapy and examined for logic, adaptiveness, and likelihood of promoting healthy behavior. The following discussions are examples from Beck and coworkers (1979):

Patient: The only way I could ever be happy is if I could be a great writer.

Therapist: What level of writing would you have to reach?

Table 46–1. Example of a daily record of dysfunctional thoughts.*

Date	Situation	Emotion(s)	Automatic Thought(s)	Rational Response	Outcome
	1. Describe actual event leading to unpleasant emotion. **or** 2. Describe stream of thoughts, daydream, or recollection leading to unpleasant emotion.	1. Specify sad/ anxious, etc. 2. Rate degree of emotion, 1–100.	1. Write automatic thought that preceded emotion. 2. Rate belief in automatic thought, 0–100%.	1. Write rational response to automatic thought. 2. Rate belief in rational response, 0–100%.	1. Rerate belief in automatic thought, 0–100%. 2. Specify and rate subsequent emotion, 1–100.
9/8	Received a letter from friend who was recently married.	Guilty 60	"I should have gone to her wedding." 90%	It was inconvenient; she wouldn't be writing if she was angry about it. 95%	10% Guilty 20
9/9	Was thinking of all the things I wanted to get done over the weekend.	Anxious 40	"I'll never get all of this done. It's too much for me." 100%	I've done more than this before, and there is no law that says I have to get it all done. 80%	25% Anxious 20
9/11	Made a mistake ordering supplies.	Anxious 60	Pictured my boss yelling at me. 100%	There is no evidence my boss will be angry; even if he is, I don't have to be upset. 100%	0% Relieved 50
9/12	Pictured myself being depressed forever.	Sad/anxious 90	"I'll never get better."	I have gotten better in the past. Just because I think something is true doesn't make it true. 80%	40% Sad/anxious 60
9/13	My date called and said he couldn't go out with me because he had to work.	Sad 95	"He doesn't like me. NO ONE could ever like me." 90%	He asked me out for next weekend, so he must like me. He probably did have to work. Even if he didn't like me, it doesn't follow that "no one could ever like me." 90%	30% Sad 50

*Reproduced, with permission, from Beck AT et al: Page 288 in: *Cognitive Therapy of Depression.* Guilford Press, 1979.

Patient: I would have to be as good as [a specific poet].
Therapist: Did this poet achieve great happiness?
Patient: No, I guess not. She killed herself.

As the therapy progresses, the focus shifts to identifying recurrent or common themes and finally to uncovering major beliefs that make the person vulnerable to depression:

Therapist: Your automatic thought was "Your children shouldn't fight and act up." And because they do, "I must be a rotten mother." Why shouldn't your children act up?
Patient: They shouldn't act up because . . . I am so nice to them.
Therapist: What do you mean?
Patient: Well, if you're nice, bad things shouldn't happen to you.
(At this point, the patient's eyes lit up.)

The course of treatment continues in this way for about 15–25 once-weekly sessions. In contrast to the more traditional psychotherapies, in cognitive therapy the clinician is active and directive and the focus is on "here and now" problems. In contrast to the more behavior-oriented therapies, cognitive therapy is concerned with altering the client's internal experiences (eg, thoughts, daydreams, feelings) rather than external behavior per se.

Beck (1985) summarized 8 studies comparing the efficacy of cognitive therapy with that of antidepressant medication. Findings showed that: (1) cognitive therapy alone was as effective as 3 trials or more effective than 2 trials of antidepressant medication; (2) the combination of cognitive therapy and drug therapy was more effective than drug therapy alone; and (3) cognitive therapy alone appears to be as effective as drug therapy plus cognitive therapy. These studies indicate that cognitive therapy achieves good results in ameliorating symptoms of moderate unipolar depression in nonpsychotic outpatients.

In an important study sponsored by the National Institute of Mental Health (Elkin et al, 1986), cognitive therapy achieved results comparable to imipramine (antidepressant medication) in reducing the symptoms of depression and improving patients' functioning. Preliminary results indicate that symptoms were eliminated completely in 50–60% of patients who received cognitive, interpersonal,* or drug therapy and in 29% of those who received a placebo plus clinical manage-

---

* For a discussion of interpersonal therapy, see Chapter 44.

ment. Imipramine reduced symptoms more quickly, but in the last 4 weeks of the 16-week treatment period, both forms of psychotherapy were as effective as the drug. However, among the patients considered "severely depressed," cognitive therapy was the least effective treatment.

Positive Imagery

Singer (1974) pioneered the research, theory, and clinical applications of positive imagery. The idea is simple: Engaging in positive imagery tends to elevate one's moods and affects, tends to increase enjoyment, and can decrease the frequency and intensity of potentially debilitating and self-defeating thoughts and feelings. The key idea is that imagery need not be explicitly related to one's difficulties or embody modeled "answers"; it just needs to be pleasant. This approach has been effective in the treatment of pain, anxiety, severe depression, and phobic behavior.

Illustrative case. The client presented for psychotherapy with the following pattern of severe anxiety and depression: On awakening each morning, she began to worry about her job, finances, and children. By the time she got to work, she was a "nervous wreck." She often returned home early because of "sickness," and more recently she began missing days of work. Though exhausted at the end of day, she had trouble falling asleep. Anxious about her situation and concerned and sad about the way things were going, she tossed and turned all night.

The treatment plan for modifying various aspects of the client's experiences, habits, and situation included the use of positive imagery: Four times a day (upon awakening and before lunch, dinner, and going to bed), the client spent at least 15 minutes with her eyes closed, thinking of the most pleasant scenes she could imagine. According to her reports during subsequent weeks of therapy, the imagery varied widely and included scenes of vacations she had taken or would like to take, funny scenes, and sexual fantasies. Some imagery was far from realistic (eg, she pictured herself floating high above the clouds). She found that these positive scenes were helpful in "setting the tone" for her days and nights; breaking the momentum generated by her depressive, anxious, and obsessive thoughts; relearning what it felt like to enjoy herself; and freeing her from the depression of what she described as "those days when my worries seemed to snowball and come down and crush me."

Extremely anxious, defensive, or resistant clients—especially those who might tend to engage in power struggles with the therapist—may find it easier to use positive imagery than to participate in other forms of treatment described above and in other chapters. With positive imagery, these patients may feel more "in control" of their treatment, feel less "performance anxiety," and experience fewer problems related to issues of authority and dependence.

Guided Imagery

Guided imagery blends a psychoanalytic approach with several cognitive-behavioral principles. Perhaps the most widely known approach is Leuner's (1969) guided affective imagery, which focuses on the working through of conflicts by use of symbolic imagery. Leuner has developed specific procedures for crisis intervention, brief therapy, and long-term analysis, but in each instance, the client creates a series of a dozen "waking dreams." Each dream has a specific motif, and the motif are in the following sequence: meadow, brook, mountain, house, edge of the woods, encounter with relatives, sexual attitudes, lion (aggressive orientation), person embodying desired characteristics (ego ideal), cave or swamp, volcano, and picture book.

The client assumes a relaxed position, and the therapist suggests the motif: "Imagine that you are in a meadow." Then the client spontaneously creates a fantasy involving the motif. Leuner notes characteristic trends of imagery for various diagnostic groups. For example, depressed clients often describe the meadow as burned or dry; compulsive clients frequently envision a constricted meadow hemmed in by a barbed-wire fence.

The approach assumes that the client's imagery symbolizes his or her unconscious dynamic structure and that working through the specific dilemmas experienced in the imagination will influence the psychic conflicts. For example, if the client confronts an overwhelming obstacle in the meadow, the therapist might ask questions leading the client to explore alternatives and find successful solutions to overcome the obstacle.*

ISSUES & MISCONCEPTIONS ABOUT BEHAVIOR-ORIENTED THERAPY

Popular misconceptions and concerns about the use of behavior-oriented therapies, as expressed by numerous investigators and outlined in the American Psychiatric Association's *Task Force Report on Behavior Therapy* (1978), are listed and briefly described below:

(1) *Behavior therapy is coercive, manipulative, and controlling.* Because behavioral techniques are often powerful, direct approaches to changing behavior, they are criticized for controlling the individual's behavior. For this reason, behavior therapists have worked with both the American Psychological Association and the Association for the Advancement of Behavior Therapy to develop ethical guidelines for informed consent, use of aversive procedures, and protection of the client's rights.

---

* For a discussion of the use of this technique to treat nonpsychiatric illness, see Chapter 51.

(2) Behavior therapy is superficial, and "symptom substitution" will occur. Proponents of the theory that many undesired behaviors are symptoms of (or epiphenomena associated with) an underlying disease argue that if *only* symptoms are addressed, then new symptoms will appear at a later date because the underlying problem (ie, disease) has been left untreated. Although this theory of causation may be true, extensive empirical data from published reports fail to support any indication of new symptoms occurring after the target behaviors have been removed. In fact, effective treatment of specific target behaviors has often resulted in improvement in other aspects of the client's lives.

(3) Behavior therapists ignore feelings and thoughts and treat humans as robots. Many of the techniques described in the previous sections are focused on the inner world of the individual (eg, images, thoughts, feelings). These private events are playing an increasingly important part in behavioral-cognitive therapies. The objectives of the behavior therapist, however, are to make the client's subjective experiences public by means of the client's self-report and self-observation and to define the experiences objectively in terms of observable phenomena or physiologic measurements. In this process, clients may become aware of their own feelings and thoughts for the first time and thus increase the likelihood of changing them.

Behavior therapy adheres to the principle of determinism, which holds that events have causes and that relationships between cause and effect follow orderly laws; however, the individual is not seen as a reflexive robot. In behavior therapy, the interaction between environment and behavior is viewed as a dynamic one. There is a reciprocal determinism that has relevance for issues such as responsibility and choice. The growing field of behavioral self-control and the increasing number of do-it-yourself strategies for control of weight, smoking, and stress indicate ways in which individuals can alter their external and internal environments. Such behavioral approaches often provide more options and actions for the individual and result in increased personal freedom and dignity.

(4) Behavior therapy is limited to a narrow spectrum of disorders. Disorders that seem particularly amenable to behavioral-cognitive psychotherapies include not only phobias but also obsessive compulsive disorders and other anxiety disorders, sexual disorders, adjustment disorder, marital problems, disorders of impulse control, unipolar depression, stammering, enuresis and hyperactivity in children, and the "habit" disorders (eg, obesity; tobacco, alcohol, and other drug dependence). In addition, the same therapeutic techniques may be used for improving social skills, assertiveness, basic self-care skills, and disruptive behaviors in severely disturbed patients.

(5) Behavior therapy denies the importance of the therapeutic relationship. To some extent this criticism is true, especially in regard to the manner in which behavior therapy was practiced in the 1950s and 1960s,

when the focus was more on manipulation of environmental factors (see Historical Context, above). Today, factors affecting the outcome of therapy, such as the expectations for treatment success, the therapeutic alliance (successful working relationship between client and therapist), and the client's motivation, have become part of the therapist's concern. Persons and Burns (1985) investigated the nature and quality of the client-therapist relationship in addition to the technical cognitive interventions. They found that a reduction in the clients' negative mood was associated with a decrease in the clients' degree of belief in their automatic thoughts; moreover, clients' good relationships with their therapists contributed additional positive changes.

(6) Behavior therapy only works with nonverbal, unintelligent, severely disturbed people. Current behavioral-cognitive approaches seem to be helpful in treating a broad spectrum of clients with a wide variety of backgrounds and personality traits. In fact, several cognitive approaches—eg, paradoxical intention, reframing (reconceptualizing problems), logical investigation of depressogenic assumptions—seem particularly effective in helping highly verbal, logical, intelligent individuals learn to recognize and control obsessional thoughts that interfere with social functioning.

(7) Behavioral-cognitive techniques are practiced only by psychologists and paraprofessionals, not by psychiatrists. This statement has some validity, although several of the well-known pioneers in these fields are psychiatrists. Behavioral techniques can often be implemented by paraprofessionals and the clients themselves. This is seen by many as an advantage, since professional time can be devoted to developing treatment strategies and performing thorough behavioral analyses. Unfortunately, most residency programs for psychiatrists do not include training in basic behavioral science, and few behavior therapists are directly involved in the programs. This is a regrettable situation, since research in behavioral science has led to a number of specific treatment programs and has provided a method of approaching problems that has great clinical value for the practice of psychiatry.

RECENT TRENDS IN BEHAVIOR & COGNITIVE THERAPIES

Two trends are clear: (1) Behavior therapy is becoming increasingly more cognitive in its approach. Perhaps the melding of the technology of behavior therapy with the clinical concerns of the cognitive therapists has prevented what Kelly (1963), an early cognitive theorist, called "the hardening of the categories." (2) Behavioral-cognitive approaches are being integrated with psychodynamic theory and practice.

These 2 trends are illustrated by the objectives of Meichenbaum's (1978) approach:

(1) Help clarify or pinpoint the nature of the client's current problem.

(2) Reduce unpleasant affect through repetition of fantasy or behavior.

(3) Teach the client to distinguish between reality and fantasy.

(4) Teach the client to make even finer distinctions among impulsive, motivational, cognitive, and behavioral aspects of his or her problem.

(5) Teach the client to control behavior or cognitions.

(6) Increase the client's ability to recognize the irrationality of his or her beliefs or behavior.

(7) Decrease expectation of disastrous consequences and increase realistic appraisal of external problems.

(8) Make the client's unconscious conscious.

The 8 components of this clinical approach have a common core reflecting the goal of behavioral-cognitive therapies—to help clients develop an increased sense of control over their inner lives and their interpersonal behavior.

REFERENCES

American Psychiatric Association: *Task Force Report on Behavior Therapy*. American Psychiatric Association, 1978.

Bandura A: *Principles of Behavior Modification*. Holt, Rinehart & Winston, 1969.

Bandura A: *Social Learning Theory*. Prentice-Hall, 1977.

Beck AT: Is behavior therapy on course? *Behav Psychother* 1985;**13**:83.

Beck AT et al: *Cognitive Therapy of Depression*. Guilford Press, 1979,

Cautela JR: Rationale and procedures for covert conditioning. In: *Advances in Behavior Therapy*. Rubin RD et al (editors). Academic Press, 1972.

Elkin I et al: Outcome findings of the NIMH collaborative research program. Presented at the National Convention of the American Psychiatric Association, May, 1986.

Gitlin B et al: Behavior therapy for panic disorder. *J Nerve Ment Dis* 1985;**173**:742.

Jacobson E: *Progressive Relaxation*. Univ of Chicago Press, 1938.

Kazdin AE: Research issues in covert conditioning. *Cognitive Ther Res* 1977;**1**:45.

Kelly GA: *A Theory of Personality: The Psychology of Personal Constructs*. Norton, 1963.

Kendall PC, Holloon S (editors): *Cognitive-Behavioral Interventions: Assessment Methods*. Academic Press, 1982.

Lanyon RI, Lanyon BP: *Behavior Therapy: A Clinical Introduction*. Addison-Wesley, 1978.

Leuner H: Guided affective imagery (GAI): A method of intensive psychotherapy. *Am J Psychother* 1969;**23**:4.

Lovaas OI, Simmons JQ: Manipulation of self-destruction in three retarded children. *J Appl Behav Anal* 1969;**2**:143.

Mahoney MJ: *Cognition and Behavior Modification*. Ballinger, 1974.

Marks I: *Cure and Care of Neuroses*. Wiley, 1981.

Marks I: *Living With Fear*. McGraw-Hill, 1978.

Meichenbaum D: *Cognitive-Behavior Modification: An Integrative Approach*. Plenum Press, 1977.

Meichenbaum D: Why does using imagery in psychotherapy lead to change. Chapter 13 in: *The Power of Human Imagination: New Methods in Psychotherapy*. Singer JL, Pope KS (editors). Plenum Press, 1978.

Paul GL, Lentz RL: *Psychological Treatment of Chronic Mental Patients*. Harvard Univ Press, 1977.

Persons JB, Burns DD: Mechanisms of action of cognitive therapy: The relative contributions of technical and interpersonal interventions. *Cognitive Ther Res* 1985;**9**:539.

Singer JL: *Imagery and Daydream Methods in Psychotherapy and Behavior Modification*. Academic Press, 1974.

Singer JL, Pope KS (editors): *The Power of Human Imagination: New Methods in Psychotherapy*. Plenum Press, 1978.

Sjoden PO, Bates S, Dockens WS: *Trends in Behavior Therapy*. Academic Press, 1974.

Thoresen CE: *The Behavioral Therapist*. Brooks/Cole, 1980.

Turner S, Calhoun KS, Adams HE: *Handbook of Clinical Behavior Therapy*. Wiley, 1981.

Wolpe J: *Psychotherapy by Reciprocal Inhibition*. Stanford Univ Press, 1958.

47

Group Psychotherapy

Nick Kanas, MD, & Dennis Farrell, MD

Group psychotherapy is a form of treatment in which beneficial changes in emotionally disturbed patients occur as a result of their interactions with other patients and at least one trained professional therapist in a group setting. Therapeutic results include both relief of symptoms and resolution of intrapsychic and interpersonal problems. The therapist's tools are clinical experience and applied theories of individual psychodynamics and interpersonal systems.

Although the activities of self-help, human potential, and consciousness-raising groups may also be considered therapeutic in a broad sense, these groups differ from psychotherapy groups in their methodology and goals, the training and qualifications of group leaders, and other characteristics (Table 47–1). Only group *psychotherapy* is appropriate or recommended as treatment for emotionally ill people, although some patients in group psychotherapy may become involved with these other types of groups as well. Participation in some of these other groups—particularly Synanon and human potential groups—may be stressful for psychiatric patients and result in increased symptoms and even psychotic reactions. For this reason, patients with emotional problems should be referred to psychotherapy groups so that a trained professional can evaluate their ability to function in the group setting.

HISTORY OF GROUP PSYCHOTHERAPY

The first psychotherapy group was described in 1907 by Joseph Pratt, a Boston internist, who developed a group method of educating and improving the morale of patients with tuberculosis. Around 1910, Jacob Moreno in Europe began using theatrical techniques to have patients "act out" problem situations in a group setting; this later became known as psychodrama. In the late 1920s and early 1930s, a number of psychiatrists began applying psychoanalytic theory to groups, emphasizing issues of transference, free association, and recapitulation of family problems.

During the late 1930s and early 1940s, Kurt Lewin began emphasizing the importance of group member interactions and introduced the notion of group dynamics, a phenomenon describing actions in a group as being more than the sum of individual interactions. The need to train more therapists in the theory of group dynamics became obvious after World War II, when large numbers of veterans requiring psychiatric assistance began to overburden the personnel resources of the mental health system. Programs to train therapists using Lewin's concepts were established at the National Training Laboratories in Maine and at the Tavis-

Table 47–1. Therapeutic group activities.

Group	Examples of Groups or Approaches	Goals	Clientele	Leader
Group psychotherapy	Psychoanalytic Interactional Transactional analysis Gestalt Psychodrama Existential Behavioral	Relief of symptoms of emotional disturbances and resolution of intrapsychic and interpersonal problems	Emotionally ill patients	Professional (MD, PhD, MSW, RN)
Self-help groups	Alcoholics Anonymous Synanon Recovery, Inc.	Support focused on a common problem	People affected by a common problem	Lay
Human potential groups	Sensitivity training Encounter T (training) groups Group-as-a-whole (Tavistock) Marathon	Personal growth and improvement of relations with other people	Anyone desiring growth and development	Often professional
Consciousness-raising groups	Women's groups Homosexual groups	Support focused on difficulties produced by societal bias	People sharing a common social characteristic	Lay

tock Clinic in England, where the work of Bion and Ezriel led to the "group-as-a-whole" approach to treatment (Kibel and Stein, 1981).

During the ensuing 30 years, numerous approaches to group psychotherapy were introduced, including transactional analysis, gestalt, interactional, existential, and behavioral approaches. Currently, techniques borrowed from a number of theoretical schools are being consolidated to devise new responses to the specific needs of patients.

EFFECTIVENESS OF GROUP PSYCHOTHERAPY

Clinical experience and anecdotal evidence support the view that group psychotherapy is effective treatment for properly selected categories of patients. Successes have been reported in both inpatient and outpatient settings with both psychotic and nonpsychotic patients. A number of theoretical approaches to group psychotherapy have been advocated (see p 546 and Table 47–4).

Evidence from controlled studies also attests to the usefulness of group psychotherapy. Since 1975, a number of reviews have concluded that group psychotherapy is effective for patients with neurotic and personality disorders; schizophrenia; alcoholism; and medical illnesses, including asthma, myocardial infarction, obesity, chronic pain, and ulcers. Group psychotherapy has been found to be as effective as or even more effective than individual psychotherapy in studies directly comparing the 2 methods.

INDICATIONS & CONTRAINDICATIONS FOR GROUP PSYCHOTHERAPY

In organizing a psychotherapy group, the therapist must take into account both diagnostic and individual psychodynamic factors.

Diagnostic Factors

A. Indications for Psychotherapy in Heterogeneous Groups: Table 47–2 shows disorders for which treatment in a heterogeneous group (ie, consisting of a variety of psychiatric disorders) is most appropriate. In such groups, the diversity of problems and issues allows for maximal interaction and breadth of discussion. In getting the group together, the therapist should consider whether one patient will be perceived by the other as "too different," since this may result in scapegoating and rejection. For example, an elderly woman in a group of young adults might be rejected by the other members even though she is in the group to work on issues unrelated to aging. If at least 2 elderly patients were in the group, the tendency to scapegoat would be lessened.

Group psychotherapy with heterogeneous groups is particularly beneficial for patients with personality and

Table 47–2. Indications and contraindications for group psychotherapy, based on diagnostic considerations.

Indications
Most personality disorders*
Neurotic disorders*
Somatoform disorders*
Major depressive episode*
Substance use disorders†
Schizophrenic disorders†
Medical illness†
Gender identity disorders†
Posttraumatic stress disorders‡
Adjustment disorders‡
Contraindications
Acute manic episode
Antisocial personality disorder
Questionable§
Organic mental disorders*
Schizoid personality disorder*
Paranoid personality disorder*
Delusional disorders*
Dissociative disorders*
Factitious disorders*
Paraphilias‡
Sexual dysfunctions‡

*Therapy in heterogeneous groups (ie, groups of patients with different disorders) is recommended.
†Therapy in homogeneous groups (ie, groups of patients with same disorder) is recommended.
‡The type of group (heterogeneous or homogeneous) depends on the individual case.
§The decision about the appropriateness of group psychotherapy is based on such factors as the patient's degree of impairment and desire for treatment and on individual psychodynamic factors.

neurotic disorders. Patients with personality disorders tend to blame others for their maladaptive interactions and lack insight into their own role in provoking interpersonal strife. Since they do not have significant degrees of anxiety or other symptoms, they are only weakly motivated to change and often come to treatment at the urging of a spouse, employer, or primary-care physician. The group psychotherapy setting is an environment in which such patients can display and then be confronted with their maladaptive interactions. At the same time, other group members can offer support and reinforcement for positive changes, and this "reward" encourages them to remain in treatment.

Illustrative case No. 1. A young advertising copywriter had lost several jobs because of her frequent failure to meet deadlines. In the group, she spoke of bad feelings about her troubled relationships with peers and authority figures and expressed perplexity about the problems. She was intelligent and showed considerable insight into other problem areas of her life, but she was oblivious to the fact that she repeatedly provoked anger and rejection by habitually coming late to the group sessions. Only after repeated confrontations with other groups members—and the therapist—did her excuses and rationalizations give way to the realization that her core problem was expressed more in her behavior than in her words.

In contrast to patients with personality disorders, patients with neurotic disorders often have a number of symptoms, such as anxiety and depression, and perceive their difficulties as coming from within. For these reasons, neurotic patients do well in individual psychotherapy, although many also benefit from group psychotherapy. Such patients use the group to gain insight into the cause of their problems and to understand the effects their symptoms may have on other people.

Illustrative case No. 2. A middle-aged man began group psychotherapy to work on feelings of depression, low self-esteem, and lack of self-assertiveness. He immediately displayed these symptoms in his behavior in the group, begging pardon for assertive expressions and adopting a submissive attitude toward more aggressive members. The group noticed these habits of behavior and said so, and with encouragement he was able to begin expressing himself more forcefully. He then told of a dream in which the therapist appeared in the role of his father, who had died when the patient was 4 years old. The patient remembered being terrified by his father's displays of fierce temper. Fear of his father was related to his fear of others as he grew up, and he adopted a self-effacing character in order to avoid provoking anger in others.

Other patients benefiting from heterogeneous group psychotherapy include those with somatoform disorders or major depressive episodes. Such patients do well in supportive group settings where the impact of their illness on others can be explored. In some cases they may also gain insight into the causes of their problems.

B. Indications for Psychotherapy in Homogeneous Groups: Table 47–2 shows disorders for which a homogeneous group format is more appropriate. All of the patients have a similar problem, and the group is oriented toward addressing that problem. Homogeneous psychotherapy groups differ from support groups involving interaction with people who share some common problem in that the approach is more insight-oriented and the leader is professionally trained. A psychotherapy group made up of alcoholics differs from a meeting of Alcoholics Anonymous in that patients in psychotherapy not only gain support and encouragement for sobriety but also focus on problems related to their alcoholism, such as intrapsychic conflict and maladaptive interpersonal relationships. Although more limited in scope than their heterogeneous counterparts, homogeneous groups quickly become cohesive and allow for greater depth in exploring a particular set of problems.

Group psychotherapy in a homogeneous group is the treatment of choice for patients with substance use disorders such as alcoholism and drug dependency. By orienting these groups around the addiction problem, several issues that affect the patients in similar ways may be discussed. Such groups are particularly useful for confronting patients who deny having the diagnosed problem, as shown in the example below.

Illustrative case No. 1. A 55-year-old man in an outpatient group consisting of alcoholics persistently denied that he was an alcoholic. Several patients began discussing how they, too, refused to believe they were alcoholics and became convinced only when physical or social problems related to drinking became so serious they could no longer be ignored or rationalized. They further stated that their drinking was not brought under control until they were able to admit they had the problem. The patient then admitted that perhaps he did drink too much, whereupon he began discussing alcohol-related difficulties in his life.

Group psychotherapy of alcoholics should emphasize abstinence as the treatment goal and deal specifically with the members' denial. The predisposing causes of alcoholism should be explored only after its manifold sequelae are thoroughly discussed. At all times, confrontation and frank discussion should be tempered with support, advice, and reinforcement of positive changes.

Although a few stable schizophrenics can be treated in heterogeneous groups, most schizophrenics do better in homogeneous groups. In heterogeneous groups consisting of both psychotic and nonpsychotic patients, it is difficult to create a group environment meeting the needs of both populations. For example, the use of uncovering techniques may help a nonpsychotic patient, but self-disclosure may produce intolerable anxiety in a schizophrenic patient. Conversely, education and reality testing may help a psychotic patient but be experienced as unbearably boring by a less disturbed group member. Schizophrenics do well in homogeneous groups emphasizing controlled expression of emotions, reality testing, and socialization and contact with others.

Illustrative case No. 2. A paranoid schizophrenic man in his late 30s was angry with his doctor for not discharging him from the hospital, which prevented him from seeing his father in another city. After announcing his conviction that "anything else I say will only be held against me," he refused to say anything further. Several patients sympathized with him but questioned whether he was ready to be discharged and rejected the notion that he would be punished for expressing his feelings. They also encouraged him to ask his doctor for a weekend pass to visit his family. After a silence, the patient admitted that he still heard voices and that maybe he was not ready for discharge. He agreed to "trust the group" and ask his doctor for a pass.

Homogeneous groups are beneficial for patients suffering from chronic pain and illness such as asthma, myocardial infarction, and cancer. In such groups, themes involving disfigurement or loss of function, the responses of loved ones, and the fear of death can be raised and dealt with in a supportive, caring manner.

Illustrative case No. 3. A 50-year-old woman with breast cancer revealed to other breast cancer patients in the group how much she feared telling her daughter about her condition. Sharing this feeling with other patients brought out similarities and differences in their responses. The patient learned that she was not alone in fearing that her daughter would shrink from her in revulsion. At the same time, she came to realize that this fear might well be exaggerated and that there were ways to talk with family members about such painful topics as cancer and the need for mutilating surgery.

Patients with gender identity disorders also benefit from homogeneous group psychotherapy where sensitive matters involving sexual themes can be openly discussed in a supportive, nonhostile environment. For treatment of some disorders, such as adjustment or posttraumatic stress disorders, either homogeneous or heterogeneous group psychotherapy may be indicated; the choice in specific cases depends on whether the patient needs help in dealing with the effects of a specific stressful event or the effects of stress in general on interpersonal functioning.

C. Contraindications to Group Psychotherapy: Group psychotherapy is not for everyone. Overstimulation in the group environment causes patients with acute manic episodes to become more hyperactive and pressured. Patients with severe antisocial personality disorders who are more interested in manipulating others than in improving their interpersonal relationships usually hinder group progress.

D. Questionable Indications for Group Psychotherapy: Table 47–2 lists several disorders for which group psychotherapy is "questionably" indicated. The decision about whether group psychotherapy is indicated depends on such factors as the degree of impairment, desire for treatment, and individual psychodynamic factors.

Individual Psychodynamic Factors

Along with general diagnostic considerations, individual psychodynamic factors must also be assessed in pondering referral for group psychotherapy. Since intrapsychic conflicts influence and are influenced by interpersonal relationships, it is helpful if patients can view their problems in terms of difficulties experienced in relationships with other. Some therapists view this capacity as a criterion of potential for gaining insight and making progress in group psychotherapy.

The process of uncovering unconscious conflicts can provoke strong feelings. For some patients, transference feelings evoked in a group setting are more intense than those that arise in individual therapy; for others, the group setting is more tolerable because transference feelings can be distributed among other group members in addition to the therapist. Patients with problems resulting from unconscious conflicts may benefit from group psychotherapy, particularly if they are unable to tolerate transference feelings evoked in individual psychotherapy.

Group psychotherapy is especially useful for patients whose psychodynamic problems lead to maladaptive interpersonal relationships, since these interactions can be observed and explored in the group. For example, authority or dependency conflicts may be observed in the way some group members relate to each other or to the group leader.

Extremely manipulative patients, inveterate malingerers, and those who are socially deviant or engage in extreme acting-out behavior do not do well in group psychotherapy except in controlled settings. Patients must have some ability to relate to others and tolerate individual differences. For this reason, patients with schizoid or paranoid personality disorder often do poorly in the group setting. Group psychotherapy patients need adequate impulse control so they can tolerate confrontation with other group members. Patients with severe organic mental disorders may become confused or anxious in group psychotherapy. Finally, a patient in acute distress and unable to tolerate the process of assimilation as a new member usually does better in individual psychotherapy, where his or her needs can be tended to more quickly and specifically.

PRACTICAL CONSIDERATIONS IN ESTABLISHING & LEADING THE GROUP

In setting up a psychotherapy group, the therapist should take into account its setting and purpose, the types of patients to be included, what their treatment goals will probably be, and whether they have complementary personality characteristics.

Numbers of Patients; Age Ranges

Most groups have 6–12 patients, and 8 is often said to be the optimal number. Having 4 or fewer patients inhibits free expression because members are afraid to disagree lest someone drop out, which would mean that the sessions would have to be discontinued. With more than 12, there is too little time for each patient.

Inpatient groups tend to be **open,** which means that new patients are admitted to the group as others are discharged. Outpatient groups may be open or closed. In **closed** groups, the makeup stays the same for long periods without addition of new members.

The age range of patients in most groups is 20–60 years, with adolescent and geriatric patients often being treated in homogeneous groups formed specifically for the purpose of dealing with the problems of people in those age groups. Some therapists advocate splitting up adults into groups of young (20–40 years) and middle-aged (40–60 years) patients.

Preparatory Sessions for Patients Entering the Group

Most therapists advocate preparatory sessions for

prospective group members. A variety of formats for these sessions can be used, ranging from a brief one-to-one discussion with the therapist to participation in a minigroup in which patients sample the group experience by undergoing a number of structured exercises. Preparation reduces the patient's anxiety over what to expect, establishes a working alliance between therapist and patient, and allows the therapist to observe the patient's reactions in a structured interpersonal setting. Careful preparation significantly reduces the number of dropouts and improves attendance at the sessions. A combined factual-experiential approach is more effective than just giving factual information about "what group psychotherapy is all about."

Whether or not a patient goes through a preparatory phase, the therapist should have some idea beforehand of the patient's style of interacting with others. One way to find out is to ask about the patient's experience with other kinds of groups (at church, at the office, etc). A more direct approach would be to draw the patient's attention to the process of interaction during the interview. The patient's response—particularly the degree of defensiveness or interest in this novel way of looking at behavior—will serve as a clue to his or her later behavior in the group.

Ground Rules

Ground rules regarding timely attendance, payment of fees, notification of planned absences, and discussion of issues before making major life changes are important aspects of the group. Patients will sometimes violate these rules for psychodynamic and interpersonal reasons. The therapist should monitor such behavior and not hesitate to bring it up in the group for general discussion.

A patient who becomes threatening or disruptive may have to be temporarily excluded from the group. The reasons should be explained to the patient and discussed with the other members. When stable and in control again, the patient may reenter the group.

Frequency & Duration of Therapy

Most psychotherapy groups meet once or twice a week, although inpatient groups and psychodynamically oriented outpatient groups may meet 3–5 times a week. A typical session lasts 1–2 hours.

The duration of therapy in inpatient groups is influenced by the average length of hospitalization, which is 2–6 weeks in most acute care units. For this reason, inpatient groups are usually characterized by rapid turnover. Outpatient groups tend to be longer-term, with some patients remaining in the group months to years, depending on their problems and treatment goals. Briefer, time-limited outpatient groups (lasting 1–4 months) generally emphasize the establishment of realistic, limited treatment goals—eg, the resolution of current problems rather than the uncovering of unconscious conflicts—and the use of didactic and supportive techniques. In these groups,

therapists tend to take an active role, encouraging patient responsibility and focusing on practical issues. Careful patient selection and pretraining are critical for the success of therapy in short-term groups.

Number of Therapists

Many group therapists prefer a **co-therapy model,** in which 2 therapists are present in the group. Both should have roughly equal training and experience so that one will not be perceived as "junior" and be scapegoated by the group. Since sessions may be disrupted or made ineffective by competition or by theoretic or technical differences of opinion between therapists, co-therapists should work to maintain a good relationship. Male-female co-therapy teams are effective in encouraging discussion of parental, gender, and sexual themes.

Advantages of co-therapy include enhanced objectivity in assessment of patients, resulting from discussion between the therapists after group sessions; the potential for increased transference feelings in the group; continuity of the group when one therapist goes on vacation or becomes ill; and better control of the group in times of crisis (eg, admission of a hostile, disruptive patient).

Combined Individual & Group Psychotherapy

Some patients undergo both individual and group psychotherapy at the same time. In some cases, the therapist is the same in both settings; in other cases, the patient has one therapist for group psychotherapy and a different one for individual psychotherapy. Most therapists prefer the former combination, since the patient can be managed without the need for time-consuming and perhaps conflictual communication with another therapist. Some group patients not receiving combined therapy resent another member's private access to the therapist; however, this competitive issue can usually be dealt with in the group.

Adding group psychotherapy for patients in individual psychotherapy is recommended if the patient does not make adequate progress in the one-to-one situation and if it appears that the group setting would allow the patient to experiment with new ways of relating to others. The challenge and stimulation of group interaction can uncover problems in personality function while at the same time providing relief from a one-to-one treatment focus.

Adding individual psychotherapy for patients in group psychotherapy is recommended if the patient has difficulty sharing problems in a group setting; if the patient wants to intensify efforts to resolve a particular problem or conflict; or if it is felt that a sudden crisis or stressful event in the patient's life can be dealt with more quickly and effectively in individual treatment.

Problems of resistance or countertransference arising in one treatment setting should be dealt with in that setting; the issue should not be avoided by recommending both individual and group psychotherapy. If there is a danger that the dissonance resulting from 2 treatment approaches might overrun fragile defenses, combined treatment should not be used.

Format of Sessions

Most psychotherapy groups are **discussion-oriented.** Patients are expected to talk about problems and other significant aspects of their personal lives. They are encouraged to divulge feelings, be open and honest, and listen to issues involving other patients. Some issues directed toward the therapist may be referred back to the group, with the therapist asking what the members think about that issue. In order to stimulate discussion, the therapist may utilize a technique called "making the rounds," whereby each patient is asked in turn to express his or her thoughts about the issue at hand. In other group psychotherapy approaches, such as transactional analysis, a lecture format may be used, with interpersonal and intrapsychic issues diagrammed on a blackboard. Videotape playback is also used in some group settings to stimulate discussion.

Some psychotherapy groups are more **action-oriented.** In psychodrama, patients are asked to assume roles (spouses, parents, etc) in acting out a specific problem. In some behavioral approaches, patients practice techniques aimed at resolution of symptoms, such as systematic desensitization (see Chapter 46). In activity groups such as music or art therapy groups, patients meet to engage in activities that serve as a basis for intrapsychic and interpersonal learning.

GROUP DYNAMICS

When people come together in groups for any purpose, forces are set in motion that affect each member. Such forces are a feature of collective human behavior and go beyond the dynamics of dyadic (in pairs) interactions. For example, a normally nonviolent, law-abiding person may commit arson and other violent crimes in the context of a mob.

The therapist must be aware of the collective forces operating in a psychotherapy group at any given moment. Since the group environment exerts strong pressures on the members, the results may be negative as well as positive. The therapist's role is to maximize the therapeutic potential of the group environment for each individual. For example, in group settings where open and honest interactions occur, the members gradually learn the importance of free exchange of ideas and feelings and can apply these principles in their daily lives. If feelings are kept bottled up during group sessions and the therapist does not encourage their expression, group work will be unproductive and patients will be less inclined to express themselves openly in daily life.

Each individual in the group is affected by his or her perceptions of what other members think and feel about various issues. In psychotherapy groups, one often finds that many (perhaps all) patients have the same perception, which can be called a **group norm.** MacKenzie (1979) has pointed out that group norms exert powerful predictive forces (pressure to conform) on the actions of individual members. If an individual's view of what is normative in a group is not in accord with reality, the discrepancy provides clues to psychodynamic and psychopathologic factors affecting that member. For example, a withdrawn, paranoid patient might perceive the group setting as hostile and nonsupportive even though most of the other members see it as a place where they can express their concerns in a friendly environment. Such discrepancies alert the therapist to important issues of individual and group dynamics, issues that become "grist for the therapeutic mill."

The therapist may sometimes wish to point out a significant characteristic of the group, such as its avoidance of a specific topic. For example, following a suicidal gesture by a group member, it would not be unusual for this topic to be avoided in the next group session; the members might talk about emotionally bland or trivial matters or behave in a pressured, anxious manner. This resistance can be overcome by a simple comment: "Many of you seem anxious today. I wonder if John's overdose has something to do with that." In most instances, the patients will begin to discuss their feelings (anger, sadness, guilt) when the subject is raised. Such **process comments** are usually offered with the intention of providing opportunities for insight into psychodynamic or interpersonal issues or for the purpose of freeing up group resistance to a topic.

PHASES OF GROUP DEVELOPMENT

The group environment is affected by several factors, including the personalities of group members; the style and therapeutic stance of the therapist; the physical setting, ie, whether inpatient or outpatient; and, perhaps most importantly, the phase of group development. A developmental sequence of phases can be observed to occur in all groups but is most obvious in long-term, closed outpatient groups. Progress from one phase to another is dependent on successful resolution of issues involving the previous phase. Group development may cease to progress if this resolution does not occur.

Although numerous phases have been described (Beck [1981] identified 9 phases), most conceptual models portray 3 main phases of group development. The **first phase** is characterized by hesitant participation and the establishment of initial group norms; the members depend on the therapist for guidance and approval. During this phase, the members should be able to perceive some common purpose in being there and declare their individual goals, while the therapist works in a quiet way to encourage the establishment of bonds between members. The **second phase** is characterized by conflict, dominance, and the establishment of a hierarchy ("pecking order") among the patients. The therapist is often seen as an appropriate figure to be rebelled against, and fantasies may be entertained of excluding the therapist from the group. Several patients may band together to attack verbally or exclude a particular patient from their discussions, thereby identifying that patient as the group scapegoat. An important task of the leader is to help the group deal constructively with these aggressive tendencies. In the **third phase,** true group cohesiveness is established along with a sense of intimacy and mutual affection and need for each other. Overdependence on a rebellion against the therapist has been worked through, and the therapist is reintegrated with the group. A great deal of productive group work can be accomplished in the third phase.

THERAPEUTIC FACTORS

The benefits of group psychotherapy may be enhanced by the therapist's recognition of factors that contribute to improvement in a patient's condition. Bloch and associates (1981) have reviewed the literature and discussed 10 factors: self-disclosure, interaction, acceptance (cohesiveness), insight, catharsis, guidance, altruism, vicarious learning, instillation of hope, and existential factors.

In 1970, Yalom described a method of studying some of these therapeutic factors, which he called curative factors. At the time of discharge, patients are given 60 statements describing 12 potentially helpful attributes of their experience in group psychotherapy and are asked to rank the statements from most helpful to least helpful. The ranking of statements is then used to create a similar ranking of the 12 curative factors (see Yalom, 1975). Table 47–3 shows a rank ordering of curative factors distilled from psychiatric patients'

responses in 2 settings: a long-term outpatient setting involving patients with nonpsychotic disorders, and an inpatient setting involving severely ill patients who required acute hospitalization. As shown in the table, the psychiatric outpatients most valued their group experience for (1) giving them feedback on interpersonal behavior, (2) allowing them an opportunity to vent repressed feelings, (3) giving them a sense of acceptance by other people, and (4) helping them discover unconscious motivations for what they do. In contrast, the psychiatric inpatients most valued their group experience for (1) giving them feelings of optimism through watching other patients improve and leave the hospital, (2) giving them a sense of acceptance by other people, (3) improving self-esteem through their ability to help others, and (4) allowing them to feel less isolated. It is apparent that what is considered curative in a group may vary depending on the type of patient in the group, the group setting, and the length of stay. The therapist should keep these issues in mind and make appropriate use of the curative factors that are most suited to the patients' needs.

TYPES OF PSYCHOTHERAPY GROUPS

Psychotherapy groups can be categorized in a number of ways: inpatient versus outpatient, experiential versus didactic, supportive versus uncovering, affective versus cognitive, etc. Table 47–4 categorizes a number of psychotherapy groups in terms of their theoretical orientation. The therapeutic goals of most of these groups are relief of symptoms and resolution of intrapsychic and interpersonal problems. However, these goals are achieved in different ways. In some groups, the projection of unconscious conflicts onto the therapist is seen as crucial, and transference interpretations are viewed as major therapeutic interventions. In other groups, patient interactions are seen as prominent group activities, since they stimulate the discussion of interpersonal issues through which patients learn more about their behavior outside of the group. The focus of some groups is on activities that occur in the group itself (**here-and-now approach**), whereas other groups emphasize past events and activities that occurred outside the group (**there-and-then approach**). Many psychotherapy groups use a combination of theoretical principles borrowed from several of the schools represented in Table 47–4. When used in an appropriate and clinically relevant manner, this eclectic approach provides the therapist with a number of techniques to meet the patients' needs.

Issues and conflicts addressed in group psychotherapy may be categorized as affecting the entire group (**group-as-a-whole approach**) or affecting an individual or part of the group. Especially in early sessions of the group—when members may display similar affects, such as depression or helplessness, together with an attitude of dependency on the leader—the focus may be on issues and events that affect the group as

Table 47–3. Curative factors in group psychotherapy, based on results of studies in which patients were asked to rank the value of their experiences.*

Group of 20 Psychiatric Outpatients		Group of 100 Psychiatric Inpatients	
Rank Order	Curative Factor	Rank Order	Curative Factor
1	Interpersonal input	1	Instillation of hope
2	Catharsis	2	Group cohesiveness
3	Group cohesiveness	3	Altruism
4	Insight (self-understanding)	4	Universality
		5	Interpersonal input
5	Interpersonal output	6	Existential factors
6	Existential factors	7	Interpersonal output
7	Universality	8	Catharsis
8	Instillation of hope	9	Insight (self-understanding)
9	Altruism		
10	Family reenactment	10	Guidance
11	Guidance	11	Family reenactment
12	Identification	12	Identification

*Methodology is described in the text. Outpatient data were reported by Yalom (1975), and inpatient data were reported by Maxmen (1973).

Table 47−4. Types of psychotherapy groups.

Theoretic Orientation of Group	Major Goals	Importance of Patient-Therapist Transference Interpretations	Importance of Group Member Interactions	Importance of Here-and-Now Emphasis	Further Reading
Psycho-analytic	Resolution of intrapsychic problems	Extremely important	Moderately important	Moderately important	Day (1981)
Interactional	Resolution of intrapsychic and interpersonal problems	Minimally important	Extremely important	Extremely important	Yalom (1975)
Transactional analysis	Resolution of intrapsychic and interpersonal problems	Minimally important	Moderately important	Moderately important	Berne (1966)
Gestalt	Resolution of intrapsychic problems	Minimally important	Minimally important	Extremely important	Peris (1969)
Psychodrama	Resolution of intrapsychic and interpersonal problems	Minimally important	Moderately important	Extremely important	Moreno (1959, 1969, 1972)
Existential	Awareness of basic problems affecting existence	Minimally important	Extremely important	Extremely important	Miller (1978)
Behavioral	Resolution of symptoms	Minimally important	Minimally important	Moderately important	Harris (1979)

a whole. As the group develops and as more differentiated and individualized responses and reactions occur, it may be necessary to intervene at the level of the individual or discuss interactions between several individuals. Theoretic approaches must be flexible enough to account for such developmental factors, and techniques should include both group and individual level interventions.

SUMMARY

Group psychotherapy is an established method of treatment in which patients may achieve relief of symptoms and resolution of intrapsychic and interpersonal problems as a result of interactions with other patients and the therapist, both in inpatient and in outpatient settings. Diagnostic considerations and individual psychodynamic factors should be taken into account in referring patients to a suitable group, and there are few absolute contraindications. Therapy groups may be heterogeneous (mixed disorders) or homogeneous (same disorder), open or closed. Adequate preparation of patients for group psychotherapy reduces the number of dropouts. Many groups use a cotherapist team approach, which offers several advantages over groups with just one therapist. Some patients benefit from being treated both individually and in a group during the same period.

Group therapists must be aware of issues involving individual psychodynamics, group dynamics, group development, and specific therapeutic factors relevant to the group. Most therapists use a combination of theoretic principles and techniques in constructing psychotherapy groups that best meet the needs of their patients.

REFERENCES

General & Historical

American Group Psychotherapy Association Standards and Ethics Committee: *A Consumer's Guide to Group Psychotherapy.* American Group Psychotherapy Association, 1973.

Kaplan HI, Sadock BJ (editors): *Comprehensive Group Psychotherapy,* 2nd ed. Williams & Wilkins, 1983.

Kibel HD, Stein A: The group-as-a-whole approach: An appraisal. *Int J Group Psychother* 1981;**31**:409.

Lieberman MA: Problems in integrating traditional group therapies with new group forms. *Int J Group Psychother* 1977;**27**:19.

Yalom ID: *Inpatient Group Psychotherapy.* Basic Books, 1983.

Yalom ID: *The Theory and Practice of Group Psychotherapy,* 2nd ed. Basic Books, 1975.

Effectiveness of Group Psychotherapy

Kanas N: Alcoholism and group psychotherapy. In: *Encyclopedic Handbook of Alcoholism.* Pattison EM, Kaufman E (editors). Gardner Press, 1982.

Kanas N: Group therapy with schizophrenics: A review of controlled studies. *Int J Group Psychother* 1986;**36**:339.

Karasu TB: Psychotherapy of the medically ill. *Am J Psychiatry* 1979:**136**:1.

Luborsky L, Singer B, Luborsky L: Comparative studies of psychotherapies. *Arch Gen Psychiatry* 1975;**32**:995.

Piper WE, Debbane EG, Garant J: An outcome study of group therapy. *Arch Gen Psychiatry* 1977;**34**:1027.

Indications & Contraindications for Group Psychotherapy

Farrell D: Psychotherapeutic approaches to medically ill patients. In: *Emotions in Health and Illness: Applications to Clinical Practice.* Van Dyke C, Temoshok L, Zegans L (editors). Grune & Stratton, 1984.

Grunebaum H, Kates W: Whom to refer for group psychotherapy. *Am J Psychiatry* 1977;**134**:130.

Kanas N: Inpatient and outpatient group therapy for schizophrenic patients. *Am J Psychother* 1985;**39**:431.

Kanas N: Multi-factor group therapy for alcoholics. *Curr Psychiatr Ther* 1982;**21**:149.

Ringler KE et al: Technical advances in leading a cancer patient group. *Int J Group Psychother* 1981;**31**:329.

Practical Considerations in Establishing & Leading the Group

Bellak L: On some limitations of dyadic psychotherapy and the role of group modalities. *Int J Group Psychother* 1980;**30**:7.

Bernard HS, Klein RS: Some perspectives on time-limited group psychotherapy. *Compr Psychiatry* 1977;**18**:579.

Day M: Psychoanalytic group therapy in clinic and private practice. *Am J Psychiatry* 1981;**138**:64.

Dick B, Lessler K, Whiteside J: A developmental framework for co-therapy. *Int J Group Psychother* 1980;**30**:273.

Duetsch CB, Kramer N: Outpatient group psychotherapy for the elderly: An alternative to institutionalization. *Hosp Community Psychiatry* 1977;**28**:440.

Farrell D: The use of active experiential group techniques with hospitalized patients. In: *Group Therapy 1976*. Wolberg LR, Aronson ML (editors). Stratton Intercontinental, 1976.

Fulkerson CCF, Hawkins DM, Alden AR: Psychotherapy groups of insufficient size. *Int J Group Psychother* 1981;**31**:73.

Ormont LR: Principles and practice of conjoint psychoanalytic treatment. *Am J Psychiatry* 1981;**138**:69.

Piper WE et al: A study of group pretraining for group psychotherapy. *Int J Group Psychother* 1982;**32**:309.

Rutan JS, Alonso A: Group therapy, individual therapy, or both. *Int J Group Psychother* 1982;**32**:267.

Wong N: Fundamental psychoanalytic concepts: Past and present understanding of their applicability to group psychotherapy. *Int J Group Psychother* 1983;**33**:171.

Group Dynamics, Development, & Therapeutic Factors

Beck AP: Developmental characteristics of the system-forming process. In: *Living Groups: Group Psychotherapy and General Systems Theory*. Durkin JE (editor). Brunner/Mazel, 1981.

Bloch S, Crouch E, Reibstein J: Therapeutic factors in group psychotherapy. *Arch Gen Psychiatry* 1981;**38**:519.

Day M: Process in classical psychodynamic groups. *Int J Group Psychother* 1981;**31**:153.

Kanas N, Barr MA: Outpatient alcoholics view group therapy. *Group* (Spring) 1982;**6**:17.

MacKenzie KR: Group norms: Importance and measurement. *Int J Group Psychother* 1979;**29**:471.

Maxmen JS: Group therapy as viewed by hospitalized patients. *Arch Gen Psychiatry* 1973;**28**:404.

Yalom ID: *The Theory and Practice of Group Psychotherapy*, 2nd ed. Basic Books, 1975.

Types of Psychotherapy Groups

Berne E: *Principles of Group Treatment*. Oxford Univ Press, 1966.

Day M: Psychoanalytic group therapy in clinic and private practice. *Am J Psychiatry* 1981;**138**:64.

Harris FC: The behavioral approach to group therapy. *Int J Group Psychother* 1979;**29**:453.

Miller J: Attaining freedom in existential group therapy. *Am J Psychoanal* 1978;**38**:179.

Moreno JL: *Psychodrama*. Vol 1, 4th ed, 1972; Vol 2, 1959; Vol 3, 1969. Beacon House.

Perls FS: *Gestalt Therapy Verbatim*. Real People Press, 1969.

Yalom ID: *The Theory and Practice of Group Psychotherapy*, 2nd ed. Basic Books, 1975.

Family Therapy

48

Rodney Shapiro, PhD

The common definition of family therapy as treatment of all or most members of a family at the same time is not strictly accurate. A number of family therapists work chiefly with nuclear family units (parents and children); others include the parents' families of origin (the parents' parents and siblings); some work only with couples; and a few—though the number is increasing—work with only one family member. Most family therapists tend to vary the attendance requirement during different phases of treatment, so that the same people do not necessarily attend all sessions. Even the composition of the therapeutic unit varies considerably. Some family therapists work alone, whereas others prefer a co-therapist, and a popular practice today is the treatment team (one or 2 therapists in a room with the family while several team members observe through a one-way mirror and call in questions and interventions during the sessions).

Leading family therapists differ sharply in their ideas and methods of treatment; eg, considerable disagreement exists about the merits of time-honored treatment practices such as facilitating good communication, encouraging the expression of affect, and developing greater self-awareness in family members.

Family therapy as presently practiced offers an array of seemingly contradictory theories and practices, but some basic assumptions clearly distinguish family therapy from other psychotherapeutic approaches. A fundamental assumption common to all models of family therapy is that disturbed psychologic functioning is not limited to a single individual but reflects disturbed interactions between persons who have significant relationships with each other. The family is the primary context in which important relationships evolve. Psychologic disturbance most likely originates during childhood as a result of participation in dysfunctional patterns of parent-parent and parent-child interactions. These disturbed patterns may persist into adulthood through the continuing influence of the family of origin as well as in the relationship patterns established by individuals with their spouses and children.

On the whole, family therapists are not much concerned with the origins of dysfunction, which are regarded as hypothetical matters not amenable to change through psychotherapy. The emphasis is rather on the here and now and on the patterns of family interaction that currently act to sustain existing problems. The therapist can evaluate problems and design interventions on the basis of data provided by family members or observable in the treatment setting. The goal of family therapy is not to change the individual per se but rather to set right the system of relationships in which the individual is involved. Changing the interpersonal context of an individual may then result in change in one or more family members.

Illustrative Case

A couple requested help because their 7-year-old son, an only child, had developed school phobia. The initial evaluation showed that the child's presenting problem was an interpersonal relationship problem involving all family members. The mother, an extremely anxious and dependent woman, had always looked to her husband for direction and support. When they met, he himself was insecure, but he compensated by asserting strong control in the relationship, and he encouraged his wife's dependence. Over several years, however, the husband became increasingly successful in business, and as he developed greater self-confidence, he began to perceive his wife as undesirably weak and demanding. When the wife realized that her husband was becoming more distant emotionally, she became even more anxious and dependent. This caused the husband to become even more distant and preoccupied with work, so that the wife's anxiety in turn increased.

The birth of the child was welcomed by both parties. The wife looked to the child for the support her husband failed to provide. The husband hoped that his son would serve as a surrogate for his wife's attentions and thus free him from her demands and alleviate his guilt about his withdrawal from her. As the child grew, he learned to tolerate his father's lack of involvement, since it seemed to ensure the continuing attention of his doting mother.

This pattern of interaction stabilized over a number of years until an unavoidable developmental shift disrupted the family's equilibrium. At age 6 years, the son began to attend primary school. The start of formal schooling represented the first major separation for mother and son. The family had actively worked to minimize the son's earlier attendance at nursery school and kindergarten, but such avoidance was no longer possible. On most mornings before school, the child complained about various ailments and "upset" feelings. More often than not, the parents permitted him to stay home. Extensive medical investigations ruled out any organic basis for the symptoms.

The parents grew increasingly distressed and felt

great conflict about the situation. On the one hand, the child's symptoms helped to stabilize the marital relationship, and both parents now felt threatened by the possibility of a disruption of the status quo. On the other hand, the parents were genuinely concerned about the consequences of their son's missed days of school. Periodically, and with much ambivalence, they would urge the boy to go to school, but his symptoms would then be worsened by marked anxiety. A conference with a pediatrician led to the referral for family therapy.

The goals of treatment were to facilitate a collaborative relationship between the parents, encourage a closer bond between father and son, help the mother achieve greater independence and autonomy, and firmly but benignly reinforce the son's school attendance as an important step toward appropriate separation from his parents. The family responded well to therapy, and these goals were realized to their satisfaction.

THE PRIMARY CONCEPTS OF FAMILY THERAPY

Family therapy is a relatively recent development in the history of psychiatry. The fundamental ideas and practices have emerged over the past 30 years, and the field is rapidly growing and diversifying.

Theodore Lidz, Murray Bowen, & Lyman Wynne

Theodore Lidz (1972) and Murray Bowen (1966) gained prominence for their extensive studies of families with an adolescent or young adult diagnosed as schizophrenic. In his work, which had a strong psychoanalytic orientation, Lidz enumerated characteristics of family functioning that were essential for normal psychosocial development. His ideas concerning the importance of clear parental roles and appropriate generational boundaries continue to influence contemporary family therapists. He was one of the first to draw attention to the influence of the father's role in determining healthy or impaired development in children. He discovered that marital relationships were invariably disturbed in families with schizophrenic offspring, and he postulated a relationship between particular modes of disturbed parental relationships and certain symptoms in children.

Murray Bowen is generally regarded as an originator and dominant figure in the history of family therapy. Beginning in 1954, he established a research project at the National Institute of Mental Health that required the hospitalization not only of schizophrenic patients but also of their entire families for study and treatment. He later incorporated his findings into an elaborate treatment approach.

A central premise in all of Bowen's work is the "undifferentiated family ego mass," or the overall state of emotional dependence between members of a given family. Bowen believed that there was a direct relationship between excessive emotional bonding and family dysfunction. He regarded differentiation of self as a necessary developmental goal for family members, and his treatment approach was designed to facilitate such differentiation.

Another major component of Bowen's work was his multigenerational model of family dynamics. He noted that problems unresolved in one generation tended to be transmitted through succeeding generations. In clinical practice, this insight meant that therapists should gain information about the patient's family origin (parents and siblings) and the earlier generation of grandparents and extended families and not just the patient's immediate family. These explorations often revealed repetitive patterns of dysfunction. Many practitioners who are influenced by Bowen's ideas emphasize the importance of having members of the patient's extended family participate in therapy sessions.

Bowen's ideas had broad appeal, and he commanded a strong following. His theories represented a fusion of psychodynamics, developmental theory, and principles of systems theory. They were comprehensive and applicable to a wide range of individual, marital, and family disorders. Above all, he provided a clear-cut treatment approach based upon his theoretical framework.

Lyman Wynne succeeded Murray Bowen as head of the Family Studies Section at the National Institute of Mental Health. He attracted a circle of outstanding researchers who generated a series of important studies on schizophrenia (Wynne and coworkers, 1958; Singer and Wynne, 1965). The term "pseudomutuality" was coined to describe a common phenomenon in families of schizophrenic patients. These families often present a facade of unity that is rigorously maintained by the prohibition of any movement toward separateness and autonomy among family members. Complex patterns of family interaction conceal individual differences, and an impervious psychologic boundary (the "rubber fence") protects the family unit from the outside world. Wynne's analysis of the interactions greatly enhanced psychiatrists' understanding of the remarkable rigidity and resistance of families with schizophrenic members.

Wynne continued his studies of schizophrenia and family processes and collaborated with Margaret Singer (1965) in producing a carefully controlled research design for studying thought disorder and communication patterns in families with schizophrenic offspring. The results of these studies demonstrated a relationship between characteristic thought disorders in schizophrenic patients and patterns of deviant communication in their parents. Wynne's ideas have influenced contemporary studies of schizophrenia and have also provided valuable insights for family therapy.

The Bateson Group

In the early 1950s, the anthropologist Gregory Bateson (1956) received a grant to study human communication and assembled a group of coworkers that included some of the future leaders in the field of family therapy, eg, Jay Haley (1959), Don Jackson (1957, 1965), and John Weakland (Watzlawick, Weakland, and Fisch, 1974). The original project was based at the Veterans Administration Hospital in Menlo Park, California. One of the group's first papers, "Toward a Theory of Schizophrenia" (1956), attracted international interest and described their concept of the "double bind," a pattern of communication they believed was characteristic of schizophrenic families. In the double bind, one family member is repeatedly required to respond to contradictory messages from a second family member. The recipient of these messages is in a "no-win" situation. The messages cannot be ignored, but no satisfactory response is possible, since the messages are contradictory (see also Chapter 27). The concept can be demonstrated by a simple example. A schizophrenic young man was hospitalized, and his mother came to visit him. She greeted him by extending her arms. He responded by hugging her, but she immediately stiffened. Interpreting that response as an indication of discomfort with bodily contact, the son backed away. As he did so, his mother reproved him by saying "What's the matter? Don't you love me anymore?"

The double bind occurs even in nonpsychotic families, but the Bateson group believed that frequent repetition of double-bind experiences was implicated in the development of schizophrenia. Subsequent studies have failed to support this contention, and in any case, schizophrenia is far too complex a disorder to be attributed to a single determinant. However, these studies were important in confirming that deviant communications are characteristic of disturbed families and that specific patterns of communication seem to reinforce family dysfunction. Numerous insights about verbal and nonverbal communication in families have had a major impact on clinical theory and practice. The work of the Bateson group was phased out in the early 1960s. Don Jackson then established the Mental Research Institute in Palo Alto, California. The publications of this group include some of the classic expositions of systems theory and clinical methods. The institute remains an influential and productive source of theory, research, and training in family therapy.

Systems Theory & Cybernetics

The development of family therapy was strongly influenced by the emergence of general systems theory (see Chapter 3). The principles of general systems theory were formulated by the biologist Ludwig von Bertalanffy. Although it is chiefly applicable to the biology of organisms, systems theory has obvious relevance for psychologic and sociologic behavior. Bertalanffy (1968) proposed a model of the human organism as an open system in constant interaction with the environment. In order to explain human behavior, therefore, one must consider the total organization of the human organism and environment (see also Chapter 3).

A particular aspect of systems theory, known as the cybernetic model, was adopted by the early Mental Research Institute theorists as a way of understanding family interaction. Cybernetics was formulated to a large extent by the mathematician Norbert Wiener as a means of conceptualizing the operating principles of diverse self-regulating systems, such as homeostatic biologic mechanisms (maintenance of certain levels of substances in the blood, eg, glucose, ions, hormones), thermostatic heating and cooling devices, and guided missiles. The basic principle is that of feedback of information. The Mental Research Institute studies noted that interactional behavior in families was regulated by communication transmitted through recurring feedback loops. As a simple example, individual X behaves in a manner that seems overly assertive to individual Y. Individual Y responds with anger. X then responds with a show of submission. Y notes the submissive response, and anger subsides. X observes the decreased anger and becomes less submissive. X and Y achieve a comfortable interactional balance, but a significant increase of assertiveness on the part of X or anger on the part of Y may trigger a new sequence of feedback loops designed to achieve equilibrium.

The cybernetic principle is important, because it illustrates a fundamental tenet of family therapy known as circular causality. Traditional theories of human psychology are based on linear causality, ie, a temporal sequence of cause leading to effect: A → B, B → C, C → D, etc. In order to understand a patient's current behavior, the therapist must explore a chain of past events stemming from the original cause. This historical perspective of cause and effect forms the basis of traditional views of the cause of psychiatric illness. The interactional model of family therapy is therefore an innovation in psychiatry in that the past is de-emphasized and the focus is on the present for understanding and treating psychologic disorders. The key assumption in family therapy is that problems or symptoms are maintained and reinforced by interactional patterns of communication and that modification of these interactional processes with treatment may produce positive changes.

Clinical Innovators

A number of clinical theorists played a major role in the development of family therapy. John Bell was one of the first clinicians to use group therapy in working with families. His writings influenced others to try clinical work with entire families. The most notable clinician in the early history of family therapy was Nathan Ackerman (1966). He was trained as a child psychiatrist and psychoanalyst, but as early as 1937 he discussed his awareness of the influence of family relationships on childhood disorders. His later writings and considerable clinical skills won him many admirers. In 1965, he established the Family Institute (subsequently renamed the Ackerman Institute), a training and treatment center in New York City that is now a major center of family therapy.

Salvador Minuchin (1967, 1974) was introduced to family therapy shortly after he emigrated to the USA in 1958. He spent several years working with black and Puerto Rican families in the slums of New York City, where he found that prevailing family therapy approaches were unsuitable. Minuchin devised a model of therapy—structural therapy—that emphasized an active role for the therapist and carefully planned strategies to achieve tangible treatment goals. Structural therapy—now one of the dominant approaches in family therapy—focuses on the relationships between all members of a family and attempts to realign the boundaries between different subgroups to improve family functioning. Minuchin headed the Philadelphia Child Guidance Clinic, whose staff included gifted theoreticians and therapists such as Jay Haley (1959, 1976, 1980) and Braulio Montalvo (see Minuchin and coworkers, 1967). The intensive training and innovative supervisory techniques became widely known because of Minuchin's writings and many personal demonstrations.

CHARACTERISTICS OF FAMILY THERAPY

Despite obvious differences among practitioners in the field of family therapy, there are principles of treatment that most therapists subscribe to. In some basic respects, family therapy includes therapeutic practices that vary radically from those used by individual or group therapists.

Comparison With Individual & Group Therapy

A. Comparison With Individual Therapy: For many years, individual therapy has been the principal way in which psychotherapy is conducted, and the essential characteristics of individual therapy continue to reflect the psychoanalytic tradition. In individual therapy, the therapist works with one person who presents with a self-recognized problem or who is identified by others as having a problem. The patient, if deemed a suitable candidate for psychoanalytically oriented psychotherapy, is expected to freely verbalize thoughts and feelings. Significant events from the past are revived and reexamined. The therapist's role is that of listener endeavoring to understand the implications of these reports. The patient is guided toward greater self-awareness as a prerequisite to changes in behavior and symptoms.

These conditions rarely occur in family therapy, where participation by one or more family members is usually required. The therapist is interested in the objective reality of family relationships; individual dynamics, defenses, and symptoms are translated into interactional terms. Since family therapists are chiefly concerned with observable behavior, they are alert to nonverbal cues and communication sequences. Current functioning is the major focus in family therapy, even though family therapists also explore develop-

mental history in the course of treatment. The goal of individual therapy is to change the individual, whereas the family therapist strives to bring about change in the family's system of relationships.

B. Comparison With Group Therapy: On initial observation, family therapy may seem like group therapy applied to a group of family members. In fact, some of the earliest practices of family therapy did borrow from group therapy. The only points of actual similarity, however, are that both group and family therapy require participation by more than one person and both are concerned in varying degrees with interpersonal relationships. The distinction between the aims of individual therapy (changing the individual patient) and family therapy (changing the system of relationships) applies to group therapy and family therapy as well; group therapy is also designed to produce change in the individual patient. Interpersonal relationships among group members do provide significant material for group therapy, but only in terms of highlighting the problems of individual participants.

There are other less apparent but highly significant differences between group and family therapy. The participants in group therapy are usually strangers to begin with; they may be urged not to see one another socially between sessions; and they may have no expectation of continuing contacts with one another beyond the life of the group. These conditions facilitate self-disclosure and confrontation, since there is no inhibiting concern that future relationships will be impaired. Furthermore, all members of the group admit to having problems; they are all "in the same boat." Their shared identity as patients also provides assurance of acceptance and encourages self-revelation.

Families, on the other hand, are bound by historical continuity, and this creates a treatment situation radically different from that of group therapy. Family members are linked by a common past, have ongoing contact, and anticipate continuing involvement in the future. Concerns about impairing relationships may severely inhibit openness and confrontation. Family members are sometimes motivated to participate in therapy because they feel they can help the person who has been identified as the patient, while they themselves are simply glad that they are not the ones who are "sick"; they may deny or be unaware of the impact their own behavior or problems may have on the identified patient. The relatives usually continue to resist being labeled as patients. These conditions make for greater resistance than is found in group therapy. A climate of support and acceptance is also less likely in family settings. Family members are all too aware of each other's faults, and criticism and even scapegoating are typical aspects of family life.

Families are generally more resistant to treatment at the outset than are patients seeking individual or group therapy. The initial obstacle poses an immediate challenge to the family therapist. It may take considerable skill to neutralize resistance and establish positive relationships with family members so that therapy can continue. On the other hand, family members are bound by deeply entrenched loyalties and obligations, and this common bond provides a powerful incentive for mutual involvement in therapy. In contrast, group therapy members experience transient relationships and less profound emotional involvement with one another.

Another difference between group and family therapy that has important clinical implications is that the therapist in the family group is literally outnumbered. Family members often share rigidly held beliefs and attitudes, and the therapist, as the representative of an alternative perspective, may not have sufficient power to influence the group. This situation is a special problem in psychotic families, which are characteristically impervious to messages from external sources. Participants in group therapy, even if all of them are psychotic, do not share a history of common beliefs, and the group therapist often finds allies among the other group members, who may help influence the ideas and behavior of any one patient.

Indications for Family Therapy

Some family therapists maintain that instead of asking when family therapy should be used, clinicians should rephrase the question and ask when family therapy is *not* indicated. These therapists assert that therapy is indicated for all problems affecting family relationships unless practical obstacles prevent attendance of family members at meetings. This view is held by a minority of purists; most practitioners believe that family therapy is the treatment of choice for several specific problems, although it is not necessarily ideal in all circumstances. Family therapists are unanimous in endorsing the value of their approach for problems of children and adolescents and for marital conflict.

Family Therapy for Children & Adolescents

In the case of children, there are 2 overriding arguments in favor of family therapy rather than individual therapy. First, it is assumed that problems of children indicate family dysfunction (as in the illustrative case presented earlier). Individual therapy for the child would therefore leave the family's problems unprobed. Second, any therapeutic success from individual therapy with the child would be short-lived unless the dysfunctional family system were also treated. In fact, the family may well resist changes that seem incompatible with the needs of the parents and the other children. It is not uncommon for parents to undermine or terminate therapy at a point when the child is manifesting signs of healthier attitudes and behavior. Some who conduct individual therapy object to family therapy for adolescents on the grounds that it impedes the adolescent's strivings for independence. They also argue that adolescents need confidentiality in order to talk freely about sex and other personal matters. Family therapists reply that adolescents with problems have failed to develop independence precisely because their families have difficulty in permitting or encouraging this phase of development. The therapist must help the entire family adjust to the increasing independence of one or more of its members. Once the family is better able to cope with the separation and individuation of the offspring, individual psychotherapy may be helpful for the adolescent now free to deal with problems in the world away from home.

Illustrative case. A 16-year-old boy whose parents had been divorced was referred for individual psychotherapy. A year earlier, the father (recently remarried) and his new wife had assumed custody from the boy's mother, who had also remarried and was now living in another state. The reasons for the referral were the boy's apathy and depression over the past year, deteriorating school grades, frequent truancy, and general noncommunicativeness.

The father, a successful professional man, was somewhat overbearing and controlling, particularly in his relationships with his wife and son. His new wife was considerably younger than he. In the initial meeting with the therapist, she repeatedly agreed with whatever her husband said. The couple refused to become involved in treatment but wanted help for their son so that—as the father put it—"he would be more pleasant to be around."

The boy responded well to psychotherapy. His noncommunicativeness evaporated, and he spoke out about his loneliness and confusion and feelings of intense hurt and anger since his parents' divorce. The family had always lived by an unspoken rule that expressions of feelings and discussions of personal issues should be avoided.

During the parents' separation and then the divorce proceedings, their discussions with the son were chiefly motivated by their competition for his allegiance. Initially, the mother had insisted the boy remain with her, but as he became withdrawn and uncooperative, she felt overwhelmed and persuaded the father to take custody, which caused the boy great distress. He felt he was being rejected by his mother and accepted grudgingly by his father. When he expressed some of these feelings, the father was outraged by what he interpreted as proof of his son's ingratitude. Following this incident, the boy suppressed such feelings, but his symptoms became worse.

After several sessions of psychotherapy, the boy's depression abated, and he reinvested his energies in schoolwork and social activities. He reported that his father seemed gratified by these changes but spent little time with him. Once past the initial crisis, however, the boy was able to explore his thoughts and feelings in more depth. He came to realize that he had often served as a buffer between his parents. His problems and symptoms had served as a focus of communication between his parents and between them and him. During his periods of improvement, he had received little attention; his stepmother was too preoccupied with her own needs, and his father was completely absorbed in work. When conflicts erupted between his father and stepmother, the boy would become difficult or demonstrate unpleasant symptoms, and this often served to distract the parents from their marital conflict.

In reflecting on these patterns of interaction, the boy became aware of the roles he had played, understood how his efforts to attract attention masked an unsatisfied hunger for affection, and felt dismayed that similar patterns were beginning in the new family system. With this increased awareness and confidence, the boy began to alter his behavior at home. He kept his distance when he sensed difficulties brewing between his father and his stepmother, and he attempted to express his thoughts and feelings directly to them. However, these changes proved unwelcome; the father interpreted the boy's increased independence as selfishness, and his attempts at confrontation were regarded as insolence. The father telephoned the therapist and angrily accused him of teaching his son "Communistic notions of rebellion." The therapist tried to reassure him about the therapy, but the father refused to consider a family meeting and withdrew his son from therapy.

The therapist later learned that the father had referred his son to a colleague who was known to have little regard for psychotherapy. The boy was placed on a regimen of antidepressant medications and brief fortnightly office visits. Six weeks later, the therapist learned that the boy had attempted suicide and was hospitalized. In looking back, he felt he should have made greater efforts to involve the entire family in therapy—that he had not acted effectively to overcome their resistance. A therapeutic alliance with the father and stepmother might have facilitated positive changes in the parents and prevented the misunderstandings that arose, although there was no guarantee that the parents would have been persuaded by further encouragement or would have benefited from treatment. The case demonstrates the risks of treating adolescents (or children) without the therapeutic collaboration of the entire family.

Family Therapy for Couples*

Few therapists would dispute the appropriateness of conjoint psychotherapy in situations of marital conflict. Treating only one of the partners may actually aggravate marital difficulties. Individual therapy may facilitate positive changes in one spouse, but the partner who has not undergone psychotherapy often remains unchanged. The spouse participating in psychotherapy may grow psychologically and no longer need or be willing to tolerate a relationship with a less mature partner. Although a traditional solution for this problem is to have each partner see a separate therapist, family therapists are critical of this arrangement, because working with only one spouse limits the therapist's overview of the total marital relationship. Rules of confidentiality discourage collaboration between therapists, and a reputable therapist would not breach

rules of professional conduct by meeting with the spouse who is undergoing treatment with another colleague. These honest constraints may inadvertently reinforce an adversarial and competitive marital relationship, however, since the partners understandably look to their own therapists for support and recognition of their individual positions, and the therapists in turn are more likely to be concerned about the welfare of their own patients and not the other party.

Maintaining a balanced relationship with both partners is difficult even when the therapist does insist on conjoint psychotherapy. Maneuvers to implicate the therapist in attacks on the spouse or attempts to ensnare the therapist into an alliance are common in marital therapy, and the therapist must exercise skill in order to avoid these traps. The risk of being manipulated is greatly increased whenever one partner is seen without the other. Some therapists do see the husband and wife separately for one or more evaluation sessions and occasionally during the remainder of treatment. The justification for separate sessions is that it facilitates personal disclosures, but this practice is not without hazard.

Illustrative case. After an initial therapy session with both partners, the wife requested a separate meeting for herself. Her husband was considering separation, and she was extremely upset. Prompted by what he considered her need for extra support, the therapist agreed. During the separate meeting, the wife repeatedly depicted her husband as harsh and unfeeling, and she wondered whether the therapist could understand what the husband was really like. Seeking to reassure her while maintaining neutrality, the therapist responded, "Yes, I do understand that you feel that way about him."

Before the couple's next scheduled therapy session, the wife called to inform the therapist that her husband was not interested in psychotherapy and asked that the therapist work individually with her. Detecting a tone of satisfaction in her voice as she said these things, the therapist insisted that both partners attend. The appointment was reinstated and the husband did attend, though he seemed angry and distant with the therapist. Inquiries revealed that following her meeting with the therapist, the wife had angrily informed her husband that the therapist had agreed with her assessment of him as harsh and unfeeling. The therapist clarified the situation, but it took effort to achieve a positive balanced relationship with both partners after this incident.

Contraindications to Family Therapy

As mentioned above, there may be circumstances—such as practical obstacles or difficulties in obtaining the cooperation of families—that militate against the use of family therapy. Geographic distance is a realistic obstacle; older patients may have outlived their families; and adult immigrants may have no family ties in their adopted country.

---

* See also Chapter 49, Marital Therapy.

There are few psychiatric contraindications to family therapy. It may be unwise to initiate family therapy if one member is in the throes of brief reactive psychosis. A paranoid individual may have such a hostile relationship with the family that attempts to bring all members together for meetings are doomed to failure. Family therapy is frequently inadvisable when the irrevocable breakup of a family has already occurred; eg, if one spouse has decided on marital separation, it may simply postpone the painful process if both partners meet at the insistence of a therapist. Sometimes a couple may actually be helped with issues of separation and divorce, particularly in relation to their children, but this must be a mutual goal in therapy. (See Chapter 49.)

CURRENT TRENDS IN FAMILY THERAPY

Many of the originators of family therapy were trained in psychoanalysis. Some retained their psychodynamic views, whereas others renounced psychoanalysis as incompatible with family therapy.

The initial schism in the field of family therapy occurred over the acceptance or rejection of psychoanalytic theory. The movement away from psychoanalysis has gathered momentum in recent years, and current trends reflect an almost complete break with psychodynamic theory and practice. Interpretation has little or no place in contemporary family therapy, and insight is regarded as irrelevant for change. The subjective states of client and therapist are largely ignored; the emphasis is on actual behavior and active treatment interventions.

Structural Family Therapy

In Salvador Minuchin's model of structural therapy (1974), the emphasis is on current functioning. The therapist initially explores the nature of the problem, translates this problem into interpersonal terms, and then devises a strategy for promoting change. Central to Minuchin's work is the concept of the family as a structural organization established by the hierarchic arrangement of relationships and the boundaries between family subgroups and members. In a well-functioning family, there is a clear hierarchic differentiation between parents, who have executive functions; and children, who have some input but much less power in decision making. The boundaries in a healthy family separate the parents from the children as one subgroup but allow sufficient interaction between the subgroups to maximize closeness and cooperation.

In dysfunctional families, there may be lopsided or chaotic hierarchic arrangements. For example, a particular child may have inordinate power, with the result that the parental coalition is weak or nonexistent. Such families are likely to experience major problems with rearing and disciplining their children. Another example of dysfunctional hierarchy is a family in which one parent has excessive power and the other parent is powerless. In dysfunctional families, boundaries between the subgroups tend to be either too rigid or too weak. When boundaries are extremely rigid—eg, between parents and children—a withdrawn quality is noted in relationships. These families do not offer closeness and a feeling of involvement, and the children are at risk of becoming delinquent or running away. Families with weak boundaries between subgroups are said to be "enmeshed." In these families, emotional dependence is so pervasive that family members may fail to achieve sufficient autonomy and differentiation to function successfully.

The goal of structural therapy is to modify the hierarchic relationships and boundaries so as to promote healthier functioning; eg, in a family in which the parental alliance is weak and one parent is overly involved with a child, treatment strategies are designed to form a parental subgroup that is separated from the child. The illustrative case at the beginning of this chapter demonstrates some of the principles of the structural approach to family therapy.

An impressive development resulted from the application of structural family therapy to the study and treatment of children suffering from diabetes, asthma, and anorexia nervosa. Minuchin and his colleagues (1978) distinguished between primary and secondary psychosomatic disorders. Primary psychosomatic disorders are those in which physiologic dysfunction is already present (eg, diabetes or allergic diathesis in patients with asthma). Existing physiologic symptoms are then exacerbated by emotional arousal due to stress. Secondary psychosomatic disorders are characterized by an absence of predisposing physiologic dysfunctions. In patients with these disorders (eg, anorexia nervosa), emotional conflicts are transformed directly into somatic symptoms.

Examination of the family systems of children with certain psychosomatic disorders reveals a characteristic pattern of personal dynamics: excessive emotional involvement of family members (enmeshment), overprotectiveness, rigidity of coping mechanisms, and ineffectiveness in resolving conflicts. A key finding is that children with certain psychosomatic illnesses are inappropriately involved in their parents' conflicts. A typical sequence of interactions recurs in these families. Conflict in the parental unit triggers stress and symptoms in the child; the child's symptoms become a focus of concern for the parents; and the conflict between the parents is temporarily diverted by the symptoms, which are both a reaction to stress and a temporary solution to stress. Family therapy is effective in breaking this cycle of interaction and bringing about improvement of symptoms.

The Minuchin group used a rigorous protocol to confirm their results. For example, in their studies of diabetic patients, they drew blood samples during family meetings in order to be able to obtain rapid readings of changes in free fatty acid levels. Increased free fatty acid levels indicate emotional arousal and signal the onset of diabetic ketoacidosis as well. This procedure furnished the group with exact data on emotional arousal associated with specific family interactions and also provided objective measurement of a positive outcome in treatment.

Strategic Family Therapy

The emphasis in strategic family therapy is on effective methods of promoting rapid change in families. The central idea of this approach is to define a problem and devise an appropriate strategy for solving that problem. Skillful methods of interviewing have been developed that rapidly and efficiently pinpoint key problem areas in families. Effective analysis should clarify the nature of interactions that reinforce and sustain the problem behaviors. A strategy is then designed to modify the interactional pattern and hence change the problem.

Although there are significant differences between the various models of strategic therapy, most focus on identifying current interactional patterns that keep a family "stuck" and on devising strategies to help the family change these patterns. The best-known approaches are the brief therapy methods of the Mental Research Institute group (Weakland, 1974) and the brilliant problem-solving techniques of Jay Haley (1976, 1980) and Chloe Madanes (1981). Mara Selvini Palazzoli (1978) led a group of psychoanalysts in developing brief strategic methods of family therapy for anorexic and psychotic adolescents. The influence of this group has been far-reaching (Hoffman, 1981).

Treatment methods used in strategic family therapy often take the form of directives given to the family that require them to do something, either during the session or at home. An intervention may be directed at having only one family member make a minor change, since strategic therapists believe that a change in any one part of a system or in one part of an interaction will result in a change in the whole system. These directives may be straightforward or paradoxic. If families appear to be reasonably compliant and likely to cooperate, the directives are usually straightforward. A simple example is that of a wife who was anxious about an impending job interview. The therapist realized that this anxiety was in part due to the wife's awareness of her husband's resistance to her taking a job outside the home. The directive given to this couple was for the husband to apply his considerable experience in the business world to the task of teaching his wife how to handle the job interview. This directive endorsed the power of the husband by putting him in charge of the symptom, and he successfully helped his wife prepare for and participate in the interview. This simple measure had in fact altered the relationship between the couple, so that the symptom was no longer "necessary."

When families are less compliant and oppose the therapist, paradoxic techniques are often successful. The idea of paradoxic therapy is based on the notion that resistant families have an interest in opposing change of any kind, from any source. The therapist, therefore suggests a directive that if contradicted by the family would paradoxically lead to positive change.

Illustrative case. A couple had worked with innumerable therapists over a 25-year period, but no apparent change had occurred. During their first session with the strategic family therapist, the couple described their unsatisfactory marital relationship but agreed that they felt hopeless about this attempt at therapy. The therapist took pains to elaborate the positive and negative aspects of the current relationship and expressed the view that it would be a mistake for the couple to change at this stage and that it would be wisest not to change at all. The couple was astonished to hear this from the therapist, since all previous therapists had struggled to promote change, with no success. The couple left the session in some bewilderment and indignation, and when they returned for the second session, they triumphantly pointed out to the therapist that they had already changed some aspects of their relationship for the better. The therapist was careful not to show his gratification but shook his head and warned the couple that attempts to make changes could have deleterious effects on their relationship. The therapist's stance paradoxically fueled the couple's determination to change even more.

Strategic treatment methods may offer dramatic results. Therein lie both their strength and their weakness. When family systems are rigid and unyielding, sometimes only paradoxic methods can alter the equilibrium of the system. On the other hand, this dramatic type of intervention may hold a seductive fascination for therapists who are somewhat manipulative and impatient with the more difficult and time-consuming processes usually necessary in psychotherapy.

SUMMARY

The current state of family therapy reveals a rift between traditional psychodynamically oriented family therapy and newer developments based on the interactional model. A few theorists believe that integration of intrapsychic concepts and family therapy is possible; most therapists regard these as conceptually incompatible. A theoretical synthesis has eluded practitioners of family therapy, but this does not mean that the therapist cannot endorse both approaches. They may represent 2 different dimensions of the same phenomenon, and both sets of data contribute to an overall understanding of family dysfunction. The psychodynamic orientation permits in-depth examination of the motivation and subjective experience of each family member, while the interactional perspective provides information about the person's social context as a source of determining individual behavior.

Although family therapy is in a state of transition, it is clear that it is a valid type of psychotherapy whose clinical effectiveness has been amply documented in several reviews. The systems theory perspective has introduced a critical dimension in revealing the interplay of family interaction and disturbed psychologic processes. The development of new family therapy techniques is influencing the practice of psychotherapy as a whole. Recent studies also suggest that family therapy may be successfully used to treat problems that do not respond to traditional treatment approaches, eg, the management of schizophrenic patients. Studies have shown that schizophrenic patients living in stressful family situations are prone to frequent relapses despite carefully monitored drug therapy. Involvement of the families of schizophrenic patients in therapy significantly reduces the frequency of relapse and the need for rehospitalization (see Chapter 27). Evidence also suggests that family therapy may be effective and appropriate in treatment of substance abuse, alcoholism, domestic violence, and delinquency. Many clinical training institutions now include family therapy as a component of the curriculum.

REFERENCES

Ackerman NW: *Treating the Troubled Family*. Basic Books, 1966.

Bateson G et al: Toward a theory of schizophrenia. *Behav Sci* 1956;**1**:251.

Bertalanffy L von: *General Systems Theory*. George Braziller, 1968.

Bowen M: The use of family therapy in clinical practice. *Compr Psychiatry* 1966;**7**:345.

Erickson MH: The use of symptoms as an integral part of hypnotherapy. In: *Advanced Techniques of Hypnosis and Therapy: Selected Papers of Milton H. Erickson, MD*. Haley J (editor). Grune & Stratton, 1967.

Glick ID, Borus JF: Marital and family therapy for troubled physicians and their families. *JAMA* 1984;**251**:1855. [And see Corrections, *JAMA* 1984;**252**:45, for a note about an error in the article.]

Goldstein M (editor): *New Developments in Interventions With Families of Schizophrenics*. Jossey-Bass, 1981.

Haley J: The family of the schizophrenic: A model system. *J Nerv Ment Dis* 1959;**129**:357.

Haley J: *Leaving Home*. McGraw-Hill, 1980.

Haley J: *Problem Solving Therapy*. Jossey-Bass, 1976.

Haley J (editor): *Advanced Techniques of Hypnosis and Therapy: Selected Papers of Milton H. Erickson, MD*. Grune & Stratton, 1967.

Hoffman L: *Foundations of Family Therapy*. Basic Books, 1981.

Jackson DD: The question of family homeostasis. *Psychiatr Q* 1957;**31 (Suppl)**:79.

Jackson DD: The study of the family. *Fam Process* 1965;**4**:1.

Lidz T: The influence of family studies on the treatment of schizophrenia. In: *Progress in Group and Family Therapy*. Sager CJ, Kaplan HS (editors). Brunner/Mazel, 1972.

Madanes C: *Strategic Family Therapy*. Jossey-Bass, 1981.

Minuchin S: *Families and Family Therapy*. Harvard Univ Press, 1974.

Minuchin S, Rosman B, Baker L: *Psychosomatic Families*. Harvard Univ Press, 1978.

Minuchin S et al: *Families of the Slums: An Exploraton of Their Structure and Treatment*. Basic Books, 1967.

Palazzoli MS et al: *Paradox and Counterparadox*. Jason Aronson, 1978.

Shapiro RJ: Alcohol and family violence. In: *Clinical Approaches to Family Violence*. Barnhill L (editor). Aspen Systems, 1982.

Shapiro RJ: Psychodynamically oriented family therapy. In: *Treatment of Emotional Disorders in Children and Adolescents*. Sholevar GP, Benson R, Blinder B(editors). Spectrum, 1980.

Singer MT, Wynne LC: Thought disorder and family relations of schizophrenics: Results and implications. *Arch Gen Psychiatry* 1965;**12**:201.

Watzlawick P, Weakland J, Fisch R: Change: *Principles of Problem Formation and Problem Resolution*. Norton, 1974.

Weakland J et al: Brief therapy: Focused problem resolution. *Fam Process* 1974;**13**:141.

Wynne LC et al: Pseudo-mutuality in the family relations of schizophrenics. *Psychiatry* 1958;**21**:205.

49

Marital Therapy

Rodney J. Shapiro, PhD

Marital therapy is a recent development in the overall history of marriage counseling. The conceptual basis of marital therapy is now strongly identified with family systems theory (see Chapter 48). The basic concepts of family therapy grew out of the studies of parents and their offspring (children, adolescents, young adults). A number of these investigations demonstrated reciprocal patterns of influence between parent-child interactions and the dynamics of the marital relationship, and it became evident that marital therapy was an essential component in work with entire families. Many family therapists have come to regard the marital relationship as the primary focus of intervention, and they consequently spend more time and effort on the couple than on the children. Family therapists conduct marital therapy as part of their work with the whole family. Marital therapy is also used when the couple is childless or the children are unavailable (eg, adult offspring who live far away from their parents) or when marital problems do not require participation of the children.

Marital therapy can be distinguished from family therapy on the basis of the unit of treatment. Marital therapy is confined to one generation (the adult dyad), whereas family therapy encompasses 2 generations (parents and children) and sometimes 3 (grandparents). All family therapists include marital therapy as part of their work, but not all marital therapists work with families. A number of therapists, though trained in family therapy, regard themselves as marital therapists because they prefer to work with couples rather than with whole families.

The term "marital therapy" is misleading in its implication that the legal definition of marriage—the joining of a man and a woman in a special kind of social and legal interdependence for the purpose of founding and maintaining a family—establishes the unit of treatment. The varying family life-styles now current require a broader focus. Marital therapy is accordingly defined in this chapter as the treatment of any unit of 2 adults, of the same sex or of opposite sexes, who consider themselves a couple by reason of cohabitation or mutual commitment.

INDICATIONS FOR MARITAL THERAPY

The Referral Process

Most therapists subscribe to the view that marital therapy is clearly indicated when problems relate directly to the marital relationship. Such problems may be obvious, eg, incessant conflict and disagreement, threats of separation, sexual difficulties. A person who seeks out a therapist, states that marital conflicts are the main concern, and indicates the partner's willingness to join in therapy is obviously seeking and expecting to receive marital therapy, and no clinician should logically refuse to see the person and the partner together, as a couple, in such circumstances or refuse to refer them to a marital therapist.

In a different situation, the patient may approach the therapist with complaints about the marital relationship but may ask for individual therapy. Underlying such a request is the patient's hope for a supportive ally to aid in coping with marital strife. Individuals frequently complain of marital difficulties but do not specifically request marital therapy. Unless the therapist prefers to practice only individual therapy, such contacts are likely to elicit either suggestions or strong recommendations from the therapist to try marital therapy.

A more complicated situation occurs when the person approaching the therapist describes several problems, some of them marital and some of a purely personal nature. Typically, the patient requests help for depression and mentions, perhaps incidentally, some difficulties in the marital relationship. The therapist who is not trained in systems theory is likely to recommend individual treatment in such a case. If marital issues then emerge as dominant problems during the course of individual therapy, the therapist will either try to work them out with the patient or refer the couple to another therapist for adjunctive marital therapy while work with the individual is continued as the primary treatment.

Unless marital therapy is specifically requested, therefore, it is unlikely to be offered or recommended by the majority of therapists who are not trained in family systems theory, although this situation is changing as the usefulness and validity of marital therapy for other kinds of problems besides marital conflict become evident.

Sex Therapy

The treatment of sexual dysfunction has become a subspecialty within the mental health field. Knowledge of the physiology and psychology of sexual functioning has been greatly expanded (see Chapter 37). Training in sex therapy is now included in the clinical training of most mental health practitioners, and many therapists have chosen to specialize in sex therapy. There has been growing recognition that sexual dysfunction is best understood as one significant component of a complex interpersonal system; in practical terms, treatment of a sexual problem must also consider the couple's interpersonal relationship. A knowledge of family systems theory and techniques of marital therapy is essential for the effective practice of sex therapy.

Illustrative case. A couple sought marital therapy on the recommendation of a urologist who had examined the husband for evaluation of long-standing impotence. Examination had ruled out any physical basis for the impotence, and an evaluation for psychotherapy was suggested. The patient's wife was invited to participate in the first interview. The wife declared that the couple's only marital problem was the husband's impotence, which she saw as a defect in her husband, and she offered several theories about the origin of the symptom. All of her conjectures related to some past failing or some flaw in the husband's character. The man became extremely withdrawn and silent during his wife's recitation. Although he was enraged by these criticisms, he was unable to express his anger directly for fear of losing control. He therefore "punished" his wife with his passivity and emotional unavailability.

Couples therapy provided an opportunity for these partners to move away from a stance of blaming and passivity and to learn to communicate more directly. Both parties were able to acknowledge and work through their own problems. As part of marital therapy, the couple received information and advice about sexual matters, and sexual exercises were prescribed as homework tasks. Therapy helped them become closer and recognize their need for each other. As their relationship improved, the impotence rapidly disappeared, and both partners were able to enjoy sex in the context of renewed intimacy.

Substance Abuse & Violence

Many people seeking psychiatric help have some substance abuse problem whether they admit it or not during the initial interview (see Chapters 25 and 26). In recent years, family therapy has proved effective in the treatment of various forms of substance abuse. Increasing use of a systems perspective in marital therapy has led to greater appreciation of the complex interpersonal context of substance abuse. For example, studies have demonstrated that families attempt to adapt to drinking problems in ways that unintentionally reinforce rather than reduce the consumption of alcohol. The most important insights have been gained in understanding the marital system of drug abusers. Shapiro (1977) and Steinglass (1981) note that the spouse of the substance abuser plays a key role in the disease and may make the essential difference in the patient's acceptance of treatment.

A serious problem closely related to substance abuse is domestic violence. Recent surveys have provided alarming statistics about the extent of child abuse, physical or sexual (over 1 million cases a year); wife battering (at least 16% of couples experience at least one violent interaction each year); and violence against parents. Traditional treatment methods have focused primarily on the victims of abuse. Shelters for women and children have proliferated in the past decade. Commendable efforts are under way to increase the availability of legal and counseling resources for victims. However, male abusers are rarely involved in treatment unless such treatment is ordered by a court of law. They are regarded as unmotivated, resistant, irresponsible, and potentially threatening to therapists. Recent studies challenge this stereotype of the male abuser (Shapiro, 1982, 1984). If approached tactfully, the majority of these men can be induced to enter into treatment. If there is no immediate threat of further violence in the family, therapy involving the couple can be highly effective. Couples therapy examines violence within the context of the marital relationship rather than concentrating on one individual as the source of violence. Interventions based on this model have proved notably successful in effecting rapid cessation and continued avoidance of violence.

Illustrative case. A couple in their mid 20s sought help for a marital crisis that had been precipitated by the wife's sudden departure from home after an argument the previous week that had ended in a physical assault by the husband. Initial evaluation revealed a pattern of conflicts and repeated episodes of battering. The husband drank heavily once or twice a month. When he was sober, the couple's disagreements rarely escalated to violence. They would either reach agreement or break off the argument without agreement, or else one party would leave the house for a time to cool down. When the husband was drinking, the disagreement usually escalated into an intense dispute that frequently included battery on the wife. To reduce the risk of further violence, the therapist suggested a rule that the couple adopted, namely, to have arguments and disagreements only when both parties were sober. The regimen included the husband's participation in an alcohol treatment program and a mutual agreement to avoid further physical violence and use therapy sessions for communicating and resolving their difficulties. In this instance, as in other cases of substance abuse and violence, it was evident that working therapeutically with both partners was more efficient and more likely to result in a satisfactory outcome than working with either one alone.

Psychiatric & Medical Disorders

Chronic depression, anxiety, psychotic disorders, borderline and narcissistic personality disorders, eating disorders, phobias, etc, are usually viewed by most clinicians as psychologic or biologic problems, and the treatment of choice is invariably *individual* psychotherapy (often with adjunctive medication). In contrast, marital and family therapists view the mental disorders as symptoms of disturbed personal interaction within a marriage or family system. An increasing number of institutions and clinicians are involving spouses and family members as part of the treatment program. Marital therapy is gaining acceptance as part of an overall treatment plan, but fundamental differences in underlying concepts result in an uneasy collaboration between clinicians espousing models of illness based on the individual and those using models based on the tenets of systems theory. An accommodation between these opposing perspectives has been achieved by permitting and even encouraging the practice of marital and family therapy in psychiatric settings, but only as long as such therapy is viewed as secondary and optional to other kinds of treatment. Marital therapy is sometimes recommended in addition to individual and pharmacologic treatment. This choice is most likely to be made when family conflict is apparent or when treatment of the individual patient is not going well.

The pioneering work of Minuchin and coworkers (1978) showed that somatic symptoms and physiologic changes (eg, in blood glucose levels) in children are closely linked to family dynamics (eg, conflicts and their resolution). Behavioral symptoms in the child (eg, running away from home) may serve as a defense that distracts the parents' attention from their own conflicts with each other. As Haley (1976) and other workers have pointed out, symptoms communicate "messages" to the partners in relationships (eg, a backache may indicate that one marital partner feels the other is a burden and a "pain" and may use the symptom to avoid work or sex). If symptoms evoke desired responses (eg, relief from responsibility or conflict), they are likely to become reinforced. Familiarity with the principles and practice of family therapy is encouraging many physicians and psychiatrists to include marital partners in their treatment of adult psychosomatic illness. Training programs in family medicine offer appropriate opportunities for teaching family therapy. A family orientation is also gaining acceptance in the treatment of serious medical illness, since the role of the spouse is often critically important in implementing a consistent treatment regimen. Catastrophic illness, disabilities, and surgical procedures are stresses that affect all members of a patient's family. Singer (1983) has shown how the management of a patient with cancer frequently includes treatment measures for both the patient and family members.

CONTRAINDICATIONS TO MARITAL THERAPY

Since family systems theory views almost all psychologic problems as symptoms representing disturbed or dysfunctional personal interaction, marital or family therapy is the treatment of choice whenever possible. Obviously, couples therapy is ruled out for single adults or widows and widowers.

An important question that frequently arises in marital therapy is whether or not to include a partner other than a spouse. Unmarried but cohabiting adults are viewed by most therapists as appropriate candidates for couples treatment. Fewer therapists agree that a noncohabiting couple should be treated as a unit. Clinicians must judge each case separately. A useful guideline is to consider conjoint therapy (see Chapter 48) for couples who seem committed to the relationship.

It is not uncommon for therapists who work with individuals to suggest marital therapy to their patients when marital conflicts seem particularly intense or when there is a crisis such as threatened separation. The expectation of these therapists is that their work will continue as the main focus of treatment and that marital therapy sessions represent but a temporary adjunct to ongoing individual therapy.

On the other hand, *family* therapists generally agree that marital therapy may be inadvisable when one or more family members are already involved in some other form of psychotherapy. Couples and family therapy is most effective when it is the sole arena for the expression and resolution of conflicts. Couples and family treatment is less effective if it is regarded as adjunctive and secondary to individual treatment. Moreover, the therapists may consciously or unconsciously compete with one another and thus undermine each other's efforts. Patients may also resist or manipulate multiple therapists. Despite these inherent risks, couples therapy can be considered as an adjunct to individual treatment in certain circumstances. The marital and individual therapists must make certain that their alliance is collaborative and noncompetitive, and both must be alert to patients' attempts to set them against each other.

TECHNIQUES OF MARITAL THERAPY

The Initial Contact

The initial contact between the patient and the therapist is particularly important, since the presenting problem may reveal marital difficulties but may not be perceived as a specific request for marital therapy. The therapist's response can be decisive in determining whether the patient will be treated on an individual basis or whether both partners will be seen conjointly, as a couple. If marital difficulties seem apparent but there is reluctance on the part of either partner to be seen conjointly, the therapist should not immediately agree to the request for an individual session or separate meetings with each spouse. Unless there is undue resistance, the couple is likely to agree to a joint meeting if the therapist insists on that format.

Clinicians who are trained in family systems theory understand that there is good reason to press for conjoint meetings from the beginning. Acceding to a patient's request to be seen alone enables the patient to take charge of an important aspect of the treatment process. Systems theory views these therapist-patient interactions as a struggle between the therapist's goals of inducing changes in behavior and symptoms and the patient's resistance to such changes. The "power" of the therapist is enhanced if it is the therapist who sets the rules from the start.

If the patient is adamant about being seen alone or convinces the therapist that the spouse will refuse to agree to a joint meeting, then an initial meeting can be arranged for the patient alone. The therapist can minimize the patient's seeming "victory" by repeatedly emphasizing personal reservations about seeing one partner without the other.

The therapist must be alert to 2 common problems that arise when sessions are held with only one member of the marital dyad. If the initial interview goes well, the patient may experience a positive connection with the therapist and may be even more reluctant to have a spouse share the treatment session. The therapist too may experience the beginning of a positive alliance and share the patient's reluctance to have a third person intrude. The second problem is that the absent partner is invariably apprehensive about what might have been said and may be even more resistant to the idea of entering treatment. Obviously, the longer the period during which only one spouse is seen, the greater will be the resistance to changing this arrangement.

Motivation for Treatment

The marital therapist must recognize and contend with another phenomenon at the outset of treatment: Marital partners rarely experience the same degree of motivation to enter therapy. Careful questioning during the initial interview will reveal and clarify this imbalance so that the therapist can develop strategies for involving the more resistant member. Typically, one partner brings the other into therapy by means of persuasion, threats, or other inducement.

Illustrative case. A woman who was receiving individual therapy was referred along with her husband for marital therapy. In the inital interview, the therapist spent some time exploring the woman's reasons for seeking marital therapy. She explained that individual therapy had helped her become aware of her dissatisfaction with her marriage. She had come to realize that her husband could not meet her needs and that she should seriously consider divorce. With the first therapist's encouragement, the patient asked her husband if he would go with her to see a marriage counselor or therapist. At first the husband refused, but he agreed when she said she would leave him if he did not consent to therapy. Knowing that the patient had given such an ultimatum alerted the second therapist to the need to win the man's confidence and involve him in therapy. The marital therapist conjectured aloud how difficult it must be for the husband to view therapy as a helpful process if he felt forced to participate. With the marital therapist's encouragement and support, the husband was initially able to vent his resentment and sense of helplessness and then felt free to admit that he was also relieved that his wife

had pressured him into seeking help. At the end of the first session, the husband astonished his wife by his genuine willingness to continue therapy.

Evaluation of the Couple

Thorough assessment of a couple presenting for treatment may take several sessions. The partners should be evaluated both as individuals and in their relationship to each other. Information should be obtained about developmental history, ego strengths and liabilities, defense mechanisms, and symptoms suggestive of possible psychologic disturbance in either individual. The relationship between the couple should receive special scrutiny. A history of the relationship always reveals recurring patterns of difficulty. The most important data, however, are derived from observations made during treatment sessions. Both verbal and nonverbal behavior patterns provide clues to the couple's characteristic styles of interaction. A capacity for closeness, clear and open communication of thoughts and feelings, and a mutual desire to solve problems are all conducive to a positive outcome of treatment.

The underlying needs that bind a couple are a source both of strength and of conflict in the relationship, and the complex dynamics are largely covert and accessible only by inference. Current knowledge about marital dynamics arises from object relations theory and systems theory (see Chapter 3). Selection of a mate is to a great extent an unconscious process influenced by internalized identifications with parents in early life. Unmet needs and disturbances in early child-parent relations are reenacted in marriage. For example, inadequate parenting often leaves the child with poor self-esteem and feelings of deprivation. Typically, these problems persist into adulthood and may motivate the adult to seek a partner to gratify these "unmet needs" (ie, provide nurturing and support). Problems then invariably arise in the marriage as the press of these unresolved childhood needs interferes with the reality-based demands of the marriage. Therapy using a systems perspective does not emphasize the role of transference and insight but concerns itself instead with the behavioral manifestations of unconscious dynamics. (An example would be a possessive and abusive husband who is motivated by unconscious fears of abandonment and rage at his mother—both stemming from early parent-child experiences.) In marital therapy, conflicts between the couple are acted out in therapy sessions, so that the covert is made overt and the therapist can intervene directly to modify interactions and thereby influence the patients' underlying motivations.

Much understanding is to be gained by exploring each partner's relationships with his or her parents and siblings (the family of origin), both during the formative years and in the present. Problems that were not resolved are likely to persist with the spouse and children. Attitudes and expectations derived from the patients' respective families may be variant or even oppositional. Current relationships between marital partners and their parents and other family members may help or hinder the marriage. Parental approval or disapproval of a son's or daughter's spouse can profoundly affect the marriage. As Framo (1981) points out, the influence of the family of origin is so pervasive that some therapists encourage the participation of members of the family of origin at different stages of couples therapy.

Marriage can be viewed as a developmental process. Blanck and Blanck (1968) note that successive phases of marriage elicit different needs and require various adaptations. A useful framework for evaluating couples is to compile a thorough history of their relationship and match their problems with specific developmental tasks. It is not uncommon to find that a couple may cope well at one stage (eg, early marriage) and not at another (eg, birth of their first child). The developmental perspective emphasizes growth and adaptation. Most marital therapists prefer this view to traditional psychiatric evaluations based on assessing psychopathology in each partner.

Treatment Plans

Evaluation of the couple should conclude with treatment recommendations. The trend in couples therapy is in the direction of short-term treatment with defined goals. The therapist works collaboratively with the couple in reaching a consensus on what they wish changed and actively guides them in formulating attainable goals. The therapist assumes responsibility for devising a treatment plan based upon the assessment of each individual, the dynamics of the relationship, the nature of the couple's problems, and the goals the partners set.

A treatment contract should be established with the couple that stipulates whether therapy is to be time-limited or open-ended and establishes frequency of sessions, rules of attendance, payment of fees, etc. Although the norm in marital therapy is for short-term (3–6 months) treatment, there are appropriate exceptions. Couples with multiple problems and serious personality disorders may require longer-term treatment and more intensive work. Regardless of the length of treatment, the frequency of sessions is seldom more than once weekly. Limiting the length and frequency of contacts discourages dependence on the therapist and encourages the couple to assume full responsibility for working toward their goals. Attendance rules usually require that both partners be present at all sessions, although the therapist may change this rule from time to time for reasons of strategy. Requirements concerning fees, cancellation policy, and so on are not essentially different from those used in individual or group therapy.

ROLE & CHARACTERISTICS OF THE THERAPIST

The Role of the Therapist

The role of the therapist working with couples is more difficult and complex than that involved in working with individuals or entire families. When working with individuals, the therapist strives to achieve a working relationship with one person that is mutually positive. In work with families, there is always the chance that some members will dislike or attack the therapist occasionally, but there are also other members who will provide support and protection. With couples, however, the challenge is to establish a positive alliance with *each* partner within a context often marked by accusations, blaming, and attempts to manipulate the therapist into taking one side or the other.

A therapist who attempts to maintain strict neutrality (along the lines of traditional psychoanalytic psychotherapy) may lose the cooperation of both partners, since they will be likely to ascribe the therapist's neutrality to a lack of interest or concern. On the other hand, should the therapist appear to empathize more with one partner than the other, the couple may still be lost to therapy if the aggrieved partner decides to leave treatment.

The marital therapist must constantly change sides, but in a way that neither antagonizes one partner to the point of leaving nor establishes a one-sided alliance with the other. The goal is not to maintain neutrality but to be able to side with each partner individually at some point in therapy. The therapist may appreciate and accept the point of view of one partner but at the same time must be vigilant to the effects this alliance has on the other partner. Some practical advice for therapists in training is never to end a session just after having strongly sided with one partner. Instead, attempts should always be made to equalize the therapist-patient alliances established during the course of the session, so that each partner can leave feeling acknowledged and understood by the therapist.

The tendency to assume positions of right and wrong is most often seen in couples therapy. The therapist must resist being drawn into arguments about what is right and what is wrong. A solid grounding in family systems theory is the therapist's best deterrent, since it is usually clear that there is neither a right nor a wrong answer when a couple's disputes are explored from the interactional point of view espoused by family systems theory. Partners who adopt **polarized positions** are said to have become snared in a repetitive sequence of interactions and are unable to experience or choose alternative ways of responding, as shown in the illustrative case below, which also shows how a seemingly simple dispute can mask complex interpersonal dynamics.

Illustrative case. A major source of conflict for the couple was the husband's apparent unwillingness to find secure employment. The wife came from a wealthy family and received a monthly allowance from her parents. The wife periodically became furious at her husband for his "laziness" in not finding "significant" work. He spent most of his time caring for their children at home and engaging in charity and volunteer work. He protested that they did not need the extra income and that he was unable to find suitable work in any case. The more the wife pressured him, the less the husband did to change the situation. At one point the wife turned to the therapist in sheer exasperation and asked, "Don't you think a grown man should have a steady job?"

The therapist's initial reaction was to agree with the wife that it was "wrong" for the husband to refuse employment and that he was clearly sponging off her. The therapist refrained from expressing an opinion, however, and sought to understand more about the interactional dynamics of the dispute. It became clear that whenever the husband did make genuine efforts to find a job, tentative as they were, the wife did not support him and in fact put obstacles in his way; she was unconsciously resisting his possible employment.

The dispute about work masked some underlying issues that could not easily be reduced to a matter of simple right or wrong. The wife had great difficulty expressing warmth and affection for either her husband or her children. The husband protected her from her deficiencies in parenting by taking care of the children during the day. One of the stabilizing influences in the marriage was the wife's certainty that her husband would never abandon her. He was a dependent and rather masochistic partner and seemed to put up with a good deal of verbal abuse. His refusal to work also enabled his wife to remain dependent on her parents, who were sympathetic to her plight and supported her.

Avoiding employment served as a defense mechanism for the husband as well, who was a dependent and vulnerable individual who related to his wife as if she were a scolding mother. His dependency needs were met by knowing that his wife seemed to need him as much as he needed her. Despite their bitter arguments, he sensed that she actually tolerated his lack of employment. His immaturity and poor self-esteem made him feel safer with children than with adults, and he looked to his children for closeness and acceptance. Having always led a sheltered life, he had profound fears of testing himself in the everyday world and subconsciously protected his self-esteem by assuring himself that he was too good for most of the jobs that were available.

Attributes & Values of the Therapist

The personal attributes and values of the therapist play a major role in influencing couples to enter therapy and in achieving a successful outcome. The therapist's age, gender, cultural background, and marital status may be significant in particular situations. A marked discrepancy in age is always difficult; couples may feel inhibited and awkward with therapists who are much younger or older than themselves, and therapists are more likely to experience counter-transference reactions in such circumstances. Gender is always a significant consideration in couples therapy. If the therapist is male, the husband may see him as a competitor, while the wife may feel that he is inca-pable of understanding the situation. Similarly, the wife may view a female therapist as a competitor, whereas the husband may believe that she is biased against men. Racial and cultural differences between therapist and client may also disrupt the therapeutic process.

Illustrative case. A therapist sought consultation for difficulties she experienced in working with a couple. She perceived the couple as extremely resistant to her efforts to help them. The consultant discovered the source of the problems to be a striking cultural and class disparity between therapist and clients. The therapist, a 38-year-old white married woman, revealed an upper-middle-class background in her reserved polite mannerisms, emotional reserve, and somewhat formal habits of speech. The couple were Mexican-Americans in their early 20s and had been living together though unmarried for about 6 months. Neither had completed high school. Both partners accepted without question the man's "macho" role in his relationships with women. The woman's major complaints related to his absences from home and suspected infidelities. He reacted angrily to what he perceived as her sexual jealousy and possessiveness. Disagreements quickly escalated into emotional outbursts, threatened violence, and verbal assaults with some obscene language. The therapist felt intimidated and threatened, and the couple interpreted her obvious discomfort as indicative of her rejection of them.

This impasse was overcome with the help of the consultant, who encouraged the therapist to examine and better understand her discomfort with the couple. She was also urged to raise the apparent differences directly with them in order to assure them that whatever their differences, she wanted to help them. The couple responded with relief when the subject came up in a session. Both the therapist and the couple were able to share their concerns, and a successful outcome was signified by honesty and good-humored teasing whenever the class differences became apparent in subsequent sessions.

Even the most thoroughly self-aware therapists are influenced by their own values and beliefs in therapy sessions. Treatment situations frequently evoke values that do not agree with the therapist's own and thereby threaten the therapist's impartiality. Therapists' experiences and views about marriage, fidelity, divorce, and sexual behavior inevitably influence their reaction to problems in these areas. Couples may sense significant differences between their life-style and that of the therapist. Some self-disclosure on the part of the therapist is appropriate and useful in marital therapy, and questions about the therapist's marital status or age and whether he or she is a parent should be readily acknowledged. Questions about sexual behavior and other more personal matters are generally irrelevant to the therapy process and may breach the boundary that should be kept intact between therapist and client. Therapists have a professional responsibility to be honest in examining how personal attitudes and feelings influence their work.

An issue that perennially arises is whether the therapist has a bias toward keeping marriages intact or encouraging their dissolution. Many couples have expectations and apprehensions about the goals of the therapist with regard to their marriages. These concerns are sometimes made explicit; more commonly, they are disguised. A common assumption is that marital therapists are in favor of keeping marriages together. Consequently, when couples are in conflict about a potential separation, the spouse wanting to maintain the relationship may see the therapist as a potential ally, whereas the one seeking separation may anticipate disapproval from the therapist.

The image of marital therapists as being in favor of marriage is not entirely their patients' projection. Marital therapy is rarely distinguished from marriage counseling, and the latter has a long history of supporting the institution of marriage. The clergy has been heavily represented in marriage counseling, and when counseling they may not subscribe to the impartial stance that is one of the prime tenets of psychotherapy.

NONTRADITIONAL COUPLE SYSTEMS

Contemporary marital therapists cannot limit their work to couples who meet the legal definition of marriage. A high divorce rate and rejection of marriage are creating considerable numbers of single adults and parents, unmarried cohabitants, and people who marry more than once. Rapidly changing social and moral values are reflected in greater tolerance for alternative life-styles and confusion about what constitutes normal family functioning. Work with nontraditional couple systems is clinically challenging and requires an innovative and flexible approach to assessment and treatment.

The Single Adult

It has been stated previously in this chapter that couples therapy may be indicated on occasion for single adults who are not living together. If the relationship is significant for the couple, then it may also be significant for assessment and therapy, and objections are few if such couples request conjoint therapy. A more difficult decision is whether to involve both partners when one of them requests individual therapy. A good strategy is to inquire about the relationship in the first session and decide with the patient at that point whether or not to invlove the partner. Even if individual therapy is indicated, there may be some point later in treatment when couples work would be beneficial.

Complications also arise when one person who is involved in an ongoing cohabitation relationship is seen in individual therapy. Traditionally trained psychodynamic psychotherapists feel confident that they can remain objective in their assessment of the patient in such situations and can avoid siding either with the patient or with the absent partner. In fact, it is highly unlikely that the therapist will be able to be objective as long as only one partner participates in treatment. For example, the therapist may make assumptions that are distorted or incorrect. When the patient describes an event that occurred with the partner, it is virtually impossible for the therapist to know what actually happened. All people, whether inadvertently or otherwise, tend to adjust their view of reality so they will seem better and feel better, and this is particularly likely to occur when they report highly charged events concerned with those they interact most closely with. When the therapist works with only one individual, various impressions and pieces of informations tend to create an image of the other partner in the therapist's mind. If the therapist never meets the partner, the impressions can never be confirmed.

If the therapist is convinced that the individual patient's problems are largely due to stresses in the relationship, then it is appropriate to insist on the advantage of conjoint therapy, and the therapist may find it beneficial to convey to the patient the difficulties of attempting to understand a relationship when one partner is absent.

The Single Parent

Working with a single parent who is involved in a significant relationship has all of the difficulties mentioned in the preceding section as well as the problem of relationships with one or more children. It is almost impossible to gain an impartial understanding of these complicated interrelationships without having both the single parent's partner and the children participate in at least some aspects of therapy.

A dominant theme in the life of single parents (most of them women) is the desire to establish a rewarding intimate domestic relationship with a person who relates well to the children. If the single parent has not found such a person or if the current partner falls short of this ideal, the parent is likely to be disillusioned and needy, and the situation is complicated for the therapist. The female single parent may idealize the therapist as an understanding and caring person, and it may be difficult for a male therapist to avoid unwittingly reinforcing that perception. The best solution to this problem of countertransference is to involve the woman's partner if he plays a significant role in her life and that of her children. If there is no such involvement, then the therapist should help the patient develop realistic expectations about potential partners and should stay alert to the need to interpret and neutralize potential transference reactions.

Couples Contemplating Separation & Divorce

Couples considering or going through separation often look to marital therapists for help. In determining whether such couples should be seen conjointly, it is first necessary to find out where they are in the separation process. When one or both partners are uncertain or ambivalent about the relationship, then it is usually appropriate to work with both partners. If one partner is definitely intent on separation or divorce, however, it may be inadvisable to insist that both parties participate in treatment.

The rejected spouse may demand that the therapist convince the partner not to leave. The spouse who has decided on separation may come for treatment only under duress and is unlikely to feel receptive to therapy, since the decision has been made to terminate, rather than work on, the relationship. In fact, if a spouse has definite plans for separation but seems willing to come in for therapy, the therapist may discover covert motives to explain this contradiction. For example, the spouse who is leaving the relationship may agree to therapy in order to relieve feelings of guilt or obtain help for the rejected partner, particularly if there are fears of strongly adverse reactions to the fact of rejection. It is not uncommon for a spouse to announce the intention to separate during the first session and use the setting to ensure immediate therapeutic help for the distraught mate. Some spouses choose the safety of a therapy visit to communicate an intent to separate because they are so fearful of the anticipated reaction of anger or even violence.

When marital separation is clearly in progress, it is unwise to insist on joint treatment in most cases. One exception to this recommendation is a couple who mutually accept the reality of separation and wish to use marital therapy as an aid in working through the separation process. The term "divorce therapy" has been coined to describe this process of working through a dissolution of marriage. Therapy may often be a means of helping couples go through a divorce. An impartial and concerned therapist can do a great deal to ensure appropriate support and understanding for each partner, help them resolve whatever differences and conflicts can be resolved, and assist them in coming to terms with problems that remain insoluble. The major feelings experienced in separation and divorce are anger, grief, and guilt. The therapist is in a position to offer both partners an opportunity to acknowledge and work through these painful feelings. Therapy with couples undergoing separation or divorce should of necessity be brief and focused. Long-term therapy, though it be offered in a sympathetic vein, may actually be counterproductive by making it more difficult for the couple to go through with separation and divorce. Therapy for couples contemplating or in the midst of separation and divorce may be especially helpful when children are involved. Couples often have confused and inconsistent ideas about how to explain the separation to their children and, more importantly, how they should continue their individual relationships with the children.

In recent years, there has been an increased and welcome collaboration between psychotherapeutic services and the legal systems involved in divorce disputes. Traditionally, in divorce proceedings, legal assistance has resulted in an adversarial contest in which each lawyer fights for the "best interests" of his or her client. Unfortunately, a lawyer's version of the client's best interests may not be in accord with the best interests of either the relationship or the children. Trained therapists functioning as mediators may facilitate the resolution of disputes about child custody and visitation arrangements. Not all couples are amenable to mediation counseling, particularly if they are already so antagonistic that working together is out of the question. For many couples, however, mediation conducted by a skillful therapist is a constructive experience that allows the divorce to take place with the least harm to the couple and their children. In some jurisdictions, judicially monitored mediation is mandatory when child custody or visitation matters are in dispute.

Homosexual Couples

Sexual behavior that was once labeled psychopathologic is now considered to be more a matter of preference or alternative life-style. Freed from the stigma of mental abnormality, many homosexual men and women feel less defensive about their relationships and more willing to seek the services of marital therapists. Homosexual couples engaged in a significant relationship deal with many of the same issues that cohabiting heterosexual couples face. Therapy is advisable only if the marital therapist is experienced in working with homosexual couples and is not influenced by negative countertransference reactions.

The question is often raised whether a heterosexual therapist can work effectively with a homesexual couple. The critical determinant is the relationship between the therapist and the couple: if they can establish a genuine positive alliance, then there is no reason why therapy should not proceed.

SUMMARY

This chapter has attempted to demonstrate both the complexity of marital therapy and its effectiveness in different situations, where its results may be as good as those associated with individual, group, or family therapy. Marital therapy requires integration of diverse concepts derived from psychodynamic theory, group dynamics, and family systems theory.

This chapter has also tried to show the wide variety of problems for which marital therapy either has relevance or is the treatment of choice. Although marital conflicts are often the main problem presented by the patient, many of the patient's other concerns may reflect a disturbance in the marital relationship. Even when the focus remains on the individual patient, involvement of the spouse can significantly enhance compliance with treatment.

The principles and techniques of marital therapy are now also being used to treat nonpsychiatric disorders as medical practitioners come to a greater appreciation of the extent to which sickness and health are influenced by family relationships.

REFERENCES

Ables B, Brandsma J: *Therapy for Couples*. Jossey-Bass, 1982.

Blanck R, Blanck G: *Marriage and Personal Development*. Columbia Univ Press, 1968.

Framo J: The integration of marital therapy with sessions with family of origin. In: *Handbook of Family Therapy*. Gurman A, Kniskern D (editors). Brunner/Mazel, 1981.

Glick D, Borus J: Marital and family therapy for troubled physicians and their families. *JAMA* 1984;**251:**1855. [And see also Corrections, *JAMA* 1984;**252:**45, for a note about an error in the article.]

Gurman A, Rice D (editors): *Couples in Conflict*. Jason Aronson, 1975.

Haley J: *Problem-Solving Therapy*. Jossey-Bass, 1976.

Kaplan HS: *Disorders of Sexual Desire*. Brunner/Mazel, 1979.

Kressel K, Deutsch M: Divorce therapy: An in-depth survey of therapists' views. *Fam Process* 1977;**16:**413.

Martin P: *A Marital Therapy Manual*. Brunner/Mazel, 1976.

Minuchin S, Rosman B, Baker L: *Psychosomatic Families*. Harvard Univ Press, 1978.

Paolino T, McCrady B: *Marriage and Marital Therapy: Psychoanalytic, Behavioral, and Systems Theory Perspectives*. Brunner/Mazel, 1978.

Shapiro RJ: Alcohol and family violence. In: *Clinical Approaches to Family Violence*. Barnhill L (editor). Aspen Systems, 1982.

Shapiro RJ: A family therapy approach to alcoholism. *J Marriage Fam Counseling* 1977;**3:**71.

Shapiro RJ: Therapy with violent families. In: *Violent Individuals and Families: A Handbook for Practitioners*. Saunders S et al (editors). Thomas, 1984.

Singer B: Psychosocial trauma, defense strategies and treatment considerations in cancer patients and their families. *Am J Fam Ther* 1983;**11:**15.

Steinglass P: Family therapy with alcoholics: A review. In: *Family Therapy of Drug and Alcohol Abuse*. Kaufman E, Kaufmann P (editors). Gardner Press, 1981.

Psychotherapy of Patients With Chronic Medical Disorders

50

Gary M. Rodin, MD

The aim of medical treatment is to improve the quality of life of sick patients. Although psychotherapy is specifically directed toward this goal, it is often overlooked as a form of treatment in general medicine. This is unfortunate, since psychologic distress is common among medical patients, and psychologic interventions not only may relieve emotional distress but also may alleviate physical symptoms.

This chapter will focus on psychotherapy in the management of patients with chronic medical disorders. Psychotherapy can be especially useful for such patients, whose suffering may extend over many years. A sensitive and informed physician can manage the emotional care of most patients with chronic illness. However, some patients may need or may request more specialized psychologic treatment requiring referral to a psychiatrist or other mental health professional. This chapter reviews the indications and contraindications for psychotherapy of such patients. Consideration will be given to the referral process and to special issues in the psychotherapy of medical patients. These issues are relevant to the psychotherapeutic management of medical patients by both primary physicians and trained psychotherapists who are treating medically ill patients. The treatment of patients with acute medical and psychiatric problems and with terminal illness is described elsewhere. (See Chapters 9, 51, and 56.)

CHARACTERISTICS OF SUPPORTIVE & EXPRESSIVE THERAPY

As described in Chapter 43, psychotherapy is usually divided into 2 major categories: supportive and expressive (or insight-oriented) psychotherapy. Both forms of therapy require that the therapist understand something of the emotional life of the patient. With the medically ill, this includes an appreciation of the meaning of the illness and of its intrapsychic, interpersonal, and environmental consequences. The traditional role of the medical practitioner in maintaining a consistent, reliable, empathic professional relationship with the patient is itself psychotherapeutic. The value of this relationship may be underestimated by

physicians who feel that they must respond to a patient's emotional distress by "doing something"—prescribing medication, offering advice, ordering further laboratory tests, etc. In fact, a supportive relationship with a physician may lessen the need for analgesics or psychotropic drugs and reduce the problem of noncompliance with treatment regimens.

Although the feeling patients may have that they are being "understood" by the therapist can be a therapeutic feature of all psychodynamic therapy, unconscious motivations and defense mechanisms are not routinely interpreted in supportive psychotherapy. Indeed, it is important in such treatment to respect the adaptive value of coping mechanisms. The capacity to deny the seriousness of an acute myocardial infarction may be associated, at least in the short term, with improved survival, although such denial may be maladaptive in the long term if it leads to noncompliance with treatment or unrealistic planning for the future.

Supportive psychotherapy is more structured, as a rule, than insight-oriented psychotherapy and is more likely to include such interventions as education, reality testing, reassurance, and advice. However, reassurance and advice may be the most commonly misused forms of supportive intervention. Reassurance is most helpful when it is based on a true appreciation of the patient's situation, including the affective component of symptoms. Premature or unrealistic reassurance is rarely comforting to the patient and may reduce the physician's credibility in harmful ways. Advice is helpful only when it is based on a realistic appraisal of the needs of the patient, particularly with regard to illness-related issues. Advice should be given sparingly in personal matters, especially since it is apt—coming from a physician—to be given undue weight. It is usually best to help patients make their own decisions rather than try to make decisions for them.

The overall aim in supportive psychotherapy is to bolster adaptive coping mechanisms, to minimize maladaptive ones, and to decrease adverse psychologic reactions such as fear, shame, and reduced self-esteem. This treatment can often be provided most effectively by an interested primary-care practitioner who has had an ongoing relationship with the patient. Expressive (insight-oriented) psychotherapy usually requires referral to a trained psychotherapist.

INDICATIONS & CONTRAINDICATIONS FOR PSYCHOTHERAPY IN PATIENTS WITH CHRONIC MEDICAL DISORDERS

Supportive psychotherapy may be indicated for patients with any chronic medical illness who are experiencing psychologic distress but who do not need or want insight therapy or for whom insight therapy would be contraindicated. This applies to most medical patients, who want symptomatic relief from emotional suffering rather than insight into the origin of their difficulties. Supportive psychotherapy may also be most appropriate for patients who have difficulty in impulse control or who are unable to tolerate intense feelings. For most patients, supportive psychotherapy is indicated during acute exacerbations of chronic disease and situations of overwhelming stress.

Expressive (insight-oriented) psychotherapy aims to promote self-understanding and intrapsychic change. Such change meliorates the patient's present life adjustment and may also diminish future vulnerability to stress. Insight-oriented therapy is indicated in a small proportion of patients. It is suitable for medical patients with identifiable psychologic or interpersonal problems, the motivation for insight, the capacity to verbalize and to understand feelings, and the ability to form a relationship. The latter is important, because the relationship with the therapist is central to this form of treatment.

By disrupting the patient's psychologic equilibrium, medical illness permits underlying conflicts and vulnerabilities to emerge. This state of temporary upheaval provides some opportunity for growth and change but may also precipitate feelings of anxiety and despair. Indeed, symptoms and signs of depression may be found in up to half of all medical patients and major affective disorders in over 10%. In addition to depression, other psychiatric disorders that may require referral for psychologic treatment include anxiety, panic and dissociative disorders, alcohol dependence, and adjustment disorders precipitated by the stress of illness. Psychotherapy for such conditions does not preclude other treatment, including pharmacotherapy.

The psychologic impact of illness is largely determined by the personality and perceptions of the patient. Lowering of self-esteem may follow the onset of a physical illness, particularly when it is serious, disabling, or visible to others. Bodily appearance and functioning are important determinants of identity and self-esteem throughout life. Disturbances in body image commonly result in feelings of weakness or personal inadequacy. Physical illness may also aggravate conflicts related to dependency and hostility. Patients who have denied feelings of dependency, either because of the need to demonstrate strength and self-sufficiency or because of difficulty trusting others, may be deeply troubled by the realistic need to depend on others when they are ill. Psychotherapy may help

such individuals accept appropriate support and deal with their fears. The sense of helplessness associated with an illness commonly stimulates feelings of anger and frustration. Patients may feel too indebted to or too dependent on those in their environment to express such feelings. Psychotherapy may provide an atmosphere of safety in which such feelings can be expressed and understood.

Some relative contraindications to insight-oriented psychotherapy of the medically ill include (1) conditions in which the emotional arousal associated with expressive therapy may be medically hazardous, eg, recent myocardial infarction; (2) medical crises or other stresses that limit the patient's capacity to tolerate anxiety or emotional disruption, which may occur during the course of insight-oriented therapy; and (3) organic brain syndromes due to cardiovascular, neurologic, metabolic, or other disorders that are associated either with cognitive impairment, which limits the capacity for verbal expression and understanding, or with emotional lability, which may be aggravated by expressive psychotherapy. Emotional exploration with such patients may be hazardous because it may precipitate a state of disorganization and distress. The cognitive and affective functions of all medical patients should be carefully assessed before insight-oriented psychotherapy is recommended.

REFERRAL FOR PSYCHOTHERAPY

Emotional disturbances are extremely common in the medically ill. Many such disturbances do not require specific treatment and are alleviated by supportive contact with the attending physician. The need to refer a patient for psychotherapy will depend on a variety of factors, including the severity of the patient's distress, the motivation for psychologic assistance, and the capacity of the attending physician to deal with such matters. Referral for psychotherapy may be unnecessarily delayed or may occur prematurely. Premature referral without careful assessment of the patient's emotional state may result when the physician is uncomfortable with emotional issues. In such cases, speedy referral to a psychiatrist or other mental health practitioner may represent avoidance by the physician of the patient's distress. At the other extreme, physicians reluctant to acknowledge the limitations of their own therapeutic influence may hesitate to refer patients for psychologic consultation or treatment. Referrals for psychotherapy may not occur because some physicians do not recognize that psychotherapy is a specific treatment modality that involves more than "chatting" with patients. Finally, physicians who are unaware of the indications for psychotherapy may feel frustrated and confused when patients who are referred do not benefit from or are not accepted into treatment.

In some cases, the physician is unaware of a patient's psychologic disturbances. Up to 50% of psychiatric disorders in medical patients are unrecognized by nonpsychiatric physicians, in part because patients refrain from expressing feelings unless the physician indicates a readiness to listen. Some physicians underestimate the significance of emotional disturbances by assuming that it is "natural" for patients who are medically ill to be upset. Too often, when it is "understandable" that a patient should be depressed, specific treatments such as psychotherapy or pharmacotherapy are not offered. Physicians may recognize that symptoms such as depression are present without appreciating that treatment may be available. Such nonintervention may be particularly hazardous with patients who are suicidal. Most patients who commit suicide have been in contact with a physician from within a few hours to a few months before death. In many cases, the significance of symptoms of depression and suicidal ideation is not appreciated. Physicians must be alert to the presence of such symptoms and to the possibility for beneficial intervention with drugs or psychotherapy on an inpatient or outpatient basis.

THE INITIATION OF PSYCHOTHERAPY

Some medical patients seek psychotherapy because of a conscious belief or unconscious wish that it will improve their health or their chances for long-term survival. This belief has been reinforced in recent years by attention in the media to the role of psychologic factors in illness and to scientific evidence that links psychologic well-being with a favorable medical outcome. However, although such benefit may occur, unrealistic expectations of benefit from psychotherapy may also contribute to traumatic disappointment. Some patients harbor magical expectations that a therapist can help them even without their participation in the process. Many of these patients are unfamiliar with the process of psychotherapy and may need education about what is required and what may reasonably be expected from psychotherapy.

Some medical patients want help to modify behavior that is affecting their health adversely, eg, noncompliance with the treatment regimen for conditions such as coronary artery disease, diabetes mellitus, or end-stage renal disease. Such concerns are valid as a focus of treatment. However, the preoccupation with illness may also be an avoidance of important underlying issues. In particular, it is convenient for some patients to attribute all of their personal difficulties to their illness, even when these difficulties have antedated the onset of illness. At the other extreme, some patients exclude the illness from their consciousness altogether. This avoidance may be an attempt to deny the significance or even the existence of the illness. Although the adaptive value of denial, especially during the acute phase of an illness, should not be underestimated, the benefits of long-term therapy will be extremely limited unless the implications of a serious illness are taken into account.

The degree to which psychotherapy in the medically ill should be extended to include aspects not directly related to the illness will depend upon a variety of factors, including the suitability of the patient for insight-oriented therapy. However, with medically ill patients, the capacity for insight and psychologic change may be difficult to determine. Some issues that arise regarding determination of the depth and focus of treatment are demonstrated by the following case.

Illustrative Case

A married woman in her 30s with insulin-dependent diabetes for 2 years sought psychotherapy because she had been unable to control her eating, and she feared that poor metabolic control posed a risk to her health. Although highly disciplined in all other areas of her life, she felt frustrated by her inability to control her appetite. She viewed the problem of dietary noncompliance as distinct from the rest of her personality, and she wanted help only in dealing with her eating problem.

After a brief period of psychotherapy during which a therapeutic relationship was established, the eating problem was satisfactorily brought under control. However, by this time, the patient came to recognize that her difficulty in regulating her diet was related to a number of underlying concerns, ie, conflicts related to dependency, helplessness, and the fear of losing control. Even more distressing than her inability to control her eating was the fear that she would become unable to control her feelings. Her initial attempt to restrict the focus of the treatment process was a means of ensuring that she would not be overwhelmed by unmanageable feelings. When this fear was addressed, she felt able to participate more fully in the therapeutic process. She recalled how the onset of her diabetes 2 years earlier was a blow to her sense of self-sufficiency. She remembered lying in bed for 2 weeks, feeling depressed and experimenting with homeopathic remedies. Subsequently, she began to cope with her illness by denying to herself and to others that her diabetes was of any significance. She worried that others would regard her as incompetent if they knew about the diagnosis. As she came to trust the therapist, she experienced a sense of sadness about her illness and was able to mourn many of the losses she had suffered.

In this case, the patient's therapy began with a limited focus on a specific dietary symptom and later included a variety of issues related and unrelated to her diabetes. Restricting the treatment to the patient's initial request would have unnecessarily limited its potential benefit.

THE THERAPEUTIC PROCESS

Psychotherapy with chronically ill medical patients basically resembles therapy with patients who are physically well. Some adjustments are necessary, however, when there is a significant exacerbation of the medical disorder, in which case the need for hospitalization may disrupt the course of psychotherapy. Furthermore, when a chronically ill patient experiences marked physical deterioration, it may be necessary to shift from insight-oriented therapy to therapy that is more supportive in nature.

Psychotherapy with medically ill patients requires flexibility on the part of the therapist. When a patient is hospitalized, treatment may continue in less than optimal circumstances. It is sometimes necessary to conduct psychotherapy at the bedside, even when there are other patients in the room. Although the patient's right to privacy must be respected, involvement of the therapist through all phases of an illness may be crucial in maintaining the therapeutic alliance. For many patients, the medical illness has already created feelings of isolation from the "normal" or "healthy" world. A therapist who discontinues treatment when the medical condition worsens may contribute to these feelings of isolation.

Emerging Feelings

Although physical illness may interfere with the course of psychotherapy, it may also be a facilitating factor. Specifically, a physical illness may heighten the patient's awareness of the passage of time and impart a sense of urgency to deal with areas of conflict. This pressure to resolve problems may diminish certain resistances that would otherwise be present. This phenomenon has been described in elderly patients and in patients of all ages in time-limited psychotherapy.

Medical patients frequently enter psychotherapy in a state of distress because their usual coping mechanisms have been eroded by the physical and psychologic effects of illness. For example, those who have tended to deny feelings of dependency are now faced with an increased need to rely on others. Some who have attempted to gain emotional independence from their parents are thrust back into a dependent relationship. Others who have avoided intense emotions experience overwhelming feelings of helplessness, anxiety, and fear. In all of these situations, illness has disrupted the psychic equilibrium and rendered the usual adaptive mechanisms ineffective. Some of the new tasks and conflicts precipitated by a physical illness are illustrated in the following case example:

Illustrative case. A 26-year-old student was referred for psychotherapy 3 months after the onset of a lymphoma. He was receiving chemotherapy and had been told that he had a good prognosis. He was later shocked when he read in a medical text that his condition might be fatal. From that time, he felt unable to plan or even think about his future until he could be more certain of the outcome of the disease. Though reserved by nature, he now found himself weeping frequently, and he was full of anxiety. When he expressed the need to discuss his feelings, his oncologist referred him for psychotherapy.

The patient described an early family life marked by tension and conflict. His father seemed volatile, and any discussion of feelings within the family resulted in eruptions of hostility. The patient responded to this dilemma by distancing himself emotionally from his family and by suppressing many of his feelings. However, his illness stimulated intense feelings that could no longer be suppressed. His emotional turmoil was further heightened when he was forced to live with his family because he could no longer fully care for himself.

The patient was fearful about his future and ashamed of his illness, which was now visible to others. His chemotherapy resulted in hair loss and a peripheral neuropathy that produced an obvious gait disturbance. Although initially awkward about communicating his feelings of fear and shame, he soon felt relieved at being able to do so. He began to perceive the therapist as an ally who could help him cope with some of the stresses of his condition and his personal life. He became able to reflect on the sources of conflict in the family and to understand some of the underlying factors. His father had been unemployed repeatedly and had become an alcoholic. He now recognized that his father was in considerable distress, and he helped to arrange a referral for his father to receive psychologic and vocational help.

The onset of serious illness in this patient disrupted the equilibrium that had been established. He was forced to confront a number of unresolved problems and to find more effective ways of coping with them. In particular, therapy helped him develop new skills in communicating his feelings and dealing with conflict. In spite of his physical weakness, it was now possible for him to modify in a beneficial way some of the destructive interactions in the family.

In the case described, the patient was able to express many feelings related to his illness and other areas of his life. However, a serious illness does not always facilitate the emergence of feelings or the resolution of emotional difficulties. In fact, the most common response to serious illness may be emotional constriction. Many patients with major medical disorders have limited access to their emotional lives and focus on the immediate concerns of their illness rather than on their feelings. Patients who fear that intolerable feelings will be aroused may be reluctant to enter psychotherapy. Since patients are better able to begin psychotherapy and to tolerate intense feelings when they are physically well, it is usually preferable to engage them in therapy early in the course of the illness, before they are too ill or discouraged.

Self-Esteem & Body Image

Bodily appearance and physical functioning are important components of identity and the sense of self throughout life. Self-esteem is inevitably affected by a serious illness, particularly in those who have been vulnerable in this area or who have relied upon vigorous good health or beauty to feel worthwhile. Indeed, when many medical patients begin psychotherapy, they are in the midst of a mourning process in which they are grieving for their lost "healthy self" and for other anticipated losses. This mourning phase early in the treatment of medically ill patients contrasts with similar feelings experienced by medically healthy patients late in psychotherapy, especially during the termination phase.

Some issues that may arise related to alterations in bodily appearance and self-esteem are depicted in the following case:

Illustrative case. A woman in her 30s with a functioning renal transplant was referred for psychotherapy with the complaint that her body was "falling apart." Although the renal transplant performed 3 years earlier was a success, the maintenance steroid medication altered her physical appearance. She had always placed great importance on her appearance and was deeply distressed by the rounding of her face and the "potbelly" the steroids had produced.

The patient reported a number of traumatic separations from her parents during childhood. She recalled consciously distancing herself emotionally from others to prevent further experiences of loss and disappointment. As an adult, she was pleasantly surprised that men found her attractive, but her relationships with men always ended before she allowed herself to feel emotionally attached. She now feared that the alterations in physical appearance would mean that men would no longer be interested in her and that she would be alone.

The first phase of psychotherapy was characterized by prolonged mourning. She recalled early experiences of separation from her parents and the associated feelings of abandonment. She now recognized with regret that her avoidance of close attachments had left her without a life partner. Although men were still interested in her, she continued to avoid them because of feelings of self-depreciation. As psychotherapy progressed, she experienced a reawakening of many feelings that had been stifled. For a time, she reported sexualized feelings in the transference and wondered about the therapist's personal life. Eventually, she became more aware of the possibilities in her personal life and began to involve herself in relationships. Although her fear of close attachments persisted, she no longer withdrew impulsively from these situations.

Idealizing the Doctor

In the case described above, the therapist was at times perceived as an idealized figure. Such idealization is common during the course of psychotherapy and may facilitate the treatment process. Idealization of the primary physician is also common among medical patients and is frequently therapeutic. This tendency to idealize authority figures is especially prominent in persons who have had difficulty maintaining self-esteem and have relied on "powerful others" in order to feel secure.

In general, physicians and psychotherapists need to accept being idealized by their patients. Optimally, idealization of the therapist during psychotherapy is tempered gradually by the minor disappointments that inevitably occur. This process of disillusionment is tolerable when it is gradual and when it is associated with a more realistic perception of the therapist and a greater ability to maintain self-esteem without such external support. Premature or excessive disappointment in the therapist or primary physician may precipitate a sense of despair. Such extreme disappointment is more likely to occur when patients with progressive medical disorders have had initial unrealistic expectations of their physicians. These patients may be filled with rage and feelings of hopelessness when their expectations prove unrealistic. Nonpsychiatric physicians and therapists should be cautious about accepting without reservation the omnipotent role conferred upon them by some patients with progressive medical conditions. The idealizations of such patients may need to be interpreted and clarified early in treatment in order to minimize traumatic disillusionment.

Intense feelings of anger and helplessness are common among medical patients and may be projected onto the therapist or primary physician, who is then perceived as hostile or ineffectual. During psychotherapy, such projections must be recognized and interpreted as part of the transference. Therapists may overlook the transference aspect of these feelings because of their own sense of frustration and impotence in the face of a progressive medical disorder. Transference feelings may also be difficult to identify when they are diluted by the patient's involvement with several people on the medical staff who are or are perceived to be of life-sustaining importance.

Some issues that may arise with regard to idealization and disillusionment in medical patients are demonstrated in the following case:

Illustrative case. A 48-year-old married woman with metastatic cancer was referred for psychotherapy because of overwhelming feelings of anxiety and depression. A year before, when the diagnosis was made, she pressed the surgeon for reassurance about her prognosis. When told that she was "one of the lucky ones," she felt optimistic, even euphoric. However, when her disease recurred 6 months later, she felt enraged that she had been "falsely encouraged." She now worried that she might "slip into a depression" and "never get better."

Before her illness, the patient's self-esteem was vulnerable, and she tended to rely on idealized others to feel secure. She had been a fearful child and would "crawl into a shell" rather than face problems. She had relied on her husband for support in later years and now feared that she might become too great a burden for him.

The patient had experienced disappointment in her physicians, whose curative powers she had idealized. There was a similar initial idealization of the psychotherapist, whom she hoped could rescue her from her plight. She pressed him as she had pressed her other physicians for encouragement about her prognosis. When further medical complications supervened, she felt as disillusioned with the therapist as she had with her other physicians, and she terminated psychotherapy.

It may not have been possible to avoid the outcome in the above case. However, earlier clarification of the patient's unrealistic expectations might have diminished her disappointment and her premature termination of psychotherapy.

Collaboration With the Primary-Care Physician

Psychotherapy with medically ill patients places special emotional and practical demands on the therapist, such as the need to collaborate with the physicians who retain responsibility for medical management of the patient. The therapist must remain aware of the patient's current medical status without assuming responsibility for it. Therapists must acknowledge resentment and other feelings toward the primary-care physician but should be careful not to collude with such feelings.

Some patients attempt to form special relationships that split the medical staff and create tension among them. This can be prevented only by frequent communication among all members of the medical staff. Because of the need for such communication, it is generally unwise for the therapist to promise absolute confidentiality. Therapists should avoid unnecessary disclosure of personal information about the patient to medical staff but should be free to communicate about matters that affect the medical course. Some issues regarding collaboration with the medical staff are depicted in the following case:

Illustrative case. A 21-year-old single diabetic woman was referred for psychiatric consultation during a hospital admission at a time when her vision was deteriorating rapidly. She agreed to the consultation, although she did not feel in need of assistance. In fact, as her vision failed, she resented the increased protectiveness of her family and others and decided to move out of the family home. From the time of onset of her diabetes at age 6 years, she believed that her parents experienced it as a burden. She felt unable to rely on them for support and withdrew from emotional contact with them.

The patient began weekly psychotherapy cautiously. Whenever she felt neglected or abused by any of her physicians, she experienced resentment that was generalized to include everyone she was involved with, including the therapist. Specifically, she objected to the medical staff's communicating with one another about her and knowing that she was seeing a psychiatrist. She was angry that communication between the therapist and the rest of the medical team about her physical status had been established as a condition of her psychotherapy.

Although the patient's concerns about confidentiality were acknowledged to be valid, the importance of the therapist's ongoing contact with the medical staff became increasingly apparent. It was sometimes difficult to determine to what extent her emotional state was affected by alterations in her metabolic control. At other times, when the factitious administration of insulin or sedative drugs was suspected, discussion and collaboration with the medical staff were essential.

The therapeutic relationship provided the patient with a limited and restricted means by which she could begin to develop some degree of trust in others. The intimacy and dependency that resulted were frightening for her, and she responded initially with detachment and attempts to split the medical staff. Only later did deep-seated fears of her unacceptability and her potential destructiveness to others emerge. Although she was sometimes able to accept interpretations about her anger, it was often necessary to let her simply ventilate her feelings.

Countertransference

Medically ill patients may provoke a variety of emotional reactions in the therapist. Some patients elicit overconcern; others arouse feelings of hostility and rejection. The therapist must identify such feelings in order to understand the patient better and to maintain an attitude of therapeutic neutrality. Neutrality in this context does not mean a lack of concern for the patient but refers to an attitude which is consistent and empathic with the patient's feelings without undue distortion by the personal reactions of the therapist. Interventions that arise from the needs of the therapist, even when well intended, may not be useful to the patient. An overly supportive attitude may develop when the therapist identifies with the patient's helplessness or attempts to counteract his or her own underlying feelings of frustration and impotence. Such support may deprive some patients of the opportunity to develop greater autonomy and self-sufficiency. Hostile feelings toward the patient may also arise for various reasons. In some cases, such negative feelings on the part of the therapist serve to maintain an emotional distance from a patient whose distress threatens to be overwhelming. In other cases, patients wish to provoke hostility in the therapist. Patients with intense rage may achieve a greater sense of control over their feelings when they can provoke similar feelings in the therapist. Both primary physicians and therapists who care for the medically ill must be able to tolerate intense feelings in themselves and in their patients in order to maintain a helpful attitude.

OUTCOME & COST-BENEFIT ANALYSIS OF PSYCHOTHERAPY WITH THE MEDICALLY ILL

Psychotherapy is often underestimated by medical practitioners as a means of improving the quality of life of medical patients. Although the benefit of psychotherapy has often been difficult to demonstrate, some of the clearest evidence has been obtained from studies of the medically ill. This benefit has been measured not only by the improvement in psychologic well-being but also by the reduced utilization of medical resources. Medical patients who participate in psychotherapy have been shown to require fewer medical investigations and treatments, either because of the effect of psychotherapy on overall health status or because of the more appropriate allocation of medical and psychologic resources.

SUMMARY

Medical illness is a stressful event in the life of any patient, although the specific meaning of the illness and the psychologic response to it may depend on a variety of factors. Supportive psychotherapy as an adjunct to treatment may be an important function of the primary-care practitioner. A small proportion of medical patients may benefit from expressive (insight-oriented) psychotherapy. This should be conducted by a specially trained psychotherapist with suitable patients. Insight-oriented therapy may be contraindicated with some medical patients because of physical debilitation or cognitive impairment.

It is common (and often therapeutic) for patients to idealize physicians and others in the helping professions. However, the stress of illness may predispose the patient to an early and fragile idealization of the therapist or primary physician. It may be necessary to interpret this idealization early in treatment to avoid traumatic disappointment and disillusionment. Mourning may also be an important feature early in therapy. Patients must grieve for anticipated losses as well as for those that have already occurred.

Medical complications or hospitalizations may disrupt the therapeutic process. The ability of the patient to tolerate affective arousal may fluctuate widely, and therapeutic interventions at any point must take this into account. In some cases, the painful reality of the physical condition interferes with the ability of the patient to form a therapeutic relationship. The transference relationship may be diluted by the need to rely on various medical staff who may have life-sustaining significance for the patient. Furthermore, the therapeutic relationship may be affected by other factors such as the breach of confidentiality that occurs when therapists work in collaboration with the medical treatment team.

Although psychotherapy may in some cases be the most important feature of management of a medically ill patient, psychotherapists more often play a secondary role. The treatment of medical complications must often assume the most urgent priority. Physical illness may also impose realistic limitations that cannot be overcome by psychologic treatment. In these and other respects, medical illness may present an ongoing challenge to the sense of competence of the therapist as well as to that of the patient.

REFERENCES

Cassel EJ: The nature of suffering and the goals of medicine. *N Engl J Med* 1982;**306:**639.

Fauman MA: Psychiatric components of medical and surgical practice. 2. Referral and treatment of psychiatric disorders. *Am J Psychiatry* 1983;**140:**760.

Forester B, Kornfeld DS, Fleiss JL: Psychotherapy during radiotherapy: Effects on emotional and physical distress. *Am J Psychiatry* 1985;**142:**22.

Freyberger H: Psychotherapeutic possibilities in medically extreme situations. *Psychother Psychosom* 1975;**26:**337.

Karasu TB: Psychotherapy with physically ill patients. Pages 258–276 in: *Specialized Techniques in Individual Psychotherapy.* Karasu TB, Bellak L (editors). Brunner/Mazel, 1980.

Köhle K, Simons C: Integrations of the psychosomatic approach into the management of the severely and fatally ill. *Psychother Psychosom* 1975;**26:**357.

Moos RH, Schaefer JA: The crisis of physical illness: An overview and conceptual approach. In: *Coping With Physical Illness.* Vol 2: *New Perspectives.* Moos RH (editor). Plenum Press, 1984.

Murphy GE: The physician's responsibility for suicide. 2. Errors of omission. *Ann Intern Med* 1975;**82:**305.

Psychotherapy Research: Methodological and Efficacy Issues. American Psychiatric Association Commission on Psychotherapies, 1982.

Rodin GM: Expressive psychotherapy in the medically ill: Resistance and possibilities. *Int J Psychiatry Med* 1984;**14:**99.

Rodin GM, Voshart K: Depression in the medically ill: An overview. *Am J Psychiatry* 1986;**143:**696.

Sifneos P: *Short-Term Psychotherapy and Emotional Crisis.* Harvard Univ Press, 1972.

Sourkes BM: *The Deepening Shade: Psychological Aspects of Life-Threatening Illness.* Univ of Pittsburgh Press, 1982.

Stein EH, Murdaugh J, MacLeod JA: Brief psychotherapy of psychiatric reactions to physical illness. *Am J Psychiatry* 1969;**125:**1040.

51

Behavioral Medicine Techniques

Daniel S. Weiss, PhD, & James H. Billings, PhD, MPH

Behavioral medicine is a broad field that deals with the application of behavioral science knowledge and techniques to problems related to *physical* health. Although the field was only defined formally in the 1970s, it includes topics once in the domain of psychosomatic medicine (see Chapter 4). Many of the techniques used in behavioral medicine are derived from theories of behaviorism (see Chapter 3) and are similar to those used in behavior therapy of patients with mental disorders (see Chapter 46). Basic concepts include learning through classical conditioning, through operant conditioning, and through modeling. What makes behavioral medicine different is its emphasis on modifying overt behavior contributing to physical (rather than mental) illness and its application of specialized techniques to manage both the somatic illness and the adverse effects of somatic treatments (eg, pain associated with dental procedures; nausea associated with cancer chemotherapy).

The principal techniques used in behavioral medicine are relaxation, imagery, hypnosis, and biofeedback. Each will be described and discussed briefly in this chapter. Relaxation is both a therapeutic technique in its own right and an important element of the others named. For example, electromyographic feedback may be used to train patients in the technique of relaxation of the facial muscles as treatment for headache. Whether this is called relaxation therapy or biofeedback therapy is a semantic distinction of no clinical significance except to point out the importance of relaxation as a therapeutic tool.

The basis of behavioral medicine is observing and changing overt behavior. The passive patient role is incompatible with the active collaboration needed to manage and modify aspects of behavior that exacerbate or sustain the problems of illness. Practitioners using behavioral medicine techniques frequently think of themselves as teachers and educators rather than therapists. In behavioral medicine, the individual is perceived as an active, attentive organism with the capacity to direct attention toward or away from phenomena. This **directed attention** appears to be the therapeutic heart of many of the techniques.

Behavioral medicine techniques may be used either as adjunctive treatments in the context of other ongoing treatment regimens, eg, relaxation training while undergoing chemotherapy, or as the primary method of treatment, eg, biofeedback for migraine headache or hypnosis for Raynaud's disease. The decision about

what is the treatment of choice cannot be made without careful evaluation of the problem and of the person. Once a careful history and problem assessment are developed, an appropriate treatment regimen containing elements of somatic, psychologic, and behavioral treatments may be selected.

In this chapter, we will discuss the use of relaxation, imagery, hypnosis, and biofeedback in the management of patients who have some dysfunctional condition. There is increasing awareness in several specialty areas (eg, cardiology) that the behavioral medicine techniques used in secondary and tertiary prevention (see Chapter 13) may have an important role in primary prevention.

Treatment Process

Boudewyns and Keefe (1982) note that despite the diversity of specific techniques, the variety of settings, and the range of expertise required to practice certain techniques, the following processes are common to all behavioral medicine: (1) problem identification, (2) measurement and analysis of the dimensions of the behavioral problem (eg, frequency, intensity) and of remaining functions, (3) matching treatment to client, (4) assessment of ongoing therapy, and (5) final evaluation of treatment outcome.

Identification and clear specification of an underlying behavioral problem are sometimes quite difficult but when finally accomplished are useful in choosing among the available behavioral techniques. Functional analysis and measurement techniques such as diaries and self-observation often will be needed to help identify the problem. A search should be made for a relationship between external events (eg, a deadline for a marketing report) and physical responses (eg, a disabling migraine headache). In some cases, the precipitant or underlying cause of the problem is clear (eg, nausea following chemotherapy); in others (eg, intermittent attacks of asthma), a detailed record of events and responses may be needed to identify a causal relationship. In any case, the treatment chosen must be tailored to the particular patient's difficulties as well as to the kind of person who is having the difficulties (see Chapter 21).

RELAXATION

Probably the most basic technique in behavioral medicine is the systematic induction of a state of relaxation. Psychologically, relaxation reduces arousal and tension, the almost universal concomitants of stress. Physiologically, the "relaxation response" (Benson, 1975) consists of slowing of the respiratory rate, reduction of blood pressure, and peripheral vasodilation.

Relaxation therapy has been used with documented success in the management of essential hypertension and headache. It is probably helpful in a wide variety of clinical conditions associated with stress, whether from threatening external events or pressures or from uncomfortable psychologic or physiologic states (see Chapter 5). In addition, relaxation is used to enhance behavior therapy (see Chapter 46) and other behavioral medicine techniques.

Self-induced relaxation is similar to the spiritual and religious meditation practiced for centuries in Eastern societies, and its effective use in modern medicine requires some element of the same kind of training. Relaxation training, like any other complex learned behavior, calls for daily practice over a period of time. The beneficial effects of relaxation exercises are realized only through consistent and unswerving use of the techniques. While it is true that relaxation responses may be induced by a skilled subject in "crisis" situations, its main usefulness is as a habitual means of maintaining a state of equanimity.

Whole-body relaxation may be used with or without relaxation to relieve muscle tension in specific parts of the body. Which techniques to choose depends upon the presenting problem, identified by the process described above. Patients for whom relaxation is mysterious, frightening, or bewildering require exercises that gradually alternate between tension and relaxation. For those who have some familiarity with the technique, only the induction of relaxation may be needed.

Audiotaped materials explaining the relaxation exercises and techniques are valuable teaching devices. Tapes are commercially available or may be prepared by the patient or therapist. A tape should include the 4 elements that Benson (1975) identifies as necessary to elicit the relaxation response: (1) a mental cue that is repeated several times silently during each exhalation; (2) a passive disregard for trying, succeeding, or being distracted, so that attention can be centered on the repetition of the cue; (3) a comfortable position that minimizes muscular activity and tension; and (4) a quiet environment with minimal distractions.

Fatigue and fear interfere with the relaxation response. The response is not the same as sleep, and relaxation is best practiced out of bed. Inability to relax because of fear of loss of control is unusual but may occur in patients with chronic psychiatric disorders.

Relaxation can be facilitated by the creative use of words that connote passivity rather than activity and have positive rather than negative association; by proper timing—allowing the individual to move at his or her own pace; and by establishment of specific times and places for practice. Setting aside a special time for relaxation exercises and nothing else may be helpful in its own right.

The basic components of the relaxation exercise are demonstrated in the office for use at home. The patient is instructed to assume a comfortable position (either seated or reclining) in a place that will be free from distraction and to adjust clothing to be comfortable. Then the patient is taught to repeat the following experience:

Close your eyes. . . . Rest your arms comfortably. . . . Let your back and shoulders rest comfortably so you can breathe easily and deeply. . . . Choose a word that is simple and calming to concentrate on as you breathe. . . . If none comes to mind, use the word "one." . . . Just allow yourself to attend to that word as you breathe. . . . Feel your neck and scalp relax. Let any tension in those muscles slip and drift away. . . . Now . . . continue to feel the relaxation flowing over you . . . down your neck . . . around your eyebrows and eyelids. . . . Allow your jaw muscles to relax. . . . Let your whole face become comfortably heavy and relaxed. . . . Now . . . slowly breathe in through your nose . . . and allow the air to fill the spaces in your lungs. . . . Feel your chest expand with air. Now . . . hold your breath. . . . Now . . . without pressure or force . . . slowly exhale through your mouth. Feel the air as it passes over your lips. Repeat the breathing cycle . . . inhale . . . hold . . . exhale and relax. Feel your body relaxing. . . . Feel the tension flow out and the calmness and warmth flow in. . . . Feel your limbs become warm and pleasantly heavy and calm. . . . Let go of the muscles in your back. . . . Feel yourself becoming deeply calm and relaxed. . . . As you repeat your breathing . . . repeat your word. . . . Inhale. . . . Exhale. . . . As you continue, feel yourself floating . . . feel the warmth and heaviness filling your body. . . . Your whole body is relaxed . . . your waist . . . your knees . . . your ankles . . . your feet. . . . Inhale . . . and exhale. . . . Now you are peacefully relaxed . . . warm and comfortably heavy. Each time you breathe, your body relaxes more deeply. . . . And yet, you are not tired. . . . You are centered . . . awake . . . aware . . . and deeply relaxed and comfortable. All your muscles are smooth and comfortable. . . . You are warm and heavy. As you breathe . . . and hold . . . and exhale . . . you become refreshed. You are relaxed . . . comfortable . . . peaceful . . . quiet. Continue to . . . inhale . . . and exhale. . . . As you relax, you feel the peace . . . the quiet. . . . You are at peace . . . refreshed. . . . Now, when you are ready . . . you may allow yourself to slowly . . . slowly . . . become aware of yourself in the room. . . . Slowly, when you are ready . . . open your eyes . . . feel yourself back in your chair. Continue to feel relaxed . . . take your warmth and comfort with you. . . . Feel relaxed . . . refreshed . . . and calm.

By reading the foregoing passage slowly and with close attention, the reader should be able to experience the beginnings of the relaxation response, which is both restful and refreshing at the same time.

IMAGERY

Techniques involving the use of imagery are related to relaxation techniques, and the 2 are frequently used in conjunction. Visual imagery is most frequently used, but auditory, kinesthetic, olfactory, and gustatory imagery may be used also. Most of what is said here about visual imagery and visualization techniques applies to all.

The ability of some people to alter the depth, vividness, and intensity of mental imagery is well documented, and there is anecdotal evidence for a relationship between visualization techniques and creative activity, peak performance, and repair and restoration of physical and mental equilibrium. Like relaxation techniques, visualization techniques take practice. Samuels and Samuels (1975) present an interesting and optimistic account of the history and uses of visualization techniques with and without the use of mind-altering drugs.

Visualization and other imagery techniques are being used today as part of integrated regimens for management of conditions such as nausea secondary to chemotherapy, preoperative anxiety, and asthma. Frequently used to deepen relaxation, visualization may be used in the induction of the relaxation response. Imagery and visualization techniques are used in psychotherapy; patients may "see pictures in their minds" and describe them more easily than they can talk abstractly about relationships or conflicts. The Lamaze program for childbirth uses visual imagery to achieve relaxation and reduction of pain.

A very controversial use of imagery is in conjunction with other therapies to promote healing of damaged tissues. The best-known example is the visualization technique used by Simonton and coworkers (1978) in treating cancer patients. Although the response was at first quite skeptical, the medical profession is now beginning to admit that some kinds of tumors may respond to physiologic changes induced by imagery techniques. Such changes may induce a remission or make the tumor more responsive to other treatment. The claims of improvement and remission that have accompanied the use of visualization may in fact result not *directly* from visualization but rather from physiologic or biochemical changes potentiated by changes induced with visualization techniques.

Some of the techniques used in visualization and other kinds of imagery overlap those used in relaxation and hypnosis. Relaxation is a prerequisite for visualization. Then, depending upon whether the imagery is to be guided by a clinician or taught to the patient for future use, the major activity is the intense focus of attention upon the image (eg, a warm beach—to promote relaxation—or a strong antibody—to promote healing). As with relaxation, the major obstacle is distraction. The trick is to let distractions enter and flow past rather than trying to resist and overcome them.

A brief example of how visualization proceeds is given by Jaffe and Bressler (1980:254):

First, using verbal language, order yourself to "manufacture and secrete saliva." By thinking about this command, see how much you can generate. Most people produce a little, but not much, for the parts of the body that produce saliva do not respond well to verbal commands.

Mental imagery represents a different approach to physiological change. Imagine that you have in your hand a big, yellow, juicy lemon. Visualize it in your mind's eye until you smell its fresh tartness. Then imagine taking a knife and slicing into the lemon. Carefully cut out a thick, juicy section. Now, take a deep bite of your imaginary lemon and begin to sense that tart, sour lemon juice splashing in your mouth, saturating every taste bud of your tongue so fully that your lips and cheeks curl. Swirl it in your mouth for another 15 to 20 seconds, bathing every corner of your mouth with its acrid taste.

As with other behavioral medicine techniques, the use of visualization should be integrated into an overall treatment program that is acceptable to the patient. Although these techniques may only be of use as adjuncts to other treatments, they may be of use with some patients with medical or psychiatric disorders.

HYPNOSIS

In spite of some lingering antipathy toward the subject, there is no doubt that hypnotic phenomena, induction of trance states, and suggestion can play important roles in the treatment of some types of anxiety and phobias and may even serve the purpose of anesthesia in some individuals. The discussion below of the mechanism of hypnosis is still open to debate.

As is true also of many of the other behavioral medicine techniques available to the clinician, hypnosis can be used in the management of a variety of complaints. The technique is especially valuable for use in children, who are often remarkably responsive to suggestion in situations associated with actual or anticipated pain. Children who acquire a facility for entering the trance state can call upon the technique later in life in situations where hypnoanesthesia might be useful (see Chapter 57).

Kroger (1977), a pioneer in the use of hypnosis in medicine and dentistry, notes that it has been useful in a variety of contexts. Anesthesia is a good example; eg, a permanent molar may be extracted painlessly with only hypnoanesthesia. Among other conditions that may benefit from hypnotic suggestion are headaches, anxiety, phobias, pain, labor, difficulties in lactation, allergic disorders, asthma, and Raynaud's disease. Properly motivated patients with problems of habitual overeating or smoking have been helped by "hypnotic suggestion"—ie, they are taught in the trance state to recite a prepared stricture against the unhygienic habit and then given the brief text to memorize and recite several times a day after self-induced hypnosis for as long as necessary. Not all patients with these or other problems will be helped by hypnosis, but if standard treatment with problems such as these is unsuccessful, referral for hypnosis may be indicated.

Clarke and Jackson (1983) discuss the relationship among the psychologic processes of thinking, perceiving, attending to, and having feelings about events in the internal and external environment. It is amply demonstrated that almost all so-called involuntary processes are modifiable if attention can be directed toward them. The authors present an integrated view of the relationship between therapeutic techniques of various kinds (eg, support, rapport, functional analysis, interpersonal interpretation) that will be used in conjunction with hypnosis. They describe what occurs during hypnotic disengagement as follows:

(1) Anxiety and arousal are reduced.

(2) Attention becomes fixed and focused rather than labile and mobile.

(3) Behavioral inertia occurs (quiescence rather than a readiness to act).

(4) Thinking becomes concrete and uncritical.

(5) The perception of control becomes directed toward the therapist rather than the self.

For these conditions to occur, formal induction by a therapist is not always necessary. Self-induction is possible, as is induction during periods of intense mental image formation, reverie, or meditation and relaxation. This again should emphasize the similarity among many of the techniques used in behavioral medicine, in which the individual is perceived as an active, attentive organism with the capacity to direct attention toward or away from phenomena.

Individuals vary in their responsiveness to different behavioral medicine techniques. When hypnosis is used to help modify anxieties, fears, habits, or symptoms, some techniques work better than others. The general description that follows applies to most cases.

Hypnosis should not be offered casually. The patient should give a suitably detailed medical and psychologic history, and the therapist should initiate a preinduction discussion during which any anxieties and misconceptions about hypnosis can be verbalized and dealt with. The aim of this phase of the hypnosis experience should be to establish rapport and raise positive expectations in the patient's mind. The therapist may discuss such things as relaxation, attention, the need to trust the hypnotist, the importance of motivation for help, and hypnosis as an experience in itself. The therapist should listen for cues suggesting that certain induction techniques (arm levitation, arm lowering, coin technique) might be resisted. It is better to choose a technique that will be comfortable for the subject than one the therapist happens to prefer.

Once a choice of technique has been made, the therapist gently and progressively suggests that the phenomenon is occurring (eg, the arm is growing heavier, the subject is getting weary holding it up, etc). Instructions for induction are best communicated directly and experientially and are not presented here. However, if induction does not occur promptly, attention may be directed to the *opposite* of the suggestion

in a subtle way. This change of direction may succeed because it now accords with the patient's actual experience (eg, the arm feels lighter, not heavier).

Once induction occurs, several techniques are available for deepening the trance state. All depend upon integration of the suggestion with what is already happening: "You will feel your arms growing more relaxed with each breath you take." These deepening procedures allow the patient to become more fully attuned to internal rather than external stimuli and thus strengthen suggestions given during hypnosis.

Termination of the hypnotic session should be done in such a way that the subject gradually reorients awareness outward, notices external stimuli, and reengages with reality. The therapist's cue for signifying that the trance has ended should be chosen to suit the patient. The cues should be clear—many clinicians use a countdown procedure. Even though the therapist may have finished the hypnotic instructions and suggestions and given an instruction to reengage, it may take 10 minutes to fully reengage. During this time, the therapist may usefully review the experience with the patient, noting what was satisfactory and unsatisfactory.

BIOFEEDBACK

The most dramatic example of behavioral medicine techniques in the treatment of somatic complaints is biofeedback. Fuller (1977) has described biofeedback as

> . . . the use of instrumentation to mirror psychophysiological processes of which the individual is not normally aware and which may be brought under voluntary control. This means giving a person immediate information about his or her own biological conditions such as: muscle tension, skin surface temperature, brain wave activity, galvanic skin response, blood pressure, and heart rate. This feedback enables the individual to become an active participant in the process of health maintenance.

The process of electronic feedback includes instrumentation that will filter and amplify a psychophysiologic signal that is then analyzed and transformed into another kind of signal capable of being "fed back" to the patient in a perceptible and comprehensible way. For example, the patient hears a tone get louder or sees a light flash more rapidly as muscle tension or heart rate increases. This process gives the patient access to changes and variations in the ongoing function of the system being monitored, since it is now possible to direct the patient's attention to the sensations that accompany the changes. This ability to associate perceived bodily experiences with processes that are ordinarily outside of conscious awareness or experience is the presumed mechanism that initiates voluntary control of the processes.

Biofeedback as a technique for treatment began in 1968, when several lines of pure research led to the discovery that in monkeys and other animals as well as humans, physiologic functions thought to be out of voluntary control were modifiable by appropriate monitoring techniques made perceptible to the subject. The important contributors to this work were Kamiya (1962) with research on the electroencephalographic alpha wave; Miller (1969) with work on conditioning heart rate, blood pressure, and vasodilation and vasoconstriction with curarized rats; Kimmel (1967) with work on the galvanic skin response; and Shearn (1962) and Frazier (1966) with independent work on changes in heart rate to avoid mild electric shock.

What this pure laboratory research spawned was a whole technology and set of useful, comprehensible, and therapeutic procedures and regimens for the treatment of disorders of purely somatic origin as well as for disorders with both somatic and psychologic components. Among the conditions that are now currently treated with biofeedback procedures are migraine headaches, insomnia, Raynaud's disease, enuresis, encopresis, chronic pain, hypertension, muscular tension, irritable bowel syndrome, peptic ulcer, esophageal spasm, fecal incontinence, and many neurologic diseases and their sequelae.

Initiation of a biofeedback treatment regimen requires the same careful consideration of diagnosis, etiology, alternative treatments, role of the complaint in the patient's life, and the impact of treatment on the patient as is required for any other treatment decision. The patient should be given a clear explanation of the procedure and its rationale. Gaarder and Montgomery (1981) classify candidates for biofeedback therapy according to types of disorders: stress syndromes (eg, tension headache), syndromes of temporary trauma with loss of learning (eg, fecal incontinence following successful rectal surgery), neurologic damage with loss or failure of learning (eg, stroke), functional derangement syndromes (eg, intermittent muscle spasms), homeostatic imbalance and dysregulation syndromes (eg, essential hypertension), and broken control loop syndromes (eg, impaired sensory input from a limb in a patient who suffered a stroke).

The basic elements of biofeedback treatment are an initial evaluation session; a baseline session that will introduce the concept of home practice; a goal-setting session that will introduce the feedback part of biofeedback; a series of treatment sessions; a phase of terminal treatment sessions; and a period of follow-up.

The type of instrumentation needed to produce biofeedback depends on the behavioral problem of the patient. The beginning practitioner must learn to identify artifacts in electrophysiologic recordings and to distinguish specific physiologic events, background levels, and spurious measurements.

The activities in a biofeedback session consist essentially of practice in control of involuntary physiologic processes. For example, to teach relaxation of the face and neck muscles to a patient with tension headache, the therapist first attaches the electronic machinery and then develops, with the patient's help, a series of instructions to attain the goals that had been set for that session. Thus, the goal might be to keep a tone below a certain threshold for 15 seconds 4 distinct times. At the conclusion of each session, specific homework is given, with the results to be reviewed the following session.

SUMMARY

Behavioral medicine has been an outgrowth of a variety of applied and basic science efforts. The emphasis is on functional analysis of the behavioral aspects of somatic and psychologic difficulties. Whether the behavior is initially accessible to modification and control or requires electronic (eg, biofeedback) or interactive (eg, hypnosis) amplification, the goal is to enable the patient to control bodily functions and psychologic responses. The approach to the patient requires a careful history, consideration of differential diagnosis, attention to contingencies and associations in the production of symptoms, emphasis on the suggestive and nonspecific factors of the helping relationship, delineation of a treatment plan, and explanations of the enhancing relationships of the available techniques (eg, relaxation with hypnosis and imagery).

With increased interest in the neurochemistry of pain, regulatory systems, and the immune system, researchers appear to be uncovering some of the mechanisms by which behavioral medicine techniques such as relaxation and visual imagery may operate. Research on the interaction of sensory and cognitive processes may provide insights into the mechanisms of biofeedback and hypnosis. The practitioner should be aware of the growing scope of behavioral medicine. The techniques are safe and may well play an increasingly importantly role in the prevention and treatment of illness and in the promotion of healthy attitudes and behavior.

REFERENCES

Benson H: *The Relaxation Response*. William Morrow, 1975.

Blanchard EB (editor): Behavioral medicine. *J Consult Clin Psychol* 1982;**50**:No. 6. [Special issue.]

Blanchard EB, Epstein LH: *A Biofeedback Primer*. Addison-Wesley, 1978.

Boudewyns PA, Keefe FJ (editors): *Behavioral Medicine in General Medical Practice*. Addison-Wesley, 1982.

Clark CC: *Enhancing Wellness*. Springer, 1981.

Clarke JC, Jackson JA: *Hypnosis and Behavior Therapy*. Springer, 1983.

Frazier TW: Avoidance conditioning of heart rate in humans. *Psychophysiology* 1966;**3**:188.

Fuller GD: *Biofeedback: Methods and Procedures in Clinical Practice*. Biofeedback Press, 1977.

Gaarder KR, Montgomery PS: *Clinical Biofeedback,* 2nd ed. Williams & Wilkins, 1981.

Horowitz MJ: *Image Formation and Psychotherapy*. Jason Aronson, 1983.

Jacobson E: *Progressive Relaxation*. Univ of Chicago Press, 1938.

Jaffe DT, Bressler DE: Guided imagery: Healing through the mind's eye. Pages 253–266 in: *Imagery*. Schorr JE et al (editors). Plenum Press. 1980.

Kamiya J: Conditioned discrimination of the EEG alpha rhythm in humans. Paper presented at the Western Psychological Association, San Francisco, 1962.

Kimmel HD: Instrumental conditioning of autonomically mediated behavior. *Psychol Bull* 1967;**67**:337.

Kroger WS: *Clinical and Experimental Hypnosis in Medicine, Dentistry, and Psychology,* 2nd ed. Lippincott, 1977.

Miller NE: Learning of visceral and glandular responses. *Science* 1969;**163**:434.

Pomerleau OF, Brady JP (editors): *Behavioral Medicine: Theory and Practice*. Williams & Wilkins, 1979.

Samuels M, Samuels N: *Seeing With the Mind's Eye*. Random House, 1975.

Schwartz GE, Weiss SM: *Proceedings of the Yale Conference on Behavioral Medicine*. US Department of Health, Education, and Welfare Publication No. (NIH) 78-1424, 1977.

Shearn DW: Operant conditioning of heart rate. *Science* 1962;**137**:530.

Simonton OC, Matthews-Simonton S, Creighton J: *Getting Well Again*. J. P. Tarcher, 1978.

Singer JL, Switzer E: *Mind-Play*. Prentice-Hall, 1980.

52

Antipsychotics & Mood Stabilizers

Leo E. Hollister, MD

The drugs considered in this chapter have both generic and specific effects. The antipsychotics are used in a wide range of mental disorders; the mood stabilizers are used in only a few disorders. **Antipsychotic** medications derive their name from their action of controlling the psychosis (or defect in reality testing) characteristic of many mental disorders, including schizophrenia, delirium, and major affective disorders. **Mood stabilizers,** such as lithium and carbamazepine, control the symptoms of mania seen in bipolar affective disorder; they are also used to prevent future episodes of mania and depression. Antipsychotic drugs can be used along with mood stabilizers in the treatment of mania, and lithium and carbamazepine have been used as adjuncts to the antipsychotic drugs in the treatment of schizophrenia. The 2 classes of drugs are discussed separately to simplify the presentation of their pharmacology.

ANTIPSYCHOTICS

The term antipsychotics is one of several applied to a group of drugs that have been used mainly for treating schizophrenia but are effective in some other psychoses as well. The preferred term in Europe is **neuroleptics,** connoting the capacity of these drugs to affect several integrating systems of the brain, including the ability to cause movement disorders. The term **major tranquilizers** has fortunately fallen into disuse, since it confounds these drugs with **minor tranquilizers** (actually sedative-hypnotics), which they resemble only superficially.

No acceptable forms of drug treatment were available for treating schizophrenia until the early 1950s, when both reserpine and chlorpromazine appeared almost simultaneously. Chlorpromazine had been developed as an antihistamine and reserpine as an antihypertensive agent. Fortuitous observations of their calming properties led to trials in psychiatric patients. Over the years, reserpine became obsolete as an antipsychotic drug, since it was not believed to be as effective as chlorpromazine and was more likely to produce mental depression. The success of chlor-

promazine led to the introduction of numerous phenothiazine derivatives. During the past 30 years, many different chemical structures have been shown to share the spectrum of pharmacologic activities associated with antipsychotic activity. No new antipsychotic drug has been introduced in the USA for over a decade.

BASIC PHARMACOLOGY OF ANTIPSYCHOTIC DRUGS

Chemical Structures

A number of chemical structures have been associated with antipsychotic properties (Fig 52–1). The drugs can be classified into 4 major groups:

A. Phenothiazine Derivatives: Three subfamilies of phenothiazines, based primarily on the side chain of the molecule, are in use. Aliphatic derivatives (eg, chlorpromazine) and some piperidine derivatives (eg, thioridazine) are the least potent. Other piperidines (eg, mesoridazine) have intermediate potency. The piperazines (eg, fluphenazine) are the most potent and, in equivalent antipsychotic doses, have reduced sedative, anticholinergic, and alpha-adrenoceptor-blocking actions. Potency refers only to the milligram doses required and has nothing to do with comparative efficacy.

B. Thioxanthene Derivatives: This group of drugs is exemplified primarily by thiothixene. In general, this group of compounds is slightly less potent than its phenothiazine homologs.

C. Butyrophenone Derivatives: This rapidly growing group, of which haloperidol is the most widely used, has a very different structure from those of the 2 preceding groups. Diphenylbutylpiperidines are closely related compounds.

D. Miscellaneous Structures: These include benzoquinolizines (tetrabenazine), dihydroindolone derivatives (molindone), phenylpiperazine derivatives (oxypertine), some tricyclic structures with a 6–7–6 ring structure (loxapine and clozapine), and a benzamide derivative (sulpiride) that is related to metoclopramide.

Pharmacokinetics

A. Metabolism: Chlorpromazine may have one

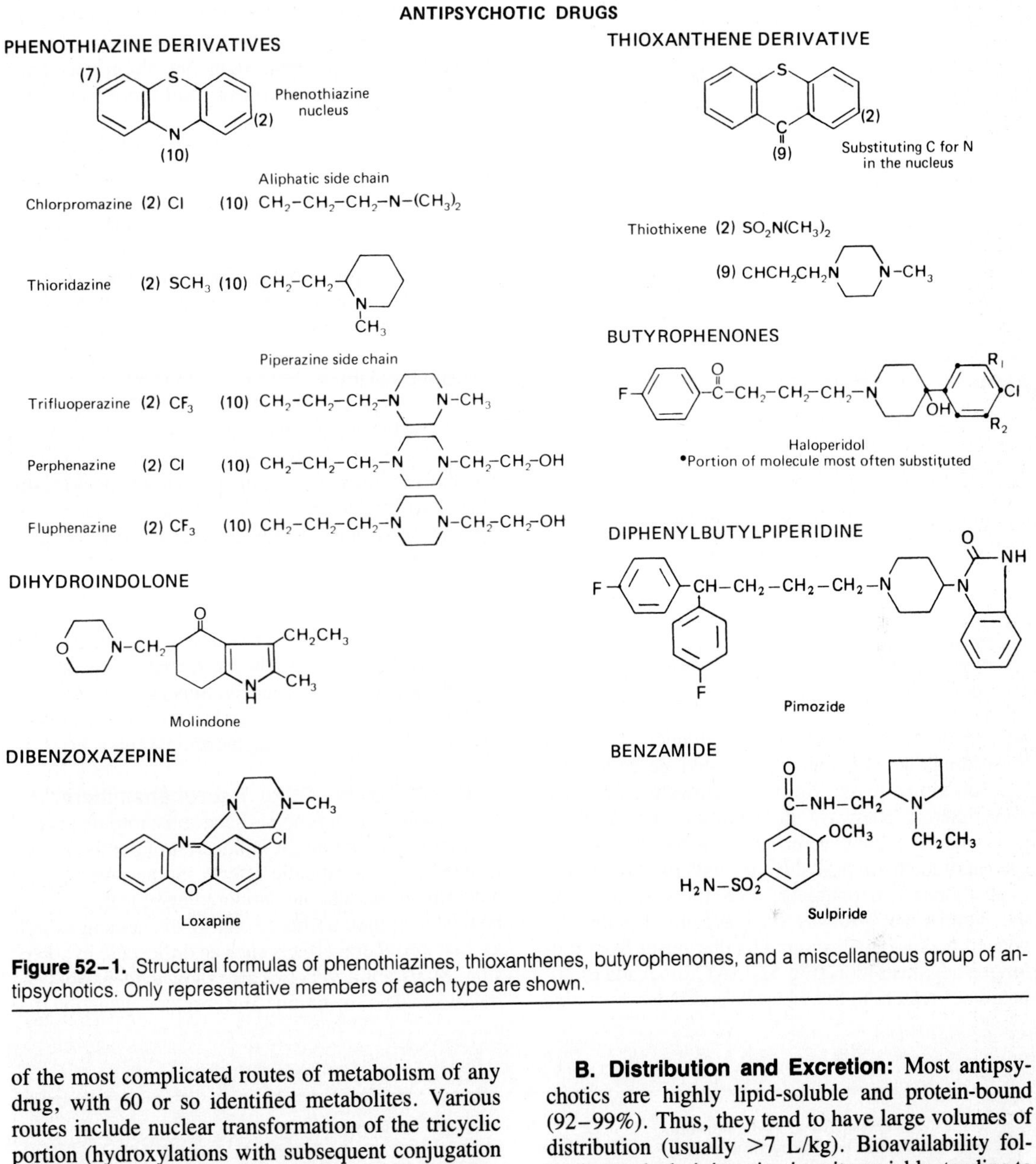

ANTIPSYCHOTIC DRUGS

Figure 52–1. Structural formulas of phenothiazines, thioxanthenes, butyrophenones, and a miscellaneous group of antipsychotics. Only representative members of each type are shown.

of the most complicated routes of metabolism of any drug, with 60 or so identified metabolites. Various routes include nuclear transformation of the tricyclic portion (hydroxylations with subsequent conjugation as well as sulfoxidation of the sulfur atom) and transformations of the aliphatic side chain (demethylations, N-oxidation, and deamination). Some of the metabolites may be active, especially the 7-hydroxy metabolite.

Thioridazine produces 2 active metabolites, mesoridazine and sulforidazine, both from sulfoxidations on the thiomethyl ring substituent. Ring sulfoxidation results in an inactive metabolite. Trifluoperazine has metabolic pathways similar to those of chlorpromazine, with the addition of opening of the piperazine moiety and formation of a free amine. The thioxanthenes are metabolized like the phenothiazines. Metabolism of haloperidol involves N-dealkylation, oxidation, and conjugation. A reduced metabolite is also active.

B. Distribution and Excretion: Most antipsychotics are highly lipid-soluble and protein-bound (92–99%). Thus, they tend to have large volumes of distribution (usually >7 L/kg). Bioavailability following oral administration is quite variable, tending to be low (25–35%) with drugs such as chlorpromazine that are extensively metabolized and higher with drugs such as haloperidol that have simpler metabolic pathways. The plasma half-lives tend to be short, ranging from 10 to 20 hours, but the clinical duration of the antipsychotic action is much longer than the short plasma half-life would indicate. Urinary metabolites of chlorpromazine may be found weeks after the last dose of chronically administered drug, suggesting that a large amount of the drug is sequestered in tissues. The importance of active metabolites in determining the clinical effects of these drugs is not known.

Pharmacodynamics

A. Effects on Dopaminergic Synapses: A

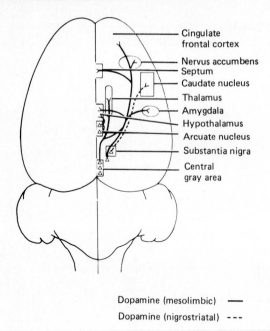

Dopamine (mesolimbic) ——
Dopamine (nigrostriatal) - - -

Figure 52–2. Diagrammatic section of brain showing the 2 principal dopaminergic tracts of the mesolimbic-frontal system and the nigrostriatal system.

number of pharmacologic and biochemical actions of these drugs suggest that they should be called **dopamine antagonists.** Fig 52–2 shows the principal dopaminergic pathways in the brain. Blockade of postsynaptic dopamine receptors in the mesolimbic system of the brain probably accounts for their ability to ameliorate schizophrenia, while the same action in the nigrostriatal pathway may account for the unwanted parkinsonism symptoms that result from prolonged administration (Fig 52–3A). Blockade of dopamine receptors in the tuberoinfundibular dopamine

pathway releases prolactin from the tonic inhibitory control of dopamine, resulting in hyperprolactinemia. Thus, the same pharmacodynamic action may have distinct psychiatric, neurologic, and endocrine consequences.

Despite their ability to block postsynaptic dopamine receptors, these drugs are only partially effective in schizophrenia. Furthermore, their effects can be easily antagonized by administering dopamine precursors, such as levodopa, or dopamine receptor agonists, such as apomorphine. These findings suggest either that dopamine receptor blockade is incomplete or that the antipsychotic action is due to some other mechanism, possibly in conjunction with the effect at dopamine synapses.

With continued use of antipsychotics, some patients develop supersensitivity of dopamine receptors, especially in the nigrostriatal system, that leads to the clinical manifestation called **tardive dyskinesia,** characterized by choreoathetoid movements resembling those associated with Huntington's disease. This change apparently occurs as a compensatory mechanism against the blockade of dopamine receptors (Fig 52–3B). Some patients, even when they are maintained on previously effective doses, experience a return or worsening of psychosis, referred to as **tardive** or **supersensitivity psychosis.** Supersensitivity of receptors in the mesolimbic system has been postulated to cause tolerance, reducing the antipsychotic effect of the drugs.

B. Effects on Other Neurotransmitters: Although some antipsychotics have antiserotonin or antinoradrenergic actions, it is uncertain how these contribute to the therapeutic effects. Some investigators have suggested that the antinoradrenergic action may be related to their ability to control excitement as well as their peripheral effects such as orthostatic hypotension. Many antipsychotics also show evidence of central blockade of histamine H_1 receptors, an action that

A. Postsynaptic dopamine receptor block by antipsychotic drugs

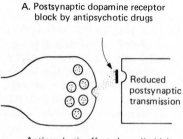

Antipsychotic effects (mesolimbic)

Extrapyramidal reactions (nigrostriatal)

B. Denervation supersensitivity

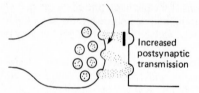

Initial disappearance of Parkinson's syndrome

Onset of tardive dyskinesia

Figure 52–3. *A:* Postsynaptic dopamine receptor blockade by antipsychotic drugs produces 2 actions: antipsychotic effects and extrapyramidal reactions. *B:* Continued treatment is thought to lead to increased dopamine stores and turnover presynaptically and new and supersensitive receptors postsynaptically. Compensatory mechanisms may eliminate initial extrapyramidal reactions (parkinsonism), but if overcompensation occurs, the symptoms may be replaced by those of tardive dyskinesia.

may relate to their sedative effects. All have varying degrees of antimuscarinic action, thioridazine being most potent. This action may reduce the intensity of parkinsonism, but it is also manifested peripherally by many common side effects, such as dry mouth, blurred vision, constipation, and difficulty in urination. Some of these effects are summarized in Table 52–1.

C. Psychologic Effects: Most antipsychotic drugs cause unpleasant reactions in nonpsychotic individuals; the combination of sleepiness, restlessness, and autonomic effects creates experiences unlike those associated with more familiar sedatives or hypnotics. Performance is impaired as judged by a number of psychomotor and psychometric tests. In general, the more active the drug or the larger the dose, the greater the impairment as shown by psychomotor tests. The crucial clinical question of the effects of such impairment on various potentially hazardous functions, such as driving, during therapeutic administration is still unsettled.

D. Neurophysiologic Effects: Antipsychotic drugs produce shifts in the pattern of electroencephalographic frequencies, chiefly in the direction of slowing and increased synchronization. The slowing (hypersynchrony) is sometimes focal or unilateral, which may lead to erroneous diagnostic interpretations. Both the frequency and the amplitude changes induced by psychotropic drugs are readily apparent and can be quantitated by sophisticated electronic techniques.

Electroencephalographic changes associated with antipsychotic drugs appear first in subcortical electrodes, supporting the view that their chief action is exerted at subcortical sites. The hypersynchrony produced by these drugs may account for their activating effect on the electroencephalogram in epileptic patients, as well as their occasional elicitation of seizures in patients with no history of seizure disorders.

E. Endocrine Effects: Antipsychotic drugs produce striking side effects on the reproductive system. Amenorrhea-galactorrhea, false-positive pregnancy tests, and increased libido have been reported in women, whereas men have been troubled by decreased libido and gynecomastia. Some of these effects are secondary to loss of the tonic inhibition of prolactin secretion by dopamine; others may be due to increased peripheral conversion of androgens to estrogens.

F. Cardiovascular Effects: Orthostatic hypotension and high resting pulse rates frequently result from use of the "low-potency" phenothiazines. Mean arterial pressure, peripheral resistance, and stroke volume are decreased, and pulse rate is increased. These are predictable from the autonomic actions of these agents (Table 52–1).

Abnormal electrocardiographic findings have been observed, especially with thioridazine. Changes include prolongation of the QT interval and abnormal configurations of the ST segment and T waves, the latter being rounded, flattened, or notched. These

Table 52–1. Unwanted pharmacologic effects of antipsychotic drugs.

Type	Manifestations	Mechanism
Autonomic nervous system	Cycloplegia, dry mouth, difficulty urinating, constipation.	Muscarinic cholinergic blockade.
	Orthostatic hypotension, impotence, failure to ejaculate.	Alpha-adrenergic blockade.
Central nervous system	Parkinson's syndrome, akathisia, dystonias.	Dopamine receptor blockade.
	Tardive dyskinesia.	Supersensitivity of dopamine receptors
	Toxic-confusional state.	Muscarinic cholinergic blockade.
Endocrine system	Amenorrhea-galactorrhea, infertility, impotence	Dopamine receptor blockade resulting in hyperprolactinemia.

changes are readily reversible upon withdrawal of the drug.

Screening Tests in Animals

Inhibition of conditioned (but not unconditioned) avoidance behavior is one of the tests most predictive of antipsychotic action. Another is the inhibition of amphetamine- or apomorphine-induced stereotyped behavior. This inhibition no doubt is related to the dopamine receptor-blocking action of the drugs, countering these 2 dopamine agonists. Other tests that may predict antipsychotic action are reduction of exploratory behavior without undue sedation, induction of a cataleptic state, inhibition of intracranial stimulation of reward areas, and prevention of apomorphine-induced vomiting. It is difficult to relate most of these tests to any model of clinical psychosis.

CLINICAL PHARMACOLOGY OF ANTIPSYCHOTIC DRUGS

Indications

A. Psychiatric Indications: The schizophrenic and other functional psychotic disorders are the primary indications for these drugs, which presently constitute the only clearly efficacious, symptomatic, pharmacologic treatment. Unfortunately, some patients do not respond at all, and virtually none show a complete response. Because some schizophrenics have a favorable course with prolonged remission after an initial episode, most physicians recommend discontinuing drug therapy after remission has been achieved following the first episode.

Schizoaffective disorders may be more similar to affective disorders than to schizophrenia. Nonetheless, the psychotic aspects of the illness require treatment with antipsychotics, which may be used in combination with other drugs, such as antidepressants or lithium.

The manic episode in bipolar affective disorder is most effectively treated with antipsychotics, although lithium alone may suffice in milder cases. As mania subsides, the antipsychotic drug may be withdrawn. Nonmanic excited states may also be managed by antipsychotics, but attempts to define the diagnosis should not be abandoned.

Psychoses associated with old age, notably Alzheimer's disease, may show some symptomatic improvement with antipsychotics. Disturbed behavior, emotional lability, and abnormal sleep-wake cycles may be improved, but the basic disorder is untouched.

Gilles de la Tourette's syndrome, characterized by unpredictable barking tics and outbursts of foul language, has been successfully managed with haloperidol and pimozide, which has been specifically approved for this indication.

The use of antipsychotics as primary treatment for depression is controversial. Because of the danger of tardive dyskinesia, most clinicians would use them only adjunctively in patients with agitated or psychotic depressions.

Acute mental disorders during withdrawal from alcohol or other drugs should not be treated with antipsychotics. Substitution of a pharmacologically equivalent drug, stabilization on that drug, and subsequent gradual withdrawal are the time-honored principles of management. Acute adverse reactions associated with the use of other social drugs may be aggravated by antipsychotics but can be managed with simple sedatives. Overdoses of amphetamine and related stimulants are best managed with haloperidol, which is also likely to help the delirium of medically or surgically ill patients.

Antipsychotics in small doses have been (wrongly) promoted for relief of anxiety associated with minor emotional disorders. The antianxiety sedatives (Chapter 54) are far better in every respect, including safety and acceptability to patients.

B. Nonpsychiatric Indications: Most antipsychotic drugs, with the exception of thioridazine, have a strong antiemetic effect. This action is due to dopamine receptor blockade, both centrally (in the chemoreceptor trigger zone of the medulla) and peripherally (on receptors in the stomach). Some drugs, such as prochlorperazine and benzquinamide, are promoted solely as antiemetics. Phenothiazines with shorter side chains have considerable H_1 receptor-blocking action and have been used for relief of pruritus or, in the case of promethazine, as preoperative sedatives. The butyrophenone droperidol is used in combination with a meperidinelike drug, fentanyl, in "neuroleptanesthesia."

Choice of Drug

A rational choice of antipsychotic drugs may be based on differences between chemical structures and the attendant pharmacologic differences, since the differences between groups are greater than the differences within groups. Thus, one might choose to be familiar with one member of each of the 3 subfamilies of phenothiazines, a member of the thioxanthene and butyrophenone groups, and perhaps 2 members of the miscellaneous group. A possible selection is shown in Table 52–2.

No basis exists for choosing drugs for use against "target symptoms," as there is no evidence of specificity in their effects. The physician whose practice often or sometimes requires prescribing drugs for long-term management of psychotic disorders does not need to know all of the drugs but should become familiar with the effects—including the side effects—of one or 2 drugs in each class. The best guide for selecting a drug for individual patients is their past responses to drugs. The trend in recent years has been away from the "low-potency" agents such as chlorpromazine and thioridazine to the "high-potency" drugs

Table 52–2. Some representative antipsychotic drugs.

Drug Class	Drug	Advantages	Disadvantages
Phenothiazines Aliphatic	Chlorpromazine[1]	Generic.	Many side effects; probably should not be used (obsolete).
Piperidine	Thioridazine[2] (Mellaril, Millazine)	Slight extrapyramidal syndrome.	800 mg/d limit; no parenteral form; (?) cardiotoxicity.
Piperazine	Fluphenazine[3] (Prolixin)	Parenteral form also available (decanoate).	(?) Increased tardive dyskinesia.
Thioxanthene	Thiothixene[4] (Navane)	Parenteral form also available.	Uncertain.
Butyrophenone	Haloperidol (Haldol)	Parenteral form also available, as well as depot form (decanoate).	Severe extrapyramidal syndrome.
Dibenzoxazepine	Loxapine (Loxitane)	(?) No weight gain.	Uncertain.
Dihydroindolone	Molindone (Moban)	(?) No weight gain.	Uncertain.

[1]Other aliphatic phenothiazines: promazine (Sparine, generic), triflupromazine.
[2]Other piperidine phenothiazines: piperacetazine (Quide), mesoridazine (Lidanar, Serentil).
[3]Other piperazine phenothiazines: acetophenazine (Tindal), perphenazine (Trilafon), carphenazine (Proketazine), prochlorperazine (Compazine, generic), trifluoperazine (Stelazine, Suprazine).
[4]Other thioxanthenes: chlorprothixene (Taractan).

such as thiothixene, haloperidol, and fluphenazine. Chlorpromazine, in fact, should probably now be considered obsolete in view of its high incidence of side effects (see below).

Well-tolerated parenteral forms of the high-potency drugs, such as fluphenazine, thiothixene, and haloperidol, are available for rapid initiation of treatment. Such dosage forms have greater bioavailability than the oral dosage forms (the latter are usually only 40–70% bioavailable), so doses should be only a fraction of what might be given orally. Depot preparations of fluphenazine decanoate and haloperidol decanoate are available for maintenance treatment in noncompliant patients. Single intramuscular doses of this drug may be adequate for long periods (1–4 weeks). However, the release characteristics of such preparations are somewhat uncertain. While their value in maintenance treatment is established for noncompliant patients, these preparations offer no advantage over oral doses in compliant patients. Thus, they should not be used routinely.

Doses & Dosage Schedules

The range of effective doses among various antipsychotics is quite broad. Even with individual drugs in each class, a wide range of doses may be used, since therapeutic margins are substantial. Some dose relationships between various antipsychotic drugs, as well as possible therapeutic ranges, are shown in Table 52–3.

There is no evidence that any antipsychotic drug is superior in overall efficacy to any other. However, some patients who fail to respond to one drug may respond to another, and for this reason, several drugs may have to be tried to find the one most effective for an individual patient. Some seemingly refractory patients have responded to larger-than-usual doses of the

Table 52–3. Dose relationships of antipsychotics.

	Minimum Effective Therapeutic Dose (mg)	Usual Range of Daily Doses (mg)
Chlorpromazine (Thorazine)	100	100–1000
Thioridazine (Mellaril, Millazine)	100	100–800
Mesoridazine (Lidanar, Serentil)	50	50–400
Piperacetazine (Quide)	10	20–160
Trifluoperazine (Stelazine, Suprazine)	5	5–60
Perphenazine (Trilafon)	10	8–64
Fluphenazine (Prolixin)	2	2–60
Thiothixene (Navane)	2	2–120
Haloperidol (Haldol)	2	2–100
Loxapine (Loxitane)	10	20–160
Molindone (Moban)	10	20–200

more potent antipsychotics, such as 200–400 mg/d of haloperidol or thiothixene. Before it is concluded that a patient will not respond to drug therapy, such doses should be tried on an experimental basis.

Antipsychotics may be given in divided daily doses initially while an effective dose level is being sought. They need not always be equally divided doses. After an effective daily dose has been defined for an individual patient, doses can be given less frequently. Once-daily doses, usually given at night, are feasible for many patients during chronic maintenance treatment. Simplification of dosage schedules leads to better compliance. Maximum dose units of many drugs are being increased by manufacturers to meet the needs of once-daily dosing.

Monitoring Plasma Concentrations

Clinical monitoring of plasma concentrations of antipsychotic agents, although technically feasible, is not warranted at this time. Attempts to define a therapeutic range of plasma concentrations are beset by many difficulties. A range of 150–300 ng/mL has been suggested for chlorpromazine, but the evidence is tenuous. Ranges of 7–20 ng/mL have been suggested for haloperidol, although some very refractory patients may benefit from levels up to 50 ng/mL.

Maintenance Treatment

Most patients with acute psychotic episodes do not have a schizophrenic disorder and do not need maintenance antipsychotic treatment. In patients with schizophrenic disorders, a small minority may remit from an acute episode and require no further drug therapy for prolonged periods. In most cases, however, schizophrenia is a chronic disorder that only partially remits, so that drug therapy must be continued indefinitely.

The issue is whether treatment should be continuous or "targeted." Continuous treatment with the lowest possible dose may be just as effective as intermittent treatment in reducing total drug exposure. As there is no way to predict who might relapse early when the drug has been completely stopped, continuous treatment reduces the risk of undoing much of the hard-won rehabilitative gains afforded by a good treatment program. The major aim of "targeted" treatment is to use drugs only when relapse is clearly evident in order to reduce total drug exposure, minimize the dulling effects of drugs, and avoid tardive dyskinesia. Crucial to the success of this approach is frequent observation of the patient for early symptoms of relapse. Thus, the choice of maintenance treatment will depend on the resources available for close follow-up of discharged patients.

Drug Combinations

Combining antipsychotic drugs confounds evaluation of the efficacy of the drugs being used. Tricyclic antidepressants may be used with antipsychotics, but only for clear symptoms of depression complicating schizophrenia. They are of no proved efficacy for alleviating the social withdrawal and blunted affect of the psychotic. Lithium is sometimes added with benefit to antipsychotic agents when patients fail to respond to the latter drugs alone. It is uncertain whether such instances represent misdiagnosed cases of mania. Sedative drugs may be added for relief of anxiety, agitation, or insomnia not controlled by antipsychotics.

The drugs most frequently combined with antipsychotics are antiparkinsonism agents. Although it has been claimed that concurrent use of these drugs reduces the bioavailability of chlorpromazine, the evidence is uncertain, and the effect is probably of little clinical consequence in any case. It has also been suggested that these drugs undo the therapeutic action of antipsychotics; but when the choice is between this theoretical possibility and the real problem of treating parkinsonism, most clinicians prefer to treat with antiparkinsonism drugs.

Adverse Reactions

Most of the unwanted effects of antipsychotics are extensions of their known pharmacologic actions, but a few are allergic and some are idiosyncratic.

A. Behavioral Effects: Antipsychotic drugs are unpleasant to take—the more so the less psychotic the patient. Many patients stop taking their drug because of the unpleasant side effects, which may be mitigated by giving small doses during the day and the major portion at bedtime. A "pseudodepression" that may be due to akinesia from these drugs usually responds to treatment with antiparkinsonism drugs. Other "pseudodepressions" may be due to using higher doses than needed in a patient who has achieved partial remission, in which case decreasing the dose may relieve the symptoms. Toxic-confusional states may occur with very high doses of drugs that have prominent anticholinergic actions. The development of supersensitivity psychosis is a matter of current concern. It appears to be far less common than tardive dyskinesia. Most reports have been anecdotal, based on an apparent need for increasing the dose of antipsychotic drug over time to attain the same degree of remission.

B. Neurologic Effects: Extrapyramidal reactions occurring early during treatment include typical Parkinson's syndrome, akathisia (uncontrollable restlessness), and acute dystonic reactions (spastic retrocollis or torticollis). Parkinson's syndrome can be treated, when necessary, with conventional antiparkinsonism drugs of the anticholinergic type or, in rare cases, by amantadine. Parkinson's syndrome may be self-limiting, so that an attempt to withdraw antiparkinsonism drugs should be made every 3–4 months. Akathisia and dystonic reactions will also respond to such treatment, but many prefer to use a sedative antihistamine with anticholinergic properties, eg, diphenhydramine, which can be given either parenterally or orally as capsules or elixir. Prophylactic use of oral diphenhydramine may be useful in patients at high risk of developing acute dystonic reactions, such as children or young adults being treated with substantial doses of high-potency drugs. Parenteral administration may be effective in reversing acute dystonia after it has occurred.

Tardive dyskinesia, as the name implies, is a late-occurring syndrome of abnormal choreoathetoid movements. It is the most important unwanted effect of antipsychotics. It has been proposed that it is caused by a relative cholinergic deficiency secondary to supersensitivity of dopamine receptors in the caudate nucleus and putamen. Older women treated for long periods are most susceptible to the disorder, although it can occur at any age and in either sex. The prevalence varies enormously, but tardive dyskinesia is estimated to occur in 20–40% of chronically treated patients. Early recognition is important, since advanced cases may be difficult to reverse. Many treatments have been proposed, but their evaluation is confounded by the fact that the course of the disorder is variable and sometimes self-limited. Most authorities agree that the first step would be to try to decrease dopamine receptor sensitivity by discontinuing the antipsychotic drug or by reducing the dose. A logical second step would be to eliminate all drugs with central anticholinergic action, particularly antiparkinsonism drugs and tricyclic antidepressants. These 2 steps are often enough to bring about improvement. If they fail, the addition of diazepam in doses as high as 30–40 mg/d may add to the response. The use of reserpine may also be considered, although one runs the risk of increasing receptor sensitivity. Other treatments that have been proposed include precursors of acetylcholine, such as lecithin or choline, propranolol, lithium, and many others.

C. Autonomic Nervous System Effects: Most patients become tolerant to the anticholinergic side effects of antipsychotic drugs. Those who are made too uncomfortable or who are impaired, as with urinary retention, should be given bethanechol, a peripherally acting cholinomimetic. Orthostatic hypotension or impaired ejaculation, common complications of therapy with chlorpromazine or mesoridazine, should be managed by switching to drugs with less marked adrenergic blocking actions.

D. Metabolic and Endocrine Effects: Weight gain is common and requires monitoring of food intake. Hyperprolactinemia in women results in the amenorrhea-galactorrhea syndrome and infertility; in men, loss of libido, impotence, and infertility may result.

E. Toxic or Allergic Reactions: Agranulocytosis is no longer a major risk except with low-potency drugs (eg, chlorpromazine or clozapine). Clozapine has enough advantages over other drugs so that the risk may be acceptable in refractory patients or in those with tardive dyskinesia. Cholestatic jaundice is now rare, even with chlorpromazine.

F. Ocular Complications: Deposits in the anterior portion of the eye (cornea and lens) are a common complication of chlorpromazine therapy. They may accentuate the normal processes of aging of the lens. Thioridazine is the only antipsychotic drug that causes retinal deposits, which in advanced cases may resemble retinitis pigmentosa. The deposits are usually associated with "browning" of vision. The maximum daily dose of thioridazine has been limited to 800 mg/d to reduce the possibility of this complication.

G. Cardiac Toxicity: Thioridazine in doses exceeding 300 mg/d is almost always associated with minor abnormalities of T waves that are easily reversible. Overdoses of thioridazine are associated with major ventricular arrhythmias, cardiac conduction block, and sudden death; it is not certain whether thioridazine can cause these same disorders when used in therapeutic doses. In view of possible additive anticholinergic and quinidinelike actions with various tricyclic antidepressants, thioridazine should not be combined with the latter drugs.

H. Effects of Use During Pregnancy: Although the antipsychotic drugs appear to be relatively safe in pregnancy, there may be a small increase in risk of dysmorphogenesis. Questions about whether to use these drugs during pregnancy and whether to abort a pregnancy in which the fetus has already been exposed must be decided individually.

I. Neuroleptic Malignant Syndrome: This early complication of treatment appears to be an idiosyncratic response. It often follows an initial large dose of antipsychotic drug. High fever, marked muscle rigidity, and autonomic signs are characteristic, but incomplete forms of the syndrome are increasingly recognized. Prompt cessation of antipsychotic drugs and vigorous cooling and rehydration are nonspecific treatments. Specific treatments include muscle relaxants (eg, baclofen and dantrolene) or dopamine agonists (eg, bromocriptine).

Drug Interactions

Pharmacodynamic interactions are more frequent than pharmacokinetic ones and are of greater importance clinically. The most important pharmacodynamic interaction of the antipsychotics is an additive depressant effect when they are used along with various other central nervous system depressants. Such drugs include conventional sedative-hypnotics, antihistamines, opiates, and alcohol. Neuroleptics have relatively little respiratory depressant action when taken by themselves, but they may have a modest additive effect when taken with other drugs that also depress respiration.

Autonomic interactions can be largely predicted from their anticholinergic and alpha-blocking actions. In addition, chlorpromazine may reverse the antihypertensive effects of drugs that work on sympathetic neurons, such as guanethidine, clonidine, bethanidine, debrisoquin, and possibly methyldopa.

Thioridazine has quinidinelike effects perhaps related to its cardiotoxicity. Other drugs with such actions include quinidine and procainamide, tricyclic antidepressants, and hydroxyzine. The use of thioridazine with any of these classes of drugs should be avoided.

Pharmacokinetic interactions are of less importance. Colloidal antacids, kaolin, and activated charcoal adsorb chlorpromazine and probably also other phenothiazines and tricyclic antidepressants. It would seem desirable to separate by at least 1–2 hours the ingestion of such antacids and the subsequent administration of any drug.

Chlorpromazine, perphenazine, haloperidol, chlorprothixene, and thioridazine inhibit the hydroxylation of imipramine and nortriptyline, and the reverse is true to some extent. Thus, concurrent administration of both types of drugs may lead to elevated plasma concentrations of both. This interaction—at least between nortriptyline and perphenazine—seems to occur only with large doses of either drug.

A possible interaction between phenothiazines (specifically thioridazine) and phenytoin might be of greater consequence. Inhibition of metabolism of phenytoin, which has a narrow therapeutic range, has led to serious clinical toxicity.

Overdoses

Poisonings with antipsychotics are rarely fatal, with the exception of those due to mesoridazine and thioridazine. In general, drowsiness proceeds to coma, with an intervening period of agitation. Neuromuscular excitability may be increased and proceed to convulsions. Pupils are miotic, and deep tendon reflexes are decreased. Hypotension and hypothermia are the rule, although fever may be present later in the course. The lethal effects of mesoridazine and thioridazine are related to their actions on the heart.

Patients should be monitored in an intensive care setting for the usual vital signs, venous pressure, arterial blood gases, and electrolytes. Attempts at gastric lavage should be made even if several hours have elapsed since the drug was taken, since gastrointestinal motility is decreased. Activated charcoal effectively binds most of these drugs, following which a saline cathartic may be given. Hypotension often responds to fluid replacement. If a pressor agent is to be used, norepinephrine or dopamine is preferred to epinephrine, whose unopposed β-adrenergic receptor-stimulant action in the presence of alpha blockade may cause vasodilatation. Seizures may be treated with either diazepam or phenytoin, the latter being given with an initial loading dose. Management of overdoses of thioridazine and mesoridazine, which are complicated by cardiac arrhythmias, is similar to that for tricyclic antidepressants (Chapter 53).

MOOD STABILIZERS

Lithium is often referred to as an "antimanic" drug, but some cases of depression also seem to respond. In many parts of the world, lithium is referred to as a "mood-stabilizing" agent because of its primary action of preventing mood swings in patients with bipolar affective (manic-depressive) disorder. Other drugs possibly effective in preventing mood swings include carbamazepine, valproic acid, and clonazepam, but carbamazepine is the only one clearly established as useful.

Bipolar affective disorder is a frequently diagnosed and very serious emotional disorder. Patients with cyclic attacks of mania have many symptoms similar to paranoid schizophrenia (grandiosity, bellicosity, paranoid thoughts, and overactivity). The gratifying response to lithium therapy of patients with bipolar disorder has made such diagnostic distinctions important.

Bipolar disorder has a strong genetic component and seems to be biologically determined. The episodes of mood swings are generally unrelated to life events. The exact biologic disturbance has not been identified, but a preponderance of catecholaminergic activity is thought to be present. Drugs that increase this activity tend to exacerbate mania, whereas those that reduce activity of dopamine or norepinephrine relieve mania. Acetylcholine may also be involved. The nature of the abrupt switch from mania to depression experienced by some patients is uncertain (see Chapter 30).

When mania is mild, lithium alone may be effective treatment. In more severe cases, it is almost always necessary to give one of the antipsychotic drugs also. After mania is controlled, the antipsychotic drug may be stopped and lithium continued as maintenance therapy.

Unlike antipsychotic or antidepressant drugs, which exert several actions on the central or autonomic nervous system, lithium ion produces only mild sedation and is devoid of adrenergic blocking or anticholinergic effects. Since it is a small inorganic ion, lithium is easily measured in body fluids such as plasma, urine, or saliva; is distributed in body water; and is not metabolized. Thus, its kinetics can be studied much more easily, and plasma or tissue concentrations can be correlated with clinical effects. A third attribute of considerable interest has been the prophylactic use of lithium in preventing both mania and depression. It is indeed remarkable that a so-called functional psychosis can be controlled so easily by such a simple chemical as lithium carbonate.

Lithium may be combined with antipsychotics when mania breaks through a prophylactic treatment program, or with antidepressants when depression becomes apparent. Although haloperidol was alleged to be a poor drug to combine with lithium, it seems in retrospect to be no different from other neuroleptics. All neuroleptics may produce more severe extrapyramidal syndromes when combined with lithium.

BASIC PHARMACOLOGY OF LITHIUM

No single mechanism accounts for the therapeutic effect of lithium. Its effects on neurotransmitters, cell membranes, cations, and water have been the major avenues of inquiry.

Lithium is thought to accelerate the presynaptic destruction of catecholamines, to inhibit release of transmitters at the synapse, and to decrease the sensitivity of the postsynaptic receptor. All of these actions would tend to correct the overactivity of catecholaminergic systems presumed to occur in mania. However, many of these actions of lithium are acute and have not been demonstrated to be sustained during chronic treatment.

Presynaptic and postsynaptic regulation of neurotransmission is intimately involved with various cations, eg, sodium, potassium, magnesium, and calcium. Neurotransmitter release is probably calcium-dependent, while the configuration of postsynaptic receptors may be altered by sodium. The passage of lithium into cells, where it exerts its major action, is intimately related to these ions as well.

Both calcium and magnesium are required to stabilize cell membranes and hence make them less fluid. Displacement by lithium of either calcium or magnesium may increase membrane permeability.

In extracellular fluid, lithium acts similarly to potassium and stimulates sodium efflux from cells, both by cation exchange and by stimulation of the Na^+-K^+ pump mechanism. Lithium also enhances the entry of choline into cells, but the significance of this action is uncertain.

The rather simple pharmacokinetic properties of lithium are summarized in Table 52–4.

CLINICAL PHARMACOLOGY OF LITHIUM

Indications

A. Bipolar Affective Disorder: Agreement is almost universal that lithium carbonate is the preferred treatment for bipolar disorder, especially in the manic phase. Because its onset of action is slow, concurrent use of antipsychotic drugs may be required for severely manic patients. The overall success rate for attaining remission from the manic phase of bipolar disorder is about 60–80%. Maintenance (prophylactic) therapy in patients with classic bipolar (manic-depressive) disorder is now well accepted. In general,

Table 52–4. Pharmacokinetics of lithium.

Absorption	Rapid. Virtually complete within 6–8 hours; peak plasma levels in 30 minutes to 2 hours.
Distribution	In total body water; slow entry into intracellular compartment. Apparent volumes of distribution of 0.5–0.9 L/kg body weight; some sequestration in bone. No protein binding.
Metabolism	None.
Excretion	Virtually entirely in urine. Lithium clearance about 20% of creatinine. Plasma half-life about 20 hours.

control with maintenance lithium is about 60–70% effective.

Some clinicians find that depressive episodes during typical bipolar illness may respond better when a tricyclic antidepressant is added to lithium maintenance during this period. Rapidly cycling manic-depressive episodes have been linked to treatment with tricyclic antidepressants. Carbamazepine may be useful in such situations or in cases in which manic episodes are not controlled by lithium alone.

B. Other Psychiatric Disorders: Acute endogenous depression is not generally considered to be an indication for treatment with lithium. On the other hand, recurrent endogenous depressions with a cyclic pattern are controlled by lithium and imipramine, both of which are superior to a placebo.

Schizoaffective disorders are characterized by a mixture of schizophrenic symptoms and altered affect in the form of depression or excitement. Antipsychotic drugs alone or combined with lithium are used in the excitement phase; tricyclic antidepressants are used if depression is present.

Alcoholism is commonly believed to have a high association with depression and mania. When the 2 conditions coexist, lithium may be useful in reducing drinking. Lithium has no established efficacy in the absence of affective symptoms.

Lithium is not regarded as useful for schizophrenia. Whether lithium added to antipsychotic drugs can enhance their efficacy in ordinary schizophrenia is an unsettled question.

An interesting application of lithium currently being investigated is the management of aggressive, violent behavior in prisoners. These men, both in and out of prison, have explosive responses to minimal provocation, possible brain damage with nonspecific abnormal electroencephalographic findings, and long histories of violent criminal behavior. Sufficient data are available to suggest that this may be an important indication for the use of lithium.

Doses & Dosage Schedules

Before treatment is started, one should obtain laboratory data such as a complete blood count, urinalysis, common biochemical tests, tests of thyroid function, and an electrocardiogram. Patients over 50 years of age should also have a creatinine clearance test. These tests serve as baseline measurements in assessing possible complications of treatment.

The patient's age, body weight, and renal function should be considered in determining initial appropriate doses of lithium carbonate. The initial volume of distribution of lithium will be the same as body water, or about 0.5 L/kg body weight for women and 0.55 L/kg for men. The proportion of body water may decrease slightly in older individuals. What is more important in older patients is a subtle decrease in renal function. Any patient over 50 years of age is likely to have a decreased creatinine clearance, which may reach 50% or less of the usual normal values without abnormal elevation of serum creatinine levels.

A daily lithium dose of 0.5 meq/kg will produce the desired serum lithium concentration in the range of 0.9–1.4 meq/L after a week of treatment if renal function is normal. Each 300-mg dose unit of lithium carbonate contains approximately 8 meq of lithium.

It is almost always necessary to give lithium in divided doses to avoid gastric distress. Medication is best taken with or shortly after meals.

Monitoring Serum Concentrations

Clinicians have relied heavily on measurements of serum concentrations for assessing both the dose required for satisfactory treatment of acute mania and the adequacy of maintenance treatment. These measurements are customarily taken 10–12 hours after the last dose, so all data in the literature pertaining to these concentrations reflect this interval.

An initial determination of serum lithium concentration should be obtained about 5 days after start of treatment, at which time steady-state conditions should obtain for the dose chosen. If the clinical response suggests a change in dosage, a simple arithmetic adjustment (present dose multiplied by desired blood level and then divided by present blood level) should produce the desired level. The serum concentration attained with the adjusted dose can be checked in another 5 days. Once the desired concentration has been achieved, levels can be measured at increasing intervals unless intercurrent illness or the introduction of a new drug into the treatment program intervenes. Recently, the tendency has been to try to treat patients with the lowest possible serum levels. The patient's clinical response takes precedence over any laboratory results; if the patient is doing well with a low level, it is maintained; if the patient shows signs of toxicity, even though the level may be "therapeutic," the drug dosage is reduced or discontinued. Maintenance treatment can often be achieved with lower levels than those required initially, probably as low as 0.5–0.6 meq/L.

Maintenance Treatment

The decision to use lithium as *prophylactic* treatment depends on many factors: the frequency and severity of previous episodes, the pattern of symptoms during episodes (eg, crescendo pattern), and the degree to which the patient is willing to follow a program of indefinite maintenance therapy. If the present attack was the patient's first, one might prefer to terminate treatment after it has subsided. Patients who have one or more episodes of illness per year are candidates for maintenance treatment. However, if the patient is unreliable, it may be better to alert the family to the initial signs of recurrence and be prepared to provide prompt treatment when needed. Some patients with mania discontinue treatment voluntarily, feeling that their spirits and initiative are suppressed by lithium.

Adverse Reactions

Many side effects associated with lithium treatment occur at varying times after treatment is started. Some are harmless, but it is important to be alert to side effects that may signify impending serious toxic reactions.

A. Neurologic and Psychiatric Effects: Tremor is one of the most frequent side effects of lithium treatment, occurring at therapeutic dose levels. Propranolol, which has been reported to be effective in essential tremor, also alleviates lithium-induced tremor. Other neurologic abnormalities that have been reported include choreoathetosis, motor hyperactivity, ataxia, dysarthria, and aphasia. Psychiatric disturbances are generally marked by mental confusion and withdrawal or bizarre motor movements.

B. Effects on Thyroid Function: Lithium probably decreases thyroid function in most patients exposed to the drug, but the effect is reversible or nonprogressive. Some patients develop frank thyroid enlargement, but only about 15% show symptoms of hypothyroidism.

C. Renal Effects: Polydipsia and polyuria are frequent but reversible concomitants of lithium treatment, occurring at therapeutic serum concentrations. The principal physiologic lesion involved is loss of the ability of the distal tubule to conserve water under the influence of antidiuretic hormone, resulting in excessive free water clearance. Resistance of lithium-induced **nephrogenic diabetes insipidus** to vasopressin has led to other attempts at management of this complication. Thiazide diuretics may be used, but the dose of lithium should be reduced by about 25% if such treatment is started.

Despite past concerns about possible **chronic interstitial nephritis** associated with long-term lithium treatment, no instances of end-stage renal failure have occurred, and decreases in creatinine clearance have been minimal. Although the kidney tubule is most vulnerable to lithium, a few cases of **minimal change glomerulopathy** with nephrotic syndrome have been reported.

Patients receiving lithium should avoid dehydration with the consequent increased concentration of lithium in urine. Periodic tests of renal concentrating ability should be carried out to detect changes.

D. Edema: Edema is a frequent side effect of lithium treatment and may be related to some effect of lithium on sodium retention. Although weight gain may be expected in patients who become edematous, water retention alone probably does not account for all of it.

E. Cardiac Toxicity: Reduced amplitude of T waves is a frequent finding during lithium treatment if the electrocardiographic tracing is examined carefully. No evidence of myocardial damage can be found when enzyme tests are done during periods of T wave abnormality, and the effect seems to be readily reversible. The sinus node may also be susceptible to toxic effects of lithium, with depression of its normal pacemaker function. The drug is definitely contraindicated in the "sick sinus" syndrome.

F. Effects of Use During Pregnancy: Renal clearance of lithium increases during pregnancy and reverts to lower levels immediately after delivery. A patient whose serum lithium concentration is in a good therapeutic range during pregnancy may develop toxic levels following delivery. Special care in monitoring lithium levels is needed at these times. Lithium is transferred to nursing infants through breast milk, in which it has a concentration about one-third to one-half that of serum. Lithium toxicity in newborns is manifested by lethargy, cyanosis, poor suck and Moro reflexes, and possibly hepatomegaly.

The issue of dysmorphogenesis is not settled. One report suggests an alarming increase in the frequency of cardiac anomalies, especially Ebstein's anomaly, in babies born to mothers receiving lithium treatment.

G. Miscellaneous Effects: Transient acneiform eruptions have been noted early in lithium treatment. Some of them subside with temporary discontinuation of treatment and do not recur with its resumption. Folliculitis is less dramatic and probably occurs more frequently. Leukocytosis is always present during lithium treatment, probably reflecting a direct effect on leukopoiesis rather than mobilization from the marginal pool. This "side effect" has now become a therapeutic effect in patients with low leukocyte counts. Disturbed sexual function has been reported in men treated with lithium.

Drug Interactions

Renal clearance of lithium is reduced about 25% in the presence of oral diuretics, and doses may have to be reduced by a similar amount. A similar reduction in lithium clearance has been noted with several of the newer nonsteroidal anti-inflammatory drugs that block synthesis of prostaglandins. It is not known whether this interaction extends to aspirin.

Overdoses

Therapeutic overdoses are more common than those due to deliberate or accidental ingestion of the drug. Therapeutic overdoses are usually due to accumulation of lithium resulting from some change in the patient's status, such as diminished serum sodium, use of diuretics, fluctuating renal function, or pregnancy. Since the tissues will have already equilibrated with the blood, the plasma concentrations of drugs may not be excessively high in proportion to the degree of toxicity; any value over 2 meq/L must be considered as indicating potential toxicity.

A primary consideration is to rid the patient of the drug. Because of the physically large amounts of drug involved in cases of acute deliberate overdosage (one may be dealing with 30–60 g), absorption is slow. Lavage should be done with a wide-bore tube, as the material tends to clump and may be difficult to remove through smaller tubes. Saline cathartics should follow lavage. Charcoal is not an effective adsorbent in this instance. As lithium is a small ion, it is dialyzed readily. Both peritoneal dialysis and hemodialysis are effective, though the latter is preferred. Dialysis should be continued until the plasma concentrations fall below the usual therapeutic range.

CARBAMAZEPINE

Carbamazepine may be used as an alternative to lithium, especially in patients who do not respond to lithium. The mode of action of carbamazepine is not clear; it must be very different from that of lithium. It may reduce the sensitization of the brain to repeated episodes of mood swing.

The doses used in the treatment of bipolar affective disorder and epilepsy are similar (roughly 800–1000 mg/d), as are the side effects.

REFERENCES

Antipsychotics

Carlsson A: Antipsychotic drugs, neurotransmitters and schizophrenia. *Am J Psychiatry* 1978;**135**:164.

Chouinard G, Jones BD: Neuroleptic-induced supersensitivity psychosis: Clinical and pharmacologic characteristics. *Am J Psychiatry* 1980;**137**:16.

Crow TJ: Molecular pathology of schizophrenia: More than one disease process? *Br Med J* 1980;**280**:66.

Dahl SG: Plasma level monitoring of antipsychotic drugs: Clinical utility. *Clin Pharmacokinet* 1986;**11**:36.

Donlon PT, Tupin JP: Successful suicides with thioridazine and mesoridazine. *Arch Gen Psychiatry* 1977;**34**:955.

Hamblin M, Creese I: Receptor binding and the discovery of psychotherapeutic drugs. *Drug Dev Res* 1981;**1**:343.

Hollister LE: Drug treatment of schizophrenia. *Psychiatr Clin North Am* 1984;**7**:435.

Hollister LE, Kim DY: Intensive treatment with haloperidol of treatment-resistant chronic schizophrenic patients. *Am J Psychiatry* 1982;**39**:1466.

Jann MW, Ereshefsky L, Saklad SR: Clinical pharmacokinetics of the depot antipsychotics. *Clin Pharmacokinet* 1985;**10**:315.

Kovelman JA, Scheiber AB: Biological substrates of schizophrenia. *Acta Neurol Scand* 1986;**73**:1.

Lehmann HE, Wilson WH, Deutsch M: Minimal maintenance medication: Effects of three dose schedules on relapse rates and symptoms in chronic schizophrenic outpatients. *Compr Psychiatry* 1983;**24**:293.

Levenson JL: Neuroleptic malignant syndrome. *Am J Psychiatry* 1985;**142**:1137.

Magliozzi JR et al: Relationship of serum haloperidol levels to clinical response in schizophrenic patients. *Am J Psychiatry* 1981;**138**:365.

Richelson E: Neuroleptic affinities for human brain receptors and their use in predicting adverse effects. *J Clin Psychiatry* 1984;**45**:331.

Schooler NR et al: Prevention of relapse in schizophrenia. *Arch Gen Psychiatry* 1980;**37**:16.

Simpson GM, Pi EH, Sramek JJ: An update on tardive dyskinesia. *Hosp Community Psychiatry* 1986;**37**:362.

Stevens JR: Schizophrenia and dopamine regulation in the mesolimbic system. *Trends Neurosci* 1979;**1**:102.

Thompson LT, Moran MG, Nies AS: Psychotropic drug use in the elderly. (2 parts.) *N Engl J Med* 1983;**308**:134, 194.

Mood Stabilizers

Albrecht J, Kampf D, Müller-Oerlinghausen B: Renal function and biopsy in patients on lithium therapy. *Pharmakopsychiatr Neuropsychopharmakol* 1980;**13**:228.

Bendz H, Andersch S, Aurell M: Kidney function in an unselected lithium population: A cross-sectional study. *Acta Psychiatr Scand* 1983;**68**:325.

Bunney WE Jr et al: Mode of action of lithium: Some biological considerations. *Arch Gen Psychiatry* 1979;**36**:898.

Consensus Development Conference. *Mood Disorders: Pharmacologic Prevention of Recurrences.* Consensus Statement. Vol 5, No. 4. National Institutes of Health, Bethesda, MD, 1984.

Danielson DA et al: Drug toxicity and hospitalization among lithium users. *J Clin Psychopharmacol* 1984;**4**:108.

Evans RW, Gualtieri CT: Carbamazepine: A neuropsychological and psychiatric profile. *Clin Neuropharmacol* 1985;**8**:221.

Goodwin FW (editor): Lithium ion. *Arch Gen Psychiatry* 1979;**36**:833.

Grof P, Lane J: Lithium: Current issues. *Prog Neuropsychopharmacol Biol Psychiatry* 1984;**8**:539.

Hansen HE, Amdisen A: Lithium intoxication: Report of 23 cases and review of 100 cases from the literature. *Q J Med* 1978;**186**:123.

Jefferson JW, Greist JH: *Primer of Lithium Therapy.* Williams & Wilkins, 1977.

Post RM et al: Dopaminergic effects of carbamazepine. *Arch Gen Psychiatry* 1986;**43**:393.

Report of the APA Task Force: The current status of lithium therapy. *Am J Psychiatry* 1975;**132**:997.

Thornhill DP: The biological disposition and kinetics of lithium. *Biopharm Drug Dispos* 1981;**2**:305.

Vestergaard P, Amdisen A, Schou M: Clinically significant side effects of lithium treatment: A survey of 237 patients in long-term treatment. *Acta Psychiatr Scand* 1980;**62**:193.

53

Antidepressants

Leo E. Hollister, MD

BASIC PHARMACOLOGY OF ANTIDEPRESSANTS

Chemical Structures

A variety of different chemical structures have been found to have antidepressant activity. The number is constantly growing, but as yet no group has been found to have a clear therapeutic advantage over the others. Table 53–1 lists some clinically used antidepressants and their trade names.

A. Tricyclics: (Fig 53–1.) Tricyclic antidepressants—so called because of the characteristic 3-ring nucleus—have been used clinically for over 2 decades. They closely resemble the phenothiazines chemically and, to a lesser extent, pharmacologically. Like the latter drugs, they were first thought to be useful as antihistamines and later as antipsychotics. The discovery of their antidepressant properties was a fortuitous clinical observation. Imipramine and amitriptyline are the prototypical drugs of the class and the most commonly used.

B. Monoamine Oxidase (MAO) Inhibitors: (Fig 53–2.) MAO inhibitors may be classified as hydrazides, exemplified by the C–N–N moiety, as in phenelzine and isocarboxazid; or nonhydrazides, which lack such a moiety, as in tranylcypromine. Tranylcypromine bears a close resemblance to dex-

Table 53–1. Usual daily doses of antidepressants.

Drug	Dose (mg)
Tricyclics	
Amitriptyline (Elavil, etc)	75–200
Clomipramine*	75–300
Desipramine (Norpramin, Pertofrane)	75–200
Doxepin (Adapin, Sinequan)	75–300
Imipramine (Tofranil, etc)	75–200
Nortriptyline (Aventyl, Pamelor)	75–150
Protriptyline (Triptil, Vivactil)	20–40
Trimipramine (Surmontil)	75–200
Monoamine oxidase inhibitors	
Isocarboxazid (Marplan)	20–50
Phenelzine (Nardil)	45–75
Tranylcypromine (Parnate)	10–30
Tetracyclics	
Maprotiline (Ludiomil)	75–300
Dibenzazepines	
Amoxapine (Asendin)	150–300
Miscellaneous	
Trazodone (Desyrel)	50–600

*In the USA, investigational use only

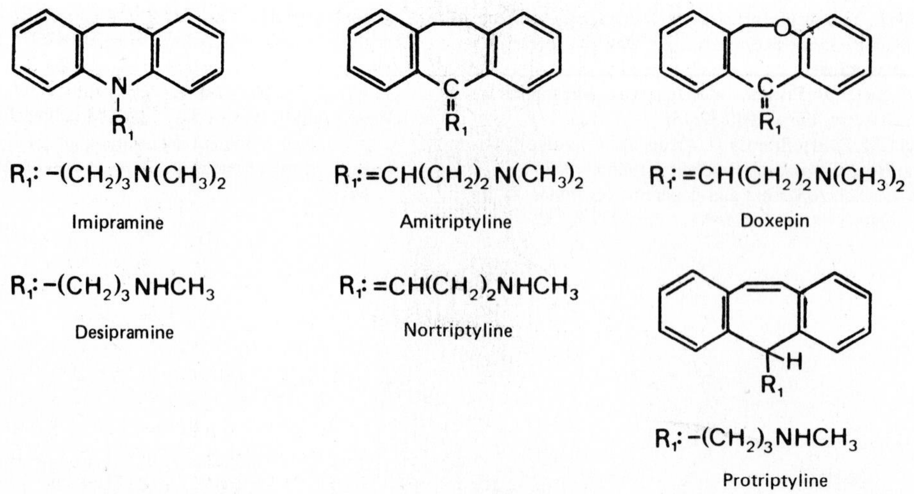

R_1: –(CH$_2$)$_3$N(CH$_3$)$_2$
Imipramine

R_1: –(CH$_2$)$_3$NHCH$_3$
Desipramine

R_1: =CH(CH$_2$)$_2$N(CH$_3$)$_2$
Amitriptyline

R_1: =CH(CH$_2$)$_2$NHCH$_3$
Nortriptyline

R_1: =CH(CH$_2$)$_2$N(CH$_3$)$_2$
Doxepin

R_1: –(CH$_2$)$_3$NHCH$_3$
Protriptyline

Figure 53–1. Structural relationships between various tricyclic antidepressants.

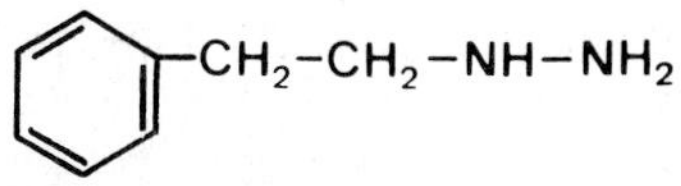

Phenelzine

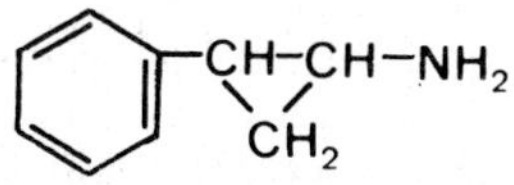

Tranylcypromine

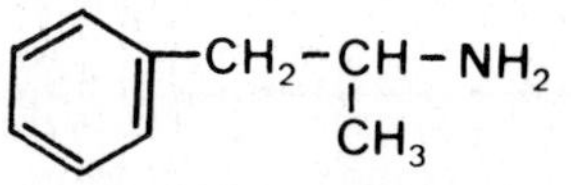

Dextroamphetamine

Figure 53–2. Some monoamine oxidase inhibitors. Phenelzine has a hydrazide configuration, while tranylcypromine has a cyclopropyl amine side chain compared with the isopropyl amine side chain of dextroamphetamine.

troamphetamine, which is itself a weak inhibitor of MAO. It retains some of the sympathomimetic characteristics of the amphetamines.

C. Sympathomimetic Stimulants: Dextroamphetamine, other amphetamines, and amphetamine surrogates such as pipradrol and methylphenidate are occasionally used as antidepressants. Although the action of amphetamines in blocking MAO has generally been regarded as too weak to confer significant antidepressant action, it may contribute to an antidepressant action in some people.

D. "Second-Generation" Drugs: (Fig 53–3.) Three new antidepressant drugs (amoxapine, maprotiline, and trazodone) are currently available in the USA, and several more may soon be approved for marketing. Some have unconventional structures, and some differ greatly from tricyclics in their pharmacologic effects, especially in their actions on aminergic neurotransmitters. No claim for increased efficacy over tricyclics has been substantiated, but claims are made that to varying degrees, these newer agents may work more quickly or have fewer adverse effects.

Amoxapine is a metabolite of the antipsychotic drug loxapine and retains some of its antipsychotic ac-

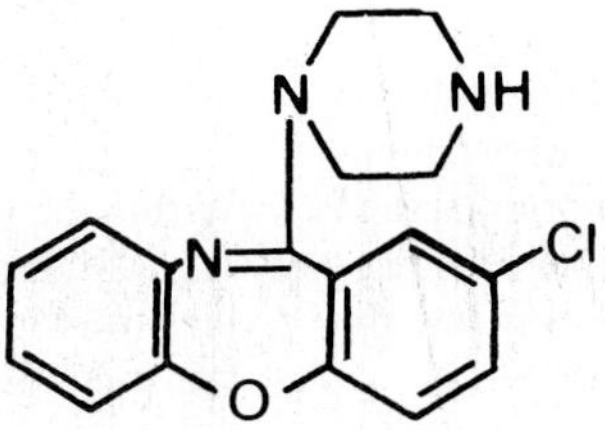

Amoxapine

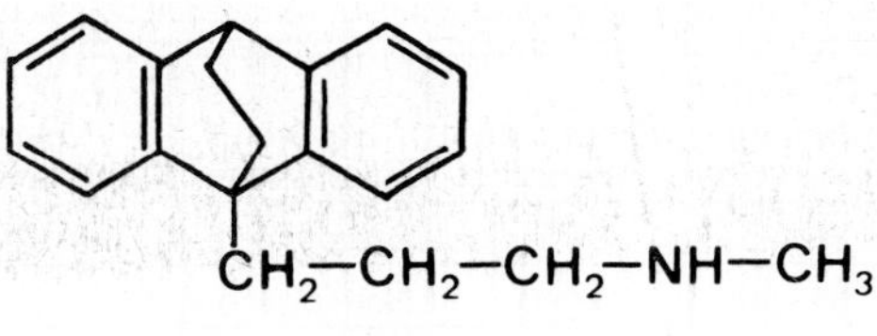

Maprotiline

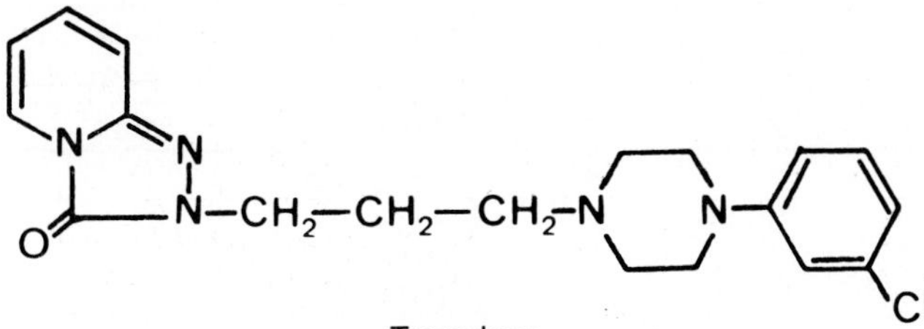

Trazodone

Figure 53–3. Some "second-generation" antidepressants.

tion. A combination of antidepressant and antipsychotic actions might make it a suitable drug for psychotically depressed patients. On the other hand, the antipsychotic action may cause akathisia, parkinsonism, amenorrhea-galactorrhea syndrome, and perhaps tardive dyskinesia. Maprotiline (a "tetracyclic" drug) is most like desipramine, even to the point of some structural resemblance. Like the latter drug, it may have less marked sedative and anticholinergic actions than the older tricyclics. Its major disadvantage is that it tends to evoke seizures at the top range of therapeutic doses. Trazodone is the most novel drug of the lot. Clinical experience has indicated unpredictable efficacy: Some patients do remarkably well, while others obtain scarcely any benefit. Many other new antidepressants are currently under clinical investigation—mainly drugs that block uptake of serotonin.

Pharmacokinetics

The pharmacokinetic parameters of various antidepressants are summarized in Table 53–2.

A. Tricyclics: Absorption of most tricyclics is incomplete, and there is significant first-pass metabolism. As a result of high protein binding and relatively high lipid solubility, volumes of distribution tend to be very large. Tricyclics are metabolized by 2 major routes: transformation of the tricyclic nucleus and alteration of the aliphatic side chain. The former route involves ring hydroxylation and conjugation to form glucuronides; the latter, primarily demethylation of the nitrogen. Monodemethylation of tertiary amines leads to active metabolites, such as desipramine and nortriptyline (Fig 53–1). The proportion of monodemethylated metabolites formed varies from one patient to another. In general, the proportion of amitriptyline to its metabolite nortriptyline favors the parent drug. The converse is the case with imipramine and its metabolite desipramine.

B. MAO Inhibitors: These drugs produce an "irreversible" inhibition of MAO that persists even after the drug is no longer detectable in plasma. In following the effectiveness of a dosage regimen, it has been more useful to measure the inhibition of MAO activity in platelets than to measure the plasma levels of the drug directly. Present feeling is that optimal antidepressant effect from these drugs requires about 60–80% inhibition of the enzyme—a degree achieved with doses of approximately 1 mg/kg/d of phenelzine.

C. "Second-Generation" Drugs: The pharmacokinetics of these drugs and of the tricyclics are similar. Although the claim for many "second-generation" drugs is faster onset of clinical action, neither a pharmacokinetic nor a pharmacodynamic explanation for this clinical effect is apparent. Some of these drugs are said to have less cardiotoxicity than tricyclics when taken in overdose quantities.

Pharmacodynamics

Drugs used to treat mental depression are not central nervous system stimulants and are actually contraindicated in organic or drug-induced central nervous system depression. Studies of the mode of action of antidepressants have largely focused on the effects on various aminergic neurotransmitters in the brain.

A. Effects on Aminergic Neurotransmitters: Soon after the introduction of reserpine in the early 1950s, it became apparent that the drug could induce depression in patients being treated for hypertension and schizophrenia as well as in normal subjects. Within the next few years, pharmacologic studies revealed that the principal mechanism of action of reserpine was to inhibit the storage of aminergic neurotransmitters such as serotonin and norepinephrine in the vesicles of presynaptic nerve endings. Reserpine induced depression and depleted stores of aminergic neurotransmitters; therefore, it was reasoned, depres-

Table 53–2. Pharmacokinetic parameters of various antidepressants.

Drug	Bioavailability (percent)	Protein Binding (percent)	Plasma $t^{1/2}$ (hours)	Active Metabolites	Volume of Distribution (L/kg)	Therapeutic Plasma Concentrations (ng/mL)
Imipramine	29–77	76–95	9–24	Desipramine	15–30	>180 total
Amitriptyline	31–61	82–96	31–46	Nortriptyline	5–10	80–200 total
Nortriptyline	32–79	93–95	18–93	10-Hydroxy	21–57	50–150
Desipramine	60–70	73–90	14–62	*	22–59	145†
Protriptyline	*	90–95	54–198	*	19–57	70–170
Doxepin	13–45	*	8–24	Desmethyl	9–33	30–150
Clomipramine	*	*	22–84	Desmethyl	7–20	240–700
Maprotiline	37–67	88	36–108	Desmethyl	15–28	200–300
Amoxapine	*	*	8	7,8-Hydroxy	*	200–400
Trazodone	*	89–95	8	m-Chlorophenylpiperazine	*	*

*No data available.
†Lower concentrations may be effective, but no data are available.
‡In the USA, investigational use only.

Table 53–3. Pharmacologic differences among several tricyclic antidepressants. (0=none, +=slight, ++=moderate, +++=high.)

Drug	Sedation	Anticholinergic Effects	Block of Amine Pump	
			For Serotonin	For Norepinephrine
Imipramine	++	++	++	++
Amitriptyline	+++	+++	+++	+
Desipramine	+	+	0	+++
Nortriptyline	++	++	+	++
Doxepin	+++	+++	Weak	
Protriptyline	0	++	Not known	

sion must be associated with decreased functional aminergic transmission. This simple syllogism provided the basis for what became known as the amine hypothesis of depression (see Chapters 11 and 30)

The amine hypothesis was buttressed by studies on the mechanism of action of various types of antidepressant drugs. Tricyclics block the amine reuptake pump, the "off switch" of aminergic neurotransmission (Table 53–3). Such an action presumably permits a longer sojourn of neurotransmitter at the receptor site. MAO inhibitors block a major degradative pathway for the aminergic neurotransmitters, which presumably permits more amines to accumulate presynaptically and more to be released. Amphetaminelike sympathomimetics also block the amine pump but are thought to act chiefly by increasing the release of catecholaminergic neurotransmitters. Thus, these 3 classes of antidepressant drugs might remedy a deficiency in aminergic neurotransmission, although by somewhat different mechanisms. Some of the "second-generation" antidepressants have similar effects on aminergic neurotransmitters, while others have mild or minimal effects.

Increased aminergic neurotransmitters in the synapse were long thought to *increase* postsynaptic responses in a deficient system. Such conclusions were based on observations of the results of acute dosage. Clinically, however, drugs are given chronically for their antidepressant action. When they are administered chronically to animals and the postsynaptic consequences are measured by the generation of cAMP, *subsensitivity* of the postsynaptic receptor is observed. Thus, the evidence now strongly suggests that downstream neurotransmission is *decreased* rather than increased.

B. Peripheral Effects: See Adverse Reactions, below.

CLINICAL PHARMACOLOGY OF ANTIDEPRESSANTS

Indications

The major indication for antidepressants is to treat depression, but a number of other uses have been established by clinical experience.

A. Depression: This indication has been kept broad deliberately, even though evidence from clinical studies strongly suggests that the drugs are specifically useful only in major depressive episodes. Major depressive episodes are diagnosed not so much by their severity as by their quality. Formerly, they were referred to as "endogenous," "vital," or "vegetative"— reflecting the characteristic disturbances of major body rhythms of sleep, hunger and appetite, sexual drive, and motor activity. The diagnosis of major depression may be uncertain in individual patients, so that on balance it is probably better to treat too many patients with tricyclics than to miss treating those who might benefit.

The decision to start treatment with an antidepressant rests on a number of variables. The more the depression conforms to the criteria for major depressive episode, melancholic type (see Chapter 30), the more likely an antidepressant will produce benefit. Prior attacks of depression, affective disorder in first-degree relatives, "vegetative" symptoms, and autonomy (the lack of any clear relationship between the degree of depression and life experiences) provide the strongest indications. A depressed mood associated with adverse life events, such as the loss of a loved one or of one's job, may turn out to be transitory. Such brief adjustment disorders with depressed mood are not indications for treatment with antidepressants. It should be remembered that anxiety is an inevitable concomitant symptom, so that every patient complaining of anxiety should be questioned about symptoms that may be more specific to depression. Too many such patients are treated, often ineffectively, with antianxiety agents rather than antidepressants. Patients with severe depressions and the potential for suicide should be hospitalized and considered for immediate treatment with electroconvulsive therapy. Antidepressants may be given concurrently and may reduce the number of electroconvulsive treatments required for remission as well as maintain remission once electroconvulsive therapy has been stopped.

B. Enuresis: Enuresis is an established indication for tricyclics. Proof of efficacy for this indication is substantial, but drug therapy is not the preferred approach. The beneficial effect of drug treatment lasts only as long as drug treatment is continued.

C. Chronic Pain: Clinicians in pain clinics have found tricyclics to be especially useful for treating a variety of chronically painful states that often cannot be definitely diagnosed. Whether such painful states represent depressive equivalents or whether such patients become secondarily depressed after some initial pain-producing insult is not clear. It is even possible that the tricyclics (sometimes phenothiazines are also used in combination) work directly on the pain pathways.

D. Other Indications: Less frequent and less well documented indications include obsessive compulsive phobic states; cataplexy associated with narcolepsy; acute panic attacks; school phobia; minimal brain damage with hyperkinesis in children; and bulimia.

Choice of Drug

Controlled comparisons of the antidepressants have usually led to the conclusion that they are roughly equivalent drugs. Although this may be true for groups of patients, individual patients may for uncertain reasons fare better on one drug than on another. Thus, finding the right drug for the patient must be accomplished empirically at present. The past history of the patient's drug experience, if available, is the most valuable guide. At times such a history may lead to the exclusion of tricyclics, as in the case of patients who have responded well in the past to MAO inhibitors.

Tricyclic antidepressant drugs are apt to be most successful in patients with clearly "vegetative" characteristics, including psychomotor retardation, sleep disturbance, poor appetite and weight loss, and loss of libido. MAO inhibitors in adequate doses may also be useful for such patients.

Tricyclics differ mainly in the degree of sedation (amitriptyline and doxepin have the most, protriptyline the least) and the amount of anticholinergic effects (amitriptyline and doxepin have the most, desipramine the least) (Table 53–3). Although it is often argued that the more sedative drugs are preferable for patients with markedly anxious or agitated depressive states while the least sedative drugs are preferable for patients with psychomotor withdrawal, this hypothesis has not been tested.

MAO inhibitors are helpful in patients described as having "atypical" depressions—a nonspecific designation scarcely helpful in their identification. Depressed patients with considerable attendant anxiety, phobic features, and hypochondriasis are the ones who respond best to these drugs. Either phenelzine or tranylcypromine may be used.

A claim made for some "second-generation" antidepressants is that they act more quickly. For patients in whom a rapid response is especially desirable, a drug such as amoxapine might be tried. Another claim is that some of the drugs (eg, trazodone) have less marked anticholinergic side effects than most tricyclics. These effects can be a limiting factor for many patients—limiting either the dose of drug tolerated or the patient's willingness to take the drug. One of the

newer agents might be considered for such patients. Finally, some of the newer drugs seem not to have the cardiotoxic effects of the tricyclics when they are taken in overdose quantities. Accordingly, patients with major heart problems might best be treated with a less hazardous drug.

Few clinicians use lithium, a mood stabilizer, as primary treatment for depression. However, some have found that lithium along with one of the other antidepressants may achieve a favorable response not obtained by the antidepressant alone. Another potential use of lithium is to prevent relapses of depression. Such antidepressant effects may be secondary to lithium's proved mood-stabilizing effect in bipolar affective disorder, as many patients with this disorder may present with depressive episodes, with mania not being apparent until later in the course.

Doses & Dosage Schedules

The usual dose ranges of antidepressants are shown in Table 53–1. Doses are almost always determined empirically; the patient's acceptance of side effects is the usual limiting factor. Tolerance to some of the objectionable side effects may develop, so that the usual pattern of treatment has been to start with small doses, increasing either to a predetermined daily dose, or to one that produces relief of depression, or to the maximum tolerated dose. The effective dose of an antidepressant varies widely depending upon many factors. Undertreatment has been thought to be a frequent cause of apparent failure of drug therapy to relieve depression.

For treatment of the acute episode, the initial doses of a tricyclic may vary from 10 to 75 mg on the first day of treatment, depending on the patient's size and tolerance for the acute effects. If a first goal is to attain a daily dose of 150 mg, increments of 25 mg may be added every second or third day until this level is reached.

The plasma half-lives of many antidepressants are long enough so that single daily doses in the early evening hours can be used (Table 53–2). The sedative and anticholinergic actions of these drugs are less bothersome when the drug is taken in the evening. However, the patient should be warned of these side effects and should construe them as evidence of the action of the drug. Patients should be warned also that noticeable improvement may be slow, perhaps taking 3 weeks or more. Inability to tolerate side effects and discouragement with treatment are 2 major causes for noncompliance and for failure of tricyclics to relieve depression.

Monitoring of Plasma Concentrations

Routine monitoring of plasma concentrations of antidepressants, while technically feasible for most drugs, is still of uncertain value. Experience with monitoring of plasma concentrations of tricyclics suggests that about 20% of patients become noncompliant at some time or other. Thus, a "poor response" in a patient for whom an adequate dosage of drug has been prescribed may be shown by measurement of the plasma drug concentration to be due merely to failure to take the drug. Blood for plasma drug level determinations should be obtained in the postabsorptive state, about 10–12 hours after the last dose. Even when sampling time is constant, the same patient may show variation in both the total plasma concentration and the proportion of parent drug versus metabolites while on a constant dose at steady-state conditions. Under no circumstances should the laboratory test results be permitted to overrule the physician's clinical judgment.

Unresponsive Patients

Almost one-third of patients receiving tricyclic antidepressants fail to respond. In evaluating a patient's resistance to treatment, one should consider the five *d's*: diagnosis, drug, dose, duration of treatment, and different treatment. Failure to respond to 2 or 3 weeks of treatment with most tricyclics at a daily dose of 150 mg, with plasma concentrations within the presumed therapeutic range, suggests the need for reassessment of the diagnosis. If the patient actually has bipolar affective disorder, lithium may be added. On the other hand, a patient with an adjustment disorder with depressed mood (reactive depression) may be overly sensitive to the side effects of the drugs and be better managed without them. It is often said that failure to respond to one tricyclic calls for a trial of therapy with another tricyclic, but there is no evidence to support that view unless the problem is related to poor tolerance of side effects. Some patients unresponsive to tricyclics are responsive to MAO inhibitors, which should be considered in all such cases. A few patients, especially elderly ones, seem to respond specifically to sympathomimetic stimulants such as dextroamphetamine. "Second-generation" drugs may be tried after failure with both tricyclics and MAO inhibitors. Finally, some patients may need a completely different type of treatment. Patients with adjustment disorders with depressed mood (reactive depression) need to deal with the precipitating event.

Electroconvulsive therapy is often viewed as a treatment of last resort for endogenous depression, but it should not be withheld from patients with this disorder who cannot be helped by drug therapy.

Drug Combinations

Combination therapy using tricyclics and MAO inhibitors has been recommended, although recent controlled trials do not suggest any special virtues for such combinations. Tricyclics should be combined with lithium or antipsychotics for treating psychotic depressions or the depressed phase of bipolar affective disorder.

Maintenance Treatment

Whether or not to undertake long-term maintenance treatment of a depressed patient depends entirely on the natural history of the disorder. If the depressive episode was the patient's first and if it responded quickly and satisfactorily to drug therapy, it is rational to gradually withdraw treatment over a period of a few months. If relapse does not occur, drug treatment can be stopped until the next attack occurs, which is unpredictable but nearly certain. On the other hand, a patient who has had several previous attacks of depression, especially if each succeeding attack was more severe and more difficult to treat, is a prime candidate for maintenance therapy.

Considerable controversy exists concerning the proper duration of treatment of a major depressive episode. Most clinicians treat with full dosage for 2–6 months, after which some discontinue therapy; others reduce the dose to one-half or one-third of the initial level. Some patients have been on maintenance treatment for years with apparent good control of their illness and no long-term adverse effects. Members of the household should be instructed in how to detect early signs of relapse; the patients themselves may be poor judges of that.

Adverse Reactions

Adverse effects of tricyclic antidepressants are summarized in Table 53–4. Most common unwanted effects are minor, but they may seriously affect the acceptance of drug treatment by the patient; the more seriously depressed the patient is, the more likely it is that unwanted effects will be tolerated. Most normal persons find that even moderate doses of these drugs cause disagreeable symptoms.

A. Sedative Effects: Although we think of antidepressants as "activators," tricyclics—with the possible exception of protriptyline—are strongly sedative. Complaints of lassitude, fatigue, and loss of energy are common, especially early in treatment. If doses are too high, the patient may sleep at inappropriate times. Sedative effects are less bothersome when a single daily dose is taken at night. MAO inhibitors—especially those with sympathomimetic actions, such as tranylcypromine—may produce mild degrees of stimulation.

B. Sympathomimetic Effects: Sympathomimetic effects of various antidepressants are usually obscured by other more prominent actions on the autonomic nervous system. However, tremor is extremely common (see Neurologic Effects, below).

C. Anticholinergic Effects: Dry mouth, constipation, urinary hesitancy, and loss of visual accommodation are the most frequent anticholinergic side effects. More extensive anticholinergic action may result in paralytic ileus or urinary retention, especially in elderly patients. Treatment with bethanechol, a peripherally acting cholinomimetic, may counter the peripheral anticholinergic action of the tricyclics.

D. Cardiovascular Effects: Palpitation, tachycardia, and orthostatic hypotension were recognized early as unwanted effects of these drugs. Later, arrhythmias and electrocardiographic abnormalities were described. Congestive heart failure and sudden death are rare complications.

E. Psychiatric Effects: Some patients may be-

Table 53–4. Side effects of tricyclic antidepressants.

Type	Minor, Early	Major
Sedative	Lassitude, fatigue.	Sleepiness; impaired consciousness with alcohol and other drugs.
Sympathomimetic	Tachycardia, tremor, sweating.	Agitation, insomnia, aggravation of psychosis.
Anticholinergic	Blurred vision, constipation, urinary hesitancy, fuzzy thinking.	Aggravation of glaucoma, paralytic ileus, urinary retention, delirium.
Cardiovascular	Orthostatic hypotension, electrocardiographic abnormalities.	Delayed cardiac conduction, arrhythmias, cardiomyopathy; sudden death.
Psychiatric	Confusion.	Central anticholinergic syndrome, withdrawal.
Neurologic	Tremor, paresthesias, electroencephalographic alterations.	Seizures, neuropathy.
Allergic/toxic		Cholestatic jaundice, agranulocytosis.
Metabolic/endocrine	Weight gain, sexual disturbances.	Gynecomastia, amenorrhea.
Birth defects		Uncertain.

come agitated and manic with tricyclics, but one should always consider the possibility that they actually have bipolar affective disorder. Confusional reactions are most often seen in patients over 40 years of age. The situation may be made worse if the patient is also receiving other drugs with anticholinergic action, such as antipsychotics or antiparkinsonism drugs.

A central anticholinergic syndrome consisting of delirium, anxiety, hyperactivity, hallucinations, disorientation, and seizures has been described for many drugs with anticholinergic action, especially when they are taken in combination. A good general rule is that any patient showing new or bizarre mental symptoms while receiving antidepressant medication should have the drug discontinued until the situation can be appraised. Most cases respond quickly to simple discontinuation of the drug.

F. Neurologic Effects: Tremor is common and is more similar to essential tremor than to the tremor of Parkinson's disease. Treatment with a beta-blocking drug such as propranolol or nadolol may be helpful. Paresthesias are less common and may herald the rare development of peripheral neuropathy. Other neurologic abnormalities are usually signs of therapeutic overdoses. Although Parkinson's syndrome has been reported, it is extremely rare. Tardive dyskinesia has not occurred.

G. Allergic or Toxic Reactions: Skin rashes are uncommon. Cholestatic jaundice and agranulocytosis have been reported but are now so rare as to hardly merit consideration.

H. Metabolic and Endocrine Effects: Weight

gain is frequent with these drugs, just as it is with the phenothiazines. It may be due in part to increased appetite with remission of depression, but a central action is probably responsible also. Some patients have complained of a craving for sweets, and beverages containing sugar are often used to relieve dry mouth.

The syndrome of inappropriate secretion of antidiuretic hormone has been reported with various tricyclics.

I. Effects of Use During Pregnancy: As is the case with so many drugs, it is not clear whether or not the antidepressant drugs have been responsible for birth defects in infants born to mothers taking the drugs early in pregnancy. The evidence is not very persuasive, and the results of national surveys are equivocal.

Drug Interactions

A. Pharmacodynamic Interactions: Some pharmacodynamic interactions of antidepressants with other drugs have already been discussed. Sedative effects may be additive with other sedatives, especially alcohol. Patients taking tricyclics should be warned that use of alcohol may lead to greater than usual impairment of driving ability. MAO inhibitors, by increasing stores of catecholamines, sensitize the patient to indirectly acting sympathomimetics such as tyramine, which is found in many fermented foods and beverages, and to sympathomimetic drugs that may be administered therapeutically, such as diethylpropion or phenylpropanolamine.

B. Pharmacokinetic Interactions: Reversal of the antihypertensive action of guanethidine is a dramatic interaction. The blood pressure not only returns quickly to high levels but may overshoot to dangerously high levels. Guanethidine is concentrated in sympathetic nerve endings by the same amine pump that is blocked by tricyclics. Thus, it is prevented from reaching its site of action. A similar reversal of action of other antihypertensives, such as methyldopa and clonidine, has been described. Although doxepin is less likely than other tricyclics to produce this interaction, because it is considerably less potent in blocking the amine pump, interaction can occur with high doses of the drug. MAO inhibitors predictably prolong the half-lives of the many drugs that are oxidatively deaminated.

Overdoses

Tricyclics are extremely dangerous when taken in overdose quantities, and depressed patients are more likely than others to be suicidal. Prescriptions should therefore be limited to amounts less than 1.25 g, or 50 dose units of 25 mg, on a "no refill" basis. If suicide is a serious possibility, the tablets should be entrusted to a family member. The drugs must be kept away from children.

Both accidental and deliberate overdoses are frequent and are a serious medical emergency. Major symptoms include (1) coma with shock and sometimes metabolic acidosis; (2) respiratory depression with a tendency to sudden apnea; (3) agitation or delirium both before and after consciousness is obtunded; (4) neuromuscular irritability and seizures; (5) hyperpyrexia; (6) bowel and bladder paralysis; and (7) a great variety of cardiac manifestations, including conduction defects and arrhythmias. Cardiac problems are the principal distinguishing features.

Management of cardiac problems is difficult. Antiarrhythmic drugs having the least depressant effect on cardiac conduction should be used. Lidocaine, propranolol, and phenytoin have been used successfully, but quinidine and procainamide are contraindicated. Physostigmine given in small (0.5-mg) intravenous boluses to a total dose of 3–4 mg may awaken the patient and reverse a rapid supraventricular arrhythmia. It is *unlikely* to be effective for ventricular arrhythmias. Continual cardiac monitoring is essential, and facilities must be at hand for resuscitation if needed. Arterial blood gases and pH should be measured frequently, since both hypoxia and metabolic acidosis predispose to arrhythmias. Sodium bicarbonate and intravenous potassium chloride may be required to restore acid-base balance and to correct hypokalemia. Electrical pacing must be used in refractory cases.

Other treatment is entirely supportive. After placement of a cuffed endotracheal tube, attempts should be made to remove residual drug from the gastrointestinal tract. Absorption may be slow because of the strong anticholinergic effects. Activated charcoal may be used to bind the drug, which may subsequently be removed by catharsis. Ventilatory assistance is of prime importance. Shock is best treated with fluids or plasma expanders, since adrenergic receptors may be blocked. Hyperpyrexia is treated by cooling. Seizures may be treated with intravenous phenytoin (which may also double as an antiarrhythmic agent) or diazepam. Patients should not be discharged until they have been conscious for a day or 2 and most abnormal signs have disappeared. Measurement of plasma concentrations of the drug may be helpful in deciding about the safety of discharge. Virtually all patients who survive recover completely with no permanent sequelae.

Intoxication with MAO inhibitors is unusual. Agitation, delirium, and neuromuscular excitability are followed by obtunded consciousness, seizures, shock, and hyperthermia. Supportive treatment is usually all that is required, although sedative phenothiazines with alpha-adrenergic receptor-blocking action, such as chlorpromazine, may be useful.

Overdoses of trazodone have been easily managed and are not life-threatening. Overdoses of maprotiline produce problems similar to those caused by tricyclic overdoses. Amoxapine produces neurologic rather than cardiac toxicity. Seizures may be difficult to control. Overdoses of amoxapine have led to death and permanent brain damage.

REFERENCES

Callaham M, Kassel D: Epidemiology of fatal tricyclic antidepressant ingestion: Implications for management. *Ann Emerg Med* 1985;**14**:1.

Costa E et al: Molecular mechanisms in the action of imipramine. *Experientia* 1983;**39**:855.

Davis JM: Overview: Maintenance therapy in psychiatry. 2. Affective disorders. *Am J Psychiatry* 1976;**133**:1.

Feinmann C: Pain relief by antidepressants: Possible modes of action. *Pain* 1985;**23**:1.

Garver DL, Davis JM: Biogenic amine hypothesis of affective disorders. *Life Sci* 1979;**24**:383.

Hollister LE: Current antidepressants. *Annu Rev Pharmacol Toxicol* 1986;**26**:23.

Hollister LE: Monitoring tricyclic antidepressant plasma concentrations. *JAMA* 1979;**241**:2530.

Hollister LE: Treatment of depression with drugs. *Ann Intern Med* 1978;**89**:78.

Hughes PL et al: Treating bulimia with desipramine: A double-blind placebo-controlled study. *Arch Gen Psychiatry* 1986;**43**:182.

Jarvik LF, Kakkar PR: Aging and response to antidepressants. Chap 4, pp 49–77, in: *Clinical Pharmacology and the Aged Patient.* Jarvik LF et al (editors). Raven, 1982.

Maxwell RA: Second-generation antidepressants: The pharmacological and clinical significance of selected examples. *Drug Dev Res* 1983;**3**:203.

Morris JB, Beck AT: The efficacy of antidepressant drugs. *Arch Gen Psychiatry* 1974;**30**:667.

Pentel PR, Benowitz NL: Tricyclic antidepressant poisoning: Management of arrhythmias. *Med Toxicol* 1986;**1**:101.

Prien RF, Kupfer DJ: Continuation drug therapy for major depressive episodes: How long should it be maintained? *Am J Psychiatry* 1986;**143**:18.

Sugrue MF: Do antidepressants possess a common mechanism of action? *Biochem Pharmacol* 1983;**32**:1811.

Tang SW, Seeman P: Effect of antidepressant drugs on serotonergic and adrenergic receptors. *Naunyn Schmiedebergs Arch Pharmacol* 1980;**311**:255.

Veith RC et al: Cardiovascular effects of tricyclic antidepressants in depressed patients with chronic heart disease. *N Engl J Med* 1982;**306**:954.

54

Drugs Used for Anxiety States & Sleep Problems

Anthony J. Trevor, PhD, & Walter L. Way, MD

I. BASIC PHARMACOLOGY OF SEDATIVE-HYPNOTICS

Drug classifications are often based on clinical uses rather than on similarities in chemical structures or mechanisms of action. Assignment of a particular compound to the sedative-hypnotic class of drugs indicates that its major therapeutic use is to cause sedation (with concomitant relief of anxiety) or to encourage sleep. These clinical uses are of such magnitude that sedative-hypnotics are among the most frequently prescribed drugs worldwide.

An effective **sedative** (or anxiolytic agent) should reduce anxiety and exert a calming effect with little or no effect on motor or mental functions. The degree of central nervous system depression caused by a sedative should be the minimum consistent with therapeutic efficacy. A **hypnotic** drug should produce drowsiness and encourage the onset and maintenance of a state of sleep that as far as possible resembles the natural sleep state. Hypnotic effects involve more pronounced depression of the central nervous system than sedation, and this can be achieved with most sedative drugs simply by increasing the dose.

Graded dose-dependent depression of central nervous system function is a characteristic of sedative-hypnotics. However, individual sedative-hypnotic drugs may differ in the relationship between the dose and the degree of central nervous system depression. Two examples of such dose-response relationships are shown in Fig 54–1. The linear slope for drug A is typical of many of the older sedative-hypnotics, particularly drugs in the barbiturate class. An increase in dose above that needed for hypnosis may lead to a state of general anesthesia. At still higher doses, such sedative-hypnotics may depress respiratory and vasomotor centers in the medulla, leading to coma and death. Deviations from a linear dose-response relationship, as shown for drug B, will require proportionately greater dosage increments in order to achieve central nervous system depressant effects more profound than those required for hypnosis. This appears to be the case for most drugs of the benzodiazepine class, and the greater margin of safety this offers is an important rea-

son for their extensive clinical use to treat anxiety states and disorders of sleep.

Chemical Classification

The benzodiazepines (Fig 54–2) are the most important sedative-hypnotics. All of the structures shown are 1,4-benzodiazepines, and most contain a carboxamide group in the 7-membered heterocyclic ring structure. A substituent in the 7 position, such as a halogen or a nitro group, is required for sedative-hypnotic activity. The structures of triazolam and alprazolam include 1,2-annelation of a triazole ring, and such drugs are sometimes referred to as triazolobenzodiazepines.

The chemical structures of some less commonly used sedative-hypnotics are shown in Fig 54–3. The barbiturates have been regarded as prototypes of the class because of their extensive use since their introduction approximately 80 years ago. The motivation to develop other sedative-hypnotics can be attributed to efforts to avoid certain undesirable features of the barbiturates, including their potential for addiction and physical dependence. Unfortunately, such efforts have not always been successful. For example, the piperidinediones such as glutethimide, introduced as

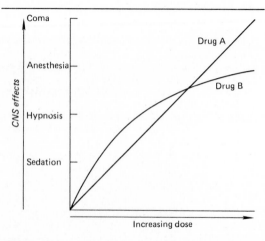

Figure 54–1. Theoretical dose-response curves for sedative-hypnotics.

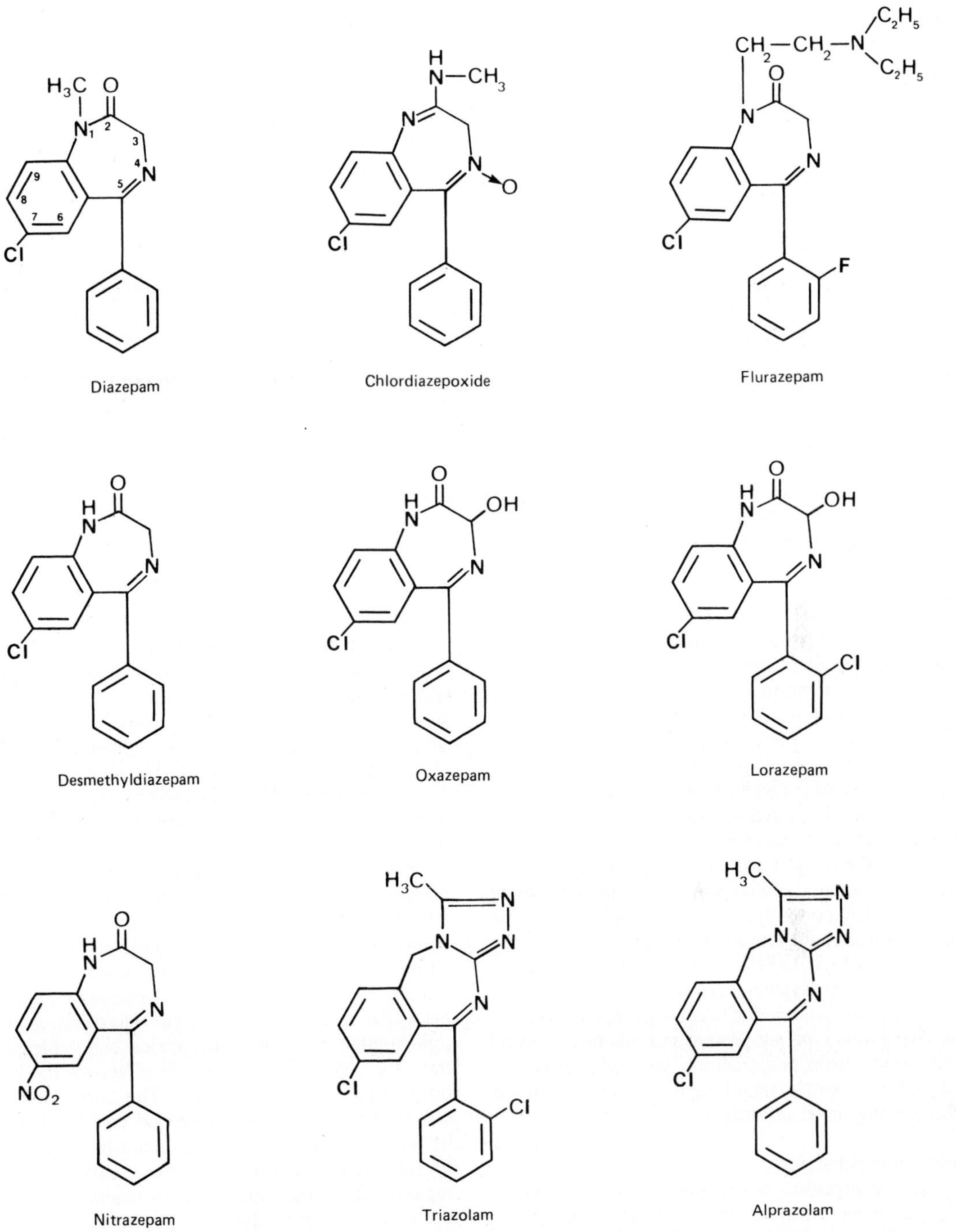

Figure 54-2. Chemical structures of benzodiazepines.

"nonbarbiturates," are in fact chemically related and virtually indistinguishable from barbiturates in their pharmacologic properties. Because of the huge market for sedative-hypnotics, such "failed attempts" have often been commercially successful. The propanediol carbamates such as meprobamate are of distinctive chemical structure but are practically equivalent to barbiturates in their pharmacologic effects, and their clinical use is rapidly declining. The sedative-hypnotic class also includes compounds of simple chemical structure, including alcohols (ethanol, chloral hydrate) and the cyclic ethers. Chlorol hydrate and its congeners, such as trichloroethanol, together with paraldehyde (not shown), continue to be used, particularly in institutionalized patients.

Other classes of drugs not included in Fig 54-3

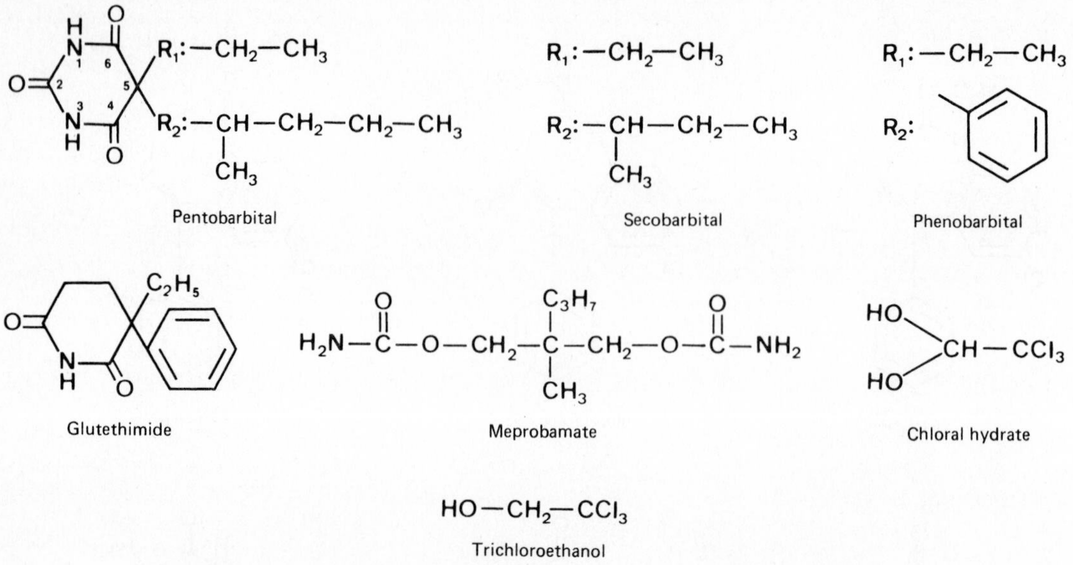

Figure 54–3. Chemical structures of barbiturates and other sedative-hypnotics.

may exert sedative effects. For example, beta-blocking drugs are effective in certain anxiety states and functional disorders, particularly those in which somatic and autonomic symptoms are prominent. Clonidine, a partial agonist at adrenergic α_2 receptors (including presynaptic autoreceptors in the brain), also appears to have anxiolytic properties. Sedative effects can also be obtained with the antipsychotic tranquilizers, the tricyclic antidepressant drugs, and antihistaminic agents. As discussed in other chapters, these agents are different from conventional sedative-hypnotics in both their effects and their major therapeutic uses. Most importantly, they do not produce general anesthesia and have low addiction liability. Since they commonly exert marked effects on the peripheral autonomic nervous system, they are sometimes referred to as "sedative-autonomic" drugs. Compounds of the antihistaminic type are present in a number of over-the-counter sleep preparations, and their autonomic properties as well as their long duration of action can result in unwanted side effects.

Pharmacokinetics

A. Absorption: When used to treat anxiety or sleep disorders, drugs of this class are usually given orally. The rates of oral absorption of sedative-hypnotics differ depending on a number of factors. Weakly basic drugs such as the benzodiazepines are absorbed most effectively at the high pH found in the duodenum, which may explain their somewhat slower onset of effect in comparison with that of the barbiturates (see below). Oral absorption of diazepam and the active metabolite of clorazepate is more rapid than that of the other commonly used benzodiazepines, whereas oxazepam is absorbed at the slowest rate. The benzodiazepine clorazepate is converted to its active form, desmethyldiazepam, by acid hydrolysis in the stomach. In the stomach (pH 1–2), weakly acidic drugs such as the barbiturates and the piperidinediones are nonionized and, since they are lipid-soluble, are usually absorbed very rapidly into the blood. One exception is glutethimide, which, because of its limited solubility in the aqueous gastric contents, may be absorbed slowly and erratically. The bioavailability of several benzodiazepines, including chlordiazepoxide and diazepam, may be unreliable after intramuscular injection.

B. Distribution: Transport of a sedative-hypnotic in the blood is a dynamic process in which drug molecules enter and leave tissues at rates dependent upon blood flow, concentration gradients, and permeabilities. Lipid solubility plays a major role in determining the rate at which a particular sedative-hypnotic enters the central nervous system. Diazepam is more lipid-soluble than chlordiazepoxide and lorazepam; thus, the central nervous system effects of the latter drugs may be slower in onset. The thiobarbiturates (eg, thiopental), in which the oxygen on C2 is replaced by sulfur, are very lipid-soluble, and a high rate of entry into the central nervous system contributes to the rapid onset of their central effects, whereas meprobamate has quite low solubility in lipids and penetrates the brain slowly even when given intravenously.

Redistribution of drug from the central nervous system to other tissues is an important feature of the biodisposition of sedative-hypnotics. Classic studies on the thiobarbiturates have shown that they are rapidly redistributed from the brain, first to highly perfused tissues such as skeletal muscle and subsequently to poorly perfused adipose tissue. These processes contribute to the termination of their major central nervous system effects. This may also be the case for other sedative-hypnotics, including the benzodiazepines, where the rate of metabolic transformation and elimination is much too slow in humans to account for the relatively short time required for dissipation of major pharmacologic effects.

Administration of sedative-hypnotics during pregnancy should be done with the recognition that the placental barrier to lipid-soluble drugs is incomplete and that all of these agents are capable of reaching the fetus. The rate of achievement of equilibrium between maternal and fetal blood is slower than that for the maternal blood and central nervous system, partly because of lower blood flow to the placenta. Nonetheless, if sedative-hypnotics are given in the predelivery period, they may contribute to the depression of neonatal vital functions.

Many sedative-hypnotics bind extensively to drug-binding sites on plasma proteins. For example, the binding of benzodiazepines to plasma albumin ranges between 80 and 97%. Since only free (nonbound) drug molecules have access to the central nervous system, the displacement of a sedative-hypnotic from plasma binding sites by another drug could modify its effects and possibly lead to drug interactions between this class and other pharmacologic agents. However, very few clinically significant interactions involving sedative-hypnotic drugs appear to be based on competition for common binding sites on the plasma proteins. One exception is chloral hydrate, which increases the anticoagulant effects of warfarin by its displacement from such binding sites.

C. Biotransformation: As noted above, redistribution to tissues other than the brain may be as important as biotransformation in terminating the central nervous system effects of many sedative-hypnotics.

However, metabolic transformation to more water-soluble metabolites is necessary for final clearance from the body of almost all drugs in this class. The microsomal drug-metabolizing enzyme systems of the liver are most important in this regard. Since few sedative-hypnotics are excreted from the body unchanged, the elimination half-life ($t_{1/2\beta}$) of most drugs in this class depends mainly on the rate of their metabolic transformation.

1. Benzodiazepines–Hepatic metabolism accounts for the clearance or elimination of all benzodiazepines. The 2 major pathways involved are microsomal oxidation, including N-dealkylation or aliphatic hydroxylation, and subsequent conjugation by glucuronyl transferases to form glucuronides that are excreted in the urine. The patterns and rates of metabolism depend on the individual drugs. One important feature of benzodiazepine metabolism is formation of active metabolites with central nervous system effects, some of which may be long-lived. As shown schematically in Fig 54–4, desmethyldiazepam, which has an elimination half-life of 40–140 hours, is an active metabolite of chlordiazepoxide, diazepam, prazepam, and clorazepate. Desmethyldiazepam in turn is biotransformed to the active compound oxazepam. Other active metabolites of chlordiazepoxide include desmethylchlordiazepoxide and demoxepam. While diazepam is metabolized mainly to desmethyldiazepam, it is also converted to temazepam (not shown in Fig 54–4) which is further metabolized in part to oxazepam. Flurazepam, which is used mainly for hypnosis, is oxidized by hepatic enzymes to 3 active metabolites, desalkylflurazepam,

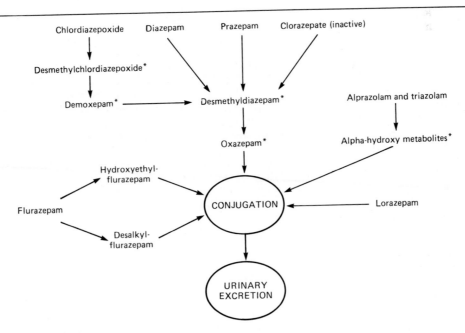

Figure 54–4. Biotransformation of benzodiazepines (*=active metabolite).

hydroxyethylflurazepam, and flurazepam aldehyde (not shown), which have elimination half-lives ranging from 30 to 100 hours. This may result in unwanted central nervous system depression, including daytime sedation. The triazolobenzodiazepines alprazolam and triazolam undergo α-hydroxylation and the resulting metabolites appear to exert weak pharmacologic effects.

The formation of active metabolites has complicated studies on the pharmacokinetics of the benzodiazepines in humans because the elimination half-life of the parent drug may have little relationship to the time course of pharmacologic effects. Those benzodiazepines for which either the parent drug or active metabolites have long half-lives are more likely to cause cumulative effects with multiple doses. Cumulative and residual effects such as excessive drowsiness should be less of a problem with such drugs as oxazepam and lorazepam, which have shorter half-lives and are metabolized directly to inactive glucuronides. Some biodispositional properties of selected benzodiazepines are given in Table 54–1.

2. Barbiturates–With the exception of phenobarbital, only insignificant quantities of the barbiturates are excreted intact. The major metabolic pathways involve oxidation by hepatic enzymes of chemical groups attached to C5, which are different for the individual barbiturates. The alcohols, acids, and ketones formed appear in the urine as glucuronide conjugates. Another type of metabolic reaction, glycosylation, involves direct attachment of glucose to N1 or N3 to form more water-soluble derivatives that can then be eliminated via the kidney. With very few exceptions, the metabolites of the barbiturates lack pharmacologic activity. The overall rate of hepatic metabolism in humans depends on the individual drug but (with the exception of the thiobarbiturates) is usually slow. The range of elimination half-life of secobarbital and pentobarbital is from 18 to 48 hours. The elimination half-life of phenobarbital in humans may be as long as 4–5 days. Multiple dosing with barbiturates with longer half-lives can lead to cumulative effects.

3. Other sedative-hypnotics–Most other sedative-hypnotics, including the piperidinediones and meprobamate, are biotransformed to more water-soluble compounds by hepatic enzymes. Trichloroethanol is the pharmacologically active metabolite of chloral hydrate and has a half-life of 6–10 hours. However, its toxic metabolite, trichloroacetic acid, is cleared very slowly and can accumulate with the nightly administration of chloral hydrate.

D. Excretion: The water-soluble metabolites of benzodiazepines and other sedative-hypnotics are excreted mainly via the kidney. In most cases, changes in renal function do not have a marked effect on the elimination of parent drugs. Phenobarbital is excreted unchanged in the urine to a certain extent (20–30% in humans), and its elimination rate can be increased significantly by alkalinization of the urine. This is partly due to increased ionization at alkaline pH, since phenobarbital is a weak acid with pK_a of 7.2. Only trace amounts of the benzodiazepines and less than 10% of a hypnotic dose of meprobamate appear in the urine unchanged.

E. Factors Affecting Biodisposition: The biodisposition of sedative-hypnotics can be influenced by several factors, particularly those that change rates of

Table 54–1. Biodispositional properties of benzodiazepines in humans.

Drug	Elimination Half-Life Range (hours)	Metabolites	Comments
Alprazolam	12–15	Active: α-hydroxyalprazolam	Rapid oral absorption.
Chlordiazepoxide	5–30	Active: desmethyl derivative, demoxepam, oxazepam	Poor intramuscular bioavailability.
Clorazepate	50–100 (metabolites)	Active: desmethyldiazepam, oxazepam	Hydrolyzed to active form in stomach.
Diazepam	50–150	Active: desmethyldiazepam, temazepam, oxazepam	Poor intramuscular bioavailability.
Flunitrazepam	12–24	Active: desmethylflunitrazepam	Large volume of distribution.
Flurazepam	24–100 (metabolites)	Active: desalkyl derivative and others	Long elimination half-lives of active metabolites.
Lorazepam	10–18	Inactive: glucuronides	Elimination not much affected by age or liver disease.
Nitrazepam	24–36	Probably inactive	Large volume of distribution.
Oxazepam	4–10	Inactive: glucuronides	Slow oral absorption may delay onset of effects.
Prazepam	30–120	Active: desmethyldiazepam	Slow oral absorption.
Temazepam	5–8	Possibly active	Slow oral absorption.
Triazolam	3–5.	Active: α-hydroxyltriazolam	Rapid oral absorption.

metabolic clearance. These include alterations in hepatic function resulting from disease, old age, or drug-induced increases or decreases in microsomal enzyme activities.

Generally, decreased hepatic function results in reduction of the clearance rates of drugs metabolized via oxidative pathways. This group includes many of the benzodiazepines, almost all of the barbiturates, the piperidinediones, and meprobamate. In very old patients or those with severe liver disease, the elimination half-lives of these drugs are usually increased significantly. If given in such cases, multiple normal doses of these sedative-hypnotics can often result in cumulative or enhanced central nervous system effects. Surprisingly, there are only a few clinical studies that document this. However, it seems prudent to lower the dose of such sedative-hypnotics in patients who are elderly or who may have limited hepatic function. Metabolism involving glucuronide conjugation appears to be less affected than oxidative metabolism by old age or liver disease.

The activity of hepatic microsomal drug-metabolizing enzymes may be increased in patients exposed to certain sedative-hypnotics on a chronic basis (enzyme induction), especially the barbiturates and carbamates. Drugs with long elimination half-lives such as phenobarbital and meprobamate are most likely to cause this effect and result in an increase in the rate of their own hepatic metabolism as well as that of certain other drugs. Self-induction of metabolism is a possible but not well-documented mechanism that contributes to the development of tolerance to sedative-hypnotics. Increased biotransformation of other pharmacologic agents by sedative-hypnotics is a potential mechanism underlying drug interactions. The benzodiazepine group of sedative-hypnotics is less likely than the barbiturates to change hepatic drug-metabolizing enzyme activity with continuous use.

Mechanisms of Action

A unitary hypothesis regarding the mechanisms of action of sedative-hypnotics has been slow to develop. As the role of gamma-aminobutyric acid (GABA) as an important inhibitory neurotransmitter in the central nervous system has been elucidated, it has become more probable that modification of its functions underlie the pharmacologic effects of several classes of drugs, including the benzodiazepines and barbiturates. Electrophysiologic studies have shown that benzodiazepines potentiate GABA-ergic neurotransmission at all levels of the neuroaxis, including the spinal cord, hypothalamus, hippocampus, substantia nigra, cerebellar cortex, and cerebral cortex. Benzodiazepines appear to increase the efficiency of GABA-ergic synaptic inhibition, which leads to a decrease in the firing rate of critical neurons in many regions of the brain. The benzodiazepines do not appear to substitute for GABA but require the presence of the neurotransmitter to elicit a response. This has led to the concept that benzodiazepines indirectly enhance GABA-ergic neurotransmission at the level of postsynaptic receptors without direct activation of GABA receptors or the associated chloride channels. The change in chloride ion conductance induced by the interaction of GABA with its receptors is enhanced by benzodiazepines, resulting in an increase in the frequency of channel-opening events. Barbiturates also facilitate the inhibitory actions of GABA at multiple sites in the central nervous system, but electrophysiologic studies show that—in contrast to benzodiazepines—they prolong rather than intensify GABA responses. At high concentrations, the barbiturates may also be GABA-mimetic, directly activating chloride ion channels. Barbiturates appear to be less selective in their actions than benzodiazepines, since they also depress the actions of excitatory neurotransmitters and exert nonsynaptic membrane effects in parallel with their effects on GABA neurotransmission. This multiplicity of sites of action of barbiturates may be the basis for their ability to induce full surgical anesthesia and for their more pronounced central depressant effects (which results in their low margin of safety) compared to benzodiazepines. The actions of other sedative-hypnotics such as meprobamate have been less well studied electrophysiologically but do not appear to be related to GABA neurotransmission.

Neurochemical studies during recent years have complemented and extended the electrophysiologic evidence for the modulation of GABA neurotransmission by benzodiazepines. High-affinity receptor sites for benzodiazepines have been demonstrated in many regions of the central nervous system, including the spinal cord, brain stem, hypothalamus, limbic structures, cerebellar cortex, and cerebral cortex. Such benzodiazepine receptors are located at GABA-ergic synapses and are functionally coupled to GABA-responsive chloride channels but are separate macromolecules from either the GABA receptor or the chloride ionophore. Possible physical and functional relationships between these components are schematically illustrated in Fig 54–5. The macromolecular complex also includes a polypeptide GABA-modulin that may modulate coupling between the GABA receptor and the benzodiazepine receptor protein. In addition, a barbiturate receptor protein (which may be identical to the chloride channel protein) is a component of the macromolecular complex. This component also contains binding sites for certain convulsant drugs such as picrotoxin.

The identification of benzodiazepine receptors in the brain has led to the characterization of 3 main types of benzodiazepine receptor ligands: (1) The clinically useful benzodiazepines which exert anxiolytic, hypnotic, and anticonvulsant effects and which appear to act as classic receptor agonists. (2) Benzodiazepine receptor *antagonists* (including the imidazodiazepine Ro 15-1788) that selectively block the actions of benzodiazepines without pharmacologic effects of their own. These molecules do not block the actions of other sedative-hypnotics such as barbiturates, meprobamate, or ethanol. Members of this second class of ligands appear to be classic antagonists, and

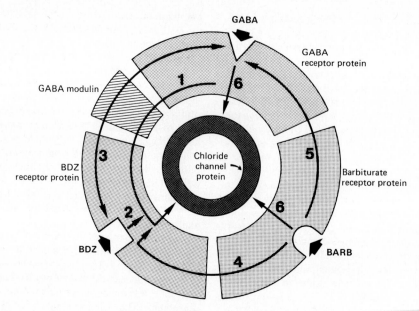

Figure 54–5. Proposed model of the GABA-benzodiazepine-chloride channel receptor complex. GABA binding to its receptor activates the chloride channel through a coupling mechanism involving GABA-modulin and the benzodiazepine (BDZ) receptor protein (1). Binding of benzodiazepines (BDZ) enhances this coupling function (2) and increases GABA binding in a reciprocal relationship (3). Binding of barbiturates (BARB) also enhances the coupling function (4), increases the affinity of GABA for its receptor (5), and may directly activate the chloride channel at high concentrations (6). GABA=gamma-aminobutyric acid.

they have potential clinical application in the treatment of benzodiazepine intoxication and overdosage. (3) A third group of *anxiogenic* benzodiazepine receptor ligands is represented by various β-carbolines, some of which are naturally occurring. These molecules can block the effects of benzodiazepine agonists, and when administered alone produce such effects as anxiety reaction, proconvulsant activity, and seizures. Such ligands have been termed "inverse agonists" and are of interest in terms of their possible role as natural endogenous mediators of anxiolytic responses.

Newer Anxiolytic Drugs

Although the benzodiazepines continue to be the agents of choice in the treatment of anxiety, their pharmacologic effects include sedation and drowsiness and synergistic central nervous system depression with other drugs, especially alcohol. Anxiolytic drugs with reduced propensity for such actions would be desirable. Several nonbenzodiazepines are presently under active investigation, including the pyrazolopyridine tracazolate, the piperazinyl pyrimidine derivative buspirone, and certain triazolopyridazines. These drugs have minimal potentiating effects on the actions of ethanol. Buspirone appears to be "anxioselective" in that it relieves anxiety with minimum sedative and muscle relaxing effects. Buspirone does not appear to exert its effects through the GABA receptor-benzodiazepine receptor-chloride ionophore complex but may interact with brain serotonin (5-HT$_{1a}$) receptors. The drug is metabolized by hepatic enzymes to 1-(2-pyrimidinyl) piperazine, which also has anxiolytic effects.

Pharmacodynamics

A. Sedation: Sedation can be defined as a decrease in responsiveness to a constant level of stimulation, with decrease in spontaneous activity and ideation. These behavioral changes occur at the lowest effective doses of the sedative-hypnotics. It is not yet clear whether antianxiety actions seen clinically are equivalent to or different from sedative effects. In ex-

Buspirone

perimental animal models, the sedative-hypnotic drugs are able to release punishment-suppressed behavior, and this disinhibition has been equated with antianxiety effects. However, the release of previously suppressed behavior may be more relevant to behavioral disinhibitory effects of these drugs, including euphoria, impaired judgment, and loss of self-control, which occur at doses slightly higher than those used to cause sedation. All sedative-hypnotic drugs are capable of releasing punishment-suppressed behavior in animals, but the benzodiazepines exert such effects at doses that do not cause general central nervous system depression. Phenothiazine antipsychotic drugs and tricyclic antidepressants are not effective in this experimental model.

B. Hypnosis: By definition, all of the sedative-hypnotics will induce sleep if high enough doses are given. Normal sleep is considered to consist of distinct stages, based on 3 physiologic measures: the electroencephalogram, the electromyogram, and the electro-oculogram (a measure of lateral movements of the eye). Based on the latter, 2 major categories can be distinguished; non-rapid eye movement (NREM) sleep, which represents approximately 70–75% of total sleep; and rapid eye movement (REM) sleep. REM and NREM sleep occur cyclically over an interval of about 90 minutes. The REM sleep stage is that in which most recallable dreams occur. NREM sleep progresses through 4 stages (1–4), with the greatest proportion (50%) of sleep being spent in stage 2. This is followed by delta or slow-wave sleep (stages 3 and 4), in which somnambulism and night terrors have been noted to occur.

The effects of drugs on the sleep stages have been studied extensively, although often with normal volunteer subjects rather than patients with sleep disorders. In the case of sedative-hypnotics, effects depend on several factors, including the specific drug, the dose, and the frequency of its administration. While some exceptions exist, the effects of sedative-hypnotics on patterns of normal sleep are as follows: (1) the latency of sleep onset is decreased (time to fall asleep); (2) the duration of stage 2 NREM sleep is increased; (3) the duration of REM sleep is decreased; and (4) the duration of slow-wave sleep is decreased.

More rapid onset of sleep and prolongation of stage 2 are presumably clinically useful effects. However, the significance of effects on REM and slow-wave sleep is not clear. Use of sedative-hypnotics for more than a week or so leads to some tolerance to their effects on sleep patterns. Withdrawal after continued use can result in a "rebound" increase in the frequency of occurrence and duration of REM sleep. It is important to recognize that claims have often been made for superiority of one sedative-hypnotic over another based on differential actions on one stage of sleep or another. Since little is known about the function of any sleep stage, statements about the desirability of a particular drug based on its effects on sleep patterns can have no validity. Clearly, clinical criteria of efficacy in alleviating a particular sleeping problem are more

useful. The ideal hypnotic—one that would promote sleep without any change in its natural pattern—has yet to be introduced.

C. Anesthesia: As shown in Fig 54–1, sedative-hypnotics in high doses will depress the central nervous system to a point known as stage III or general anesthesia. However, the suitability of a particular agent as an adjunct in anesthesia depends mainly on the physicochemical properties that determine its rapidity of onset and duration of effect. Among the barbiturates, thiopental and methohexital are very lipid-soluble, penetrating brain tissue rapidly following intravenous administration. Rapid tissue redistribution accounts for the short duration of action of these drugs, which are therefore useful in anesthesia practice.

Although certain of the benzodiazepines have been used intravenously in anesthesia, none of them have proved successful as induction agents capable of producing surgical anesthesia by themselves. This statement is supported by the fact that the MAC (minimum alveolar concentration) of another anesthetic cannot be reduced to zero by the substitution of a benzodiazepine. Diazepam and midazolam have been studied in this regard and are incapable of producing adequate surgical anesthesia. Not surprisingly, most of the benzodiazepines given in large doses may cause a persistent postanesthetic depression. This is probably related to their relatively long half-lives and the formation of active metabolites. It is possible that newer benzodiazepines with much shorter half-lives will be more useful in clinical practice.

D. Anticonvulsant Effects: Most of the sedative-hypnotics are capable of inhibiting the development and spread of epileptiform activity in the central nervous system, but some selectivity exists in that certain drugs do so without marked central nervous system depression, so that normal mentation and activity are relatively unaffected. Of the barbiturates, phenobarbital and metharbital (converted to phenobarbital in the body) are effective in the treatment of grand mal and jacksonian epilepsy. Certain benzodiazepines also have selective actions: diazepam is used in status epilepticus and in the treatment of seizures induced by local anesthetics, and nitrazepam is used in certain infantile spasms and myoclonic seizures.

E. Muscle Relaxation: Some sedative-hypnotics, particularly members of the carbamate and benzodiazepine groups, exert inhibitory effects on polysynaptic reflexes and internuncial transmission, and at high doses may depress transmission at the skeletal myoneural junction. Selective actions of this type leading to muscle relaxation can be readily demonstrated in animals, and this has led to claims of usefulness for relaxing contracted voluntary muscle in joint disease or muscle spasm. Unfortunately, there is little clinical evidence to support such claims at dose levels that do not also cause significant depression of the central nervous system, leading to changes in mental or motor functions. What positive evidence does exist concerns specialized clinical situations such as the treatment with diazepam of spasticity in patients with cerebral palsy.

F. Effects on Respiration and Cardiovascular Function: At hypnotic doses in healthy patients, the effects of sedative-hypnotics on respiration are comparable to changes during natural sleep. However, sedative-hypnotics even at therapeutic doses can produce significant respiratory depression in patients with obstructive pulmonary disease. Effects on respiration are dose-related, and depression of the medullary respiratory center is the usual cause of death due to overdose of sedative-hypnotics.

At doses up to those causing hypnosis, no significant effects on the cardiovascular system are observed in healthy patients. However, in hypovolemic states, congestive heart failure, or other diseases impairing cardiovascular function, normal doses of sedative-hypnotics may cause cardiovascular depression, probably as a result of actions on the medullary vasomotor centers. At toxic levels, myocardial contractility and vascular tone may both be depressed by central and peripheral effects, leading to circulatory collapse. Respiratory and cardiovascular effects become more apparent when sedative-hypnotics are given intravenously.

Tolerance; Psychologic & Physical Dependence

Tolerance, a decrease in responsiveness to a drug following continuous exposure, is a common feature of the sedative-hypnotics. In some instances, it may result in a need to increase the dose to maintain symptomatic improvement or to promote sleep. It is important to recognize that **cross-tolerance** occurs between the sedative-hypnotics described here and also with ethanol—a feature of some clinical importance, as explained below. The mechanisms of development of tolerance to sedative-hypnotics are not well understood. An alteration in rates of metabolic inactivation with chronic administration may be partly responsible (metabolic tolerance), but changes in responsiveness of the central nervous system (pharmacodynamic tolerance) are more important.

The perceived desirable properties of relief of anxiety, euphoria, disinhibition, and promotion of sleep have led to the compulsive misuse of virtually all of the drugs classed as sedative-hypnotics. The consequences of abuse of these agents can be defined in both psychologic and physiologic terms. The psychologic component may initially parallel simple neurotic behavior patterns hard to differentiate from those of the inveterate coffee drinker or cigarette smoker. When the pattern of sedative-hypnotic use becomes compulsive, more serious complications develop, including physical dependence and tolerence.

Physical dependence can be described as an altered physiologic state that requires continuous drug administration to prevent the appearance of an abstinence or withdrawal syndrome. As described more fully later, in the case of sedative-hypnotics this syndrome is characterized by states of increased excitability that may even progress to convulsions. All sedative-hypnotics are capable of causing physical dependence when used on a chronic basis. However, the severity of withdrawal symptoms differs between individual drugs and depends also on the magnitude of the dose used immediately prior to cessation of use. When higher doses of sedative-hypnotics are used, abrupt withdrawal will lead to more serious withdrawal signs. Differences in the severity of withdrawal symptoms between individual sedative-hypnotics relate in part to biodisposition properties, since drugs with long half-lives are eliminated slowly enough to accomplish gradual withdrawal with few physical symptoms. The use of drugs with very short half-lives for hypnotic effects may lead to signs of withdrawal even between doses. For example, triazolam, a benzodiazepine with a half-life of about 4 hours, has been reported to cause daytime anxiety when used to treat sleep problems.

II. CLINICAL PHARMACOLOGY

TREATMENT OF ANXIETY STATES

Throughout history, the psychologic and behavioral responses to stress have been a significant part of human experience, and many ingenious approaches have been devised for relieving the various symptoms of anxiety. Before considering the clinical use of sedative-hypnotics, it is important to analyze the patient's symptoms carefully. If the patient presents with anxiety as a primary complaint, other psychiatric problems must be suspected. These may best be managed by psychotherapy or, when the situation warrants, by the use of pharmacologic agents such as the tricyclic antidepressants or antipsychotic drugs. Frequently, however, anxiety is secondary to organic disease states— acute myocardial infarction, angina pectoris, gastrointestinal ulcers, etc—which themselves require specific therapy. Another class of secondary anxiety states (situational anxiety) results from circumstances that may only have to be dealt with once or a few times, including anticipation of frightening medical or dental procedures and family illness or other tragedy. Even though situational anxiety tends to be self-limiting, the *short-term* use of sedative-hypnotics may be appropriate for the treatment of this and certain disease-associated anxiety states. Similarly, the acute use of a sedative-hypnotic as a premedicant prior to surgery or some unpleasant medical procedure is rational and proper (Table 54–2).

Historically, the rationale for the treatment of anxiety with sedative-hypnotics was quite empirical, since evidence for efficacy from well-controlled, blind clinical studies did not become available until the last decade. Difficulties in establishing efficacy can be re-

Table 54–2. Clinical uses of sedative-hypnotics.

Table 54–2. Clinical uses of sedative-hypnotics.

For relief of anxiety.
Hypnosis.
For sedation and amnesia before medical and surgical procedures.
Treatment of epilepsy and seizures states.
Intravenous administration, as a component of balanced anesthesia.
For control of ethanol or other sedative-hypnotic withdrawal states.
For muscle relaxation in specific neuromuscular disorders.
As diagnostic aids or for treatment in psychiatry.

lated to many nonpharmacologic factors that influence the success of therapy, including personal expectations, personality of the therapist, environmental factors, and the placebo response. Although anxiety symptoms can now be ameliorated by drug therapy, it is not always easy to demonstrate the superiority of one drug over another. Thus, a preference for a particular drug for a specific situation is often based on factors other than pharmacologic effect. An exception to this generalization is alprazolam, which is particularly effective in the treatment of panic disorders and agoraphobia and may be more selective in this regard than other benzodiazepines.

Although phenobarbital, meprobamate, and certain sedative-autonomic drugs (hydroxyzine, diphenhydramine) continue to be used, the most commonly used drugs for treatment of anxiety are the benzodiazepines. The selection of benzodiazepines is based on several sound pharmacologic principles: (1) a relatively high therapeutic index (see drug B in Fig 54–1), since hypnotic and anesthetic doses are considerably higher than those causing sedation; (2) a low risk of drug interactions based on enzyme induction; (3) slow elimination rates, which may favor persistence of useful central nervous system effects; and (4) a low risk of physical dependence, with minor withdrawal symptoms.

Disadvantages of the benzodiazepines include the tendency to develop psychologic dependence, the formation of active metabolites, and their higher cost. *As is true of all drugs of the sedative-hypnotic class, the benzodiazepines exert additive central nervous system depression when administered with other drugs, including ethanol.* The patient should be warned of this possibility to avoid impairment of performance of any task requiring mental alertness and motor coordination.

Perhaps the most important guide to therapy is to use the drug selected with appropriate restraint to minimize adverse effects. A dose should be prescribed that does not impair mentation or motor functions during working hours. Some patients may tolerate the drug better if most of the daily dose is given at bedtime, with smaller doses during the day. Prescriptions should be written for short periods, since there is little justification for long-term therapy. The physician should make an effort to assess the efficacy of therapy from the patient's subjective responses. Plasma drug

concentrations are too variable to be useful as a guide to dosage. Combinations of antianxiety agents should be avoided, and people taking sedatives should be cautioned about drinking alcohol and concurrent use of over-the-counter medications.

The clinical use of beta-blocking drugs (eg, propranolol) as antianxiety agents has been suggested in a number of situations. The sympathetic nervous system overactivity associated with anxiety appears to be satisfactorily relieved by the beta-blockers, and a slight improvement in the nonsomatic components of anxiety may also occur. Of the various studies comparing the effects of beta-blocking drugs with those of benzodiazepines, none has demonstrated any significant therapeutic differences, and in fact, when somatic or autonomic symptoms are absent, the benzodiazepines are more consistently effective. Thus, the best performance noted with beta-blockers has been when somatic symptoms have been a prominent part of the anxiety state. These somatic symptoms include tremor, palpitation, dizziness, excess sweating, and other signs of autonomic overactivity, frequently in association with a sense of fear or panic. Even though there are suggestions that these compounds affect central nervous system actions, it is believed that most of the effects are peripheral in action. This conclusion is based on the fact that even beta-blockers that do not pass the blood-brain barrier have effective antianxiety actions. Propranolol given in doses of 80–240 mg daily is usually effective in diminishing somatic symptoms. The antihypertensive drug clonidine has also been used in the treatment of anxiety states, including panic attacks. Concomitant treatment with drugs that exert alpha-adrenoceptor-blocking actions (including tricyclic antidepressants) may decrease the effects of clonidine. Withdrawal from clonidine after protracted use, especially at high doses, has led to life-threatening hypertensive crisis.

TREATMENT OF SLEEP PROBLEMS

The complaint of insomnia embraces a wide variety of sleep problems that include difficulty in falling asleep, frequent awakenings, short duration of sleep, and "unrefreshing" sleep. Insomnia is a serious complaint calling for careful evaluation to uncover posible causes (organic, psychologic, situational, etc) that can perhaps be managed without hypnotic drugs. Nonpharmacologic therapies sometimes useful include proper diet and exercise, avoiding stimulants before retiring, ensuring a comfortable sleeping place, and retiring at a regular time each night. In some cases, however, the patient will need and should be given a sedative-hypnotic for a limited period. It should be noted that the discontinuance of any drug in this class can lead to rebound insomnia. *Note: Long-term use of hypnotics is irrational and dangerous medical practice.*

The hypnotic drug selected should be one that provides sleep of fairly rapid onset (decreased sleep latency) and sufficient duration, with minimal "hangover" effects such as drowsiness, dysphoria, and mental or motor depression. Drugs with a favorable therapeutic index such as benzodiazepines are generally preferred. However, many benzodiazepines have slow elimination rates and are biotransformed to active metabolites—properties that are undesirable because they lead to cumulative and hangover effects. Triazolam has the shortest half-life of the currently available benzodiazepines used for the management of sleep problems and theoretically should exert minimal hangover effects when used on an acute basis. If hypnotics are used every night, tolerance can occur, leading to dose increases by the patient to produce the desired effect. It should be recalled that if physical dependence develops, the shorter-acting drugs are associated with more intense withdrawal signs when discontinued. The drugs commonly used for sedation and hypnosis are listed in Table 54–3 together with recommended doses.

OTHER THERAPEUTIC USES

Table 54–2 summarizes several other important clinical uses of drugs in the sedative-hypnotic class. For sedative and possible amnestic effects during medical or surgical procedures such as endoscopy and bronchoscopy, as well as premedication prior to anesthesia, oral formulations of shorter-acting drugs are preferred. When drug administration is under close supervision, the danger of accidental or intentional overdosage is less than in the outpatient situation, and a barbiturate may be as appropriate as any sedative-hypnotic. Meprobamate and, more recently, the benzodiazepines have frequently been used as central muscle relaxants, though evidence for general efficacy without accompanying sedation is lacking. Sedative-hypnotics are occasionally used as diagnostic aids in neurology and psychiatry.

CLINICAL TOXICOLOGY OF SEDATIVE-HYPNOTICS

Direct Toxic Actions

Many of the common adverse effects of drugs in this class are those resulting from dose-related depression of central nervous system functions. In ambulatory patients, relatively low doses may lead to drowsiness, impaired judgment, and diminished motor skills, sometimes with a significant impact on driving skills, job performance, and personal relationships. Hangover effects are not uncommon following use of drugs with long half-lives for sleep problems in such patients. The most common reversible cause of confusional states in the elderly is overuse of sedative-hypnotics. At higher doses, toxicity may present as lethargy or a state of exhaustion or, alternatively, gross symptoms equivalent to those of ethanol intoxication. The titration of useful therapeutic effects against such side effects is usually more difficult with sedative-hypnotics that exhibit steep dose-response relationships of the type shown in Fig 54–1 (drug A), including the barbiturates and piperidinediones. Unwanted depression of central nervous system functions also occurs more frequently when therapy is continued for longer periods and when drugs with long half-lives and active metabolites are used. The physican should be aware of variability among patients in terms of doses causing adverse effects. A relatively small dose in one individual may result in unwanted central nervous system depression that would require 2 or 3 times that dose in another patient. Variability is even more common in patients with cardiovascular or respiratory disease and hepatic impairment or in old age.

Sedative-hypnotics are the drugs most frequently involved in deliberate overdosage situations, in part because of their general availability as the most commonly prescribed pharmacologic agents. The benzodiazepines are generally considered to be "safer" drugs in this respect, since they have flatter dose-response curves. Epidemiologic studies on the incidence of drug-related deaths support this general assumption—

Table 54–3. Dosages of drugs used commonly for sedation and hypnosis.

Sedation		Hypnosis	
Drug	**Dosage**	**Drug**	**Dosage (at Bedtime)**
Alprazolam (Xanax)	0.25–0.5 mg 2–3 times daily	Chloral hydrate	500–1000 mg
Chlordiazepoxide (Librium)	10–20 mg 2–3 times daily	Flurazepam (Dalmane)	15–30 mg
Clorazepate (Tranxene)	5–7.5 mg twice daily	Lorazepam (Ativan)	2–4 mg
Diazepam (Valium)	5 mg twice daily	Methaqualone* (Quaalude)	150–250 mg
Lorazepam (Ativan)	1–2 mg once or twice daily	Pentobarbital	100–200 mg
Oxazepam (Serax)	15–30 mg 3–4 times daily	Secobarbital	100–200 mg
Phenobarbital	15–30 mg 2–3 times daily	Temazepam (Restoril)	10–30 mg
Prazepam (Centrax)	10–20 mg 2–3 times daily	Triazolam (Halcion)	0.5–1 mg

*Methaqualone has been discontinued, but illicit use of the drug will probably continue.

eg, 0.3 deaths per 1 million tablets of diazepam prescribed versus 11.6 deaths per 1 million capsules of secobarbital in a recent study. Of course, many factors other than the specific sedative-hypnotic could influence such data—particularly the presence of other central nervous system depressants, including ethanol. In fact, most serious cases of drug overdosage, intentional or accidental, do involve polypharmacy; and when combinations of agents are taken, the practical "safety" of benzodiazepines may be less than the foregoing would imply.

The lethal dose of any sedative-hypnotic is variable. If discovery of the ingestion is made early and a conservative treatment regimen is started, the outcome is rarely fatal, even following very high doses. On the other hand, for most sedative-hypnotics, with the exception of benzodiazepines, a dose as low as 10 times what is required for hypnosis may be fatal if the patient is not discovered or does not seek help in time. With severe toxicity, the respiratory depression from central actions of the drug may be complicated by aspiration of gastric contents in the unattended patient—an even more likely occurrence if ethanol is present. Loss of brain stem vasomotor control, together with direct myocardial depression, further complicates successful resuscitation. In such patients, treatment consists of mechanical respiration; maintenance of plasma volume, renal output, and cardiac function; and perhaps use of a positive inotropic drug such as dopamine, which preserves renal blood flow. Hemodialysis or hemoperfusion may be used to hasten elimination of some of these drugs.

Adverse effects of the sedative-hypnotics that are not referable to their central nervous system actions occur infrequently. Hypersensitivity reactions, including skin rashes, occur only occasionally with most drugs of this class. Reports of teratogenicity leading to fetal deformation following use of piperidinediones and certain benzodiazepines justify caution in the use of these drugs during pregnancy. Because barbiturates enhance porphyrin synthesis, they are absolutely contraindicated in patients with a history of acute intermittent porphyria.

Alterations in Drug Response

Depending on dosage and duration of use, tolerance may occur to many of the pharmacologic effects of sedative-hypnotics. This can be demonstrated experimentally in humans by changes in the effects of chronic use of these drugs on the electroencephalogram and other characteristics of the stages of sleep. Clearly, it must occur with respect to other effects, since it is known that chronic abusers sometimes ingest quantities of sedative-hypnotics many times the conventional dosage without experiencing severe toxicity. However, it should not be assumed that the degree of tolerance achieved is identical for all pharmacologic effects, and there is evidence that lethal dose ranges are not altered significantly with chronic use of sedative-hypnotics. Cross-tolerance between the different sedative-hypnotics, including ethanol, could

lead to an unsatisfactory therapeutic response when standard doses of a drug are used in a patient with a recent history of abuse of these agents.

With chronic use of sedative-hypnotics, especially as doses are increased, a state of physical dependence can occur. This may develop to a degree unparalleled by chronic use of any other drug group, *including the opiates,* since withdrawal from a sedative-hypnotic can have severe and life-threatening manifestations. Withdrawal symptoms range from restlessness, anxiety, weakness, and orthostatic hypotension to hyperactive reflexes and generalized seizures. The severity of withdrawal symptoms depends to a large extent on the dosage range used immediately prior to discontinuance but also on the particular drug. For example, barbiturates such as secobarbital or pentobarbital (in doses < 400 mg/d) or diazepam (< 40 mg/d) may produce only mild symptoms of withdrawal when discontinued. On the other hand, the use of more than 800 mg/d of barbiturates or 50–60 mg/d of diazepam for 60–90 days is likely to result in seizures if abrupt withdrawal is attempted. Symptoms of withdrawal are usually more severe following discontinuance of sedative-hypnotics with shorter half-lives. Symptoms are less pronounced with longer-acting drugs, which may partly accomplish their own withdrawal by virtue of their slow elimination. Cross-dependence, defined as the ability of one drug to suppress abstinence symptoms from discontinuance of another drug, is quite marked among sedative-hypnotics. This provides the rationale for therapeutic regimens in the management of withdrawal states. Thus, longer-acting drugs such as phenobarbital and diazepam can be used to alleviate withdrawal symptoms of shorter-acting drugs, including ethanol.

Drug Interactions

The most frequent drug interactions involving sedative-hypnotics are interactions with other central nervous system depressant drugs, leading to additive effects. These interactions have some therapeutic utility with respect to the use of these drugs as premedicants or anesthetic adjuvants. However, they can lead to serious adverse effects, including enhanced depression with concomitant use of many other drugs. Obvious additive effects can be predicted with use of alcoholic beverages, narcotic analgesics, anticonvulsants, phenothiazines, and other sedative-hypnotic drugs. Less obvious but just as important is enhanced central nervous system depression with a variety of antihistamines, antihypertensive agents, and antidepressant drugs of the tricyclic class.

Interactions involving changes in the activity of hepatic drug-metabolizing enzyme systems can occur, especially following continuous use of barbiturates and meprobamate. For example, in humans, barbiturates have been shown to increase metabolic degradation rates of dicumarol, phenytoin, digitalis compounds, and griseofulvin, effects that could lead to decrease in response to these agents. Cimetidine has recently been reported to double the elimination half-life of diazepam, presumably via inhibition of hepatic metabolism. As mentioned above, chloral hydrate may displace warfarin from plasma proteins to cause enhanced anticoagulant effects.

REFERENCES

Allquander C: Dependence on sedative and hypnotic drugs. *Acta Psychiatr Scand [Suppl]* 1978;**270:**1.

Breimer DD: Clinical pharmacokinetics of hypnotics. *Clin Pharmacokinet* 1977;**2:**93.

Burrows GD, Norman TR, Davies B: *Antianxiety Agents.* Vol 2 of: *Drugs in Psychiatry,* Elsevier, 1984.

Choi DW, Farb DH, Fischbach GD: Chlordiazepoxide selectively potentiates GABA conductance of spinal cord and sensory neurons in culture. *J Neurophysiol* 1981;**45:**621.

Consensus Conference: Drugs and insomnia: The use of medications to promote sleep. *JAMA* 1984;**251:**2410.

Council on Scientific Affairs: Hypnotic drugs and treatment of insomnia report. *JAMA* 1981;**245:**749.

Danneberg P, Weber KH: Chemical structure and biological activity of the diazepines. *Br J Clin Pharmacol* 1983;**16:**2315.

Goldberg ME et al: Novel non-benzodiazepine anxiolytics. *Neuropharmacology* 1983;**22:**1499.

Greenblatt DJ et al: Benzodiazepines: A summary of pharmacokinetic properties. *Br J Clin Pharmacol* 1981;**11:(Suppl 1):**11S.

Greenblatt DJ et al: Clinical pharmacokinetics of the newer benzodiazepines. *Clin Pharmacokinet* 1983;**8:**233.

Greenblatt DJ et al: Current status of benzodiazepines. *N Engl J Med* 1983;**309:**354.

Haefely W, Polc P: Electrophysiological studies on the interaction of anxiolytic drugs with GABAergic mechanisms. Pages 113–145 in: *Anxiolytics: Neurochemical, Behavioral and Clinical Perspectives.* Malick JB, Enna SJ, Yamamura HI (editors). Raven Press, 1983.

Mendelson WB: *The Use and Misuse of Sleeping Pills: A Clinical Guide.* Plenum Press, 1980.

Middlemiss DN et al: Beta-adrenoreceptor antagonists in psychiatry and neurology. *Pharmacol Ther* 1981;**12:**419.

Mohler H, Richards JG: Receptors for anxiolytic drugs. Pages 15–40 in: *Anxiolytics: Neurochemical, Behavioral and Clinical Perspectives.* Malick JB, Enna SJ, Yamamura HI (editors). Raven Press, 1983.

Olsen RW: GABA-benzodiazepine-barbiturate receptor interactions. *J Neurochem* 1981;**37:**1.

Rosenbaum JF: The drug treatment of anxiety. *N Engl J Med* 1982;**306:**401.

Sepinwall J, Cook L: Behavioral pharmacology of antianxiety drugs. Chap 6, pp 345–393, in: *Biology of Mood and Antianxiety Drugs.* Vol 13 of: *Handbook of Psychopharmacology.* Iversen LL, Iversen SD, Snyder SH (editors). Plenum Press, 1978.

Skolnick P, Panl SM: The mechanism(s) of action of the benzodiazepines. *Med Res Rev* 1981;**1:**3.

Snyder SH: Drugs and neurotransmitter receptors in the brain. *Science* 1984;**224:**22.

Solomon F et al: Sleeping pills, insomnia, and medical practice. *N Engl J Med* 1979;**300:**803.

Study RE, Barker JL: Diazepam and (−)pentobarbital: Fluctuation analysis reveals different mechanisms for potentiations of GABA responses in cultured central neurons. *Proc Natl Acad Sci USA* 1981;**78:**7180.

Tallman JF et al: Receptors for the age of anxiety: Pharmacology of the benzodiazepines. *Science* 1980;**207:**274.

An Overview of Consultation/Liaison Psychiatry

55

Howard H. Fenn, MD, & Herbert Ochitill, MD

Consultation is a common process in medical practice whereby a specialist—the consultant—offers advice about a case to a colleague requesting assistance—the consultee. Since the "caseload" of psychiatric problems in general medical settings exceeds the capacity of psychiatrists or other mental health professionals to deal with it, psychiatric consultation maximizes scarce mental health resources. Consultation may permit primary-care providers to continue to manage all but the most difficult patients without making a referral or transferring responsibility to a mental health professional. Some patients will not accept referral or transfer; others cannot afford mental health treatment, especially when their insurance benefits are limited. Furthermore, psychiatric consultation is a way of providing expert advice that multiplies the effect of mental health knowledge beyond the immediate problem or case. It improves the consultee's ability to recognize the need for psychologic management in future cases, which enhances early intervention and prevention of more serious problems. It also provides the consultee with expertise that can be applied to settings and situations in which mental health consultation is not readily available. Finally, it helps the consultees to use the recommendations in ways that are congruent with their individual styles in dealing with patients.

This chapter will present an overview of the consultation role of psychiatrists. It will provide guidelines to the general process of psychiatric consultation and details about its application in 2 major settings: the community at large and the health care system in particular. Community-based psychiatric consultation involves the schools, courts, jails, welfare agencies, and churches. Health system–based consultation involves the outpatient clinic, doctor's office, and general hospital. Consultation in the general hospital is discussed in the next chapter.

The following illustrative case identifies stages at which mental health consultation might have been helpful to a patient in a variety of settings. Although direct treatment of psychiatric illness is important, the case emphasizes how interventions outside the limits of the direct service model might have affected the outcome of a difficult psychiatric problem.

Illustrative case. A 15-year-old boy was belligerent toward his teachers, disruptive in class, and increasingly truant. He ran away from home and was arrested several times for fighting and being drunk in public. At each court appearance the juvenile court judge warned him about the consequences of future misbehavior, but the youngster seemed indifferent to admonition. On more than one occasion he showed up drunk at his minister's office, distressed about a beating his alcoholic father had given him or his mother. He would rail against his father and praise his mother for enduring mistreatment in order to keep the family of 8 together.

The patient's fighting and drinking also brought him into contact with the health care system. He was taken to the hospital emergency room for knife wounds incurred during gang fights. At other times he arrived in a wild state, threatening the security staff recklessly. He appeared unconcerned about any danger to himself. On one occasion he was admitted to the intensive care unit in a comatose condition after he overdosed on alcohol and diazepam in an apparent suicide attempt.

The adult participants were unable to intervene effectively or soon enough for several reasons. They found it difficult to understand the patient's illogical and self-destructive behavior. He did things that aroused anger and placed him in an adversarial position with respect to other people. His erratic behavior also occurred in many places, so that no one person was able to comprehend the whole picture or know what to expect when he suddenly appeared.

If professionals involved in the case had sought psychiatric consultation to help them understand the young man, they would have been able to develop interventions based upon their own strengths and appropriate roles.

One teacher, for example, reacted to this student's defiance by demanding that the boy behave or leave the class. A school psychologist could have helped the instructor appreciate the student's underlying need for concern as well as control. Together they could have considered alternative interventions. The instructor might have had the youngster return to class after school hours for punishment, avoiding a confrontation. This would have satisfied both the adolescent's need to talk to an admired male parent figure and the need to be disciplined.

The judge was relatively lenient at first, in the hope that warnings alone would have some effect. A court-appointed psychiatric consultant could have helped the judge understand why, in the context of the defendant's home situation, this approach might not be successful. To the boy, the court's ineffective response was no different from his parents' indifference. That encouraged his escalating delinquency, which increased the judge's frustration and increased the likelihood that he would eventually deliver a severe sentence. Such a sentence would solidify the boy's identity as a criminal. Earlier punishment supplemented by mandatory outpatient psychiatric follow-up with the patient and his family might have helped.

The minister felt so eager to help and felt so sorry for the boy that he was willing to see him under any circumstances. A mental health consultant could have pointed out the need to see the boy only when he was sober. This would have encouraged the boy to adopt more socially acceptable behavior.

Psychiatric consultation in the health care setting might have identified the boy's suicidal thinking before he made a serious suicide attempt. Consultation with the intensive care unit staff members in cases such as this one would help them find ways to effectively manage the patient after the crisis is over and might promote their understanding of the mixed feelings of concern and resentment often evoked by patients who try to kill themselves.

DEFINITIONS

In **consultation psychiatry,** or mental health consultation, the mental health professional helps professionals in other fields (teachers, social workers, etc) solve mental health problems that arise in their professional work situation. The focus is on the immediate problem the consultee presents, and the goals are both to remedy or improve the current situation and to increase the consultee's psychologic skills.

In **liaison psychiatry,** mental health professionals offer their expertise in an ongoing fashion to a group of professionals who work together and share a common group of patients or problems. The group is often based in the health care setting, such as a medical ward, an intensive care unit, or an outpatient clinic. However, mental health liaison work may also be done in schools, in the courts, and in the workplace. The continuing relationship allows the expert to learn more about the needs of the on-site personnel in a more systematic way. The 2 parties become familiar enough with each other so that the psychiatrist can seek out cases during regular rounds or staff conferences rather than wait for referrals. Liaison psychiatry has a greater potential than case-by-case consultation for enhancing the staff's early recognition of psychiatric problems.

Because a consultant on one case may go on to develop a productive liaison relationship with a medical team or unit staff, the term **consultation/liaison psychiatry** is used frequently.

The following differences help distinguish consultation from other interpersonal techniques in psychiatry. In **psychiatric education,** a student follows a prearranged curriculum and a fixed set of exercises, organized by the teacher, in order to acquire a specific body of knowledge. The teacher also evaluates the student's performance. In consultation, consultees learn from the specific case or problem they have chosen to present and are not evaluated by the consultant. In **supervision,** a relationship exists between a more experienced and a less experienced professional from the same discipline. The supervisor accepts responsibility for the supervisee's performance and may discuss the latter's intrapsychic and interpersonal dynamics as they are relevant to the work. A consultation relationship usually occurs between professionals of different disciplines, and the personality of the consultee is rarely addressed.

Dynamic psychotherapy, an interaction between a suffering person and a healing professional, is designed to relieve suffering by helping the patient gain greater self-awareness, especially regarding unconscious thoughts and feelings. The therapist interprets a patient's defenses, transference, and resistances, something that would never be done with a consultee. Instead, a consultee's defenses are supported, and transference is minimized by focusing on the work problem.

The psychiatrist in **administration** establishes policy, delegates responsibility for implementing it, and takes responsibility for its outcome. Relationships are based upon lines of authority. In consultation, the consultee is not bound to carry out directives or even to continue the relationship.

In **collaboration,** professionals work together on the same project, making joint decisions and contributing to the work. Although consultants may perform some of the tasks of preliminary data gathering and interviewing, in general they do not carry out their own recommendations. Exceptions to this approach are discussed in the next chapter.

PRINCIPLES OF CONSULTATION PRACTICE

The following guidelines, derived from practice in community settings, form the basis of good psychiatric consultation practice.

(1) The consultee must be accepted as a competent professional. This attitude forms the basis for a trusting coequal relationship, increasing the quality and honesty of communication between consultant and consultee.

(2) An attempt should be made to understand the environment in which the consultee is functioning. Problems can be understood best in the larger context of the social and physical environment in which they occur. Similarly, recommendations and interventions should be appropriate to the social system or environment in which the problem has arisen.

(3) Specific ways of handling problems should be suggested, since explanations and emotional support are rarely enough.

(4) The consultee must be allowed to accept or reject proffered advice. Consultees will adopt suggestions that can be incorporated into their personal styles of problem solving. In this way, the consultee actively applies newly gained knowledge, which should increase the usefulness of the consultation interchange and reinforce the knowledge so that it can be used again. Consultants in the health care setting who do not endorse this "noninterventionist" approach advocate asserting authority or taking over the management of cases they feel might test the limits of the consultee's skill too severely. They argue that the primary goal, as in any medical consultation, is good patient care, and that the consultee can learn by seeing this process in action. The argument makes sense in the context of the teaching hospital, where many of the staff are resident physicians.

(5) The consultant should avoid focusing on the consultee's psychologic problems. When the consultee displaces personal conflicts and feelings onto the work situation, the successful consultant does not "interpret" but instead emphasizes the work problem. Fear of being "psychoanalyzed" by a consultant impairs communication between the consultee and consultant. The consultant should avoid the appearance of personal scrutiny and judgmental assessment of the consultee.

COMMUNITY CONSULTATION SERVICES

It is well established that most persons with emotional disorders do not seek care in the mental health system (see Chapter 13). Consultation psychiatry provides a means for making available to a wider segment of the community the techniques for assessment, treatment, and prevention of mental disorders. By providing consultation services to various agencies and institutions, mental health professionals are able to vastly increase the scope of their efforts. Groups at high risk for onset or recurrence of emotional disorder thus become more apt to be identified and treated.

The availability of consultation services also offers a vehicle for improvement of the general effectiveness of personnel and programs outside of the mental health care system. Mental health consultation has been used to solve human relations problems in the welfare system, the criminal justice system, schools, and various types of community organizations. Better performance by community agencies contributes to the general welfare of the community.

HISTORICAL BACKGROUND OF COMMUNITY CONSULTATION SERVICES

The success of public health efforts in the 1900s provided the expectations and theoretical groundwork for the later development of community-based consultation in psychiatry. The **mental hygiene movement**—which started in 1908 with the organization of the National Committee for Mental Hygiene—and the **child guidance movement** of the 1920s held up prevention of mental illness as an achievable goal and identified juvenile courts, schools, hospitals, family service agencies, and jails as settings where much could be done to achieve it. When Erich Lindemann (1944) at Harvard studied survivors of the Coconut Grove fire in 1944, he demonstrated how future emotional distress could be prevented with well-timed interventions. Caplan's work (1970) since then has provided a theoretical basis and guide to the practice of preventive psychiatry in the community.

The federal government, starting with the formation of the National Institute of Mental Health in 1946, endorsed the notion that mental health, like public health, was a concern of the community. The 1963 Community Mental Health Centers Act encouraged the establishment of consultation and education services as integral parts of every mental health center. Recent legislation has reinforced the importance of prevention but has de-emphasized consultation.

MODELS IN COMMUNITY MENTAL HEALTH

Descriptive models for community consultation have been useful in planning procedures for intervention by mental health consultants. One scheme relates each category of consultation to a distinctive set of goals and operations.

Case Consultation

A. Client-Centered: This is the most common type of mental health consultation. The consultee seeks assistance in dealing with what are perceived as a client's psychiatric problems. The consultee asks about a specific case and is seeking an assessment leading to specific recommendations for use with a particular client. The consultant addresses this primary need and hopes that the process will also help the consultee approach similar problems more effectively in the future.

The consultant in a client-centered situation spends relatively little time with the consultee, using most of the allotted time to assess the client and develop an impression and a set of recommendations. To the degree the consultant hopes to influence the consultee's future work, time with the consultee may be increased. As psychiatrists have increasing cumulative contact with the professional staff of the community agency, they can reduce their direct involvement with clients and rely increasingly on the experience and judgment of certain consultees. In a few instances, cases will be presented to a consultant given little or no opportunity for direct evaluation of the client. The purpose in such cases is still "client-centered," however—ie, to provide specific feedback about a particularly difficult case even though the client is minimally available to the consultant.

B. Consultee-Centered: The emphasis in consultee-centered case consultations is on review of factors that are causing problems in the professional's work with the client. The goal is to improve the consultee's ability to deal with the kind of problems presented by the case; effecting changes in the client is of secondary importance. The assumption is that the consultee's difficulties with the case figure prominently in the request for consultation.

The consultee's statement of the difficulties and understanding of the case are reviewed. Information from others (including the client) is sought in order to enhance the consultant's understanding of the consultee's problems. The distinction between this activity and supervision of the consultee is not always clear. However, the consultant—unlike the supervising professional—has no general responsibility for the work performance of the consultee.

Administrative Consultation

A. Program-Centered: When a program director or administrator asks a consultant to review and make recommendations regarding problems that have arisen in an ongoing program or problems in planning a new program, the consultant enters an area of activity very distinct from case consultation. The intent is to explore organizational problems.

The consultant studies the program or organization—its structure, staffing, purposes, and functions. The consultant's report contains recommendations that deal specifically with the problems presented. The questions may emphasize an administrator's interest in how emotional or psychologic factors have impeded program development. Administrators may want to know how best to take into account emotional factors when designing a new program.

B. Consultee-Centered: When the administrative skills of the consultee become the focus of the consultant's efforts, the activity is regarded as consultee-centered. The information the consultant obtains about the organization of the agency is used to upgrade the consultee's organizational problem-solving ability.

Because of the goals of this activity, the consultant spends most of the available time becoming acquainted with the organizational perspective of the consultee. The duration of consultant activity in consultee-centered consultation is often longer than in program-centered consultation.

CONSULTATION TO COMMUNITY AGENCIES

There has been considerable growth since World War II in the use of consultation services by community agencies and institutions, most notably the schools and the criminal justice system. Consultation has expanded into new areas, such as work with religious organizations and pastoral counselors.

Despite extensive activity, there has been insufficient evaluation of the impact of consultant services on community functions. The need for clear justifications of expenditures for consultant services will increase as fiscal constraints on mental health care tighten.

The Criminal Justice System

The psychiatric consultant provides case-centered and administrative consultation to the various agencies that make up the criminal justice system (see Chapter 58). Psychiatric assessment, intervention, or referral can occur at each step along the judicial route: pretrial hearing; pre- and postsentencing assessment; probationary period; incarceration in institutions for the criminally insane and for criminal offenders; and the period of parole.

During the pretrial phase, the salient issue is the individual's competence to participate in the judicial process. Generally, a brief assessment should be made of the defendant's ability to comprehend the proceedings and assist a lawyer in his or her defense. There is little interest in the individual's psychiatric status per se and none in improving the psychiatric skills of the professionals associated with the court.

The consultant may be called on to testify in court about the accused's mental state and at that time may be exposed to the rigors of the adversarial process in cross-examination.

In dealing with the criminal justice system (jails, prisons, detention halls, institutions for the criminally insane), the consultant must realize that the chief goal of the consultee facility is humane confinement and only secondarily to effect attitudinal or behavioral changes in the inmates. Although concerns about the mental health and welfare of inmates may provoke requests for consultation, more often the consultant is asked to advise about the prevention and management of hostile and assaultive behavior. Staff workers may be inclined to see any disturbed behavior as manipulative or "mean" rather than as a manifestation of mental disorder. There is great external pressure on correctional agencies to keep an orderly house, and identifying and managing emotional disorders is not perceived as one of their functions. The tension between helping and controlling is often high; the staff's inclination in dealing with behavioral disturbances is to increase "discipline."

Parole and probation officers who identify emotional disturbances among their caseload may seek client-centered consultation.

The juvenile justice system deals with young people who have troubled backgrounds and disturbed behavior. Greater emphasis is placed on the potential and need for behavioral change among youthful offenders than is the case with adult offenders. The mental health consultant engages in several kinds of activity: assistance in judgment of the juvenile's competence, assessment of mental status and intellectual potential, and recommendations for treatment and placement.

Public Welfare Agencies

Social service agencies emphasize the importance of encouraging individuals and families to achieve maximal self-sufficiency. In an attempt to improve their capacity to respond to the emotional needs of their client population, public welfare agency administrators and caseworkers have looked to community psychiatrists for assistance. The activities of these agencies consist in large part in providing family and child welfare services.

Welfare agencies serve the aged, the blind, families with dependent children, and persons with severe disability resulting from mental or physical disorders. Any of these people may have major psychosocial problems and psychiatric disturbances. Geriatric psychiatry calls attention to the special emotional needs of the elderly, and the caseworker often is one of the few individuals to have periodic contact with aged welfare recipients. Severely disabled blind people or hearing-impaired people have great difficulties achieving independence. Single-parent families with several dependents living in poor neighborhoods are at risk for emotional disorder based, at the very least, on the struggle to obtain the necessities of life. Finally, persons with a disabling mental disorder are benefited by a strong relationship between the caseworker and the treating mental health professional.

The consultant plays a complex role in assisting the consultee to identify disturbed individuals and those at risk of developing behavioral disturbances; in aiding the caseworker to distinguish psychiatric disorder from "problems in living"; and in helping workers to review their feelings about public relief for the poor and the legitimacy of the needs of those served. Consultation can be invaluable in helping workers deal with and give appropriate assistance and support to clients with severe psychiatric disorders.

Schools

Consultants work in the school system in a number of settings. The staff of a day-care center may wish to give more attention to the emotional needs of preschoolers. Special education teachers in an elementary school may want help in designing a class format that anticipates the behavioral difficulties associated with their students' handicaps. Guidance counselors in an urban high school may ask that psychiatric consultation be made available to assist them in their work.

In these settings, the primary objectives of consultees are to educate the students and, especially in the elementary school years, to promote their social and emotional development. Developmental issues and their relationship to learning ability are important. In addition to objectives related to the students themselves, teachers and administrators want classroom interaction that enhances education and are looking for ways to improve student group behavior. As with other agencies that serve children, the school becomes involved with the family. In this way, personnel in the school system become aware of family problems, including emotional ones.

Recent trends in education have implications for psychiatric consultation. There has been increasing pressure on the schools to raise and then enforce minimum scholastic requirements for promotion and graduation. The public clamors for discipline in the schools, prompted partly by the growing number of assaults by students on teachers and other students. These concerns are compounded by public awareness of drug and alcohol abuse by school-age children. All of these problems have led to an interest in psychiatric consultation services on the part of parents, school administrators, educators, and other mental health professionals within the school system.

Religious Organizations

Members of the clergy serve not only their own congregations and communicants but many members of the community through church-sponsored activities. Perhaps no other group of community workers serves as well as an immediate resource for many troubled individuals and families. Religious workers of all faiths contribute to the emotional welfare of their communities and in this way help to minimize the development or recurrence of mental disorder. Religious organizations provide psychologic, social, and material support. When mentally troubled people seek help from pastoral workers rather than from the mental health system, the pastoral counselor becomes the de facto primary mental health care provider.

The problems that come to the attention of this class of mental health care providers include alcoholism, failing marriages, and social isolation of the sick and elderly. The church and its agencies may formally define their mission in these terms or may deal ad hoc with the problems as they arise. Pastoral workers have varied degrees of experience and training. Workers in the outreach ministries are often lay volunteers.

Counseling is one of several important activities undertaken by the clergy. Consultation may focus on such disparate activities as the cleric's administration of a counseling project or the intent and impact of his or her ministry. Traditionally, the minister is obligated to become involved in people's problems even without invitation. This provides great opportunities for beneficial intervention.

The psychiatric consultant must demonstrate to the pastoral consultee the importance of a more informed assessment and more skillful management of the emotional problems that come to his or her attention. At the same time, the consultant must convey a sense of respect for the consultee's counseling objectives and religious frame of reference, including ethical and moral connotations.

CRISIS CONSULTATION

Crisis theory and intervention strategies are an important part of the work of the community mental health clinician. The consultant is often called upon to help the consultee master or survive a crisis. Crises may operate as destructive forces or may offer the potential for beneficial change. Crisis situations are fluid and thus responsive to intervention.

All crises have elements of surprise and uncertainty. A crisis is a profoundly disturbing situation posing a threat to the capacity of the client, worker, or system to function in an organized, effective fashion. Crisis consultation usually involves a client with an acute, severe disturbance and represents a challenge to the coping ability of the consultant. Occasionally, a consultee may have a sense of crisis under what may seem to be less than urgent circumstances. However, the consultee's sense of crisis is the required element in crisis consultation even when the consultant does not share the consultee's perception of the gravity of the situation.

The surprise and uncertainty characteristic of crisis situations are a barrier to comprehension and appropriate action. These features generate pressures on the consultant that must be appreciated before the consultant undertakes to function in crisis consultation. There may be a demand for an immediate response before information is gathered and analyzed and a coherent management strategy developed.

In working with the staff during a crisis consultation, the consultant must sort out the sources of staff anxiety and determine whether they are personal, organizational, or clinical. Even when the request is conveyed as if a client-centered consultation were being sought, all sources of tension should be reviewed with the consultee. The personal tension a staff worker may contribute to the crisis may be partially relieved by contact with the psychiatrist. Since the worker and the consultant may have different objectives, the consultant must try to correct inappropriate expectations. Familiarity with the staff is invaluable in resolving these issues.

Even when tempted (and able) to resolve a crisis unilaterally, the consultant should avoid "taking over." Though the consultee may not want to get involved with handling clinical material, the opportunity should be taken to increase the consultee's skills for the benefit of future clients. At the very least, the consultee should be encouraged to observe the consultant interacting with the client.

The consultant helps staff members to become more sensitive to the signs of impending behavioral crisis in their clients. The staff should develop greater appreciation of its capacity to assess, manage, and prevent crises. Ideally, as the staff spends more time with a consultant, the ability to identify problems and prevent crises improves.

Staff autonomy in mastering a crisis is a function of the availability of mental health services. Consultants should clearly define their accessibility and should be familiar with mental health resources for the population served by the agency. Naturally, those agencies with least access to emergency psychiatric care have the greatest incentive to improve their own crisis management skills.

Illustrative case. A Protestant minister who was motivated to provide psychologic counseling to his congregation received a frantic phone call from a young woman who had just received laboratory confirmation of her unwanted pregnancy. She was unmarried and still living at home, and she described herself as feeling "morbidly guilty" and "terribly confused, with nowhere to turn." She mentioned thoughts of suicide as "the only answer now." He urged her to come to the rectory immediately.

The minister had attended a few sessions with other religious advisors and pastoral workers at a neighborhood mental health clinic where group discussions led by a psychiatrist had explored the clerical role in mental health counseling. Suddenly fearful that he might mishandle the "crisis" that would soon present itself at his door, he placed an urgent call to the psychiatrist and explained what had happened. The psychiatrist agreed that the situation might call for more expertise than the minister possessed at his present level of training and offered to participate in the interview. The offer was gratefully accepted.

The psychiatrist arrived a few minutes after the young woman, and she agreed to let him hear her story. The psychiatrist unobtrusively took on the major role during the interview while the minister looked on. The matter was concluded when the young woman made a series of appointments to see the psychiatrist privately.

For the clergyman, this experience was unique. It came at a time when a program of education and consultation had been initiated. The problem facing this helping professional was acute and related to the psychologic distress of a parishioner. Though events challenged the coping capacities of all 3 persons involved—the young woman, the clergyman, and the psychiatrist—the crisis provided an opportunity for improving the minister's skills.

HEALTH SYSTEM–BASED CONSULTATION

The practice of consultation in the health care setting has benefited from several recent developments in psychiatry: (1) *DSM-III* offers a more reliable nosology, so that primary-care physicians can have a better understanding of the diagnostic criteria for psychiatric disorders. (2) Better techniques for identifying and treating syndromes such as the panic/phobic disorders have widened the scope of what the psychiatrist has to offer nonpsychiatrists. (3) Research into the psychophysiologic and psychosocial factors associated with disease has broadened the theoretical base of clinical work outside psychiatry. (4) The emphasis on a systems approach to patient care has compelled psychiatrists to view each patient as a whole, without neglecting the biologic or social spheres. This method allows for a better understanding of medical and surgical patients and makes medical problems more interesting to the psychiatrist. These advances also have increased the interest of nonpsychiatrists in psychiatry. The barrier between psychiatry and other specialties has been lowered, leaving a membrane permeable to the exchange of information between physicians with different kinds of training and varied scientific biases.

LIAISON APPROACH

Psychiatric liaison activities are increasing in importance in health care settings. The needs for psychiatric intervention among hospitalized patients are too great to be satisfied by individual case consultation alone. These needs demand active case detection and continuing staff education. The guidelines of consultation psychiatry have been complemented by the following principles of liaison psychiatry: (1) Become involved early in the course of medical treatment. This may necessitate active screening of patients at high risk for psychologic problems. (2) Develop working relationships with primary-care physicians in clinical, research, and educational activities. (3) Follow patients and families through the course of hospitalization. (4) Adopt the role of ombudsman, allying oneself with patients and becoming a spokesperson for their needs.

Two general methods of liaison psychiatry are in use today in health care settings. One is **geographic,** in which mental health professionals confine their activities to a specific area such as a ward or clinic. This fosters a good relationship with the permanent staff, such as nurses and paraprofessionals. Another approach is by **specialty,** in which the psychiatrist works only with a certain group of medical or surgical colleagues. This naturally encourages identification with the doctors from that particular specialty.

Many innovative programs in liaison psychiatry have flourished in different centers across the country. At Mount Sinai Hospital in New York, a psychiatrist and a nonpsychiatrist physician together conduct weekly teaching rounds and serve as role models. The nonpsychiatrist physician gradually assumes more responsibility for teaching biopsychosocial issues. At the University of Alabama, psychiatrists are part of an interdisciplinary clinical team in the family medicine

service. Groups at the University of West Virginia and the University of Virginia have developed a program in which residents are trained in psychiatry and medicine. Medical students and residents rotate through a ward that integrates medical and psychiatric care.

Another approach to liaison psychiatry that focuses primarily on physicians in training has emerged at the University of California, San Francisco. Third-year medical students spend 2 hours a week of every clerkship in a patient-oriented seminar devoted to the psychiatric aspects of medical practice. The required course is taught by physicians from that particular specialty and by psychiatrists. This course was inspired by George Engel's success at the University of Rochester in teaching psychosocial concepts and medicine together. There the liaison mental health professional is a nonpsychiatrist physician who has had training in the principles and concepts of psychology.

SYSTEMS APPROACH

The systems approach encourages understanding of the total patient by integrating the biologic, psychologic, and social spheres into the formulation of any clinical situation (see Chapter 3). It has particular appeal to the consultation/liaison psychiatrist because it imposes a framework of organization on the immense amount of data that confronts the consultation/liaison practitioner. It allows the clinician to consider data from any system level (ie, biologic, psychologic, or social data) that may be pertinent, and this affords a comprehensive approach to interventions. Clinical approaches to problems at each level can be developed.

Leigh and Reiser (1980) use a patient evaluation grid (PEG) as one way of conceptualizing the systems approach. The grid (Fig 55–1) shows the patient's problems in 3 spheres and 3 distinct time frames: current, recent, and past (background). One can in this way visualize the course of a problem through time and see the relationships between the social, psychologic, and biologic levels. Another model for organizing systems arranges the data into a matrix (Table 55–1) that lists significant factors affecting both the consultee and the patient. This model prompts the consultant to consider the interactions between patient and consultee in recommending interventions. In Fig 55–1 and Table 55–1, these systems approaches are used to illustrate the case of the "belligerent boy" described at the beginning of the chapter.

At the **environmental (social)** level, as shown in Table 55–1, the patient's family refuses to acknowledge the father's violence and drinking or to listen to the patient's complaints. This forces the patient to express his feelings in another setting and to do so with actions rather than with words. The trouble this causes the teacher, as when the student disrupts class, motivates the consultation request. The consultant must consider the constraints inherent in the classroom set-

	Current	Recent	Past (Background)
Environmental (social) factors	Patient runs away from home.	Father beats mother.	Father and mother have long-standing marital conflicts.
Behavioral and psychologic factors	Patient feels depressed and guilty.	Patient feels anger toward parents and only expresses feelings when intoxicated.	Patient represses feelings.
Biologic factors	Patient shows early signs of alcohol dependence.	Patient has frequent episodes of intoxication.	Patient has family history of alcoholism.

Figure 55–1. Patient evaluation grid (PEG), modified and adapted from Leigh and Reiser (1980). In the example shown, significant elements of the illustrative case of the "belligerent boy" are noted in the boxes. (See case details in text and Table 55–1.) Use of the grid helps the consultant organize a plan for evaluation and formulation of interventions.

ting, such as the strong need for order and the rights of the other students, in fashioning a recommendation to see the student after class.

At the **behavioral** level, the patient provokes authorities to anger and challenges them to control him. They react according to their unique personality styles and roles, as when the judge reprimands the patient and threatens punishment, assuming that this response will alter the boy's behavior. In fact, the patient sees the judge's inaction as impotent and disinterested, causing him to escalate his delinquent behavior in order to elicit action. The consultant recommends, instead, that the judge provide appropriate discipline for the patient's misbehavior along with mandatory counseling.

Such interactions occur at an unconscious **psychologic** level also. The patient feels unhappy, holds his parents responsible, and expresses this in self-destructive behavior around adult authority figures. The minister, in turn, feels a sense of responsibility toward the patient and perhaps a twinge of guilt that he has not done enough. This makes him want to listen to the patient under any circumstances instead of setting limits to the drinking. The patient perceives that the minister is "bending over backward" as if responsible for the patient's behavior. It becomes difficult for the patient then to accept responsibility and to sort out his feelings toward his parents. The consultant identifies this dynamic relationship and uses the consultee's reactions to explain the patient's psychology. This helps the consultee view the situation less personally.

The **biologic** level of the matrix shows that the patient may be demonstrating important neurovegetative clinical signs of depression (poor concentration, decreased energy) and early evidence of alcohol dependence. However, the patient's stormy behavior may divert the attention of the various consultees from this important category of clinical information.

SUMMARY

The purpose of consultation/liaison psychiatry is to improve the ability of non–mental health practitioners to identify and deal with clients in need of psychiatric help. The ultimate goal is the prevention of mental illness or, at least, the reduction of severe illness caused by psychiatric problems. The consultant in psychiatry approaches the task from the framework of certain guiding principles and focuses upon those areas where the consultee wants help. **Case consultation** is usually done in clinical situations involving patients and their families. **Client-centered** case consultation provides evaluation and recommendations that focus only upon the patient. **Consultee-centered** case consultation focuses upon the abilities of the consultee in dealing with particular situations. In **administrative consultation,** the work of the consultee involves directing a pro-

Table 55–1. Matrix for organizing evaluation and interventions in psychiatric consultations.*

Factors	Data Derived From Patient's History and Examination	Data Derived From Consultation With Others (Teacher, Judge, Minister)	Consultant's Interventions
Environmental (social)	**Characteristics of the patient's family system:** 1. Father becomes drunk and beats mother and patient. 2. Mother remains with father in order to keep family together. 3. Situation is not discussed; both parents ignore patient's distress.	**Characteristics of consultees' social system:** 1. School dictates that teacher maintain order in class. 2. Criminal justice system empowers judge to protect society from delinquent behavior. 3. Church directs clergy to provide unqualified support to distraught parishioners.	**Environmental interventions:** 1. Tell teacher to deal with patient after class. 2. Recommend that judge remove patient from delinquent peer group. 3. Help minister provide a social situation in which the rules about drinking are different from those of the patient's family. 4. Facilitate or provide family therapy.
Behavioral	**Patient's behavior:** 1. He runs away from home and drinks when upset. 2. He provokes fights and challenges authority figures. 3. He expresses his feelings when intoxicated.	**Consultees' behavior:** 1. Teacher meets patient's challenge with a counterchallenge to leave class. 2. Judge reprimands patient and delays punishment. 3. Minister continues to see patient when latter is drunk.	**Behavioral interventions:** 1. Help the teacher develop a relationship within the structure of "afterclass punishment." 2. Recommend that judge react to misbehavior with commensurate penalty plus psychiatric follow-up. 3. Encourage minister to see patient only when the latter is sober and can talk rationally.
Psychologic	**Patient's underlying psychologic characteristics:** 1. He is unable to tolerate feelings of hate toward mother and experiences guilt for these. 2. He redirects anger toward himself by drinking and recklessness. 3. He masters angry feelings toward father by identifying with father's drinking. 4. He wishes to communicate depressive feelings to parents but cannot.	**Consultees' psychologic reactions:** 1. Teacher is angry and wishes to retaliate. 2. Judge either overreacts or underreacts to patient's provocation. 3. Minister feels responsible for patient's behavior.	**Psychologic interventions:** 1. Provide an explanation of patient's underlying psychodynamics. 2. Facilitate data gathering and development of hypotheses. 3. Encourage detachment from personal involvement and sense of responsibility. 4. Reduce unrealistic expectations of changing patient's behavior.
Biologic	**Patient's biologic manifestations:** 1. Poor concentration. 2. Decreased energy. 3. Frequent episodes of intoxication (acute organic brain syndrome). 4. Beginnings of physiologic addiction to alcohol.	**Consultees' concerns related to patient's biologic manifestations:** 1. Patient's stormy behavior diverts attention from underlying concomitants of depression: poor concentration, decreased energy level, poor appetite, etc.	**Biologic interventions:** 1. Facilitate better nutrition by limiting alcohol abuse. 2. Work up underlying depression and its biologic concomitants.

*The example shows data from the illustrative case of the "belligerent boy," which is discussed in the text and in Fig 55–1.

gram. **Program-centered** administrative consultation analyzes the particular organization and provides recommendations for dealing with its problems. **Consultee-centered** administrative consultation focuses upon the consultee's administrative skills. Each of these models can be applied to settings in the community, such as the schools, religious organizations, public welfare agencies, the criminal justice system, and particular sites in the health care system. In the latter setting, the **liaison** approach is often used, in which a mental health professional works in an ongoing fashion with a group of health care providers. Such a group may be based in a ward or clinic, the **geographic** model; or may have in common a set of skills or similar patients, the **specialty** model. In these contacts, the consultation/liaison psychiatrist often makes use of a **systems** approach to clinical issues, in which the biologic, social, psychologic, and behavioral aspects of the patient's life are considered in arriving at recommendations. The following chapter will discuss consultation psychiatry as practiced in the setting most familiar to medical students and physicians in training—the general hospital.

REFERENCES

Anderson RG, Robinson C, Ruben HL: Mental health training and consultation: A model for liaison with clergy. *Hosp Community Psychiatry* 1978;**29**:800.

Barsky A, Brown H: Psychiatric teaching and consultation in a primary care clinic. *Psychosomatics* 1982;**23**:9.

Berlin IN: Learning mental health consultation. *Ment Hygiene* 1964;**48**:257.

Bertalanffy L von: *General Systems Theory: Foundations, Development, Applications.* George Braziller, 1968.

Bindman AJ: The clinical psychologist as a mental health consultant. In: *Progress in Clinical Psychology.* Abt LE, Reiss BJ (editors). Grune & Stratton, 1966.

Bindman AJ: Mental health consultation: Theory and practice. *J Consult Psychol* 1959;**23**:473.

Caplan G: *The Theory and Practice of Mental Health Consultation.* Basic Books, 1970.

Deutsch A: The mental hygiene movement and its founder. Chapter 15 in: *The Mentally Ill in America,* 2nd ed. Deutsch A (editor). Columbia Univ Press, 1952.

Edelstein P, Ross WD, Schultz JR: The biopsychosocial approach: Clinical examples from a consultation-liaison service. (3 parts.) *Psychosomatics* 1982;**23**:15, 141, 233.

Engel GL: The clinical application of the biopsychosocial model. *Am J Psychiatry* 1980;**137**:535.

Fitzgerald JF, Peske MA, Goodwin RC: Competency evaluations in Connecticut. *Hosp Community Psychiatry* 1978; **29**:450.

Garrick TR, Stotland NL: How to write a psychiatric consultation. *Am J Psychiatry* 1982;**139**:849.

Goldberg RJ, Van Dyke C: Psychiatric consultation: When to request and what to expect. *RI Med J* 1982;**64**:115.

Kaplan HI, Freedman AM, Sadock BJ (editors): *Comprehensive Textbook of Psychiatry/IV,* 4th ed. Williams & Wilkins, 1985.

Leigh H, Reiser MF: *The Patient: Biological, Psychological, and Social Dimensions of Medical Practice.* Plenum Press, 1980.

Lindemann E: Symptomatology and management of acute grief. *Am J Psychiatry* 1944;**101**:141.

Lipowski ZJ: Psychiatric consultation: Concepts and controversies. *Am J Psychiatry* 1977;**134**:523.

Mendelsohn M, Meyer E: Psychiatric consultation with patients on medical and surgical wards: Patterns and processes. *Psychiatry* 1961;**23**:197.

Neil JR, Sandifer MG: *Practical Manual of Psychiatric Consultation.* Williams & Wilkins, 1980.

Pasnau RO: Consultation-liaison psychiatry at the crossroads: In search of a definition for the 1980s. *Hosp Community Psychiatry* 1982;**33**:989.

Rosen DH, Blackwell B: Teaching psychiatry in medicine. *Arch Intern Med* 1982;**142**:1113.

Strain JJ: Collaborative efforts in liaison psychiatry. Chapter 12 in: *Handbook of Clinical Health Psychology.* Millon I, Green G, Meagher R (editors). Plenum Press, 1982.

Strain JJ: Needs for psychiatry in the general hospital. *Hosp Community Psychiatry* 1982;**33**:996.

Consultation/Liaison Psychiatry in the General Hospital

56

Craig Van Dyke, MD, & Richard Goldberg, MD

Consultation/liaison psychiatry is the practical application of psychiatric knowledge and techniques to the care of medical patients in a general hospital. While commonly assumed to be synonymous with psychosomatic medicine, consultation/liaison psychiatry is actually more diverse and requires a knowledge of general psychiatry as well as a familiarity with medical and surgical diseases and their treatments, neuroanatomy and neurobehavioral disorders, pharmacology, and systems theory.

As the bridge between psychiatry and medicine, consultation/liaison psychiatry has always occupied a strategic position. At present, while psychiatry is striving to be included in the mainstream of medicine, this strategic position is more critical than ever. Implicit in this position is consultation/liaison psychiatry's responsibility to both medicine and psychiatry. From medicine's perspective, we must make psychiatry relevant by assisting in the care of patients and by training medical students and residents. From the other perspective, we must assist psychiatry in its endeavor to return to its medical origins. This may take the form of training psychiatric residents to treat the emotional and cognitive problems of medical and surgical patients or emphasizing that the brain has an anatomy and physiology and is not a "black box." Perhaps the most important role is maintaining those physicianly attitudes and feelings that are present in every medical student who becomes a psychiatrist.

In clinical practice, consultation/liaison psychiatrists treat medical and surgical patients with emotional and cognitive problems. Epidemiologic studies (vonAmmon Cavanaugh, 1983) reveal that 30–65% of medical inpatients have significant psychiatric symptoms, with the most frequent diagnoses being anxiety, depression, and organic mental disorder. Contributing further to the incidence of psychiatric problems in medical patients is the high rate of physical illness in psychiatric patients, who may represent a disproportionately large segment of the population seeking medical treatment. As an example, in one study (Davies, 1965) it was noted that 58% of all patients in a psychiatric clinic had a physical illness. Others have found shortened survival in patients suffering from schizophrenia, mania, and depression. While suicide accounted for part of the high death rate, other causes of death were accidents, infections, and circulatory disorders.

With the recent development and application of brief cognitive screening tests (see Chapter 18), there is increasing appreciation that medical and surgical patients have a high rate of cognitive impairments. For example, about 30% of patients in acute medical inpatient units have cognitive deficits (vonAmmon Cavanaugh, 1983; De Paulo and Folstein, 1978). The rate may be twice as high in neurology inpatient units. However, since many of these brief cognitive screening examinations do not systematically assess constructional or language skills, the true incidence of cognitive impairment in medical populations is probably greater than reported.

Despite a high incidence of emotional and cognitive disturbances, only 2–12% of medical and surgical patients are evaluated by a psychiatric consultant (Lipowski, 1967; Moses and Barzilay, 1967; Schwab and coworkers, 1966). The reasons for this are not completely clear, but a number of factors may be at work. If the psychiatric symptoms are understandable in the context of the patient's illness, the primary physician may feel no need to request a psychiatric consultation. When a patient with cancer develops depressive symptoms, the primary physician may feel the reaction is appropriate and that no treatment is required, or that if treatment is required the primary physician should be able to provide it. Primary physicians may also believe that a psychiatric consultant might have nothing positive to offer and might even upset the patient. Another critical factor is that in many cases, primary physicians simply fail to recognize emotional and cognitive problems in their patients.

This chapter focuses on inpatient consultation/liaison psychiatry and is intended to make the primary physician a better consumer of the services. Eight common clinical problems for which psychiatric consultation is indicated will be described, as well as liaison activities with intensive care and hemodialysis units.

CONSULTATION PROCEDURE

A primary-care physician may request a consultation by a personal call to the consultant or by submitting a written request. Usually, but not always, the patient has been prepared for the visit.

Following the primary physician's request for consultation, the psychiatric consultant's first task is to define as precisely as possible the questions being asked by the consultee. Sometimes this is quite easy, as with the patient who has attempted suicide, was hospitalized, and may require evaluation of the need for suicide precautions or further psychiatric treatment. At other times the questions being asked are quite vague; eg, the consultee may believe that the patient's emotional response to the medical illness is inappropriate but is unable to state the problem more precisely. A preliminary discussion between the consultee and consultant can sharpen the focus of the consultation. Following this, the consultant reviews the chart, with special emphasis on any drugs the patient is taking. For inpatients, discussion with the nursing staff may be helpful. A discussion with the family often provides important supplemental information.

The consultant then interviews the patient, preferably in private. Consultants must make it clear at the outset that they are psychiatrists and discuss any feelings the patient has about being interviewed by a psychiatrist. Patients are then asked to verbalize their understanding of the medical or surgical problem and the difficulties it has created. During the interview, a formal mental status examination should be performed. The essence of the consultation process, however, is to gather information about the problems that led to the consultation request. While this may seem obvious, it is not uncommon for inexperienced consultants to gather extensive information about the patient's life and psychodynamics without investigating the "chief complaint" of the primary physician.

The consultant should then formulate a differential diagnosis and discuss it with the primary physician along with whatever has been learned about the specific issues for which the consultation was requested. Discussion of these issues should also occur with the nursing staff for inpatients. For example, a depressed medical patient with suicidal ideation should be discussed at length with the nursing staff so that they will understand the context of the patient's depression and the specific precautions to be taken.

The consultation note should be brief, and specifically labeled as a *psychiatric* consultation, with date, time, and sources of information. Details of the patient's history and information about the specific problem for which the consultation was requested should be stated. Discretion is called for, since medical records have less privacy protection than psychiatric records. It is critical to omit superfluous information that may be embarrassing or lead to inappropriate labeling of the patient. The mental status examination should be recorded in detail, since it represents the most objective information in the note. It is particularly helpful as baseline information that can be referred to when the patient is seen later. Finally, a working diagnosis and a differential diagnosis are recorded.

The heart of the consultation note is the recommendations, and these must address the consultee's questions. The recommendations should be stated as specifically as possible. It is not sufficient to state that the patient should be evaluated for certain conditions and started on certain medications. Rather, the specific tests and details of the drug regimen should be stated, along with the target symptoms and potential adverse effects. Follow-up examination by the consultant is an integral part of all consultations. This allows the patient, consultee, and consultant to evaluate the impact of the initial recommendations and to make appropriate modifications.

PSYCHIATRIC CONSULTATION

The 8 categories discussed below do not necessarily reflect traditional diagnostic categories, and most are not medical or psychiatric syndromes. All can be considered complex clinical situations that include interacting biologic, psychologic, and social factors.

ORGANIC MENTAL DISORDERS

A significant number of hospital patients have an organic mental disorder that remains unrecognized or masquerades as some other problem such as depression or noncompliant behavior. Organic mental disorder should be the first consideration in any evaluation of impaired mood, thought, or behavior. In its most dramatic form, gross delirium is easily recognized by noting the patient's impaired attention, perceptual disturbances, agitation, and disorientation. Visual hallucinations, which many clinicians associate with schizophrenia, are actually more common in organic mental disorders such as delirium tremens and toxic encephalopathy. It is not uncommon for consultees to mistakenly ascribe even obvious organic delirium to some psychogenic cause. There are, of course, many less severe cases in which mild delirium or dementia is characterized by impaired intellect, memory, or personality change. In many situations, the consultant will recognize the presence of organic mental disorder only by performing a specific mental status examination (see Chapter 18). Assessment of language and other higher functioning is often neglected but critical for the detection of aphasia, apraxia, and agnosia.

The recognition of organic mental disorder is important because it often has a specific cause and treatment. Furthermore, failure to provide treatment may lead to permanent deficits and mislabeling of the patient's symptoms. The common denominator in organic mental disorder is impairment of cerebral function. Specific causes include metabolic derangements, drug toxicity or withdrawal, vascular compromise, infections, intracranial tumors, and neuronal degeneration. The consultant must be prepared to review the medical evaluation of the patient with special emphasis on the presence of neurologic findings. The psychiatric consultant must also review all laboratory evaluations and neurodiagnostic tests, such as lumbar puncture, electroencephalography, and cranial CT scan, and be prepared to make recommendations for further tests. In the hospital setting, most cases of organic mental disorder are either partially or entirely reversible. The most frequent cause is a metabolic imbalance, such as alterations in renal, pancreatic, hepatic, cardiovascular, or pulmonary function. A comprehensive drug review is crucial. This may be supplemented by toxicology screening and serum levels of potentially psychoactive substances. Although a great many drugs may produce psychiatric symptoms as adverse side effects, the most common offenders are the central nervous system depressants, digitalis, cimetidine, levodopa, corticosteroids, and antihypertensive and atropinic agents.

Primary treatment consists of correction of the underlying medical abnormality. In addition, certain adjunctive measures are useful. Neuroleptics in small doses may be useful in controlling the agitation of the confused patient and are often superior to benzodiazepines, which may further confuse patients with organic mental disorder. Environmental changes can minimize patient confusion. Such manipulations include provision of calendars, clocks, night-lights (to minimize "sundowning"), familiar objects from home, and frequent orientation by staff and family. Clear, straightforward, and consistent communication from the staff and family also helps patients organize their experience. Precautions must also be instituted for individuals at risk for hurting themselves (eg, falling out of bed, getting lost) as a result of their cognitive impairment.

DEPRESSION

Depressed mood is probably the most common reason for psychiatric consultations. When such depression is a response to the stresses of medical illness, it may respond to improvement in the patient's clinical condition or to reassurance by the primary physician. However, when symptoms become severe and interfere with the patient's daily activities or participation in treatment, psychiatric evaluation should be requested. Aside from depressed mood or crying, the depressed medical patient may be noncompliant with treatment, functioning at a more severely impaired level than is warranted by the medical condition, or preoccupied with somatic symptoms.

There is a tendency to assume that depressed mood in a medical patient represents an understandable adjustment reaction that does not warrant treatment. ("Wouldn't you be depressed if you had lupus?") This may lead to needless suffering, since the depression may respond to treatment. For example, approximately 50% of patients are persistently depressed following stroke. Although it might be reasonable to

think that the degree of disability is the main risk factor for development of depression, in fact it is not. The location of the lesion plays a much greater role. Patients with left hemispheric stroke, especially involving the anterior pole, are at greatest risk for developing depression. Such depression can be treated with antidepressant medication. Assuming that a feeling of depression in medical patients is an adjustment reaction can lead to diagnostic errors. In one study (Levine and coworkers, 1978) of 100 cancer patients referred to the psychiatric service for evaluation of depression, 26% proved to have organic mental disorder misdiagnosed as depression.

Sleep disturbances may be due to pain or paroxysmal nocturnal dyspnea; appetite disturbance to nausea; fatigue to anemia; and impaired concentration to the effects of drugs such as theophylline. Ignoring these possibilities can lead to an overdiagnosis of depression.

As in other settings, the treatment of depression in medically ill patients involves both psychotherapy and antidepressant medications. Supportive psychotherapy assists many patients and their families in coping with the illness. Antidepressant drugs are useful in treating depressed medical patients and can improve mood, appetite, and sleep patterns. Many of these agents must be used cautiously in patients with cardiac conduction abnormalities (especially bundle branch blocks); in patients with organic mental disorder, who may become more confused; and in those for whom anticholinergic side effects would be detrimental. Many of these drugs cause orthostatic hypotension and must be used carefully in patients who cannot tolerate a decrease in blood pressure. Monoamine oxidase inhibitors should be used with extreme caution in this population, because the drugs have numerous interactions with food substances and with other drugs.

The evaluation of suicidal potential is a major function of the psychiatric consultant. The possibility of suicide must be evaluated in all depressed medical patients. The consultant must decide whether the patient requires suicide precautions (constant observation, plastic dining utensils, etc) and what type of psychiatric follow-up is indicated after recovery in cases of self-inflicted medical or surgical problems.

PATIENT MANAGEMENT PROBLEMS

Psychiatric consultation may be requested to assist in management of (1) the agitated, disruptive patient; (2) the patient whose noncompliance may have serious consequences (eg, the patient who insists upon leaving the hospital against medical advice); and (3) the patient whose personality problems interfere with clinical management (eg, patients who are excessively demanding, seductive, or paranoid) (see Chapter 36). The psychiatric consultant is not an alternative to the hospital security personnel, although this sometimes seems to be a prevailing expectation. The physically threatening patient is better managed initially by calling upon properly trained security officers, or police officers from the community if necessary.

The evaluation of patient management problems involves consideration of biologic, psychologic, and social factors as they interact in a particular clinical setting. Since many patient management problems arise out of some underlying medical process, recognition and correction of that problem are of primary concern. Metabolic imbalance, drug intoxications, and drug withdrawal syndromes are frequent causes of agitation. The consultant should make specific recommendations for immediate management, including the indications and contraindications for use of restraints or medications to control agitation. The consultant should decide whether antipsychotic drugs or benzodiazepines are indicated and in what dosages. The consultant is also expected to offer guidelines regarding the legal implications (if any) of treating such patients (see Chapter 58).

The consultant must assess to what extent a patient's personality style might be contributing to a dysfunctional response to illness. At times, brief psychiatric intervention helps the patient adjust to the situation by identification of specific anxieties concerning illness and hospitalization. Specific issues, if pertinent, should be discussed with the staff along with appropriate management guidelines (eg, limit setting for regressed patients). For many patients, control is a major concern. These patients often engage in power struggles with the staff over their own diagnosis and treatment. Conceding to these patients as much "control" as possible if it does no harm (eg, letting the patient decide which arm the blood is drawn from) minimizes conflict over more critical matters (eg, agreeing to take medications or consent to surgical procedures). Schizophrenia and bipolar affective disorder are not frequent causes of problems in medical patient management.

Social dysfunction contributes to patient management problems in many cases. The psychiatric consultant must often function as a social system consultant by suggesting ways in which medical treatment protocols can be modified to avoid or overcome management problems. When several specialists are involved in the care of the patient, poor communication, diffusion of clinical responsibility, and some mismanagement may result. If patients know that there are conflicting opinions about what should be done for them, they may become anxious, angry, or depressed. One solution is for the psychiatric consultant to suggest that a consensus be reached and executed by the primary physician in charge of the case.

This section has distinguished biologic, personality, and social systems for the sake of discussion; however, it is important to consider their interactions in disruptive or excessively anxious patients. Many instances of abrupt departure against medical advice (and other problems with disruptive patients) emerge through the interplay of an underlying organic mental disorder (eg, drug withdrawal) and dysfunction of the interaction between the patient and the treatment team. Evaluation and intervention in all 3 systems is frequently required to resolve such problems without interfering with clinical care.

SYMPTOMS WITH NO APPARENT MEDICAL CAUSE

Psychiatric consultation is often requested for evaluation of patients who have chronic somatic complaints or impaired sensory, motor, or autonomic function for which no medical explanation can be found. The frustration such a patient engenders in the primary clinician is often what prompts the consultation request. The consultant may be asked whether the patient has a conversion disorder. Conversion disorder is characterized by the presence of a psychologic conflict, out of the awareness of the patient, that produces anxiety, and the involuntary "conversion" of this anxiety into a somatic sign or symptom that symbolically expresses and resolves the psychologic conflict. Hypnosis or amobarbital interviews may be useful both in evaluating and in treating this condition.

Other categories of psychiatric illness may also lead to physical signs and symptoms with no apparent medical basis. Both depressed and schizophrenic patients may present somatic preoccupations that are quite confusing until the psychiatric diagnosis is made. Certain patients, usually women, have lifelong patterns of multiple somatic complaints, sometimes called Briquet's syndrome or somatization disorder (see Chapter 32). Patients with factitious disorders consciously simulate a medical illness or a specific sign or symptom (see Chapter 40). This simulation may represent a life-style devoted to simulating medical illness (Munchausen's syndrome, or chronic factitious illness). These patients differ from malingerers, who pretend to have medical problems to achieve a specific conscious goal (eg, to gain narcotics or disability compensation). Recognition of these psychologic conditions should alert the staff to withhold invasive diagnostic and therapeutic efforts. Treatment can then be focused on psychosocial issues.

The consultation psychiatrist should watch for medical illnesses presenting as psychiatric syndromes. Systemic lupus erythematosus, multiple sclerosis, seizure disorders, and degenerative central nervous system diseases may be puzzling because the somatic signs and symptoms and the associated emotional symptoms are often wrongly attributed to psychiatric illness. Although treatment must be directed first toward the medical condition, it is occasionally necessary to treat the psychiatric symptoms as well (eg, antipsychotic medication for the psychosis associated with systemic lupus erythematosus).

In the course of psychiatric evaluation of these patients, 2 recurrent issues need clarification. The first is "secondary gain" (eg, sympathy, or exemption from certain social expectations or responsibilities). Since all illnesses offer some degree of secondary gain, this mechanism should not be assumed uncritically to "explain" the signs or symptoms. The psychiatric consultant should help the patient and the family prevent secondary gain from impeding recovery.

The second issue is the diagnosis of "histrionic personality disorder." It is not true that patients with this disorder are more likely than others to have conversion disorders. The problem is that these histrionic and seductive patients present their somatic signs and symptoms (which may in fact have a medical explanation) in a less-than-believable fashion. Long-term follow-up of patients with the diagnosis of conversion reaction reveals that about 25% have a medical disorder that accounts for the symptoms (Watson and Buranen, 1979). Presumably, the initial presentation of these patients is in the early stages of their medical disease, when it is difficult or impossible to make the proper diagnosis.

PAIN

Patients may continue to complain of pain despite analgesic management that is usually effective. This difficult clinical problem may give rise to requests for psychiatric consultation. Such consultation requires an awareness that pain is a complex phenomenon involving an interplay of biologic and psychosocial factors.

The consultant should review these patients with the primary physician, with emphasis on the potential biologic basis for the pain and the current treatment strategies. The patient is then evaluated for certain psychiatric disorders that are associated with unusual or refractory pain syndromes. Depression should be considered, since its association with chronic pain may lead to increased preoccupation with the pain and louder complaints. Other syndromes to consider include schizophrenia, somatoform pain disorder, and factitious disorders (see above).

Psychosocial factors may also play a role in refractory pain syndromes. Pain may have a special meaning for the patient or may be "modeled" after the pain of a person who was emotionally close to the patient. At times it may mimic the pain a close relative experienced in a terminal illness. Cultural background, unresolved mourning, and secondary gain may play a role in the pain syndrome (see Chapter 32).

Patients with chronic pain often make escalating demands for pain medication that make primary physicians feel uncomfortable. Although it has been estimated that iatrogenic "addiction" is relatively rare in medical patients, physicians often perceive these demands as evidence of drug dependence and request consultation. Because physicians wish to avoid having their patients become "addicted" to narcotics, pain is often undertreated. Undermedication often leads to increased protestations of pain. If the patient's complaint has a "dramatic" emphasis, the physician and staff may discount its true nature, so that a vicious cycle may ensue with the patient receiving less and less analgesic medication in spite of increasing complaints. The psychiatric consultant must have a thorough knowledge of analgesic management and be able to recognize pain problems due to undermedication. Cases of "refractory pain" are often adequately managed by simply increasing the analgesic dosage. This is especially true in the case of acute pain or the pain of terminal cancer.

Over the past few years, techniques for pain control other than narcotic analgesics have been developed for chronic pain. Nonsteroidal analgesics are effective alternatives to narcotics for many patients. Tricyclic antidepressants, often in lower doses than used to treat depression, have been effective for chronic pain. The mechanism of their action is unknown, but it appears to be distinct from their antidepressant effects. Supportive psychotherapy, guided imagery, and hypnosis can also be effective for about one-fourth of patients (see Chapters 32, 46, and 51).

For many years, placebos had a role in the evaluation and treatment of chronic pain. The basis for their use was the mistaken notion that response to placebos indicated a functional, or nonorganic, cause. In fact, all that response to a placebo tells the physician is that the patient is a placebo responder. Evidence that analgesia produced by placebos can be reversed by the narcotic antagonist naloxone suggests that placebos act at least in part through physiologic mechanisms (see Chapter 10).

SUBSTANCE ABUSE

The consultation psychiatrist has a role in the evaluation, treatment, and referral of patients with substance abuse problems who are being treated in a medical setting. Narcotic abusers are not uncommon on surgical wards, where they are usually being treated for abscesses, cellulitis, or injuries. These patients tolerate pain poorly and are quite demanding of the staff's attention. It is helpful to remember that 20 mg of methadone once or twice a day is required to block withdrawal symptoms in most of these patients. After recovery from their medical or surgical problems, referral to the appropriate substance abuse treatment facility is indicated.

Withdrawal from alcohol or sedative drugs (especially barbiturates) is actually more life-threatening than withdrawal from narcotics. The psychiatric consultant must be prepared to help in the assessment of patients with nonnarcotic substance abuse and to assist in the pharmacologic management of delirium tremens and other sedative drug withdrawal syndromes (see Chapter 25).

Inasmuch as patients with alcohol-related medical problems account for 15–40% of admissions to hospitals (Kissin, 1977), it is surprising how poorly this problem is evaluated and treated. Other than quantifying the incoming patient's alcohol consumption over the recent past, no other inquiries are usually made. However, it is important to ask about the circumstances at onset or recurrence of drinking, periods of abstinence, attempts at treatment and their outcome, and any history of blackouts or delirium tremens. Referral to alcohol treatment programs should be vigorously pursued.

MANAGEMENT OF OTHER PSYCHIATRIC DISORDERS

A patient with a major psychiatric disorder may be admitted for management of a medical or surgical illness. Since these patients (those with schizophrenia and major affective or anxiety disorders) may be taking a number of psychotropic medications (antipsychotic drugs, antidepressants, lithium carbonate), the psychiatrist should offer consultation on drug interactions and medically relevant side effects. Specific advice on patient management may allow the staff and the patient to become more comfortable with each other. Psychotic patients, for example, need to have reality pointed out to them and their misperceptions corrected (eg, that the antibiotic medication is treating their pneumonia, not poisoning them). The consultant may also act as the liaison between the hospital and other psychiatric referral facilities to provide useful information about the patient's previous psychiatric history and treatment.

FORENSIC ISSUES

The psychiatric consultant is often requested to make a judgment about the competence of a patient to refuse or consent to a medical or surgical procedure. Part of this process consists of evaluating whether the patient has a psychiatric disorder (emotional or cognitive) that impairs judgment. Competence is the ability to give informed consent, ie, to understand the nature, benefits, and risks of treatment and the consequences of refusing it. The standard of competence varies with the risk/benefit ratio of the procedure. A patient with moderate organic mental disorder may be competent to consent to a CT scan but not to major surgery. The determination of competence is a judicial decision, though psychiatric opinion often serves as the basis for decisions. *Psychiatric consultants should become familiar with the state laws and court decisions governing these situations.*

Most "forensic" cases for which the consultant is called represent patient management problems rather than actual legal issues. For example, the problem of the cancer patient refusing chemotherapy can usually be dealt with by a clinical approach to the patient's experience rather than recourse to a legal procedure. Patients refusing treatment should be evaluated for the presence of organic mental disorder and depression and asked about concerns regarding their situation. Court permission is usually required to treat patients' medical conditions against their will (beyond provision of emergent, lifesaving measures). Psychiatrists should distinguish clinical and medicolegal issues

from an ethical dilemma, about which they may have no expertise.

While the laws differ in some jurisdictions, commitment is not generally a recourse for patients who refuse medical treatment. Patients can be committed if there is an imminent risk that they will harm themselves or others because of a mental disorder. However, this means being actively suicidal, not simply refusing medical treatment. Even in the rare instance when refusal of medical treatment is an active suicide attempt, commitment may allow the physicians to treat the mental condition against the patient's will but not the medical condition.

PSYCHIATRIC LIAISON ACTIVITY

For a psychiatrist, liaison practice implies an ongoing relationship with a medical unit (ward, outpatient clinic, etc). Implicit in this relationship is the psychiatrist's intimate working knowledge of the medical setting. The liaison psychiatrist develops a trusting relationship with the medical staff and can assist them in decisions about the care of their patients. This type of psychiatric input has shortened the length of stay for certain types of medical patients (Levitan and Kornfeld, 1981). The liaison psychiatrist has a major commitment to teaching the medical staff about those aspects of psychiatry that are pertinent to patient care. Liaison also creates the possibility for conducting research on the prevalence, consequences, and management of psychiatric disorders of medical patients.

Psychiatrists have developed liaison relationships with various types of clinical units. Liaison activities with intensive care and hemodialysis units are discussed here. The former is representative of the problems in acute care and the latter of problems in the chronic care setting.

INTENSIVE CARE UNITS

The problems the psychiatric consultant faces in intensive care units are frequently more dramatic than what takes place in general medical and surgical units. The emphasis on technology makes the intensive care unit an alien environment, where incorporation of the human element seems difficult. The care system is more complex, and the personnel may feel they are too busy with "really important lifesaving activities" to bother with psychosocial issues. The psychiatrist and the consultee may also fear that a psychiatric consultation may make the patient worse. After all, patients in intensive care units are in a medically precarious condition, and it is plausible that "upsetting" them with psychologic issues might lead to a life-threatening drop in blood pressure, arrhythmia, or some other medical catastrophe. Although this issue is not resolved, the literature generally supports the view that important psychologic issues can be helpfully raised in the intensive care setting. Finally, it is difficult to interview the patient in an intensive care unit, because of the lack of privacy and the presence of life-support systems. Communicating with an intubated patient requires patience and perseverance. However, the psychiatrist's work depends upon verbal exchange with patients, and the difficult conditions encountered in the intensive care unit should not dissuade the consultant from making the effort if the consultation is felt to be a critical element in treatment.

Patient Issues

In one study of a coronary care unit (Cassem and Hackett, 1971), the most frequent reasons for consultation were anxiety, depression, and management of behavior (eg, agitation, psychosis). Anxiety was due to fear of impending death because of pain, breathlessness, weakness, or the occurrence of new complications. Depression resulted from diminished self-esteem caused by the heart attack. Most management problems stemmed from denial of illness and inappropriate euphoric, hostile, or sexual behavior. Consultation requests for each problem typically occurred at different intervals after admission, with a peak of anxiety on days 1 and 2, a peak of depression on days 3 and 4, and a bimodal distribution for abnormal behaviors.

The consultant also needs a working knowledge of how to assess a patient's personality type and how this personality interacts with a particular medical situation to create a behavioral management problem (see Chapter 36). Despite the psychologically traumatic nature of most medical catastrophes, the capacity of people to adjust is remarkably high. Problem patients usually have a history of personality or emotional difficulties. As a basic principle of consultation psychiatry, the patient's psychologic defenses should be supported whenever possible and psychotropic medications used appropriately when needed. Coping skills and strengths should be discovered and reinforced. For example, successful denial in the acute phase of myocardial infarction may be associated with longer survival. It is important for the consultant to know the natural history of response to life-threatening illness and the issues that are unique to each disorder. For example, patients who have had a myocardial infarction may at first fear dying in their sleep. Following recovery, their concerns may be about sexual performance. Patients surviving cardiac arrest frequently suffer from insomnia, violent dreams, ongoing fantasies about dying, and a tendency to exaggerate physical disability.

It is important for the consultant to have a systems perspective on patient-staff interactions. This calls for skill in interpreting patient behavior to the staff, in helping the staff examine their own reactions, and in proposing more constructive ways for the staff to relate to the patient.

The consultant should be aware that transferring out of a special unit creates stress for many patients, both psychologically and physically. While it is true that leaving an intensive care unit is a welcome sign of clinical improvement, this is not always true for patients leaving a coronary care unit, many of whom become anxious about transferring to a lower level of care where cardiac rhythm is not so closely monitored. In the latter situation, careful explanation can be quite helpful. In addition, the consultant's involvement with patients in special units is helpful in establishing a relationship for subsequent intervention. This is crucial in preventing psychosocial morbidity (eg, difficulty returning to work) that can follow such experiences. For example, 10–15% of patients who survive their first myocardial infarction are not working a year later (Doehrman, 1977). The primary causes of this work disability are psychologic and social factors.

Family Issues

Although the family must endure and deal with its own distress during a life-threatening illness of one of its members, it can help with the emotional problems of the patient. Their presence in the room or nearby is usually both reassuring and orienting. If family members are "at a loss for words" or feel uncomfortable trying to provide support in such trying circumstances, the consultant should assist the primary physician or nursing staff in explaining the patient's condition to the family, screening the family for maladaptive responses, or providing an opportunity to begin the process of mourning. The consultant must be careful not to displace the primary physician or nursing staff, since they usually have a long-standing relationship with the family.

Staff Issues

Work in the intensive care unit is stressful but not clearly more so than work in other clinical settings. There are unique issues that the intensive care unit staff must contend with, such as the noisy and crowded environment. The pace can be quite hectic, and the margin for error is narrow. During the actual performance of technical procedures, there is often little stress. However, anxiety is prominent in ambiguous clinical or ethical situations such as decisions about terminating life-support systems. A series of unavoidable deaths may leave the staff feeling discouraged and frustrated.

The intensive care unit places unique demands on the nursing staff. There is great prestige and personal satisfaction in working in such an environment and performing many procedures (eg, treating arrhythmias or initiating cardiopulmonary resuscitation) that in other clinical settings are outside the purview of nursing. The nurses must also contend with the many physicians caring for the patient and their differing opinions about diagnosis and treatment. It is difficult for the nurse to provide psychologic support to the patient one moment and carry out an invasive and painful procedure the next.

There is widespread agreement that staff support groups, led by a liaison psychiatrist, are helpful in coping with the stress of working in a coronary care unit or intensive care unit. Four characteristics of successful support groups in the intensive care unit are (1) identification and acknowledgment of feelings; (2) sharing of these feelings; (3) review of the experience with criticism, support, and praise; and (4) application of what is learned to future situations.

The groups are effective in diminishing inappropriate guilt and fantasies of omnipotence. The groups allow the staff a protective setting where grief over the loss of patients can be expressed. Identification of psychosocial problems and effective communication are other functions these groups serve.

HEMODIALYSIS UNITS

The advent of hemodialysis allowed the first truly effective treatment for end-stage renal disease. However, in the USA, it was not available to all patients with this condition until September 1972, when the necessary monies were allocated by Medicare legislation. In response to this legislation, dialysis centers were developed, and many physicians and others shifted their attention to the care of these patients. In 1985, it was estimated that 85,000 patients were being treated in dialysis programs and that the annual cost to the federal government was $2 billion.

Patient Issues

As with patients in intensive care units, anxiety about death is an issue for patients receiving hemodialysis. In addition, there are many psychologic issues associated with being maintained chronically by a machine. Patients may have difficulty resolving distortions about their body image now that they are attached to a machine and dependent on it for life. The lives of these patients also cycle continuously from treatment to treatment. As time for the next treatment approaches, patients may begin suffering from signs of increasing uremia, with nausea, lethargy, fatigue, and slowed mentation or inattention. During or immediately after treatment, patients may suffer from a dysequilibrium syndrome characterized by headache, nausea, muscle cramps, and irritability and occasionally by disorientation, delirium, obtundation, and convulsions. Although the cause is not known, this syndrome has been attributed to rapid shifts in fluids and electrolytes. After recovery from the acute effects of treatment, patients may enjoy a brief period of well-being before symptoms of progressive uremia again become manifest and it is time for the next treatment. Add to this cycle the severe restrictions on the amount of sodium, potassium, and fluids that may be ingested and it is obvious that the quality of life for many patients is not to be envied.

For many patients receiving hemodialysis, it is difficult to keep a job, enjoy leisure activities, and function normally in the family. Hemodialysis creates a conflict for these patients. On one hand, they are encouraged to be as independent as possible in work, family, and social activities; on the other, they must spend a significant proportion of their time in a dependent role, being cared for by the medical staff and attached to a hemodialysis machine.

Dialysis patients suffer from a number of other physical and psychologic problems. Most are anemic. Many suffer from decreased libido, and men are often impotent as well. Obviously, with all of these problems and losses, depression is common, and these patients have a higher risk of suicide. Finally, in some patients who have been on hemodialysis for a number of years, a progressive "dialysis dementia" occurs. The condition is without focal neurologic signs and is characterized by behavioral and speech disturbances, cognitive deterioration, and myoclonus. There is no known cause or treatment, and death usually results within 1–2 years. Psychiatrists have a role in assessing emotional or behavioral disturbances in dialysis patients and in suggesting methods of treatment. For example, brief individual or group psychotherapy helps patients cope with psychosocial problems.

Staff Issues

As in all chronic care situations, the staff must cope with treating the same patients over long periods of time. The medical staff has the chronic responsibility for keeping patients alive who for the most part never get better (the exception being patients who undergo successful renal transplantation surgery). Adding to the staff's sense of responsibility and frustration are those patients who are noncompliant with their dietary restrictions or medications (often to the point of being self-destructive) and those who are extremely passive and dependent and expect the staff to do everything for them.

Given the relative stability of the patient population, it is not surprising that hemodialysis units develop their own distinctive ethos. Psychiatrists are helpful in leading staff support groups and serving as systems consultants. In this role, psychiatrists help the staff deal with the complexities of caring for patients on a long-term basis. Psychiatrists can also assist the staff in their assessment of a patient's suitability for other forms of dialysis, such as home hemodialysis or chronic ambulatory peritoneal dialysis.

PSYCHIATRIC CONSULTATION TEAM

Consultation psychiatrists may work alone or in conjunction with other mental health professionals. While such collaboration is not new, there remains much confusion over the shared and unique contributions of the psychiatrist, psychologist, social worker, and nurse in hospital consultation.

One model that integrates various disciplines involves formation of a multidisciplinary team. The concept of the team, however, implies a coordinated interdisciplinary effort. The interdisciplinary team concept does not imply simply that there are 4 professions (psychiatry, psychology, social work, and nursing) competing for overlapping territory and role functions. When the unique contributions of each team member have not been properly identified, there are strained feelings, competitiveness, political hostility, and confusion—all affecting patient care adversely. While it is true that some of the same clinical functions can be performed as well by one professional as another, it is by understanding the unique contributions of each team member that an effective clinical force is created and directed toward helping patients.

The Psychiatrist

The unique contribution of the psychiatrist is the ability to provide differential biopsychosocial diagnoses of disorders of mood, thought, and behavior. The ability to evaluate organic mental disorders, including neurologic syndromes, and knowledge of the effects of medication on the central nervous system are crucial to the understanding of psychologic impairments in medical patients. The psychiatrist must be in a position to review cases interviewed by nonphysician members of the mental health care team and make certain that medical evaluation has been adequate. Such case review and coordination can be facilitated by the use of a standardized psychiatric data base that allows team members from other disciplines to gather information in a standardized fashion. The psychiatrist has the advantage of being able to interact with other physicians on a colleague-to-colleague basis and can integrate other mental health professionals into the health care team.

The Psychologist

Psychologists with training in behavioral medicine have skills that are very useful in the consultation context. They are specially trained to provide behavioral interventions such as self-regulatory therapies (relaxation and biofeedback) and behavior modification. These skills are pertinent to specific situations with medical patients, eg, reduction of pain associated with complications of the disease or with repetitive procedures such as chemotherapy and bone marrow biopsies (see Chapter 51).

There is growing awareness that medical patients have a high incidence of cognitive deficits. A psychologist with skills in neuropsychologic assessment is therefore of great use to the team (see Chapter 20). Psychologists also are the team members with the best training in research methodology.

The Social Worker

The problems of medical patients cannot be understood without appropriate consideration of their social environment, vocation, and financial resources. Social workers, with training in couples or family therapy, may be particularly effective in helping family members cope with the impact of the patient's illness.

Although discharge planning is not solely the responsibility of the social worker, many of the details involved in discharge planning, such as locating appropriate nursing home placements, are often left to social workers. However, as important as this is to patient care, the social worker on the mental health team has a unique task that goes beyond that of technical facilitator. For example, a request for assistance with discharge planning may present an opportunity to identify significant psychologic distress. A professional social worker trained in the psychosocial aspects of medical care can recognize the real issue and not be misled into providing a service that misses the patient's actual needs.

The Psychiatric Nurse Clinical Specialist

The nurse clinical specialist is a registered nurse who has taken a master's degree in specialized nursing care (in this case, psychiatry) and is the team member who knows most about the daily realities of the hospital, especially those pertaining to nursing care. Morale within the nursing staff may strongly influence the care provided. The nurse clinical specialist is in the best position to have access to such information and to be able to interact with the medical system in a corrective fashion. Certain patients are especially difficult. In the management of these difficult patients, no other member of the team can interact as well with the nurses to effect a proper approach to patient assessment and management. By virtue of their medical background and close involvement with patients, nurse clinicians are in a unique position to monitor the response to treatment. Psychiatric liaison nurses are able to intervene effectively at many levels because of their medical, surgical, and psychiatric experience and their understanding of the nursing system in the hospital.

SUMMARY

Consultation/liaison psychiatry in the general hospital involves the comprehensive evaluation and treatment of medical and surgical patients. Psychiatrists in this field are in the unique position of being able to consider the interaction of biologic, psychologic, and social factors in the diagnosis and treatment of patients. As the major link between psychiatry and medicine, consultation/liaison psychiatrists are playing a major role in the establishment of a biopsychosocial model of medical care.

REFERENCES

Abramowicz M (editor): Drugs that cause psychiatric symptoms. *Med Lett Drugs Ther* 1984;**26**:75.

Cassem NH, Hackett TP: Psychiatric consultation in a coronary care unit. *Ann Intern Med* 1971;**75**:9.

Davies DW: Physical illnes in psychiatric out-patients. *Br J Psychiatry* 1965;**111**:27.

De Paulo JR, Folstein MF: Psychiatric disturbances in neurological patients: Detection, recognition, and hospital course. *Ann Neurol* 1978;**4**:225.

Doehrman SR: Psycho-social aspects of recovery from coronary heart disease: A review. *Soc Sci Med* 1977;**11**:199.

Gilman AG, Goodman LS, Gilman A (editors): *Goodman and Gilman's The Pharmacological Basis of Therapeutics,* 7th ed. Macmillan, 1985.

Goldberg RJ, Tull RM: *The Psychosocial Dimensions of Cancer.* Free Press, 1983.

Guggenheim FG, Weiner MF (editors): *Manual of Psychiatric Consultation and Emergency Care.* Jason Aronson, 1984.

Hackett TP, Cassem NH (editors): *Massachusetts General Hospital Handbook of General Hospital Psychiatry.* Mosby, 1978.

Karasu TB, Steinmuller RI (editors): *Psychotherapeutics in Medicine.* Grune & Stratton, 1978.

Kissin B: Medical management of the alcoholic patient. In: *Treatment and Rehabilitation of the Chronic Alcoholic.* Kissin B, Begleiter H (editors). Plenum Press, 1977.

Kornfeld DS et al: Delirium after coronary artery bypass surgery. *J Thorac Cardiovasc Surg* 1978;**76**:93.

Levine PM, Siberfarb PM, Lipowski ZJ: Mental disorders in cancer patients. *Cancer* 1978;**42**:1385.

Levitan SJ, Kornfeld DF: Clinical and cost benefits of liaison psychiatry. *Am J Psychiatry* 1981;**138**:790.

Lipowski Z: Review of consultation psychiatry and psychosomatic medicine. 2. Clinical aspects. *Psychosom Med* 1967;**29**:201.

Lowinsen JH, Ruiz P (editors): *Substance Abuse: Clinical Problems and Perspectives.* Wiliams & Wilkins, 1981.

Moses R, Barzilay J: The influence of psychiatric consultation on the course of illness of the general hospital patient. *Compr Psychiatry* 1967;**8**:16.

Schwab J et al: Medical patients' reactions to referring physicians after psychiatric consultation. *JAMA* 1966;**195**:1120.

Temoshok L, Van Dyke C, Zegans LS (editors): *Emotions in Health and Illness: Theoretical and Research Foundations.* Grune & Stratton, 1983.

vonAmmon Cavanaugh S: The prevalence of emotional and cognitive dysfunction in a general medical population: Using the MMSE, GHQ, and BDI. *Gen Hosp Psychiatry* 1983;**5**:15.

Watson CG, Buranen C: The frequency and identification of false-positive conversion reactions. *J Nerv Ment Dis* 1979;**167**:243.

Weiner H: *Psychobiology and Human Disease.* Elsevier, 1977.

Child & Adolescent Psychiatry

57

Charles M. Binger, MD

Despite generations of social concern, research, and legislative action pertaining to the health and welfare of children and adolescents, their major health and mental health needs are not being met. In the USA, 27% of the population are under the age of 18, and an estimated 10% of this group are in need of mental health care. Those requiring professional help include (1) children and adolescents with major mental and emotional problems such as pervasive developmental disorders, autism, mental retardation, organic mental disorders, schizophrenia, severe depression, delinquency, drug abuse, psychosomatic disorders, and learning disorders; (2) those who suffer from disorders that result in less severe impairment but who nevertheless require professional help; and (3) those at risk for psychiatric disorders, such as children with physical handicaps or chronic illnesses, foster children, institutionalized young people, children of migrant parents or divorced parents, physically and sexually abused children, those whose parents suffer from psychiatric disorders, and children who have lost a parent or sibling.

About 4500 child psychiatrists were practicing in the USA in 1987. The Graduate Medical Education National Advisory Committee of the Department of Health and Human Services estimated that 8000–10,000 child psychiatrists will be needed by the year 2000 and reported that the shortage in the field of child psychiatry is greater than in any of the 33 other medical specialities examined. This emphasizes not only the need for attracting qualified physicians to the field but also the importance of collaboration of child psychiatrists with the wide range of professionals—including pediatricians, family practitioners, social workers, clinical psychologists, family counselors, and teachers—currently working with emotionally disturbed young people.

All professionals who work with children, adolescents, and their families require special knowledge and skills beyond training that focuses on adults. A child is not a small adult, and the needs of children differ from those of adults (see Chapters 6 and 7). Physiologic, psychologic, and cognitive growth is accompanied by new vulnerabilities to biologic, psychologic, and social stresses. Children and adolescents unable to cope with stressful periods of development may not seek help or even know that help is available or needed; thus, it is important for professionals and other adults to identify early signs of emotional problems in young people and refer them for treatment.

HISTORY OF CHILD & ADOLESCENT PSYCHIATRY

The recognition that emotional disturbances can occur in children is probably a 20th century phenomenon, beginning with Freud's detailed clinical description of phobia in a 5-year-old boy.

Adolf Meyer was influential in advancing the field of child psychiatry in America, and on his recommendation, William Healy was appointed in 1908 to direct the first child guidance center in the USA (the now famous Chicago Institute of Juvenile Research). Healy brought together an interdisciplinary team whose approach involved psychoanalysis, psychologic testing, and detailed individual case studies of juvenile delinquents. Child guidance clinics based on the Chicago model developed throughout the USA with support by the Commonwealth Fund. These were mostly community clinics that dealt with a variety of disorders in children and adolescents.

Prior to the 1920s, several scientific fields—eg, psychiatry, education, criminology, psychology, and pediatrics—were involved with child research. However, the body of knowledge from research and clinical practice was not well enough integrated to warrant recognition of child psychiatry as an organized specialty. By the early 1920s, child psychiatry was a recognized professional field of interest and was on its way to becoming a specialty medical discipline.

In 1924, the American Orthopsychiatric Association was formed as an interdisciplinary organization of physicians, psychologists, social workers, and educators. It offered a forum for the communication of experiences and skills in caring for disturbed children and their families. The organization continues to serve in this capacity and publishes the *American Journal of Orthopsychiatry*.

In 1948, the American Association of Psychiatric Clinics for Children was formed from a group of 54 child guidance clinics. This organization developed the first standards for training professionals and treating emotional problems in children.

The American Academy of Child Psychiatry, formed in 1953, evolved from a small group of senior practitioners and academicians into a national organization representing the scientific, clinical, and political bases of Amercian child psychiatry. Its growth is reflected in regional organizations established throughout the USA and adjoining countries. In 1986, the name of the academy was changed to the American Academy of Child and Adolescent Psychiatry to more fully delineate the scope of training, clinical activities, and research undertaken by its members. The Academy publishes the bimonthly *Journal of the American Academy of Child and Adolescent Psychiatry*.

Procedures for certification in the subspecialty of child psychiatry were established in 1959 by the American Board of Psychiatry and Neurology. The field has advanced rapidly—expanding its range of therapies, clinical services, scientific studies, and clinical research and evolving from a discipline based primarily on community child guidance clinics to one broadly established in the private sector of medicine, university health centers, public institutions, and community mental health agencies.

TRAINING IN CHILD PSYCHIATRY

In the USA, following a 3- to 4-year medical school education leading to the MD degree, the child psychiatrist trainee spends the first postgraduate year in a hospital internship program. This may be in any of the medical or surgical specialities but is usually spent in either a combined psychiatry-internal medicine or psychiatry-pediatrics program. The second and third postgraduate years are spent in a psychiatric residency program focused on caring for adults in both inpatient and outpatient settings. The fourth and fifth years are devoted to a specialized child and adolescent psychiatry program. The graduate is then eligible to take the board examination in psychiatry, which in turn determines eligibility for the examination in child psychiatry. With this extensive training in adult inpatient and outpatient psychiatry, plus specialized training in child and adolescent psychiatry, the child psychiatrist is truly a "general psychiatrist."

The 2-year child psychiatry training program offers balanced clinical experience that includes working with infants, children, adolescents, and parents and collaboration with professionals in many fields. The outpatient experience includes crisis intervention, brief treatment, comprehensive diagnostic evaluation and treatment planning, and long-term outpatient psychotherapy. Inpatient experience involves caring for seriously disturbed children and adolescents. In these settings, the trainee is exposed to a wide range of psychopathologic problems, and clinical experience includes therapeutic programs such as individual therapy, play therapy, family therapy, group therapy, and drug therapy. In addition, trainees are involved in pediatric consultation and consultation with various community institutions and agencies (schools, child care agencies, domestic relations court, youth guidance services, etc).

The training program also provides for experience in teaching, administration, and research. Training methods include individual supervision, treatment reviews, and clinical conferences. Seminars are offered in normal growth and development; biologic aspects of child psychiatry; etiology and pathogenesis of developmental, mental, and neurologic disorders in children, adolescents, and parents; concepts of diagnostic assessment and treatment planning; psychotherapy and various other approaches to treatment of children, adolescents, and parents; basic concepts of research; pediatric and community consultation; social and legal aspects of child psychiatry; and the techniques of teaching and administration.

TREATMENT SETTINGS & RESPONSIBILITIES

A recent survey by the American Academy of Child Psychiatry dispelled the notion that child psychiatrists work principally in large metropolitan areas and showed that they practice in large and small metropolitan areas as well as rural communities. Currently, because there is a shortage of child psychiatrists, opportunities for practice exist in virtually every region of the country in large or small communities.

Most child psychiatrists are involved in a variety of professional activities simultaneously. This most often includes private office practice with adults, children, adolescents, and families. In addition, child psychiatrists with a private office practice treat children in hospitals and residential and day-care settings. They frequently act as consultants to pediatricians, school administrators, and a variety of professionals in social agencies, and they may work with family court or juvenile court functionaries or the police in child custody disputes, cases of child abuse and neglect, and criminal proceedings in juvenile court. Child psychiatrists also teach in general and child psychiatry training programs. Other child psychiatrists work mainly in specific settings such as community mental health programs, health maintenance organizations, etc.

APPROACHES TO DIAGNOSIS & DEVELOPMENT OF THE TREATMENT PLAN

In the initial diagnostic process, which usually takes 3–4 weeks, the child is assessed in the context of the family. As a rule, the family is first seen together, and then each family member is seen in individual sessions. A detailed developmental history is taken of the child and family members, and their difficulties—as well as their strengths and coping capacities, which may markedly influence treatment—are assessed. Further information is obtained from professionals involved with the child, such as the pediatrician, a teacher, a school psychologist or school administrator, and social service workers. Through this diagnostic process, which may also be viewed by the family as a brief course of therapy, an understanding is gained of how the child's difficulties affect the parents and how the parents' own conflicts alter or influence their response to the child.

As part of the diagnostic process, the child is frequently seen by a clinical psychologist, a specialist in educational testing, a pediatrician or pediatric neurologist, and a speech and hearing specialist. It is the function of the child psychiatrist to collaborate with a variety of specialists, to synthesize and integrate their findings with clinical data obtained during the physical examination and psychiatric evaluation, and to share the findings with the family members and other professionals who are working with the family—all of which leads toward implementation of a comprehensive treatment plan.

Illustrative Case No. 1

A 10½-year-old boy was referred to a child psychiatrist by the school social worker. The child had failed to progress academically despite placement in a class for children with learning disabilities. His behavior was disruptive at school, and at home he showed signs of low self-esteem.

The first interview was with the mother and stepfather, who had been married since the patient was 6 years old. The patient's biologic father had left home when the patient was 2 years old, and the mother and stepfather had dated for about a year before marrying. At the time of the marriage, the family consisted of the patient (age 6), the mother, the stepfather, and the stepfather's son by a previous marriage (age 14).

The patient's birth and delivery had been normal. The mother felt that his early development had also been normal except for a delay in speech (he was 3 years old when he spoke his first words), but his nursery school teacher thought his overall development was delayed. In elementary school, the patient had learning and behavior problems and received several failing marks. He was placed in a special class but was not progressing adequately there.

During the family interviews, significant additional details came to light. During the past 2 years, the patient had been sexually abused several times by his adolescent stepbrother. He at first had been too fearful and ashamed to tell his parents. Doing so led to considerable stress between the parents, and the teenager was sent to live with his mother. The parents continued to experience tension as a result of this decision. For the past 4 years, the patient had had "imaginary companions" with whom he talked a good part of the day. He was physically clumsy and had no friends. During the course of several interviews, the patient talked very slowly but candidly with the therapist while engaging in play activities. He chose simple words but was able to communicate in a comprehensible manner. He understood that he was seeing a psychiatrist because of his poor school performance, and he spoke out about his school difficulties, poor self-image ("I'm dumb"), sadness, and difficulty making friends.

Psychologic testing demonstrated that the patient was functioning at a level bordering on mild mental retardation and that he had learning problems related to cognitive and visual-motor integration (see Chapter 20). Projective tests (see Chapter 21) showed themes of violation, humiliation, and penetration. Except for his slight clumsiness, he showed no abnormalities in pediatric and neurologic examinations. Hearing and language evaluation revealed normal hearing but great difficulty in the areas of receptive and expressive language. In summary, the results of the history and examinations suggested (1) a marked language disorder that had affected cognitive abilities and (2) emotional difficulties secondary to the language and learning handicaps and to a 2-year period of stressful sexual involvement with the older stepbrother.

The initial treatment plan proposed to the parents included the following: school placement in a special class for language-handicapped children; individual psychotherapy for the patient, focusing on his internal emotional conflicts; and psychotherapy for the parents, focusing on their marital difficulties. A program of exercises to help the patient overcome his clumsiness and poor self-image was also recommended.

In the above case in which the child was referred to a child psychiatrist for evaluation of learning difficulties, immediate considerations included sociocultural factors that could inhibit learning; physical illness that could directly affect learning or could have prevented the child from attending school regularly; and brain damage, mental retardation, cognitive deficits, hearing deficits, language difficulties, severe emotional disorders, life stresses, and inadequate educational experience. All of these factors were evaluated in the context of diagnostic and therapeutic interviews with the child and family and in collaboration with numerous professionals. The clinical data were then synthesized, and a comprehensive treatment plan was developed and shared with the parents and with professionals in the community in a manner that encouraged implementation of the plan.

Illustrative Case No. 2

A 16-year-old girl was referred by her family physician from a nearby community. The chief complaints were of recurrent episodes of confusion, depersonalization, paranoid delusions, loosening of associations, fearfulness, withdrawal from the parents, hyperactivity, and depression. The first episode occurred 4 months prior to referral. The episodes appeared to be associated with menstrual periods, but symptoms did not completely resolve between periods. The patient had not responded to counseling in her local community.

In the course of a 4-week evaluation, the patient and both parents were seen together in 2 family diagnostic-therapeutic interviews, and each was seen individually on 3 separate occasions. The initial differential diagnostic considerations included seizure disorder, premenstrual syndrome, psychotic depressive reaction, schizophrenic reaction, brief reactive psychosis, toxic drug reaction, and neurologic disease.

During the initial family interview, the patient was calm and coherent and expressed concern about having missed 4 months of school. Her parents were anxious and bewildered. They stated that their daughter had always been a well-behaved, modest young woman but that they had not dared let her return to school for fear that she might commit suicide. In subsequent interviews, it became apparent that this was a family in which no member was allowed to express feelings of anger or sadness directly. The parents had not had intercourse in 2 years and were on the verge of divorce. The wife saw her husband as domineering, and he saw her as depressed and withdrawn. During the past 2 years, a series of life stresses had occurred: Older relatives on both sides had fallen seriously ill; a close friend of the patient and mother was killed in a car accident, and both of them were still grieving her loss; and the mother was diagnosed as having mitral valve prolapse and was receiving medication for cardiac arrhythmia.

The patient was anxious and concerned about her mother. In individual confidential interviews, each of the family members began to look more closely at their feelings and the stresses affecting their lives. As the evaluation progressed through the 4-week period, significant changes began to occur. The parents began to communicate better with each other, and their relationship improved. The patient became more expressive of her feelings, both positive and negative, and began to function more autonomously as an individual. She disclosed that several months before the onset of symptoms, she had had a relationship with and felt sexually attracted to an older man. She had also tried marihuana for the first time.

Laboratory studies and physical and neurologic examinations, including CT scan and an electroencephalogram, showed no abnormal findings. A gynecologic consultant rejected a diagnosis of premenstrual syndrome.

During the evaluation period, the patient returned to school. She went through 2 menstrual periods with no recurrence of symptoms, and her parents became less anxious about her.

By the time evaluation was completed, the patient was functioning well in school and at home. There had been significant alterations in family dynamics. The daughter had been serving as the focus of problems—had been offered and had accepted the role of "patient"—in a rigid family system in which the parents were locked in a struggle over sexuality, intimacy, and self-esteem. This was a time when the daughter was experiencing similar conflicts in her own process of development. The role of patient was abandoned when she and her parents acknowledged the problems and were able to look more closely at their feelings and reactions to the many stresses in their lives. Recommendations were made for continuation of family therapy in the local community. There was no need for medication. The focus on menstrual periods was thought to be symbolic rather than physiologic.

In follow-up at 6 months and 1 year, the patient was still functioning well in school and at home.

The patient in this case presented with atypical psychosis. The child psychiatrist elicited a history of the psychodynamic and stress events contributing to the onset of symptoms and evaluated the family and individual psychodynamics. The patient was referred for examinations and consultations, and the findings were shared with the family and community professionals involved in the case. A treatment plan was then implemented and was successful.

METHODS OF THERAPY

The particular methods used for the treatment of a specific child or adolescent are based on the clinical findings of the above-mentioned diagnostic process and resulting treatment plan. Multiple methods are frequently used simultaneously. Some of these methods are carried out by the child psychiatrist, while some are done in collaboration with other professionals as part of the comprehensive treatment plan. Most child psychiatrists work simultaneously with the parents, since the patient's difficulties are interwoven with family dynamics and the psychodynamics of each family member.

Concomitant Individual Psychotherapy

In this form of therapy, the psychiatrist works individually with the parents and the patient, with due regard for their expectations about confidentiality. Individual therapy focuses on internal conflicts arising out of past life experiences and current difficulties; school, work, or marital problems; and concerns about other family members. Most older children and adolescents are able to participate in this type of therapy, which is based on verbalization of conflicts, feelings, and emotions.

Play Therapy

Children have difficulty verbalizing internal conflicts, feelings, emotions, and fantasies, but they are often able to communicate internal material using the symbolic language of play. With help provided by verbal interaction with the therapist, internal conflicts can often be brought to the fore and resolved.

Family Therapy

The child psychiatrist usually meets with the entire family as a group but may meet with several members of the family together (both parents without the child; one parent with the child). The approach is frequently based on the concept of **transactional analysis,** which postulates that family events have no discrete significance outside of a larger context of interdependent subsystems. The child psychiatrist may use family therapy in addition to or sometimes instead of individual psychotherapy.

Group Therapy

Activity and verbalization techniques have been developed for group therapy of children at different stages of development. The assumptions underlying the activity therapy are that children will manifest and resolve conflicts in action as they do in play and that such actions are accessible to analysis and interpretation. In the verbalization approach, children are encouraged to discuss their current difficulties and the problems they encounter within the group. With very young children, play therapy can be used as part of group therapy.

Hypnosis

Hypnosis is a useful adjunct in the management of children with a variety of clinical problems and diagnoses. It is most commonly used in the treatment of sleep and appetite disorders, habit disorders (such as nail biting), and psychogenic amnesia. Hypnosis has been effective in relieving pain associated with severe burns or other injuries. In recent years, hypnosis has also been used to treat children with behavior disorders as well as phobic and other anxiety disorders.

Behavior Therapy

Behavior therapy attempts to apply information about the way in which maladaptive behavior has been learned to the task of unlearning it. This is usually in contrast to the psychodynamic viewpoint, which is that behavior cannot be changed without uncovering and resolving underlying conflicts. Behavior therapy approaches to particular symptoms are often useful in combination with insight-oriented psychotherapy.

Drug Therapy

Drug therapy is useful in the treatment of specific disorders in childhood and adolescence, such as psychotic disorders, multiple tics, hyperactivity, depression, and severe anxiety. The psychologic implications of the use of drugs must be considered, and drugs should not be used alone but in conjunction with other forms of therapy.

Collaborative Therapy

In collaborative psychotherapy, family members are seen by different mental health specialists. A child psychiatrist may see the child in individual play therapy while a social worker works with the parents conjointly in marital therapy. Within this structure, there is usually ongoing collaboration between the therapists.

When educational problems are present—as is often the case with emotionally disturbed children and adolescents—treatment must include appropriate educational measures such as special tutoring, placement in special classes, or speech therapy. The child psychiatrist usually works in collaboration with the child's teachers and other counselors.

Other examples of professionals with whom the child psychiatrist collaborates are pediatricians, family physicians, social workers, and probation officers.

Psychiatric Hospitalization, Residential Treatment, Day-Care Treatment, & Alternative Home Placement

Children are admitted to the hospital for psychiatric evaluation and treatment if behavior is so severely disturbed that outpatient evaluation and treatment are difficult or impossible. Hospital admission may be required for children and adolescents who manifest extremely aggressive or hyperactive behavior, serious depression with suicidal ideas or attempts, bizarre and withdrawn psychotic behavior, anorexia nervosa, deprivation dwarfism, multiple tics, or severe conduct disorders. The psychiatric inpatient unit must provide a supportive environment in which a variety of therapeutic approaches can be utilized by collaborating professionals to meet specific needs. These include individual and family therapy; recreational, musical, art, and occupational therapy; special education; drug therapy; and behavior therapy. Within this setting, the child psychiatrist has the major responsibility for developing, implementing, and coordinating a comprehensive treatment plan.

Following inpatient treatment, many children are able to return home. Others require alternative home placement such as foster homes or therapeutic group homes. While some resume normal activities and continue treatment on an outpatient basis, others need a more structured therapeutic program provided by a day-care treatment center. Children with chronic disorders may need prolonged treatment in a residential treatment setting.

Illustrative Case

A 12-year-old boy was referred by a neurologist to a child psychiatric ward for immediate admission because of recurrent episodes of "pseudoseizures" during which the patient exhibited violent behavior toward his 6-year-old brother and declared that he wanted to kill him. He appeared not to remember these episodes. On admission to the ward, the patient appeared to be remorseful about his "seizures."

The history revealed that the patient's parents had experienced marital difficulties for a number of years and had separated several times. The patient's early growth and development had been normal; however, when he entered elementary school, he had learning problems diagnosed as attention deficit disorder. He was given stimulant medication but showed no improvement, and his behavioral difficulties increased. When he was 6 years old, his younger brother was born. When he was 10 years old, his mother gave birth to a baby boy who did well for 2 months and then died a "crib death." Both parents reacted strongly to the baby's death, and the mother eventually became severely depressed and suicidal and had to be hospitalized for several months. The patient did not actively grieve but blamed himself for the baby's death. Several months later, he began having violent outbursts during which he threatened to kill his younger brother. He became extremely aggressive also with peers, and learning and behavioral difficulties in school increased, as did the intensity of his outbursts. Parental conflicts kept pace with the patient's worsening behavioral problem.

Neurologic and pediatric consultation upon the patient's admission to the hospital disclosed nothing that might justify a diagnosis of seizure disorder. Psychologic testing showed the patient to be of low to average intelligence with a variety of perceptual-motor deficits that interfered with learning. Testing produced evidence of underlying depression, which included self-depreciative thoughts and suicidal ideation. There was no evidence of thought disorder.

Throughout the hospital stay, the child psychiatrist saw the parents and the patient together in family interviews and had individual psychotherapy sessions with each family member. The diagnostic impression was that the patient was suffering from unresolved grief and a long-standing emotional disorder related to family conflicts. He also had chronic learning difficulties related to limited intelligence, perceptual-motor deficits, and emotional difficulties.

The patient made steady progress in a specialized inpatient program that included recreational and occupational therapy, special education, appropriate limit setting, behavior therapy (with a point system based on behavior modification concepts), and drug therapy (antidepressants) along with individual psychotherapy. His chronic emotional problems, unresolved grief, and resultant depression began to ease, and after he made significant improvement, he returned home in 3 months. The family continued in outpatient family therapy, and the patient was admitted to a specialized therapeutic day-care program that offered special education facilities. The patient made steady progress, and after a year he was placed in a regular school class. Throughout this period, the child psychiatrist was responsible for the development and implementation of a treatment plan, which involved psychotherapy and collaborating with a variety of consultants and members of the hospital and day-care treatment team: nurses, recreational and occupational therapists, and teachers.

FUTURE DIRECTIONS

The American Academy of Child and Adolescent Psychiatry sponsored an extensive study to define the current status of child psychiatry and recommend directions for the future, and the report, *Child Psychiatry: A Plan for the Coming Decades (Project Future),* published in 1983, has had a significant impact on training and activities of professionals in the field.

The report concludes that there is a need to improve and expand psychiatric care for children and adolescents—particularly those who are or may become severely ill, maladapted, or disabled—and their families. Child psychiatrists are urged to assume greater responsibility for the direct psychiatric and medical care of such patients. The report emphasizes that the training of child psychiatrists, which includes training in general psychiatry and in medicine, provides the specialized knowledge and skills necessary to assume a leadership role in the psychiatric and medical evaluation and treatment of children and adolescents with severe emotional or adaptational problems, mental and physical disabilities, or neurologic deficits.

It is recommended also that child psychiatrists provide assistance to other physicians and health care professionals through pediatric consultation and liaison activities and by consulting and collaborating with personnel of schools and social agencies. Child psychiatrists are urged to investigate preventive strategies to lower the incidence of psychiatric illness of children at risk.

The report makes a variety of recommendations for didactic and clinical training to enhance skills in evaluating and caring for seriously disturbed and handicapped patients and providing consultation in such cases. Continued training with less severely disturbed patients is also recommended. Child psychiatrists should be trained to deal with legal issues and problems and to perform forensic psychiatric assessments. This would involve psychiatrists in the juvenile court system as well as with courts hearing cases of child abuse and neglect, child custody, and commitment of children to institutions.

A major emphasis of the report is on research. All child psychiatry trainees should become familiar with research methods and findings, and postresidency research programs should be developed to provide training for those who wish to participate in research. The field offers extensive opportunities for research, especially in nosology, epidemiology, the pathogenesis of psychopathologic disorders in childhood and adolescence, the impact of catastrophic life events, biologic correlates of behavior (see Chapter 10), and methods of treatment.

REFERENCES

Adams P: The influence of new information from social sciences on concepts, practice and research in child psychiatry. *J Am Acad Child Psychiatry* 1982;**21:**533.

Anders T: The child psychiatrist and research. *J Am Acad Child Psychiatry* 1982;**21:**570.

Child Psychiatry: A Plan for the Coming Decades (Project Future). American Academy of Child Psychiatry, 1983.

Henderson PB: *Essentials in the Education and Training of Child Psychiatrists.* American Academy of Child Psychiatry, 1977.

Leon R: Child psychiatry and academia. Pages 442–446 in: *Basic Handbook of Child Psychiatry.* Vol 4. Noshpitz J (editor). Basic Books, 1979.

McDermott J, McGuire C, Berner E: Roles and functions of child psychiatrists. In: *Report on the Project on Certification in Child Psychiatry.* American Board of Psychiatry and Neurology, 1976.

Mrazek DA, Prugh D: Critical incidents and child psychiatry training. *J Am Acad Child Psychiatry* 1980;**19:**311.

Rosen B: Distribution of child psychiatry services. Pages 485–500 in: *Basic Handbook of Child Psychiatry.* Vol 4. Noshpitz J (editor). Basic Books, 1979.

Sabshin M: The future of the psychiatrist. Chapter 6 in: *Mental Health in the 21st Century.* Williams T, Johnson J (editors). Lexington Books, 1980.

Silver LB: The crisis in child psychiatry recruitment in the United States—circa 1980. *J AM Acad Child Psychiatry* 1980;**19:**711.

Silver LB et al: Governmental peer review of training programs in child psychiatry. *Am J Psychiatry* 1977;**134:**11.

58

Forensic Psychiatry

Bernard L. Diamond, MD

Forensic psychiatry is a general term that denotes the interface between law and psychiatry. This chapter will discuss the field of forensic psychiatry under the following headings: the psychiatric expert witness; criminal law and psychiatry, including insanity, the guilty but mentally ill offender, diminished capacity, and competency to stand trial; involuntary hospitalization and conservatorship; the rights of patients, including informed consent, the right to treatment, the right to refuse treatment, confidentiality, and privileged communication; and special issues.

THE PSYCHIATRIC EXPERT WITNESS

The law and its institutions function in society as decision-making and dispute-resolving instruments. Depending on the nature of the disputed issue, the decisions may be made by the executive (administrative), legislative, or judicial branch of government, and in some cases by direct vote of the people. Rational decision making in courts of law requires that facts and other types of information be made available to the judge or jury sitting as "trier of fact." Certain kinds of judicial decisions call for input of technical information beyond the scope of knowledge of the layperson.

Information required for legal fact finding is most commonly obtained from witnesses. **Ordinary witnesses** at trial are called to provide factual information about which they have direct personal knowledge; generally speaking (there are exceptions), they are not permitted to express their opinions. When specialized or technical information is needed, the parties must call **expert witnesses** to provide technical data and to express their relevant opinions.

There are 2 kinds of psychiatric testimony (expert witnesses). A psychiatrist who has examined or treated a patient may be called as a witness and asked to provide information about the patient's condition and treatment, including, at times, opinions about causation and prognosis. A different situation exists when a psychiatrist is asked to perform an examination or testify as an expert specifically for legal purposes.

The psychiatrist called on to present clinical testimony should be willing to testify if the patient wishes the psychiatrist to do so, or if the privilege of confidentiality has been waived by the patient, or if the psychiatrist is legally required to testify. The psychia-

trist should maintain adequate records and properly prepare to give testimony. Preparation should include close familiarity with the details of the patient's clinical condition and treatment and some knowledge of the pertinent legal issues. A preliminary conference with the attorney acting for the patient is often useful. The attorney may wish a written report before the court appearance.

The psychiatrist may be required to give testimony in the form of a **deposition.** A deposition is a device for taking sworn testimony before trial for use at trial. Its purpose is to preserve testimony for later use in cases where the witness might not be available at trial for any reason. A deposition may take place in the doctor's own office or at any convenient place. Usually, only the opposing attorney and a court reporter are present. However, witnesses giving deposition testimony are under oath just as if they were in court. They may or may not be required to give testimony again in court before a judge and jury. It is important that there be no discrepancies between the testimony in the deposition and that given later in the trial court.

A **subpoena** is an order, backed by the authority of a judge, for the witness to appear at a deposition or in court. It usually also requires that the physician produce the patient's clinical records, or that the records be made available to the attorney, in which case a personal appearance is not required. Failure to comply with a subpoena is punishable as contempt of court. A subpoena to appear at a deposition or in court will specify a particular time and place. In the case of depositions, reasonable requests for changes in time and place of appearance will usually be granted by the attorney for the requesting party. The psychiatrist may not have to be subpoenaed if there is an agreement to testify voluntarily. The arrangements for time and place can then be agreed on between the attorney and the doctor.

The psychiatrist who testifies as an expert in court or in a deposition or who prepares a report for any legal purpose is entitled to a reasonable fee. In all cases it should be understood clearly how much will be paid, when payment will be made, and who is responsible for payment. Although lawyers are permitted to take most civil cases on a contingent fee basis, it is not ethical for doctors to agree to a contingent fee for professional services and testimony. It is not improper, if circumstances warrant, to request partial payment in advance.

Expert witnesses should be prepared to give their professional qualifications. A prepared resume is helpful, including education, postgraduate training, licensing, specialty board certification, membership in professional organizations, publications, honors and awards, and any other information relevant to establishing the psychiatrist's credentials as an expert.

In providing forensic psychiatric testimony, psychiatrists are in quite a different role. They may or may not have performed a clinical examination of the litigant, or if they did, the examination was performed solely for legal purposes. Usually it is not the patient who seeks the examination, and control over the findings is not retained by either the psychiatrist or the subject of the examination. It is generally preferable to perform an appropriate clinical examination whenever possible. However, a forensic psychiatrist may sometimes be called on to provide testimony on purely hypothetical issues or to give opinions about scientific or clinical issues relevant to the legal questions.

Forensic expert testimony requires much more legal knowledge than ordinary clinical testimony. Special training is advisable, and it is now possible to obtain certification as an expert witness from the American Board of Forensic Psychiatry. In order to sit for the board examinations, the candidate must first be certified in psychiatry by the American Board of Psychiatry and Neurology and must have additional training, experience, and specialized practice in forensic work.

Difficult ethical problems may arise in the practice of forensic psychiatry. A person being examined by a "doctor" may be confused about the function of the forensic specialist and may assume the existence of a traditional clinical relationship, believing that the examination is for the patient's benefit or that what the patient and specialist say is confidential. It is imperative that the psychiatrist in such a situation explain his or her role to the subject and disclose the purposes of the examination, the limits of confidentiality, what is likely to happen to the information derived, and what may be the possible consequences. There have been instances where psychiatrists have attempted to obtain incriminating information from suspects, sometimes coercing or eliciting confessions under the guise of therapy. Psychiatrists have deliberately deceived defendants by concealing their role and giving false assurances of confidentiality. Such conduct is not only unethical and unprofessional, but it may form the basis of successful appeal of the defendant's conviction.

In 1985, the US Supreme Court made an important decision in *Ake v Oklahoma,* holding that when a state allows the defense of insanity, the state must provide funds for the employment of a psychiatric expert for an indigent defendant. In its discussion of the role of the psychiatric expert, the Court made it clear that such an expert is part of the defense team and may participate actively in the trial on behalf of the defense, rejecting the concept of the expert as an uninvolved and impartial participant in the legal process.

The psychiatric expert witness should strive toward objectivity, honesty, and a high standard of ethical practice. Because expert witnesses are important participants in our adversary system of justice, they cannot avoid being placed in an adversarial position and should not claim an attitude of impartiality that does not exist. Often the public reputation of the forensic psychiatrist is that of the "hired gun," willing to accommodate opinions and testimony to the needs of the lawyer who pays the most. This image, and the consequent detriment to the psychiatric profession as a whole, can only be avoided by the most scrupulous ethical and professional integrity.

CRIMINAL LAW & PSYCHIATRY

Insanity

Many of the decisions that must be made in the area of criminal law depend upon the psychologic attributes of the defendant. Traditionally, Anglo-American systems of criminal justice rely heavily on blameworthiness. Persons who commit criminal acts are held responsible only to the extent that they deserve blame for what they have done. Blameworthiness implies that the criminal act was the result of a willful decision by one exercising a power of free will. Hence, a crime must consist of the union of the guilty act (*actus reus*) and the guilty mind or intent (*mens rea*).

This basically theologic system of criminal responsibility has been gradually modified, so that today in the USA, a mental element—*mens rea*—in its original free-will sense is not a necessary feature of the definition of every crime. However, in the case of most common-law crimes such as murder, robbery, and theft, American law follows the traditional model. To convict a defendant of a crime it must be proved, beyond a reasonable doubt, that the defendant committed the criminal act and possessed, at the time of the act, the mental state or "criminal intent" required by the statutory definition of the crime charged.

This system of criminal law is often called *mens rea* law. A system of law in which people are held responsible for their acts without consideration of their mental state or blameworthiness is known as "strict liability" law. One may challenge the relevancy, utility, and efficiency of *mens rea* law in modern society. However, it is deeply rooted in our religious, social, and political heritage, and it is not likely to be replaced in the foreseeable future with a system of criminal law dominated by strict liability.

Accordingly, in every criminal trial, a decision must be made concerning this psychologic element of the crime. An insane defendant is deemed to be incapable, because of mental disease or defect, of possessing any degree of *mens rea;* hence, an insane person is not capable of committing any crime, regardless of what he or she has done—thus the verdict, "Not guilty by reason of insanity." In short, an insane person is not to be blamed for his or her actions, which are the result of mental disease rather than exercise of free will, and he or she cannot be held criminally responsible.

Juries are reluctant to find a defendant not guilty by reason of insanity even though the evidence might indicate that to be a just and proper verdict. Most insanity acquittals have been in trials to a judge without a jury, where the prosecution has agreed with the defense lawyer that the defendant was insane.

Even otherwise well informed professionals such as judges, attorneys, legislators, and physicians have exaggerated notions about the frequency of insanity verdicts. When asked to estimate the number of felony defendants found not guilty by reason of insanity, they usually estimate from 10 to 30% or more. The actual incidence is between 0.1% and 0.5%.

In ancient law, only the most obviously deranged persons were considered to be insane. The terms *furiosus, non compos mentis,* etc, denoted total deprivation of reason and will. Insanity was thought to be recognizable by any layperson, and no expert testimony was needed.

The good and evil test was introduced into English law as early as the 14th century, when it was used to define the criminal responsibility of children. By the 16th century, it was applied as a criterion for the criminal responsibility of adults. By the early 19th century, the good and evil test had been recast into the "knowledge of right and wrong" test. There is nothing to indicate that the change represented a substantive alteration.

In January 1843, a young Scotsman, Daniel M'Naghten, assassinated the secretary to the Prime Minister of England. He had intended to kill the Prime Minister, Sir Robert Peel, but shot the secretary instead. In a sensational trial, M'Naghten was declared not guilty by reason of insanity. Queen Victoria, the Prime Minister, the press, and the public could not accept what seemed to be exculpation of a defendant they were convinced was a political assassin. An investigation by the House of Lords culminated in the summoning of the 15 Chief Justices of England to Parliament. The justices were asked to respond to a series of questions about the laws of England relevant to the acquittal by reason of insanity of defendants such as M'Naghten. Their response to these questions has been immortalized in the criminal law throughout the English-speaking world as the "M'Naghten rules of insanity."

The principal rule incorporated into the criminal laws of the USA and most countries that derive their legal systems from English common law is as follows (West and Walk, 1977:79):

> . . . [T]o establish a defense on the ground of insanity, it must be clearly proved that, at the time of the committing of the act, the party accused was labouring under such a defect of reason, from disease of the mind, as not to know the nature and quality of the act he was doing, or, if he did know it, that he did not know he was doing what was wrong. The mode of putting the latter part of the question to the jury on these occasions has generally been whether the accused at the time of doing the act knew the difference between right and wrong. . . .

Although this formula presented to the House of Lords did not carry the legal authority of an appellate decision, it fitted in so well with traditional concepts of morality and responsibility that it was almost immediately adopted by most American states and has tended to dominate all legal concepts of criminal responsibility of the mentally ill. The concepts that went into the M'Naghten rules were not new, as has sometimes been thought; they simply restated in contemporary language legal principles already established in the USA and England.

Even by 1843 standards, knowledge of right and wrong as a criterion of criminal responsibility was outdated by existing concepts of psychopathology, since it considered only abnormalities of cognition, ignoring defects of will and impulse control. Most of the efforts subsequently to broaden the applicability of the insanity defense have consisted of adding some type of *volitional* factor as an alternative to the purely cognitive principle of the M'Naghten formula. The volitional test was at first defined as "irresistible impulse" and later as "ability to adhere to the right" or as "ability to conform one's actions to the requirements of the law."

In 1869 and 1871, the New Hampshire Supreme Court held that if the jury determines, as issues of fact, that the defendant is suffering from a mental disease or defect and that the criminal act is a result or product of the mental disease or defect, the defendant must be found not guilty by reason of insanity. In 1895 and 1897, the United States Supreme Court held that a defendant is insane if, because of mental disease or defect, he or she was unable at the time of the offense to distinguish right from wrong or if, though able to make that distinction, the defendant's powers of will were so destroyed that he or she could not control the actions. The Supreme Court also ruled that when the issue of insanity is raised by the defendant, the prosecutor has the burden of proving beyond a reasonable doubt that the defendant is sane. Later, in 1952, the Court held that these decisions were binding only on federal courts and need not be followed by the states.

In 1954, Judge David Bazelon of the District of Columbia Court of Appeals wrote the famous *Durham* decision:

> The rule . . . is not unlike that followed by the New Hampshire court since 1870. It is simply that an accused is not criminally responsible if his unlawful act was the product of mental disease or mental defect.

Although hailed at the time as a great advance of the law, other jurisdictions were reluctant to follow. This was especially so after the District of Columbia Court of Appeals held that this rule applied to defendants with a diagnosis of antisocial personality who were not otherwise mentally ill. A substantial number of defendants were found insane in the District who would not have been deemed so elsewhere.

The American Law Institute (ALI) developed in the 1950s a "Model Penal Code" in an attempt to bring some uniformity to the widely disparate criminal law codes of the states. Included was a proposal for a rule of responsibility of the mentally ill that included both cognitive and volitional factors:

> A person is not responsible for criminal conduct if at the time of such conduct as a result of mental disease or defect he lacks substantial capacity either to appreciate the criminality [wrongfulness] of his conduct or to conform his conduct to the requirements of law.

To prevent the so-called sociopathic (antisocial) personality from using the defense of insanity, there is a clause that has not always been accepted in jurisdictions where the ALI rule has been adopted:

> The terms "mental disease or defect" do not include an abnormality manifested only by repeated criminal or otherwise antisocial conduct.

Although the psychiatrists who participated in the drafting of the ALI rule would have preferred the *Durham* rule, many state and federal courts adopted ALI as the standard, and finally, in 1972, the District of Columbia Court of Appeals relinquished *Durham* in favor of a slightly modified ALI rule. Public and legislative outcry after the insanity acquittal of John Hinckley for the attempted assassination of President Reagan has prompted both the American Psychiatric Association and the American Bar Association to retreat from their former support of the ALI rule. Both organizations have now recommended the adoption of the "Bonnie rule" (after Professor Richard J. Bonnie of the University of Virginia, who first proposed it):

> A person is not responsible for criminal conduct if, at the time of such conduct, and as a result of mental disease or defect, that person was unable to appreciate the wrongfulness of such conduct.

In 1984, Congress enacted the Insanity Defense Reform Act of 1985, which applies to all federal crimes and is essentially the same as the Bonnie rule:

> It is an affirmative defense to a prosecution under any Federal statute that, at the time of the commission of the acts constituting the offense, the defendant, as a result of a severe mental disease or defect, was unable to appreciate the nature and quality or the wrongfulness of his acts. Mental disease or defect does not otherwise constitute a defense. 18 USCA Sect. 20(a) (Supp 1986).

For the first time, a uniform rule of responsibility for all federal jurisdictions was established by legislative action rather than judicial decision.

A persistent concern of the public is the possibility of early release of a dangerously mentally ill person after he or she has been acquitted by reason of insanity. It is widely feared that such persons will kill again, and sometimes the fear proves justified. In the 19th century, a verdict of not guilty by reason of insanity resulted in confinement for life in a mental institution. But with the development of modern treatment methods, including psychotropic drugs, periods of hospital confinement generally have been greatly shortened. The difficulties of making accurate predictions of potential for future violent behavior have aggravated this problem.

It is not possible to return to the old system of indefinite confinements, for appellate courts have generally held that the period of hospital confinement of a defendant who has been committed after having been found not guilty by reason of insanity can be no longer than the period of imprisonment for the crime charged. If a defendant recovers from his or her illness and is evaluated as not dangerous by the time the trial is completed, the defendant must be set free after his or her acquittal on grounds of insanity at the time of the offense. Generally, release from confinement after an insanity acquittal is contingent on recovery to the point of no longer being dangerous rather than recovery from the mental illness itself.

Except for the District of Columbia, federal law makes no provision for the hospitalization of defendants acquitted by reason of insanity. Such "patients" are ordinarily transferred to the custody of their own state hospital system, where they can then be involuntarily hospitalized in accordance with civil commitment proceedings. In many states, such a commitment can be only for a short period.

Guilty But Mentally Ill

Alaska, Connecticut, Georgia, Illinois, Indiana, Kentucky, Michigan, and New Mexico have adopted a new verdict of "guilty but mentally ill" while still retaining the verdict of not guilty by reason of insanity.

Although the guilty but mentally ill verdict may suggest by its terms that the convicted offender will receive treatment for the mental illness, such treatment is not mandatory. Furthermore, this verdict does not mitigate the sentence and may even enhance the sentence, since a parole or release board may be reluctant to release an offender with a record of mental illness after a minimum period of imprisonment.

Many who advocate this verdict hope that it will reduce or eliminate successful insanity defenses, since it gives the jury an alternative verdict. However, experience in Michigan with the guilty but mentally ill verdict has not been associated with a decrease in the number of acquittals based on insanity.

Despite the popular appeal of this verdict, both the American Psychiatric Association (in 1982) and the American Bar Association (in 1986) expressed their opposition to the addition of guilty but mentally ill to the possible verdicts of the criminal law. If such a verdict does not provide assurance of psychiatric care and treatment and does not mitigate the severity of the criminal sentence, it is difficult to see what value it has other than to create the false appearance that some special consideration is being given to a mentally ill defendant.

Diminished Capacity

The diminished capacity defense, as it has developed in California, is derived from laws concerned with the criminal responsibility of intoxicated persons. For centuries, Anglo-American law has struggled to reconcile the principle of *mens rea* with the problem of the offender who is voluntarily intoxicated at the time of the criminal act. By law, a person so intoxicated that he or she no longer has normal powers of will should be at least partly excused from responsibility for a criminal act committed during that state.

Voluntary intoxication could not be used, however, to avoid responsibility for all crime, nor could it negate the existence of a **general intent,** but it might in some cases establish that a specific intent could not have been present.

For example, the "general intent" crime of assault requires only the minimum awareness that one is striking out at another person. Intoxication is not a defense to a crime of general intent. However, the more serious crime of assault with intent to do bodily harm requires proof both of the unlawful act and of the existence of the specific "intent to do bodily harm." If the offender were sufficiently intoxicated at the time of the offense, the offender might successfully claim that he or she could not have formed that specific intent. Thus, such an offender might be found guilty only of the lesser offense of simple assault; if the offender had been sober, he or she would have been guilty of the more serious crime.

Finding a defendant guilty of a lesser included offense because of absence of the specific intent required by the definition of the greater crime is known as **diminished responsibility** or **diminished capacity.** In 1939, the California Supreme Court ruled that psychiatric testimony relevant to mental or emotional abnormalities must be admissible at trial for a specific intent crime. A mental illness far short of what would be required to establish exculpation under the not guilty by reason of insanity standard might still be sufficient to negate a specific intent such as malice or premediation. For example, a jury might find that the specific intent of premeditation is negated by the defendant's limited ability to rationally plan the criminal act. It might then find the defendant guilty of second-degree murder rather than first-degree murder. Or it might find that the specific intent of malice is negated by the defendant's impairment (by mental or emotional illness) of his or her power of self-control; this would result in a verdict of manslaughter rather than murder.

The principle has long existed in the criminal law of reducing the degree of a homicide in cases involving extreme passion or provocation. Thus, in crimes of passion, the offender may be guilty of manslaughter instead of murder. However, before this defense will succeed, the passion or provocation must have been of such a degree and of such a nature that a "reasonable man" would have succumbed to the criminal act. Evidence that the defendant was particularly vulnerable to provocation or susceptible to "passion" would not be admissible. The standard must be that of the "reasonable man," and the special qualities of the defendant are not relevant.

The diminished capacity defense eliminates the "reasonable man" standard. What matters is the actual state of mind of the particular defendant. Evidence of psychopathology and other mental qualities are relevant.

The defense of diminished capacity makes practical sense if there are appropriate psychiatric treatment facilities within a prison system and the period of confinement required by the conviction for the lesser included crime is not greatly longer than would result from the involuntary hospitalization after the not guilty by reason of insanity verdict. It is useful also in cases where the mental illness is of a kind and degree that usually does not result in an insanity verdict.

In June 1982, by popular initiative vote, the diminished capacity defense was abolished in California. However, the defense is slowly gaining headway in other states and is sometimes advocated as a complete substitute for the insanity defense.

Competency to Stand Trial

Due process in criminal trials requires that the defendant be able to understand what is happening and to participate in a meaningful way in the trial process. A defendant cannot be tried in absentia, either literally or figuratively. Competency to stand trial is assumed unless the issue is raised before the trial starts. Although the issue of insanity can be raised only by the defense, the question of competency can be raised by the defense, the prosecution, or the judge. When the issue is raised, the judge will either appoint psychiatrists to examine the defendant or will commit the defendant to a hospital for evaluation.

A hearing is then held to determine if the defendant is competent to be tried. The defendant is entitled to a jury trial on this issue if he or she wishes. In contrast to the legal issues concerned with criminal responsibility, the criteria for determining competency to stand trial are identical in all jurisdictions in the USA. In *Dusky v United States,* 362 US 402 (1960), the United States Supreme Court ruled as follows:

> . . . [T]he test must be whether he has sufficient present ability to consult with his lawyer with a reasonable degree of rational understanding—and whether he has a rational as well as factual understanding of the proceedings against him.

Most state laws specify that the incompetency must be the result of mental disease or defect. However, the Supreme Court decision does not so limit the test, and some authorities believe that the existence of mental illness or defect is not essential to a finding of incompetency.

If found to be incompetent to stand trial, the defendant is then usually committed to a mental institution for treatment. When competency is restored, the defendant may then go to trial and may be found guilty unless it is determined that the defendant was insane at the time of the offense.

Because determining incompetency is simpler than

a full-scale criminal trial and no proof is required that the defendant actually committed the crime, there has been a tendency to use competency procedures as a permanent disposition of offenders who might otherwise have been found to be insane. The defendant would be committed to a state hospital and, if never reevaluated as competent, could be involuntarily hospitalized indefinitely.

In *Jackson v Indiana,* 406 US 715, 738 (1972), the United States Supreme Court radically altered this situation. The appeal concerned a mentally retarded deaf-mute with limited ability to communicate who had been charged with 2 trivial offenses. Although he was harmless, Indiana law required that he be committed to a state hospital for the criminally insane until he became competent. In his case, that meant confinement for life for trivial offenses he might not even have committed. The Court stated, as a matter of law:

. . . [A] person charged by a State with a criminal offense who is committed solely on account of his incapacity to proceed to trial cannot be held more than the reasonable period of time necessary to determine whether there is a substantial probability that he will attain that capacity in the foreseeable future.

The *Jackson* decision has required revision of most state laws on the commitment of incompetent defendants, including limiting the period of confinement to no longer than the maximum period that could be imposed after a guilty verdict or plea of guilty. No longer can a determination of incompetency be used as a means of permanent disposition of a defendant, and institutions are under pressure to restore competency by adequate treatment and return the defendant for trial at the earliest possible time.

INVOLUNTARY HOSPITALIZATION & CONSERVATORSHIP

Until the 1960s, the involuntary hospitalization of mental patients was accomplished by complex formal legal proceedings that resulted in near-total loss of the civil, legal, and personal rights of ordinary citizens. Commitments were indefinite and remained in effect until the patient was restored to competency by a second legal procedure.

Because of the expense and complexity of the legal requirements, the actual proceedings were often greatly foreshortened in the interest of convenience at the expense of right. Judges sometimes served as "rubber stamps," indiscriminately approving whatever recommendations were made by examining physicians who may have had no training or experience in psychiatry and may have obtained their appointment to the "lunacy commission" as a political reward.

Most patients, especially if they were depressed or passive, received little legal guidance or protection. A paranoid, demanding, or aggressive patient might demand a jury trial, which would involve protracted legal proceedings. In many cases, to avoid that expense, commitment proceedings simply would be dropped and the patient released.

By the mid 1960s, new forms of commitment procedures were being devised. The leading example was the Lanterman-Petris-Short Mental Health Act of California, which became effective in 1969. The goals of the new laws were as follows: (1) to eliminate altogether, or to reduce to the absolute minimum, legal procedures for short-term commitments; (2) to eliminate all involuntary hospitalizations based solely on the existence of a mental disease or the need for care and treatment; (3) to permit involuntary hospitalization only if the patient is dangerous to self or others or is unable to provide for basic living requirements; (4) to eliminate all indefinite, purely custodial commitments; and (5) to maximize opportunities for effective treatment and early restoration of patients to their communities.

Where previous commitment periods were measured in months and years, these new procedures spoke only of hours and days of involuntary confinement. Furthermore, the patient was not to be deprived of any legal or civil rights and was not automatically assumed to be incompetent.

After an initial 72-hour period of observation, patients could be involuntarily detained for 2 weeks if found to be dangerous to themselves or others or to be gravely disabled. This 2-week extension required no legal procedures and was accomplished solely on the certification of the staff of the mental health facility. A patient who continued to be actively suicidal could be detained for an additional 2-week period. But after that, the patient must consent to voluntary treatment or be released.

No commitment provisions were made for long-term hospitalization for disabled patients. Instead, the concept of conservatorship was developed. A conservatorship differs from a guardianship in important ways. When made the ward of a guardian, one loses all rights of self-determination. One becomes like a child whose parent assumes responsibility for care and decisions. A conservator, however, acquires only limited powers over the conservatee. In a mental health conservatorship, the conservator usually has the authority to admit the conservatee to a mental hospital as a voluntary patient and to act as a substitute decision maker in consenting for treatment. The period of conservatorship is limited by statute; in California, it is 1 year, and the patient is entitled to legal counsel and a jury trial in superior court. The only ground for granting a mental health conservatorship is that the patient be gravely disabled. Grave disability is defined as inability, because of mental disease, to provide food, clothing, and shelter for oneself. The fact of grave disability must be proved beyond a reasonable doubt.

Most mental health laws permit commitment for periods of months for persons found to be dangerous to others. In California, 6 months is permitted, and commitment must be in superior court with legal counsel, a jury if requested, and proof beyond a reasonable doubt.

Because commitment to a mental institution is a civil procedure, many states originally required only the ordinary civil standard of proof, ie, a preponderance of the evidence. However, in 1979, in a case originating in Texas, the United States Supreme Court ruled that involuntary hospitalization required proof by "clear and convincing evidence." This is a higher standard of proof than the preponderance of evidence but not as high as beyond a reasonable doubt. Some states, California included, nevertheless retained their stricter standards for longer commitments and conservatorships.

Some states have additional commitment procedures for the involuntary hospitalization of special types of cases. There are (or have been) commitment procedures for sexual psychopaths (mentally disordered sex offenders) and so-called psychopathic delinquents. California pioneered the development of commitment procedures for sexual psychopaths (later termed mentally disordered sex offenders [MDSO]) but has now repealed all such laws. The national trend is away from such specialized commitments. However, there are now new commitment procedures for "mentally disordered violent offenders" (MDVO). Such laws permit the confinement of such offenders to continue after their prison terms have expired.

All states and the District of Columbia—but not other federal jurisdictions—have provisions for the commitment of offenders determined to be incompetent to stand trial or not guilty by reason of insanity.

Commitments of all types were originally for indefinite periods of time. But one by one, each type of commitment has been subject to time limitations either by legislative or judicial action. Today in some states in the USA, no indeterminate commitments of any kind are permitted. When the commitment is associated with criminal procedures, the period of confinement cannot be greater than it would have been if the defendant had been convicted of the crime. If involuntary hospitalization is still necessary at the expiration of the time limit, additional legal procedures are required.

A new concept is outpatient commitment for less serious conditions or offenses. **Outpatient commitment** requires patients to attend a clinic as often as needed for therapy or regulation of medication but does not otherwise restrict their activities. Failure to comply with treatment is reportable to the legal authorities and can lead to custodial confinement and involuntary treatment measures. Outpatient commitment may prove to be far less expensive to the community and more acceptable to patients and their families.

THE RIGHTS OF PATIENTS

The Right to Treatment

Although commitments for involuntary hospital-

ization are usually for the purpose of providing treatment, until recently there was no way to require a state to provide such treatment. Many state institutions for the mentally ill and the mentally retarded provided neither adequate treatment nor humane physical facilities for their involuntary patients.

Dr Morton Birnbaum, a lawyer and physician in general practice, first suggested, in 1960, that involuntarily institutionalized patients have a constitutional right to treatment and that this could be a means of forcing states to meet at least the minimum standards for care and treatment.

It was not until 1972 that this constitutional right to treatment was established in federal court. In the leading class-action case of *Wyatt v Stickney,* 314F Supp 373 (1972), it was held that the physical conditions and lack of treatment in both the state hospital and the institution for the mentally retarded in Alabama were so bad that the constitutional rights of the inmates were being violated.

Judge Johnson of the Federal District Court first gave the Commissioner of Mental Health, Dr Stickney, the opportunity to improve conditions in the Alabama institutions. Dr Stickney was forced to report back to the court that the Alabama Legislature and the Governor were unwilling to appropriate the necessary funds. After extensive hearings in which many experts testified, Judge Johnson then set forth, in his decision, the precise details of the standards for mental health care and physical facilities for involuntary patients that would meet constitutional standards. He then ordered Alabama to conform to those standards.

The *Wyatt* decision was upheld on appeal, so the constitutional right to treatment for involuntary patients is now established throughout the USA. Unfortunately, this decision does not establish a right to treatment for *voluntary* patients.

The United States Supreme Court accepted for review a somewhat parallel case, that of *O'Connor v Donaldson,* 422 US 563 (1975). Florida state law provided that a person may be committed to a state hospital merely on the basis of the existence of mental illness. After many years of confinement and after failure to obtain relief from state courts, Donaldson sued the superintendent of the hospital (O'Connor) and his ward doctor in federal court for violation of his civil rights. He was a Christian Scientist and had refused medication but was willing to receive other forms of therapy. At no time had he been dangerous to himself or others. He was awarded damages by the trial jury. The Fifth Circuit Court of Appeals sustained the award, ruling that Florida law permitting commitment on the basis of the existence of a mental illness alone was unconstitutional and also that Donaldson's constitutional right to treatment had been violated by the hospital's failure to provide alternative treatment to medication.

The United States Supreme Court upheld the principle that mental illness alone can never justify restricting a person's liberty. There must always be something more, such as a condition dangerous to oneself or others. However, the Court found that it was not necessary to reach the issue of the constitutionality of the right to treatment in Donaldson's case. Chief Justice Burger, in a separate opinion, made it clear that he did not believe there is a legal right to treatment that can be enforced on the states.

Although the constitutional right to treatment is now incorporated into existing law, there is concern that should it come before the United States Supreme Court and the views of former Chief Justice Burger should prevail, this progressive concept will be destroyed.

Informed Consent & the Right to Refuse Treatment

It is a basic principle of law that adults of sound mind must consent to medical or surgical procedures. They have the right to refuse all treatment even when their refusal is foolish and contrary to the judgment of their physicians and families.

In recent years, there has been considerable emphasis on the right of informed consent. Without adequate information on which to base a decision, consent is without legal force, and it is a professional obligation of physicians to provide their patients with the information required to make rational decisions. To perform a medical or surgical procedure on a patient without consent is a battery, a misdemeanor (although the consent in low-hazard procedures may be implied by the patient's cooperation). To obtain consent without properly informing a patient may constitute negligence.

The leading cases on medical informed consent are *Canterbury v Spence*, 464 F 2d 772 (DC Cir 1972), and *Cobbs v Grant*, 8 Cal 3d 229 (1972). Both courts insist that informed consent is a legal duty and its fulfillment is to be judged by legal standards instead of by the standards of practice of the medical community. This represents a significant change whose implications are still not fully appreciated by the medical profession, for many doctors unwittingly fail to provide the legal minimum of information to their patients.

The patient must be given adequate information about the nature, risks, and benefits of the proposed treatment. For the patient to make a rational choice, he or she must also be given similar information about alternative treatments. Hazards of extremely low incidence need not be mentioned. If the patient does not wish to be informed and says so to the doctor, he or she need not be given further information.

Denial of the opportunity to weigh the risks and alternatives for oneself and to make a personal decision is proper only when the patient is a minor, is incompetent, or is in a condition of emergency. If competency is questioned, the court must be petitioned to so state and to appoint a conservator to make the required decision.

For a minor, informed consent must be obtained from the parent or guardian unless there is a specific statutory exception. The exceptions—such as the mi-

nor's right to consent to obstetric care or to treatment for communicable disease, or to receive information about use of contraceptives—vary greatly from state to state, and *it is of critical importance that psychiatrists be familiar with the consent laws of the state in which they practice*. A few states have special provisions for minors to consent, in certain limited circumstances, to psychotherapy or drug or alcohol treatment without their parents' knowledge.

Emergencies are generally defined by the law as life-and-death situations that demand immediate action. If a patient is unconscious and requires immediate treatment, consent is not necessary.

If a patient is mentally incompetent, the right of informed consent generally passes to the nearest available relative or to a designated substitute decision maker, such as a conservator. A serious problem exists with many modern commitment laws. Accepting the principle that involuntary hospitalization should not also result in unlimited legal disability and loss of rights, short-term commitment laws do not declare a patient incompetent. It can be argued that even though a psychotic patient is certified for involuntary hospitalization and treatment, the patient has not necessarily lost the right of informed consent and the right to refuse treatment. To override that right may require a complicated legal procedure to adjudge the patient incompetent.

At present, hospital psychiatrists generally assume that laws authorizing involuntary hospitalization for purposes of treatment authorize that treatment to be given without informed consent and despite the patient's objection. That assumption may be incorrect.

Several important lawsuits (in Massachusetts, New Jersey, and California) have challenged the right of the psychiatrist to treat such patients unless they have consented or unless they have been declared incompetent. This issue has not been resolved, and a variety of conflicting appellate decisions exist. Some authorities interpret the United States Supreme Court decision in *Youngberg v Romeo* to mean that committed patients have no right to refuse necessary medications. The Court did not rule on this issue but held that courts should defer to the professional judgment of physicians in determining standards for treatment.

There is a clear trend toward close legal scrutiny of the problems of consent of persons in coercive situations. In 1973, in *Mackey v Procunier*, the Ninth Circuit Court of Appeals held that giving a prisoner succinylcholine as part of an experimental behavior modification program was "impermissible tinkering with the mental processes." The same year, in *Knecht v Gilman*, the Eighth Circuit Court of Appeals held that the administration of apomorphine as an example of "aversive stimuli" was cruel and unusual punishment. In 1980, the United States Supreme Court held that a prisoner may be transferred from a prison to a mental hospital for treatment without informed consent only after a formal hearing with reasonable due process safeguards. The minimum procedural requirements are considerably stricter than some states now impose for short-term involuntary hospitalization of nonprisoners. It can be anticipated that these minimum procedures will eventually become mandatory for all persons.

Confidentiality & Privileged Communication

There is no disagreement that effective psychotherapy requires a trusting relationship between patient and therapist. The foundation of that trust is the patient's belief that the therapist will maintain the confidentiality of their communications. If the therapist is required by law to breach that confidentiality, therapy becomes difficult, if not impossible. An enforced demand for breach of confidentiality with respect to one patient's communications may affect all patients, for the others may cease to believe—and rightly—that their confidences will be kept confidential.

The obligation of confidentiality between doctor and patient is usually required by professional practice regulations and by the ethical standards of professional organizations. However, of greater importance are the statutory provisions establishing immunity to the subpoena power for certain types of confidential communications.

Neither the criminal law nor the civil law could function adequately if courts did not have the right to compel witnesses to testify. This compulsion is accomplished by means of the subpoena (meaning "under penalty"), which is an order to appear as a witness in court or at a deposition. Doctors are usually served with a *subpoena duces tecum,* which requires that they also produce their relevant records and documents. Although the power to issue subpoenas belongs to the judge (or sometimes to a legislative committee or other governmental investigative agency), it is customary to issue subpoenas routinely at the request of an attorney representing a party to the action.

It has been established since ancient times that the preservation of certain relationships requires confidentiality and that the social importance of preserving these relationships outweighs the requirements of law and justice. The confidential communications of such a protected relationship are called **privileged communications.**

Traditionally, privilege has existed for communications between priest and penitent, attorney and client, and husband and wife. Privilege for the confidential communications of physicians and patients has traditionally existed in most European countries. Contrary to what most doctors believe, it never existed in Anglo-American common law. Protection of confidential communications between physicians and patients in the USA is therefore entirely statutory. The protection provided for physician-patient communications is in many cases so slight that it is useless in the instances where it is needed most. For example, many state laws provide no protection if the patient is involved in any type of criminal proceeding.

As the practice of psychotherapy became wide-spread in the 1950s, it became increasingly apparent that additional protection was necessary for the psychotherapist-patient relationship. There seemed to be little possibility of strengthening the physician-patient privilege, and even if that could be accomplished, it would not help nonmedical psychotherapists. The solution was to draft special psychotherapist-patient privileged communication laws. By the 1960s, Georgia, Connecticut, California, and a few other states had enacted psychotherapist-patient privilege laws.

Although the psychotherapist-patient privilege is far broader than the physician-patient privilege in that it provides protection in criminal as well as civil cases, the protection is far from absolute. The statutes provide many exceptions. For example, a patient who puts his or her mental state at issue in litigation thus waives the right of privilege for relevant records and the therapist's testimony. If a patient is believed to be dangerous to the person or property of others, the therapist may be privileged or even required to breach confidentiality. In addition, statutes such as those for the reporting of child abuse, communicable disease, and gunshot or other wounds—and judicial decisions such as the result in California's *Tarasoff* case—may require breaches of confidence. It is not unusual for there to be unresolved conflicts in the law, where one law permits therapists to maintain confidentiality and another requires them to breach it.

The *Tarasoff* decision (17 Cal 3d 425 [1976]) imposes upon a psychotherapist who knows (or should know) that a patient is dangerous to a specific potential victim the duty to protect the victim by notifying the police or by warning the victim. Although commitment laws may grant immunity from suit for any action taken in connection with the involuntary hospitalization of a patient, they do not give immunity for failure to comply with the *Tarasoff* duty. New Jersey has now adopted *Tarasoff,* and other states may well follow this precedent. The Ninth Circuit Court of Appeals has accepted the *Tarasoff* duty for federal jurisdictions and has emphasized that failure to properly diagnose the dangerousness of a patient is clearly malpractice (*Jablonski by Pahls v United States,* 712 F 2d 391 [9th Cir 1983]). In 1986, the California legislature simplified the *Tarasoff* obligation to warn the victim and limited the liability of the therapist.

The right of privilege belongs solely to the patient, who may waive this right without the consent of the therapist. All attempts to provide joint control over the privilege for both therapist and patient (as exists for the priest-penitent relationship) have failed.

Increasingly, legislatures are requiring the therapist to breach confidentiality even if there is only a suspicion of child abuse or child molestation. Reporting of dependent and elderly adult abuse is required in some states.

It is of critical importance that psychotherapists familiarize themselves with the laws regulating confidentiality and privilege in the state within which they practice. There are great differences between states, and one cannot extrapolate the law of one state with the assumption that it will provide a reliable guide to the law of one's own jurisdiction.

SPECIALIZED AREAS IN FORENSIC PSYCHIATRY

There are increasing numbers of legal areas where the skills of the forensic psychiatrist are utilized. Because most of these require specialized legal and medical knowledge, the average psychiatrist is not likely to be involved in them. Hence, they will be discussed only superficially in this chapter.

The law has been hesitant to permit the recovery of damages for **emotional distress.** However, now the law is tending to become less restrictive, and all sorts of claims are being made for psychologic and emotional harm alleged to have been inflicted by the negligence of others. As a result, forensic psychiatrists are frequently called on to evaluate such claims and to testify as expert witnesses in these personal injury trials. This area of tort law is still very complex, and one should not participate as such an expert unless one is thoroughly familiar with the legal issues.

Workers' compensation law is another area that has tended to attract the interest of forensic psychiatrists. It is now well settled that the stress of employment may sometimes cause or aggravate mental or emotional illness. When this occurs, the worker is entitled to be compensated in proportion to the disability as one would be for a physical injury incurred on the job. The stresses of employment may also be relevant to disability retirement claims. These cases must be carefully evaluated by a psychiatrist, the degree of disability assessed, reports written, and often testimony given in hearings.

Psychiatric malpractice is another growing field. There is a steady increase in the number of malpractice suits filed against psychiatrists. The level is not yet a cause for concern, but each case requires a specialized inquiry and often will require expert testimony on a wide variety of issues.

Child custody issues may require psychiatric expertise on questions of the "best interests of the child," the child-parent relationship, psychologic needs of children at different stages of development, fitness of parents, and the impact of parental psychologic disturbance on the child. As "no-fault" divorce laws become widespread, there is a tendency for legal battles that would have previously been fought on questions of morality, blame, money, and property to shift to the arena of child custody. This results in an increased need for forensic skills in child psychiatry.

As the behavioral sciences have become more involved in the justice system, there are frequent needs for experts to participate in evidentiary hearings on particular issues. Expert testimony may be needed on questions such as the validity of hypnosis for the enhancement of memory of witnesses; the ability of psychiatrists to predict dangerousness; the psychology of entrapment; the effects of racial discrimination; the stress of combat in the armed forces; and many other issues.

Despite the serious problem of credibility of psychiatric expert testimony in criminal trials, there seems to be an endless need for the expertise of the forensic psychiatrist. In the complex modern world, it is inevitable that the processes of the law will require an ever-increasing input of technical expertise. In the past, psychiatry has tended to dominate forensic behavioral science. This is changing rapidly: Psychologists with proper credentials and experience are accepted as experts on insanity, child custody, and other legal issues; and sociologists, anthropologists, linguists, criminologists, and penologists are all beginning to appear in court to offer useful opinion for the benefit of the trier of fact in reaching difficult decisions. However, the basic principle of expert testimony remains unchanged: that the witness be truly an expert in training, experience, and knowledge.

REFERENCES

American Bar Association: Criminal justice mental health standards. Chapter 7 in: *American Bar Association Standards for Criminal Justice*. Little, Brown, 1986.

American Medical Association Committee on Medicolegal Problems: Insanity defense in criminal trials and limitation of psychiatric testimony. (Committee report.) *JAMA* 1984; **251:**2967.

American Psychiatric Association: Statement on the insanity defense. *Am J Psychiatry* 1983;**140:**681.

Birnbaum M: The right to treatment. *J Am Bar Assoc* 1960; **46:**499.

Brooks AD: *Law, Psychiatry and the Mental Health System.* Little, Brown, 1974. [Supplement, 1980.]

Diamond BL: Criminal responsibility of the mentally ill. *Stanford Law Rev* 1961;**14:**59.

Diamond BL: The fallacy of the impartial expert. *Arch Crim Psychodynamics* 1959;**3:**221. [Reprinted in: Allen RC, Fer-

ster EZ, Rubin JG: *Readings in Law and Psychiatry,* rev ed. Johns Hopkins Press, 1975.]

Diamond BL: Isaac Ray and the trial of Daniel McNaughten. *Am J Psychiatry* 1954;**112:**39.

Goldstein J, Freud A, Solnit AJ: *Before the Best Interests of the Child.* Free Press, 1979.

Goldstein J, Freud A, Solnit AJ: *Beyond the Best Interests of the Child.* Free Press, 1973.

Platt A, Diamond BL: The origins of the "right and wrong" test of criminal responsibility and its subsequent development in the United States: An historical survey. *Calif Law Rev* 1966;**54:**1227.

Slovenko R: *Psychiatry and Law.* Little, Brown, 1973.

West DJ, Walk A (editors): *Daniel McNaughton: His Trial and the Aftermath.* Gaskell, 1977.

Legal Cases

Addington v Texas, 441 US 418 (1979).

Ake v Oklahoma, 407 US 68 (1985).

Brawner v United States, 471 F 2d 969 (DC Cir 1972).

Canterbury v Spence, 464 F 2d 772 (DC Cir 1972).

Carter v General Motors et al, 361 Mich 577, 106 NW 2d 105 (1960).

Cobbs v Grant, 8 Cal 3d 229, 104 Cal Rptr 505, 502 P 2d 1 (1972).

Davis v United States, 160 US 469 (1895) and 165 US 373 (1897).

Dillon v Legg, 68 Cal 2d 728, 69 Cal Rptr 72, 441 P 2d 912 (1968).

Durham v United States, 214 F 2d 862 (DC Cir 1954).

Dusky v United States, 362 US 402 (1960).

Frye v United States, 293 F 1013 (DC App 1923).

Jablonski by Pahls v United States, 712 F 2d 391 (9th Cir 1983).

Jackson v Indiana, 406 US 715, 738 (1972).

Knecht v Gilman, 488 F 2d 1136 (8th Cir 1973).

Mackey v Procunier, 477 F 2d 877 (9th Cir 1973).

O'Connor v Donaldson, 422 US 563 (1975).

Rennie v Klein, 653 F 2d 836 (3d Cir 1981).

Roger v Okin, 634 F 2d 650 (1st Cir 1980).

State of New Hampshire v Jones, 50 NH 3269 (1871).

State of New Hampshire v Pike, 49 NH 399 (1869).

Tarasoff v Regents of the University of California, 17 Cal 3d 425, 131 Cal Rptr 14, 551 P 2d 334 (1976).

Vitek v Jones, 445 US 480 (1980).

Wyatt v Stickney, 314 F Supp 373 (MD Ala ND 1972); *Wyatt v Aderholt*, 503 F 2d 1305 (5th Cir 1974).

Youngberg v Romeo, 457 US 307 (1982).

Suicide, Homicide, & Other Psychiatric Emergencies

59

Roland Levy, MD

Every physician must be prepared to make a prompt diagnosis and provide efficient treatment for psychiatric emergencies. This chapter emphasizes actual or attempted homicide and suicide, since these are the most serious psychiatric emergencies the physician is called upon to deal with. Careful assessment and prompt institution of appropriate management may significantly affect the outcomes in such cases and may prevent harm to the medical staff. Other psychiatric emergencies are mentioned, and references are given to more complete discussions in other chapters in this text.

The physician should be familiar with the state or local reporting requirements relating to self-injury or injuries to others by means of "a knife, gun, pistol, or other deadly weapon" (California Penal Code Section 11160).

Definitions

A. Psychiatric Emergency: A psychiatric emergency is a disturbance in thoughts, feelings, or actions requiring immediate treatment. Whether the disturbance is termed an emergency depends on the patient's physical and psychologic status and on the physician's frame of reference and understanding of the events requiring action.

B. Crisis: A crisis is a stressful situation perceived as a threat to the self and indicating a decisive turning point toward either improvement or deterioration.

C. Crisis Intervention: This term is often used in community psychiatry to denote brief therapeutic techniques using various personnel and incorporating the following concepts. A "crisis" is a situation that presents a challenge to the patient, family, and community and has been created by an altered set of circumstances. If the patient and his or her social system successfully master the crisis, there is opportunity for enrichment of the personality and development of better adaptive responses. Should the result be a failure to meet the challenge, maladaptive responses occur that may worsen individual or group deficits. The period of the crisis is an opportune time to mobilize the patient and family to seek help and to become involved with longer-term assistance.

SUICIDE

In the USA, suicide ranks as the eighth major cause of death, with over 20,000 recorded suicides each year. Conservative estimates are that attempted suicide is 10 times more frequent than successful suicide. These figures do not include unconsciously motivated fatal "accidents" or numerous other self-destructive behaviors (eg, alcoholism).

About twice as many women attempt suicide as men. Successful suicides, however, are 2–4 times more frequent in men. Suicidal behavior is more common with advancing age; in persons who are widowed, divorced, separated from their spouses, or otherwise isolated, uprooted, or lonely; in persons of lower socioeconomic status; in Protestants; and in foreign-born immigrants. Guns are the most commonly used means of successful suicide (50% of men and 25% of women). Men are more likely than women to commit suicide by violent means (Table 59–1).

The clinician evaluating the risk of suicide should try to determine whether the patient has formed a definite plan for suicide; eg, Has the patient made out a will, changed an insurance policy, or decided on the method, time, and place for the act? The clinician must assess previous suicide attempts and obtain a family history of suicide. In evaluating mental status, the clinician should ask about feelings of rejection and uselessness and whether the patient is working. Coexisting depression with associated anxiety or acute worsening of depression is a danger signal, as is a rapid superficial improvement in depression, which may be a sign that a plan for suicide has been devised. Increasing hostility may also be a clue to impending suicide. Financial worries (real or imagined) with ideas of impending poverty are often associated with suicide. People with painful illnesses, particularly if associated with prolonged sleep disturbance, are at greater risk of suicide. Individuals with a recent history of alcoholism or drug abuse are also definite suicidal risks.

Clues to Suicide

People who are contemplating suicide often provide clues that must be carefully assessed.

A. Verbal Clues: The individual may sometimes make direct statements about wanting to die or "end it all." Less direct ways of expressing suicidal ideation

Table 59–1. Suicide rate per 1000 population among 3800 attempted suicides, by high- and low-risk categories of risk-related factors.*

Factor	High-Risk Category	Suicide Rate	Low-Risk Category	Suicide Rate
Age	45 years of age and older	24	Under 45 years of age	9.4
Sex	Male	19.9	Female	9.2
Race	White	14.3	Nonwhite	8.7
Marital status	Separated, divorced, widowed	12.5	Single, married	8.6
Living arrangements	Alone	48.4	With others	10.1
Employment status†	Unemployed, retired	16.8	Employed ‡	14.3
Physical health	Poor (acute or chronic condition in the 6 months preceding the attempt)	14	Good ‡	12.4
Mental condition	Nervous or mental disorder, mood or behavioral symptoms, including alcoholism	19.1	Presumably normal, including brief situational reactions ‡	7.2
Medical care (within 6 months)	Yes	16.4	No ‡	10.8
Method	Hanging, firearms, jumping, drowning	28.4	Cutting or piercing, gas or carbon monoxide, poison, combination of other methods, other	12
Season	Warm months (April–September)	14.2	Cold months (October–March)	10.9
Time of day	6:00 AM–5:59 PM	15.1	6:00 PM–5:59 AM	10.5
Where attempt was made	Own or someone else's home	14.3	Other type of premises, out of doors	11.9
Time interval between attempt and discovery	Almost immediately; reported by person making attempt	10.9	Later	7.2
Intent to commit suicide (self report)	No ‡	14.5	Yes	8.5
Suicide note	Yes	16.7	No ‡	12.3
Previous attempt or threat	Yes	25.2	No ‡	11

*Reproduced, with permission, from Tuckman J, Youngman WF: A scale for assessing suicide risk of attempted suicides. *J Clin Psychol* 1968;**24**:17.
†Does not include homemakers and students.
‡Incudes cases for which information on this factor was not given in the police report.

are, "It's too much to bear!" "You'd be better off without me!" "I'd be better off dead!" A patient who asks, "How does one leave his body to science?" or who says, "I have a friend who's real depressed and talks about suicide a lot" is sending messages in very simple code.

B. Behavioral Clues: A direct behavioral clue is ingestion of a small amount of some potentially lethal drug. Putting one's affairs in order, arranging for a casket, and giving away prized possessions are indirect clues.

C. Situational Clues: Situational clues are inherent in life experiences associated with major stress, eg, an impending surgical procedure, a diagnosis of chronic fatal illness, or a recent loss—the death of a loved one, loss of a job, eviction, retirement, etc.

D. Syndromic Clues: Syndromic clues are certain constellations of emotions that are commonly associated with suicide. Depression is the most common one, but there are others. Suicide also occurs in people who are not depressed but are disoriented; eg, in acute delirium, suicidal behavior may be an attempt to flee

some imagined threat. Individuals with psychotic disorders associated with impaired impulse control may attempt suicide in response to hallucinations commanding them to do so. Suicide also occurs in defiant people, who may view suicide as a means of taking an active, resistive stance in the face of some real or imagined threat to their self-esteem. Suicide by a dependent, dissatisfied individual is often a masked hostile gesture toward some other individual or group perceived as not having fulfilled dependency needs. ("Now you'll feel sorry!")

Assessing the Risk of Suicide

The physician must stay alert to the possibility of suicide in patients presenting for treatment. Most people who attempt suicide have been seen by a physician a few months before, and most successful suicides have signaled their intent to loved ones and others and have expressed a need for help, often in the preceding 24 hours. The physician must regard suicide attempts or verbalized suicidal thoughts as emergencies, since even so-called "hysterical" and "manipulative" patients may succeed in self-destructive acts.

The following steps are recommended for the assessment of suicidal risk:

(1) Ascertain the patient's characteristic mode of reacting to stress and whether suicide has ever been considered or attempted in response to a stressful event.

(2) Evaluate presenting symptoms as possible somatic manifestations of depression, particularly anxiety, insomnia, fatigue, constipation, loss of appetite, or menstrual irregularities.

(3) If the patient has considered suicide in the past, explore the following:

(a) The frequency and extent of suicidal ideas.

(b) The contemplated means of committing suicide.

(c) The feelings associated with suicide and with the means of suicide, eg, fear, resignation.

(d) The availability of means for committing suicide, eg, gun, poison.

(e) The relationship of suicidal ideation to ordinary acts of everyday life.

(f) The patient's ability to imagine how loved ones would be affected by the suicide.

Assessing the Degree of Suicidal Risk

If the physician has determined that the patient is a suicidal risk, the severity of risk must be assessed. The following types of suicidal behavior are discussed in order of increasing risk:

(1) Transient thoughts about dying. People with transient ideas of death may entertain fantasies such as, "They'll miss me when I'm gone." Such common notions are usually of little significance. Concern and caution are warranted, however, if the patient is an adolescent or an emotionally unstable adult.

(2) Sustained thoughts about dying and recurrent wishes for death. Sustained ideas about death and recurrent death wishes may function as a painful habit that enables the person to deal with stress. Suicidal gestures such as superficial wrist cutting or nonlethal ingestion of drugs may occur occasionally.

(3) Frustrated feelings and impulsive behavior. A patient may have little hope for support from the environment and may feel that most forms of relief have been exhausted. The patient is therefore frustrated and close to anger much of the time. The anger may be turned inward or outward, leading to the possibility of a suicidal or homicidal act.

(4) Court of last resort. A person may feel that he or she has depleted all emotional resources. Such an individual no longer feels rage, frustration, or despair, and death is viewed as a way of avoiding further anguish.

(5) The logical decision to die. A person may approach suicide from a logical and philosophic point of view. Such a person sees death as inevitable and asks, "So why not now?" This type of individual is at the highest risk of suicide but rarely comes to the attention of the physician.

Suicide Prevention

The concept underlying and justifying suicide prevention efforts is that people contemplating suicide may nonetheless want to be prevented from doing so. Even those who do not want to be "rescued" or dissuaded from their suicidal purpose should be, since proper treatment and environmental adjustments can often restore such people to better health. Astute observation can almost always uncover clues to suicidal intentions. Almost all suicidal behavior stems from a sense of isolation and anguish. The function of suicide is to terminate unbearable existence. A single significant relationship may be sufficient to sustain an individual in an otherwise intolerable situation.

Many persons considered to be suicidal risks do not require hospitalization. Those in high-risk categories should be hospitalized. In doubtful cases, the decision about hospitalization is based on the physician's assessment of the adequacy of the patient's external support system and the integrity of the patient's impulse control mechanism. Lack of an effective support system and poor impulse control in patients otherwise at low risk for suicide may call for hospitalization.

People with suicidal ideas should not be offered the means of acting on them. When such a patient is hospitalized with suicide precautions, there should be no access to an unsecure window, stairwell, etc. Potential instruments of suicide such as shoelaces, belts, coat hangers, caustic cleansers, and cutlery should be kept from the patient. Some patients need constant close observation.

Although some general measures apply to the management of all suicidal persons, specific measures depend on the specific underlying diagnosis, since treatment differs depending on whether the patient has a major affective disorder, schizophrenia, delirium, or dysthymic disorder. Appropriate treatment may include psychotherapy, pharmacologic therapy, and, in some cases, electroconvulsive therapy.

Illustrative case No. 1. A 20-year-old unmarried college student living at home with her parents and younger siblings was brought to the emergency room after a nearly fatal drug overdose. The family had come to the USA from a Middle Eastern country 3 years previously. The patient stated that her suicide attempt was in response to her father's demands that she keep the cultural values of their native country rather than adopt those of the new culture. She resented his "dictatorial" approach and envied the freedom of her American peers. The patient showed no evidence of psychosis and was felt to be suffering from adjustment disorder. Treatment centered on several emergency family sessions. The father was approached as the head of the family and was helped to express his concerns and fears about the family's exposure to new cultural attitudes. He was able to see how his attitudes were reflected in his children's conflicts, and he reluctantly agreed to allow them greater freedom. The children learned to view their father not as a tyrant but rather as a man in culture shock still trying to be a good father. After the initial hostility had subsided, an agreement was reached that both "sides" were able to feel comfortable with. The patient was discharged after one day in the hospital, and the family was referred to an outpatient psychiatric clinic for further family therapy.

Illustrative case No. 2. A 58-year-old divorced surgeon experienced a manic episode. He had a history of depression that began in late adolescence, and his last episode of depression had occurred 10 years before. During the manic episode, he lost all of his hospital affiliations, incurred several malpractice suits, and accumulated huge debts, all in several weeks. He was hospitalized and treated with lithium, and his excitement subsided. He then became suicidally depressed. The depression responded favorably to the addition of tricyclic antidepressant medication to the regimen. After the patient was discharged from the hospital, the dosage of the tricyclic antidepressant was reduced and finally discontinued. Maintenance treatment with lithium alone was subsequently successful.

Illustrative case No. 3. A 72-year-old retired married man had experienced the onset of depression 2 years previously. He was agitated and had regressed, and his wife could not cope with him. Antidepressant medications were tried but had to be stopped because of their side effects. The patient consented to electroconvulsive therapy and underwent a series of 9 treatments that resulted in complete remission of symptoms.

Suicide in Adolescents

In recent years, the rate of suicide among adolescents has risen to alarming proportions. The evaluation of adolescent patients must be conducted with special care. Adolescents generally tend to be more impulsive than adults, and the suicidal adolescent is less likely to be suffering from depression than an adult. Behavioral changes often precede a suicide attempt, but the adolescent is less likely than an adult to show characteristic anxiety, sleep disturbance, loss of appetite, or other symptoms often associated with depression. In such teenagers, it is common for the underlying psychiatric condition to be schizophrenia rather than an affective disorder.

Illustrative case. A 16-year-old boy was admitted to the hospital after swallowing several of his mother's antihypertensive pills. The history revealed progressive social withdrawal over the past year, and school records showed a significant decline in academic performance for 2 years. The patient admitted having auditory hallucinations in the form of derogatory voices, and he also had ideas of reference. Antipsychotic medications relieved both his hallucinations and his depression.

HOMICIDE

Homicide is the killing of a human being by another human being. Murder, as defined by California Penal Code Section 187, is "the killing of a human being, or a fetus, with malice aforethought." In this discussion the term "homicide" is used without regard to legal distinctions (justifiable, excusable, with or without malice, etc).

Most homicides occur at night, with the highest incidence between 8:00 PM Saturday and 2:00 AM Sunday. Fifty percent of homicides occur on weekends or holidays; most of them occur in the home; the victim and perpetrator are frequently members of the same family; and the victim may be the perpetrator. Homicide is committed 5 times more often by men than by women, although in recent years the incidence of homicides perpetrated by women has been increasing.

The risk of homicide is increased in persons with psychosis characterized by persecutory delusions, and the risk is especially high when the delusions have come to focus on one individual. The homicide risk is increased also in individuals with a history of violence, hatred of authority, or antisocial personality traits. Evidence of rivalry, jealousy, or sexual conflicts; a recent history of withdrawal, brooding, and moodiness; and a history of alcoholism or drug abuse are other significant risk factors.

Most homicidal acts are not premeditated but occur during periods of heightened emotional tension that coincide with the ready availability of some sort of weapon. Anything that impairs impulse control increases the risk of violent assault, eg, "premedicated" murder after the use of alcohol or street drugs by the perpetrator.

Illustrative case No. 1. A 54-year-old municipal employee believed that his supervisor and fellow workers were ridiculing him by making sexual gestures and remarks and creating obstacles to performance of his job. Three physicians prescribed barbiturates and amphetamines to relieve his symptoms of anxiety and depression, and the patient obtained refills from several pharmacies. His wife was aware of his misuse of medication but did not notify any of the physicians. After a negative performance review one day, the patient shot his supervisor and 2 coworkers. Medical testimony at the patient's trial emphasized impaired judgment resulting from his state of chronic intoxication. He was found guilty of second-degree murder.

Illustrative case No. 2. A 26-year-old man with no history of psychiatric or criminal problems struck up an acquaintance with a woman at a bus stop. They arranged to meet the following day in a park. Shortly before the appointed time, the patient ingested some LSD. As the couple was walking in a secluded area, the patient suddenly became convinced that the woman was turning into a man. He attempted to tear off her clothes to validate that belief, and when she resisted, he physically assaulted her. He was apprehended and charged with attempted murder and assault with intent to commit rape.

OTHER PSYCHIATRIC EMERGENCIES

Acute Nonpsychotic Disorders

Emergencies may occur in 3 types of nonpsychotic disorders: anxiety disorders, including panic attacks and conversion reactions of a dissociative type, as well as fugue states; personality disorders; and antisocial states, in which aggressive behavior occurs frequently (see Chapters 31, 33 and 36).

Illustrative case No. 1. An 18-year-old man was brought to the emergency room after he threatened his mother with a knife when she refused to give him money. He had a long history of depression and antisocial behavior—theft, assault, robbery—and had been incarcerated in juvenile facilities several times. He was released after a brief period of observation, since his mother refused to press charges and he was neither psychotic nor depressed.

Illustrative case No. 2. A 22-year-old male college student was brought to the emergency room for evaluation after a sudden onset of paralysis and aphonia following a motor vehicle accident. The other driver had been tailgating him for a mile and then smashed his car from behind. After medical examination failed to account for the symptoms, sodium pentobarbital was administered intravenously, and the symptoms quickly disappeared. The patient then related that just before the onset of paralysis and aphonia, he had experienced a feeling of murderous rage toward the other driver.

Delirium

Delirium is common in patients presenting to emergency rooms, especially in association with alcohol or drug intoxication. Any stimulant or depressant drug may cause delirium when taken in sufficient quantities. Of special importance is phencyclidine psychosis, since individuals who have ingested this drug often exhibit episodes of extreme violence, and the reaction lasts longer than those due to other hallucinogens (see Chapter 25). Delirium may also be caused by other factors, eg, head trauma, cardiovascular disorders, metabolic disorders, and infections (see Chapters 24 and 56).

Illustrative case. A 68-year-old woman was brought to the hospital by her brother, who had been called by the manager of her apartment building. She had been wandering the halls and bothering other tenants and had not been caring for herself. Laboratory studies revealed severe hypothyroidism. Thyroid hormone replacement therapy led to gradual improvement in the patient's mental status.

Dementia

Persons suffering from dementia are not usually highly aggressive. They do have a lowered threshold of emotional control, however, and may become assaultive when they find themselves in situations they do not understand.

Illustrative case. An 86-year-old man was admitted to the hospital after he assaulted his 89-year-old sister. She reported that over the past several years, he had shown progressive deterioration in intellectual function. He completely denied his failing abilities and became assaultive when his sister tried to help him prepare a meal. Examination revealed senile dementia.

Acute Psychotic Disorders

Impulse control may be tenuous in individuals experiencing an acute psychotic episode, and they may be extremely assaultive as a result. The paranoid delusions associated with paranoid schizophrenia and other paranoid psychotic disorders may lead patients to act out, and the delusions are a special cause for concern if patients feel that a specific person in the environment is the source of the persecution.

The excitement that may erupt during a catatonic episode occurs less frequently than agitation caused by paranoid delusions, but it is unpredictable and usually associated with extreme violence.

Illustrative case No. 1. A 40-year-old single man with a long history of paranoid schizophrenia made an appointment at a medical clinic for evaluation of chronic urologic complaints. After the examination, he was told that there were no physical abnormalities. A few minutes later, the patient thought he heard the doctor discussing his case in a demeaning way with a group of nurses. In a rage, he pulled out a gun and shot the physician.

Individuals in the manic phase of bipolar disorder may be assaultive if they feel someone is interfering with their activities. Manic patients are not always jovial and humorous and may in fact be extremely agitated and aggressive. Aggressive behavior may also occur during episodes of depression; in fact, psychotically depressed people may be homicidal. The victim is often a loved one with whom the patient has identified and on whom the patient's misery is projected. ("You're just like me, and we're both miserable. I'll kill you and then myself, and then we'll both be free from all of this.") The act is committed in order to save the other person from "a life of misery."

Illustrative case No. 2. During a recurrent manic attack, a 31-year-old man became impatient while waiting for a bus. He approached a car stopped at an intersection, pulled the driver out, drove off at high speed, and hit another vehicle. In the emergency room, he had to be physically restrained while the physician gave treatment for severe lacerations.

Illustrative case No. 3. A 42-year-old woman who had been married for some time became pregnant for the first time. Three months after delivery of a healthy child, she experienced severe depression with suicidal ideation. In her state of hopelessness, she drowned the child in the bathtub and then slashed her wrists.

Untoward Consequences of Medication

Emergencies may arise as a consequence of medications being used to treat a psychiatric condition. Antipsychotic medications, particularly high-potency preparations, may cause dramatic dystonic states, catatonia, and neuroleptic malignant syndrome (see Chapters 24 and 52). Lithium therapy must be closely monitored to avoid toxicity. The tricyclic antidepressants prescribed for major depression may be used in a suicide attempt. Monoamine oxidase inhibitors may produce serious hypertensive reactions resulting from interaction with exogenous tyramine and similar sympathomimetic substances (see Chapter 53).

Adjustment Disorder & Posttraumatic Stress Disorder

Adjustment disorder represents a transient response to overwhelming environmental stress in individuals without apparent underlying psychiatric illness. Adjustment disorder is characterized by impaired social or vocational functioning and by symptoms that exceed the normally expected reaction. Such symptoms may develop in persons who suffer a major loss or in those who are victims of violence (eg, rape, spouse beating, or child abuse).

Posttraumatic stress disorder (stress response syndrome) is a reaction to an identifiable stress outside the normal range of experience (eg, car crash, natural disaster). The pattern of response consists of an initial outcry (an emotional response that is almost a reflex), followed by denial (emotional numbing, avoidance of ideas connected to the stressor, and behavioral constriction), an intrusive phase (unbidden ideas and feelings that are difficult to dispel), and a phase of working through and completion.

In both adjustment disorder and posttraumatic stress disorder, prompt crisis intervention may facilitate resolution of symptoms and prevent development of a more chronic psychiatric disorder (see Chapters 31 and 35).

GENERAL APPROACH TO VIOLENT OR ACUTELY EXCITED PATIENTS

The physician attempting to deal with a violent patient should use a calm, systematic approach. The patient's behavior should be accepted as a symptom of the illness, and no patient should ever be rejected or ridiculed. Patients who become violent in the emergency room are often those who have been kept waiting; these patients interpret the wait as a sign that others do not consider them important or do not feel they need immediate treatment. The physician should act promptly and decisively, introduce himself or herself, and explain the plan of treatment: "Mr Allen, I'm Dr Rodriguez of the emergency department staff. I'd like to talk to you for a few minutes and then do a physical examination." The physician should then obtain a history and perform the examination. Information from friends and relatives is often needed in order to develop an appropriate plan of treatment.

The physician should make sure that backup help is available for management of patients who are obviously psychotic or aggressive. The area should be free of objects that could be used as weapons. The medical staff should never turn their backs or let the patient come between them and the door; the door should be readily accessible both to the patient and to the interviewer. If a violent patient escapes security guards, the police should be called immediately.

Threatening calls or letters should never be ignored, since to do so may actually encourage the caller or writer to escalate the activity.

When a violent patient presents in the office or emergency room, it is appropriate to acknowledge realistic fear but not panic. The physician must exercise self-control in order to control the patient and the situation. Facing the patient at a discreet distance with arms crossed is a nonthreatening stance that nevertheless enables the physician to avoid or deflect blows. The physician should not attempt to deal unaided with a violent patient. Agitated patients confronted with ample force are less likely to become assaultive.

Potentially assaultive patients should be discreetly searched for weapons in the emergency room by being asked to change to hospital clothing.

If restraints are needed, they should be used promptly and applied as gently as possible. An early show of authority and control may prevent injuries and allow the physician to proceed with treatment. Destructive behavior must be prevented not only because of the property damage or personal injuries to others that might occur but also because of the guilt feelings and lowered self-esteem the patient inevitably faces when self-control is restored.

The physician should never threaten a patient; never openly disagree with a hostile patient; and never make insincere promises; never ridicule a patient; and never do anything that would hurt a patient's pride. If the physician intends to obtain psychiatric consultation, medication should be avoided, if possible, so that the psychiatric staff can better assess the patient's baseline condition. It is best not to assume that a violent patient has a psychogenic problem until various organic causes of the psychologic disturbance have been seriously considered.

SUMMARY

Dealing with psychiatric emergencies requires considerable knowledge and skill. The physician must be able to reach an accurate diagnosis quickly and begin appropriate treatment without delay. The crisis should be resolved promptly and in a way that eases the transition to the next phase of treatment. How the physician behaves during the emergency phase will strongly influence what happens later.

REFERENCES

Bulletin of Suicidology. Vols 1–8. National Clearinghouse for Mental Health Information, Rockville, Maryland, 1967–1971.

Hayes JR, Roberts TK, Solway SS (editors): *Violence and the Violent Individual.* Spectrum Publications, 1981.

Neuroleptic malignant syndrome. *Lancet* 1984;**1**:545.

Psychiatric emergencies. Chap 9, pp 197–228, in: *Legal Implications of Emergency Care.* Appleton-Century-Crofts, 1969.

Psychiatric emergencies. Chapter 27 in: *Modern Synopsis of Comprehensive Textbook of Psychiatry/IV,* 4th ed. Kaplan HI, Freedman AM, Sadock BJ (editors). Williams & Wilkins, 1985.

Rund DA, Hutzler JC: *Emergency Psychiatry.* Mosby, 1983.

Sandus S et al: *Violent Individuals and Families.* Thomas, 1984.

Tuckman J, Youngman WF: A scale for assessing suicide risk of attempted suicides. *J Clin Psychol* 1968;**24**:17.

60

Occupational Psychiatry

Carroll M. Brodsky, MD, PhD

Occupational psychiatry is concerned with the prevention, assessment, and treatment of mental disorders and disability in the workplace. As this subspecialty field has evolved, there has been increasing recognition of the important role work plays in maintaining as well as disrupting mental health. Physical and emotional stressors in the workplace have been identified and found to produce both organic and functional mental disorders, and the mental states of workers have been shown to affect their own safety and productivity as well as that of their coworkers. The workplace environment is conducive to research, since large numbers of workers are exposed to similar interpersonal, social, and physical factors (eg, noise, chemicals), and the effects of any single factor can be measured by comparing exposed to unexposed groups.

Employers are concerned with prevention of mental health problems in workers because these problems disrupt work, reduce productivity, affect morale, and are costly in terms of employees' medical care and rehabilitation. Terminating the employment of a disturbed worker and training a replacement are also costly and disruptive procedures. Employers thus look to occupational psychiatrists to develop techniques of selecting people who are better able to meet the requirements of their jobs.

The field of occupational psychiatry has also developed in response to the need for forensic consultation about the relationship between events in the workplace and the worker's mental health, since medicolegal decisions require specialized knowledge about work, its requirements, and its impact on health.

CONCEPTS OF WORK & STRESS

Psychiatrists' interests have broadened to include questions about the "culture" of the workplace and its physical, social, and psychologic conditions and about individual and cultural attitudes toward work.

Most workplaces focus on producing goods or providing services at a profit and do not include among their primary missions the furtherance of an individual's job satisfaction or growth as a person or as a worker, except as these further the organization's goals. Ordinarily, an employer will not assume the traditionally "parental" functions of offering support, care, and growth enhancement unless doing so is in the organization's enlightened best interests or made necessary by law or by contracts negotiated between workers and management.

Each workplace has its own "culture" with its own communication patterns, status patterns, and values. Understanding the culture contributes to determining the characteristics (eg, personalities) of those who can function well in it and the reactions of those who cannot. Each workplace also has patterns of reward and condoned harassment (sexual, racial, ethnic, and age- or seniority-related) and has initiation rites that are discomforting to new workers, especially if they do not understand the nature and functions of such practices.

Occupational psychiatry is concerned with work-related stresses that precipitate various maladaptive reactions in vulnerable individuals. The concept of "stress" is widely discussed in lay and professional circles in both medical and psychologic terms, and the psychiatrist in the workplace will be confronted with the word in a variety of forms: "The stress caused my problem." "I was stressed." "I suffer from stress." "There is stress all over the place." "I could feel the stress in my stomach."

Individuals with work stress usually experience an unpleasant awareness of their internal or external environment when they are at work, anticipating going to work, or just thinking about work. An individual may experience work stress without awareness, however, and in this case its presence may be suspected by others who note changes in the individual's behavior or mental or physical status. The person working under strong competitive pressure may enjoy the activity and not perceive it as stressful but may nonetheless suffer physical harm because the body is under stress.

The occupational psychiatrist must consider the following in evaluating workers for stress: (1) Most people work because they must, and many would probably not work if they did not have to. (2) Many jobs require that workers perform their tasks in environments that may be dirty, noisy, hot or cold, dangerous, crowded or isolated, or under- or overventilated—all of which are stressful when the worker finds them unpleasant. (3) Many workers hate their jobs because of the physical risks imposed; because the work is boring or demeaning, tiring, or even painful; or because oppressive employers make unreasonable demands for high performance at low pay. Workers may also hate their jobs because they are overqualified for them; because they feel they have not done as much with their lives as they might have; or because they feel they can never please all of the people who undertake to judge their performance. Some are distracted or concerned by problems that have nothing to do with their jobs and may find their jobs stressful because their energy is being diverted to other uses.

TRAINING OF OCCUPATIONAL HEALTH CARE PROFESSIONALS

Occupational psychiatry trains medical and mental health professionals to practice in and consult with work organizations, assess prospective employees' mental and emotional fitness for specific kinds of jobs, and treat persons in the work force who have mental disorders. Because occupational psychiatrists use the same treatment techniques employed by other psychiatrists, including psychotropic drugs, individual psychotherapy, and work-group therapy (similar to family therapy), their general training does not differ greatly from that of other psychiatrists. The special training of the occupational psychiatrist includes learning about work cultures, work organizations, potentially harmful physical factors, and federal, state, and local laws relating to work, including regulations limiting the employer's options to reject an applicant or discharge an employee and regulations relating to disability.

Occupational psychiatrists share with other social and behavioral scientists the obligation to provide information to educators responsible for training students to become workers. Just as many people cannot adjust to military discipline, many who enter the work force find they are unprepared for work discipline.

PRINCIPLES OF MANAGING PROBLEMS IN THE WORKPLACE

The Psychiatrist-Patient Relationship

Treatment of mental disorders arising in the workplace is the same as elsewhere in psychiatry, with the exception that the psychiatrist-patient (or psychologist-patient) relationship may be different, a fact that should be made clear to the patient. Workers who come to health care professionals expect that their communications will be confidential and that the professional will take a history, conduct an examination, make a diagnosis, and initiate treatment. Frequently, however, the occupational mental health professional will have only one function: to diagnose the condition or evaluate the level of disability and report the findings to the employer. Workers who have not been informed of the nature of the interaction will complain when they learn that their statements were not held in confidence and that they will not be treated by the examiner. Therefore, the worker's oral or written "informed consent" should be obtained before evaluation is undertaken, and a notation should be made in the records.

Some workers believe that any health care professional employed or retained by the employer is a "company doctor" who will be concerned only with the employer's best interests, at the worker's expense if necessary. Psychiatrists can ease such apprehensions by explaining how their role differs from the usual doctor-patient relationship. In some cases, the need for specialized facilities or services (eg, substance abuse treatment programs) may justify referral to another mental health professional or residential treatment center in the community.

Most workers now have some type of private health insurance or government-subsidized workers' compensation or national health care. Work-related physical or mental disorders usually entitle the worker to full compensation for costs of care, including psychiatric hospitalization and treatment. The employer customarily receives reports on the worker's diagnosis, the present level of disability, an assessment of the causes of disability, a review of the treatment being given, and the progress being made.

Referral Pathways

Workers may present themselves to an occupational psychiatrist, sometimes with complaints of depression, anxiety, confusion, or other emotional problems caused by or interfering with work. They often have difficulty in recognizing or articulating psychologic problems and thus present with vague or somatic complaints. In other cases, family members may be concerned about what seem to be work-related psychologic problems and contact the psychiatrist directly.

A worker may be referred by a supervisor or employer because of absenteeism, forgetfulness or confusion, a perceived drop in productivity, proneness to accidents or suspected sabotage, or suspected or evident abuse of alcohol or drugs. Coworkers may report that the individual's behavior is "different," bizarre, or confused and characterized by unsafe practices or assaultive or threatening behavior that affects the safety and performance of other workers.

A worker who has been exposed to toxic chemicals may be referred to a company psychiatrist for a prophylactic checkup and assessment of possible psychologic symptoms or for follow-up for unusual behavior at work or at home.

Diagnosis & Testing

The diagnostic process in the workplace is the same as elsewhere (with physical examinations and special studies as described in other chapters), except that special consideration is given to the contribution of noxious factors at work. Attributing an illness or injury to work initiates a medicolegal process, and determining the cause of the disorder may be important later in the process. The psychiatrist should consider the specific types of physical and psychologic traumas experienced by the individuals in addition to all substances to which they have been exposed. Published data on the toxic effects of some of these substances, especially their effects on mental function, may be incomplete. Thus, it is important to consider epidemiologic factors such as the occurrence of similar symptoms or complaints in coworkers.

Psychologic testing is useful in confirming a suspected diagnosis of mental disorder or determining if the worker's test performance is similar to that of persons with brain damage. Judgments about the probable outcome of surgery in patients with certain pain syndromes (eg, low back pain) can be enhanced by psychologic tests, and such tests can be helpful in following a patient's progress and determining degrees of recovery.

Frequently, however, the meaning of test findings is obscured by the absence of baseline data, and results of prior testing should be obtained if they are available. These are important, for example, in determining whether the worker's IQ has been affected or whether mental impairment is of recent organic origin. Medical, educational, military, and personnel records may contain earlier test scores as well as histories of mental disorder or impairment and problems in performance. Descriptions of jobs completed successfully or special skills (eg, hobbies, sports) also provide baseline data on mental function.

Treatment

Guidelines for management of special problems in the workplace are discussed below, as are specific programs implemented by employers and state and federal agencies. Individual and group counseling procedures are discussed in other chapters.

Evaluation for Disability & Return to Work

There is sometimes a conflict between the employer's need for the worker's services and the worker's need for treatment. Although some jobs may be held for a particular worker almost indefinitely, others are not. Workers may urge the physician to release them for work before they have recovered sufficiently, and employers may demand medical clearance for return to work too soon. Workers may try to persuade a physician to authorize protracted certification of disability after recovery, and employers reluctant to permit a worker's return may do the same. The psychiatrist or psychologist should consider the worker's condition and the impact on his or her health status of return to work while keeping in mind the worker's wishes and needs and the likelihood of success or failure on returning to work.

A. Recognition of Deviant Disability Behavior:

1. Long-term claims of disability–Some workers continue to claim they are disabled long after objective findings have resolved. In such cases, the physician and psychiatrist should consider that the worker might be unmotivated to return to work because he or she is angry with the employer, has low morale, finds work physically or psychologically stressful, is concerned about further illness or injury,

or is focusing on the damage resulting from the injury or illness. The worker may have decided to change occupations or retire or may be benefiting from secondary gains such as attention, sedative drugs, hope for compensation, and role changes.

2. Disability disclaimers–Some workers do not complain of illness even when they have symptoms. This group includes 2 identifiable clinical subpopulations: (1) those who tend to deny illness generally and who attach benign labels to their bodily sensations and continue with their activities for as long as they can; and (2) those whose positions require that they project an image of strength, health, and invulnerability (eg, politicians and professional athletes) and who return to work long before they should, even though they know they might be hurting themselves. In such cases, physicians must recognize the psychologic and social forces that are operating, explore them with the worker, and give advice about the medical risks. Physicians should not release an employee to return to work prematurely and should keep the employer informed of the feasibility and timing of the employee's return to work.

B. Guidelines for Return to Work: After maximum recovery has occurred, the occupational psychiatrist must answer the following questions: Is the worker capable of doing the job? If not, is other work available in that workplace, and will the pay be comparable to what was earned before? Even if the old job is available, should the worker return to it? Will the worker be more susceptible to illness or injury than before? On balance, will it be better to return to a job that has some harmful component because being unemployed will be even more harmful? In cases of mental health disability, will coworkers harass or reject the mentally ill worker?

Workers recovering from myocardial infarction, for example, are concerned that the physical or mental stress of work might have caused or hastened the coronary occlusion and that further stresses might cause recurrence or death. They may be angry at their employers for having subjected them to these stresses and at themselves for having stayed on the job for so long. They may be fearful about returning to work but worried about how to support themselves and their families if they do not work.

The physician must inform patients about the risk factors for their particular conditions, especially as they relate to returning to work, retiring, or changing jobs. Although the physician may offer a clinical opinion, it is the patient who must decide which course of action to pursue.

Completing Occupational Psychiatry Reports

The types of information required in medical reports vary among disability programs. In writing a report, the physician and psychiatrist should generally consider what specific questions they are attempting to answer, what information the receiver of the report is entitled to have, and who else will have access to the report. Permissions for release of information should be obtained from the patient whenever necessary.

A report on the diagnosis or treatment (or both) of a mental disorder should include the worker's complaints and symptoms; findings on psychiatric examination (eg, the worker's mental status); treatment recommended or given; the projected duration of treatment; and the presence of disability, its estimated duration and relationship to work, and any future work limitations. The report should avoid offering speculations about conscious and unconscious forces that may have combined to produce the worker's present mental state.

MANAGEMENT OF SPECIAL PROBLEMS

Stress
(See also Chapter 5.)

The occupational psychiatrist can help employers identify and rectify some of the sources of counterproductive work stress that do not stem from the core operations of the business. Stress may be "necessary" if the business is going to "succeed"—sell its products, make profits, and meet its goals with the resources available. Stress is "unnecessary" and counterproductive when it can be traced to harassment or uncivility by other workers or supervisors or by oppressive employer practices of any kind.

Occupational psychiatrists, in much the same way as military chaplains, can affect work reactions by using their special status to help supervisors and workers modify maladaptive practices and by serving as negotiators and mediators for those who have interpersonal conflicts. They are often welcomed by both sides in a work dispute, because the company offers no reasonable alternative means of settling such disputes.

Physicians and other mental health professionals can help workers by encouraging them to examine all sources of stress in their lives. Reluctance to discuss work problems may be due to a perception of the complaining worker as a "whiner" who cannot handle adult responsibility. Work and concerns about work do cause physical and mental symptoms, and the mental health professional should examine those problems with the troubled worker rather than assume the existence of deep, underlying problems. Workers may have many sources of anxiety in their lives, and helping them resolve work problems will remove one important component of distress.

The following is an attempt to outline an overall approach to help a distressed worker survive and overcome his or her problems:

(1) Encourage the employee to present his or her problems for discussion. Recognize that the employee's views might differ from those of coworkers and superiors.

(2) Urge the employee to assess areas outside of work—family relationships, recreation and social life, general health and well-being, and lifestyle—and to consider their contribution to current distress at work. Attend to changes in the employee's life, such as divorce, death, or other losses that might serve as transition points from health to illness.

(3) Urge the employee to develop alternative ways of dealing with stress and to consider their advantages and disadvantages. If some obvious alternative is overlooked, ask about it. Offer no advice that might increase distress or might tend to impose a decision the employee is not ready to make (resign, take legal action, accept the situation, etc.)

(4) Determine whether the degree of distress is sufficient to warrant the use of sedating or tranquilizing medications or hospitalization.

(5) Arrange for follow-up. Continue to provide support by exploring further with the employee the sources of work stress and available stress-management techniques.

(6) Establish programs that assist new workers' transition into the workplace and that encourage present workers to accept new workers.

(7) Sensitize supervisors to the psychologic impact of their communications and to workers' needs for informal feedback as well as for regular, written performance evaluations.

Burnout

Job burnout is a state of exhausted motivation to continue daily efforts to sustain a high level of job performance. Some workers experience what may be called "instant burnout"—ie, they are disappointed with the job from the start, feeling that the work was not what they expected, so that they feel foolish or perhaps betrayed. Some workers never undergo the burnout experience and upon retirement are able to say honestly that they always had a sense of job satisfaction and no regrets about their career choice.

Job burnout may begin with a shift in the worker's goals, eg, the desire for a job with more status and responsibility or higher pay. Workers sometimes believe they cannot change jobs because of financial commitments or because it is too late to seek additional training. Burnout also occurs when a worker believes that the goals of the organization are not as lofty and worthwhile as once perceived. For example, police officers describe their disillusionment in terms of complaints about corruption, brutality, political control of the police force, or the courts' unwillingness to "back them up." Teachers often attribute burnout to the students' unwillingness to learn, the parents' indifference, the administration's unwillingness to discipline disruptive or assaultive students, the lack of special programs for educationally gifted or handicapped students, and the lack of community support for teachers' activities. Burnout occurs when the goals of the organization change, eg, if pride in the quality of services or products must be sacrificed in order to increase production and sales or make a deadline.

Burnout may be problem with workers who feel unappreciated because they are passed over for promotion or are denied an increase in pay or because their efforts are otherwise unrecognized. It can occur even when workers continue to enjoy their work but feel their salaries are not commensurate with what workers in other jobs are earning. Inflation can contribute to burnout by reducing the buying power of salaries that had been adequate before.

Job burnout is often a symptom of spontaneously occurring depression or of depression that is a reaction to problems in nonwork areas, such as family life. Dissatisfaction with marriage and children and their problems as teenagers can make work seem useless except as drudgery performed for a wage.

Job burnout is reversible. A raise in pay, a new assignment, and a conscious effort by someone in a higher position to congratulate a worker for a good performance may rekindle job enthusiasm. Most often the worker needs help in evaluating the causes of burnout. The approach of the occupational psychiatrist in helping patients with burnout is similar to that outlined above for management of stress.

Absenteeism

Frequent missed days of work because of colds, headaches, and other minor ailments always raise a question of malingering. Absences on Fridays or Mondays that might have been designed to extend a weekend trip—or, in the case of Monday absences, might be due to alcoholic overindulgence over the weekend—are regarded with suspicion by employers concerned with maintaining production schedules.

Illness is an excuse most people use on occasion to avoid or postpone unpleasant duties. The "sick role" is a social cushion that offers welcome temporary relief from responsibility. Workers often late for work may prefer to stay home and "call in sick" rather than invent ingenious excuses for being late. A worker who stays home to be with a sick child may prefer to explain the absence as due to personal illness. Disaffected employees may take unwarranted sick leave as an act of defiance or a way of punishing an employer for real or fancied wrongs.

Many organizations have rules requiring medical justification for frequent absences or absences longer than 1 or 2 days. These rules should be enforced uniformly so that no worker can argue that a request for medical justification was a discriminatory act.

Occupational health personnel should not raise the question of malingering in cases of absenteeism but should try to understand what is happening and help the worker find acceptable ways of dealing with the problems that may be the occasion for missed days. Medical treatment should not be offered to workers who claim they are ill when there are no corroborative symptoms or signs of illness, since treatment merely serves to reinforce the illness behavior.

Mass Psychogenic Illness

During occasional outbreaks of mass psychogenic illness or epidemic hysteria, a number of workers simultaneously manifest symptoms such as dizziness, weakness, or difficulty in breathing or may faint or have "fits." The affected workers frequently relate the onset of their symptoms to something in the work environment, such as a strange odor or exposure to some industrial chemical or toxic waste product. As rumors of the illness spread and new cases continue to be reported, worker anxiety and absenteeism may escalate even to the point of necessitating plant shutdown. These outbreaks affect mostly women in a mainly female work force but spare the female supervisors. The affected workers are often subject to both physical stress factors (accelerated work pace, poor lighting, noise) and psychologic ones (boredom, absence of social interaction), and peer and supervisory relationships might be important in setting the stage for such an outbreak.

Many outbreaks of psychogenic illness have occurred among hospital workers. Such epidemics are probably reactions to fears of infectious disease. (One of the earliest such epidemics, the "Royal Free Hospital Disease in 1955," was reported to be associated with a fear of poliomyelitis.) Some outbreaks seem to spread by "psychologic contagion" after one worker develops mysterious, undiagnosed physical symptoms.

Physicians confronted with an outbreak of similar symptoms among many workers should not make any assumptions or diagnoses based solely on the presence of many cases. They should not assume that the symptoms are the result of individual or group "hysteria," nor should they assume that the cause is toxic or infectious until they have examined each patient and made *individual* diagnoses.

If there is no evidence of a disorder due to known physical agents, one should consider whether psychogenic factors might be producing the symptoms. In all instances, treatment should be based on diagnoses.

In most instances, symptoms of mass psychogenic illness resolve shortly after onset. Physicians should remember that they can cause symptoms to become fixed if they tell patients that they might have a disease that could result in death or prolonged disability.

Although mass illness behavior conjures up visions of plague, legionnaires' disease, poisoning, etc, if physicians cannot find any physical disorder in the individual patients, they should not assume that an epidemic of physical disorder is present.

Patients involved in a mass illness phenomenon are frightened and believe they might be the victims of physical disease that is more dangerous because it has not been diagnosed. Physicians should not discuss the symptoms as being "psychologic" or "all in your head," but instead they should inform such patients that physical findings confirming disease are absent and indicate that they will continue to examine the patients for physical changes until the symptoms disappear or an identifiable physical disorder manifests itself.

Patients whose symptoms resolve might need some follow-up care in order to help them understand their experience. Those whose symptoms persist in the absence of a physical disorder should be studied in order to determine what psychologic factors, conscious or unconscious, may be delaying their recovery.

Mental Disorders & Substance Use Disorders

Many psychotic individuals and others with mental illness work regularly, with little absenteeism. Examples are patients who are schizophrenic, paranoid, or profoundly depressed; those who abuse alcohol or drugs; and those who have organic mental disorders.

Physicians and other mental health professionals face difficult dilemmas when asked if a person identified as mentally ill or as a recovering substance abuser should be hired, permitted to remain on the job, permitted to return to work, or required to choose between coming back or losing disability benefits. In general, the response of the health care professional will be based on assessment of the following: risks to the safety and welfare of the mentally ill worker, the employee's coworkers, and the public (eg, if the worker drives a bus or truck or is a public safety officer); risks of damage to equipment or to operations of the workplace (eg, workers in electric power plants); the worker's need for further treatment if the work schedule interferes with it; and the worker's ability to work safely if maintained on psychotropic drugs.

A. Hiring: See Preemployment Screening, below.

B. Remaining on the Job: Workers with mental disorders or substance use disorders can usually remain on the job if the following conditions are met: (1) They are productive; ie, there is no evidence that their problem impairs job performance. (2) They are supported by coworkers and superiors who are willing to assist them through crises. (3) Their symptoms do not offend or frighten others. (4) They are not hospitalized because of behavior outside of work and removed from the workplace by relatives or civil authorities. (5) Their jobs do not involve responsibility for the welfare and safety of others.

C. Returning to the Job: In addition to the considerations outlined above and on p 669, health care professionals must consider what their own liability might be if they recommend return to work and the worker is then injured on the job or causes injury to another worker and the episode is attributed to bad judgment in recommending reinstatement. The professional faces a similar dilemma in evaluating a person who is not psychotic but is maintained on medications known to reduce mental acuity, concentration, alertness, etc.

Industrial Accidents

An increased interest in the phenomena associated with industrial accidents has contributed to the development of occupational psychiatry and psychology as special fields of interest. In the late 19th century, physicians noted that some workers with a compensable work-related injury recovered more slowly (and sometimes not at all) than persons with comparable injuries sustained in non-work-related activities. Furthermore, these workers presented their symptoms more dramatically than the nonworkers. Physicians devised diagnostic labels for specific injuries with symptoms not justified by physical findings on examination (eg, "railway spine" for those who claimed injury from an accident on a train).

As workers' compensation laws were passed in more countries and in some states of the USA (first in New York in 1910), the physical and psychologic reactions accompanying such injuries engaged the attention of psychiatrists dealing with these workers. The psychiatric syndromes displayed were frequently dramatic, similar to those studied by Charcot and Freud, and seemed reversible only by resolution of pending litigation or other source of secondary gain. In other cases, there seemed to be no way to modify the symptoms, and it was suggested that the illness behavior was supported by other gains or was congenial to the individual's personality structure.

In the early days of what might be called the workers' compensation movement in law and industry, the injured worker presented chiefly with physical symptoms; psychiatric disability was rarely claimed or even acknowledged to exist as a work-related hazard. More recently, the workers' compensation programs (see below) have compensated workers claiming psychiatric disability unrelated to physical injury, and the number of such claims has increased. This has raised concerns about the compensation system, because the physician called upon to evaluate such claims must rely on symptoms not verifiable by objective tests.

The most common work-related psychiatric syndromes are the posttraumatic stress disorders (posttraumatic neuroses), variants of depressive disorders, and a number of somatoform disorders, including conversion disorders, factitious disorders, and malingering.

A. Prevention: Theoretically, all industrial accidents are preventable. Safety engineers and industrial hygienists look for hazards in the workplace in order to reduce illness and injury. The major hazards include equipment failure due to metal fatigue or improper installation; inadequate safety devices on equipment (guards, etc); wet and slippery surfaces on floors, stairs, and ladders; and failure of workers or others to follow safety rules as a result of carelessness or distraction (eg, forgetting to make sure no one is near a machine before a switch is thrown), ignorance about safety measures, or refusal to follow established safety measures. The dangers inherent in any workplace are enhanced by the negligence of managers and workers. Peer pressure should be brought to bear on substance-abusing employees who endanger their coworkers through diminished alertness or impulsive risk-taking.

The occupational psychiatrist can make the workplace safer by investigating the causes of accidents that do occur and explaining to managers and workers the psychologic factors that may have contributed to an accident; by identifying workers who have attentional deficits and therefore increase the risk of injury to themselves and others; and by working with management, labor, plant safety engineers, and agencies concerned with safety (eg, the Occupational Safety and Health Administration [OSHA] and insurance companies) to create a safe work environment. This includes permitting workers to report health and safety hazards without fear of reprisals from coworkers or supervisors.

B. Treatment: Treatment will be specific to the injury, but the manner in which treatment is offered and delivered will affect the time of recovery. Employers' reactions to the injured workers are among the data by which workers judge whether employers care about them and if the loyalty employers demand is reciprocated. The following suggestions for the psychologic support and management of injured workers are based on complaints about treatment from workers who have experienced unduly prolonged periods of convalescence from physical or psychologic work injuries:

1. Accept the worker's statement that an injury has occurred.

2. Do not try to minimize the seriousness of the injury; wait until examination has determined its severity.

3. If possible, have someone accompany the worker to the medical facility.

4. Stay with the worker until a relative arrives or until the worker is released and can be returned to the job or taken home.

5. Call or visit the worker. Do not ask about returning to work unless the worker or the physician indicates that a sufficient degree of recovery has occurred. Set up a regular inquiry schedule.

6. Make a point of asking returning workers if they can do their jobs. If the answer is no or if the worker is unsure, try to assign light duties until recovery is complete.

Some workers cannot or will not return to their former jobs. They may be suffering from posttraumatic stress disorder or may feel the job is too dangerous. Because they are reluctant to admit they are frightened or unwilling to risk another injury, workers sometimes continue to complain of symptoms and receive unnecessary treatment, often resulting in iatrogenic illness.

SPECIAL ROLES OF OCCUPATIONAL PSYCHIATRISTS

Preemployment Screening

Interviews and psychologic tests may be used to identify persons with mental disorders (eg, psychoses) or severe personality disorders who may be unsuited for a particular job. Not hiring these individuals is sometimes in the best interest of the applicant as well as the employer and other workers. The examiner's judgment is only advisory, and federal and state laws or union contracts may prohibit rejecting an applicant on grounds of psychologic incapacity.

Sensitive military and civilian jobs such as in defense, space, or nuclear programs or industries sup-

plying equipment for these programs impose special requirements for psychologic stability, and occupational psychiatrists may be asked to assist in the selection process for these positions by interviewing candidates, reviewing the results of psychologic testing, and assessing health, school, or work performance records.

Assistance During Transition Periods

Changes in the workplace are unavoidable in changing times, and the occupational psychiatrist should know the workers and the workplace well enough to predict the impact of changes in schedules, work requirements, places of work, and supervisors as well as the impact of layoffs, plant relocation, corporate mergers, or technologic advances such as automation. The psychiatrist can assist management by serving as an "adaptation engineer" to help workers deal with adjustment disorders.

Special problems are involved in integrating the workplace—introducing women, men, homosexuals, or members of ethnic groups who have not worked in that setting before—and both the old and the new workers must be helped to adapt to changes.

Workplace Education & Research

Formal seminars and informal sessions with managers, executives, and workers may increase their understanding about stress, coping processes, feelings of loss that accompany change, and even the psychodynamics of mental illnesses. Sessions may also teach techniques for effective interpersonal communication. Questions asked during seminars or discussions may be phrased in general terms, but they usually reflect conscious or unconscious problems of the questioner and should be dealt with accordingly.

The research role of the occupational psychiatrist includes gathering epidemiologic data on the distribution of mental disorders in the workplace and identifying problems in the job environment that adversely affect adjustment at home or at work.

Health Promotion Programs

Growing anxiety about the financial consequences of rising health care and disability costs has prompted employers to expand their cost-containment programs and supplement long-standing employee assistance programs with "wellness" or health promotion programs. The shift toward the view that health promotion is the concern of the employer and in the best interests both of the employees and of the company is taking place in larger companies, which have substantial commitments to employee health benefits. Workers themselves are becoming more health conscious, showing more concerns about the effects of smoking, toxic substances, stress, and nutrition.

The primary emphasis of health promotion programs is on health—reinforcing the intent and will of basically healthy workers to remain so and facilitating self-correction by people developing health problems.

Health promotion programs deal with a wide range of health issues, such as cardiovascular fitness, weight loss and nutrition, smoking cessation, hypertension control, stress management, and general life-style reappraisal and overhaul. Employers evaluate the cost-effectiveness of the programs in terms of participation rates, adherence rates, and success rates. The primary focus of employee assistance programs is on illness and on remedial services aimed at restoring the health and productivity of workers with well-advanced problems (eg, substance abuse and evident mental disorders).

Data regarding cost-benefit ratios for both programs generally suggest that recovered costs exceed program costs in terms of reduced absenteeism, turnover, and medical costs and reduced workers' compensation and long-term disability disbursements. Less measurable benefits include favorable employee response to perceived good will (reflected in higher morale, job satisfaction, and productivity), enhanced image and reputation of the company, and advantages in personnel recruitment. Some industrial insurance companies reward organizations that use employee assistance or health promotion programs by reducing their health coverage premiums.

Cost benefits have been obvious in smoking cessation and hypertension control. Fitness and exercise programs also show cost benefits. Inasmuch as most health promotion programs are aimed broadly at control of "risk factors," absenteeism and turnover rates may be favorably influenced by such intangibles as the fellowship that comes with shared activities and learning about health and discussing it as well as by absolute control of risk factors.

While in practice health promotion programs are generally not planned and carried out in coordination with employee assistance programs, both are often found in large organizations, and there is a positive relationship between the proportion of the work force using employee assistance programs and the proportion participating in health promotion programs. Occupational psychiatrists can facilitate a comprehensive approach to the mental and physical health of workers by emphasizing the needs of certain target groups and encouraging employers to adopt appropriate programs. The psychiatrist can also emphasize that the success of such programs will depend on how well they can accommodate the needs of the workers, the structure and requirements of the workplace, and the program characteristics, all of which must fit creatively into the "culture" of the work organization.

Entitlement Programs

Many disabled workers are unaware of the benefits to which they are entitled and do not obtain the financial aid or rehabilitation and treatment available to them. The benefits vary according to the type of entitlement program and the type of disability and its cause (eg, related to work or military service or not related to work).

Occupational psychiatrists and psychologists are involved in the following major benefit programs:

A. Workers' Compensation Programs: Although state workers' compensation statutes may vary to some extent in different parts of the country, an effort is being made to make them uniform. In some states, benefits are granted or denied on the recommendation of the treating physician alone, while other states provide for a more complex system of determining that an injury occurred, that its disabling effects persist, or that continuing medical care is required. Workers' compensation laws are "no fault," which means that negligence of the employee or of the employer is not a factor in determining whether the worker will be compensated for work-related injury or illness.

The key provisions of these laws are as follows: (1) The worker is compensated for injury that occurs in the course of or arises out of employment. The worker's named beneficiary receives death benefits if the worker is killed. (2) Medical care is provided for the consequences of the injury even if the injury was only an aggravating factor that exacerbated an existing condition. (3) If the worker is unable to return to the job, the employer and its insurers must bear the costs of retraining for other employment, including self-employment. (4) Permanent disability payments are provided when further recovery seems unlikely to occur.

Physicians who attend injured workers must file complete reports (on official forms) of every occupational injury or illness within 5 days after the first visit. Subsequent reports to the agency must include descriptions of the treatment given and its results and the physician's best estimate of the duration of the disability.

If mental health professionals are concerned that such reports would jeopardize the treatment relationship, the patient can be referred to an independent examiner for determination of degree of disability and the need for continuing treatment.

B. Social Security Disability Programs: The federal Social Security Administration manages the Social Security Disability Insurance (SSDI) and the Supplemental Security Income (SSI) programs, which are financed by tax revenues and are designed to provide monthly benefits to eligible disabled persons.

Both programs define disability as an "inability to engage in any substantial gainful activity by reason of a medically determinable physical or mental impairment which can be expected to result in death or has lasted or can be expected to last for a continuous period of not less than 12 months."

SSDI provides benefits for disabled workers who have contributed to the Social Security trust fund through a specific tax on their income and who therefore have an "earned right" to disability insurance benefits. To qualify, a worker must have earned a certain number of work credits within a specified period that varies according to the worker's age, and there is a waiting period before benefits can be collected.

SSI provides a minimum income level for the needy aged, blind, and disabled, and the client qualifies because of financial need rather than because of an "earned right."

Physicians provide medical evidence that allows a claims examiner to evaluate an individual's level of impairment and the impact of the impairment on ability to work, but the decision whether the impairment constitutes a disability is legally an administrative and not a medical one.

Rehabilitation Programs

A number of rehabilitation resources for disabled workers are available in most communities. If the disability resulted from a work-related illness or injury, the employer is liable for costs of rehabilitating the worker for other employment or for self-employment. If disability is not work-related, state and private rehabilitation agencies are available. Occupational mental health professionals often participate actively in rehabilitation efforts.

Factors that adversely influence the success of rehabilitation programs include the following: (1) older age and lower educational achievement; (2) unwillingness to contemplate subsistence at a lower living standard because of reduced income; (3) unwillingness to relocate to an area where jobs are available for which the worker can be retrained; (4) unrealistic expectations of entering new fields (law, television writing) requiring skills the worker does not have and cannot be taught; (5) preference for the simplicity and ease of the unemployed life-style; (6) altered self-image as a "disabled" or weak person, lacking in strength or stamina; and (7) fear of failure upon returning to work, in some cases amounting to phobic dread of even leaving the house.

Retirement Programs & Planning

Ideally, retirement planning should begin when the individual takes his or her first "regular" job. Many people choose employers because of retirement provisions, and some workers leave higher-paying jobs in order to work for the government or organizations offering greater job security and better retirement benefits. Others strive for the highest take-home pay and rely on personal investments, Social Security benefits, and union pension plans for support after retirement. Frequently, they are disheartened when they learn how meager their retirement incomes will be. Many studies have suggested that an adequate income is the single most important factor in a successful retirement.

Given the wide range of retirement situations—from the formal retirement of the 30-year military person who will have full medical and commissary privileges as well as a pension approximating his or her highest level of working income, to the seasonal or migrant worker whose work life ends without an "official" retirement—one can provide only general principles for assisting the potential retiree and the troubled retired person.

Education about retirement should begin in high school. Such discussion will not only inform potential workers about their own futures but will acquaint them with the living situations of the vast numbers of older retired workers. This educational process should continue during the time of employment.

Managers responsible for administering retirement benefits should provide each worker with a projection of retirement benefits, including medical benefits. Although benefits will change over the years, workers can more accurately estimate their future income and manage their finances more intelligently if they know their potential retirement status.

Before workers retire, occupational psychiatrists can assist in establishing fitness programs to improve or maintain the workers' physical and mental well-being during the retirement years. Individual programs should change as workers grow older, and the occupational psychiatrist can help workers make the transition to fitness activities that are age-appropriate and are likely to be carried on after retirement. Older employees who come to believe they should give up the exertions of youth (an attitude of surrender to aging and death) should be offered support and instruction to facilitate healthy changes in attitude and behavior.

Planning for retirement means being aware of the nature of the changes involved. Many workers are unsophisticated about the interpersonal difficulties they may experience after retirement. There will be an additional 8 or more hours to be filled every day, usually at home with the spouse. Widowed or unmarried retired workers may be lonely and start drinking. If the spouse is still working, there may be tensions related to that, with the working spouse urging the retired one to get another job or take on more of the housekeeping responsibilities. If the spouse is not working, a new pattern of interaction must be established to permit each partner some solitude and privacy. Marriages have broken up after retirement because the partners are unable to adapt to so much unfamiliar "togetherness."

Workers should be warned against making radical changes in life-style, eg, selling the house and buying a recreational vehicle the size of a studio apartment. Some people imagine that after retirement they will travel from place to place, always in good weather, making new friends. The possibilities for disappointment of such expectations are as abundant as they are obvious, and workers preparing for retirement should be urged to test during short vacations their assumptions about anticipated changes in their life-style.

There is almost as much defensive denial about retirement as there is about dying. Professionals and workers discuss retirement as an abstraction, but few "clinical" retirement activity services are offered except by the insurance companies interested in selling their plans. Both providers and prospective recipients of retirement benefits may prefer to discuss these benefits in vague terms rather than describe the specific benefits, calculate their individual applications, and explore options that can increase these benefits. The reluctance to discuss matters related to retirement stems in part from a tendency to postpone thinking about them when one is just beginning a job. Some employers have stated in the media that they would not hire younger workers who seemed concerned about retirement benefits; knowing this, many workers are uneasy about inquiring about these benefits early in their careers.

Workers coming to the ends of their careers often become reflective during counseling. Many have a tendency to use counseling as a "debriefing" session in which to ponder opportunities they may have missed, the reasons for their choices, and their satisfactions or regrets. Mental health professionals should not undertake this kind of "debriefing" unless they are prepared to follow through until the retiring worker has reached some resolution of these feelings. Retirement is a time of relief and rejoicing for some and of self-recrimination, anger, and depression for others.

The approach of retirement may confront a worker with the prospect of loss of independence and productivity, especially if personal career aspirations were unfulfilled, and the psychiatrist can be helpful during this transition time.

Forensic Consultations

Psychiatrists and psychologists are often asked to give expert testimony at hearings or trials involving work-related issues. Guidelines for preparing to testify can be listed as follows:

A. Preparing:
1. Review all of the pertinent records and reports.
2. Form conclusions that are as definite as possible and be able to explain their basis.
3. Make diagnoses according to criteria in *DSM-III-R* whenever possible.
4. Become familiar with the law pertaining to the legal controversy.

B. Testifying:
1. Be sure the question is understood before answering.
2. Respond as simply as possible.
3. Do not permit others to restate responses in ways that alter meaning.
4. Keep in mind that words—not tone and volume—are recorded by court reporters; therefore, words must be chosen for emphasis or to convey conviction.
5. Avoid technical language except when using the terms of *DSM-III-R*, which can be referred to by others.
6. Do not entertain theories about the case that have not been thoroughly developed or thought through prior to testifying.
7. Avoid advocacy.

SUMMARY

The roles of occupational psychiatrists will vary with the industries in which they work, the size of the facilities, and the relationship between management and labor in the facilities. The scope of their activities will vary with the trust they engender among members of both groups. Their roles will continue to evolve, and they themselves can structure those roles. Like liaison psychiatrists, occupational psychiatrists can interest other health professionals in preventing mental illness and in attending to preventive health principles in their evaluations and treatments of injured workers and those with occupational illnesses. Through their behavior, they can affect the environment of the workplace, making it a more benign and gratifying place for all who work there.

REFERENCES

Barth PS, Hunt HA: *Workers' Compensation and Work-Related Illnesses and Diseases*. MIT Press, 1980.

Brodsky CM: Genesis of a problem population. Pages 119–123 in: *Communication and Social Interaction*. Ostwald PF (editor). Grune & Stratton, 1977.

Brodsky CM: *The Harassed Worker*. Lexington Books, 1976.

Brodsky CM: Work stress in correctional institutions. *J Prison Jail Health* 1982;**2**:74.

Cataldo MF, Coates TJ (editors): *Health and Industry: A Behavioral Medicine Perspective*. Wiley, 1986.

Colligan MJ, Murphy LR: A review of mass psychogenic illness in work settings. Pages 33–55 in: *Mass Psychogenic Illness: A Social Psychological Analysis*. Colligan MJ, Pennebaker JW, Murphy LR (editors). Lawrence Erlbaum Associates, 1982.

Cooper CL, Payne R (editors): *Current Concerns in Occupational Stress*. Wiley, 1980.

Eisenstat RA, Felner RD: Toward a differentiated view of burnout: Personal and organizational mediators of job satisfaction and stress. *Am J Community Psychol* 1984;**12**:411.

Lezak M: *Neuropsychologic Assessment*, 2nd ed. Oxford Univ Press, 1983.

Manuso JSJ (editor): *Occupational Clinical Psychology*. Praeger, 1983.

Pollock W, Stack RH: *1982 Survey of National Corporations on Health Care Cost Containment*. National Association of Employers on Health Care Alternatives, 1983.

Preventing Illness and Injury in the Workplace. Office of Technology Assessment, Washington, DC, 1985.

Parkinson RS et al: *Managing Health Promotion in the Workplace: Guidelines for Implementation and Evaluation*. Mayfield, 1982.

Rom WM (editor): *Environmental and Occupational Medicine*. Little, Brown, 1983.

Shain M, Suurvali H, Boutilier M: *Healthier Workers: Health Promotion and Employee Assistance Programs*. Lexington Books, 1986.

Glossary of Psychiatric Signs & Symptoms

The diagnostic process in psychiatry begins with a careful history, physical examination, and mental status examination. Observations take the form of signs and symptoms. This section is a glossary of terms used to define and describe these signs and symptoms.

Affect: Emotions or feelings as they are expressed by the patient and observable by others. Affect is an objective sign observable on mental status examination—in contrast to mood (see below), which is a subjective experience reported by the patient. Affect is characterized in several ways: (1) By the type of emotion expressed and observed: anger, sadness, elation, etc. (2) By the intensity and the range of emotion expressed: flat, blunted, constricted, or broad. In **flat** affect, there is no expression of feeling; the face is immobile and the voice monotonous. In **blunted** affect, the expression of feeling is severely reduced. In **constricted** affect, the expression of feelings is clearly reduced, but to a lesser degree than in the case of blunted affect. **Broad** affect describes the normal condition in which a full range of feelings is expressed. (3) By its appropriateness: **Inappropriate** affect is apparent emotion discordant with accompanying thought or speech (eg, laughing while telling a story most people would find horrifying). (4) By consistency of emotion: **Labile** affect shifts rapidly between different emotional states such as crying, laughing, and anger.

Ambivalence: The condition of having 2 strong but opposite feelings or ideas. The individual cannot decide to respond one way or the other, with the result that there is difficulty in taking any action. A feature of obsessive compulsive disorder and schizophrenia.

Anhedonia: Loss of interest in pleasure-seeking activities. A feature of depressive disorder.

Anorexia: Loss of or diminished appetite. A feature of depressive disorder.

Anxiety: A dysphoric (unpleasant) state similar to fear when there is no apparent source of danger. A feeling of apprehension, anticipation, or dread of possible danger. Anxiety is sometimes defined by the physiologic state of autonomic arousal, alertness, vigilance, and motor tension. Free-floating anxiety is anxiety in the absence of an identifiable object of dread. Phobia (see below) is severe anxiety aroused by a specific object or circumstance even though the subject knows the feeling "doesn't make sense."

Autistic thinking: Thought derived from fantasy. External reality is accorded subjective and fantasied meanings. Preoccupation with the private world may lead the autistic individual to withdraw from external reality.

Automatic obedience: Obedience to commands without exercising critical judgment. A feature of catatonia.

Blocking: Disruption of thought evidenced by an interruption or momentary disruption of speech. It appears that the individual tries to remember what he or she was thinking or saying.

Catalepsy: A condition in which the subject "freezes" in almost any abnormal posture in which he or she is placed (left arm extended, etc). A feature of catatonia.

Catatonia: A syndrome characterized by cataleptic posturing, stereotypy, mutism, stupor, negativism, automatic obedience, echolalia, and echopraxia. There are 2 subtypes: excited and retarded. Catatonia was formerly thought to be a subtype of schizophrenia. It is now thought to be a feature of affective disorders (chiefly mania), schizophrenia, organic mental disorder, and other psychoses.

Cerea flexibilitas ("waxy flexibility"): A specific type of catalepsy in which the examiner encounters resistance ("like bending a soft wax rod") upon attempting to move parts of the subject's body. A feature of catatonia.

Circumstantiality: A disturbance of communication in which the train of associations is interrupted by frequent digressions before the central idea is finally presented. The digressions are irrelevant or marginally relevant to what is being said. Seen in a wide variety of pathologic states, or may be a normal if annoying language habit.

Clang associations: The rhyming or punning associations of one word with another with no logical connection. *Example:* "My head is rock candy. Dandy. Randy. Sandy. Piece of the rock. Mutual of Omaha." Seen in manic episodes, schizophrenia, and other psychotic states.

Clouding of consciousness: In *DSM-III*, impaired awareness of the environment. Defined elsewhere as the least severe impairment of consciousness on the continuum from full alertness to coma.

Compulsion: The need to repeat some action in a ritualistic, stereotyped manner, uncontrollable by an act of will. The act frequently has symbolic meaning. The subject knows there is no true connection between the motor behavior and the fantasied wish or fear. The compulsive act may seem unpleasant, tedious, or distressful, but resistance is associated with mounting anxiety that can be relieved only by performing the act. Seen in obsessive compulsive disorder and schizophrenia.

Concrete thinking: Thinking characterized by diminished capacity to form abstractions. The subject is unable to think metaphorically or hypothetically. Thought is limited to one dimension of meaning. Words and figures of speech are taken literally, and the nuances of implied meaning are not used or not appreciated. Common in organic mental disorder and schizophrenia.

Confabulation: The fabrication of events or data that either fill in gaps in a story or constitute entire fictions in response to questions that cannot be factually answered because of organic memory impairment. A feature of amnestic syndrome.

Confusion: A disturbance of consciousness with loss of orientation to person, place, or time. (See Disorientation.) Confusion may be due to impaired memory loss (as in dementia) or to deficit in attention (as in delirium).

Delirium: A disturbance of consciousness resulting from organic brain disease (usually acute) and characterized by clouding of consciousness, restlessness, confusion, psychomotor retardation or agitation, and affective lability. It has a rapid onset and a fluctuating, waxing and waning course, and there is an associated disturbance of sleep.

Delusion: (See also Hallucination, Ideas of reference, and Paranoia.) A false belief or idea firmly held despite abundant contradictory evidence. A defect of reality testing. (A belief is not delusional if it is shared by other members of a culture or large group.) A delusion is always evidence of psychosis. *Examples:* (1) Delusions of **being controlled,** ie, that thoughts, feelings, or behaviors are controlled by external forces. (2) Delusions of **grandeur,** ie, that one is influential and important, perhaps having occult powers, or that one actually is some powerful figure out of history ("Napoleonic complex"). (3) Delusions of **persecution,** ie, that one is being followed, harassed, threatened, or plotted against. (4) Delusions of **reference,** ie, that external events or "portents" have personal significance, such as special messages or commands. A person with delusions of reference believes that strangers on the street are talking about him or her, the television commentator is sending coded messages, etc.

Dementia: Deterioration (due to organic brain syndrome) from a previous level of intellectual functioning involving personality change and resulting in impairment of memory, abstract thinking, judgment, and impulse control. Clouding of consciousness does not occur. Dementia may be chronic (with insidious onset) or acute and reversible or irreversible.

Depersonalization: The experience of feeling strange, unreal, and detached from the environment or from oneself, ie, of being outside one's body, or that parts of the body are very large or very small or not under one's control, etc. Seen in a wide variety of disorders, including depression, anxiety, schizophrenia, epilepsy, and hypnagogic states. It may be a normal finding in adolescents. (See Derealization.)

Derailment: "Getting off the track" with respect to speech, volition, or thought. Moving in random fashion from one topic, thought, or behavior to another.

Derealization: The experience of feeling that the immediate environment is unreal or changed. (Depersonalization and derealization occur together and are probably aspects of the same phenomenon.)

Dereistic thinking: Failure to take the facts of reality into account, so that thoughts derive mainly from fantasy rather than experience and logical inference.

Disorientation: (1) Not oriented to **time,** ie, not knowing what day, month, season, or year it is; (2) not oriented to **place,** ie, not knowing the name of the building one is in or the kind of building, or the city, state, or country where one is presently located; or (3) not oriented to **person,** ie, not knowing who one is. Disorientation is one of the diagnostic criteria for delirium and is seen in delirium and organic memory disturbances.

Echolalia: Repetition of another person's speech. (See next item.)

Echopraxia: Imitation of another person's movements. (Echolalia and echopraxia are seen in pervasive developmental disorders, organic mental disorders, catatonia, and other psychotic disorders.)

Flight of ideas: A series of thoughts verbalized rapidly with abrupt shifts of subject matter with no apparent logical reason. Flight of ideas is associated with pressure of speech (see below). It is often difficult to differentiate flight of ideas from loosening of associations (see below). Classically, the connections between associations in flight of ideas are thought to be more coherent than in loosening of associations. However, in its severe form, flight of ideas can result in complete disorganization and incoherence. Seen in mania as well as in organic mental disorders, schizophrenia, and other psychotic and nonpsychotic states.

Folie à deux ("madness for two"): A disorder characterized by the sharing of delusional (usually persecutory) ideas by 2 or more (folie à plusieurs) individuals living in close association usually in a family relationship. One member of the pair (or group) seems always to influence and dominate the others. The delusional ideas may lead to strange types of behavior such as preparing for the end of the world.

Formication: See Hallucination, tactile, below.

Fugue: Sudden, unexpected "flights" or wandering away from home or workplace and assumption of a new identity. There is amnesia for the previous identity and no memory of the fugue when it is over.

Hallucination: A false sensory perception of what is not there. An illusion (see below) differs in being a perceptual distortion of something that is there. A delusion (see above) differs in being a disorder of thought. A delusion is always a sign of psychosis, since it represents a defect in reality testing. A hallucination is not always a sign of psychosis; eg, one who "sees" pink elephants but knows they are not really there is not psychotic. One who "feels" bugs crawling on his or her skin and believes the bugs are really there is not only hallucinating but is also psychotic. *Examples:* (1) **Auditory** hallucinations—false perceptions of sounds (voices, music, buzzing, motor noises, murmuring). (2) **Gustatory** hallucinations—false perceptions of taste. (3) **Olfactory** hallucinations—false perceptions of smell. (4) **Somatic** hallucinations—false sensations of something happening in or to the body such as the sensation of knives piercing the body or a feeling of electricity in the arms. (Usually associated with a delusion consistent with the feeling.) (5) **Tactile** hallucinations—false sensations of touch. (Usually associated with a delusion consistent with the sensation.) **Formication** (from L *formica*, "ant"), a particular type of tactile hallucination, is the sensation of bugs crawling on or under the skin. (6) **Visual** hallucinations—false visual perceptions with eyes open in a lighted environment. (Visual images with the eyes closed are not true hallucinations. **Hypnagogic** and **hypnopompic** hallucinations—images experienced during the "twilight" stages while falling asleep and waking up, respectively—are not true hallucinations.)

All of the above hallucinations can occur in schizophrenia, affective disorders, and organic mental disorders. Auditory and somatic hallucinations are common in functional disorders. Visual hallucinations are suggestive of organic mental disorders but are seen in functional disorders. Gustatory, olfactory, and tactile hallucinations strongly suggest organic mental disorders. Tactile hallucinations are common in drug and alcohol withdrawal and intoxication states.

Ideas of reference: Similar to delusions of reference (see above) but held with less conviction.

Illusion: (See also Hallucination.) A distorted perception of a material object.

Incoherence: Speech that is incomprehensible because of severe loosening of associations, distortions of grammer or syntax, or the use of idiosyncratic word definitions.

Insomnia: Difficulty sleeping—either **initial insomnia,** difficulty in falling asleep; **middle insomnia,** waking up in the middle of the night and going back to sleep with difficulty; or **terminal insomnia,** awakening early without being able to go back to sleep.

Loosening of associations: (See also Flight of ideas and Tangentiality.) A disorder of thinking and speech in which ideas shift from one subject to another with remote or no apparent reasons. The speaker is unaware of the incongruity. A classic sign of schizophrenia but may be seen also in any psychotic state.

Mood: The subjective experience of feeling or emotion as described by the patient in the history. Mood is a pervasive and sustained emotion. Distinct from affect (see above), which is a feeling state noted by the examiner during the mental status examination. Mood is characterized by the type of emotion the patient describes, eg, sadness, feeling blue, happiness, elation, anger, and anxiety. Mood is **dysphoric** if the experience is unpleasant, eg, characterized by irritability, anger, or depression. Mood can be elevated, expansive, or **euphoric,** eg, characterized by increasing feelings of well-being, energy, and positive self-regard.

Mood-congruent: A term applied to hallucinations or delusions whose content is consistent with the predominant mood. Mood-congruent hallucinations or delusions in mania, for example, typically involve grandiosity, inflated self-esteem, confidence of one's personal powers, and identifications with famous persons or deities. Mood-congruent hallucinations or delusions in depression involve themes of worthlessness, guilt, defectiveness, disease, death, nihilism, and deserved punishment.

Mood-incongruent: A term applied to hallucinations or delusions whose content has no apparent relationship to the predominant mood. Examples are persecutory delusions, delusions of reference, delu-

sions of control, thought insertion, thought withdrawal, and thought broadcasting, in which the content has no apparent relation to the mood-congruent themes mentioned above. Mood-incongruent hallucinations and delusions are seen in schizophrenia and sometimes in mania and depression.

Mutism: Not speaking. A feature of catatonia.

Negativism: Extreme opposition, resistance to suggestion. A feature of catatonia.

Neologisms: Invented "new words," with new meanings, often formed by combining elements of other words. A feature of schizophrenia and other psychotic disorders.

Obsession: Recurring ideas, images, or wishes that dominate thought. The content may be unacceptable and actively resisted but intrudes into consciousness agian and again. A feature of obsessive compulsive disorder and some cases of schizophrenia.

Panic attacks: Anxiety attacks, characterized by palpitations, a sense of imminent doom, fear of losing control, tightness in the chest, hyperventilation, light-headedness, nausea, and peripheral paresthesias. There are no cardiopulmonary, endocrine, or other physical disorders that might account for the symptoms. Seen in a wide variety of psychotic and nonpsychotic disorders as well as in normal people subjected to sufficient stress.

Paranoia: A psychotic disorder characterized by delusions of grandeur and persecution, suspiciousness, hypersensitivity, hyperalertness, jealousy, guardedness, resentment, humorlessness, litigiousness, and sullenness. *DSM-III* classifies the paranoid disorders as paranoia, shared paranoid disorder (folie à deux; see above), acute paranoid disorder, and atypical paranoid disorder. Paranoid schizophrenia is listed separately as a subtype of schizophrenia. (1) **Paranoid ideation** is a consistent finding in paranoid patients, who are convinced that people are thinking "bad thoughts" about them, that they are being followed, that they are the object of evil conspiracies, etc. It includes ideas of reference, ideas of persecution, grandiose ideas, and ideas of jealousy. Paranoid ideation differs from paranoid delusions in that the ideas are held with less conviction than delusions. (2) **Paranoid style** is a character style featuring hypervigilance, litigiousness, rigidity, humorlessness, jealousy, sullenness, suspiciousness, and hyperattention to evidence in the environment that corroborates paranoid suspicions.

Perseveration: Repetitive behavior or repetitive expression of a particular word, phrase, or concept during the course of speech. Perseveration is seen in organic mental disorders, schizophrenia, and other psychotic disorders.

Phobia: (See also Anxiety.) An admittedly irrational fear of a particular object or situation, so that the person's life is dominated by avoidance behavior.

Posturing: The assumption of various abnormal bodily positions, often a feature of catatonia.

Poverty of content of speech: Speech that is persistently vague, overly concrete or abstract, repetitive, or stereotyped.

Poverty of speech: Speech that is decreased in amount and nonspontaneous, consisting mainly of brief and unelaborated responses to questions.

Pressure of speech: (See also Flight of ideas.)

Speech that is rapid and unstoppable, as if the speaker is driven to keep speaking. Speech is often loud and emphatic and hard to interrupt. It can dominate conversations or go on when no one is listening or responding. A feature of mania and seen also in other psychotic conditions, organic mental disorders, and nonpsychotic conditions associated with stress.

Psychomotor agitation: Motor restlessness and hyperactivity associated with tension, anxiety, and irritability.

Psychomotor retardation: Decreased motor activity, slowed speech, poverty of speech, delayed response to questions, and low, monotonous voice tones associated with feelings of fatigue.

Psychosis: A level of disordered thinking in which the person is unable to distinguish reality from fantasy because of impaired ability to test reality. Psychosis may be transient (hours or days) or persistent (months or years). The characteristic deficit in psychosis is not "loss of touch with reality" but loss of the ability to process experience appropriately, ie, to differentiate what data are coming from the outside world and what information originates in one's inner world of preconceptions, expectations, and emotions. Psychosis can be defined as an impairment of **reality testing. Reality sense** can be impaired in the absence of psychosis. One may "sense" that people are following him or her when that is not the case, and may experience hallucinations. One may have a quite distorted view of his or her strengths or weaknesses. As long as these hypotheses, no matter how bizarre, can be tested against objective evidence and rejected or at least doubted as a result of that rational process, psychosis can be ruled out. As reality testing—the capacity to challenge bizarre perceptions—becomes further impaired, the subject becomes less able or willing to look at or be swayed by external evidence. "Ideas" solidify as delusions, which progressively become more bizarre and complex. Thought becomes more and more preoccupied with fantasy and the subjective world as external cues are progressively ignored. The boundary between nonpsychotic and psychotic ideation and perception is not sharp. There is a spectrum from minimally distorted to grossly distorted nonpsychotic thinking, from mild impairment to severe impairment of reality testing, and from mild psychosis with circumscribed delusions to the extremely bizarre and disorganized psychotic state.

Reality sense: (See Psychosis, above.) One's feelings, thoughts, and perceptions about the way things are.

Reality testing: (See Psychosis, above.) The process of testing one's thoughts or hypotheses against cues identified in the external world.

Schneiderian first-rank symptoms: Symptoms believed by Kurt Schneider (1957), a German psychiatrist, to be pathognomonic of schizophrenia in the absence of organic disease: (1) Certain kinds of **auditory hallucinations**—hearing one's thoughts spoken aloud, hearing voices conversing with one another, or hearing voices keeping a running commentary on one's behavior. (2) **Somatic hallucinations**—frequently of a sexual nature, accompanied by delusional beliefs consistent with the sensations. The physical sensations are commonly attributed by

the person to external causes, forces, energies, or hypnotic suggestion. (3) **Thought withdrawal**—the belief that other people are taking one's thoughts away. (4) **Thought insertion**—the belief that someone else is implanting thoughts into one's head. (5) **Thought broadcasting**—the belief that one's thoughts are known by others, as if everyone else could read one's mind. (6) **Delusional perceptions**—attaching abnormal significance, usually with self-reference, to a genuine perception. For example, the subject interprets a stop sign as an exhortation from another world to "stop being such a bad person." (7) **Delusions of being controlled**—the belief that one's actions, feelings, and impulses are really derived from, influenced by, or directed by external people or forces.

Stereotypy: An isolated, purposeless movement performed repetitively. A feature of catatonia and seen also in schizophrenia. Intoxication with amphetaminelike drugs will also produce stereotypic behavior.

Stupor: Stupor is a particular level of diminished consciousness (ie, one stage more alert than coma) in which mental and physical activity is minimal as a result of organic impairment. Stupor can also refer to a functional state in which the patient appears to be unaware of the environment, unresponsive and motionless but aware of the surroundings. A feature of catatonia and seen also in severe depression and schizophrenia.

Tangentiality: A disturbance of communication in which the subject "takes off on a tangent" away from a central idea or question and does not return. It may be a digression or an introduction of a new theme. It is related to loosening of associations and speech derailment in that there is a jump from one thought or topic to another. Tangentiality has been used synonymously with loosening of associations; however, the latter is characterized by repeated derailments with many associations that seem disconnected. Tangential thinking can be quite coherent as long as it successfully evades the central theme. A feature of a wide variety of pathologic and normal states.

Thought broadcasting, thought insertion, thought withdrawal: See Schneiderian first-rank symptoms, above.

Thought disorder: Any disturbance of thinking that affects language, communication, thought content, or thought process. A **disorder of thought content** is characterized by delusions or marked illogicality. A **formal thought disorder** is a disorder in form of process of thinking, as distinguished from content of thought. Formal thought disorder is characterized by a failure to follow semantic, syntactic, or logical rules. It may range from simple blocking and mild circumstantiality to loosening of associations and loss of reality testing. Classically, formal thought disorder is the hallmark of schizophrenia. However, because the meaning of formal thought disorder is not clearly delineated, it is not used as a descriptive term by *DSM-III*.

Vegetative signs: In describing signs of depression, the term refers to disturbances of sleep, loss of appetite, weight loss, constipation, and loss of sexual interest. Vegetative functions refer to autonomic physiologic functions related to growth, nutrition, or homeostasis of the organism.

Index